Dietary Reference Intakes:

Vitamins

Life Stage Group	Vitamin A (µg/d)[a]	Vitamin C (mg/d)	Vitamin D (µg/d)[b,c]	Vitamin E (mg/d)[d]	Vitamin K (µg/d)	Thiamin (mg/d)	Riboflavin (mg/d)	Niacin (mg/d)[e]	Vitamin B$_6$ (mg/d)	Folate (µg/d)[f]	Vitamin B$_{12}$ (µg/d)	Pantothenic Acid (mg/d)	Biotin (µg/d)	Choline (mg/d)[g]
Infants														
0–6 mo	400*	40*	10	4*	2.0*	0.2*	0.3*	2*	0.1*	65*	0.4*	1.7*	5*	125*
6–12 mo	500*	50*	10	5*	2.5*	0.3*	0.4*	4*	0.3*	80*	0.5*	1.8*	6*	150*
Children														
1–3 y	300	15	15	6	30*	0.5	0.5	6	0.5	150	0.9	2*	8*	200*
4–8 y	400	25	15	7	55*	0.6	0.6	8	0.6	200	1.2	3*	12*	250*
Males														
9–13 y	600	45	15	11	60*	0.9	0.9	12	1.0	300	1.8	4*	20*	375*
14–18 y	900	75	15	15	75*	1.2	1.3	16	1.3	400	2.4	5*	25*	550*
19–30 y	900	90	15	15	120*	1.2	1.3	16	1.3	400	2.4	5*	30*	550*
31–50 y	900	90	15	15	120*	1.2	1.3	16	1.3	400	2.4	5*	30*	550*
51–70 y	900	90	15	15	120*	1.2	1.3	16	1.7	400	2.4[h]	5*	30*	550*
>70 y	900	90	20	15	120*	1.2	1.3	16	1.7	400	2.4[h]	5*	30*	550*
Females														
9–13 y	600	45	15	11	60*	0.9	0.9	12	1.0	300	1.8	4*	20*	375*
14–18 y	700	65	15	15	75*	1.0	1.0	14	1.2	400[i]	2.4	5*	25*	400*
19–30 y	700	75	15	15	90*	1.1	1.1	14	1.3	400[i]	2.4	5*	30*	425*
31–50 y	700	75	15	15	90*	1.1	1.1	14	1.3	400[i]	2.4	5*	30*	425*
51–70 y	700	75	15	15	90*	1.1	1.1	14	1.5	400	2.4[h]	5*	30*	425*
>70 y	700	75	20	15	90*	1.1	1.1	14	1.5	400	2.4[h]	5*	30*	425*
Pregnancy														
14–18 y	750	80	15	15	75*	1.4	1.4	18	1.9	600[j]	2.6	6*	30*	450*
19–30 y	770	85	15	15	90*	1.4	1.4	18	1.9	600[j]	2.6	6*	30*	450*
31–50 y	770	85	15	15	90*	1.4	1.4	18	1.9	600[j]	2.6	6*	30*	450*
Lactation														
14–18 y	1,200	115	15	19	75*	1.4	1.6	17	2.0	500	2.8	7*	35*	550*
19–30 y	1,300	120	15	19	90*	1.4	1.6	17	2.0	500	2.8	7*	35*	550*
31–50 y	1,300	120	15	19	90*	1.4	1.6	17	2.0	500	2.8	7*	35*	550*

Note: This table (taken from the DRI reports, see www.nap.edu) presents Recommended Dietary Allowances (RDAs) in **bold type** and Adequate Intakes (AIs) in ordinary type followed by an asterisk (*). An RDA is the average daily dietary intake level sufficient to meet the nutrient requirements of nearly all (97–98 percent) healthy individuals in a group. It is calculated from an Estimated Average Requirement (EAR). If sufficient scientific evidence is not available to establish an EAR, and thus calculate an RDA, an AI is usually developed. For healthy breastfed infants, an AI is the mean intake. The AI for other life stage and gender groups is believed to cover the needs of all healthy individuals in the groups, but lack of data or uncertainty in the data prevent being able to specify with confidence the percentage of individuals covered by this intake.

[a] As retinol activity equivalents (RAEs). 1 RAE = 1 µg retinol, 12 µg β-carotene, 24 µg α-carotene, or 24 µg β-cryptoxanthin. The RAE for dietary provitamin A carotenoids is two-fold greater than retinol equivalents (RE), whereas the RAE for preformed vitamin A is the same as RE.

[b] As cholecalciferol. 1 µg cholecalciferol = 40 IU vitamin D.

[c] Under the assumption of minimal sunlight.

[d] As α-tocopherol. α-Tocopherol includes RRR-α-tocopherol, the only form of α-tocopherol that occurs naturally in foods, and the 2R-stereoisomeric forms of α-tocopherol (RRR-, RSR-, RRS-, and RSS-α-tocopherol) that occur in fortified foods and supplements. It does not include the 2S-stereoisomeric forms of α-tocopherol (SRR-, SSR-, SRS-, and SSS-α-tocopherol), also found in fortified foods and supplements.

[e] As niacin equivalents (NE). 1 mg of niacin = 60 mg of tryptophan; 0–6 months = preformed niacin (not NE).

[f] As dietary folate equivalents (DFE). 1 DFE = 1 µg food folate = 0.6 µg of folic acid from fortified food or as a supplement consumed with food = 0.5 µg of a supplement taken on an empty stomach.

[g] Although AIs have been set for choline, there are few data to assess whether a dietary supply of choline is needed at all stages of the life cycle, and it may be that the choline requirement can be met by endogenous synthesis at some of these stages.

[h] Because 10 to 30 percent of older people may malabsorb food-bound B$_{12}$, it is advisable for those older than 50 years to meet their RDA mainly by consuming foods fortified with B$_{12}$ or a supplement containing B$_{12}$.

[i] In view of evidence linking folate intake with neural tube defects in the fetus, it is recommended that all women capable of becoming pregnant consume 400 µg from supplements or fortified foods in addition to intake of food folate from a varied diet.

[j] It is assumed that women will continue consuming 400 µg from supplements or fortified food until their pregnancy is confirmed and they enter prenatal care, which ordinarily occurs after the end of the periconceptional period—the critical time for formation of the neural tube.

Dietary Reference Intakes: RDA, AI*

Life Stage Group	Calcium (mg/d)	Chromium (µg/d)	Copper (µg/d)	Fluoride (mg/d)	Iodine (µg/d)	Iron (mg/d)	Magnesium (mg/d)	Manganese (mg/d)	Molybdenum (µg/d)	Phosphorus (mg/d)	Selenium (µg/d)	Zinc (mg/d)	Potassium (g/d)	Sodium (g/d)	Chloride (g/d)
Infants															
0–6 mo	200*	0.2*	200*	0.01*	110*	0.27*	30*	0.003*	2*	100*	15*	2*	0.4*	0.12*	0.18*
6–12 mo	260*	5.5*	220*	0.5*	130*	**11**	75*	0.6*	3*	275*	20*	**3**	0.7*	0.37*	0.57*
Children															
1–3 y	**700**	11*	**340**	0.7*	**90**	**7**	**80**	1.2*	**17**	**460**	**20**	**3**	3.0*	1.0*	1.5*
4–8 y	**1,000**	15*	**440**	1*	**90**	**10**	**130**	1.5*	**22**	**500**	**30**	**5**	3.8*	1.2*	1.9*
Males															
9–13 y	**1,300**	25*	**700**	2*	**120**	**8**	**240**	1.9*	**34**	**1,250**	**40**	**8**	4.5*	1.5*	2.3*
14–18 y	**1,300**	35*	**890**	3*	**150**	**11**	**410**	2.2*	**43**	**1,250**	**55**	**11**	4.7*	1.5*	2.3*
19–30 y	**1,000**	35*	**900**	4*	**150**	**8**	**400**	2.3*	**45**	**700**	**55**	**11**	4.7*	1.5*	2.3*
31–50 y	**1,000**	35*	**900**	4*	**150**	**8**	**420**	2.3*	**45**	**700**	**55**	**11**	4.7*	1.5*	2.3*
51–70 y	**1,000**	30*	**900**	4*	**150**	**8**	**420**	2.3*	**45**	**700**	**55**	**11**	4.7*	1.3*	2.0*
>70 y	**1,200**	30*	**900**	4*	**150**	**8**	**420**	2.3*	**45**	**700**	**55**	**11**	4.7*	1.2*	1.8*
Females															
9–13 y	**1,300**	21*	**700**	2*	**120**	**8**	**240**	1.6*	**34**	**1,250**	**40**	**8**	4.5*	1.5*	2.3*
14–18 y	**1,300**	24*	**890**	3*	**150**	**15**	**360**	1.6*	**43**	**1,250**	**55**	**9**	4.7*	1.5*	2.3*
19–30 y	**1,000**	25*	**900**	3*	**150**	**18**	**310**	1.8*	**45**	**700**	**55**	**8**	4.7*	1.5*	2.3*
31–50 y	**1,000**	25*	**900**	3*	**150**	**18**	**320**	1.8*	**45**	**700**	**55**	**8**	4.7*	1.5*	2.3*
51–70 y	**1,200**	20*	**900**	3*	**150**	**8**	**320**	1.8*	**45**	**700**	**55**	**8**	4.7*	1.3*	2.0*
>70 y	**1,200**	20*	**900**	3*	**150**	**8**	**320**	1.8*	**45**	**700**	**55**	**8**	4.7*	1.2*	1.8*
Pregnancy															
14–18 y	**1,300**	29*	**1,000**	3*	**220**	**27**	**400**	2.0*	**50**	**1,250**	**60**	**12**	4.7*	1.5*	2.3*
19–30 y	**1,000**	30*	**1,000**	3*	**220**	**27**	**350**	2.0*	**50**	**700**	**60**	**11**	4.7*	1.5*	2.3*
31–50 y	**1,000**	30*	**1,000**	3*	**220**	**27**	**360**	2.0*	**50**	**700**	**60**	**11**	4.7*	1.5*	2.3*
Lactation															
14–18 y	**1,300**	44*	**1,300**	3*	**290**	**10**	**360**	2.6*	**50**	**1,250**	**70**	**13**	5.1*	1.5*	2.3*
19–30 y	**1,000**	45*	**1,300**	3*	**290**	**9**	**310**	2.6*	**50**	**700**	**70**	**12**	5.1*	1.5*	2.3*
31–50 y	**1,000**	45*	**1,300**	3*	**290**	**9**	**320**	2.6*	**50**	**700**	**70**	**12**	5.1*	1.5*	2.3*

Note: This table (taken from the DRI reports, see www.nap.edu) presents Recommended Dietary Allowances (RDAs) in **bold type** and Adequate Intakes (AIs) in ordinary type followed by an asterisk (*). An RDA is the average daily dietary intake level sufficient to meet the nutrient requirements of nearly all (97-98 percent) healthy individuals in a group. It is calculated from an Estimated Average Requirement (EAR). If sufficient scientific evidence is not available to establish an EAR, and thus calculate an RDA, an AI is usually developed. For healthy breastfed infants, an AI is the mean intake. The AI for other life stage and gender groups is believed to cover the needs of all healthy individuals in the groups, but lack of data or uncertainty in the data prevent being able to specify with confidence the percentage of individuals covered by this intake.

Data from: Reprinted with permission from the Dietary Reference Intakes series, National Academies Press. Copyright 1997, 1998, 2000, 2001, 2005, 2011 by the National Academies of Sciences, courtesy of the National Academies Press, Washington, DC. These reports may be accessed via www.nap.edu.

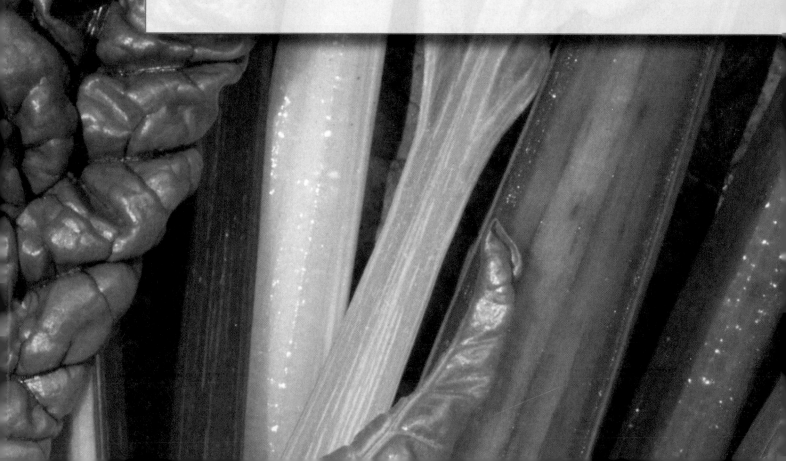

HELPING STUDENTS NAVIGATE NUTRITION'S TOUGH TOPICS

FOR A DEEPER UNDERSTANDING

Mapping Tough Concepts with a Clear Learning Path

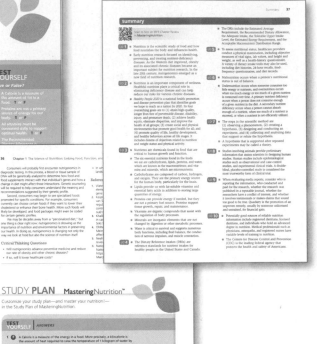

UPDATED! Study Plan tied to Learning Outcomes

All chapters, including In Depth chapters, now include numbered learning outcomes that link to the end-of-chapter Study Plan. Within the Study Plan, each summary point and review question is tied to a learning outcome, helping students to identify areas that they need to review. These Study Plans are further enhanced with activities within MasteringNutrition.

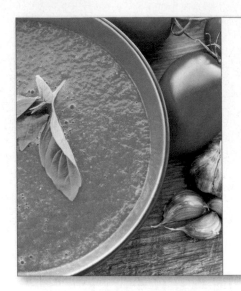

UPDATED!
Food Equity, Sustainability, and Quality chapter

Recognizing new research and emerging topics, the chapter formerly titled Global Hunger has been recast to cover food security, equity, and the environment, giving it a timely new approach. In addition, the chapter now follows the food safety chapter, with the text then ending with the three lifecycle chapters.

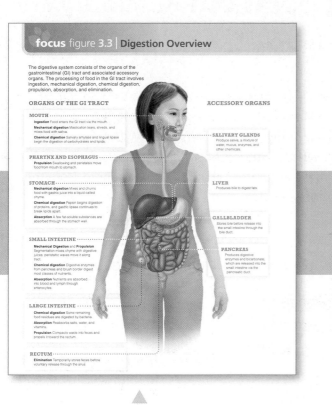

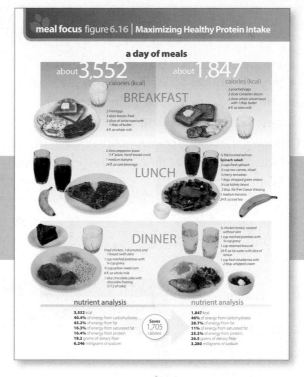

UPDATED! Additional Focus Figures

New Focus Figures on tough topics have been added, including the scientific method, Vitamin D and calcium regulation, and hormonal control of appetite. These colorful full-page figures teach key concepts in nutrition through bold, clear and detailed visual presentations. These dynamic figures also have corresponding coaching activities in Mastering Nutrition.

Focus Figures include introductory text that explains how the figure is central to concepts that students will cover throughout the text.

* Students get clear directions via text and stepped-out art that guide the eye through complex processes, breaking them down into manageable pieces that are easy to teach and understand.
* Focus Figures provide dynamic illustrations—often paired with photographs—that make topics come alive.
* Full-page format enables micro-to-macro levels of explanation for complex topics.

Meal Focus Figures

Students get a visual comparison of possible meal choices, ranging from high- and low-density meals to meals high in refined carbohydrates vs fiber-rich meals. Each figure offers an easy-to-understand comparison of the key nutrients for that topic as well as clear images of the foods being assessed. New coaching activities complement each figure in MasteringNutrition.

Continuous Learning
Before, During & After Class with
MasteringNutrition™ with MyDietAnalysis

The MasteringNutrition online homework, tutorial, and assessment system includes content specific to introductory nutrition courses, delivering self-paced tutorials that focus on your course objectives, provide individualized coaching, and respond to each student's progress.

MyDietAnalysis is now available as single sign on to MasteringNutrition. For smartphone users, a new mobile website version of MyDietAnalysis is available. Students can track their diet and activity intake accurately, anytime and anywhere, from their mobile devices.

BEFORE CLASS

Dynamic Study Modules and eText 2.0 provide students with a preview of what's to come.

NEW! Dynamic Study Modules enable students to study effectively on their own in an adaptive format. Students receive an initial set of questions with a unique answer format asking them to indicate their confidence.

Once completed, Dynamic Study Modules include explanations using material taken directly from the text.

NEW! Interactive eText 2.0 complete with embedded media is mobile friendly and ADA accessible.
* Now available on smartphones and tablets.
* Seamlessly integrated videos and other rich media.
* Accessible (screen-reader ready).
* Configurable reading settings, including resizable type and night reading mode.
* Instructor and student note-taking, highlighting, bookmarking, and search.

DURING CLASS

Learning Catalytics and Engaging Media

Learning Catalytics, a "bring your own device" student engagement, assessment, and classroom intelligence system, allows students to use their smartphone, tablet, or laptop to respond to questions in class.

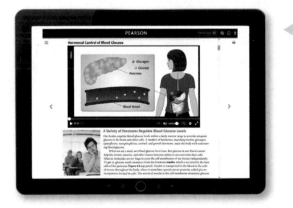

AFTER CLASS

Easy-to-Assign, Customize, and Automatically Graded Assignments

The breadth and depth of content available to you to assign in Mastering is unparalleled, allowing you to quickly and easily assign homework to reinforce key concepts.

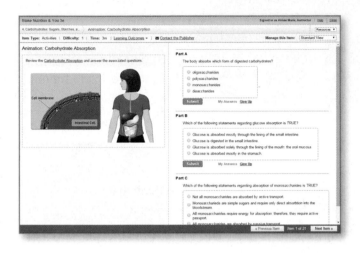

◄ **UPDATED!** Nutrition Animations have been updated and made compatible for Mastering and mobile devices. These animations address tough topics and common misconceptions and feature a more contemporary look to appeal to today's students. Corresponding activities within Mastering with wrong-answer feedback have also been updated.

NEW! *ABC News* Lecture Launcher videos cover up-to-date hot topics that occur in the nutrition field that bring nutrition to life and spark discussion. These are accompanied by multiple-choice questions with wrong-answer feedback. ▶

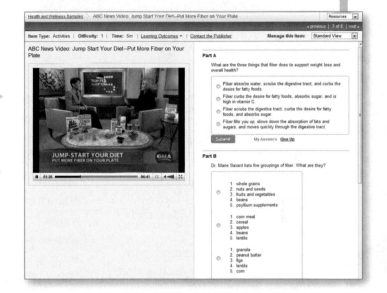

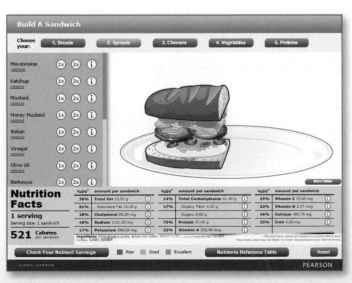

◄ **UPDATED!** 18 NutriTools Build-A-Meal Coaching Activities allow students to apply nutrition concepts to improve their health through interactive mini-lessons that provide hints and feedback. The Build a Meal, Build a Pizza, Build A Salad, and Build A Sandwich tools have been carefully rethought to improve the user experience, making them easier to use. They are now HTML5 compatible.

Everything You Need to Teach
In One Place

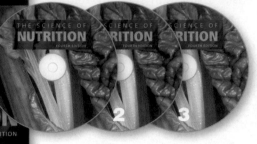

Teaching Toolkit DVD for *The Science of Nutrition*

The *Teaching Toolkit* DVD provides everything that you need to prep for your course and deliver a dynamic lecture, in one convenient place. These valuable resources are included on three disks:

DISK 1
Robust Media Assets for Each Chapter

- *ABC News* Lecture Launcher videos
- Nutrition Animations
- PowerPoint Lecture Outlines
- Media-Only PowerPoint® slides for easy importing of videos and animations
- PowerPoint clicker questions and Jeopardy-style quiz show questions
- Files for all illustrations and tables and selected photos from the text

DISK 2
Comprehensive Test Bank

- Test Bank in Microsoft Word, PDF, and RTF formats
- Computerized Test Bank, which includes all the questions from the test bank in a format that allows you to easily and intuitively build exams and quizzes

DISK 3
Additional Innovative Supplements for Instructors and Students

For Instructors

- Instructor Resource and Support Manual in Microsoft Word and PDF formats
- Step-by-step MasteringNutrition tutorials
- Video introduction to Learning Catalytics™
- *Great Ideas in Teaching Nutrition*

For Students

- *Eat Right! Healthy Eating in College and Beyond*
- Food Composition Table

User's Quick Guide for *The Science of Nutrition*

This easy-to-use printed supplement accompanies the Teaching Toolkit and offers easy instructions for both experienced and new faculty members to get started with the rich Toolkit content and MasteringNutrition.

THE SCIENCE OF
NUTRITION

FOURTH EDITION

Janice L. Thompson, PhD, FACSM

University of Birmingham | University of New Mexico

Melinda M. Manore, PhD, RD, CSSD, FACSM

Oregon State University

Linda A. Vaughan, PhD, RD

Arizona State University

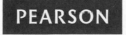

Senior Acquisitions Editor: Michelle Cadden
Project Manager: Tu-Anh Dang-Tran
Program Manager: Susan Malloy
Development Editor: Laura Bonazzoli
Art Development Editor: Kim Brucker
Editorial Assistant: Heidi Arndt
Development Manager: Cathy Murphy
Program Management Team Lead:
Mike Early
Project Management Team Lead: Nancy Tabor
Production Management and Composition:
   Lumina Datamatics
Design Manager: Mark Ong

Cover and Interior Designer: Tamara Newnam
Art House: Lachina
Rights & Permissions Project Manager:
   William Opaluch
**Rights & Permissions Management and
   Research:** QBS, Amanda Larkin
Senior Procurement Specialist:
   Stacey Weinberger
Executive Product Marketing Manager:
   Neena Bali
Field Marketing Manager: Mary Salzman
Cover Photo Credit: Wally Eberhart/
Getty Images

Library of Congress Cataloging-in-Publication Data

Thompson, Janice L., author.
The science of nutrition / Janice L. Thompson, PhD, FACSM, University of Birmingham |
University of New Mexico, Melinda M. Manore, PhD, RD, CSSD, FACSM, Oregon State University,
Linda A. Vaughan, PhD, RD, Arizona State University. —Fourth edition.
      pages cm
Includes bibliographical references and index.
ISBN 978-0-13-417509-6 (pbk.)
   1. Nutrition—Textbooks.   I. Manore, Melinda, 1951- author.   II. Vaughan, Linda A. (Linda Ann)
author.   III. Title.
TX354.T47 2015
363.8—dc23
                                                                         2015033058

                                                 2   16

                                                 ISBN 10: 0-13-417509-3;
                                                 ISBN 13: 978-0-13-417509-6 (Student edition)
                                                 ISBN 10: 0-13-439335-X;
www.pearsonhighered.com   ISBN 13: 978-0-13-439335-3 (Instructor's Review Copy)

PEARSON

Dedication ━━━━━━━━━

This book is dedicated to my amazing family, friends, and colleagues—you provide constant support, encouragement, and unconditional love. It is also dedicated to my students and the communities with which I work—you continue to inspire me, challenge me, and teach me. —**JLT**

This book is dedicated to my wonderful colleagues, friends, and family—your guidance, support, and understanding have allowed this book to happen. —**MMM**

This book is dedicated to my strong circle of family, friends, and colleagues. Year after year, your support and encouragement sustain me. —**LAV**

About the Authors

Janice L. Thompson, PhD, FACSM University of Birmingham • United Kingdom

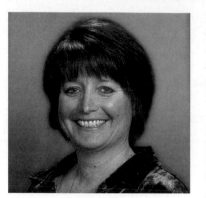

Janice Thompson earned a doctorate in exercise physiology and nutrition at Arizona State University. She is currently Professor of Public Health Nutrition and Exercise at the University of Birmingham in the School of Sport and Exercise Sciences. Her research focuses on designing and assessing the impact of nutrition and physical activity interventions to reduce the risks for obesity, cardiovascular disease, and type 2 diabetes in high-risk populations. She also teaches nutrition and research methods courses and mentors graduate research students.

Janice is a Fellow of the American College of Sports Medicine (ACSM), a member of the Scientific Committee of the European College of Sports Science, and a member of the American Society for Nutrition (ASN), the British Association of Sport and Exercise Science (BASES), and the Nutrition Society. Janice won an undergraduate teaching award while at the University of North Carolina, Charlotte, a Community Engagement Award while at the University of Bristol, and the ACSM Citation Award for her contributions to research, education, and service to the Exercise Sciences. In addition to *The Science of Nutrition*, Janice coauthored the Pearson textbooks *Nutrition: An Applied Approach* and *Nutrition for Life* with Melinda Manore.

Janice loves hiking, yoga, traveling, and cooking and eating delicious food. She likes almost every vegetable except fennel and believes chocolate should be listed as a food group.

Melinda M. Manore, PhD, RD, CSSD, FACSM Oregon State University

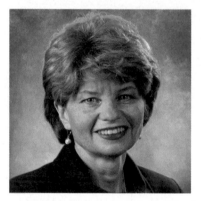

Melinda Manore earned a doctorate in human nutrition with minors in exercise physiology and health at Oregon State University (OSU). She is the past chair of the Department of Nutrition and Food Management and is currently a professor of nutrition at OSU. Prior to her move there, she was a professor at Arizona State University. Melinda's area of expertise is nutrition and exercise, particularly the role of diet and exercise in health and prevention of chronic disease, exercise performance, and weight control. She has a special focus on the energy and nutritional needs of active women and girls across the life cycle.

Melinda is an active member of the Academy of Nutrition and Dietetics (AND) and the American College of Sports Medicine (ACSM). She is the past chair of the AND Research Dietetic Practice Group; served on the AND Obesity Steering Committee; and is an active member of the Sports, Cardiovascular, and Wellness Nutrition Practice Group. She is a fellow of ACSM and has served as vice president and on the Board of Trustees.

Melinda is also a member of the American Society of Nutrition (ASN) and the North American Association for the Study of Obesity (NAASO). She is the past chair of the U.S. Department of Agriculture (USDA) Nutrition and Health Committee for Program Guidance and Planning and currently is chair of the USDA, ACSM, AND Expert Panel Meeting, *Energy Balance at the Crossroads: Translating Science into Action*. She serves on the editorial board of numerous research journals and has won awards for excellence in research and teaching. Melinda also coauthored the Pearson textbooks *Nutrition: An Applied Approach* and *Nutrition for Life* with Janice Thompson.

Melinda is an avid walker, hiker, and former runner who loves to garden, cook, and eat great food. She is also an amateur birder.

Linda A. Vaughan, PhD, RD Arizona State University

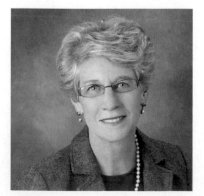

Linda Vaughan is a professor and the director of the School of Nutrition and Health Promotion at Arizona State University. Linda earned a doctorate in agricultural biochemistry and nutrition at the University of Arizona. She currently teaches, advises graduate students, and remains involved in research as time permits. Her area of specialization is older adults and life cycle nutrition.

Linda is an active member of the Academy of Nutrition and Dietetics (AND), the American Society of Nutrition (ASN), and the Arizona Dietetic Association. She has served as chair of the Research and Dietetic Educators of Practitioners practice groups of the AND. Linda has received numerous awards, including the Arizona Dietetic Association Outstanding Educator Award (1997) and the Arizona State University Supervisor of the Year award (2004). In addition to being a coauthor of *The Science of Nutrition*, Linda is also a key contributor to the Pearson textbooks *Nutrition: An Applied Approach* and *Nutrition for Life* by Janice Thompson and Melinda Manore.

Linda enjoys swimming, cycling, and baking bread in her free time.

Welcome to The Science of Nutrition, Fourth Edition!

As nutrition researchers and educators, we know that the science of nutrition is constantly evolving. Our goal as authors is to provide students and instructors with the most recent and scientifically accurate nutrition information available.

Learning to Avoid Nutrition Confusion

What should I eat? In this age of information saturation, many different answers to that question are available 24 hours a day, from multiple sources: via the Internet, social media, television, and radio; in books, newspapers, and magazines; and on billboards, posters, and the sides of vending machines—even food packages offer nutrition advice. From research studies with contradictory findings to marketing claims for competing products, potential sources of confusion abound.

You're probably not fooled by the ads for diets and supplements in your e-mail inbox, but what kinds of nutrition messages *can* you trust? Which claims are backed up by scientific evidence, and of those, which are relevant to you? How can you evaluate the various sources of nutrition information and find out whether the advice they provide is accurate and reliable? How can you navigate the Internet to find reliable nutrition facts and avoid nutrition myths? How can you develop a way of eating that's right for you—one that supports your physical activity, allows you to maintain a healthful weight, and helps you avoid chronic disease? And if you're pursuing a career in nutrition or another healthcare field, how can you continue to obtain the most current and valid information about food and physical activity as you work with individual clients?

Why We Wrote This Book

The Science of Nutrition began with the conviction that both students and instructors would benefit from an accurate, clear, and engaging textbook that links nutrients with their functional benefits. As instructors, we recognized that students have a natural interest in their bodies, their health, their weight, and their success in sports and other activities. We developed this text to demonstrate how nutrition relates to these interests. *The Science of Nutrition* empowers you to reach your personal health and fitness goals while teaching you about the scientific evidence linking nutrition with disease. This information will be vital to your success as you build a career in nutrition or another health-related discipline.

You'll also learn how to debunk nutrition myths and how to distinguish nutrition fact from fiction. Throughout the chapters, material is presented in lively narrative that is scientifically sound and that continually links the evidence with these goals. Information on current events, and recent and ongoing research, keeps the inquisitive spark alive, illustrating how nutrition is very much a "living" science and a source of spirited ongoing debate.

The content of this text is designed for nutrition and other science and healthcare majors, but is also applicable and accessible to students in the liberal arts. We present the *science* of nutrition in a conversational style with engaging features that encourage you to apply the material to your own life and to the lives of your future clients, patients, or students. To support visual learning, the writing is supplemented by illustrations and photos that are attractive, effective, and level-appropriate. As teachers, we are familiar with the myriad challenges of presenting nutrition information in the classroom. We have therefore developed an exceptional ancillary package with a variety of tools to assist instructors in successfully meeting these challenges. We hope to contribute to the excitement of teaching and learning about nutrition: A subject that affects every one of us, a subject so important and relevant that correct and timely information can make the difference between health and disease.

Hallmark Text Features

A multitude of popular features have been updated throughout this new edition, challenging you to think about how the recommendations of different nutritional experts (and others who may be less than expert, such as some media sources) apply to your unique health issues, activity level, energy requirements, food preferences, and lifestyle. **Nutrition Myth or Fact?** boxes, which now appear near the end of each chapter preceeding the Study Plan section, explore the science supporting or challenging common beliefs about foods, while the **Highlight** boxes explore research across a range of important, specific nutritional issues. **Nutrition Label Activity** feature boxes help you understand how to interpret food label information, so that you can make better nutritional choices. **You Do the Math** feature boxes give you a hands-on chance to practice important calculations that reveal key nutrition information.

Four visually vibrant **In Depth** "mini chapters" cover the key areas of alcohol, vitamins and minerals, phytochemicals, and disordered eating, and offer instructors flexibility in incorporating them into their course. The Vitamins and Minerals In Depth specifically provides an overview of micronutrient basics prior to the first functional chapter.

In providing these features, in addition to the new features listed in a later section, we hope that by the time you finish this book you'll feel more confident and engaged in making decisions about your diet and physical activity.

*Nutri-*Case | **You Play the Expert!**

In addition to the aforementioned features, our **Nutri-Case** scenarios provide you with the opportunity to evaluate the nutrition-related beliefs and behaviors of five people representing a range of backgrounds and nutritional challenges. As you encounter them, keep in mind that these case scenarios are for instructional purposes, not intended to suggest that students using this text are qualified to offer nutritional advice to others. In the real world, only properly trained and licensed health professionals are qualified to provide nutritional counseling. Take a moment to get acquainted with our Nutri-Case characters here.

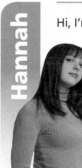

Hannah

Hi, I'm Hannah. I'm 18 years old and in my first year at Valley Community College. I'm 5′ 6″ and right now I weigh 171 lbs. I haven't made up my mind yet about my major. All I know for sure is that I don't want to work in a hospital like my mom! I got good grades in high school, but I'm a little freaked out by college so far. There's so much homework, plus one of my courses has a lab, plus I have to work part-time because my mom doesn't have the money to put me through school. Sometimes I feel like I just can't handle it all. And when I get stressed out, I eat. I've already gained 10 pounds and I haven't even finished my first semester!

Theo

Hi, I'm Theo. Let's see, I'm 21, and my parents moved to the Midwest from Nigeria 11 years ago. I'm 6′ 8″ tall and weigh in at 200 lbs. The first time I ever played basketball, in middle school, I was hooked. I won lots of awards in high school and then got a full scholarship to the state university, where I'm a junior studying political science. I decided to take a nutrition course because, last year, I had a hard time making it through the playing season, plus keeping up with my classes and homework. I want to have more energy, so I thought maybe I'm not eating right. Anyway, I want to figure out this food thing before basketball season starts again.

Liz

I'm Liz, I'm 20, and I'm a dance major at the School for Performing Arts. I'm 5'4" and currently weigh about 103 lbs. Last year, two other dancers from my class and I won a state championship and got to dance in the New Year's Eve celebration at the governor's mansion. This spring, I'm going to audition for the City Ballet, so I have to be in top condition. I wish I had time to take a nutrition course, but I'm too busy with dance classes, rehearsals, and teaching a dance class for kids. But it's okay, because I get lots of tips from other dancers and from the Internet. Like last week, I found a website especially for dancers that explained how to get rid of bloating before an audition. I'm going to try it for my audition with the City Ballet!

Judy

I'm Judy, Hannah's mother. I'm 38 years old and a nurse's aide at Valley Hospital. I'm 5'5" and weigh 200 lbs. Back when Hannah was a baby, I dreamed of going to college so I could be a registered nurse. But then my ex and I split up, and Hannah and me, we've been in survival mode ever since. I'm proud to have raised my daughter without any handouts, and I do good work, but the pay never goes far enough and it's exhausting. I guess that's partly because I'm out of shape, and my blood sugar's high. Most nights, I'm so tired at the end of my shift that I just pick up some fast food for supper. I know I should be making home-cooked meals, but like I said, I'm in survival mode.

Gustavo

Hello. My name is Gustavo. I'm 69 years young at the moment, but when I was 13 years old I came to the United States from Mexico with my parents and three sisters to pick crops in California. Now I manage a large vineyard. They ask me when I'm going to retire, but I can still work as hard as a man half my age. Health problems? None. Well, maybe my doctor tells me my blood pressure is high, but that's normal for my age! I guess what keeps me going is thinking about how my father died 6 months after he retired. He had colon cancer, but he never knew it until it was too late. Anyway, I watch the nightly news and read the papers, so I keep up on what's good for me, "Eat less salt" and all that stuff. I'm doing great! I'm 5'5" tall and weigh 166 lbs.

Throughout this text, you'll read about these five characters as they grapple with various nutrition-related challenges in their lives. As you do, you might find that they remind you of people you know, and you may discover you have something in common with one or more of them. Our hope is that by applying the information you learn in this course to their situations, you will deepen your understanding of the importance of nutrition in your own life.

New in the Fourth Edition

The Fourth Edition of *The Science of Nutrition* includes a wealth of dynamic new features and innovations. Key among these is the **MasteringNutrition™** online homework, tutorial, and assessment system, which delivers self-paced tutorials and activities that provide individualized coaching, focus on course objectives, and offer tools enabling instructors to respond individually to each student's progress. The proven Mastering system provides instructors with customizable, easy-to-assign, automatically graded assessments that motivate students to learn outside of class and arrive prepared for lecture. Key MasteringNutrition features include the following:

- **Interactive eText 2.0**—now available on smartphones and tablets—is Americans with Disabilities Act (ADA) accessible (screen-reader ready). This new eText 2.0 seamlessly integrates videos and animations, offers configurable reading settings (including resizable type and night reading mode), and allows instructor and student note-taking, highlighting, bookmarking, and search.

- **Focus Figure** and **Meal Focus Figure Coaching Activities** that guide students through key nutrition concepts with interactive mini-lessons.

- **Nutrition Animations** have been updated and made compatible for Mastering and mobile devices. Corresponding activities with wrong-answer feedback have also been updated.

- *ABC News* **Videos** with quizzing bring nutrition to life and spark discussion with up-to-date hot topics that occur in the nutrition field. Multiple-choice questions provide wrong-answer feedback to redirect students to the correct answer.

- **18 NutriTools Coaching Activities** allow students to apply nutrition concepts to improve their health through interactive mini-lessons that provide hints and feedback. The Build a Meal, Build a Pizza, Build a Salad, and Build a Sandwich tools have been carefully rethought to improve the user experience, making them easier to use. They are now HTML5 compatible.

- **Single sign-on for MyDietAnalysis**, a software system that allows students to complete a diet assignment. Students keep track of their food intake and exercise and enter the information to create a variety of reports (e.g., the balance between fats, carbohydrates, and proteins in their diet; how many calories they're eating; whether they're meeting the Recommended Dietary Allowances [RDAs] for vitamins and minerals; etc.). **MyDietAnalysis activities** have been added within Mastering that incorporate the use of MyDietAnalysis. A mobile version gives students 24/7 access via their smartphones to easily track food, drink, and activity on the go.

- **Dynamic Study Modules** enable students to study effectively on their own in an adaptive format. Students receive an initial set of questions with a unique answer format asking them to indicate their confidence level.

- **Learning Catalytics**™ is an interactive, student response tool that uses students' smartphones, tablets, or laptops to engage them in more sophisticated tasks and thinking. Now included with **MasteringNutrition™** with eText, Learning Catalytics enables you to generate classroom discussion, guide your lecture, and promote peer-to-peer learning with real-time analytics.

- **MP3s** related to chapter content, with multiple-choice questions that provide wrong-answer feedback.

- **Access to** *Get Ready for Nutrition,* providing students with extra math and chemistry study assistance.

- **A Study Area** that is broken down into learning areas and includes videos, animations, MP3s, and other resources.

Focus Figures illuminate some of the toughest topics for students to learn and understand. New topics for these full-page figures include the scientific method, Vitamin D and calcium regulation, and hormonal control of appetite. New to this edition, **Meal Focus Figures** graphically depict the differences in sets of meals, such as a comparison of nutrient density or a comparison of two high-carbohydrate meals, to engage students with useful information.

Each chapter now offers students a **Study Plan** to guide them through the chapter. Each chapter begins with numbered learning outcomes, which are then referenced in the relevant section of the chapter. At the end of each chapter, the relevant learning outcome is again referenced in the chapter summary and review questions, offering students a clear learning path through the chapter. Corresponding activities in Mastering reinforce the connections. The end-of-chapter study plan also now repeats the Test Yourself questions from the chapter opener while providing the answers.

Chapter 16, now titled Food Equity, Sustainability, and Quality: The Challenge of "Good" Food, is a major revision of the previous global hunger chapter. This timely new approach focuses on issues most relevant to students today. The chapter is now earlier in the book following the food safety chapter, with the text concluding with the three chapters covering nutrition throughout the life cycle.

The visual walkthrough at the front of the book provides additional information on the new features in the Fourth Edition. Specific changes to each chapter include the following:

Chapter 1

- Highlight on the concept of a kilocalorie now incorporated into the narrative text.
- Added a new Focus Figure on Dietary Reference Intakes (Focus Figure 1.9).
- Added a new Focus Figure on the scientific method (Focus Figure 1.10).
- Updated Nutrition Myth or Fact? (previously Nutrition Debate) on nutrigenomics.
- Added a new figure on epigenetics in the nutrigenomics Nutrition Myth or Fact?.
- Updated all applicable references.

Chapter 2

- Added definitions and distinguished between whole foods, processed foods, and functional foods.
- Added a new section on "Other Eating Plans," which includes a brief overview of the Exchange Lists and the Dietary Approaches to Stop Hypertension (DASH) diet, including adding web links at the end of the chapter.
- Added a new section, "High-Tech Tools," to help students analyze their diets. This section includes information on various web-based tools and apps.
- Added a new paragraph on grocery store nutrition guidance systems, including a nutrition online link to the Nu-Val system.
- Added a new section discussing the recent Food and Drug Administration (FDA) requirements that all restaurants, movie theatres, and vending machines include calorie counts and basic nutrition information by 2016.
- Replaced previous Figure 2.4 on nutrient density with a new Focus Figure 2.4, "Optimizing Nutrient Density.."
- Retired all of the ethnic diet pyramids and revised the Mediterranean eating plan within the plate design (now Figure 2.6).
- Incorporated updated information on the Mediterranean diet as part of the text narrative.
- Introduced MiPlato as a Spanish-language alternative to MyPlate (now Figure 2.10).
- Updated and expanded the Nutrition Myth or Fact? (previously Nutrition Debate) on the DGAs and MyPlate, including updated research examining whether people are using them, discussing existing conflicts of interest that may be influencing the recommendations, and including a discussion and figure of two alternative graphics, the Healthy Eating Plate and the Power Plate.
- Updated all applicable references.

Chapter 3

- Expanded discussion of hormones involved in hunger/satiety responses.
- Moved Figure 6.12 of enzymes from Chapter 6, Proteins, in previous edition, to this chapter (now Figure 3.5).
- Added content on role of lingual lipase in chemical digestion.
- Updated information on mechanisms of gastroesophageal reflux disease (GERD) and slightly revised figure.
- Addressed current status of research on non-celiac gluten sensitivity.

- Added a brief discussion of colon cancer.
- Replaced Nutri-Case on Liz and food allergies with Nutri-Case on Judy and eating cues.
- Replaced Nutrition Debate on screening for celiac disease with a Nutrition Myth or Fact? on the microbiome, probiotics, and prebiotics.
- Updated all applicable references.

Chapter 4

- Added information on fructans (including inulin) within the section discussing fiber.
- Expanded Highlight examining the question, "Are All Forms of Sugar the Same?."
- Added new Meal Focus Figure 4.15 on maximizing fiber intake.
- Updated section on the effect of high sugar intake on risks for obesity and diabetes.
- Updated section on the recent evidence examining consumption of diet soft drinks and weight loss/gain.
- Expanded the section on diabetes, including damage caused to blood vessels, discussion of prediabetes, discussion and table with values for normal glucose, impaired fasting glucose, and diabetes (including HbA1c values).
- Added new Focus Figure 4.18 on diabetes.
- Nutrition Myth or Fact? (formerly Nutrition Debate) was expanded to explore the role of sugar more broadly (and not just high-fructose corn syrup) in the obesity epidemic.
- Updated all applicable references.

Chapter 4.5

- Updated all statistics regarding alcohol-related deaths, complications, and other related issues.
- Added a link to help students calculate Calorie content of alcoholic beverages.
- Expanded section "Taking Control of Your Alcohol Intake."
- New Figure 3 on calculating Calorie content of alcoholic beverages.
- Updated all applicable references.

Chapter 5

- Updated Highlight, "Is Margarine More Healthful Than Butter?"
- Updated Figures 5.1, 5.5, 5.9, 5.15.
- Updated discussion of the role of dietary fat in chronic disease, including trans fats and cholesterol.
- Added new Focus Figure 5.16 on atherosclerosis.
- Added new Focus figure 5.18 on lipoprotein transport and distribution.
- Added new Nutrition Myth or Fact? (formerly Nutrition Debate), "Are Saturated Fats Bad or Benign?"
- Added discussion on eating more sustainably when selecting fish.
- • Added new figure 5.9, part a, on bile emulsifying fats.
- Added new Meals Focus Figure 5.14 on reducing saturated fats.
- Expanded the Nutrition Label Activity on how much fat in food so that it is more comprehensive.
- Updated references.

Chapter 6

- Updated sections on the effect of consuming excess protein on heart disease, kidney function, and bone loss.
- Updated section on the role of nuts in lowering risk for type 2 diabetes and heart disease.
- Expanded section on whether amino acid supplements help build muscle mass and increase muscle strength.

- Enhanced list of ways to increase legume intake.
- Added new Focus Figure 6.16 on meals high and low in healthy protein sources.
- Added new Nutrition Myth or Fact? (formerly Nutrition Debate) on whether there is a need to increase current protein recommendations.
- Updated all applicable references.

Chapter 7

- Added new introductory story for the chapter.
- Added a brief overview of cholesterol synthesis.
- Updated Figures 7.10 and 7.25.
- Updated Highlight on carnitine.
- Updated the Nutrition Myth or Fact? (formerly Nutrition Debate) on dietary thermogenics.
- Updated the Highlight on carnitine.
- Updated all applicable references.

Chapter 7.5

- Added section on ultra-trace minerals.
- Added discussion on nutrient competition for absorption.
- Changed vitamin D guidelines from IU to μg.
- Updated all applicable references.

Chapter 8

- Revised learning objectives.
- Updated figures.
- Updated Highlight, "Can Chromium Supplements Enhance Body Composition?"
- Updated Nutrition Myth or Fact? (formerly Nutrition Debate), "Treating PMS with Vitamin B_6 and Folic Acid: Does It Work? Is it Risky?"

Chapter 9

- Added new chapter-opening story.
- Added new discussion of alkaline water.
- Updated Figure 9.2.
- Added new Focus Figure 9.5 on fluid and electrolyte balance.
- Added cashew milk to discussion of (cow's) milk alternatives.
- Added discussion of ultra-trace minerals.
- Added new Nutrition Myth or Fact? (formerly Nutrition Debate) on the sodium controversy.
- Updated all applicable references.

Chapter 10

- Restructured chapter headings to more closely link the learning outcomes with textual information and review questions.
- Added new Focus Figure 10.5 on vitamin A's role in vision.
- Updated Highlight feature on vitamin C and the common cold.
- Moved disorders linked to tobacco use from Highlight box to text.
- Expanded section on the link between free radicals, antioxidants, and cardiovascular disease.
- Updated and expanded Nutrition Myth or Fact? (formerly Nutrition Debate) on multivitamins and mineral supplements and added information on botanicals and herbs.
- Updated all applicable references.

Chapter 10.5

- Half of this In Depth chapter was updated and rewritten so that it focuses on four main ideas, reflected in the four learning outcomes.
- All of the research studies cited have been updated (except for the acknowledged classics), including the Highlight box on peanut butter and jelly sandwiches.

Chapter 11

- Reorganized all section headings to improve flow and enable linkage with learning objectives.
- Clarified that it is red bone marrow that is involved in the production of most blood cells.
- Revised the sections discussing the roles of parathyroid hormone (PTH) and vitamin D on calcium absorption from the kidney and the role of the sarcoplasmic reticulum in releasing calcium to stimulate muscle contraction.
- Added new Focus Figure 11.5 on vitamin D and calcium regulation.
- Revised Figure 11.9 to include evidence that vitamin D conversion is inhibited in the winter months in geographic areas above the 37 degree latitude line.
- Expanded and moved content on calcium supplements to the new Nutrition Myth or Fact? (formerly Nutrition Debate), "Preserving Bone Mass: Are Supplements the Solution?"
- Incorporated new research on the role of exercise in osteoporosis prevention and treatment and on the risks and benefits of medications currently used to treat osteoporosis.
- Updated all applicable references.

Chapter 12

- Updated information on iron absorption from mixed diets.
- Added new information on vitamin K and its various forms.
- Updated information on anemia worldwide and World Health Organization (WHO) 2025 plans for a 50% reduction of anemia in women of reproductive age.
- Updated section on the role of nutrients in immune response.
- Added new information on the worldwide problem of child malnutrition and its impact on the immune system.
- Updated information on the role of zinc in human health.
- Expanded the discussion of the components of blood.
- Updated Nutrition Myth or Fact? (formerly Nutrition Debate), "Zinc and the Common Cold."
- Updated all applicable references.

Chapter 13

- Substantially reorganized the chapter, revised chapter headings and learning objectives, and deleted repetitive information to improve flow and readability.
- Added new Focus Figure 13.5 on energy balance.
- Expanded information on complications of bariatric surgery.
- Updated and expanded information on weight loss medications.
- Added information on mindful eating.
- Expanded sections on the associations of environmental factors and poverty with obesity.
- Expanded section on the multifactorial nature of obesity.
- Added new Focus Figure 13.9 on the complex factors contributing to obesity.
- Revised obesity surgery figure (Figure 13.10) to include sleeve gastrectomy.
- Added new Meal Focus Figure 13.11 on managing calorie intake.
- Moved Nutrition Debate on whether it costs more to eat right to Chapter 16 where it is now a Highlight box.

- Updated Nutrition Myth or Fact? (formerly Nutrition Debate) on whether higher carbohydrate, lower fat diets have been overrated, and added information on the Paleo Diet to this feature and also to the chapter text.
- Updated all applicable references.

Chapter 13.5

- Added learning outcomes.
- Updated Highlight, "Muscle Dysmorphia: The Male Eating Disorder?"
- Updated segment on various types of disordered eating that can be part of a syndrome.
- Updated new DSM-5.

Chapter 14

- Revised phrasing of section headings to make them more direct and applicable to the content being covered.
- Added new Figure 14.1 on health benefits of physical activity.
- Updated Figure 14.3 to include examples of activities, providing a more complete illustration of the Frequency, Intensity, Time, and Type (FITT) principle.
- Added new Focus Figure 14.7 on what fuels our activities.
- Added new Meal Focus Figure 14.10 on maximizing carbohydrates to support activity.
- Added new information and references related to intrinsic and extrinsic motivation to being active, high-intensity interval training (HIT), recent evidence to support the benefits of the 2008 Physical Activity Guidelines, and the benefits of consuming food sources high in carbohydrate and protein to enhance muscle glycogen storage and performance.
- Updated and tightened up the Nutrition Myth or Fact? (formerly Nutrition Debate) on ergogenic aids.

Chapter 15

- Updated all research throughout.
- Added brief discussions of hepatitis A virus (HAV) and *Toxoplasma gondii.*
- Moved discussion of bovine spongiform encephalopathy (BSE)/variant Creutzfeldt–Jakob disease (vCJD) from box to narrative and updated and condensed.
- Expanded discussion of STECs.
- Replaced FightBac figure with Foodsafety.gov logo.
- Replaced table of cooking temperatures with narrative bullets, updated.
- Discussed FDA preliminary determination on partially hydrogenated oils (PHOs) as no longer generally recognized as safe.
- Added discussion of the top five reasons for genetic modification of crops, including herbicide tolerance and insect resistance.
- Added separate discussion of the health risks of POPs and expanded the discussion of plasticizers, dioxins, and concerns about the carcinogenicity of glyphosate.
- Added brief discussion of the FDA's imposition of a voluntary ban on the use of antibiotics in livestock for other than medical purposes.
- Updated the USDA's definition and description of organic foods, and added a brief discussion of the issue of their higher cost.
- Moved discussion of environmental food issues such as sustainability to Chapter 16.
- Revised and updated Tables 15.1 on government agencies, Table 15.2 on bacteria, and Table 15.4 on the Environmental Working Group's dirty dozen and clean fifteen.
- Entirely revised and expanded the Nutrition Myth or Fact? (formerly Nutrition Debate) on genetically modified organisms (GMOs).
- Updated all applicable references.

Changes to Chapter 16

- This new chapter, "Food Equity, Sustainability, and Quality: The Challenge of 'Good' Food," replaces the last edition's Chapter 19, "Global Nutrition."
- New topics include disparities in availability of high-quality, nourishing food; factors thought to contribute to the poverty-obesity paradox; the unsafe working conditions on many U.S. farms; and the inequitable wages paid to many farm and food-service workers.
- Updated and significantly expanded the section on food sustainability and the effects of our current system of food production, dominated by industrial agriculture, on food diversity and the environment that had been covered in narrative of the third edition, in Chapter 15.
- Added new discussion of the role of the food industry in shaping nutrition recommendations and consumer choices through lobbying, marketing, etc.
- Expanded discussion of global, national, and local initiatives that are increasing the availability of nourishing food and included a look at some simple steps individuals can take, such as buying fair-trade foods or reducing beef consumption, which can help begin to meet the challenge of "good" food.
- Updated and expanded Nutrition Myth or Fact? (formerly Nutrition Debate in Chapter 6) on meat consumption and global warming, including a new section from a 2014 analysis identifying the resources used and emissions released to produce 1,000 kcal of beef versus 1,000 kcal of food crops (wheat, rice, and potatoes).

Chapter 17

- Added discussion of the effects of obesity on fertility.
- Added discussion of pregnancy concerns for older women.
- Expanded the discussion of *Listeria monocytogenes* infection during pregnancy.
- Changed the Nutri-Case to support the teaching point on the increased risk for type 2 diabetes in children of a mother who had gestational diabetes.
- Added a discussion on the safety of artificial sweeteners in pregnancy.
- Added a discussion of the use of prescription and over-the-counter (OTC) drugs and herbal supplements during pregnancy.
- Added a discussion of lower rates of breastfeeding in obese mothers and contributing factors.
- Added a flow chart on consequences of fetal adaptation to undernourishment to the Nutrition Myth or Fact? (formerly Nutrition Debate) on long-term effects of the fetal environment.
- Updated all applicable reference.

Chapter 18

- Expanded discussion on the responsibilities of parents in supporting healthful diets for their children/families, including their role in the management of their children's weight.
- Replaced MyPyramid graphic with MyPlate Daily Food Plan.
- Updated discussion on the role of breakfast related to nutrient intake and weight management.
- Expanded discussion of the short- and long-term metabolic consequences of obesity.
- Updated information related to School Lunch and Breakfast programs, food insecurity among children.
- Added explanations of "class 2" and "class 3" obesity among children and adolescents.
- Expanded the Nutrition Myth or Fact? (formerly Nutrition Debate) on bariatric surgery in adolescents.
- Updated all applicable references.

Changes to Chapter 19

- Expanded discussion on consequences of inactivity among older adults.
- Updated dietary protein recommendations for older adults.
- Expanded discussion of bariatric surgery in older adults.
- Added a new section on dehydration among older adults.
- Added new dietary recommendations to reduce the risk of Alzheimer's disease.
- Added new discussion on pressure ulcers in elderly.
- Added new discussion on the impact of "crushing" drugs for easier administration of drugs for older adults.
- Updated and expanded discussion of food insecurity among older adults.
- Updated descriptions of federal food assistance programs.
- Added new Centers for Disease Control and Prevention (CDC) guidelines on physical activity for older adults in the "Seniors on the Move" Highlight.
- Updated Nutrition Myth or Fact? (formerly Nutrition Debate) on living longer through a low-energy diet.
- Updated all statistics related to aging.
- Updated all applicable references.

Appendices, Front Matter, and Back Matter

- Appendix A, "The USDA Food Guide Evolution," and Appendix I, "Organizations and Resources," have been moved online. Remaining appendices have been renumbered.

Supplemental Resources for Instructors and Students

For the Instructor

Intructor Review Copy
978-0-13-439335-3 / 0-13-439335-X

Instructor Resource and Support Manual
978-0-13-432699-3 / 0-13-432699-7

This popular and adaptable resource, available on the Teaching Toolkit DVD, enables instructors to create engaging lectures and additional activities via chapter summaries, learning objectives, chapter outlines, key terms, in-class discussion questions, and activity ideas, including a diet analysis activity and a Nutrition Debate activity for each chapter, in addition to a list of all web resources by chapter.

Teaching Toolkit DVD
978-0-13-424386-3 / 0-13-424386-2

This rich teaching resource offers everything you need to create lecture presentations and course materials, including JPEG and PowerPoint® files of the art, tables, and selected photos from the text, and "stepped-out" art for selected figures from the text, as well as animations for the majors nutrition course.

   The DVD allows for "click and play" in the classroom—no downloading required—and includes the following:

Media Assets for Each Chapter

- *ABC News* Lecture Launcher videos
- Nutrition Animations
- PowerPoint Lecture Outlines

- Media-Only PowerPoint® slides for easy importing of videos and animations
- PowerPoint clicker questions and Jeopardy-style quiz show questions
- Files for all illustrations and tables and selected photos from the text

Comprehensive Test Bank

- Test Bank in Microsoft Word, PDF, and RTF formats
- Computerized Test Bank, which includes all the questions from the printed test bank in a format that allows you to easily and intuitively build exams and quizzes

Additional Supplements

For Instructors

- Instructor Resource and Support Manual in Microsoft Word and PDF formats
- Step-by-step MasteringNutrition tutorials
- Video introduction to Learning Catalytics™
- *Great Ideas in Teaching Nutrition*

For Students

- *Eat Right! Healthy Eating in College and Beyond*
- Food Composition Table

TestGen® Test Bank
978-0-13-432698-6 / 0-13-432698-9

The Test Bank, provided in MasteringNutrition and the Teaching Toolkit DVD, contains multiple-choice, true/false, and essay questions for content from each chapter, in addition to new Bloom's Taxonomy levels and correlations to the start-of-chapter Learning Objectives.

Great Ideas: Active Ways to Teach Nutrition
978-0-321-59646-8 / 0-321-59646-3

This updated, revised booklet compiles the best ideas from nutrition instructors across the country on innovative ways to teach nutrition topics with an emphasis on active learning. Broken into useful pedagogic areas including targeted and general classroom activities, and an overview of active learning principles, this booklet provides creative ideas for teaching nutrition concepts, along with tips and suggestions for classroom activities that can be used to teach almost any topic.

MyDietAnalysis Website
www.mydietanalysis.com
ISBN: 0-321-73390-8

MyDietAnalysis was developed by the nutrition database experts at ESHA Research, Inc. and is tailored for use in college nutrition courses. It offers an accurate, reliable, and easy-to-use program for your students' diet analysis needs. MyDietAnalysis features a database of nearly 20,000 foods and multiple reports. Available online, the program allows students to track their diet and activity and generate and submit reports electronically. MyDietAnalysis is also available at no additional cost as a single sign-on to MasteringNutrition with all new copies of the textbook.

For online users, a mobile website version of MyDietAnalysis is available, so students can track their diet and activity intake accurately, anytime and anywhere, from their mobile device.

Food Composition Table
978-0-321-66793-9 / 0-321-66793-X

Entries from the USDA Nutrient Database for Standard Reference are provided, offering the nutritional values of over 1,500 separate foods in an easy-to-follow format.

Course Management Options for Instructors

MasteringNutrition™

www.masteringnutrition.pearson.com/www.pearsonmylabandmastering.com
MasteringNutrition™
The MasteringNutrition online homework, tutorial, and assessment system delivers self-paced tutorials and activities that provide individualized coaching, focus on your course objectives, and are responsive to each student's progress. The Mastering system helps instructors maximize class time with customizable, easy-to-assign, and automatically graded assessments that motivate students to learn outside of class and arrive prepared for lecture.

For the Student

Food Composition Table
978-0-321-66793-9 / 0-321-66793-X

Entries from the USDA Nutrient Database for Standard Reference are provided, offering the nutritional values of over 1,500 separate foods in an easy-to-follow format.

MyDietAnalysis Website
www.mydietanalysis.com
MyDietAnalysis was developed by the nutrition database experts at ESHA Research, Inc. and is tailored for use in college nutrition courses. It offers an accurate, reliable, and easy-to-use program for your students' diet analysis needs. MyDietAnalysis features a database of nearly 20,000 foods and multiple reports. Available online, the program allows students to track their diet and activity and generate and submit reports electronically. MyDietAnalysis is also a included at no additional cost as a single sign on to MasteringNutrition with all new copies of the textbook.

For online users, a mobile website version of MyDietAnalysis is available, so students can track their diet and activity intake accurately, anytime and anywhere, from their mobile device.

MasteringNutrition™
www.masteringnutrition.pearson.com/www.pearsonmylabandmastering.com

MasteringNutrition™
The MasteringNutrition online homework, tutorial, and assessment system delivers self-paced tutorials and activities that provide individualized coaching, focus on your course objectives, and are responsive to each student's progress. The Mastering system helps instructors maximize class time with customizable, easy-to-assign, and automatically graded assessments that motivate students to learn outside of class and arrive prepared for lecture.

Eat Right! Healthy Eating in College and Beyond
978-0-805-38288-4 / 0-805-38288-7

This handy, full-color, 80-page booklet provides students with practical guidelines, tips, shopper's guides, and recipes, so that they can start putting healthy eating guidelines into action. Written specifically for students, topics include healthy eating in the cafeteria, dorm room, and fast-food restaurants; eating on a budget; weight-management tips; vegetarian alternatives; and guidelines on alcohol and health.

Acknowledgments

It is eye-opening to write a textbook and to realize that the work of so many people contributes to the final product. There are numerous people to thank, and we'd like to begin by extending our thanks to the fabulous staff at Pearson for their incredible support and dedication to this book. Publisher Frank Ruggirello committed extensive resources to ensure the quality of each new edition of this text, and his ongoing support and enthusiasm helped us maintain the momentum we need to complete this project. Our acquisitions editor, Michelle Cadden, provided unwavering vision, support, and guidance throughout the process of writing and publishing this book. We could never have completed this text without the exceptional writing and organizational skills of Laura Bonazzoli, our developmental editor and cowriter. In addition to enhancing the quality of this textbook through her enthusiasm and creativity, Laura was responsible for writing the new chapter on food equity, sustainability, and quality. We also express our sincere gratitude to our project manager, Tu-Anh Dang-Tran. We know that managing all the aspects of a textbook is a bit like herding cats. Tu-Anh worked tirelessly to improve the text and steer us on our course, and kept us sane with her patience, sense of humor, and excellent editorial instincts. We are also indebted to art development editor Kim Brucker, who contributed to the art enhancements in this edition. Heidi Arndt, editorial assistant extraordinaire, provided superior editorial and administrative support that we would have been lost without. Our thanks also to Marie Beaugureau, Laura Southworth, and Deirdre Espinoza, for their support and guidance in previous editions.

Multiple talented players helped build this book in the production and design process as well. The resourceful Nancy Kincade and Tracy Duff and their colleagues at Lumina Datamatics kept manuscripts moving throughout the process and expertly tracked the many important details in this complex project. We'd also like to thank Nancy Tabor, project management team lead, for her guidance and assistance; and Mark Ong, design manager, who guided designer Tamara Newnam through the interior and cover designs and selection of the beautiful chapter-opening photos.

We can't go without thanking the marketing and sales teams who have been working so hard to get this book out to those who will benefit most from it, especially executive product marketing manager Neena Bali and the excellent Pearson marketing and market development teams for their enthusiastic support and innovative ideas.

Our goal of meeting instructor and student needs could not have been realized without the team of educators and editorial staff who worked on the substantial supplements package for *The Science of Nutrition*. Aimee Pavy, content producer, expertly supervised all aspects of the media program, including MasteringNutrition. Chelsea Logan expertly guided every aspect of the Teaching Toolkit DVD, and Kirsten Forsberg was our project manager for the Instructor Support Manual. Thanks to our supplements authors and contributors, with special appreciation to Laura Bonazzoli for the Test Bank revisions, and Southern Editorial for their work on the Instructor Resource Manual. Our gratitude to all for their valuable contributions to this edition.

We would also like to thank the many colleagues, friends, and family members who helped us along the way. Janice would specifically like to thank her supportive and hard-working colleagues at the University of Birmingham. "Their encouragement and enthusiasm keep me going through seemingly endless deadlines. My family and friends have been so incredibly wonderful throughout my career. Mom, Dianne, Pam, Steve, Aunt Judy, and cousin Julie are always there for me to offer a sympathetic ear, a shoulder to cry on, and endless encouragement. Although my Dad is no longer with us, his unwavering love and faith in my abilities inspired me to become who I am. I am always amazed that my friends and family actually read my books to learn more about nutrition—thanks for your never-ending support! You are incredible people who keep me sane and healthy and help me to remember the most important things in life."

Melinda would specifically like to thank her husband, Steve Carroll, for the patience and understanding he has shown through this process—once again. He has learned that there is always another chapter due! Melinda would also like to thank her family, friends, and professional colleagues for their support and listening ear through this whole process. They have all helped make life a little easier during this incredibly busy time.

Linda would like to acknowledge the unwavering support of her family and friends, a solid network of love and understanding that keeps her afloat. She would also like to thank Janice and Melinda for providing the opportunity to learn and grow through the process of writing this book.

Janice L. Thompson

Melinda M. Manore

Linda A. Vaughan

Reviewers

We extend our sincere gratitude to the following reviewers for their invaluable assistance in guiding the revision of and improvements in this text.

Lori Zienkewicz
Mesa Community College

Lisa Morse
Arizona State University

Simin Levinson
Arizona State University

Sherri Arthur
Oklahoma City Community College

Wendy Buchan
California State University, Sacramento

Eugene Fenster
Metropolitan Community College

Lisa Blackman
Tarrant County College

Christopher Wendtland
Monroe Community College

Candice Hines-Tinsley
Chaffey College

Alyce Fly
Indiana University Bloomington

Brief Contents

Contents

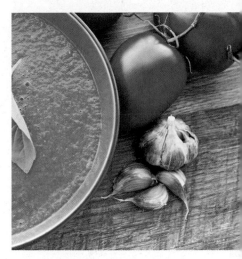

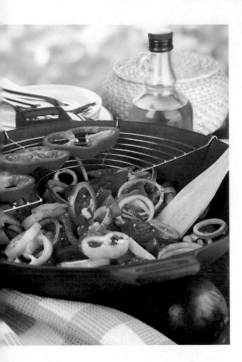

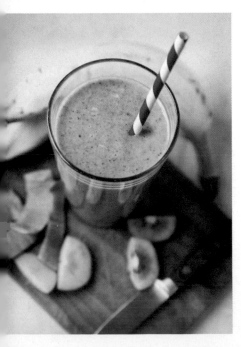

4 Carbohydrates: Plant-Derived Energy Nutrients 110

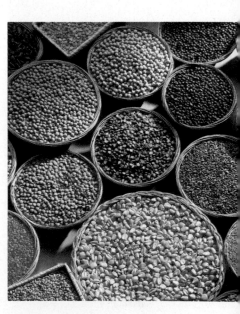

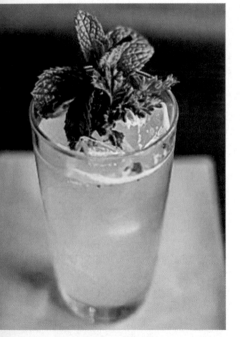

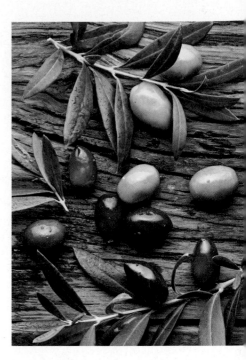

6 Proteins: Crucial Components of All Body Tissues 210

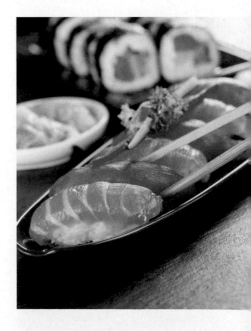

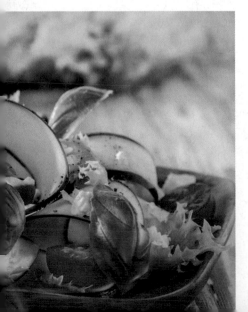

7 Metabolism: From Food to Life 250

Why Is Metabolism Essential for Life? 252

Anabolism and Catabolism Require or Release Energy 252

Energy Stored in Adenosine Triphosphate Fuels the Work of All Body Cells 253

What Chemical Reactions Are Fundamental to Metabolism? 254

In Dehydration Synthesis and Hydrolysis Reactions, Water Reacts with Molecules 255

In Phosphorylation Reactions, Molecules Exchange Phosphate 256

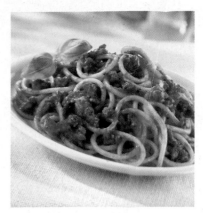

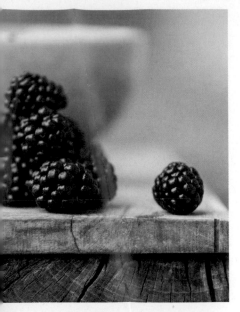

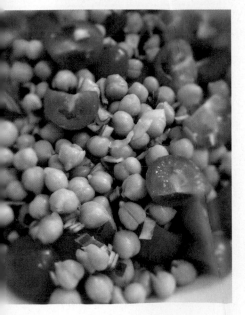

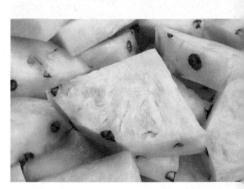

9 Nutrients Involved in Fluid and Electrolyte Balance 340

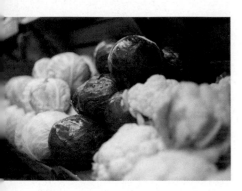

10 Nutrients Involved in Antioxidant Function and Vision 378

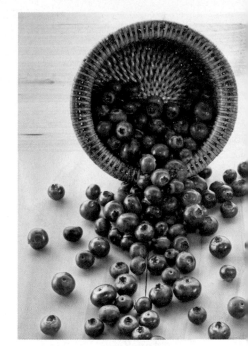

10.5 IN**DEPTH**
Phytochemicals: Another Advantage of Plants 418

11 Nutrients Involved In Bone Health 424

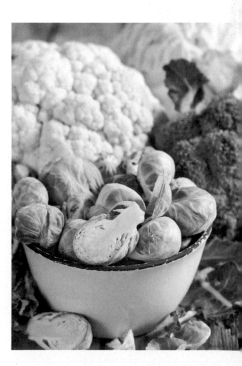

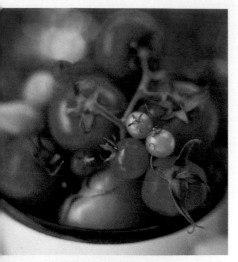

12 Nutrients Involved in Blood Health and Immunity 462

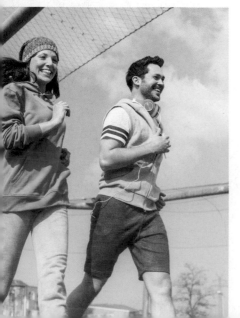

13 Achieving and Maintaining a Healthful Body Weight 496

13.5 IN**DEPTH**
Disordered Eating 540

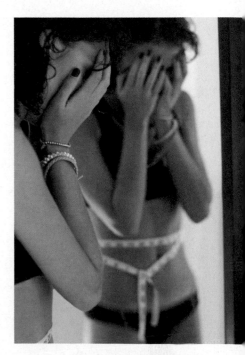

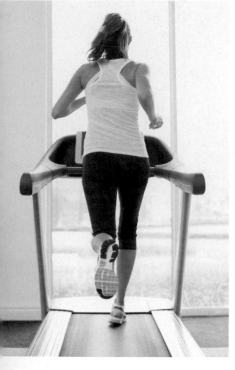

14 Nutrition and Physical Activity: Keys to Good Health 552

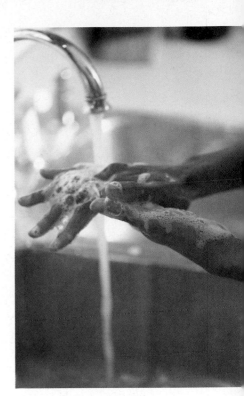

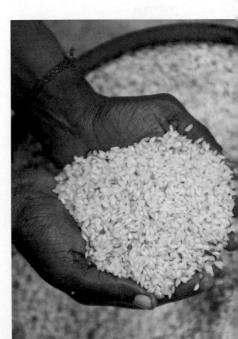

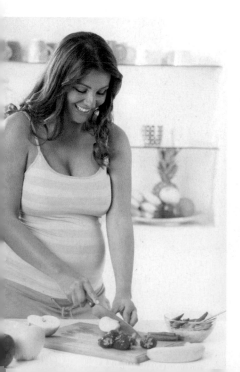

17 Nutrition Through the Life Cycle: Pregnancy and the First Year of Life 654

18 Nutrition Through the Life Cycle: Childhood and Adolescence 706

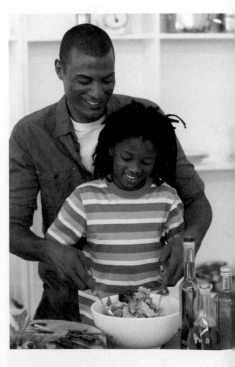

19 Nutrition Through the Life Cycle: The Later Years 742

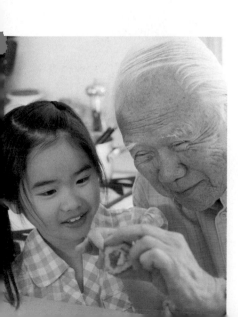

Appendices

Special Features

NUTRITION MYTH OR FACT?

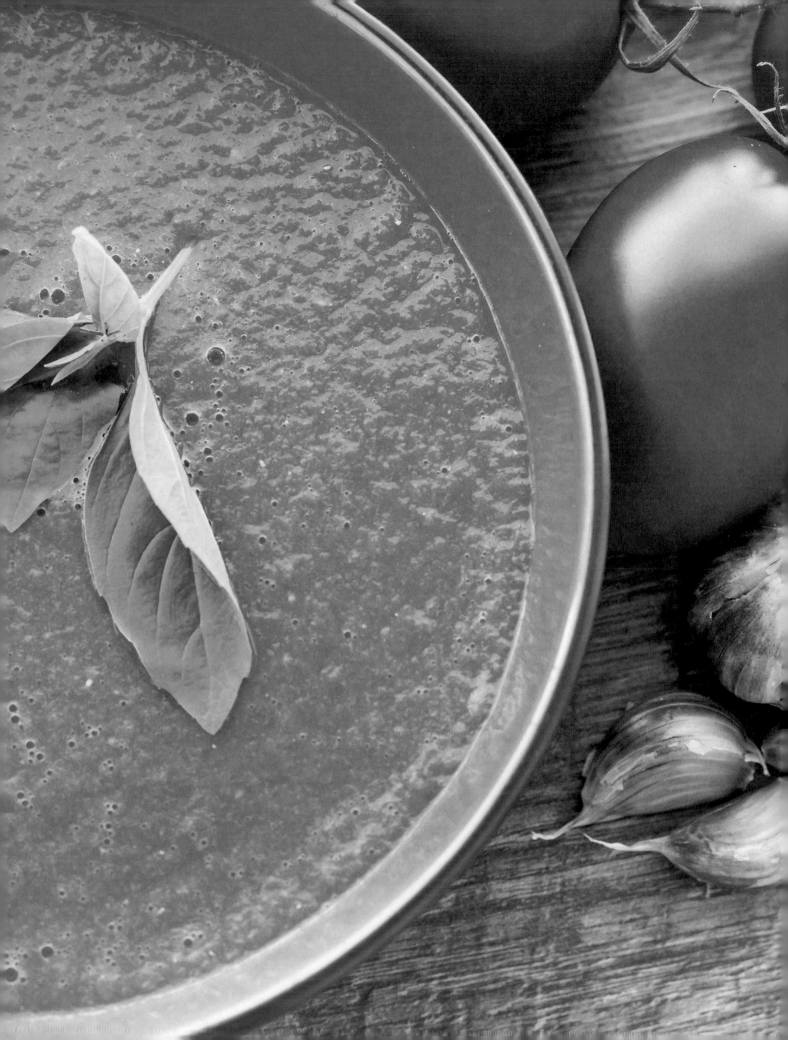

1 The Science of Nutrition: Linking Food, Function, and Health

Learning Outcomes

After studying this chapter, you should be able to:

1 Define the term *nutrition* and describe the history of nutrition science, *pp. 4–6*.

2 Discuss why nutrition is important to health, *pp. 6–9*.

3 Identify the six classes of nutrients essential for health and describe their functions, *pp. 9–15*.

4 Distinguish among the six types of Dietary Reference Intakes for nutrients, *pp. 15–18*.

5 Describe the tools nutritional professionals and other healthcare providers use for gathering data related to an individual's nutritional status and diet, *pp. 18–21*.

6 Explain how nutrition professionals classify malnutrition, *pp. 21–22*.

7 Discuss the four steps of the scientific method, *pp. 22–26*.

8 Compare and contrast the various types of research studies used in establishing nutrition guidelines, *pp. 26–27*.

9 Describe various approaches you can use to evaluate the truth and reliability of media reports, websites, and other sources of nutrition information, *pp. 28–30*.

10 List at least four sources of reliable and accurate nutrition information and state why they are trustworthy, *pp. 30–33*.

TEST YOURSELF

True or False?

1 A Calorie is a measure of the amount of fat in a food. **T** *or* **F**

2 Proteins are not a primary source of energy for our body. **T** *or* **F**

3 All vitamins must be consumed daily to support optimal health. **T** *or* **F**

4 The Recommended Dietary Allowance is the maximum amount of nutrient that people should consume to support normal body functions. **T** *or* **F**

5 Results from observational studies do not indicate cause and effect. **T** *or* **F**

Test Yourself answers are located in the Study Plan.

MasteringNutrition™

Go to **www.masteringnutrition .pearson.com** (or **www .pearsonmylabandmastering .com**) for chapter quizzes, pre-tests, interactive activities, and more!

Marilyn is 58 years old and works as a clerk at a small gift shop. During the last year, she has noticed that she is becoming increasingly tired at work and feels short of breath when performing tasks that she used to do easily, such as stocking shelves. This morning, she had her blood pressure checked for free at a local market and was told by the woman conducting the test that the reading was well above average. Assuming the woman's white lab coat meant that she was a healthcare professional, Marilyn asked her whether or not high blood pressure could explain her fatigue. The woman replied that fatigue was certainly a symptom and advised Marilyn to see her physician. When Marilyn explained that she tried to avoid trips to the doctor because her health insurance plan had a high deductible, the woman said, "Well, I'm not a physician, but I *am* a nutritionist, and I can certainly tell you that the best thing you can do to reduce your high blood pressure is to lose weight. We're running a special all month on Fiber Lunch, our most popular weight-loss supplement. You take it 30 minutes after your midday meal and it cleans out your digestive tract, keeping you from absorbing a lot of the food you eat. I can personally recommend it, because it helped me lose 30 pounds."

Marilyn wasn't convinced that she needed to lose weight. Sure, she was stocky, but she'd been that way all her life, and her fatigue had only started in the past year. But then she remembered that lately she'd been having trouble getting her rings on and off and that her shoes were feeling tight. So maybe the nutritionist was right and she should lose a few pounds. And hadn't she seen an ad for Fiber Lunch in her favorite women's magazine, or maybe on their website? Noticing Marilyn wavering, the nutritionist added, "A few weeks after I started taking Fiber Lunch, my blood pressure went from sky-high to perfectly normal." She certainly looked slender and healthy, and her personal testimonial convinced Marilyn to spend $12 of her weekly grocery budget on the smallest bottle of the supplements.

What do you think of the advice Marilyn received? Was the nutritionist's assessment of her nutritional status adequate? Was the treatment plan sound? Just what is a "nutritionist," anyway? In this chapter, we'll begin to answer these questions as we explore the role of nutrition in human health, identify the six classes of nutrients, and describe what constitutes a professional nutritional assessment. You'll also learn how to evaluate nutrition-related research studies, as well as how to distinguish science from scams. But first, let's take a quick look at the evolution of nutrition as a distinct scientific discipline.

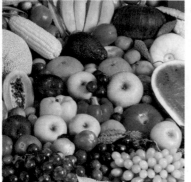

The study of nutrition encompasses everything about food.

LO 1 Define the term *nutrition* and describe the history of nutrition science.

What Is the Science of Nutrition and How Did It Evolve?

Although many people think that *food* and *nutrition* mean the same thing, they don't. **Food** refers to the plants and animals we consume. It contains the energy and nutrients our body needs to maintain life and support growth and health. **Nutrition,** in contrast, is a science. Specifically, it is the science that studies food and how food nourishes our body and influences our health. It identifies the processes by which we consume, digest, metabolize, and store the nutrients in foods and how these nutrients affect our body. Nutrition also involves studying the factors that influence our eating patterns, making recommendations about the amount we should eat of each type of food, maintaining food safety, and addressing issues related to the production of food and the global food supply.

When compared with other scientific disciplines, such as chemistry, biology, and physics, nutrition is a relative newcomer. The cultivation, preservation, and preparation of food have played a critical role in the lives of humans for millennia, but in the West, the recognition of nutrition as an important contributor to health has developed slowly only during the past 400 years.

It started when researchers began to observe an association between diet and illness. For instance, in the mid-1700s, long before vitamin C itself had been identified, researchers discovered that the vitamin C–deficiency disease *scurvy*, which causes joint pain, tissue breakdown, and even death, could be prevented by consuming citrus fruits. By the mid-1800s, the three energy-providing nutrients—carbohydrates, lipids, and proteins—had been identified, as well as a number of essential minerals. Nutrition was coming into its own as a developing scientific discipline.

food The plants and animals we consume.

nutrition The scientific study of food and how it nourishes the body and influences health.

Still, vitamins were entirely unrecognized, and some fatal diseases that we now know to be due to vitamin deficiency were then thought to be due to infection. For instance, when Dutch physician Christian Eijkman began studying the fatal nerve disease *beriberi* in the 1880s, he conducted experiments designed to ferret out the causative bacterium. Finally, Eijkman discovered that replacing the polished white rice in a patient's diet with whole-grain brown rice cures the disease. Still, he surmised that something in the brown rice conferred resistance to the beriberi "germ." It was not until the 20th century that the substance missing in polished rice—the B-vitamin *thiamin*—was identified and beriberi was definitively classified as a deficiency disease. Another B-vitamin, niacin, was discovered through the work of Dr. Joseph Goldberger in the early 1900s. The accompanying *Highlight* box describes Dr. Goldberger's daring work.

Nutrition research continued to focus on identifying and preventing deficiency diseases through the first half of the 20th century. Then, as the higher standard of living after World War II led to an improvement in the American diet, nutrition research began pursuing a new objective: supporting wellness and preventing and treating **chronic diseases**— that is, diseases that come on slowly and can persist for years, often despite treatment.

chronic disease A disease characterized by a gradual onset and long duration, with signs and symptoms that are difficult to interpret and that respond poorly to medical treatment.

HIGHLIGHT

Solving the Mystery of Pellagra

In the first few years of the 20th century, Dr. Joseph Goldberger successfully controlled outbreaks of several fatal infectious diseases, from yellow fever in Louisiana to typhus in Mexico. So it wasn't surprising that, in 1914, the Surgeon General of the United States chose him to tackle another disease thought to be infectious that was raging throughout the South. Called pellagra, the disease was characterized by a skin rash, diarrhea, and mental impairment. At the time, it afflicted more than 50,000 people each year, and in about 10% of cases it resulted in death.

Goldberger began studying the disease by carefully observing its occurrence in groups of people. He asked, if it is infectious, then why would it strike children in orphanages and prison inmates yet leave their nurses and guards unaffected? Why did it overwhelmingly affect impoverished mill workers and share croppers while leaving their affluent (and well-fed) neighbors healthy? Could a dietary deficiency cause pellagra? To confirm his hunch, he conducted a series of trials in which he fed afflicted orphans and prisoners, who had been

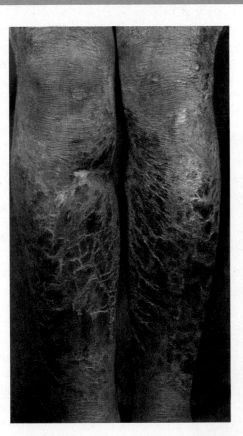

Pellagra is often characterized by a scaly skin rash.

consuming a limited, corn-based diet, a variety of nutrient-rich foods, including meats. They recovered. Moreover, orphans and inmates who did not have pellagra and ate the new diet did not develop the disease. Finally, Goldberger recruited 11 healthy prison inmates, who in return for a pardon of their sentence agreed to consume a limited, corn-based diet. After 5 months, six of the 11 developed pellagra.

Still, many skeptics were unable to give up the idea that pellagra was an infectious disease. So to prove that pellagra was not spread by germs, Goldberger, his colleagues, and his wife deliberately injected and ingested patients' scabs, nasal secretions, and other bodily fluids. They remained free of the disease.

Although Goldberger could not identify the precise component in the new diet that cured pellagra, he eventually found an inexpensive and widely available substance, brewer's yeast, that when added to the diet prevented or reversed the disease. Shortly after Goldberger's death in 1937, scientists identified the precise nutrient that was deficient in the diet of pellagra patients: niacin, one of the B-vitamins, which is plentiful in brewer's yeast.

Source: Kraut, A. *Dr. Joseph Goldberger and the War on Pellagra.* National Institutes of Health, Office of NIH History. http://history.nih.gov/exhibits /Goldberger/index.html.

wellness A multidimensional, lifelong process that includes physical, emotional, and spiritual health.

Chronic diseases of particular interest to nutrition researchers include obesity, cardiovascular disease, type 2 diabetes, and various cancers. This new research has raised as many questions as it has answered, and we still have a great deal to learn about the relationship between nutrition and chronic disease.

In the closing decades of the 20th century, an exciting new area of nutrition research began to emerge. Reflecting our growing understanding of genetics and epigenetics, *nutrigenomics* seeks to uncover links among our genes, our environment, and our diet, and to generate nutrition information tailored to our genetic makeup. But is this promise of personalized nutrition ever likely to be fulfilled? Check out the ***Nutrition Myth or Fact?*** at the end of this chapter to find out.

RECAP

Food refers to the plants and animals we consume, whereas *nutrition* is the scientific study of food and how food affects our body and our health. In the past, nutrition research focused on the prevention of nutrient-deficiency diseases, such as scurvy and beriberi; currently, a great deal of nutrition research is dedicated to identifying dietary patterns that can lower the risk for chronic diseases, such as type 2 diabetes and heart disease. Nutrigenomics is an emerging focus of nutrition research. ∎

LO 2 Discuss why nutrition is important to health.

How Does Nutrition Contribute to Health?

Proper nutrition can help us improve our health, prevent certain diseases, achieve and maintain a desirable weight, and maintain our energy and vitality. When you consider that most people eat on average three meals per day, this results in more than 1,000 opportunities a year to affect our health through nutrition. The following section provides more detail on how nutrition supports health and wellness.

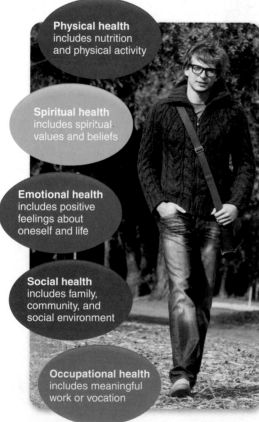

Physical health includes nutrition and physical activity

Spiritual health includes spiritual values and beliefs

Emotional health includes positive feelings about oneself and life

Social health includes family, community, and social environment

Occupational health includes meaningful work or vocation

FIGURE 1.1 Many factors contribute to an individual's wellness. Primary among these are a nutritious diet and regular physical activity.

Nutrition Is One of Several Factors Supporting Wellness

Traditionally, **wellness** was defined simply as the absence of disease. However, as we have learned more about our health and what it means to live a healthful lifestyle, our definition has expanded. Wellness is now considered to be a multidimensional process, one that includes physical, emotional, social, occupational, and spiritual health (**Figure 1.1**). Wellness is not an end point in our lives but rather is an active process we engage in with every day.

In this book, we focus on two critical aspects of wellness: nutrition and physical activity. These two are so closely related that you can think of them as two sides of the same coin: our overall state of nutrition is influenced by how much energy we expend doing daily activities, and our level of physical activity has a major impact on how we use the nutrients in our food. We can perform more strenuous activities for longer periods of time when we eat a nutritious diet, whereas an inadequate or excessive food intake can make us lethargic. A poor diet, inadequate or excessive physical activity, or a combination of these also can lead to serious health problems. Finally, several studies have suggested that healthful nutrition and regular physical activity can increase feelings of well-being and reduce feelings of anxiety and depression. In other words, wholesome food and physical activity just plain feel good!

A Healthful Diet Can Prevent Some Diseases and Reduce Your Risk for Others

Nutrition appears to play a role—from a direct cause to a mild influence—in the development of many diseases (**Figure 1.2**). As we noted earlier, poor nutrition is a direct cause of deficiency diseases, such as scurvy and beriberi. Thus, early nutrition research focused on identifying the causes of nutrient-deficiency diseases and means to prevent them. These discoveries led nutrition experts to develop guidelines for nutrient intakes that are high enough to prevent deficiency diseases, and to lobby for the fortification of foods with nutrients of concern. These measures, along with a more abundant and reliable food supply, have ensured that most nutrient-deficiency diseases are no longer of concern in developed countries. However, they are still major problems in many developing nations.

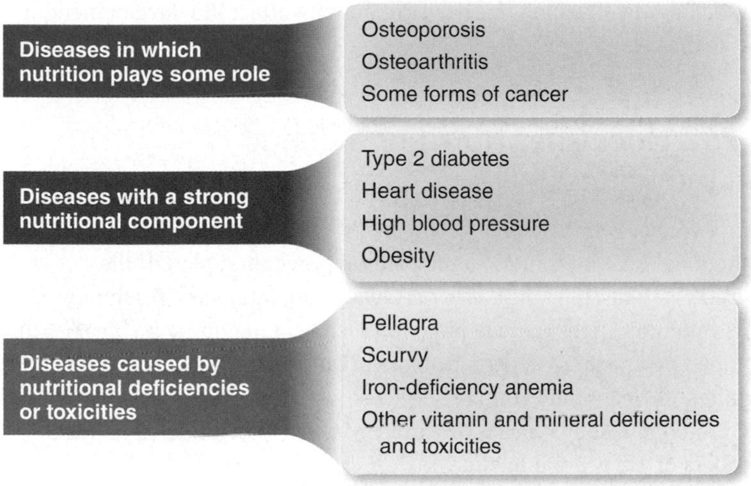

Diseases in which nutrition plays some role	Osteoporosis Osteoarthritis Some forms of cancer
Diseases with a strong nutritional component	Type 2 diabetes Heart disease High blood pressure Obesity
Diseases caused by nutritional deficiencies or toxicities	Pellagra Scurvy Iron-deficiency anemia Other vitamin and mineral deficiencies and toxicities

FIGURE 1.2 The relationship between nutrition and human disease. Notice that, whereas nutritional factors are only marginally implicated in the diseases of the top row, they are strongly linked to the development of the diseases in the middle row and truly causative of those in the bottom row.

In addition to directly causing disease, poor nutrition can have a more subtle influence on our health. For instance, it can contribute to the development of brittle bones, a disease called *osteoporosis,* as well as to the progression of some forms of cancer. These associations are considered mild; however, poor nutrition is also strongly associated with three chronic diseases that are among the top ten causes of death in the United States (**Figure 1.3**).

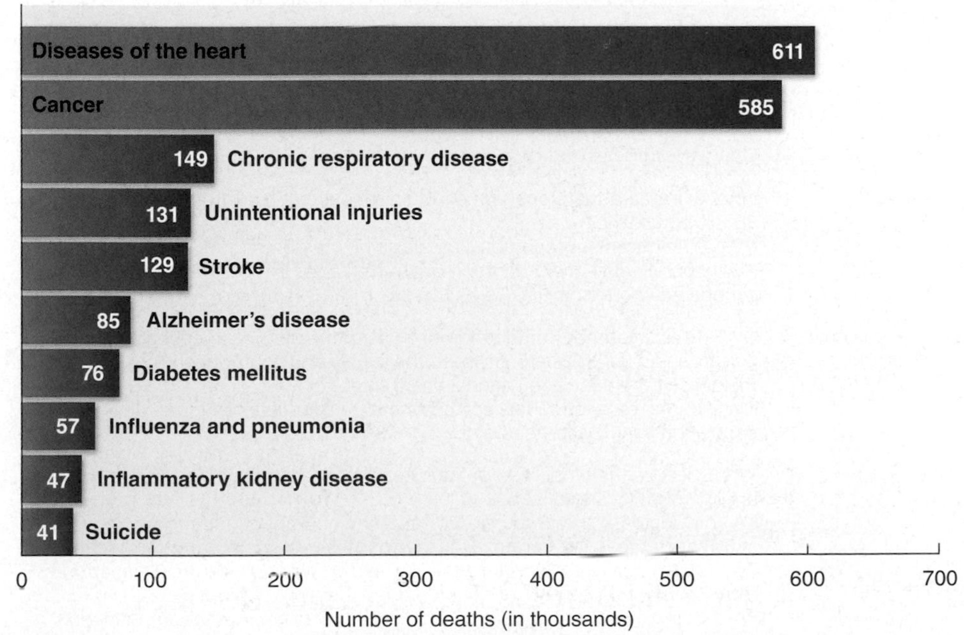

	Number of deaths (in thousands)
Diseases of the heart	611
Cancer	585
Chronic respiratory disease	149
Unintentional injuries	131
Stroke	129
Alzheimer's disease	85
Diabetes mellitus	76
Influenza and pneumonia	57
Inflammatory kidney disease	47
Suicide	41

FIGURE 1.3 Of the 10 leading causes of death in the United States in 2012, three—heart disease, stroke, and diabetes—are strongly associated with poor nutrition. (*Source:* K. D. Kochanek, S. L. Murphy, J. Xu, and E. Arias. "Mortality in the United States, 2013," *NCHS Data Brief* No. 178 [December, 2014].)

1994

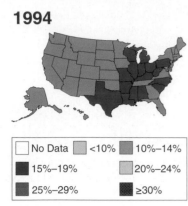

☐ No Data	☐ <10%	☐ 10%–14%
■ 15%–19%	☐ 20%–24%	
■ 25%–29%	■ ≥30%	

2010

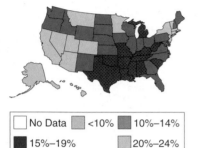

☐ No Data	☐ <10%	☐ 10%–14%
■ 15%–19%	☐ 20%–24%	
■ 25%–29%	■ ≥30%	

FIGURE 1.4 These diagrams illustrate the increase in obesity prevalence across the United States from 1994 to 2010, the last year during which there was a significant increase in rates. Obesity is defined as a body mass index greater than or equal to 30, or approximately 30 lb overweight for a 5'4" woman. (*Source:* Graphics from Centers for Disease Control and Prevention, Obesity Prevalence Maps 1985 to 2010.)

These are heart disease, stroke, and diabetes. Recent research indicates that poor diets and physical inactivity account for 10% of deaths and disability worldwide.[1]

It probably won't surprise you to learn that the primary link between poor nutrition and mortality is obesity. Fundamentally, obesity is a consequence of consuming more energy than is expended. At the same time, obesity is a well-established risk factor for heart disease, stroke, type 2 diabetes, and some forms of cancer. Unfortunately, the **prevalence** of obesity, or the percentage of the population that is affected with obesity at a given time, has dramatically increased throughout the United States from the 1970s through about 2010 (**Figure 1.4**). Fortunately, over the last few years, the rate has leveled off. Throughout this text, we will discuss in detail how nutrition and physical activity affect the development of obesity and other chronic diseases.

Healthy People 2020 Identifies Nutrition-Related Goals for the United States

Because of its importance to the wellness of all Americans, nutrition has been included in *Healthy People*, the national health promotion and disease prevention plan of the United States. It is revised every decade, and *Healthy People 2020*, launched in January 2010, identifies the goals and objectives that we hope to reach as a nation by the year 2020.[2] This agenda was developed by a team of experts from a variety of federal agencies under the direction of the Department of Health and Human Services. Input was gathered from a large number of individuals and organizations, including hundreds of national and state health organizations and members of the general public.

The four overarching goals of *Healthy People* are to "(1) attain high-quality, longer lives free of preventable disease, disability, injury, and premature death; (2) achieve health equity, eliminate disparities, and improve the health of all groups; (3) create social and physical environments that promote good health for all; and (4) promote quality of life, healthy development, and healthy behaviors across all life stages." These broad goals are supported by hundreds of specific goals and objectives, including 22 related to nutrition and weight status (NWS). There are also 15 objectives addressing physical activity (PA), which is, of course, related to nutrition. **Table 1.1** identifies a few of the nutrition and physical activity objectives from *Healthy People 2020*.

TABLE 1.1 Nutrition and Physical Activity Objectives from *Healthy People 2020*

Topic	Objective Number and Description
Weight status	NWS-8. Increase the proportion of adults who are at a healthy weight from 30.8% to 33.9%. NWS-9. Reduce the proportion of adults who are obese from 34.0% to 30.6%. NWS-10.2. Reduce the proportion of children aged 6 to 11 years who are considered obese from 17.4% to 15.7%.
Food and nutrient composition	NWS-14. Increase the contribution of fruits to the diets of the population aged 2 years and older. NWS-15. Increase the variety and contribution of vegetables to the diets of the population aged 2 years and older. NWS-15. Increase the variety and contribution of vegetables to the diets of the population aged 2 years and older.
Physical activity	PA–1. Reduce the proportion of adults who engage in no leisure-time physical activity from 36.2% to 32.6%. PA–2.1. Increase the proportion of adults who engage in aerobic physical activity of at least moderate intensity for at least 150 minutes per week, or 75 minutes per week of vigorous intensity, or an equivalent combination from 43.5% to 47.9%. PA–2.3. Increase the proportion of adults who perform muscle-strengthening activities on 2 or more days of the week from 21.9% to 24.1%.

Data adapted from: "Healthy People 2020" (U.S. Department of Health and Human Services).

prevalence The percentage of the population that is affected with a particular disease at a given time.

RECAP

Nutrition is an important component of wellness and is strongly associated with physical activity. Nutrition appears to play a role—from a direct cause to a mild influence—in the development of many diseases. *Healthy People 2020* is a health promotion and disease prevention plan for the United States that includes numerous objectives related to nutrition and weight status and physical activity.

nutrients Chemicals found in foods that are critical to human growth and function.

organic A substance or nutrient that contains the elements carbon and hydrogen.

inorganic A substance or nutrient that does not contain carbon and hydrogen.

LO 3 Identify the six classes of nutrients essential for health and describe their functions.

What Are Nutrients?

We enjoy eating food because of its taste, its smell, and the pleasure and comfort it gives us. However, we rarely stop to think about what our food actually contains. Foods are composed of many chemical substances, some of which are not useful to the body and others of which are critical to human growth and function. These latter chemicals are referred to as **nutrients**. The six groups of nutrients found in foods are (**Figure 1.5**)

- Carbohydrates
- Lipids (including fats and oils)
- Proteins
- Vitamins
- Minerals
- Water

As you may know, the term *organic* is commonly used to describe foods that are grown with little or no use of chemicals. But when scientists describe individual nutrients as **organic,** they mean that these nutrients contain the elements *carbon* and *hydrogen*, which are essential components of all living organisms. Carbohydrates, lipids, proteins, and vitamins are organic. Minerals and water are **inorganic**. Both organic and inorganic nutrients are equally important for sustaining life but differ in their structures, functions, and basic chemistry. You will learn more about these nutrients in subsequent chapters; a brief review is provided here.

Macronutrients Provide Energy

Carbohydrates, lipids, and proteins are the only nutrients in foods that provide energy. By this we mean that these nutrients break down and reassemble into a fuel that the body uses to support physical activity and basic physiologic functioning. Although taking a multivitamin and a glass of water might be beneficial in some ways, it will not provide you with the energy you need to do your 20 minutes on the stair-climber! Along with water, the energy nutrients are also referred to as **macronutrients**. *Macro* means "large"; thus, macronutrients are those nutrients needed in relatively large amounts to support normal function and health.

Alcohol is found in certain beverages and foods, and it provides energy—but it is not considered a nutrient. This is because it does not support the regulation of body functions or the building or repairing of tissues. In fact, alcohol is considered to be both a drug and a toxin. (Details about alcohol are provided in In Depth 4.5 on pp. 152–163.)

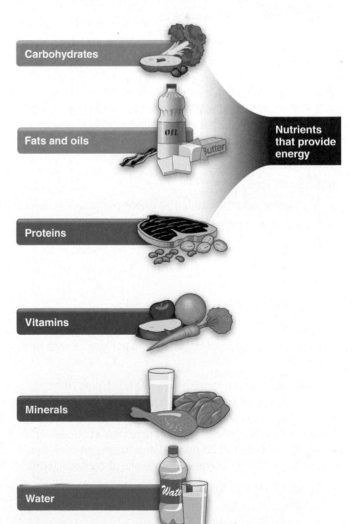

SIX GROUPS OF ESSENTIAL NUTRIENTS

Carbohydrates

Fats and oils

Nutrients that provide energy

Proteins

Vitamins

Minerals

Water

FIGURE 1.5 The six groups of nutrients found in the foods we consume.

Nutrition scientists in the United States typically use the metric system of measurement, but the U.S. customary system is also commonly used, especially in information for the public. Thus, it is important for anyone learning about nutrition to learn how to express and calculate both metric and nonmetric units. Refer to the *You Do the Math* box "Cooking with Metrics" to see how to cook a delicious meal using new skills. For help converting between customary and metric measures, see Appendix D.

macronutrients Nutrients that the body requires in relatively large amounts to support normal function and health. Carbohydrates, lipids, proteins, and water are macronutrients.

Energy Is Measured in Kilocalories

The energy in foods is measured in units called *kilocalories* (*kcal*). A kilocalorie is the amount of heat required to raise the temperature of 1 kilogram (about 2.2 lb) of water by 1 degree Celsius. We can say that the energy found in 1 gram of carbohydrate is equal to 4 kcal.

YOU Do the Math — Cooking with Metrics

Theo is planning to cook a romantic Valentine's Day dinner for his girlfriend, Heidi. Heidi loves roast chicken, so, Theo has searched the Internet to find a recipe for roast chicken that appears relatively quick and easy and contains ingredients that are affordable. Theo finds a recipe that seems perfect, but it comes from a website based in the United Kingdom, where metric units are used in cooking. Here is the ingredient list:

- 1 whole chicken, approximately 1.6 kg
- 2 medium onions
- 2–3 carrots, approximately 150 grams
- 8 small new potatoes, approximately 600 grams total
- 2 sticks of celery
- 1 bulb of garlic
- olive oil
- sea salt and freshly ground black pepper
- 1 lemon
- a small bunch of fresh thyme, rosemary, bay, or sage or a mixture

Cooking temperature for this recipe is listed as 240°C. Theo uses the metric conversions included in Appendix D of this textbook, Calculations and Conversions, to assist him in estimating the weight of the chicken (in pounds and ounces) and the carrots and potatoes (in ounces) and to convert oven temperature to Fahrenheit. Here are the results of his calculations:

1. Converting the weight of the chicken into pounds and ounces:
   a. 1 kg is equivalent to 2.2 pounds. By multiplying the weight of the chicken in kilograms by 2.2,

Theo will get the weight of the chicken in pounds—1.6 kg × 2.2 lb/kg = 3.52 lb.
   b. To calculate the number of ounces, Theo knows that there are 16 ounces in 1 lb. He multiplies the fraction of 1 lb (in this case, 0.52) by 16 ounces = 0.52 × 16 = 8.32, or approximately 8 ounces. Thus, Theo is looking to buy a chicken that weighs approximately 3 lb 8 ounces.

2. Converting the weight of the carrots and potatoes from grams into ounces:
   a. To perform this calculation, Theo knows that 1 gram = 0.035 ounce. He multiplies the weight of the carrots or potatoes in grams by 0.035 to get their weight in ounces.
   b. For the carrots—150 grams × 0.035 ounce/gram = 5.25 ounces of carrots
   c. For the potatoes—600 grams × 0.035 = 21 ounces of potatoes

3. To calculate the cooking temperature in Fahrenheit, Theo needs to multiply °C by 9, then divide by 5. Then he needs to add 32 to this value:

   [(°C × 9)/5] + 32 = [(200°C × 9)/5] + 32 = (1,800/5) + 32 = 360 + 32 = 392°F

   The closest setting to this on Theo's oven is 400°F, so he will cook the chicken at this temperature.

4. Now try these steps yourself to calculate the metric equivalents in a recipe from the United States calling for 12 ounces of haddock, 4 ounces of shallots, and a baking temperature of 400°F.

Kilo- is a prefix used in the metric system to indicate 1,000 (think of *kilometer*). Technically, 1 kilocalorie is equal to 1,000 calories. A kilocalorie is also sometimes referred to as a *large calorie* or as a *Calorie*, written with a capital C. Because they're designed for the public, nutrition labels typically use the term *calories* to indicate kilocalories. Thus, if the wrapper on an ice cream bar states that it contains 150 calories, it actually contains 150 kcal.

In this textbook, we use the term *energy* when referring to the general concept of energy intake or expenditure. We use the term *kilocalories* (*kcal*) when discussing units of energy. We use the term *Calories* with a capital "C" when presenting information about foods and food labels.

Both carbohydrates and proteins provide 4 kcal per gram, alcohol provides 7 kcal per gram, and fats provide 9 kcal per gram. Thus, for every gram of fat we consume, we obtain more than twice the energy derived from a gram of carbohydrate or protein.

Nutrition
M I L E S T O N E

In **1782**, the French chemist Antoine Lavoisier invented a device that could measure the heat produced by chemical reactions, including those taking place in an animal. He called his device a *calorimeter*, from the Latin word *calor*, meaning "heat." Using his calorimeter, Lavoisier made the first measurements of the energy (thermal energy, or heat) produced by the consumption of various types of foods. Today, we measure this heat in units called Calories.

Carbohydrates Are a Primary Fuel Source

Carbohydrates are the primary source of fuel for the human body, particularly for neurologic functioning and physical exercise (**Figure 1.6**). A close look at the word *carbohydrate* reveals the chemical structure of this nutrient. *Carbo-* refers to carbon, and *-hydrate* refers to water. You may remember that water is made up of hydrogen and oxygen. Thus, carbohydrates are composed of chains of carbon, hydrogen, and oxygen.

Carbohydrates are found in a wide variety of foods: rice, wheat, and other grains, as well as vegetables and fruits. Carbohydrates are also found in *legumes* (foods that include lentils, beans, and peas), seeds, nuts, and milk and other dairy products. Fiber is also classified as a type of carbohydrate. (Carbohydrates and their role in health are the focus of Chapter 4.)

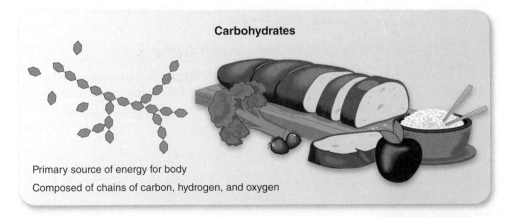

Carbohydrates

Primary source of energy for body
Composed of chains of carbon, hydrogen, and oxygen

FIGURE 1.6 Carbohydrates are a primary source of energy for our body and are found in a wide variety of foods.

Lipids Provide Energy and Other Essential Nutrients

Lipids are another important source of energy for the body (**Figure 1.7**). Lipids are a diverse group of organic substances that are largely insoluble in water. In foods, they are found in solid fats and liquid oils. Lipids include triglycerides, phospholipids, and sterols. Like carbohydrates, lipids are composed mainly of carbon, hydrogen, and oxygen (and in phospholipids, phosphorus and sometimes nitrogen); however, they contain proportionately much less oxygen and water than do carbohydrates. This quality partly explains why they yield more energy per gram than either carbohydrates or proteins.

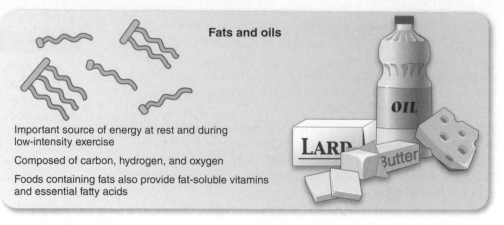

FIGURE 1.7 Lipids are an important energy source during rest and low-intensity exercise. Foods containing lipids also provide other important nutrients.

Triglycerides (more commonly known as fats) are by far the most common lipid in foods. They are composed of an alcohol molecule called *glycerol* attached to three acid molecules called *fatty acids*. As we'll discuss throughout this book, triglycerides in foods exert different health effects according to the type of fatty acids they contain. Some fatty acids are associated with an increased risk of chronic disease, whereas others—including essential fatty acids—protect our health. Triglycerides are an important energy source when we are at rest and during low- to moderate-intensity exercise. The human body is capable of storing large amounts of triglycerides as adipose tissue, or body fat. These fat stores can be broken down for energy during periods of fasting, such as while we are asleep. Foods that contain lipids are also important for the absorption of fat-soluble vitamins.

Phospholipids are a type of lipid that contains phosphate. The body synthesizes phospholipids, and they are found in a few foods. Cholesterol is a form of lipid that is synthesized in the liver and other body tissues. It is also available in foods of animal origin, such as meat and eggs. Plant sterols are present in some plant-based foods such as vegetable oils. (Chapter 5 provides a thorough review of lipids.)

Proteins Support Tissue Growth, Repair, and Maintenance

Proteins also contain carbon, hydrogen, and oxygen, but they differ from carbohydrates and lipids in that they contain the element *nitrogen* (**Figure 1.8**). Within proteins, these four elements assemble into small building blocks known as *amino acids*. We break down dietary proteins into amino acids and reassemble them to build our own body proteins—for instance, the proteins in muscles and blood.

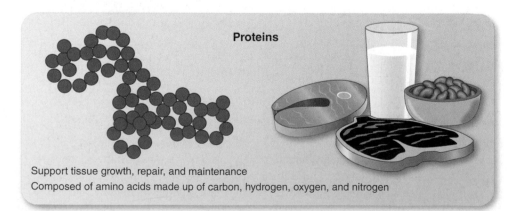

FIGURE 1.8 Proteins contain nitrogen in addition to carbon, hydrogen, and oxygen. Proteins support the growth, repair, and maintenance of body tissues.

YOU Do the Math

Calculating the Energy Contribution of Carbohydrates, Lipids, and Proteins

One of the most useful skills to learn as you study nutrition is determining the percentage of the total energy someone eats that comes from carbohydrates, lipids, or proteins. These data are an important first step in evaluating the quality of an individual's diet. Fortunately, a simple equation is available to help you calculate these values.

To begin, you need to know how much total energy someone consumes each day, as well as how many grams of carbohydrates, lipids, and proteins. You also need to know the kilocalorie (kcal) value of each of these nutrients: the energy value for carbohydrates and proteins is 4 kcal per gram, the energy value for alcohol is 7 kcal per gram, and the energy value for lipids is 9 kcal per gram. Working along with the following example will help you perform the calculations:

1. Let's say you have completed a personal diet analysis for your mother, and she consumes 2,500 kcal per day. From your diet analysis you also find that she consumes 300 g of carbohydrates, 90 g of lipids, and 123 g of proteins.

2. To calculate her percentage of total energy that comes from carbohydrates, you must do two things:

   a. Multiply her total grams of carbohydrate by the energy value for carbohydrate to determine how many kilocalories of carbohydrate she has consumed.

   300 g of carbohydrate $\times$ 4 kcal/g = 1,200 kcal of carbohydrate

   b. Take the kilocalories of carbohydrate she has consumed, divide this number by the total number of kilocalories she has consumed, and multiply by 100. This will give you the percentage of total energy that comes from carbohydrate.

   (1,200 kcal/2,500 kcal) $\times$ 100 = 48% of total energy from carbohydrate

3. To calculate her percentage of total energy that comes from lipids, you follow the same steps but incorporate the energy value for lipids:

   a. Multiply her total grams of lipids by the energy value for lipids to find the kilocalories of lipids consumed.

   90 g of fats $\times$ 9 kcal/g = 810 kcal of lipids

   b. Take the kilocalories of lipids she has consumed, divide this number by the total number of kilocalories she consumed, and multiply by 100 to get the percentage of total energy from lipids.

   (810 kcal/2,500 kcal) $\times$ 100 = 32.4% of total energy from lipids

4. Now try these steps to calculate the percentage of the total energy she has consumed that comes from proteins.

These calculations will be useful throughout this course as you learn more about how to design a healthful diet. Later in this book, you will learn how to estimate someone's energy needs and determine the appropriate amount of energy to consume from carbohydrates, fats, and proteins.

Although proteins can provide energy, they are not usually a primary energy source. Proteins play a major role in building new cells and tissues, maintaining the structure and strength of bone, repairing damaged structures, and assisting in regulating metabolism and fluid balance.

Proteins are found in many foods. Meats and dairy products are primary sources, as are seeds, nuts, and legumes. We also obtain small amounts of protein from vegetables and whole grains. (Proteins are explored in detail in Chapter 6.)

Now that you've been introduced to the three energy nutrients, refer to the **You Do the Math** box (see above) to learn how to calculate the different energy contributions of carbohydrates, lipids, and proteins in one day's diet.

Micronutrients Assist in the Regulation of Physiologic Processes

Vitamins and minerals are referred to as **micronutrients**. That's because we need relatively small amounts of these nutrients to support normal health and body functions.

micronutrients Nutrients needed in relatively small amounts to support normal health and body functions. Vitamins and minerals are micronutrients.

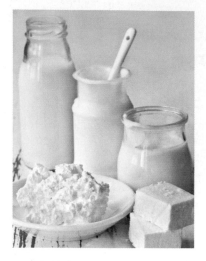

Fat-soluble vitamins are found in a variety of fat-containing foods, including dairy products.

Vitamins are organic compounds that assist in the regulation of the body's physiologic processes. Contrary to popular belief, vitamins do not contain energy (or kilocalories); however, they do play an important role in the release and utilization of the energy found in carbohydrates, lipids, and proteins. They are also critical in building and maintaining healthy bone, blood, and muscle; in supporting our immune system so we can fight illness and disease; and in ensuring healthy vision.

Vitamins are classified as two types: **fat-soluble vitamins** and **water-soluble vitamins** (Table 1.2). This classification reflects how vitamins are absorbed, transported, and stored in our body. As our body cannot synthesize most vitamins, we must consume them in our diet. Both fat-soluble and water-soluble vitamins are essential for our health and are found in a variety of foods. Learn more about vitamins in In Depth 7.5 on pp. 292–303. Individual vitamins are discussed in detail later in this text (Chapters 8 through 12).

TABLE 1.2 Overview of Vitamins

Type	Names	Distinguishing Features
Fat soluble	A, D, E, K	Soluble in fat Stored in the human body Toxicity can occur from consuming excess amounts, which accumulate in the body
Water soluble	C, B-vitamins (thiamin, riboflavin, niacin, vitamin B_6, vitamin B_{12}, pantothenic acid, biotin, folate)	Soluble in water Not stored to any extent in the human body Excess excreted in urine Toxicity generally only occurs as a result of vitamin supplementation

Minerals include sodium, calcium, iron, and over a dozen more. They are classified as inorganic because they do not contain carbon and hydrogen. In fact, they do not "contain" other substances at all. Minerals are single elements, so they already exist in the simplest possible chemical form. Thus, they cannot be broken down during digestion or when our body uses them to promote normal function; and unlike certain vitamins, they can't be destroyed by heat or light. All minerals maintain their structure no matter what environment they are in. This means that the calcium in our bones is the same as the calcium in the milk we drink, and the sodium in our cells is the same as the sodium in our table salt.

Minerals have many important physiologic functions. They assist in fluid regulation and energy production, are essential to the health of our bones and blood, and help rid the body of harmful by-products of metabolism. Minerals are classified according to the amounts we need in our diet and according to how much of the mineral is found in the body. The two categories of minerals in our diet and body are the **major minerals** and the **trace minerals** (Table 1.3). Learn more about minerals in In Depth 7.5 on pages 292–303. Individual minerals are discussed in detail later in this text (Chapters 8 through 12).

fat-soluble vitamins Vitamins that are not soluble in water but soluble in fat. These include vitamins A, D, E, and K.

water-soluble vitamins Vitamins that are soluble in water. These include vitamin C and the B-vitamins.

major minerals Minerals we need to consume in amounts of at least 100 mg per day and of which the total amount in our body is at least 5 g (5,000 mg).

trace minerals Minerals we need to consume in amounts less than 100 mg per day and of which the total amount in our body is less than 5 g (5,000 mg).

TABLE 1.3 Overview of Minerals

Type	Names	Distinguishing Features
Major minerals	Calcium, phosphorus, sodium, potassium, chloride, magnesium, sulfur	Needed in amounts greater than 100 mg/day in our diet Amount present in the human body is greater than 5 g (5,000 mg)
Trace minerals	Iron, zinc, copper, manganese, fluoride, chromium, molybdenum, selenium, iodine	Needed in amounts less than 100 mg/day in our diet Amount present in the human body is less than 5 g (5,000 mg)

Water Supports All Body Functions

Water is an inorganic macronutrient that is vital for our survival. We consume water in its pure form; in juices, soups, and other liquids; and in solid foods, such as fruits and vegetables. Adequate water intake ensures the proper balance of fluid both inside and outside our cells and assists in the regulation of nerve impulses and body temperature, muscle contractions, nutrient transport, and excretion of waste products. (Chapter 9 focuses on water.)

RECAP

The six essential nutrient groups found in foods are carbohydrates, lipids, proteins, vitamins, minerals, and water. Carbohydrates, lipids, and proteins are energy nutrients. Carbohydrates are the primary energy source; lipids provide fat-soluble vitamins and essential fatty acids and act as energy-storage molecules; and proteins support tissue growth, repair, and maintenance. Vitamins are organic compounds that assist with regulating a multitude of body processes. Minerals are inorganic elements that have critical roles in virtually all aspects of human health and function. Water is essential for survival and supports all body functions. ■

What Are the Current Dietary Intake Recommendations and How Are They Used?

LO 4 Distinguish among the six types of Dietary Reference Intakes for nutrients.

Now that you know what the six classes of nutrients are, you are probably wondering how much of each a person needs each day. We identify specific nutrient intakes in relevant chapters later in this text. For now, you need to become familiar with the set of intake standards used to shape nutrition recommendations in the United States and Canada.

The Dietary Reference Intakes Identify a Healthy Person's Nutrient Needs

In the past, the dietary standards in the United States were referred to as the *Recommended Dietary Allowances* (*RDAs*), and the standards in Canada were termed the *Recommended Nutrient Intakes* (*RNIs*). These standards defined recommended intake values for various nutrients and were used to plan diets for both individuals and groups. As noted earlier, they were adopted with the goal of preventing nutrient-deficiency diseases; however, in developed countries, these diseases are now extremely rare. Thus, nutrition scientists have developed a new set of reference values aimed at preventing and reducing the risk of chronic disease and promoting optimal health. These new reference values in both the United States and Canada are known as the **Dietary Reference Intakes (DRIs)** (**Focus Figure 1.9**, page 16). These standards include and expand upon the former RDA values; for example, they set new recommendation standards for nutrients that do not have RDA values, and they establish an upper level of safety for some nutrients.

The DRIs are dietary standards for healthy people only; they do not apply to people with diseases or those who are suffering from nutrient deficiencies. Like the RDAs and RNIs, they identify the amount of a nutrient needed to prevent deficiency diseases in healthy individuals, but they also consider how much of this nutrient may reduce the risk for chronic diseases in healthy people. The six DRI values are presented in the following sections (also see Focus Figure 1.9).

Dietary Reference Intakes (DRIs) A set of nutritional reference values for the United States and Canada that applies to healthy people.

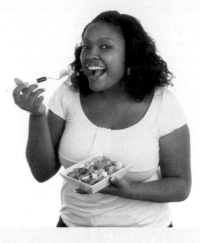

Dietary Reference Intakes (DRIs) are specific reference values for each nutrient issued by the United States National Academy of Sciences, Institute of Medicine. They identify the amounts of each nutrient that one needs to consume to maintain good health.

DRIs FOR MOST NUTRIENTS

EAR The Estimated Average Requirement (EAR) is the average daily intake level estimated to meet the needs of half the people in a certain group. Scientists use it to calculate the RDA.

RDA The Recommended Dietary Allowance (RDA) is the average daily intake level estimated to meet the needs of nearly all people in a certain group. Aim for this amount!

AI The Adequate Intake (AI) is the average daily intake level assumed to be adequate. It is used when an EAR cannot be determined. Aim for this amount if there is no RDA!

UL The Tolerable Upper Intake Level (UL) is the highest average daily intake level likely to pose no health risks. Do not exceed this amount on a daily basis!

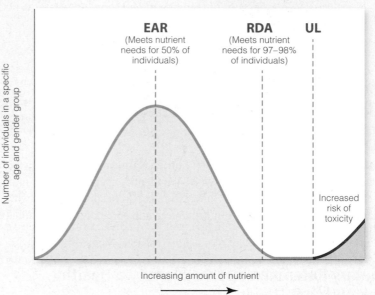

DRIs RELATED TO ENERGY

AMDR The Acceptable Macronutrient Distribution Range (AMDR) is the recommended range of carbohydrate, fat, and protein intake expressed as a percentage of total energy.

EER The Estimated Energy Requirement (EER) is the average daily energy intake predicted to meet the needs of healthy adults.

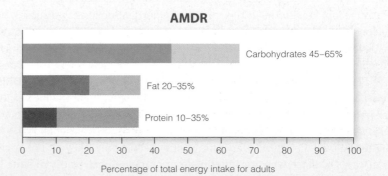

The Estimated Average Requirement Guides the Recommended Dietary Allowance

The first step nutrition researchers take in determining a population's nutrient requirements is to calculate the **Estimated Average Requirement (EAR)**. The EAR represents the average daily nutrient intake level estimated to meet the requirement of half of the healthy individuals in a particular life stage or gender group.[3] As an example, the EAR for iron for women between the ages of 19 and 30 years represents the average daily intake of iron that meets the requirement of half of the women in this age group. Scientists use the EAR to define the RDA for a given nutrient. Obviously, if the EAR meets the needs of only half the people in a group, then the recommended intake will be higher.

The Recommended Dietary Allowance Meets the Needs of Nearly All Healthy People

Recommended Dietary Allowance (RDA) was the term previously used to refer to *all* nutrient recommendations in the United States. The RDA is now considered one of many reference standards within the larger umbrella of the DRIs. The RDA represents the average daily nutrient intake level that meets the nutrient requirements of 97% to 98% of healthy individuals in a particular life stage and gender group.[3] The graph in Figure 1.9 compares the RDA to the EAR. For example, the RDA for iron is 18 mg per day for women between the ages of 19 and 50. This amount of iron will meet the nutrient requirements of almost all women in this age group.

   Again, scientists use the EAR to establish the RDA. In fact, if an EAR cannot be determined for a nutrient, then this nutrient cannot have an RDA. When this occurs, an Adequate Intake (AI) value is determined.

The Adequate Intake Is Based on Estimates of Nutrient Intakes

The **Adequate Intake (AI)** value is a recommended average daily nutrient intake level based on observed or experimentally determined estimates of nutrient intake by a group of healthy people.[3] These estimates are assumed to be adequate and are used when the evidence necessary to determine an RDA is not available. Many nutrients have an AI value, including vitamin K, chromium, fluoride, and certain types of fats. More research needs to be done on human requirements for the nutrients assigned an AI value, so that an EAR, and subsequently an RDA, can be established.

   In addition to establishing RDA and AI values for nutrients, an upper level of safety for nutrients, or Tolerable Upper Intake Level, has also been defined.

The Tolerable Upper Intake Level Is the Highest Level That Poses No Health Risk

The **Tolerable Upper Intake Level (UL)** is the highest average daily nutrient intake level likely to pose no risk of adverse health effects to almost all individuals in a particular life stage and gender group.[3] This does not mean that we should consume this intake level or that we will benefit from meeting or exceeding the UL. In fact, as our intake of a nutrient increases in amounts above the UL, the potential for toxic effects and health risks increases. The UL value is a helpful guide to assist you in determining the highest average intake level that is deemed safe for a given nutrient. Note that there is not enough research to define the UL for all nutrients.

The Estimated Energy Requirement Is the Intake Predicted to Maintain a Healthy Weight

The **Estimated Energy Requirement (EER)** is defined as the average dietary energy intake that is predicted to maintain energy balance in a healthy individual. This dietary intake is

Estimated Average Requirement (EAR) The average daily nutrient intake level estimated to meet the requirement of half of the healthy individuals in a particular life stage or gender group.

Recommended Dietary Allowance (RDA) The average daily nutrient intake level that meets the nutrient requirements of 97% to 98% of healthy individuals in a particular life stage and gender group.

Adequate Intake (AI) A recommended average daily nutrient intake level based on observed or experimentally determined estimates of nutrient intake by a group of healthy people.

Tolerable Upper Intake Level (UL) The highest average daily nutrient intake level likely to pose no risk of adverse health effects to almost all individuals in a particular life stage and gender group.

Estimated Energy Requirement (EER) The average dietary energy intake that is predicted to maintain energy balance in a healthy individual.

Acceptable Macronutrient Distribution Range (AMDR) A range of intakes for a particular energy source that is associated with reduced risk of chronic disease while providing adequate intakes of essential nutrients.

malnutrition A nutritional status that is out of balance; an individual is either getting too much or not enough of a particular nutrient or energy over a significant period of time.

defined by a person's age, gender, weight, height, and level of PA that is consistent with good health.[4] Thus, the EER for an active person is higher than the EER for an inactive person, even if all other factors (age, gender, and so forth) are the same.

The Acceptable Macronutrient Distribution Range Is Associated with Reduced Risk for Chronic Diseases

Carbohydrates, proteins, and many types of fats have an RDA. In addition, the **Acceptable Macronutrient Distribution Range (AMDR)** identifies a range of intake for the three energy nutrients that is both adequate and associated with a reduced risk of chronic disease.[4] The AMDR is expressed as a percentage of total energy (or total kcal). The AMDR also has a lower and upper boundary; if we consume nutrients above or below this range, there is a potential for increasing our risk for poor health. The AMDRs for carbohydrate, fat, and protein are listed in Focus Figure 1.9.

Diets Based on the Dietary Reference Intakes Promote Wellness

The primary goal of dietary planning is to develop an eating plan that is nutritionally adequate, meaning that the chances of consuming too little or too much of any nutrient are very low. By eating a diet that provides nutrient intakes that meet the RDA or AI values, a person is more likely to maintain a healthy weight, support his or her daily physical activity, and prevent nutrient deficiencies and toxicities.

The DRI values are listed in several tables at the back of this book; they are also identified with each nutrient as it is introduced throughout this text. Find your own life stage group and gender in the left-hand column; then simply look across to see each nutrient's value that applies. Using the DRI values in conjunction with diet-planning tools, such as the *Dietary Guidelines for Americans* or the *USDA Food Guide,* will ensure a healthful and adequate diet. (Chapter 2 provides details on how you can use these tools to develop a healthful diet.)

RECAP

The DRIs are standards for nutrients established for healthy people in a particular life stage or gender group. The EAR represents the nutrient intake level that meets the requirement of half of the healthy individuals in a group. The RDA represents the level that meets the requirements of 97% to 98% of healthy individuals in a group. The AI is based on estimates of nutrient intake by a group of healthy people when there is not enough information to set an RDA. The UL is the highest daily nutrient intake level that likely poses no health risk. The EER is the average daily energy intake that is predicted to maintain energy balance in a healthy adult. The AMDR is a range of intakes associated with reduced risk of chronic disease and adequate intakes of essential nutrients.

LO 5 Describe the tools nutritional professionals and other healthcare providers use for gathering data related to an individual's nutritional status and diet.

LO 6 Explain how nutrition professionals classify malnutrition

How Do Nutrition Professionals Assess the Nutritional Status of Clients?

Before nutrition professionals can make valid recommendations about a client's diet, they need to have a thorough understanding of the client's current nutritional status, including his or her weight, ratio of lean body tissue to body fat, and intake of energy and nutrients. A client's nutritional status may fall anywhere along a continuum from healthy to imbalanced. **Malnutrition** refers to a situation in which a person's nutritional status is out of balance; the individual is either getting too much or too little of a particular nutrient or energy over a significant period of time.

The results of the nutritional-status assessment are extremely important, because they will become the foundation of any dietary or other lifestyle changes that are recommended and will provide a baseline against which the success of any recommended changes are evaluated. For instance, if assessments reveal that an adolescent client is 20 lb underweight and consumes less than half the recommended amount of calcium each day, these baseline data are used to support a recommendation of increased energy and calcium intake and to evaluate the success of these recommendations in the future.

Nutrition professionals and other healthcare providers use a variety of tools to determine the nutritional status of clients. As you read about these in the following section, keep in mind that no one method is sufficient to indicate malnutrition. Instead, a combination of tools is used to confirm the presence or absence of nutrient imbalances.

Tests Conducted during a Physical Examination Elicit Objective Data

Physical examinations should be conducted by a trained healthcare provider, such as a physician, nurse, nurse practitioner, or physician assistant. The tests conducted during the examination, which vary according to the client's medical history, disease symptoms, and risk factors, are *objective;* that is, they yield data that can be empirically verified.

Vital Sign Assessment and Laboratory Tests Provide Clues to Nutritional Status

Typical tests include checking of vital signs (pulse, blood pressure, body temperature, and respiration rate), auscultation of heart and lung sounds, and laboratory analysis of blood and/or urine samples. Nutritional imbalances may be detected by examining the client's hair, skin, tongue, eyes, and fingernails.

A person's age and health status determine how often he or she needs a physical examination. It is typically recommended that a healthy person younger than 30 years of age have a thorough exam every 2 to 3 years. Adults between the ages of 30 and 50 should have an examination every 1 to 2 years, and people older than 50 years of age should have a yearly exam. However, individuals with established diseases or symptoms of malnutrition may require more frequent examinations.

Anthropometric Assessments Include Measurements of Height and Weight

Anthropometric assessments are, quite simply, measurements of human beings (*anthropos* is a Greek word meaning "human"). The most common anthropometric measurements are height and body weight. Other measurements that may be taken include head circumference in infants and circumference of limbs and the waist.

Accurate anthropometric measurements require that the healthcare provider taking the measurement be properly trained and use the correct tools. Measurements are then compared with standards specific for a given age and gender. This allows healthcare providers to determine if a person's body size or growth is normal for his or her age and gender. Repeated measurements can also be taken on the same person over time to assess trends in nutritional status and growth.

Although not technically considered an anthropometric assessment tool, body composition may also be measured. That is, the healthcare provider will use one of several available methods to determine the ratio of fat tissue to nonfat tissue (lean body mass) of which the client's body is composed. (Specific details about body composition assessment are discussed in Chapter 13.)

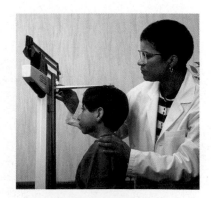

Measuring height is a common anthropometric assessment, and when repeated over time it can help determine a person's nutritional status.

Health-History Questionnaires Elicit Subjective Information

Health-history questionnaires are tools that assist in cataloging a person's history of health, illness, drug use, exercise, and diet. These questionnaires are typically completed just prior to the physical examination by a nurse or other healthcare professional, or the patient may be asked to complete one independently. The questions included in health-history questionnaires usually relate to the following:

- Demographic information, including name, age, contact information, and self-reported height and body weight
- Current medication status, potential drug allergies, and history of drug use
- Family history of disease
- Personal history of illnesses, injuries, and surgeries
- History of menstrual function (for females)
- Exercise history
- Socioeconomic factors, such as education level, access to shopping and cooking facilities, marital status, and racial/ethnic background

In addition, a trained nutrition professional can administer one of a number of specific questionnaires to assess a person's nutrient and energy intakes. Examples include a diet history, 24-hour dietary recalls, food-frequency questionnaires, and diet records. As you read about each of these tools, bear in mind that they are all *subjective;* that is, they rely on a person's self-report. The accuracy of the data cannot be empirically verified, as it can, for example, by repeating a measurement of a person's weight. Of these tools, the one or two selected by nutrition professionals will depend on what questions they wish to answer, the population they are working with, and the available resources. Following is a brief description of each.

> Want to learn more about the ABCD's of nutritional assessment? Go to http://education-portal.com and type in "Assessing Your Nutrition" into the search bar. Go to the first link and press "Watch Lesson" to begin.

A Diet History Uses an Interview or Questionnaire

A diet history is typically conducted by a trained nutrition professional. Diet history information is gathered using either an interview process or a questionnaire. Generally included in the diet history are the patient's current weight, usual weight, and body weight goals; factors affecting appetite and food intake; typical eating patterns (including time, place, dietary restrictions, frequency of eating out, and so forth); disordered eating behaviors (if any); economic status; educational level; living, cooking, and food-purchasing arrangements; medication and/or dietary supplement use; and physical activity patterns. A diet history can help identify any nutrition or eating problems and highlight a person's unique needs.

Twenty-Four-Hour Dietary Recalls Assess Recent Food Intake

The 24-hour dietary recall is used to assess recent food intake. A trained nutrition professional interviews the person and records his or her responses. The person recalls all of the foods and beverages consumed in the previous 24-hour period. Information that the person needs to know to provide an accurate recall includes serving sizes, food-preparation methods, and brand names of convenience foods or fast foods that were eaten. The 24-hour recall has serious limitations, including the fact that it does not give an indication of a person's typical intake; other limitations include reliance on a person's memory and his or her ability to estimate portion sizes.

Food-Frequency Questionnaires Estimate Typical Intakes over a Predefined Period

Food-frequency questionnaires can assist in determining a person's typical dietary pattern over a predefined period of time, such as 1 month, 6 months, or 1 year. These questionnaires include lists of foods with questions regarding the number of times these foods are eaten during the specified time period. Some questionnaires only assess qualitative information, meaning they include only a list of typical foods that are eaten and not amounts eaten. Semi-quantitative questionnaires are also available; these assess specific foods eaten and the quantity consumed.

Diet Records Involve Listing All Foods and Beverages Consumed

A diet record is a list of all foods and beverages consumed over a specified time period, usually 3 to 7 days. The days selected for recording the person's diet should be representative of typical dietary and activity patterns.

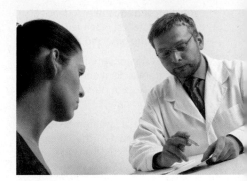

Diet records are a specific type of questionnaire, usually involving some training from a nutrition professional to ensure accuracy.

The client is responsible for filling out the record accurately, and both training and take-home instructions are essential. The record is more accurate if all foods consumed are weighed or measured, labels of all convenience foods are saved, and labels of supplements are provided. Providing a food scale and measuring utensils can also assist people in improving the information they provide on diet records.

Although diet records can provide a reasonably good estimate of a person's energy and nutrient intakes, they are challenging to complete accurately and in sufficient detail. Because of this burden, people may change their intake to simplify completing the diet record. They may also change their intake simply because they know it will be analyzed; for example, a client who typically eats ice cream after dinner might forego this indulgence for the duration of the diet record. In addition, analyses are time-consuming and costly.

Think back to the advice that the nutritionist gave to Marilyn in our chapter-opening scenario. Now that you have learned about both subjective and objective methods for assessing a person's nutritional status, you probably recognize that the nutritionist failed to perform even a rudimentary nutritional assessment; instead, she based her weight-loss recommendation solely on a measurement of Marilyn's blood pressure! Later in this chapter, we'll explain what the term *nutritionist* really means and discuss the importance of working within one's scope of practice. But for now, let's look at an example of how healthcare professionals use subjective and objective assessments to determine malnutrition.

A Finding of Malnutrition Requires Further Classification

If the results of nutrition assessment lead to a finding of malnutrition, the nutrition professional classifies the finding further as overnutrition or undernutrition:

- **Overnutrition** occurs when a person consumes too much energy or too much of a given nutrient over time, causing conditions such as obesity, heart disease, or nutrient toxicity. Overnutrition is further classified as overweight or obesity (see Chapter 13).
- **Undernutrition** refers to a situation in which someone consumes too little energy or too few nutrients over time, causing significant weight loss, nutrient deficiency, or a nutrient-deficiency disease.

Nutrient deficiencies are further classified as primary or secondary:

- **Primary deficiency** occurs when a person does not consume enough of a nutrient in the diet; thus, the deficiency occurs as a direct consequence of an inadequate intake.
- **Secondary deficiency** occurs when a person cannot absorb enough of a nutrient in his or her body, when too much of a nutrient is excreted from the body, or when a nutrient is not utilized efficiently by the body. Thus, a secondary deficiency is secondary to, or a consequence of, some other disorder.

overnutrition A situation in which too much energy or too much of a given nutrient is consumed over time, causing conditions such as obesity, heart disease, or nutrient-toxicity symptoms.

undernutrition A situation in which too little energy or too few nutrients are consumed over time, causing significant weight loss or a nutrient-deficiency disease.

primary deficiency A deficiency that occurs when not enough of a nutrient is consumed in the diet.

secondary deficiency A deficiency that occurs when a person cannot absorb enough of a nutrient, excretes too much of a nutrient from the body, or cannot utilize a nutrient efficiently.

subclinical deficiency A deficiency in its early stages, when few or no symptoms are observed.

covert A sign or symptom that is hidden from a client and requires laboratory tests or other invasive procedures to detect.

overt A sign or symptom that is obvious to a client, such as pain, fatigue, or a bruise.

Symptoms of a nutrient deficiency are not always obvious. A deficiency in its early stages, when few or no symptoms are observed, is referred to as a **subclinical deficiency**. The signs of a subclinical deficiency are typically **covert,** meaning they are hidden and require laboratory tests or other invasive procedures to detect. Once the signs and symptoms of a nutrient deficiency become obvious, they are referred to as **overt**. In the following example, notice that several nutrition assessment tools are used together to determine the presence of a nutrient deficiency.

Bob is a 70-year-old man who has come to his healthcare provider to discuss a number of troubling symptoms. He has been experiencing numbness and tingling in his legs and feet, loses his balance frequently, has memory loss and occasionally feels disoriented, and has intermittent periods of blurred vision. A health history is taken and reveals that Bob has mild hypertension, but he has been regularly physically active and was in good health until the past 6 months. A physical examination shows him to be underweight for his height, with pale skin, and experiencing tremors in his hands. His memory is also poor upon examination. Bob's physician orders some laboratory tests and refers him to the clinic's dietitian, who takes a diet history. During the history, Bob reveals that, a year ago, he began wearing dentures that have made it difficult for him to chew properly. He reports that over time he "gave up on eating anything tough, especially meat." When asked if he eats fish, he says that he has never eaten it, as he does not like the taste. Also, he avoids consuming dairy products because they cause stomach upset, intestinal gas, and diarrhea. When asked if he takes any supplements, Bob explains that he is on a limited income and cannot afford them.

Laboratory test results reveal that Bob is suffering from a deficiency of vitamin B_{12}. This deficiency is primary in nature, as Bob is not consuming meats, fish, or dairy products, which are the primary sources of vitamin B_{12} in our diet. He also does not take a supplement containing vitamin B_{12}. By the time Bob visited his healthcare provider, he was suffering from a clinical deficiency and was showing overt signs and symptoms.

RECAP

Malnutrition refers to a person's nutritional status being out of balance. To determine if malnutrition exists, healthcare providers conduct a physical examination, including vital signs assessment, lab tests, and anthropometric measures, and a health-history questionnaire. The client may also be asked to complete a diet history, a 24-hour dietary recall, a food-frequency questionnaire, or a diet record. If the results of nutrition assessment lead to a finding of malnutrition, the nutrition professional classifies the finding further as overnutrition or undernutrition. Overnutrition occurs when a person consumes too much energy or too much of a nutrient, and develops overweight or obesity. Undernutrition is a situation in which someone consumes too little energy or too few nutrients over time. Nutrient deficiencies are further categorized as primary or secondary. Either type, in its early stages, can be subclinical.

LO 7 Discuss the four steps of the scientific method.

LO 8 Compare and contrast the various types of research studies used in establishing nutrition guideline.

How Can You Interpret Research Study Results?

"Eat more carbohydrates! Fats cause obesity!"
"Eat more protein and fat! Carbohydrates cause obesity!"

Do you ever feel overwhelmed by the abundant and often conflicting advice in media reports and on the Internet related to nutrition? If so, you are not alone. In addition to the "high-carb, low-carb" controversy, we've been told that calcium supplements are essential to prevent bone loss and that calcium supplements have no effect on bone loss; that high fluid intake prevents constipation and that high fluid intake has no effect on constipation; that coffee and tea can be bad for our health and that both can be beneficial! How can you navigate this sea of changing information? What constitutes valid, reliable evidence, and how can you determine whether or not research findings apply to you?

To become a more informed critic of product claims and nutrition news items, you need to understand the research process and how to interpret the results of different types of studies. Let's begin.

Research Involves Applying the Scientific Method

When confronted with a claim about any aspect of our world, from "The Earth is flat" to "Carbohydrates cause obesity," scientists, including nutritionists, must first consider whether or not the claim can be tested. In other words, can evidence be presented to substantiate the claim, and if so, what data would qualify as evidence? Scientists worldwide use a standardized method of looking at evidence called the *scientific method*. This method ensures that certain standards and processes are used in evaluating claims. The scientific method usually includes the following steps, which are described in more detail below and summarized in **Focus Figure 1.10**:

- The researcher makes an *observation* and description of a phenomenon.
- The researcher proposes a *hypothesis*, or educated guess, to explain why the phenomenon occurs.
- The researcher develops an *experimental design* that will test the hypothesis.
- The researcher *collects and analyzes data* that will either support or reject the hypothesis.
- If the data do not support the original hypothesis, then an *alternative hypothesis* is proposed and tested.
- If the data support the original hypothesis, then a *conclusion* is drawn.
- The experiment must be *repeatable*, so that other researchers can obtain similar results.
- Finally, a *theory* is proposed offering a conclusion drawn from repeated experiments that have supported the hypothesis time and time again.

Observation of a Phenomenon Initiates the Research Process

The first step in the scientific method is the observation and description of a phenomenon. As an example, let's say you are working in a healthcare office that caters to mostly older adult clients. You have observed that many of these clients have high blood pressure, but some have normal blood pressure. After talking with a large number of clients, you notice a pattern developing in that the clients who report being more physically active are also those with lower blood pressure readings. This observation leads you to question the relationship that might exist between physical activity and blood pressure. Your next step is to develop a *hypothesis,* or possible explanation for your observation.

A Hypothesis Is a Possible Explanation for an Observation

A **hypothesis** is also sometimes referred to as a research question. In this example, your hypothesis might be "Adults over age 65 with high blood pressure who begin and maintain a program of 45 minutes of aerobic exercise daily will experience a decrease in blood pressure." Your hypothesis must be written in such a way that it can be either supported or rejected. In other words, it must be testable.

An Experiment Is Designed to Test the Hypothesis

An *experiment* is a scientific study that is conducted to test a hypothesis. A well-designed experiment should include several key elements:

- The *sample size*, or the number of people being studied, should be adequate to ensure that the results obtained are not due to chance alone. Would you be more likely to believe a study that tested 5 people or 500?
- Having a *control group* is essential for comparison between treated and untreated individuals. A control group is a group of people who are as much like the treated group as possible except with respect to the *condition* being tested. For instance,

hypothesis An educated guess as to why a phenomenon occurs.

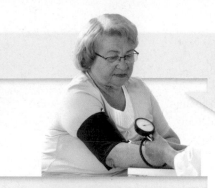

OBSERVATIONS

A pattern is observed in which older adults who are more active appear to have lower blood pressure than those who are less active.

HYPOTHESIS

Adults over age 65 with high blood pressure who participate in a program of 45 minutes per day of aerobic exercise will experience a decrease in blood pressure.

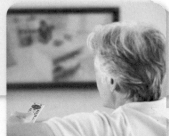

EXPERIMENT
Randomized Clinical Trial

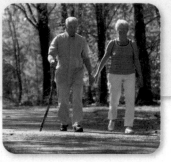

Modified hypothesis

Control group:
No exercise

OBSERVATIONS

Experimental group:
45 minutes of daily aerobic exercise

Data support hypothesis
Average blood pressure was reduced by 8 mmHg for systolic blood pressure and 5 mmHg for diastolic blood pressure in the experimental group.
The control group experienced a slight increase in blood pressure.

Data do not support hypothesis

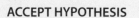

Reject
hypothesis

Modify hypothesis

REPEAT EXPERIMENT

ACCEPT HYPOTHESIS

A hypothesis supported by repeated experiments over many years may be accepted as a theory.

THEORY

in your study, 45 minutes daily of aerobic exercise would be the condition; the experimental group would consist of people over age 65 with high blood pressure who perform the exercise, and the control group would consist of people of the same age with high blood pressure who do not perform the exercise. Using a control group helps a researcher judge if a particular treatment has worked or not.

■ A good experimental design also attempts to control for other factors that may coincidentally influence the results. For example, what if someone in your study is on a diet, smokes, or takes blood pressure–lowering medication? Because any of these factors can affect the results, researchers try to design experiments that have as many constants as possible. In doing so, they increase the chance that their results will be *valid*. To use an old saying, you can think of validity as "comparing apples to apples."

Data Are Collected and Analyzed to Determine Whether They Support or Reject the Hypothesis

As part of the design of the experiment, the researcher must determine the type of data to collect and how to collect them. For example, in your study the data being collected are blood pressure readings. These values could be collected by a person or a machine, but because the data will be closely scrutinized by other scientists, they should be as accurate as technology allows. In this case, an automatic blood pressure gauge would provide more reliable and consistent data than blood pressure measurements taken by research assistants.

Once the data have been collected, they must be interpreted or analyzed. Often, the data will begin to make sense only after being organized and put into different forms, such as tables or graphs, to reveal patterns that at first are not obvious. In your study, you can create a graph comparing blood pressure readings from both your experimental group and your control group to see if there is a significant difference between the blood pressure readings of those who exercised and those who did not.

Most Hypotheses Need to Be Refined

Remember that a hypothesis is basically a guess as to what causes a particular phenomenon. Rarely do scientists get it right the first time. The original hypothesis is often refined after the initial results are obtained, usually because the answer to the question is not clear and leads to more questions. When this happens, an alternative hypothesis is proposed, a new experiment is designed, and the new hypothesis is tested.

An Experiment Must Be Repeatable

One research study does not prove or disprove a hypothesis. Ideally, multiple experiments are conducted over many years to thoroughly test a hypothesis. Indeed, repeatability is a cornerstone of scientific investigation. Supporters and skeptics alike must be able to replicate an experiment and arrive at similar conclusions, or the hypothesis becomes invalid. Have you ever wondered why the measurements used in scientific textbooks are always in the metric system? The answer is repeatability. Scientists use the metric system because it is a universal system and thus allows repeatability in any research facility worldwide.

Unfortunately, media reports on the findings of a research study that has just been published rarely include a thorough review of the other studies conducted on that topic. Thus, you should never accept one report in a newspaper or magazine as absolute fact on any topic.

A Theory May Be Developed Following Extensive Research

If the results of multiple experiments consistently support a hypothesis, then scientists may advance a **theory**. A theory represents a scientific consensus (agreement) as to why a particular phenomenon occurs. Although theories are based on data drawn from repeated experiments, they can still be challenged and changed as the knowledge within a scientific discipline evolves. For example, at the beginning of this chapter, we said that the prevailing theory held that beriberi was an infectious disease. Experiments were conducted over

theory A scientific consensus, based on data drawn from repeated experiments, as to why a phenomenon occurs.

several decades before their consistent results finally confirmed that the disease is due to thiamin deficiency. We continue to apply the scientific method to test hypotheses and challenge theories today.

RECAP

The steps in the scientific method are (1) observing a phenomenon, (2) creating a hypothesis, (3) designing and conducting an experiment, and (4) collecting and analyzing data that support or refute the hypothesis. If the data are rejected, then an alternative hypothesis is proposed and tested. If the data support the original hypothesis, then a conclusion is drawn. A hypothesis that is supported after repeated experiments may be called a theory.

Various Types of Research Studies Tell Us Different Stories

Understanding the role of nutrition in health involve constant experimentation. Depending on how the research study is designed, we can gather information that tells us different stories. Let's take a look at the various types of research.

Animal Studies Can Inform Human Studies

In many cases, studies involving animals provide preliminary information that assists scientists in designing human studies. Animal studies also are used to conduct research that cannot be done with humans. For instance, researchers can cause a nutrient deficiency in an animal and study its adverse health effects over the animal's life span, but this type of experiment with humans is not acceptable. Drawbacks of animal studies include ethical concerns and the fact that the results may not apply directly to humans.

Over the past century, animal studies have advanced our understanding of many aspects of nutrition, from micronutrients to obesity. Still, some hypotheses can only be investigated using human subjects. The three primary types of studies conducted with humans are observational studies, case-control studies, and clinical trials.

Observational Studies Assess Relationships between Dietary Habits and Disease Trends

Epidemiological studies examine patterns of health and disease conditions in defined populations. Epidemiological studies commonly report the *prevalence* and *incidence* of disease. As defined earlier in the chapter, prevalence refers to the actual percentage of the population that has a particular disease at a given period of time. **Incidence** refers to the rate of new (or newly diagnosed) cases of a disease within a period of time. **Observational studies** are a type of epidemiological study used to assess dietary habits, disease trends, and other health phenomena of large populations and determining the factors that may influence these phenomena. However, these studies can only indicate *relationships* between factors; they do not prove or suggest that the data are linked by cause and effect. For example, smoking and low vegetable intake appear to be related in some studies, but this does not mean that smoking cigarettes causes people to eat fewer vegetables or that eating fewer vegetables causes people to smoke.

Case-Control Studies Are More Complex Observational Studies

Case-control studies are more complex observational studies with additional design features that allow scientists to gain a better understanding of things that may influence disease. They involve comparing a group of individuals with a particular condition (for instance, 1,000 elderly people with high blood pressure) to a similar group without this condition (for instance, 1,000 elderly people with normal blood pressure). This comparison allows the researcher to identify factors other than the defined condition that differ between the two groups. For example, researchers may find that 75% of the people in their

epidemiological studies Studies that examine patterns of health and disease conditions in defined populations.

incidence The rate of new (or newly diagnosed) cases of a disease within a period of time.

observational studies Types of epidemiological studies that indicate relationships between nutrition habits, disease trends, and other health phenomena of large populations of humans.

case-control studies Complex observational studies with additional design features that allow us to gain a better understanding of factors that may influence disease.

normal blood pressure group are physically active but that only 20% of the people in their high blood pressure group are physically active. Again, this would not prove that physical activity prevents high blood pressure. It would merely suggest a significant relationship between these two factors.

Clinical Trials Are Tightly Controlled Experiments Examining Cause and Effect

Clinical trials are tightly controlled experiments in which an intervention is given to determine its effect on a certain disease or health condition. Interventions include medications, nutritional supplements, controlled diets, and exercise programs. In clinical trials, people in the experimental group are given the intervention, but people in the control group are not. The responses of the two groups are compared. In the case of the blood pressure experiment, researchers could assign one group of elderly people with high blood pressure to an exercise program and assign a second group of elderly people with high blood pressure to a program where no exercise is done. Over the next few weeks, months, or even years, researchers could measure the blood pressure of the people in each group. If the blood pressure of those who exercised decreased and the blood pressure of those who did not exercise rose or remained the same, the influence of exercise on lowering blood pressure would be supported.

Two important questions to consider when evaluating the quality of a clinical trial are whether the subjects were randomly chosen and whether the researchers and subjects were blinded:

- *Randomized trials:* Ideally, researchers should *randomly* assign research participants to intervention groups (who get the treatment) and control groups (who do not get the treatment). Randomizing participants is like flipping a coin or drawing names from a hat; it reduces the possibility of showing favoritism toward any participants and ensures that the groups are similar on the factors or characteristics being measured in the study. These types of studies are called *randomized clinical (controlled) trials*.
- *Single- and double-blind experiments:* If possible, it is also important to *blind* both researchers and participants to the treatment being given. A *single-blind experiment* is one in which the participants are unaware of or *blinded* to the treatment they are receiving, but the researchers know which group is getting the treatment and which group is not. A *double-blind experiment* is one in which neither researchers nor participants know which group is really getting the treatment. Double blinding helps prevent the researcher from seeing only the results he or she wants to see, even if these results do not actually occur. In the case of testing medications or nutrition supplements, the blinding process can be assisted by giving the control group a placebo. A *placebo* is an imitation treatment that has no effect on participants; for instance, a sugar pill may be given in place of a vitamin supplement. Studies like this are referred to as placebo-controlled *double-blind randomized clinical trials*.

There has been substantial interest in the "placebo effect." This refers to some people experiencing improved health—for instance, pain reduction—despite the fact that they have received only a placebo. Although the placebo effect does not occur for all people or across the range of health conditions and diseases affecting the population, it is an intriguing phenomenon that researchers continue to explore to better understand how personal beliefs and attitudes can impact one's response to research and medical treatments.

Want to learn more about the placebo effect and how it may lead to improvements in health? Go to www.cbsnews.com and type "Placebo Phenomenon" to be directed to the video.

RECAP

Studies involving animals provide preliminary information that assists scientists in designing human studies. Types of epidemiological studies in humans include observational studies and case-control studies. Clinical trials are conducted in humans to determine cause and effect of a given treatment or intervention. Each type of study can be used to gather a different kind of data.

clinical trials Tightly controlled experiments in which an intervention is given to determine its effect on a certain disease or health condition.

LO 9   Describe various approaches you can use to evaluate the truth and reliability of media reports, websites, and other sources of nutrition information.

How Can You Use Your Knowledge of Research to Help You Evaluate Nutrition Claims?

How can all of this research information assist you in becoming a better consumer and critic of media reports and Internet sites? By having a better understanding of the research process and the types of research conducted, you are more capable of discerning the truth or fallacy within media reports. One of the most important points to consider when examining any media report is the issue of conflict of interest.

Watch for Conflict of Interest and Bias

You probably wouldn't think it strange to see an ad from your favorite brand of ice cream encouraging you to "Go ahead. Indulge." It's just an ad, right? But what if you were to read about a research study in which people who ate your favorite brand of ice cream improved the density of their bones? Could you trust the study results more than you would the ad?

To answer that question, you'd have to ask several more, such as who conducted the research and who paid for it. Specifically:

- Was the study funded by a company that stands to profit from certain results?
- Are the researchers receiving a stipend (payment), goods, personal travel funds, or other perks from the research sponsor, or do they have investments in companies or products related to their study?

If the answer to either of these questions were yes, a **conflict of interest** would exist between the researchers and the funding agency. A *conflict of interest* refers to a situation in which a person is in a position to derive personal benefit and unfair advantage from actions or decisions made in their official capacity. Whenever a conflict of interest exists, it can seriously compromise the researchers' ability to conduct impartial research and report the results in an accurate and responsible manner. That's why, when researchers submit their results for publication in scientific journals, they are required to reveal any conflicts of interest they may have that could be seen as affecting the integrity of their research. In this way, people who review and eventually read and interpret the study are better able to consider if there are any potential researcher *biases* influencing the results. A bias is any factor—such as investment in the product being studied or gifts from the product manufacturer—that might influence the researcher to favor certain results.

Recent media investigations have reported widespread bias in studies funded by pharmaceutical companies testing the effectiveness of their drugs for medical treatment. In addition, journals in both the United States and Europe have been found less likely to publish negative results (that is, study results suggesting that a therapy is not effective). Also, clinical trials funded by pharmaceutical companies are more likely to report positive results than are trials that were independently financed.[5] This lack of *transparency*, or failure to openly present all research findings, has serious implications: if ineffectiveness and side effects are not fully reported, healthcare providers may be prescribing medications that are ineffective or even harmful.

The seriousness of this issue has inspired researchers around the world to demand a global system whereby all clinical trials are registered and all research results are made accessible to the public. The development of such a system would allow for independent review of research data and help healthcare providers and patients make decisions that are fully informed. As a first step, the U.S. Food and Drug Administration in 2009 launched a Transparency Initiative with the goal of making available to the public useful and understandable information about FDA activities and decision making.

conflict of interest A situation in which a person is in a position to derive personal benefit and unfair advantage from actions or decisions made in their official capacity.

Evaluate the Sources and Content of the Claims

In addition to conflict of interest and bias, make sure you investigate the author of the report, the references cited in it, and the content of its claims:

- Who is reporting the information? Many people who write for popular magazines, newspapers, and the Internet are not trained in science and are capable of misinterpreting research results. But even trained scientists and physicians can misreport research results for financial gain. For instance, if the report is published on the website of a healthcare provider who sells the product or service that was studied, you should be skeptical of the reported results.
- Is the report based on reputable research studies? Did the research follow the scientific method, and were the results reported in a reputable scientific journal? Ideally, the journal is peer reviewed; that is, the articles are critiqued by other specialists working in the same scientific field. A reputable report should include the reference, or source of the information, and should identify researchers by name. This allows the reader to investigate the original study and determine its merit. Some reputable nutrition journals are identified later in this chapter.
- Is the report based on testimonials about personal experiences? Are sweeping conclusions made from only one study? Be aware of personal testimonials, as they are fraught with bias. In addition, one study cannot answer all of our questions or prove any hypothesis, and the findings from individual studies should be placed in their proper perspective.
- Are the claims in the report too good to be true? Claims about curing diseases or treating many conditions with one product, for example, should cause you to question the validity of the report.

As you may know, **quackery** is the promotion of an unproven remedy, usually by someone unlicensed and untrained, for financial gain. Marilyn, the woman with high blood pressure from our opening story, was a victim of quackery. She probably would not have purchased that weight-loss supplement if she had understood that it was no more effective in promoting weight loss than a generic fiber supplement costing less than half the price.

> To learn more about how to spot quackery, go to www.quackwatch.com, enter "spot quack" in the search box, and then click on "Critiquing Quack Ads."

Evaluate a Website's Credibility

The Internet is increasingly becoming the repository of almost all credible scientific information, including health and nutrition information. But it's simultaneously the source of some of the most unreliable and even dangerous pseudoscience. How can you determine if the information published on a website is credible? Here are some tips to assist you in separating Internet fact from fiction:

- Look at the credentials of the people sponsoring and providing information for the website. Is the individual, group, or company responsible for the website considered a qualified professional in the area of emphasis? Are the names and credentials of those contributing to the website available? Are experts reviewing the content of the website for accuracy and currency?
- Look at the date of the website. Is it fairly recent? Because nutrition and medical information are constantly changing, websites should be updated frequently, and the date of the most recent update should be clearly identified on the site.
- Look at the web address. The three letters following the "dot" in a World Wide Web address can provide some clues as to the credibility of the information. Government addresses (ending in ".gov"), academic institutions (ending in ".edu"), and professional organizations (ending in ".org") are typically considered to be relatively credible sources of information. However, lecture notes, PowerPoint slides, student assignments, and similar types of documents that can be found on university websites may not be current,

quackery The promotion of an unproven remedy, such as a supplement or other product or service, usually by someone unlicensed and untrained.

accurate, or credible sources of information. Addresses ending in ".com" designate commercial and business sites. Many of these are credible sources, but many are not. It is important to check the qualifications of those contributing to the site and to consider if their primary motivation is to encourage you to buy a product or service.

■ Look at the bottom line. What is the message being highlighted on the site? Is it consistent with what is reported by other credible sources? If the message contradicts what would be considered as common knowledge, then you should question its validity and intent. An additional clue that a website may lack credibility includes strong and repeated claims of conspiracy theories designed to breed distrust of existing reputable sites.

These suggestions can also be applied to spam. If you have an e-mail account, you're probably familiar with spam ads that make promises such as "Weight-loss miracles for only $19.99!" Do you delete them unread? Or are you tempted to open them to see if you might find something worth exploring?

Throughout this text we provide you with information to assist you in becoming a more educated consumer regarding nutrition. You will learn about labeling guidelines, the proper use of supplements, and whether various nutrition topics are myths or facts. Armed with the information in this book, plus plenty of opportunities to test your knowledge, you will become more confident when evaluating nutrition claims.

RECAP

When evaluating media reports, consider whether a conflict of interest exists, who is reporting the information, who conducted and paid for the research, whether or not the research was published in a reputable journal, and whether it involves testimonials or makes claims that sound too good to be true. Quackery is the promotion of an unproven remedy, usually by someone unlicensed and untrained, for financial gain. When evaluating websites, check the site's credentials, date, address, and underlying message. ■

*Nutri-*Case

Liz

"Am I ever sorry I caught the news last night right before going to bed! They had a report about this study that had just come out saying that ballet dancers are at some superabnormally high risk for fractures! I couldn't sleep thinking about it, and then today in dance class, every move I made, I was freaking out about breaking my ankle. I can't go on being afraid like this!"

What information should Liz find out about the fracture study to evaluate its merits? Identify at least two factors she should evaluate. Let's say that her investigation of these factors leads her to conclude that the study is trustworthy—what else should she bear in mind about the research process that would help her take a more healthy perspective when thinking about this single study?

 LO 10 List at least four sources of reliable and accurate nutrition information and state why they are trustworthy.

Nutrition Advice: Who Can You Trust to Help You Choose Foods Wisely?

Over the past few decades, as researchers have discovered more and more links between nutrition and health, the public has become increasingly interested in understanding how nutrition affects them personally. One result of this booming interest has been a barrage of nutrition claims on television infomercials; on websites; in magazines; on product packages; and via many other forums. Most individuals do not have the knowledge or training to interpret and evaluate the reliability of this information and thus are vulnerable to misinformation and potentially harmful quackery.

Nutrition professionals are in a perfect position to work in a multitude of settings to counsel and educate their clients and the general public about sound nutrition practices. The following discussion identifies some key characteristics of reliable sources of nutrition information.

Trustworthy Experts Are Educated and Credentialed

It is not possible to list here all of the types of health professionals who provide reliable and accurate nutrition information. The following is a list of the most common groups:

- *Registered dietitian (RD):* To become a **registered dietitian (RD)** requires, minimally, a bachelor's degree, completion of a supervised clinical experience, a passing grade on a national examination, and maintenance of registration with the Academy of Nutrition and Dietetics (formerly the American Dietetic Association). There is now an optional change to the RD designation—*RD/Nutritionist.* This designation indicates that anyone who has earned an RD is also a qualified nutritionist, but not all nutritionists are RDs (see below). Individuals who complete the education, experience, exam, and registration are qualified to provide nutrition counseling in a variety of settings. For a reliable list of RDs in your community, contact the Academy of Nutrition and Dietetics (see **Web Links**).

- *Licensed dietitian:* A licensed dietitian is a dietitian meeting the credentialing requirement of a given state in the United States to engage in the practice of dietetics.[6] Each state has its own laws regulating dietitians. These laws specify which types of licensure or registration a nutrition professional must obtain in order to provide nutrition services or advice to individuals. Individuals who practice nutrition and dietetics without the required license or registration can be prosecuted for breaking the law.

- *Professional with an advanced degree (a master's degree [MA or MS] or doctoral degree [PhD]) in nutrition:* Many individuals hold an advanced degree in nutrition and have years of experience in a nutrition-related career. For instance, they may teach at community colleges or universities or work in fitness or healthcare settings. Unless these individuals are licensed or registered dietitians, they are not certified to provide clinical dietary counseling or treatment for individuals with disease. However, they are reliable sources of information about nutrition and health.

- *Physician:* The term *physician* encompasses a variety of healthcare professionals. A medical doctor (MD) is educated, trained, and licensed to practice medicine in the United States. However, MDs typically have very limited experience and training in the area of nutrition. Medical students in the United States are not required to take any nutrition courses throughout their academic training, although some may take courses out of personal interest. On the other hand, a number of individuals who started their careers in nutrition go on to become MDs and thus have a solid background in nutrition. Nevertheless, if you require a dietary plan to treat an illness or a disease, most MDs will refer you to an RD. In contrast, an osteopathic physician, referred to as a doctor of osteopathy (DO), may have studied nutrition extensively, as may a naturopathic physician, a homeopathic physician, or a chiropractor. Thus, it is prudent to determine a physician's level of expertise rather than assuming that he or she has extensive knowledge of nutrition.

In contrast to the above, the term *nutritionist* generally has no definition or laws regulating it. In some cases, it refers to a professional with academic credentials in nutrition who may also be an RD.[6] In other cases, the term may refer to anyone who thinks he or

For a list of registered dietitians in your community, visit the Academy of Nutrition and Dietetics at www.eatright.org.

registered dietitian (RD) A professional designation that requires a minimum of a bachelor's degree in nutrition, completion of a supervised clinical experience, a passing grade on a national examination, and maintenance of registration with the Academy of Nutrition and Dietetics (in Canada, the Dietitians of Canada). RDs are qualified to work in a variety of settings.

she is knowledgeable about nutrition. There is no guarantee that a person calling himself or herself a nutritionist is necessarily educated, trained, and experienced in the field of nutrition. It is important to research the credentials and experience of any individual calling himself or herself a nutritionist. In the chapter-opening scenario, how might Marilyn have determined whether or not the "nutritionist" was qualified to give her advice?

Government Sources of Information Are Usually Trustworthy

Many government health agencies have come together to address the growing problem of nutrition-related disease in the United States. These agencies, funded with taxpayer dollars, provide financial support for research in nutrition and health, and organize and disseminate the most recent and reliable research-based nutrition information and recommendations. A few of the most recognized and respected of these government agencies are discussed here.

The Centers for Disease Control and Prevention Protects the Health and Safety of Americans

The **Centers for Disease Control and Prevention (CDC)** is considered the leading federal agency in the United States that protects human health and safety. Located in Atlanta, Georgia, the CDC works in the areas of health promotion, disease prevention and control, and environmental health. The CDC's mission is to promote health and quality of life by preventing and controlling disease, injury, and disability. Among its many activities, the CDC supports two large national surveys that provide important nutrition and health information.

The **National Health and Nutrition Examination Survey (NHANES)** is conducted by the National Center for Health Statistics and the CDC. The NHANES tracks the food and nutrient consumption of Americans. Nutrition and other health information is gathered from interviews and physical examinations. The database for the NHANES survey is extremely large, and an abundance of research papers have been generated from it. To learn more about the NHANES, see the *Web Links* at the end of this chapter.

The **Behavioral Risk Factor Surveillance System (BRFSS)** was established by the CDC to track lifestyle behaviors that increase our risk for chronic disease. The world's largest telephone survey, the BRFSS gathers data at the state level at regular intervals. Although the BRFSS includes questions related to injuries and infectious diseases, it places a particularly strong focus on the health behaviors that increase our risk for some of the nation's leading killers: heart disease, stroke, cancer, and diabetes. These health behaviors include:

- Not consuming enough fruits and vegetables
- Being overweight
- Using tobacco and abusing alcohol
- Not getting medical care that is known to save lives, such as screening exams

These behaviors are of particular interest because it is estimated that 50% to 60% of deaths in the United States can be attributed to smoking, alcohol misuse, lack of physical activity, and an unhealthful diet.

The National Institutes of Health Is the Leading Medical Research Agency in the World

The **National Institutes of Health (NIH)** is the world's leading medical research center, and it is the focal point for medical research in the United States. The NIH is one of the agencies of the Public Health Service, which is part of the U.S. Department of Health and Human Services. The mission of the NIH is to uncover new knowledge that leads to better health for everyone. This mission is accomplished by supporting medical research throughout the world and by fostering the communication of this information. Many institutes within the NIH conduct research into nutrition-related health issues. Some of these institutes are:

Centers for Disease Control and Prevention (CDC) The leading federal agency in the United States that protects the health and safety of people. Its mission is to promote health and quality of life by preventing and controlling disease, injury, and disability.

National Health and Nutrition Examination Survey (NHANES) A survey conducted by the National Center for Health Statistics and the CDC; this survey tracks the nutrient and food consumption of Americans.

Behavioral Risk Factor Surveillance System (BRFSS) The world's largest telephone survey that tracks lifestyle behaviors that increase our risk for chronic disease.

National Institutes of Health (NIH) The world's leading medical research center and the focal point for medical research in the United States.

- National Cancer Institute (NCI)
- National Heart, Lung, and Blood Institute (NHLBI)
- National Institute of Diabetes and Digestive and Kidney Diseases (NIDDK)
- National Center for Complementary and Alternative Medicine (NCCAM)

To find out more about the NIH, see the **Web Links** at the end of this chapter.

Professional Organizations Provide Reliable Nutrition Information

A number of professional organizations represent nutrition professionals, including healthcare providers, scientists, and educators. These organizations publish cutting-edge nutrition research studies and educational information in journals that are accessible at most university and medical libraries. Some of these organizations are:

- *The Academy of Nutrition and Dietetics:* This is the largest organization of food and nutrition professionals in the world. The mission of this organization is to promote nutrition, health, and well-being. (The Canadian equivalent is Dietitians of Canada.) The Academy of Nutrition and Dietetics publishes a professional journal called the *Journal of the Academy of Nutrition and Dietetics* (formerly the *Journal of the American Dietetic Association*).
- *The American Society for Nutrition (ASN):* The ASN is the premier research society dedicated to improving quality of life through the science of nutrition. The ASN fulfills its mission by fostering, enhancing, and disseminating nutrition-related research and professional education activities. The ASN publishes a professional journal called the *American Journal of Clinical Nutrition.*
- *The Society for Nutrition Education (SNE):* The SNE is dedicated to promoting healthy, sustainable food choices in communities through nutrition research and education. The primary goals of the SNE are to educate individuals, communities, and professionals about nutrition education and to influence policy makers about nutrition, food, and health. The professional journal of the SNE is the *Journal of Nutrition Education and Behavior.*
- *The American College of Sports Medicine (ACSM):* The ACSM is the leading sports medicine and exercise science organization in the world. The mission of the ACSM is to advance and integrate scientific research to provide educational and practical applications of exercise science and sports medicine. Many members are nutrition professionals who combine their nutrition and exercise expertise to promote health and athletic performance. *Medicine and Science in Sports and Exercise* is the professional journal of the ACSM.
- *The Obesity Society (TOS):* TOS is the leading scientific society dedicated to the study of obesity. It is committed to improving the lives of people with obesity, nurturing careers of obesity scientists and healthcare providers, and promoting interdisciplinary obesity research, management, and education. The official TOS journal is *Obesity Journal.*

RECAP

A registered dietitian is qualified to provide nutrition counseling. The CDC is the leading federal agency in the United States that protects human health and safety. The CDC supports two large national surveys that provide important nutrition and health information: the NHANES and the BRFSS. The NIH is the leading medical research agency in the world. The Academy for Nutrition and Dietetics, the American Society for Nutritional Sciences, the SNE, the ACSM, and TOS are examples of professional organizations that provide reliable nutrition information. ■

Nutrition Myth OR Fact?

Nutrigenomics: Personalized Nutrition or Pie in the Sky?

Agouti mice are specifically bred for scientific studies. These mice are normally yellow in color, obese, and prone to cancer and diabetes, and they typically have a short life span. When agouti mice breed, these traits are passed on to their offspring. Look at **Figure 1.11**; do you see a difference? The mouse on the right is obviously brown and of normal weight, but what you can't see is that it did not inherit its parents' susceptibility to disease and therefore will live a longer, healthier life. What caused this dramatic difference between parent and offspring? The answer is diet!

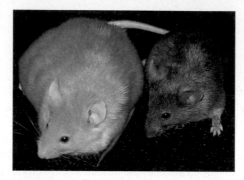

FIGURE 1.11 Prompted only by a change in her diet before she conceived, an inbred agouti mouse (left) gave birth to a young mouse (right) that differed not only in appearance but also in its susceptibility to disease.

of the agouti gene. In essence, they turned it off. When the mothers conceived, their offspring still carried the agouti gene on their DNA, but their cells no longer used the gene to make proteins. In short, the gene was no longer expressed; thus, the traits, such as obesity, that were linked to the agouti gene did not appear in the offspring. These Duke University studies were some of the first to directly link a dietary intervention to a genetic modification and contributed significantly to the emerging science of *nutrigenomics* (*nutritional genomics*).

Genetics and Epigenetics

In 2003, researchers at Duke University reported that, when they changed the mother's diet just before conception, they could "turn off" the agouti gene, and any offspring born to that mother would appear normal.[1] A *gene* is a segment of DNA, the substance responsible for inheritance, or the passing on of traits from parents to offspring. An organism's *genome* is its complete set of DNA, which is found packed into the nucleus of its body cells. Genes are precise regions of DNA that encode instructions for assembling specific proteins. In other words, genes are *expressed* in proteins; for instance, one way that the agouti gene is expressed is in the pigment proteins that produce yellow fur. (Genes and proteins are discussed in more detail in Chapter 6.)

The Duke University researchers interfered with normal gene expression in their agouti mice by manipulating the mice's diet. Specifically, they fed the mother mice a diet that was high in methyl donors, compounds that can transfer a methyl group (CH_3) to another molecule. This transfer, called methylation, is one of several *epigenetic* mechanisms; that is, mechanisms that alter gene expression without changing the DNA sequence itself. In epigenetics, factors such as methyl donors bind to regions on the proteins (called histones) around which DNA spools. (See the accompanying **FIGURE 1.12**.) When they do, they affect how tightly or loosely the DNA and its histones are wound: The genes in loosely wound DNA are accessible to the cell for use in protein synthesis, whereas the genes in tightly bound regions cannot be read.

This activation or deactivation of genes can trigger changes in inheritable characteristics. In the agouti mice, the methyl donors in the mothers' diet triggered deactivation

What Is Nutrigenomics?

Nutrigenomics studies the interactions among genes, the environment, and nutrition. Until the late 20th century, scientists believed that the genes a person is born with determined his or her traits rigidly, but we now know that genetic expression is influenced—perhaps significantly—by chemicals present in the foods we most commonly eat and the substances in our environment to which our cells are commonly exposed. These include chemicals present in tobacco, drugs, alcohol, and environmental toxins. This helps explain why the appearance and health of identical twins—who have the same DNA—commonly change as the twins age.

In addition, as we saw with the agouti mice, nutrigenomics has shown that the food chemicals we expose our genes to can affect their expression not only in our own bodies but also in our offspring. In the Duke University study, switching off the agouti gene caused beneficial changes in the offspring mice. But sometimes flipping the switch can be harmful, as when paternal exposure to radiation causes changes in sperm cells that increase the likelihood of birth defects in the offspring.

Several commonly observed phenomena are now thought to be due at least in part to nutrigenomic mechanisms. For example, it has long been noted that some people will lose weight on a specific diet and exercise program, whereas others following the same diet and exercise program will gain weight. Some people who smoke develop cardiovascular disease or cancer, whereas others do not. And in some people, moderate alcohol consumption appears to reduce the risk of cardiovascular disease, whereas in other people, it does not. These varying results are now thought to depend to a certain extent on how these factors affect the individual's epigenome.[2,3]

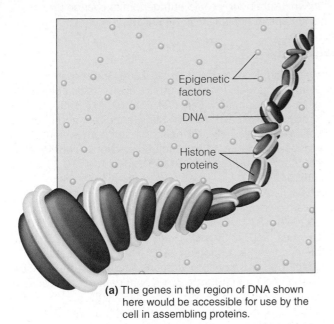

(a) The genes in the region of DNA shown here would be accessible for use by the cell in assembling proteins.

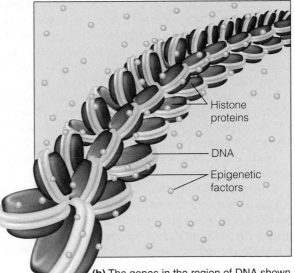

(b) The genes in the region of DNA shown here are so tightly wound around the histone proteins that the cell would not be able to access them and use them.

FIGURE 1.12 The epigenome includes the histone proteins around which the DNA strand is spooled and the epigenetic factors that surround it. The binding of epigenetic factors to the histone proteins causes physical and functional changes. (a) When DNA is loosely wrapped around its histones, its genes are more accessible for use in protein synthesis. (b) When DNA is tightly wound around its histones, its genes are inaccessible; thus, these genes are not expressed as proteins.

Promises of Nutrigenomics

Recently, a working group of the American Society for Nutrition published a list of urgent research needs, one of which was for research into nutrigenomics to help determine how specific nutrients interact with genes and proteins and to provide information on individualized nutrient requirements.[4] These goals reflect two fundamental promises of nutrigenomics. The first is that once we better understand specific nutrient–gene interactions, including how nutrients might influence cellular communication, use and storage of energy, and other processes, nutrigenomics may help people reduce their risk of developing diet-related diseases and possibly even treat existing conditions through diet alone.[5]

The second promise is personalized nutrition. In this future world, you would provide a tissue sample to a healthcare provider, who would send it to a lab for genetic analysis. The results would guide the provider in creating a diet tailored to your genetic makeup. By identifying both foods to eat and foods to avoid, this personalized diet would help you turn on beneficial genes and turn off genes that could be harmful. Although research into personalized nutrigenomics is ongoing, evidence to date is inconclusive, and we are still very far from personalized nutrition.[5]

Challenges of Nutrigenomics

If the promises of nutrigenomics strike you as pie in the sky, you're not alone. Many researchers caution, for example, that dietary "prescriptions" to prevent or treat chronic diseases would be extremely challenging, because multiple genes may be involved, as well as countless nutritional and environmental factors. In addition, genetics researchers currently believe that there are about 21,000 to 25,000 genes in human DNA, but that these genes represent only a fraction of the DNA in body cells.[6] The remaining regions of DNA are considered noncoding but are thought to have other functions, many of which may influence nutrition and health. Moreover, the pathways for genetic expression are extremely complex, and turning on a gene may have a beneficial effect on one body function but a harmful effect on another. To complicate the matter further, other factors such as age, gender, and lifestyle will also affect how different foods interact with these different genetic pathways. In short, the number of variables that must be considered in order to develop a "personalized diet" is staggering.

This daunting complexity has not stopped companies from offering naïve consumers nutrigenomics products and services ranging from at-home testing kits to "personalized" diets. Currently, we lack convincing evidence that these products and services are useful, and regulation of the nutrigenomics industry is a growing concern.

When Will Nutrigenomics Become a Viable Healthcare Option?

Delivering on the promises of nutrigenomics will require a multidisciplinary approach involving researchers in genetics, nutrition, chemistry, molecular biology, physiology, pathology, sociology, ethics, and many more. The number and complexity of interactions these scientists will have to contend with are so great that decades may pass before nutrigenomics is able to contribute significantly to human health.

Consumers will probably first encounter nutrigenomics in diagnostic testing. In this process, a blood or tissue sample of DNA will be genetically analyzed to determine how food and food supplements interact with that individual's genes and how a change in diet might affect those interactions. Genetic counseling will be required to help consumers understand the meaning and recommendations suggested by their genetic profile.

Second, consumers may begin to see specialized foods promoted for specific conditions. For example, consumers currently can choose certain foods if they want to lower their cholesterol or enhance their bone health. More such foods will likely be developed, and food packages might even be coded for certain genetic profiles.

We may be decades away from a "personalized diet," but one thing is clear right now: nutrigenomics is showing us the importance of nutrition and environmental factors in preserving our health. In doing so, nutrigenomics is changing not only the way we look at food but also the science of nutrition itself.

Critical Thinking Questions

- Will nutrigenomics advance preventive medicine and reduce our rate of obesity and other chronic diseases?
- If so, will it lower healthcare costs?

- In what other ways could nutrigenomics change the landscape of healthcare in America?

References

1. Waterland, R. A., and R. L. Jirtle. 2003. Transposable elements: targets for early nutritional effects on epigenetic gene regulation. *Mol. Cell. Biol.* 23(15):5293–5300.
2. Keijer, J., F. P. Hoevenaars, A. Nieuwenhuizen, and E. M. van Schothorst. 2014. Nutrigenomics of body weight regulation: a rationale for careful dissection of individual contributors. *Nutrients* 6(10):4531–4551. doi: 10.3390/nu6104531.
3. Khalil, C. A. 2014. The emerging role of epigenetics in cardiovascular disease. *Ther. Adv. Chronic. Dis.* 5(4):178–187.
4. Ohlhorst, S. D., R. Russell, D. Bier, D. M. Klurfeld, Z. Li, J. R. Mein …, and E. Konopka. 2013. Nutrition research to affect food and a healthy lifespan. *Adv. Nutr.* 4(5):579–584.
5. Neeha, V. S., and P. Kinth. 2013. Nutrigenomics research: a review. *J. Food Sci. Technol.* 50(3):415–428.
6. National Human Genome Research Institute. 2014. National DNA Day. Updated March, 2014. https://www.genome.gov/26525485. Accessed March 14, 2015.

STUDY **PLAN**   MasteringNutrition™

Customize your study plan—and master your nutrition!— in the Study Plan of MasteringNutrition.

TEST YOURSELF | *ANSWERS*

1. **F** A Calorie is a measure of the energy in a food. More precisely, a kilocalorie is the amount of heat required to raise the temperature of 1 kilogram of water by 1 degree Celsius.

2. **T** Carbohydrates and lipids are the primary energy sources for the body.

3. **F** Most water-soluble vitamins need to be consumed daily. However, we can consume foods that contain fat-soluble vitamins less frequently because our body can store these vitamins.

4. **F** The RDA is the average daily nutrient intake level that meets the nutrient requirements of 97% to 98% of healthy individuals in a particular life stage and gender group.

5. **T** Observational studies indicate relationships between nutrition and factors such as disease, but they do not indicate cause and effect.

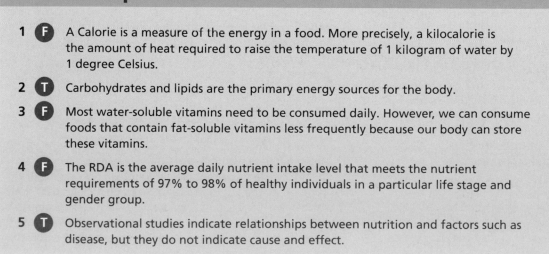

summary

Scan to hear an MP3 Chapter Review in **MasteringNutrition**.

LO 1 ■ Nutrition is the scientific study of food and how food nourishes the body and influences health.

■ Early nutrition research focused on identifying, preventing, and treating nutrient-deficiency diseases. As the Western diet improved, obesity and its associated chronic diseases became an important subject for nutrition research. In the late 20th century, nutrigenomics emerged as a new field of nutrition research.

LO 2 ■ Nutrition is an important component of wellness. Healthful nutrition plays a critical role in eliminating deficiency disease and can help reduce our risks for various chronic diseases.

■ *Healthy People 2020* is a national health promotion and disease prevention plan that identifies goals we hope to reach as a nation by 2020. Its four overarching goals are to (1) attain high-quality, longer lives free of preventable disease, disability, injury, and premature death; (2) achieve health equity, eliminate disparities, and improve the health of all groups; (3) create social and physical environments that promote good health for all; and (4) promote quality of life, healthy development, and healthy behaviors across all life stages. It includes dozens of objectives related to nutrition and weight status and physical activity.

LO 3 ■ Nutrients are chemicals found in food that are critical to human growth and function.

■ The six essential nutrients found in the foods we eat are carbohydrates, lipids, proteins, and water, which are known as the macronutrients; and vitamins and minerals, which are micronutrients.

■ Carbohydrates are composed of carbon, hydrogen, and oxygen. They are the primary energy source for the human body, particularly for the brain.

■ Lipids provide us with fat-soluble vitamins and essential fatty acids in addition to storing large quantities of energy.

■ Proteins can provide energy if needed, but they are not a primary fuel source. Proteins support tissue growth, repair, and maintenance.

■ Vitamins are organic compounds that assist with the regulation of body processes.

■ Minerals are inorganic elements that are not changed by digestion or other metabolic processes.

■ Water is critical to survival and supports numerous body functions, including fluid balance, the conduction of nervous impulses, and muscle contraction.

LO 4 ■ The Dietary Reference Intakes (DRIs) are reference standards for nutrient intakes for healthy people in the United States and Canada.

■ The DRIs include the Estimated Average Requirement, the Recommended Dietary Allowance, the Adequate Intake, the Tolerable Upper Intake Level, the Estimated Energy Requirement, and the Acceptable Macronutrient Distribution Range.

LO 5 ■ To assess nutritional status, healthcare providers conduct a physical examination, including objective measures of vital signs, lab values, and height and weight, as well as a health-history questionnaire. A variety of dietary intake tools may also be used, including diet histories, 24-hour recalls, food-frequency questionnaires, and diet records.

LO 6 ■ Malnutrition occurs when a person's nutritional status is out of balance.

■ Undernutrition occurs when someone consumes too little energy or nutrients, and overnutrition occurs when too much energy or too much of a given nutrient is consumed over time. A primary nutrient deficiency occurs when a person does not consume enough of a given nutrient in the diet. A secondary nutrient deficiency occurs when a person cannot absorb enough of a nutrient, when too much of a nutrient is excreted, or when a nutrient is not efficiently utilized.

LO 7 ■ The steps in the scientific method are (1) observing a phenomenon, (2) creating a hypothesis, (3) designing and conducting an experiment, and (4) collecting and analyzing data that support or refute the hypothesis.

■ A hypothesis that is supported after repeated experiments may be called a theory.

LO 8 ■ Studies involving animals provide preliminary information that assists scientists in designing human studies. Human studies include epidemiological studies such as observational and case-control studies, and experimental clinical trials. A double-blind, placebo-controlled study is considered the most trustworthy form of clinical trial.

LO 9 ■ When evaluating media reports, consider who is reporting the information, who conducted and paid for the research, whether the research was published in a reputable journal, whether the researchers have a conflict of interest, and whether it involves testimonials or makes claims that sound too good to be true. Quackery is the promotion of an unproven remedy, usually by someone unlicensed and untrained, for financial gain.

LO 10 ■ Potentially good sources of reliable nutrition information include registered dietitians, licensed dietitians, and individuals who hold an advanced degree in nutrition. Medical professionals such as physicians, osteopaths, and registered nurses have variable levels of training in nutrition.

■ The Centers for Disease Control and Prevention (CDC) is the leading federal agency that protects the health and safety of Americans.

- The National Health and Nutrition Examination Survey (NHANES) is a survey conducted by the CDC and the National Center for Health Statistics that tracks the nutritional status of people in the United States.
- The Behavioral Risk Factor Surveillance System (BRFSS) was established by the CDC and is the world's largest telephone survey; the BRFSS gathers data at the state level on the health behaviors and risks of Americans.
- The National Institutes of Health (NIH) is the leading medical research agency in the world. The mission of the NIH is to uncover new knowledge that leads to better health for everyone.

review questions

LO 1 1. Early nutrition research focused on
a. improving agricultural yields.
b. classifying plants as edible or inedible.
c. identifying and preventing nutrient-deficiency diseases.
d. investigating associations between diet and chronic disease.

LO 2 2. Which of the following statements is true?
a. Scurvy is caused by a nutrient deficiency.
b. Osteoporosis is caused by a nutrient deficiency.
c. Heart disease is caused by a nutrient toxicity.
d. A poor diet causes diabetes.

LO 3 3. Vitamins A and C, thiamin, calcium, and magnesium are considered
a. water-soluble vitamins.
b. fat-soluble vitamins.
c. energy nutrients.
d. micronutrients.

LO 4 4. To maintain good health, you should aim to consume
a. the EAR for vitamin C.
b. the RDA for vitamin C.
c. the UL for vitamin C.
d. within the AMDR for vitamin C.

LO 5 5. Which of the following assessment methods provides objective data?
a. Measurement of height
b. History of illnesses, injuries, and surgeries
c. Assessment of fatigue
d. Twenty-four-hour dietary recall

LO 6 6. As a result of a severe digestive disorder, Jane has lost 20% of her body weight and states she is "exhausted all the time." Jane is experiencing
a. overnutrition.
b. primary deficiency.
c. subclinical deficiency.
d. overt signs and symptoms.

LO 7 7. Which of the following statements about the scientific method is true?
a. "One hundred inactive residents of the Sunshine Care Home have high blood pressure, and 32 inactive residents have normal blood pressure" is an example of a valid hypothesis.
b. "A high-protein diet increases the risk for porous bones" is an example of a valid hypothesis.
c. If an experiment yields data that support a hypothesis, that hypothesis is confirmed as fact.
d. If the results of multiple experiments consistently support a hypothesis, it is confirmed as fact.

LO 8 8. An independent research team was hired by a beverage company to conduct a study into the effectiveness of a new vitamin-herb bottled tea on reducing the incidence of colds. The team recruited volunteers and divided them by surname into two groups of 100 participants each. Volunteers whose surname began with a letter of the alphabet from A through M drank the tea once daily. Those whose surname began with N through Z drank once daily a beverage that had a similar color and flavor but no active ingredient. Researchers phoned all participants with a surname beginning in A–M on Mondays and all participants with a surname beginning in N–Z on Tuesdays once a week for 6 months and asked them whether or not they had experienced a cold. This is an example of a (an)
a. observational study.
b. case-control study.
c. randomized clinical trial.
d. double-blind placebo-controlled study.

LO 9 9. The study described in question 8 was funded by a company that stood to profit from results supporting their product's effectiveness. This is an example of
a. peer review.
b. a conflict of interest.
c. transparency.
d. quackery.

LO 10 10. Sources of reliable and accurate nutrition information include
a. the nutritionist on the staff of your local supermarket.
b. the personal trainer at your campus fitness center.
c. the website of the National Institutes of Health.
d. an advertisement for a weight-loss program you read in the health section of the *New York Times*.

true or false?

LO 3 11. **True or false?** Fat-soluble vitamins provide energy.

LO 4 12. **True or false?** The RDA represents the highest daily nutrient intake level that is not associated with health risks.

LO 5 13. **True or false?** A food-frequency questionnaire elicits subjective data.

LO 8 14. **True or false?** An epidemiological study is a clinical trial in which a large population participates as members of the experimental and control groups.

LO 10 15. **True or false?** Nutrition-related reports in the *Journal of the Academy of Nutrition and Dietetics* are likely to be trustworthy.

LO 4 16. Compare the EAR with the RDA.

LO 8 17. Explain the role of the control group in a clinical trial.

LO 9 18. Imagine that you are in a gift shop and meet Marilyn, from the chapter-opening scenario. Learning that you are studying nutrition, she tells you of her experience and states that the supplements "didn't seem to do much of anything." She asks you, "How can I find reliable nutrition information?" How would you answer?

math review

LO 3 19. You are following a recipe that calls for 200 grams of raisins. How many ounces of raisins is this?

LO 4 20. Kayla meets with a registered dietitian recommended by her doctor to design a weight-loss diet plan. She is shocked when a dietary analysis reveals that she consumes an average of 2,200 kcal and 60 grams of fat each day. What percentage of Kayla's diet comes from fat, and is this percentage within the AMDR for fat?

Answers to Review Questions and Math Review can be found online in the MasteringNutrition Study Area.

web links

www.healthypeople.gov
Healthy People 2020
Search this site for a list of objectives that identify the most significant preventable threats to health in the United States and that establish national goals to reduce these threats.

www.eatright.org
The Academy of Nutrition and Dietetics (formerly the American Dietetic Association)
Obtain a list of registered dietitians in your community from the largest organization of food and nutrition professionals in the United States. Information about careers in dietetics is also available at this site.

www.cdc.gov
Centers for Disease Control and Prevention (CDC)
Visit this site for additional information about the leading federal agency in the United States that protects the health and safety of people.

www.cdc.gov/nchs
National Center for Health Statistics
From the CDC site, click the "National Data" link to learn more about the National Health and Nutrition Examination Survey (NHANES) and other national health surveys.

www.nih.gov
National Institutes of Health (NIH)
Find out more about the National Institutes of Health, an agency under the U.S. Department of Health and Human Services.

www.nutrition.org
American Society for Nutrition (ASN)
Learn more about the American Society for Nutrition and its goal to improve quality of life through the science of nutrition.

www.acsm.org
American College of Sports Medicine (ACSM)
Obtain information about the leading sports medicine and exercise science organization in the world.

www.obesity.org
The Obesity Society
Learn about this interdisciplinary society and its work to develop, extend, and disseminate knowledge in the field of obesity.

www.iom.edu/Global/Topics/Food-Nutrition
Institute of Medicine of the National Academies
Learn about the Institute of Medicine's history of examining the nation's nutritional well-being and providing sound information about food and nutrition.

www.ncbi.nlm.nih.gov/pubmed
PubMed
Search the more than 24 million citations for biomedical literature, including journals and online books.

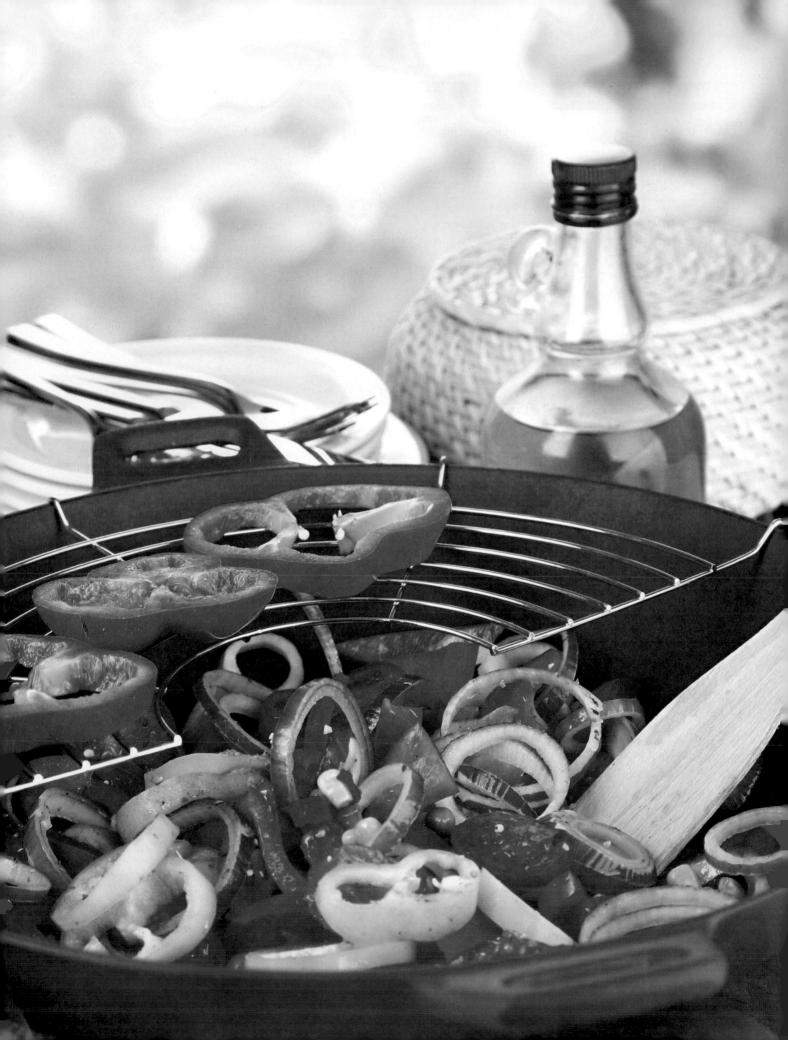

2 Designing a Healthful Diet

Learning Outcomes

After studying this chapter, you should be able to:

1 Define the components of a healthful diet, *pp. 42–43.*

2 Read a food label and use the Nutrition Facts panel to determine the nutritional adequacy of a given food, *pp. 44–47.*

3 Distinguish among label claims related to nutrient content, health, and body structure or function, *pp. 47–49.*

4 Explain the concept of nutrient density and identify a variety of nutrient-dense foods, *pp. 50–52.*

5 Discuss five key messages of the *Dietary Guidelines*, including choices to make more often and choices to limit, *pp. 50–54.*

6 Identify the five food groups included in the USDA Food Patterns and the key message for each group, *pp. 54–55.*

7 Compare MyPlate to the Mediterranean diet, *pp. 55–56.*

8 Define *empty* Calories and discuss the role that empty Calories and serving size play in designing a healthful diet, *p. 56.*

9 Discuss several ways that technology can help you design and maintain a healthful diet, *p. 61.*

10 List at least four ways to practice moderation and apply healthful dietary guidelines when eating out, *pp. 62–63.*

TEST YOURSELF

True or False?

1 A healthful diet should always include vitamin supplements. **T** *or* **F**

2 All foods sold in the United States must display a food label. **T** *or* **F**

3 A cup of coffee with cream and sugar has about the same number of Calories as a café mocha. **T** *or* **F**

4 The top nutritional guidelines in the United States encourage abstinence from alcohol. **T** *or* **F**

5 It is possible to eat healthfully when dining out. **T** *or* **F**

Test Yourself answers are located in the Chapter Review.

MasteringNutrition™

Go online for chapter quizzes, pre-tests, interactive activities, and more!

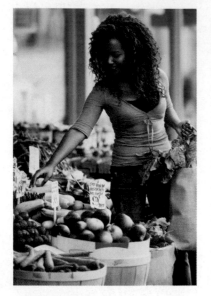

Each person needs to determine his or her own pattern of healthful eating.

Shivani and her parents moved to the United States from India when Shivani was 6 years old. Although delicate in comparison to her American peers, Shivani was healthy and energetic, excelling in school and riding her new bike in her suburban neighborhood. By the time Shivani entered high school, her weight had caught up to that of her American classmates. Now a college freshman, she has joined the almost 17% of U.S. teens who are obese.[1] Shivani explains, "In India, the diet is mostly rice, lentils, and vegetables. Many people are vegetarians, and many others eat meat only once or twice a week, and very small portions. Desserts are only for special occasions. When we moved to America, I wanted to eat like all the other kids: hamburgers, french fries, sodas, and sweets. I gained a lot of weight on that diet, and now my doctor says my cholesterol, my blood pressure, and my blood sugar levels are all too high. I wish I could start eating like my relatives back in India again, but they don't serve rice and lentils in the campus dining halls."

What influence does diet have on health? What exactly qualifies as a "poor diet," and what makes a diet healthful? Is it more important to watch how much we eat or what kinds of foods we choose? What do the national dietary guidelines advise, and do they apply to "real people" like you?

Many factors contribute to the confusion surrounding healthful eating. First, as we discussed in Chapter 1, nutrition is a relatively young science, emerging around 1900, with the discovery of the first vitamin in 1897. The initial Recommended Dietary Allowance (RDA) values for the United States were published in 1941. Thus, new findings on the benefits of foods and nutrients are discovered almost daily. These new findings contribute to regular changes in how a healthful diet is defined. Second, because the popular media typically report the results of only selected studies, usually the most recent, we often lack a complete picture of all the research conducted in any given area. Third, there is no one right way to eat that is healthful and acceptable for everyone. We are individuals with unique needs, food preferences, and cultural influences. Thus, there are literally millions of different ways to design a healthful diet to fit individual needs.

Given all this potential confusion, it's a good thing there are nutritional tools to guide people in designing a personalized, healthful diet. In this chapter, we introduce these tools, including food labels, the *Dietary Guidelines for Americans*, the U.S. Department of Agriculture Food Patterns (and its accompanying graphic, MyPlate), and others. Before exploring the question of how to design a healthful diet, however, it is important to understand what a healthful diet *is*.

LO 1 Define the components of a healthful diet.

What Is a Healthful Diet?

A **healthful diet** provides the proper combination of energy and nutrients. It has four characteristics: it is adequate, moderate, balanced, and varied. No matter if you are young or old, overweight or underweight, healthy or coping with illness, if you keep in mind these characteristics of a healthful diet, you will be able to consciously select foods that provide you with the appropriate combination of nutrients and energy each day.

A Healthful Diet Is Adequate

An **adequate diet** provides enough of the energy, nutrients, and fiber to maintain a person's health. A diet may be inadequate in only one area. For example, as noted, many people in the United States do not eat enough vegetables and therefore are not consuming enough of the fiber and micronutrients found in vegetables. However, their intake of other types of foods may be adequate or even excessive. In fact, some people who eat too few vegetables are overweight or obese, which means that they are eating a diet that exceeds their energy needs.

healthful diet A diet that provides the proper combination of energy and nutrients and is adequate, moderate, balanced, and varied.

adequate diet A diet that provides enough of the energy, nutrients, and fiber to maintain a person's health.

On the other hand, a generalized state of undernutrition can occur if an individual's diet contains an inadequate level of several nutrients for a long period of time. To maintain a thin figure, some individuals may skip one or more meals each day, avoid foods that contain any fat, and limit their meals to only a few foods, such as a bagel, a banana, or a diet soda. This type of restrictive eating pattern practiced over a prolonged period can cause low energy levels, loss of bone and hair, impaired memory and cognitive function, menstrual dysfunction in women, and even death.

A diet that is adequate for one person may not be adequate for another. For example, the energy needs of a small woman who is lightly active are approximately 1,700 to 2,000 kilocalories (kcal) each day, while a highly active male athlete may require more than 4,000 kcal each day to support his body's demands. These two individuals differ greatly in their activity level and in their quantity of body fat and muscle mass, which means they require very different levels of fat, carbohydrate, protein, and other nutrients to support their daily needs.

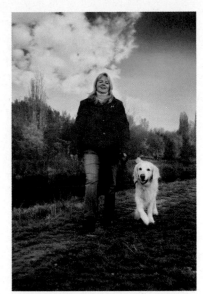

A Healthful Diet Is Moderate

Moderation is one of the keys to a healthful diet. **Moderation** refers to eating any foods in moderate amounts—not too much and not too little. If a person eats too much or too little of certain foods, health goals cannot be reached. For example, some people drink as much as 60 fluid ounces (three 20-oz bottles) of soft drinks on some days. Drinking this much contributes an extra 765 kcal of energy to a person's diet. In order to allow for these extra kilocalories and avoid weight gain, an individual would need to reduce food intake, which could lead to cutting healthful food choices out of his or her diet. In contrast, people who drink mostly water or other beverages containing little or no energy can consume a greater amount of more nourishing foods that will support their wellness.

A Healthful Diet Is Balanced

A **balanced diet** contains the combinations of foods that provide the proper proportions of nutrients. As you will learn in this course, the body needs many types of foods in varying amounts to maintain health. For example, fruits and vegetables are excellent sources of fiber, vitamin C, potassium, and magnesium. Meats are not good sources of fiber and these nutrients, but they are excellent sources of protein, iron, zinc, and copper. By eating the proper balance of all healthful foods, including fruits, vegetables, and meats or meat substitutes, we can be confident that we are consuming the balanced nutrition we need to maintain health.

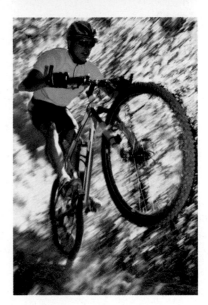

A diet that is adequate for one person may not be adequate for another. A woman who is lightly active will require fewer kilocalories of energy per day than a highly active male.

A Healthful Diet Is Varied

Variety refers to eating many different foods from the different food groups on a regular basis. With thousands of healthful foods to choose from, trying new foods on a regular basis is a fun and easy way to vary your diet. Eat a new vegetable each week or substitute one food for another, such as raw spinach on your turkey sandwich in place of iceberg lettuce. Selecting a wide variety of foods increases the likelihood of consuming the multitude of nutrients the body needs. As an added benefit, eating a varied diet prevents boredom and avoids the potential of getting into a "food rut." Later in this chapter, we provide suggestions for eating a varied diet.

moderation Eating any foods in moderate amounts—not too much and not too little.

balanced diet A diet that contains the combinations of foods that provide the proper nutrient proportions.

variety Eating a lot of different foods each day.

RECAP

A healthful diet provides adequate nutrients and energy, and it includes sweets, fats, and salty foods in moderate amounts only. A healthful diet includes an appropriate balance of nutrients and a wide variety of foods. ■

LO 2 Read a food label and use the Nutrition Facts panel to determine the nutritional adequacy of a given food.

LO 3 Distinguish among label claims related to nutrient content, health, and body structure or function.

How Can Reading Food Labels Help You Improve Your Diet?

To design and maintain a healthful diet, it's important to read and understand food labels. It may surprise you to learn that a few decades ago there were no federal regulations for including nutrition information on food labels! The U.S. Food and Drug Administration (FDA) first established such regulations in 1973. These regulations were not as specific as they are today and were not required for many of the foods available to consumers. Throughout the 1970s and 1980s, consumer interest in food quality grew substantially, and many watchdog groups were formed to protect consumers from unclear labeling and false claims made by some manufacturers.

Public interest and concern about how food affects health became so strong that in 1990 the U.S. Congress passed the Nutrition Labeling and Education Act. This act specifies which foods require a food label, provides detailed descriptions of the information that must be included on the food label, and describes the companies and food products that are exempt from publishing complete nutrition information on food labels. For example, detailed food labels are not required for meat or poultry, as these products are regulated by the U.S. Department of Agriculture (USDA), not the FDA. In addition, foods such as coffee, fresh produce, and most spices are not required to follow the FDA labeling guidelines, as they contain insignificant amounts of all the nutrients that must be listed in nutrition labeling.

Five Components Must Be Included on Food Labels

Five primary components of information must be included on food labels (**Figure 2.1**).

1. **A statement of identity:** The common name of the product or an appropriate identification of the food product must be prominently displayed on the label. This information tells us very clearly what the product is.
2. **The net contents of the package:** The quantity of the food product in the entire package must be accurately described. Information may be listed as weight (such as grams), volume (fluid ounces), or numerical count (4 each).
3. **Ingredient list:** The ingredients must be listed by their common names, in descending order by weight. This means that the first product listed in the ingredient list is the predominant ingredient in that food. This information can be useful in many situations, such as when you are looking for foods that are lower in fat or sugar or when you are attempting to identify foods that contain whole-grain flour instead of processed wheat flour.
4. **The name and address of the food manufacturer, packer, or distributor:** This information can be used if you want to find out more detailed information about a food product and to contact the company if there is something wrong with the product or you suspect that it caused an illness.
5. **Nutrition information:** The Nutrition Facts panel contains the nutrition information required by the FDA. This panel is the primary tool to assist you in choosing more healthful foods. An explanation of the components of the Nutrition Facts panel follows.

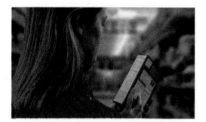

Learning how to read food labels is a skill that can help you meet your nutritional goals.

Nutrition Facts panel The label on a food package containing the nutrition information required by the FDA.

How to Read and Use the Nutrition Facts Panel

Focus Figure 2.2 (page 46) shows an example of the recently re-designed **Nutrition Facts panel.** You can use the information on this panel to learn more about an individual food, and you can use the panel to compare one food to another. Let's start at the top of the panel and work our way down to better understand how to use this information.

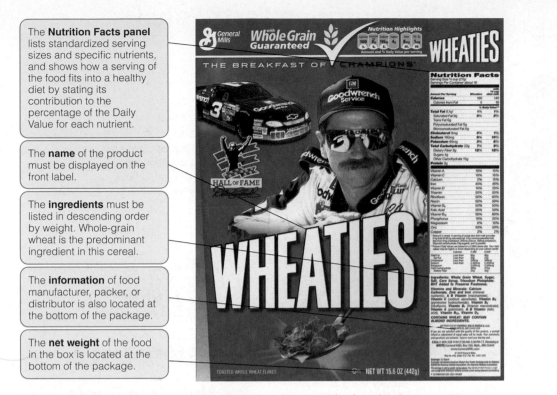

The **Nutrition Facts panel** lists standardized serving sizes and specific nutrients, and shows how a serving of the food fits into a healthy diet by stating its contribution to the percentage of the Daily Value for each nutrient.

The **name** of the product must be displayed on the front label.

The **ingredients** must be listed in descending order by weight. Whole-grain wheat is the predominant ingredient in this cereal.

The **information** of food manufacturer, packer, or distributor is also located at the bottom of the package.

The **net weight** of the food in the box is located at the bottom of the package.

FIGURE 2.1 The five primary components that are required for food labels. (*Source:* © ConAgra Brands, Inc. Reprinted by permission.)

1. **Serving size and servings per container:** describes the serving size in a common household measure (such as cup), a metric measure (grams), and the number of servings contained in the package. Serving size is standardized making comparison shopping easier. However, keep in mind that the serving size listed on the package may not be the same as the amount *you* eat. To assist consumers, the amount per serving size is clearly listed, and for packages of foods that are commonly consumed in one sitting, this information reflects the amount in the entire package. It is important to factor in how much of the food you eat when determining the amount of nutrients that this food contributes to your actual diet.

2. **Calories and Calories from fat per serving:** describes the total number of Calories in larger, bolder print. The total number of Calories that come from fat per one serving of that food has been removed. However, additional information provided will allow you to determine the amount of fat, added sugars, and other key nutrients the food contains.

3. **Percent daily values (%DVs):** This section has been reorganized to list the %DV on the left, followed by the nutrient name and the grams of the nutrient in the food. The %DV tells you how much a serving of food contributes to your overall intake of nutrients listed on the label. For example, 10 grams of fat constitutes 15% of an individual's total daily recommended fat intake. Because we are all individuals with unique nutritional needs, it is impractical to include nutrition information that applies to each person consuming a food. That would require thousands of labels! Thus, when defining the %DV, the FDA based its calculations on a 2,000-Calorie diet. Even if you do not consume 2,000 Calories each day, you can still use the %DV to figure out whether a food is high or low in a given nutrient. For example, foods that contain less than 5% DV of a nutrient are considered low in that nutrient, while foods that contain more than 20% DV are considered high in that nutrient. If you are trying to consume

percent daily values (%DVs) Information on a Nutrition Facts panel that identifies how much a serving of food contributes to your overall intake of nutrients listed on the label; based on an energy intake of 2,000 Calories per day.

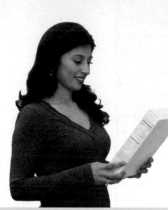

The U.S. Food and Drug Administration (FDA) is proposing new changes to the 20-year-old nutrition labels on packaged foods. The changes to the nutrition label provide information to help compare products and make healthy food choices.

Current Label

GRANOLA

Nutrition Facts

Serving Size 2/3 cup (55 g)
Servings Per Container About 8

Amount Per Serving

Calories 230	Calories from Fat 72

	% Daily Value*
Total Fat 8 g	**12%**
Saturated Fat 1 g	**5%**
Trans Fat 0 g	
Cholesterol 0 mg	**0%**
Sodium 160 mg	**7%**
Total Carbohydrates 37 g	**12%**
Dietary Fiber 4 g	**16%**
Sugars 1 g	
Protein 3 g	
Vitamin A	10%
Vitamin C	8%
Calcium	20%
Iron	45%

* Percent Daily Values are based on a 2,000 calorie diet. Your daily value may be higher or lower depending on your calorie needs.

		Calories:	2,000	2,500
Total Fat	Less than		65 g	80 g
Sat Fat	Less than		20 g	25 g
Cholesterol	Less than		300 mg	300 mg
Sodium	Less than		2,400 mg	2,400 mg
Total Carbohydrate			300 g	375 g
Dietary Fiber			25 g	30 g

SERVINGS

- Serving sizes are standardized, making comparison shopping easier.

NEW
- Servings and serving sizes are larger and bolder.
- "Amount per serving" will be changed to "Amount per (serving size)" such as "Amount per cup."

CALORIES

- Calories per serving and the number of servings in the package are listed.

NEW
- Calories are larger to stand out more.
- "Calories from fat" is removed.

DAILY VALUES

- Daily Values are general reference values based on a 2,000 Calorie diet.
- The %DV can tell you if a food is high or low in a nutrient or dietary substance.

NEW
- Daily Values are listed first.
- A shorter footnote that more clearly explains %DV will be included.
- The %DV for added sugars will be included on labels of packaged foods.

ADDED SUGARS

NEW
- Added sugars are listed.

VITAMINS & MINERALS

- Vitamin A, vitamin C, calcium, and iron are required.
- Other vitamins and minerals are voluntary.

NEW
- Vitamin D and potassium are required, in addition to calcium and iron.
- Vitamins A and C are voluntary.
- Actual amounts of each nutrient are listed as well as the %DV.

Proposed New Label

GRANOLA

Nutrition Facts

8 servings per container

Serving size	2/3 cup (55 g)

Amount per 2/3 cup

Calories 230

% DV*	
12%	**Total Fat** 8 g
5%	**Saturated Fat** 1 g
	Trans Fat 0 g
0%	**Cholesterol** 0 mg
7%	**Sodium** 160 mg
12%	**Total Carbs** 37 g
14%	Dietary Fiber 4 g
	Sugars 1 g
	Added Sugars 0 g
	Protein 3 g
10%	**Vitamin D** 2 mcg
20%	**Calcium** 260 mg
45%	**Iron** 8 mg
5%	**Potassium** 235 mg

* Footnote on Daily Values (DV) and calories reference to be inserted here.

more calcium in your diet, select foods that contain more than 20% DV for calcium. In contrast, if you are trying to consume lower-fat foods, select foods that contain less than 5% or 10% fat. By comparing the %DV between foods for any nutrient, you can quickly decide which food is higher or lower in that nutrient without having to know anything about how many Calories you need. The additional change to this section is that it is required to include the %DVs for added sugars, vitamin D, calcium, iron, and potassium; inclusion of vitamins A and C are now voluntary. The actual amount of added sugars and these micronutrients is now listed, in addition to their %DV.

4. **Footnote (lower part of panel):** tells you that the %DVs are based on a 2,000-Calorie diet and that your needs may be higher or lower. The remainder of the footnote includes a table with values that illustrate the differences in recommendations between a 2,000-Calorie and 2,500-Calorie diet; for instance, someone eating 2,000 Calories should strive to eat less than 65 g of fat per day, whereas a person eating 2,500 Calories should eat less than 80 g of fat per day. The table may not be present on the package if the food label is too small. When present, the footnote and the table are always the same because the information refers to general dietary advice for all Americans rather than to a specific food.

Food Labels Can Display a Variety of Claims

Have you ever noticed a food label displaying a claim such as "This food is low in sodium" or "This food is part of a heart-healthy diet"? The claim may have influenced you to buy the food, even if you weren't sure what it meant. So let's take a look.

The FDA regulates two types of claims that food companies put on food labels: nutrient claims and health claims. Food companies are prohibited from using a nutrient or health claim that is not approved by the FDA.

The Daily Values on the food labels serve as a basis for nutrient claims. For instance, if the label states that a food is "low in sodium," that food contains 140 mg or less of sodium per serving. **Table 2.1** (p. 48) defines terms approved for use in nutrient claims.

Food labels are also allowed to display certain claims related to health and disease. The health claims that the FDA allows at the present time are listed in **Table 2.2** (p. 49). To help consumers gain a better understanding of nutritional information related to health, the FDA has developed a Health Claims Report Card (**Figure 2.3**), which grades the level of

Want to find out more about how to use food labels to maintain a healthy weight? Go to **www.fda.gov** and type in the search bar "Make Your Calories Count."

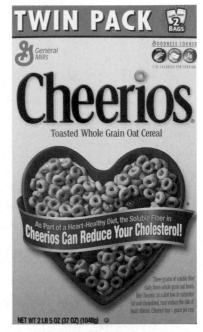

This Cheerios label is an example of an approved health claim.

Health Claims Report Card

FDA category | | Required disclaimer

A	**High** Significant scientific agreement	Applies to claims listed in Table 2.2 No disclaimer needed
B	**Moderate** Evidence is not conclusive	"… although there is scientific evidence supporting the claim, the evidence is not conclusive."
C	**Low** Evidence is limited and not conclusive	"Some scientific evidence suggests … however, FDA has determined that this evidence is limited and not conclusive."
D	**Extremely Low** Little scientific evidence supporting this claim	"Very limited and preliminary scientific research suggests … FDA concludes that there is little scientific evidence supporting this claim."

FIGURE 2.3 The U.S. Food and Drug Administration's Health Claims Report Card. (*Source:* Data from "Assessing Consumer Perceptions of Health Claims," by Neal Hooker and Ratapol P. Teratanavat, from the Federal Drug Administration website. Updated April 4, 2010.)

TABLE 2.1 U.S. Food and Drug Administration (FDA)–Approved Nutrient-Related Terms and Definitions

Nutrient	Claim	Meaning
Energy	Calorie free	Less than 5 kcal per serving
	Low Calorie	40 kcal or less per serving
	Reduced Calorie	At least 25% fewer kcal than reference (or regular) food
Fat and cholesterol	Fat free	Less than 0.5 g of fat per serving
	Low fat	3 g or less fat per serving
	Reduced fat	At least 25% less fat per serving than reference food
	Saturated fat free	Less than 0.5 g of saturated fat AND less than 0.5 g of *trans* fat per serving
	Low saturated fat	1 g or less saturated fat and less than 0.5 g *trans* fat per serving AND 15% or less of total kcal from saturated fat
	Reduced saturated fat	At least 25% less saturated fat AND reduced by more than 1 g saturated fat per serving as compared to reference food
	Cholesterol free	Less than 2 mg of cholesterol per serving AND 2 g or less saturated fat and *trans* fat combined per serving
	Low cholesterol	20 mg or less cholesterol AND 2 g or less saturated fat per serving
	Reduced cholesterol	At least 25% less cholesterol than reference food AND 2 g or less saturated fat per serving
Fiber and sugar	High fiber	5 g or more fiber per serving*
	Good source of fiber	2.5 g to 4.9 g fiber per serving
	More or added fiber	At least 2.5 g more fiber per serving than reference food
	Sugar free	Less than 0.5 g sugars per serving
	Low sugar	Not defined; no basis for recommended intake
	Reduced/less sugar	At least 25% less sugars per serving than reference food
	No added sugars or without added sugars	No sugar or sugar-containing ingredient added during processing
Sodium	Sodium free	Less than 5 mg sodium per serving
	Very low sodium	35 mg or less sodium per serving
	Low sodium	140 mg or less sodium per serving
	Reduced sodium	At least 25% less sodium per serving than reference food
Relative Claims	Free, without, no, zero	No or a trivial amount of given nutrient
	Light (lite)	This term can have three different meanings: (1) a serving provides one-third fewer kcal than or half the fat of the reference food; (2) a serving of a low-fat, low-Calorie food provides half the sodium normally present; or (3) lighter in color and texture, with the label making this clear (for example, "light molasses")
	Reduced, less, fewer	Contains at least 25% less of a nutrient or kcal than reference food
	More, added, extra, or plus	At least 10% of the Daily Value of nutrient as compared to reference food (may occur naturally or be added); may only be used for vitamins, minerals, protein, dietary fiber, and potassium
	Good source of, contains, or provides	10–19% of Daily Value per serving (may not be used for carbohydrate)
	High in, rich in, or excellent source of	20% or more of Daily Value per serving for protein, vitamins, minerals, dietary fiber, or potassium (may not be used for carbohydrate)

*High-fiber claims must also meet the definition of low fat; if not, then the level of total fat must appear next to the high-fiber claim.
Source: "Food Labeling Guide," from FDA.gov.

functional foods Foods that may have biologically active ingredients with the potential to provide health benefits beyond providing energy and nutrients necessary to sustain life.

whole foods Foods in their natural state such as nuts, oats, and blueberries, that can also be classified as functional foods.

confidence in a health claim based on current scientific evidence. For example, if current scientific evidence is not convincing, a particular health claim may have to include a disclaimer, so that consumers are not misled.

Food manufacturers often make health claims for so-called **functional foods.** These are foods that may have biologically active ingredients with the potential to provide health benefits beyond providing energy and nutrients necessary to sustain life.[2] Also called *nutraceuticals,* functional foods include **whole foods,** such as nuts, oats, and blueberries,

TABLE 2.2 U.S. Food and Drug Administration–Approved Health Claims on Labels

Disease/Health Concern	Nutrient	Example of Approved Claim Statement
Osteoporosis	Calcium	Regular exercise and a healthy diet with enough calcium help teens and young adult white and Asian women maintain good bone health and may reduce their high risk of osteoporosis later in life.
Coronary heart disease	Saturated fat and cholesterol Fruits, vegetables, and grain products that contain fiber, particularly soluble fiber Soluble fiber from whole oats, psyllium seed husk, and beta glucan soluble fiber from oat bran, rolled oats (or oatmeal), and whole-oat flour Soy protein Plant sterol/stanol esters Whole-grain foods	Diets low in saturated fat and cholesterol and rich in fruits, vegetables, and grain products that contain some types of dietary fiber, particularly soluble fiber, may reduce the risk of heart disease, a disease associated with many factors.
Cancer	Dietary fat Fiber-containing grain products, fruits and vegetables Fruits and vegetables Whole-grain foods	Low-fat diets rich in fiber-containing grain products, fruits, and vegetables may reduce the risk of some types of cancer, a disease associated with many factors.
Hypertension and stroke	Sodium Potassium	Diets containing foods that are a good source of potassium and that are low in sodium may reduce the risk of high blood pressure and stroke.*
Neural tube defects	Folate	Healthful diets with adequate folate may reduce a woman's risk of having a child with a brain or spinal cord defect.
Dental caries	Sugar alcohols	Frequent between-meal consumption of foods high in sugars and starches promotes tooth decay. The sugar alcohols in [name of food] do not promote tooth decay.

*Required wording for this claim. Wordings for other claims are recommended model statements but are not required verbatim.
Source: "Food Labeling Guide," from FDA.gov.

as well as **processed foods,** including fortified, enriched, or enhanced foods. Examples of processed functional foods include orange juice with added calcium and vitamin D, or bread enriched with folate. Sometimes, the health-promoting substances are developed in a functional food by altering the way in which the food is produced. For example, eggs with higher levels of omega-3 fatty acids (fats that help protect against heart disease) result from feeding hens a special diet. And fruits and vegetables can be genetically engineered to contain higher levels of nutrients.

In addition to nutrient and health claims, labels may also contain structure–function claims, generic statements about a food's impact on the body's structure and function. Structure–function claims cannot refer to a specific disease or symptom. Examples of structure–function claims include "Builds stronger bones," "Improves memory," "Slows signs of aging," and "Boosts your immune system." These claims can be made without approval from the FDA, and require no proof; thus, there are no guarantees that any benefits identified in structure–function claims are true about that particular food.

RECAP

The ability to read and interpret food labels is important for designing and maintaining a healthful diet. Food labels must list the identity of the food, the net contents of the package, the contact information for the food manufacturer or distributor, the ingredients in the food, and a Nutrition Facts panel providing information about Calories, certain nutrients, and fiber. Food labels may also contain claims related to nutrients, health, and body structure and function.

processed foods Includes foods that are fortified, enriched, or enhanced, such as orange juice with added calcium and vitamin D, or bread enriched with folate.

*Nutri-*Case

Gustavo

"Until last night, I hadn't stepped inside of a grocery store for 10 years, maybe more. But then my wife fell and broke her hip and had to go to the hospital. On my way home from visiting her, I remembered that we didn't have much food in the house, so I thought I'd do a little shopping. Was I ever in for a shock. I don't know how my wife does it, choosing between all the different brands, reading those long labels. She never went to school past sixth grade, and she doesn't speak English very well, either! I bought a frozen chicken pie for my dinner, but it didn't taste right. So I got the package out of the trash and read the label on the back, and that's when I realized there wasn't any chicken in it at all! It was made out of tofu! This afternoon, my daughter is picking me up, and we're going to do our grocery shopping together!"

Given what you've learned about FDA food labels, what parts of a food package should Gustavo read before he makes a choice? What else can he do to make his grocery shopping easier? Imagine that, like Gustavo's wife, you have only limited skills in mathematics and reading. In that case, what other strategies might you use when shopping for nutritious foods?

 LO 4 Explain the concept of nutrient density and identify a variety of nutrient-dense foods.

LO 5 Discuss five key messages of the *Dietary Guidelines*, including choices to make more often and choices to limit.

How Do the *Dietary Guidelines for Americans* Promote a Healthful Diet?

The ***Dietary Guidelines for Americans*** are a set of principles developed by the USDA and the U.S. Department of Health and Human Services (HHS) to promote health, reduce the risk for chronic diseases, and reduce the prevalence of overweight and obesity among Americans through improved nutrition and physical activity.[3] They are updated approximately every 5 years, and the current Guidelines can be found at http://health.gov/dietaryguidelines/2015. The 2015 Guidelines incorporate five recommendations focused on the development of healthful eating patterns in people 2 years of age and older. These key recommendations are:

1. Follow a healthful eating pattern across the lifespan.
2. Focus on variety, nutrient density, and amount.
3. Limit Calories from added sugars and saturated fats and reduce sodium intake.
4. Shift to healthier food and beverage choices.
5. Support healthful eating patterns for all.

Eat Healthfully at Every Life Stage

The 2015 Guidelines are based on the idea that that a healthful eating pattern is an adaptable framework that allows individuals to enjoy foods that are appealing and health-promoting in light of their age, developmental status, health requirements, and personal, cultural, and traditional preferences. All food and beverage choices matter because they have an impact on overall health. The goal is to choose a healthful eating pattern at an appropriate Calorie level to help achieve and maintain an optimal body weight, support nutrient adequacy, and reduce the risk of chronic disease.

These Guidelines promote the physical activity recommendations included in the *2008 Physical Activity Guidelines for Americans*, which are discussed in more detail in Chapter 14. Briefly, they emphasize a minimum of doing the equivalent of 150 minutes of moderate intensity activity each week.

Focus on Variety and Nutrient Density

An important strategy for balancing your Calories is to consistently choose **nutrient-dense foods** and beverages—that is, foods and beverages that supply the highest level of nutrients for the least amount of Calories (energy). **Meal Focus Figure 2.4** compares 1 day of meals

Dietary Guidelines for Americans A set of principles developed by the U.S. Department of Agriculture and the U.S. Department of Health and Human Services to assist Americans in designing a healthful diet and lifestyle.

nutrient-dense foods Foods that provide the highest level of nutrients for the least amount of energy (Calories).

a day of meals

low NUTRIENT DENSITY	high NUTRIENT DENSITY

BREAKFAST

low NUTRIENT DENSITY

1 cup puffed rice cereal with
½ cup whole milk
1 slice white toast with
1 tsp. butter
6 fl. oz grape drink

high NUTRIENT DENSITY

1 cup cooked oatmeal with
½ cup skim milk
1 slice whole-wheat toast with
1 tsp. butter
6 fl. oz grapefruit juice

LUNCH

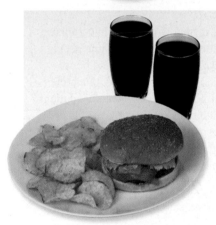

Cheeseburger

3 oz regular ground beef
1.5 oz cheddar cheese
1 white hamburger bun
2 tsp. Dijon mustard
2 leaves iceberg lettuce
1 snack-sized bag potato chips
32 fl. oz cola soft drink

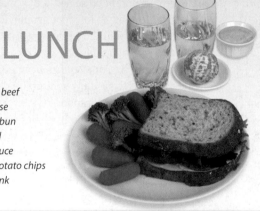

Turkey sandwich

3 oz turkey breast
2 slices whole-grain bread
2 tsp. Dijon mustard
3 slices fresh tomato
2 leaves red leaf lettuce
1 cup baby carrots with
broccoli crowns
20 fl. oz (2.5 cups) water
1 peeled orange
1 cup nonfat yogurt

DINNER

Green salad

1 cup iceberg lettuce
¼ cup diced tomatoes
1 tsp. green onions
¼ cup bacon bits
1 tbsp. regular Ranch salad dressing
3 oz beef round steak, breaded and fried
½ cup cooked white rice
½ cup sweet corn
8 fl. oz (1 cup) iced tea
3 chocolate sandwich cookies
1 12-oz can diet soft drink
10 Gummi Bears candy

Spinach salad

1 cup fresh spinach leaves
¼ cup sliced tomatoes
¼ cup diced green pepper
½ cup kidney beans
1 tbsp. fat-free Italian salad dressing
3 oz broiled chicken breast
½ cup cooked brown rice
½ cup steamed broccoli
8 fl. oz (1 cup) skim milk
1-1/2 cup mixed berries

nutrient analysis

3,319 kcal
11.4% of energy from saturated fat
11.6 grams of dietary fiber
3,031 milligrams of sodium
83 milligrams of vitamin C
18.2 milligrams of iron
825 milligrams of calcium

Provides
more
nutrients
and fewer
calories!

nutrient analysis

1,753 kcal
3% of energy from saturated fat
53.1 grams of dietary fiber
2,231 milligrams of sodium
372 milligrams of vitamin C
15.2 milligrams of iron
1,469 milligrams of calcium

that are high in **nutrient density** to meals that are low in nutrient density. As you can see in this figure, skim milk is more nutrient dense than whole milk, and a peeled orange is more nutrient dense than a soft drink. This example can help you select the most nutrient-dense foods when planning your meals.

Another tool for selecting nutrient-dense foods is in your supermarket! Have you ever wondered why there are numbers or stars on the shelf labels under everything from produce to canned goods? They are there to help shoppers make more healthful choices. Higher numbers or more stars indicate foods with a higher nutrient density. For example, in one system, kale gets the highest possible numerical score, whereas a can of spaghetti and meatballs scores near the bottom. Although a few nutritional guidance systems are in use in U.S. supermarkets, by far the most common is the NuVal system.

> Learn more about the NuVal system at www.nuval.com.

Limit Sodium, Fat, Sugars, and Alcohol

The *Dietary Guidelines* suggest that we reduce our consumption of the following foods and food components. Doing so will help us maintain a healthy weight and lower our risk for chronic diseases.

Sodium

Excessive consumption of sodium, a major mineral found in salt, is linked to hypertension (high blood pressure) in some people. Eating a lot of sodium also can cause some people to lose calcium from their bones, which can increase their risk for bone loss and bone fractures. Although table salt contains sodium and the major mineral chloride, much of the sodium we consume comes from processed and prepared foods. Key recommendations include keeping your daily sodium intake below 2,300 milligrams (mg) per day. This is the amount in just 1 teaspoon of table salt! People with hypertension and other medical conditions may be advised by their physicians to reduce their sodium intake even further. Some ways to decrease your sodium intake include the following:

- Eat fresh, plain frozen, or canned vegetables without added salt.
- Limit your intake of processed meats, such as cured ham, sausage, bacon, and most canned meats.
- When shopping for canned or packaged foods, look for those with labels that say "low sodium."
- Add little or no salt to foods at the table.
- Limit your intake of salty condiments, such as ketchup, mustard, pickles, soy sauce, and olives.

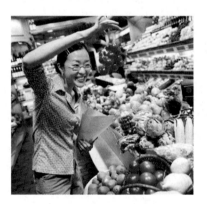

When grocery shopping, try to select foods that are moderate in total fat, sugar, and salt.

Fat

Fat is an essential nutrient and therefore an important part of a healthful diet; however, because fats are energy dense, eating a diet high in total fat can lead to overweight and obesity. In addition, eating a diet high in cholesterol and saturated fat (a type of fat abundant in meats and other animal-based foods) is linked to an increased risk for heart disease. For these reasons, less than 10% of your total daily Calories should come from saturated fat, and *trans* fats should be avoided as much as possible. You can achieve this goal by replacing solid fats, such as butter and lard, with vegetable oils, as well as by eating meat less often and fish or vegetarian meals more often. Finally, replace full-fat milk, yogurt, and cheeses with low-fat or nonfat versions.

Sugars

Limit foods and beverages that are high in added sugars, such as sweetened soft drinks and fruit drinks, cookies, and cakes. Added sugars should make up less than 10% of your daily Calories. High-sugar foods contribute to overweight and obesity, and they promote tooth decay. Moreover, doughnuts, cookies, cakes, pies, and other pastries are typically made with unhealthful fats and are high in sodium.

nutrient density The relative amount of nutrients per amount of energy (number of Calories).

Alcohol

Alcohol provides energy, but not nutrients. In the body, it depresses the nervous system and is toxic to liver and other body cells. Drinking alcoholic beverages in excess can lead to serious health and social problems; therefore, those who choose to drink are encouraged to do so sensibly and in moderation: no more than one drink per day for women and no more than two drinks per day for men, and only by adults of legal drinking age. Adults who should not drink alcohol are those who cannot restrict their intake, women of childbearing age who may become pregnant, pregnant and lactating women, individuals taking medications that can interact with alcohol, people with certain medical conditions, and people who are engaging in activities that require attention, skill, or coordination.

Consume More Healthful Foods and Nutrients

Another goal of the *Dietary Guidelines* is to encourage people to increase their consumption of healthful foods rich in nutrients, while keeping their Calorie intake within their daily energy needs. Key recommendations for achieving this goal include the following:

- Increase your intake of fruits and vegetables. Each day, try to eat a variety of vegetables from all subgroups, including dark green, red and orange, legumes (beans and peas), starchy, and others.
- Make sure that at least half of all grain foods—such as breads, cereals, pasta, and rice—that you eat each day are made from whole grains.
- If dairy is tolerated, choose fat-free or low-fat milk and milk products, which include milk, yogurt, cheese, and fortified soy beverages.
- When making protein choices, choose protein foods that are lower in solid fat and Calories, such as lean cuts of beef or skinless poultry. Try to eat more fish and shellfish in place of traditional meat and poultry choices. Also choose eggs, beans and peas, soy products, and unsalted nuts and seeds.
- Choose foods that provide an adequate level of dietary fiber as well as nutrients of concern in the American diet, including potassium, calcium, and vitamin D. These nutrients help us maintain healthy blood pressure and reduce our risks for certain diseases. Healthful foods that are good sources of these nutrients include fruits, vegetables, beans and peas, whole grains, and low-fat milk and milk products.

Follow Healthful Eating Patterns

There is no one healthful eating pattern that everyone should follow. Instead, the recommendations made in the *Dietary Guidelines* are designed to accommodate diverse cultural, ethnic, traditional, and personal preferences and to fit within different individuals' food budgets. The Guidelines offer several flexible templates, including the U.S.-Style, Mediterranean-Style, and Vegetarian-Style eating patterns.

Building a healthful eating pattern also involves following food safety recommendations to reduce your risk for foodborne illnesses, such as those caused by microorganisms and their toxins. The four food-safety principles emphasized in the *Dietary Guidelines* are:

- *Clean* your hands, food contact surfaces, and vegetables and fruits.
- *Separate* raw, cooked, and ready-to-eat foods while shopping, storing, and preparing foods.
- *Cook* foods to a safe temperature.
- *Chill* (refrigerate) perishable foods promptly.

Table 2.3 provides examples of how you can change your current diet and physical activity habits to meet some of the recommendations in the *Dietary Guidelines*.

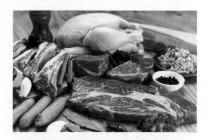

Another important tip is to avoid unpasteurized juices and milk products; raw or undercooked meats, seafood, poultry, and eggs; and raw sprouts.

TABLE 2.3 Ways to Incorporate the *Dietary Guidelines for Americans* into Your Daily Life

If You Normally Do This:	Try Doing This Instead:
Watch television when you get home at night.	Do 30 minutes of stretching or lifting of hand weights in front of the television.
Drive to the store down the block.	Walk to and from the store.
Go out to lunch with friends.	Take a 15- or 30-minute walk with your friends at lunchtime 3 days each week.
Eat white bread with your sandwich.	Eat whole-wheat bread or some other bread made from whole grains.
Eat white rice or fried rice with your meal.	Eat brown rice or try wild rice.
Choose cookies or a candy bar for a snack.	Choose a fresh nectarine, peach, apple, orange, or banana for a snack.
Order french fries with your hamburger.	Order a green salad with low-fat salad dressing on the side.
Spread butter or margarine on your white toast each morning.	Spread fresh fruit compote on whole-grain toast.
Order a bacon double cheeseburger at your favorite restaurant.	Order a turkey burger or grilled chicken sandwich without the cheese and bacon, and add lettuce and tomato.
Drink nondiet soft drinks to quench your thirst.	Drink iced tea, ice water with a slice of lemon, seltzer water, or diet soft drinks.
Eat salted potato chips and pickles with your favorite sandwich.	Eat carrot slices and crowns of fresh broccoli and cauliflower dipped in low-fat or nonfat Ranch dressing.

RECAP

The goals of the *Dietary Guidelines for Americans* are to promote health, reduce the risk for chronic diseases, and reduce the prevalence of overweight and obesity among Americans. The five main messages are to eat healthfully across the lifespan; to focus on variety and nutrient density; to limit sodium, saturated fat, added sugars, and alcohol; to consume more healthful foods and nutrients; and to follow healthful eating patterns. ■

 LO 6 Identify the five food groups included in the USDA Food Patterns and the key message for each group.

LO 7 Compare MyPlate to the Mediterranean diet.

LO 8 Define *empty* Calories and discuss the role that empty Calories and serving size play in designing a healthful diet.

LO 9 Discuss several ways that technology can help you design and maintain a healthful diet.

How Can the USDA Food Patterns Help You Design a Healthful Diet?

The USDA Food Patterns were developed to help Americans incorporate the *Dietary Guidelines* into their everyday lives. They identify daily amounts of foods, and nutrient-dense choices, to eat from the five major food groups and their subgroups. The food groups emphasized in the USDA Food Patterns are grains, vegetables, fruits, dairy, and protein foods. The food groups are represented in the plate graphic with segments of five different colors. **Figure 2.5** illustrates each of these food groups and provides detailed information on the nutrients they provide and recommended servings each day.

MyPlate Incorporates Many of the Features of the Mediterranean Diet

MyPlate is both the visual representation of the USDA Food Patterns and an interactive, personalized guide to diet and physical activity (**Figure 2.6**, page 56). You can access MyPlate on the Internet to assess your current diet and physical activity level and to plan appropriate changes. MyPlate and its accompanying website help Americans:

- Eat in moderation to balance Calories.
- Eat a variety of foods.
- Consume the right proportion of each recommended food group.

MyPlate The visual representation of the USDA Food Patterns.

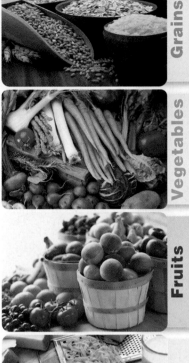

Grains

Make half your grains whole. At least half of the grains you eat each day should come from whole-grain sources.

Eat at least 6 oz of whole-grain bread, cereal, crackers, rice, or pasta every day.

Whole-grain foods provide fiber-rich carbohydrates, riboflavin, thiamin, niacin, iron, folate, zinc, protein, and magnesium.

Vegetables

Vary your veggies. Eat a variety of vegetables and increase consumption of dark-green and orange vegetables, as well as dry beans and peas.

Eat at least 2½ cups of vegetables each day.

Vegetables provide fiber and phytochemicals, carbohydrates, vitamins A and C, folate, potassium, and magnesium.

Fruits

Focus on fruits. Eat a greater variety of fruits (fresh, frozen, or dried) and go easy on the fruit juices.

Eat at least 2 cups of fruit every day.

Fruits provide fiber, phytochemicals, vitamins A and C, folate, potassium, and magnesium.

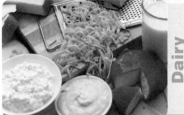

Dairy

Get your calcium-rich foods. Choose low-fat or fat-free dairy products, such as milk, yogurt, and cheese. People who can't consume dairy foods can choose lactose-free dairy products or other sources, such as calcium-fortified juices and soy and rice beverages.

Get 3 cups of low-fat dairy foods, or the equivalent, every day.

Dairy foods provide calcium, phosphorus, riboflavin, protein, and vitamin B_{12} and are often fortified with vitamins D and A.

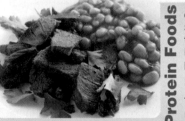

Protein Foods

Go lean with protein. Choose low-fat or lean meats and poultry. Switch to baking, broiling, or grilling more often, and vary your choices to include more fish, processed soy products, beans, nuts, and seeds. Legumes, including beans, peas, and lentils, are included in both the protein and the vegetable groups.

Eat about 5½ oz of lean protein foods each day.

These foods provide protein, phosphorus, vitamin B_6, vitamin B_{12}, magnesium, iron, zinc, niacin, riboflavin, and thiamin.

FIGURE 2.5 Food groups of the USDA Food Patterns.

- Personalize their eating plan.
- Increase their physical activity.
- Set goals for gradually improving their food choices and lifestyle.

MyPlate incorporates many features of the Mediterranean diet, which has been associated with a reduced risk for cardiovascular disease. There is actually not a single Mediterranean diet because the Mediterranean region includes Portugal, Spain, Italy, France, Greece, Turkey, and Israel. Each of these countries has different dietary patterns; however, there are many similarities. Aspects of the diet seen as more healthy than the typical U.S. diet include the following:

- Red meat is eaten only monthly, and eggs, poultry, fish, and sweets are eaten weekly, making the diet low in saturated fats and refined sugars.
- The primary fat used for cooking and flavor is olive oil, making the diet higher in monounsaturated fats and lower in saturated fats.

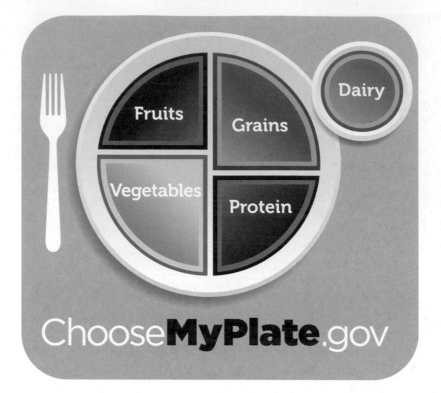

FIGURE 2.6 The USDA MyPlate graphic is an interactive food guidance system based on the *Dietary Guidelines for Americans* and the Dietary Reference Intakes from the National Academy of Sciences. Eating more fruits, vegetables, and whole grains and choosing foods low in fat, sugar, and sodium from the five food groups in MyPlate will help you balance your Calories and consume a healthier overall diet. (*Data from:* MyPlate graphic, U.S. Department of Agriculture.)

- Foods eaten daily include grains, such as bread, pasta, couscous, and bulgur; fruits; beans and other legumes; nuts; vegetables; and cheese and yogurt. These choices make this diet high in vitamins and minerals, fiber, beneficial plant chemicals called phytochemicals, and probiotics and prebiotics (discussed in Chapter 3).
- Wine is included, in moderation.

As you'll discover, MyPlate does not make specific recommendations for protein food choices. In contrast, the Mediterranean diet recommends beans, other legumes, and nuts as daily sources of protein; fish, poultry, and eggs weekly; and red meat only about once each month. Also, for dairy choices, the Mediterranean diet recommends cheese and yogurt in moderation and suggests drinking water or wine (in moderation) rather than milk. As you can see in **Figure 2.7**, it is easy to create a healthy Mediterranean-style eating plan using the principles of MyPlate.

Limit Empty Calories

One concept emphasized in the USDA Food Patterns is that of **empty Calories.** These are Calories from solid fats and/or added sugars that provide few or no nutrients. The USDA recommends that you limit the empty Calories you eat. Foods that contain the greatest amount of empty Calories include cakes, cookies, pastries, doughnuts, soft drinks, fruit drinks, cheese, pizza, ice cream, sausages, hot dogs, bacon, and ribs. High-sugar foods, such as candies, desserts, gelatin, soft drinks, and alcoholic beverages, are called *empty Calorie foods*. However, a few foods that contain empty Calories from solid fats and added sugars also provide important nutrients. Examples are sweetened applesauce, sweetened breakfast cereals, regular ground beef, and whole

empty Calories Calories from solid fats and/or added sugars that provide few or no nutrients.

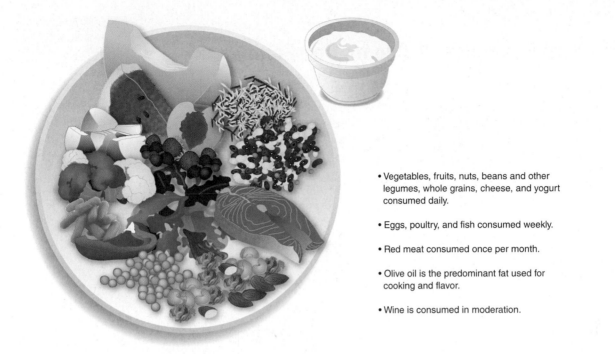

- Vegetables, fruits, nuts, beans and other legumes, whole grains, cheese, and yogurt consumed daily.

- Eggs, poultry, and fish consumed weekly.

- Red meat consumed once per month.

- Olive oil is the predominant fat used for cooking and flavor.

- Wine is consumed in moderation.

FIGURE 2.7 MyPlate can be easily used to design a Mediterranean-style eating plan.

milk. To reduce your intake of empty Calories but ensure you get adequate nutrients, choose the unsweetened, lean, or nonfat versions of these foods.

Watch Your Serving Size

The USDA Food Patterns also helps you decide *how much* of each food you should eat. The number of servings is based on your age, gender, and activity level. A term used when defining serving sizes that may be new to you is **ounce-equivalent (oz-equivalent).** It is defined as a serving size that is 1 ounce, or that is equivalent to an ounce, for the grains and meats and beans sections. For instance, both a slice of bread and ½ cup of cooked brown rice qualify as ounce-equivalents.

What is considered a serving size for the foods recommended in the USDA Food Patterns? **Figure 2.8** (page 258) identifies the number of cups or oz-equivalent servings recommended for a 2,000-Calorie diet and gives examples of amounts equal to 1 cup or 1 oz-equivalent for foods in each group. As you study this figure, notice the variety of examples for each group. For instance, an oz-equivalent serving from the grains group can mean one slice of bread or two small pancakes. Because of their low density, 2 cups of raw, leafy vegetables, such as spinach, actually constitute a 1-cup serving from the vegetables group. Although an oz-equivalent serving of meat is actually 1 oz, ½ oz of nuts also qualifies. One egg, 1 tablespoon of peanut butter, and ¼ cup cooked legumes are also each considered 1 oz-equivalents from the protein group. Although it may seem inconvenient to measure food servings, understanding the size of a serving is crucial to planning a nutritious diet.

Using the USDA Food Patterns (and their visual representation, MyPlate) does have some challenges. For example, no nationally standardized definition for a serving size

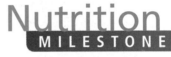

Nutrition
MILESTONE

Did you know that in the United States food guides in one form or another have been around for over 125 years? That's right! Back in 1885, a college chemistry professor named Wilber Olin Atwater helped bring the fledging science of nutrition to a broader audience by introducing scientific data boxes that became the basis for the first known U.S. food guide. Those early dietary standards focused on defining the nutrition needs of an "average man" in terms of his daily consumption of proteins and Calories. These became food composition tables defined in three sweeping categories: protein, fats, and carbohydrate; mineral matter; and fuel values. As early as 1902, Atwater advocated for three foundational nutritional principles that we still support today; the concepts of variety, proportionality, and moderation in food choices and eating. (Check out the Study Area of MasteringNutrition for related information on the development of the USDA Food Guide.)

ounce-equivalent (oz-equivalent) A serving size that is 1 ounce, or equivalent to an ounce, for the grains and the protein foods sections of MyPlate.

Serving Size Examples: 1 Cup or 1 oz-Equivalent

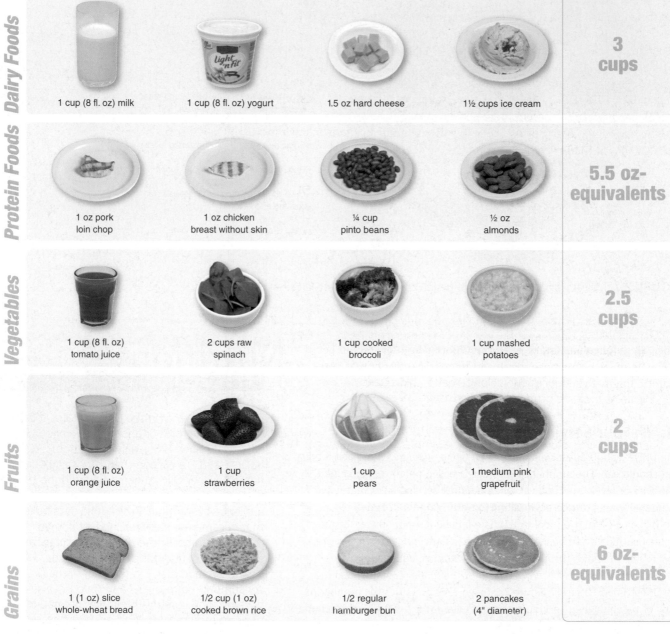

				Recommended Serving for 2,000 kcal/day
Dairy Foods	1 cup (8 fl. oz) milk	1 cup (8 fl. oz) yogurt	1.5 oz hard cheese	1½ cups ice cream	**3 cups**
Protein Foods	1 oz pork loin chop	1 oz chicken breast without skin	¼ cup pinto beans	½ oz almonds	**5.5 oz-equivalents**
Vegetables	1 cup (8 fl. oz) tomato juice	2 cups raw spinach	1 cup cooked broccoli	1 cup mashed potatoes	**2.5 cups**
Fruits	1 cup (8 fl. oz) orange juice	1 cup strawberries	1 cup pears	1 medium pink grapefruit	**2 cups**
Grains	1 (1 oz) slice whole-wheat bread	1/2 cup (1 oz) cooked brown rice	1/2 regular hamburger bun	2 pancakes (4" diameter)	**6 oz-equivalents**

FIGURE 2.8 Examples of serving sizes in each food group of MyPlate for a 2,000-kcal food intake pattern. You can use the following visualizations of common household objects to help you estimate serving sizes: 1.5 oz of hard cheese is equal to four stacked dice, 3 oz of meat is equal in size to a deck of cards, and one-half of a regular hamburger bun is the size of a yo-yo.

exists for any food. Thus, a serving size as defined in the USDA Food Patterns may not be equal to a serving size identified on a food label. For instance, the serving size for crackers suggested in the USDA Food Patterns is three to four small crackers, whereas a serving size for crackers on a food label can range from five to 18 crackers, depending on the size and weight of the cracker.

Also, for food items consumed individually—such as muffins, frozen burgers, and bottled juices—the serving sizes in the USDA Food Patterns are typically much smaller than the items we actually buy and eat. In addition, serving sizes in restaurants, cafés, and movie theaters have grown substantially over the past 30 years (**Figure 2.9**). This "super-sizing" phenomenon, now widespread, indicates a major shift in accepted eating behaviors and is an important contributor to the rise in obesity rates around the world. For over 10 years it has been recognized[4] that the discrepancy between USDA serving size standards and the portion size of many common foods sold outside the home is staggering— chocolate chip cookies have been reported as seven times larger than USDA standards, a serving of cooked pasta in a restaurant can be almost five times larger, and steaks are more than twice as large.[5] Thus, when using diet-planning tools, such as the USDA Food Patterns, learn the definition of a serving size for the tool you're using and *then* measure your food intake to determine whether you are meeting the guidelines. If you don't want to gain weight, it's important to become informed about portion size.

How much physical activity do you think you'd need to perform in order to burn off the extra Calories in a larger portion size? Try the ***You Do the Math*** and find out.

How Much Exercise Is Needed to Combat Increasing Food Portion Sizes?

Although the causes of obesity are complex and multifactorial, it is speculated that one reason obesity rates are rising globally is due to a combination of increased energy intake, reflecting expanding food portion sizes, and reduced overall daily physical activity. This math activity should help you better understand how portion sizes have increased over the past 20 years and how much physical activity you would need to do to expend the excess energy resulting from these larger portion sizes.

The two set of photos in **Figure 2.9** give examples of foods whose portion sizes have increased substantially. A bagel 20 years ago had a diameter of approximately 3 inches and contained 140 kcal. A bagel today is about 6 inches in diameter and contains 350 kcal. Similarly, a cup of coffee 20 years ago was 8 fl. oz and was typically served with a small amount of whole milk and sugar. It contained about 45 kcal. A standard coffee mocha commonly consumed today is 16 fl. oz and contains 350 kcal; this excess energy comes from the addition of a sweet flavored syrup and whole milk.

On her morning break at work, Judy routinely consumes a bagel and a coffee mocha. Judy has type 2 diabetes, and her doctor has advised her to lose weight. How much physical activity would Judy need to do to "burn" this excess energy? Let's do some simple math to answer this question.

1. Calculate the excess energy Judy consumes from both of these foods:

   a. Bagel: 350 kcal in larger bagel − 140 kcal in smaller bagel = 210 kcal extra

   b. Coffee: 350 kcal in large coffee mocha − 45 kcal in small regular coffee = 305 kcal extra

   Total excess energy for these two larger portions = 515 kcal

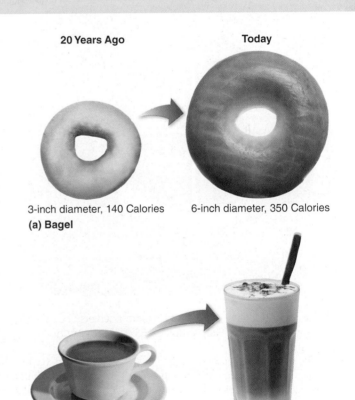

20 Years Ago   **Today**

3-inch diameter, 140 Calories   6-inch diameter, 350 Calories
(a) Bagel

8 fluid ounces, 45 Calories   16 fluid ounces, 350 Calories
(b) Coffee

FIGURE 2.9 Examples of increases in food portion sizes over the past 30 years. (a) A bagel has increased in diameter from 3 inches to 6 inches; (b) a cup of coffee has increased from 8 fl. oz to 16 fl. oz and now commonly contains Calorie-dense flavored syrup as well as steamed whole milk.

2. Judy has started walking each day in an effort to lose weight. Judy currently weighs 200 lb. Based on her relatively low fitness level, Judy walks at a slow pace (approximately 2 miles per hour); it is estimated that walking at this pace expends 1.2 kcal per pound of body weight per hour. How long does Judy need to walk each day to expend 515 kcal?

a. First, calculate how much energy Judy expends if she walks for a full hour by multiplying her body weight by the energy cost of walking per hour = 1.2 kcal/lb body weight × 200 lb = 240 kcal.

b. Next, you need to calculate how much energy she expends each minute she walks by dividing the energy cost of walking per hour by 60 minutes = 240 kcal/hour ÷ 60 minutes/hour = 4 kcal/minute.

c. To determine how many minutes she would need to walk to expend 515 kcal, divide the total amount of energy she needs to expend by the energy cost of

walking per minute = 515 kcal ÷ 4 kcal/minute = 128.75 minutes.

Thus, Judy would need to walk for approximately 104 minutes, or about 1 hour and 45 minutes, to expend the excess energy she consumes by eating the larger bagel and coffee. If she wanted to burn off all of the energy in her morning snack, she would have to walk even longer, especially if she enjoyed her bagel with cream cheese!

Now use your own weight in these calculations to determine how much walking you would have to do if you consumed the same foods:

a. 1.2 kcal/lb × (your weight in pounds) = _____ kcal/hour (If you walk at a brisk pace, use 2.4 kcal/lb.)

b. _____ kcal/hour ÷ 60 minutes/hour = _____ kcal/minute

c. 515 extra kcal in bagel and coffee ÷ _____ kcal/minute = _____ minutes

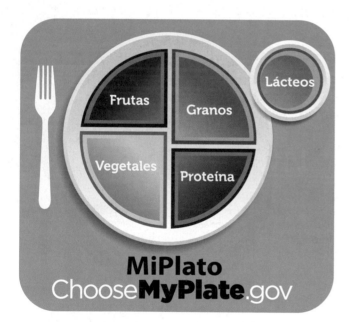

FIGURE 2.10 MiPlato is the Spanish language version of MyPlate. (Data from: MiPlato graphic, U.S. Department of Agriculture.)

Despite their efforts to improve their nutrition and physical activity recommendations for Americans, the USDA and HHS have met with some criticism for the *Dietary Guidelines for Americans* and the MyPlate graphic. Refer to the **Nutrition Myth or Fact?** essay at the end of this chapter to learn more about this controversy.

Consider Ethnic Variations and Other Eating Plans

As you know, the population of the United States is culturally and ethnically diverse, and this diversity influences our food choices. **Figure 2.10** is a Spanish-language version of MyPlate. Like the English-language version, it recommends food groups, not specific food choices. As we illustrated with the Mediterranean Diet, MyPlate easily accommodates foods that we may consider part of an ethnic diet. You can also easily incorporate into MyPlate foods that match a vegetarian diet or other lifestyle preferences.

Another eating plan you can use to design a healthful diet is the DASH diet, which stands for "Dietary Approaches to Stop Hypertension." This low-sodium diet is similar to MyPlate and the Mediterranean Diet in its emphasis on fruits, vegetables, and whole grains. The DASH diet plan is discussed in more detail in Chapter 9.

The **exchange system** is another tool that can be used to plan a healthful diet. This system was originally designed for people with diabetes by the American Dietetic Association (now known as the Academy of Nutrition and Dietetics) and the American Diabetes Association. It has also been used successfully in weight-loss programs. Exchanges, or portions, are organized according to the amount of carbohydrate, protein, fat, and Calories in each food. There are six food groups, or exchange lists, and these lists contain foods that are similar in Calories, carbohydrate, fat, and protein content. The six exchange lists are starch/bread, meat and meat substitutes, vegetables, fruits, milk, and fat. In

---

addition to these lists, there are other categories that can assist you in meal planning, including free foods (any food or drink less than 20 Calories per serving), combination foods (foods such as soups, casseroles, and pizza), and special-occasion foods (desserts such as cakes, cookies, and ice cream). Refer the **Web Links** at the end of this chapter for more details about exchange lists for meal planning.

Get Some High-Tech Help

You've learned how to design a healthful diet by reading food labels and following the *Dietary Guidelines for Americans* and the USDA Food Patterns. Here, we provide an overview of tools that can help you analyze your diet and determine the nutrient content of foods with or without labels.

Many diet analysis programs are available to help you evaluate the quality of your diet. One example of a web-based tool available to the public is MyPlate Supertracker (see the **Web Links** at the end of this chapter). This tool allows you to analyze your current dietary intake and physical activity and to create personalized healthy eating and physical activity plans. It also provides access to information on the nutrient content of over 8,000 foods as well as tips to support you in making healthier choices. Using MyPlate Supertracker, you can track your current food intake and physical activity and compare it to targets you've set.

Students using this textbook also have access to MyDietAnalysis, a diet analysis software package developed by the nutrition database experts at ESHA Research. MyDietAnalysis is tailored for use in college nutrition courses, and it features a database of nearly 20,000 foods and multiple report options. This program is accurate, reliable, and easy-to-use in calculating the quality of your dietary intake.

In addition, anyone can access the USDAs Nutrient Database for Standard Reference to find nutrient information on over 8,000 foods (see **Web Links** at the end of this chapter). You can also search on a specific nutrient (for instance, iron) to find out how much of that nutrient is present in a vast number of foods. The database even provides information on components of foods that are not classified as essential nutrients and are thus not typically included in diet analysis programs. These include, for example, caffeine, certain phytochemicals, and binders like oxalic acid that can inhibit nutrient absorption. The USDA's Nutrient Database is updated annually, and any errors are identified, corrected, and highlighted for users.

Now even your cell phone can help you to eat more healthfully! Numerous apps are now available to help people plan and keep track of healthy dietary changes. Some have you scan a barcode to get a broad nutritional profile of the food. Others help you track Calories or food additives, or to create a healthful shopping list or meal plans. Some send you a daily nutrition tip. What's more, many of these apps are free—as long as you don't mind putting up with the on-screen ads.

> To find reviews of more than two dozen nutrition-related apps, visit the Academy of Nutrition and Dietetics at www .eatrightpro.org. In the search bar, type "App reviews."

RECAP

The USDA Food Patterns can be used to plan a healthful, balanced diet that includes foods from the grains group, vegetables group, fruits group, dairy group, and protein foods group. The MyPlate graphic and website incorporates aspects of the Mediterranean diet. To follow the USDA Food Patterns successfully, it's important to limit your consumption of empty Calories and monitor your portion sizes. DASH diet and the exchange system are two examples of healthful food plans. The exchange system was originally designed for people with diabetes. Exchanges, or portions, are organized according to the amount of carbohydrate, protein, fat, and Calories in each food. Various dietary analysis software packages and apps for smartphones and other mobile devices are high-tech ways to design and maintain a healthy diet.

LO 10 List at least four ways to practice moderation and apply healthful dietary guidelines when eating out.

From 2016, nutritional labeling is required in chain restaurants and other food retail outlets, including Calorie information for standard menu items.

Can Eating Out Be Part of a Healthful Diet?

How many times each week do you eat out? Data from the USDA indicate that buying foods away from home now accounts for about half of all food expenditures,[6] and U.S. consumers eat away from home an average of almost five times per week.[7] Full-service restaurants and fast-food outlets are the most common sources of foods eaten away from home. Given that almost 35% of all adults in the United States are classified as obese,[1] it is imperative that we learn how to eat more healthfully when eating out.

The Hidden Costs of Eating Out

Table 2.4 compares foods served at McDonald's and Burger King restaurants. As you can see, a regular McDonald's hamburger has only 240 kcal, whereas the Big Mac has 530 kcal. A meal of a Big Mac, large french fries, and a small McCafé Chocolate Shake provides 1,600 kcal. This meal has enough energy to support an entire day's needs for a small, lightly active woman! Similar meals at Burger King and other fast-food chains are also very high in Calories, not to mention total fat and sodium.

Fast-food restaurants are not alone in serving large portions. Most sit-down restaurants also serve large meals, which may include bread with butter, a salad with dressing, sides of vegetables and potatoes, and free refills of sugar-filled drinks. Combined with a high-fat appetizer like potato skins, fried onions, fried mozzarella sticks, or buffalo wings, it is easy to eat more than 2,000 kcal at one meal!

After years of lobbying by health and nutrition professionals, the U.S. FDA has agreed to require nutrition labeling in chain restaurants and many other retail food outlets beginning in 2016. Calorie information must be posted for standard menu items on menus and menu boards, along with a brief statement about suggested daily energy intake. Other nutrient information, such as calories from fat, sodium content, and so forth must be made available in writing upon request.

TABLE 2.4 Nutritional Value of Selected Fast Foods

Menu Item	Kcal	Fat (g)	Fat (% kcal)	Sodium (mg)
McDonald's				
Hamburger	240	8	30	480
Cheeseburger	290	11	34	680
Quarter Pounder with cheese	520	26	45	1,110
Big Mac	530	27	46	960
French fries, small	230	11	43	130
French fries, medium	340	16	42	190
French fries, large	510	24	42	290
Coke, large	280	0	0	5
McCafé Chocolate Shake (small)	560	16	26	240
McCafé Chocolate Shake (large)	850	23	24	380
Burger King				
Hamburger	230	9	35	460
Cheeseburger	270	12	40	630
Whopper	650	37	51	910
Double Whopper	900	56	56	980
Bacon Double Cheeseburger	390	21	48	790
French fries, small	340	15	40	480
French fries, medium	410	18	40	570
French fries, large	500	22	40	710

A number of restaurant chains across the country have been printing nutrition information on their menus for several years, and some communities have taken the additional step of enforcing mandatory menu labeling in restaurants. Have these actions influenced Americans to make healthier food choices when eating out? Recent reviews of the research conducted in this area indicate that Calorie-labeling has not resulted in any consistent or substantive changes in food choices made by adults or children.[8,9] It also has not appeared to significantly increase the number of healthful menu options or reduce the Caloric-content of foods offered. Although some restaurants have reduced the Calories, fat, and sodium content of menu items, in most cases these foods still exceed the levels recommended for promoting health.

There is some evidence that providing contextual or interpretive information may affect Calorie consumption. For example, a study conducted in adolescents examined consumption of sugar-sweetened beverages. Researchers provided easy-to-understand information about Calories, number of teaspoons of sugar, and number of minutes that one would need to run or walk to expend the Calories in the beverage. Posting this information reduced the size and number of sugar-sweetened beverages that the adolescents purchased, and these changes persisted for 6 weeks after the signs were removed.[10]

The Healthful Way to Eat Out

With a little education, you can maintain a healthful diet and still enjoy eating out. Most restaurants, even fast-food restaurants, offer lower-fat menu items that you can choose. For instance, eating a regular McDonald's hamburger, a side salad, and a diet beverage or water provides 285 kcal and 9 g of fat (38.4% of kcal from fat). Adding their low-fat Balsamic salad dressing would add another 25 kcal and 1 g of fat. Other fast-food restaurants also offer smaller portions, sandwiches made with whole-grain bread, grilled chicken or other lean meats, and side salads. Many sit-down restaurants offer "lite" menu items, such as grilled chicken and a variety of vegetables, which are usually a much better choice than eating from the regular menu.

Check out the **_You Do the Math_** box (on page 64) for an example of how to make more healthful food choices when eating out. In addition, here are some other suggestions on how to eat out in moderation. Practice some of these suggestions every time you eat out:

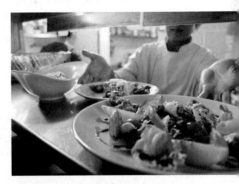

Eating out can be part of a healthful diet if you're careful to choose wisely.

- Avoid all-you-can-eat buffet-style restaurants.
- Avoid appetizers that are breaded, fried, or filled with cheese or meat, or skip the appetizer altogether.
- Order a healthful appetizer instead of a larger meal as your entrée.
- Order your meal from the children's menu.
- Share an entrée with a friend.
- Order broth-based soups instead of cream-based soups.
- If you order meat, select a lean cut and ask that it be grilled or broiled rather than fried or breaded.
- Instead of a beef burger, order a chicken burger, fish burger, or veggie burger.
- Order a meatless dish filled with vegetables and whole grains. Avoid dishes with cream sauces and a lot of cheese.
- Order a salad with low-fat or nonfat dressing served on the side.
- Order steamed vegetables on the side instead of potatoes or rice. If you order potatoes, make sure you get a baked potato (with very little butter or sour cream on the side).
- Order beverages with few or no Calories, such as water, tea, or diet drinks. Avoid coffee drinks made with syrups, as well as those made with cream, whipping cream, or whole milk.
- Don't feel you have to eat everything you're served. If you feel full, take the rest home for another meal.
- Skip dessert or share one dessert with a lot of friends, or order fresh fruit for dessert.
- Watch out for those "yogurt parfaits" offered at some fast-food restaurants. Many are loaded with sugar, fat, and Calories.

By following the suggestions in this list, you can eat out regularly and still maintain a healthful body weight.

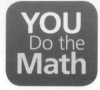

Determining the Healthiest Food Choices When Eating Out

Theo's friend and teammate, Jake, has put on extra weight over the basketball season. He had hoped to start more games this season, but their coach has made it clear that Jake needs to improve his fitness and lose the extra weight to be competitive as a starter.

Jake typically makes healthful food choices when he's on campus or at home, as he has a wide range of meals to choose from in the dining hall, and his family serves healthy foods when he visits them. But Jake really struggles to eat right when the team is on the road, as they typically frequent fast-food outlets or sit-down restaurants that serve meals high in Calories, saturated fat, and salt. Jake knows that Theo is taking a nutrition class and asks him for help in selecting healthier menu items when they are ordering their meals on the road. Theo is happy to help. Fortunately, the fast-food restaurant where they stop for dinner has posted at the counter the nutrition values (Calories, total fat [g and %Daily Value], saturated fat [g and %Daily Value], and sodium [g]) for their menu items. They agree that Jake should order a chicken sandwich, as Theo has learned that chicken has a much lower fat content than beef.

The menu items that Jake selected are:

fat, and sodium. As Theo examines these totals, he realizes that the %Daily Values for fat and saturated fat are based on a 2,000-Calorie-per-day intake—as Jake is a highly active male, this value is neither helpful nor appropriate. To determine the % of Calories from fat in the chicken sandwich, Theo does the following calculations:

a. Multiply the total fat (g) in the sandwich by 9 Calories (kcal)/g = 29 g × 9 Calories/g = 261 Calories from fat.

b. Divide the Calories from fat by the total Calories in the sandwich and multiply by 100 = (261 Calories ÷ 620 Calories) × 100 = 42% of total Calories comes from fat in the sandwich.

c. Multiply the saturated fat (g) in the sandwich by 9 Calories/g = 15 g × 9 Calories/g = 135 Calories from saturated fat.

d. Divide the Calories from saturated fat by total Calories in the sandwich = (135 Calories ÷ 620 Calories) = 21.8% of total Calories comes from saturated fat in the sandwich.

Menu Item	Calories	Total Fat (g)	Total Fat (%Daily Value)	Saturated Fat (g)	Saturated Fat (%Daily Value)	Sodium (g)
Chicken club sandwich	620	29	45%	15	37%	1,200
Large french fries	500	25	38%	3.5	17%	350
Ketchup (4 packets)	60	0	0%	0	0%	440
Side salad	20	0	0%	0	0%	10
Salad dressing (1 packet)	170	15	23%	2.5	12%	530
Total	1,370	69	Not applicable	21	Not applicable	2,530

Jake's goal is to select food items that are lower in total Calories, % of Calories from fat, % of Calories from saturated fat, and sodium. As Theo examines these totals, he realizes that the %Daily Values for fat and saturated

After thinking about these figures for % of Calories from fat and saturated fat, Jake decides to select a healthier sandwich that is lower in fat. He selects a grilled chicken club sandwich, at it has only 460 Calories, 16 g of fat, and 6 g of saturated fat.

Now you do the math to calculate the % total Calories from fat and % total Calories from saturated fat in the grilled chicken club sandwich.

What other changes could Jake make to his menu selections to reduce his total intake of Calories, fat, saturated fat, and sodium?

RECAP

Many restaurants serve very large portions of foods high in empty Calories. Healthful ways to eat out include choosing smaller menu items, ordering meats that are grilled or broiled, avoiding fried foods, choosing items with steamed vegetables, avoiding energy-rich appetizers and desserts, and eating less than half of the food you are served.

Nutrition Myth OR Fact?

Nutrition Advice from the U.S. Government: Is Anyone Listening?

The National Nutrition Monitoring and Related Research Act (1990) requires the federal government to publish a research-based report every 5 years to provide nutrition and dietary guidelines for the general public. The *2015-2020 Dietary Guidelines for Americans* were released in January 2016 by the U.S. Department of Health and Human Services (HHS) and the U.S. Department of Agriculture (USDA) to replace the 2010 Guidelines. They continue to be accompanied by the MyPlate graphic and website (www.chooseMyPlate.gov) that offer practical tools in support of the Guidelines. The Guidelines and tools were designed to be user-friendly to help people eat more healthfully, achieve an optimal body weight, and reduce their risk for chronic diseases.

But are the *Dietary Guidelines* based on scientific consensus? Do people actually consult them for meal-planning, shopping, or eating out? Moreover, is there any evidence that the Guidelines and MyPlate make a difference in improving the health of Americans?

To begin to answer these questions, let's review the changes made in revising the 2010 Guidelines into the 2015 version:[1]

- Instead of focusing solely on food groups and nutrients, the updated Guidelines recommend following a healthful eating pattern. They define an *eating pattern* as "the combination of food and beverages that constitute an individual's complete dietary intake over time." An eating pattern describes a person's customary way of eating or a combination of foods and beverages that are recommended for consumption.
- The Guidelines remind consumers that every food and beverage choice influences their health.
- The updated Guidelines advise limiting intake of added sugars to less than 10% of total daily energy intake.
- They also suggest consuming less than 10% of total energy from saturated fat. In recognition of the health benefits of unsaturated fats, the 2010 upper limit for total energy intake from fat is gone.
- The 2010 recommendation to limit dietary cholesterol intake to 300 mg per day is also gone; the recommendation now states that individuals should consume as little dietary cholesterol as possible.

Despite these updates, concerns are being expressed about the failure of the 2015-2020 Guidelines to include all of the recommendations put forth in the report of the Dietary Guidelines Advisory Committee, the committee that reviewed the current scientific evidence about the impact of diet on health. Two omissions of concern are:[1]

- A recommendation to reduce consumption of red and processed meat. This recommendation was made because of the association of red and processed meat intake with increased risk for cardiovascular disease and some cancers, as well as to support a more sustainable and secure food supply. (For more on the environmental costs of beef production, see Chapter 16.)

- A recommendation to reduce consumption of sugar-sweetened beverages. This recommendation reflects the association of high intake of sugar-sweetened beverages with increased risks for obesity and type 2 diabetes.

A further concern is the potential for conflicts of interest to arise within the USDA when developing the guidelines. Do industry groups such as the National Cattlemen's Beef Association and the American Beverage Association "purchase" recommendations—or limitations on recommendations—that favor their profits over public health? Experts have argued that, to protect their profit margin, large special interests from the food and agricultural industries exert undue influence over the Guidelines, and that this influence has prompted USDA officials to disregard or minimize scientific evidence related to the benefits or health risks of various foods.[1]

Two alternatives to MyPlate have been developed that address these concerns: the Harvard School of Public Health developed a Healthy Eating Plate (www.hsph.harvard.edu), and the Physicians Committee for Responsible Medicine has proposed the Sustainable Power Plate (www.pcrm.org).

The Healthy Eating Plate highlights using healthy oils and avoiding *trans* fat, consuming virtually all grains as whole grains, consuming more vegetables, selecting healthy protein sources from fish, poultry, beans and nuts, and drinking water, tea, or coffee with little or no added sugar. It also emphasizes daily physical activity. The Sustainable Power Plate illustrates a plant-based eating pattern that emphasizes fruits, vegetables, whole grains, and legumes.

Because the release of MyPlate and these alternatives has been so recent, no studies are yet available comparing their effectiveness in reducing risks for obesity and related chronic diseases.

No matter what the strengths and limitations of the *Dietary Guidelines* and MyPlate might be, a bigger question arises—is anyone listening? Research examining this question in the context

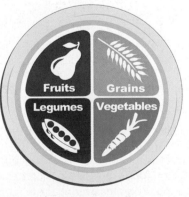

The Sustainable Power Plate

The Sustainable Power Plate was developed by the Physicians Committee for Responsible Medicine as an alternative to MyPlate.

of the 2005 Guidelines found that less than half of Americans 16 years of age and older had even heard of them.[2] A more recent study exploring this question after the publication of the 2010 Guidelines and MyPlate (2011) found that, despite media coverage, awareness of these tools was less than 25% in those sampled, including only about 6% in college students![3].

The goal of the *Dietary Guidelines* and MyPlate is to help reduce the alarmingly high obesity and chronic disease rates in the United States. A primary assumption is that people will use these tools to design their diets. However, the evidence currently available suggests that only a small percentage of the population is even aware of them. Clearly, more research is needed to determine whether Americans make an attempt to follow the recommendations, and if so, whether these changes have a positive impact on public health. Until more evidence of their impact is gathered and assessed, the debate about their value will continue.

Critical Thinking Questions

1. How would you re-design and market MyPlate to make it more useful and accessible to the general public?
2. Do you think any federal guidelines can make a difference in how Americans eat? If so, why? If not, how might the money used to develop these guidelines be better spent?
3. Conduct your own research into how well the current Guidelines reflect the recommendations put forth in the Scientific Report of the 2015 Dietary Guidelines Advisory Committee. Compare the Guidelines[4] with the Scientific Report.[5] Identify at least two areas of discrepancy not discussed here and propose how the current Guidelines could be modified to eliminate these discrepancies.

References

1. Phares, E.H. 2016. New Dietary Guidelines remove restriction on total fat and set limit for added sugars but censor conclusions of the scientific advisory committee. *The Nutrition Source,* 7 January 2016. Available at: http://www.hsph.harvard.edu/nutritionsource/2016/01/07/new-dietary-guidelines-remove-restriction-on-total-fat-and-set-limit-for-added-sugars-but-censor-conclusions/.
2. Wright, J. D. and C. Y. Wang. 2011. Awareness of Federal Dietary Guidance in persons aged 16 years and older: results from the National Health and Nutrition Examination Survey 2005–2006. *J. Am. Diet. Assoc.* 111:295–300.
3. Epstein, S. B., K. Jean-Pierre, S. Lynn, and A. K. Kant. 2013. Media coverage and awareness of the 2010 Dietary Guidelines for Americans and MyPlate. *Am. J. Health Prom.* 28(1):e30–e39.
4. U.S. Department of Health and Human Services and U.S. Department of Agriculture. *2015–2020 Dietary Guidelines for Americans.* 8th Edition. December 2015. Available at http://health.gov/dietaryguidelines/2015/guidelines/.
5. Scientific Report of the 2015 Dietary Guidelines Advisory Committee. Advisory Report to the Secretary of Health and Human Services and the Secretary of Agriculture. 2015. Available at: http://health.gov/dietaryguidelines/2015-scientific-report/.

STUDY **PLAN** | Mastering Nutrition™

Customize your study plan—and master your nutrition!— in the Study Area of MasteringNutrition.

TEST YOURSELF | *ANSWERS*

1 **F**   A healthful diet can be achieved by food alone; particular attention must be paid to adequacy, variety, moderation, and balance. However, some individuals may need to take vitamin supplements under certain circumstances.

2 **F**   Detailed food labels are not required for meat or poultry, as these products are regulated by the U.S. Department of Agriculture, and coffee and most spices are not required to have food labels, as they contain insignificant amounts of all the nutrients that must be listed on food labels. Fresh produce and seafood are exempt, with a voluntary nutrition labeling program covering these foods to include labels on shelves and posters.

3 **F**   A cup of black coffee with a tablespoon of cream and a teaspoon of sugar has about 45 kcal. In contrast, a café mocha might contain from 350 to 500 kcal, depending on its size and precise contents.

(Continued)

4 **F** The *Dietary Guidelines for Americans* recommend that people who choose to drink should do so sensibly and in moderation. Moderation is defined as no more than one drink per day for women and no more than two drinks per day for men.

5 **T** Although eating out poses many challenges, it is possible to eat a healthful diet when dining out. Ordering and/or consuming smaller portion sizes, selecting foods that are lower in fat and added sugars, and selecting eating establishments that serve more healthful foods can help.

summary

Scan to hear an MP3 Chapter Review in **MasteringNutrition**.

LO 1 ■ A healthful diet is adequate, moderate, balanced, and varied.

LO 2 ■ The U.S. Food and Drug Administration (FDA) regulates the content of food labels; food labels must contain a statement of identity, the net contents of the package, the contact information of the food manufacturer or distributor, an ingredient list, and nutrition information.

■ The Nutrition Facts panel on a food label contains important nutrition information about serving size; servings per package; total Calories and Calories of fat per serving; a list of various macronutrients, vitamins, and minerals; and the %Daily Values for the nutrients listed on the panel.

LO 3 ■ The FDA regulates nutrient and health claims found on food labels; however, claims that a food contributes to body structure or function are not regulated.

LO 4 ■ The Dietary Guidelines are general directives to promote health, reduce the risk for chronic diseases, and reduce the prevalence of overweight and obesity among Americans through improved nutrition and physical activity. A key message is to balance Calories to maintain weight by consistently choosing nutrient-dense foods; that is, foods that supply a high level of nutrients for a low number of Calories.

LO 5 ■ Other key messages of the DGAs include eating whole-grain foods, fruits, and vegetables daily; and limiting sodium, fat, sugars, and alcohol. It is also important to follow healthful eating patterns such as the USDA Food Patterns and MyPlate, and to practice food safety.

LO 6 ■ The USDA Food Patterns provide a conceptual framework for the types and amounts of foods that make up a healthful diet. The groups in the USDA Food Patterns include grains, vegetables, fruits, dairy foods, and protein foods. The key messages are: Make half your grains whole. Vary your veggies. Focus on fruits. Get your calcium-rich foods. Go lean with protein.

LO 7 ■ MyPlate is the graphic representation of the USDA Food Patterns. Like the Mediterranean diet, it encourages the consumption of fruits, vegetables, and whole grains. MyPlate includes milk daily, however, whereas the Mediterranean diet includes more yogurt and cheese. Also, MyPlate does not make specific recommendations for protein foods, whereas the Mediterranean diet emphasizes legumes and nuts daily, and fish, poultry, and eggs weekly.

LO 8 ■ The USDA Food Patterns defines empty Calories as Calories from solid fats and/or added sugars that provide few or no nutrients. The USDA recommends that you limit your consumption of empty Calories.

■ Specific serving sizes are defined for foods in each group of the USDA Food Patterns. However, there is no standard definition for a serving size, and the serving sizes defined in the Food Patterns are generally smaller than those listed on food labels or in the servings generally sold to consumers.

LO 9 ■ Many diet analysis programs are available to help you evaluate the quality of your diet. One example of a web-based tool available to the public is MyPlate Supertracker. Students using this text also have access to MyDietAnalysis software, and many nutrition-related apps are now available for smartphones and other mobile devices.

LO 10 ■ Eating out can be challenging because of the high fat content and large serving sizes of many fast-food and sit-down restaurant menu items.

■ Behaviors that can improve the quality of your diet when eating out include choosing lower-fat meats that are grilled or broiled, eating vegetables and salads as side or main dishes, asking for low-fat salad dressing on the side, skipping high-fat desserts and appetizers, and drinking low-Calorie or non-Caloric beverages.

review questions

LO 1 **1.** An adequate diet is defined as a diet that
   a. provides enough energy to meet minimum daily requirements.
   b. provides enough of the energy, nutrients, and fiber needed to maintain a person's health.
   c. provides a sufficient variety of nutrients to maintain a healthful weight and to optimize the body's metabolic processes.
   d. contains combinations of foods that provide healthful proportions of nutrients.

LO 2 **2.** The Nutrition Facts panel identifies which of the following?
   a. all of the nutrients and Calories in the package of food
   b. the Recommended Dietary Allowance for each nutrient found in the package of food
   c. a footnote identifying the Tolerable Upper Intake Level for each nutrient found in the package of food
   d. the %Daily Values of selected nutrients in a serving of the packaged food

LO 3 **3.** On a package of crackers, the phrase *reduced fat*
   a. is an example of an FDA-approved nutrient claim.
   b. is an example of a USDA-approved health claim.
   c. and *low fat* have the same meaning.
   d. guarantees that a food has less than 0.5 g of fat per serving.

LO 4 **4.** What does it mean to choose foods for their nutrient density?
   a. Dense foods, such as peanut butter or chicken, are more nutritious choices than transparent foods, such as fruit juice or candy, which should be limited.
   b. Foods with a lot of nutrients per Calorie, such as fish, are more nutritious choices than foods with fewer nutrients per Calorie, such as candy, which should be limited.
   c. Foods darker in color, such as whole-grain bread, should be chosen and lighter colored foods, such as white sandwich bread, should be avoided.
   d. Fat makes foods dense, and thus foods high in fat should be avoided.

LO 5 **5.** The *Dietary Guidelines for Americans* recommend which of the following?
   a. choosing and preparing sodium-free foods
   b. consuming two alcoholic beverages per day
   c. increasing your intake of fruits and vegetables
   d. following the Mediterranean diet

LO 6 **6.** The USDA Food Patterns recommend that you
   a. make half your grains whole; that is, make at least half of your grain choices whole grain foods.
   b. go lean with green; that is, make lean vegetable choices.
   c. vary your dairy; that is, choose milk, yogurt, and a variety of cheeses every day.
   d. drink at least two to three servings of fruit juice each day.

LO 7 **7.** MyPlate
   a. recommends eating red meat only monthly.
   b. recommends eating fish weekly.
   c. recommends eating legumes and nuts as daily sources of protein.
   d. does not make specific recommendations for protein food choices.

LO 8 **8.** Empty Calories are defined as
   a. the extra amount of energy a person can consume each day after meeting all essential needs through eating nutrient-dense foods.
   b. Calories from the water content of foods and beverages.
   c. Calories from solid fats and added sugars that provide few or no nutrients.
   d. Calories in any portion of food larger than the serving size indicated on the packaging.

LO 9 **9.** An online tool that allows Americans to analyze their current diet and physical activity and create personalized healthy eating and physical activity plans is
   a. the NuVal System.
   b. the exchange system
   c. MyPlate Supertracker
   d. MyDietAnalysis.

LO 10 **10.** Which of the following statements about eating out is true?
   a. It is not possible to eat healthfully while eating out.
   b. Calorie-labeling on restaurant menus has been shown to increase the likelihood that patrons will make more healthful, lower-Calorie menu choices.
   c. When ordering meat, it is more healthful to ask that it be fried or breaded rather than grilled or broiled.
   d. One way to reduce the Calorie content of a restaurant meal is to order an appetizer instead of an entrée.

true or false

LO 2 **11. True or false?** A food label must include a list of ingredients in descending order by weight.

LO 3 **12. True or false?** Structure–function claims on food labels must be approved by the FDA.

LO 6 **13. True or false?** The USDA Food Patterns classify beans, peas, and lentils in both the vegetables group and the protein foods group.

LO 8 **14. True or false?** The USDA has written a standardized definition for a serving size for most foods.

LO 10 **15. True or false?** One strategy for eating out more healthfully would be to order pasta with a cheese sauce instead of a tomato sauce.

short answer

LO 1 16. Defend the statement that no single diet can be appropriate for every human being.

LO 2 17. You work for a food company that is introducing a new variety of soup. Design a label for this new soup, including all five label components required by the FDA.

LO 3 18. If the label on a box of cereal claims that the cereal is "high in fiber," at least how much fiber does it provide per serving?

LO 7 19. You are chatting with your nutrition classmate, Sylvia, about her attempts to lose weight.

"I tried one of those low-carb diets," Sylvia confesses, "but I couldn't stick with it because bread and pasta are my favorite foods! Now I'm on the Mediterranean diet. I like it because it's a low-fat diet, so I'm sure to lose weight; plus, I can eat all the bread and pasta I want!" Do you think Sylvia's assessment of the Mediterranean diet is accurate? Why or why not?

LO 8 20. Explain why the USDA Food Patterns identify a range in the number of suggested daily servings of each food group instead of telling us exactly how many servings of each food to eat each day.

math review

LO 10 21. Hannah goes to a sandwich shop near the university at least once a week to buy what she considers a healthy lunch, which includes a chicken breast sandwich, garden salad (with Ranch dressing), and a diet cola. Recently, the shop started posting the Calorie and fat content of its menu items. Hannah discovers the following about the Calorie and fat content of the items in her "healthy lunch":

- Chicken sandwich—317 Calories, 4 g fat
- Garden salad—49 Calories, 1 g fat

- Ranch dressing (1 packet)—280 Calories, 28 g fat
- Diet cola—0 Calories, 0 g fat

Based on this information, what is the total Calorie and fat content of Hannah's lunch? What is the percentage of Calories from fat for this lunch? Which food item is contributing the highest amount of fat to Hannah's lunch, and what can she do to make a healthier change to this lunch?

Answers to Review Questions and Math Review can be found online in the MasteringNutrition Study Area and in the back of the book.

web links

www.fda.gov
U.S. Food and Drug Administration (FDA)
Learn more about the government agency that regulates our food and first established regulations for nutrition information on food labels.

www.cnpp.usda.gov/dietaryguidelines
2010 Dietary Guidelines for Americans
Use these guidelines to make changes in your food choices and physical activity habits to help reduce your risk for chronic disease.

http://www.choosemyplate.gov/
The USDA's MyPlate Home Page
Use the SuperTracker on this website to assess the overall quality of your diet and level of physical activity based on the USDA MyPlate.

http://www.nhlbi.nih.gov/health/educational/ wecan/eat-right/portion-distortion.htm
National Institutes of Health (NIH) Portion Distortion Quiz
Take this short quiz to see if you know how today's food portions compare to those of 30 years ago.

www.diabetes.org
American Diabetes Association
Find out more about meal-planning exchange lists.

www.eatright.org
Academy of Nutrition and Dietetics
Visit the Public Information Center section of this website for additional resources to help you achieve a healthful lifestyle.

ndb.nal.usda.gov/
U.S. Department of Agriculture National Nutrient Databases
Search this site to find nutrition information on over 8,000 foods, and to find foods that are high in a particular nutrient of interest.

www.hsph.harvard.edu/
Harvard School of Public Health
Scroll down to "The Nutrition Source" on this site to learn more about the Healthy Eating Plate, an alternative to the USDA MyPlate.

www.pcrm.org
Physicians' Committee for Responsible Medicine
Visit this site to view the Power Plate, a vegetarian alternative to the USDA MyPlate. Click on "Health and Nutrition" and select "Vegetarian and Vegan Diets" for details.

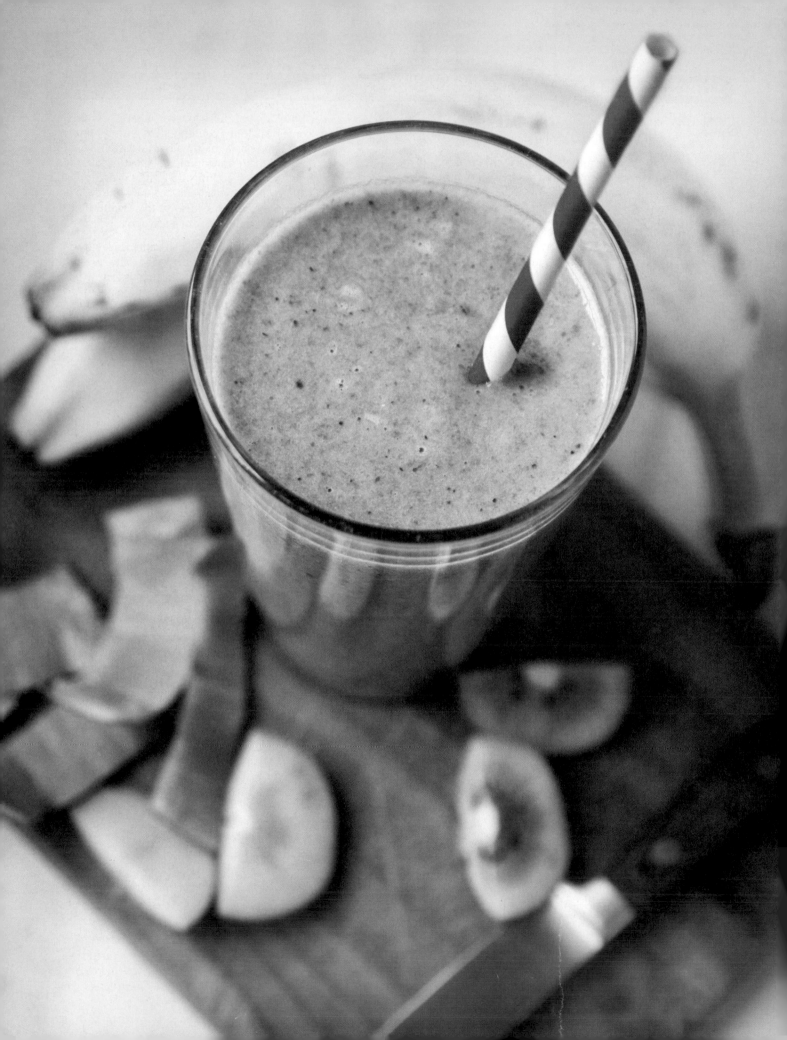

3 The Human Body: Are We Really What We Eat?

Learning Outcomes

After studying this chapter, you should be able to:

1 Distinguish between appetite and hunger, describing the physiologic mechanisms and other influences behind both conditions, *pp. 72–76*.

2 Describe the contribution of each organ of the gastrointestinal tract to the digestion, absorption, and elimination of food, *pp. 76–81*.

3 Explain how the pH of the stomach's internal environment contributes to the stomach's role in digestion, *pp. 82–85*.

4 Identify the primary role of enzymes and of hormones in accomplishing chemical digestion, *pp. 87–88*.

5 Discuss the roles of the gallbladder, pancreas, and liver in accomplishing chemical digestion, *pp. 88–90*.

6 Explain how the anatomy of the small intestine's lining contributes to its absorptive function, *pp. 90–91*.

7 List and describe the four types of absorption that occur in the small intestine, *pp. 90–92*.

8 Identify three gastrointestinal tract movements and three divisions of the nervous system that contribute to gastrointestinal function, *pp. 94–95*.

9 Describe the causes, symptoms, and treatments of gastroesophageal reflux disease, peptic ulcers, food allergies, celiac disease, vomiting, inflammatory bowel diseases, and functional gastrointestinal disorders, *pp. 96–98*.

10 Compare the incidence of colorectal cancer with that of other cancers of the gastrointestinal system, and explain the role of screening in reducing colorectal cancer deaths, *p. 104*.

TEST YOURSELF

True or False?

1 Sometimes you may have an appetite even though you are not hungry. **T** *or* **F**

2 Your stomach is the primary organ responsible for telling you when you are hungry. **T** *or* **F**

3 If you eat only small amounts of food, over time, your stomach will permanently shrink. **T** *or* **F**

4 The entire process of the digestion and absorption of one meal takes about 24 hours. **T** *or* **F**

5 Most ulcers result from a type of infection. **T** *or* **F**

Test Yourself answers are located in the Study Plan.

MasteringNutrition™

Go online for chapter quizzes, pre-tests, interactive activities, and more!

wo months ago, Andrea's lifelong dream of becoming a lawyer came one step closer to reality: she moved out of her parents' home in the Midwest to attend law school in Boston. Unfortunately, the adjustment to a new city, new friends, and her intensive course work was more stressful than she'd imagined, and Andrea has been experiencing insomnia and exhaustion. What's more, her always "sensitive stomach" has been getting worse: after every meal, she gets cramps so bad that she can't stand up, and twice she has missed classes because of sudden attacks of pain and diarrhea. She suspects that the problem is related to stress and wonders if she is going to experience it throughout her life. She is even thinking of dropping out of school if that would make her feel well again.

Almost everyone experiences brief episodes of abdominal pain, diarrhea, or other symptoms from time to time. Such episodes are often caused by eating too much or too quickly, food poisoning, or an infection such as influenza. But do you know anyone who experiences these symptoms periodically for days, weeks, or even years? If so, has it made you wonder why? What are the steps in normal digestion and absorption of food, and at what points can the process break down?

We begin this chapter with a look at some of the factors that make us feel as if we want to eat. We then discuss the **gastrointestinal (GI) system;** that is, the body system responsible for digestion of food, absorption of nutrients, and elimination of wastes. Finally, we look at some disorders that affect these processes.

Why Do We Feel the Urge to Eat?

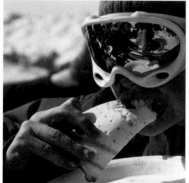

You've just finished eating at your favorite Thai restaurant. As you walk back to the block where you parked your car, you pass a bakery window displaying several cakes and pies, each of which looks more enticing than the last, and through the door wafts a complex aroma of coffee, cinnamon, and chocolate. You stop. You know you're not hungry, but you go inside and buy a slice of chocolate torte and an espresso, anyway. Later that night, when the caffeine from the chocolate and espresso keeps you awake, you wonder why you succumbed.

Two mechanisms prompt us to seek food: **hunger** is a physiologic drive for food that occurs when the body senses that we need to eat. The drive is *nonspecific*; when you're hungry, a variety of foods could satisfy you. If you've recently finished a nourishing meal, then hunger probably won't compel you toward a slice of chocolate torte. Instead, the culprit is likely to be **appetite,** a psychological desire to consume *specific* foods. It is aroused when environmental cues—such as the sight of chocolate cake or the smell of coffee—stimulate our senses, prompting pleasant emotions and often memories.

People commonly experience appetite in the absence of hunger. That's why you can crave cake and coffee even after eating a full meal. On the other hand, it is possible to have a physiologic need for food yet have no appetite. This state, called *anorexia,* can accompany a variety of illnesses from infectious diseases to mood disorders. It can also occur as a side effect of certain medications, such as the chemotherapy used in treating cancer patients. Although in the following sections we describe hunger and appetite as separate entities, ideally the two states coexist: we seek specific, appealing foods to satisfy a physiologic need for nutrients.

The Hypothalamus Prompts Hunger in Response to Various Signals

Because hunger is a physiologic stimulus that drives us to find food and eat, often we experience it as an unpleasant sensation. The primary organ producing that sensation is the brain. That's right—it's not our stomachs, but our brains that tell us when we're hungry. The region of brain tissue that is responsible for prompting us to seek food is called the

LO 1 Distinguish between appetite and hunger, describing the physiologic mechanisms and other influences behind both conditions.

Hunger is a physiologic stimulus that prompts us to find food and eat.

gastrointestinal (GI) system The body system responsible for digestion, absorption, and elimination. It includes the organs of the GI tract and the accessory organs.

hunger A physiologic sensation that prompts us to eat.

appetite A psychological desire to consume specific foods.

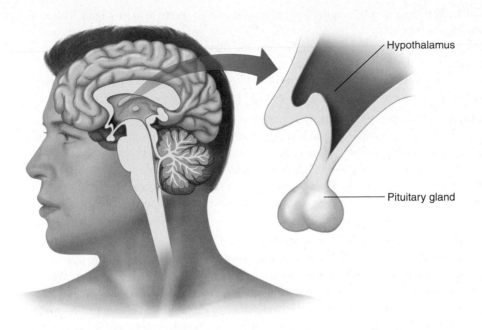

FIGURE 3.1 The hypothalamus triggers hunger by integrating signals from nerve cells throughout the body, as well as from messages carried by hormones.

Hypothalamus

Pituitary gland

hypothalamus (**Figure 3.1**). It's located just above the pituitary gland and brain stem in a region of the brain responsible for regulating many types of involuntary activity.

The hypothalamus contains a cluster of nerve cells known collectively as the feeding center. Stimulation of the feeding center triggers feelings of hunger that drive us to eat. In contrast, signals from a cluster of cells called the satiety center (*satiety* means fullness) inhibit the feeding center cells. This prompts us to stop eating.

The feeding and satiety centers work together to regulate food intake by integrating signals from three sources: nerve cells in the gastrointestinal system, chemical messenger molecules called hormones, and the amount and type of food we eat. Let's examine these three types of signals.

The Role of Nerve Cells

One important hunger-regulating signal comes from nerve cells lining the stomach and small intestine that detect changes in pressure according to whether the organ is empty or distended with food. The cells relay these data to the hypothalamus. For instance, if you have not eaten for many hours and your stomach and small intestine do not contain food, this information is sent to the hypothalamus, which in turn prompts you to experience the sensation of hunger.

Nerve cells in the mouth, pharynx (throat), and esophagus (the tube leading to the stomach) also contribute to feelings of hunger and satiety. Chewing and swallowing food, for example, stimulates these nerve cells, which then relay data to the satiety center in the hypothalamus. As a result, we begin to feel full.

The Role of Hormones

Hormones are molecules, usually proteins or lipids, that are secreted into the bloodstream by one of the many *endocrine glands* of the body. In the bloodstream, they act as chemical messengers, binding to and triggering a response in target cells far away from the gland in which they were produced. The relative levels of different hormones in the blood help regulate body functions. Hormones important in hunger and satiety include the following.

Insulin and Glucagon These hormones are produced in the pancreas and are responsible for maintaining blood glucose levels. *Glucose*, a simple sugar, is the body's most readily available fuel supply. It's not surprising, then, that its level in our blood is an important signal regulating hunger. When we have not eaten for a while, our blood glucose levels

hypothalamus A region of the brain below (*hypo*-) the thalamus and cerebral hemispheres and above the pituitary gland and brain stem where visceral sensations such as hunger and thirst are regulated.

hormone A chemical messenger that is secreted into the bloodstream by one of the many endocrine glands of the body. Hormones act as regulators of physiologic processes at sites remote from the glands that secreted them.

fall, prompting a decrease in the level of insulin and an increase in glucagon. This chemical message is relayed to the hypothalamus, which then prompts us to eat in order to supply our bodies with more glucose. After we eat, the hypothalamus picks up the sensation of distention in the stomach and intestine, and the rise in blood glucose levels as our body begins to absorb nutrients from our meal. These signals trigger an increase in insulin secretion and a decrease in glucagon, and the feeling of satiety.

Ghrelin and Cholecystokinin   The hormone ghrelin is produced by the stomach. Immediately after a meal, ghrelin levels plummet. As time since our last meal elapses, ghrelin levels begin to rise. A fast-acting hormone, ghrelin triggers the hypothalamus to strongly induce us to eat. As you might suppose, when we dramatically restrict our food intake, ghrelin levels surge. Opposite in action to ghrelin is the hormone cholecystokinin (CCK), which is produced in the small intestine in response to food entry. CCK causes stimulation of the satiety center.

Leptin   The hormones we've discussed so far act in short-term regulation of food intake. But our body produces other hormones that regulate food intake over time. One of the most important of these is leptin, a protein produced by our adipose cells (fat cells). When we consume more Calories than we burn, the extra Calories are converted to fat and stored in adipose tissue. The more adipose tissue our body carries, the more leptin we produce. Leptin acts on the hypothalamus to suppress hunger. Unfortunately, obese people appear to be leptin-resistant.

The Role of Amount and Type of Food

Foods containing protein have the highest satiety value, in part because they increase the secretion of satiety hormones and reduce the secretion of ghrelin.[1] This means that a ham-and-egg breakfast will cause us to feel satiated for a longer period of time than will pancakes with maple syrup, even if both meals have exactly the same number of Calories. High-fat meals have a higher satiety value than high-carbohydrate meals.

Another factor affecting hunger is how bulky the meal is—that is, how much fiber and water are within the food. Bulky meals tend to stretch the stomach and small intestine, which sends signals back to the hypothalamus telling us that we are full, so we stop eating. Beverages tend to be less satisfying than semisolid foods, and semisolid foods have a lower satiety value than solid foods. For example, if you were to eat a bunch of grapes, you would feel a greater sense of fullness than if you drank a glass of grape juice providing the same number of Calories.

Environmental Cues Trigger Appetite

Whereas hunger is prompted by internal signals, appetite is triggered by aspects of our environment. The most significant factors influencing our appetite are sensory data, social and cultural cues, and learning (**Figure 3.2**).

The Role of Sensory Data

The sight, smell, taste, texture, and sound of foods stimulate sensory receptors, which transmit signals to the brain. Foods that are artfully prepared, arranged, or ornamented appeal to our sense of sight. Food producers know this and spend millions of dollars annually in the United States to promote and package their products in an appealing way. The aromas of foods can also be powerful stimulants. Much of our ability to taste foods actually comes from our sense of smell. This is why foods are not as appealing when we have a stuffy nose due to a cold. Texture, or "mouth feel," is also important, as it stimulates nerve endings sensitive to touch in our mouths and on our tongues. Even our sense of hearing can be stimulated by foods, from the fizz of cola to the crunch of corn chips.

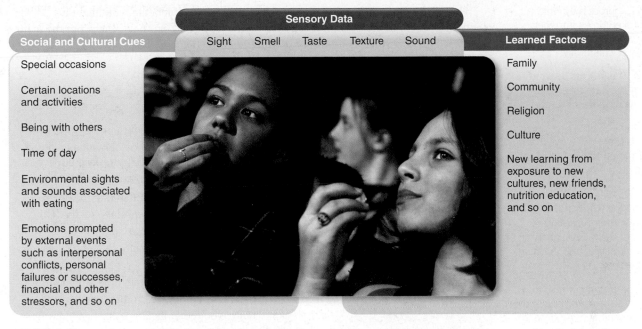

Social and Cultural Cues	Sensory Data					Learned Factors
	Sight	Smell	Taste	Texture	Sound	

Social and Cultural Cues

Special occasions

Certain locations and activities

Being with others

Time of day

Environmental sights and sounds associated with eating

Emotions prompted by external events such as interpersonal conflicts, personal failures or successes, financial and other stressors, and so on

Learned Factors

Family

Community

Religion

Culture

New learning from exposure to new cultures, new friends, nutrition education, and so on

FIGURE 3.2 Appetite is a drive to consume specific foods, such as popcorn at the movies. It is aroused by social and cultural cues and sensory data and is influenced by learning.

The Role of Social and Cultural Cues

The brain's association with certain social events, such as birthday parties or holiday gatherings, can stimulate our appetite. Many people feel an increase or a decrease in appetite according to whom they are with; for example, they may eat more when at home with family members and less when out on a date. For some people, certain activities, such as watching a movie or studying, can trigger appetite. In some cases, appetite masks an emotional response to an external event. For example, after receiving a failing grade or arguing with a close friend, a person might experience a desire for food rather than a desire for emotional comfort. Many people crave food when they're frustrated, worried, or bored; or when they are at a gathering where they feel anxious or awkward. Others subconsciously seek food as a "reward." For example, have you ever found yourself heading out for a burger and fries after handing in a term paper?

The Role of Learning

Do you eat stewed octopus? Cactus? What about grasshoppers? If you'd grown up in certain parts of the world, you probably would. That's because your preference for particular foods is largely a learned response. The family, community, religion, and/or culture in which you're raised teach you what plant and animal products are appropriate to eat. If your parents fed you cubes of plain tofu throughout your toddlerhood, then you are probably still eating tofu now. That said, early introduction to foods is not essential: we can learn to enjoy new foods at any point in our life.

Food preferences also change when people learn what foods are most healthful in terms of nutrient density and the prevention of chronic diseases. Since reading the preceding chapters (Chapters 1 and 2), has your diet changed at all?

We can also "learn" to dislike foods we once enjoyed. For example, if we experience an episode of food poisoning after eating undercooked scrambled eggs, we might develop a strong distaste for all types of cooked eggs. Many adults become vegetarians after learning about the treatment of animals in slaughterhouses: they might have eaten meat daily when young but no longer have any appetite for it.

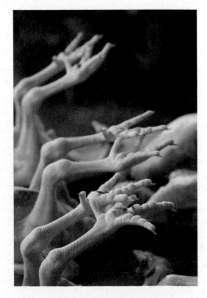

Food preferences are influenced by the family and culture in which you are raised.

digestion The process by which foods are broken down into their component molecules, either mechanically or chemically.

absorption The process by which molecules of food are taken from the gastrointestinal tract into the circulation.

elimination The process by which the undigested portions of food and waste products are removed from the body.

gastrointestinal (GI) tract A long, muscular tube consisting of several organs: the mouth, pharynx, esophagus, stomach, small intestine, and large intestine.

sphincter A tight ring of muscle separating some of the organs of the GI tract and opening in response to nerve signals indicating that food is ready to pass into the next section.

accessory organs of digestion The salivary glands, liver, pancreas, and gallbladder, which contribute to GI function but are not anatomically part of the GI tract.

Now that you know the difference between hunger and appetite, you might be wondering which of these states most often motivates you to eat. If so, check out the feature box *Highlight: Do You Eat in Response to External or Internal Cues?* (p. 77).

Judy | *Nutri*-Case

"Ever since I was diagnosed with type 2 diabetes, I've felt as if there's a 'food cop' spying on me. Sometimes I feel like I have to look over my shoulder when I pull into the Dunkin' Donuts parking lot. My doctor says I'm supposed to eat fresh fruits and vegetables, fish, brown bread, brown rice . . . I didn't bother telling him I don't like that stuff and I don't have the money to buy it or the time to cook it even if I did. Besides, that kind of diet is for movie stars. All the real people I know eat the same way I do."

What do you think? Is the diet Judy's doctor described really just for "movie stars"? Of the many factors influencing why and what we eat, identify at least two that might be affecting Judy's food choices. If you were to learn that Judy had not finished high school, would that fact have any bearing on your answer? If so, in what way?

RECAP

Hunger is a physiologic drive for food triggered by the hypothalamus in response to cues about stomach and intestinal distention and the levels of certain hormones. Appetite is a psychological desire to consume specific foods. It is triggered when external stimuli arouse our senses, and it often occurs in combination with social and cultural cues. Our preference for certain foods is largely learned from the culture in which we were raised, but our food choices can change with exposure to new foods or new learning experiences. ∎

LO 2 Describe the contribution of each organ of the gastrointestinal tract to the digestion, absorption, and elimination of food.

LO 3 Explain how the pH of the stomach's internal environment contributes to the stomach's role in digestion.

What Happens to the Food We Eat?

When we eat, the food we consume is digested; then the useful nutrients are absorbed; and, finally, the waste products are eliminated. But what does each of these processes really entail? In the simplest terms, **digestion** is the process by which foods are broken down into their component molecules, either mechanically or chemically. **Absorption** is the process in which these products of digestion move through the wall of the intestine. **Elimination** is the process by which the undigested portions of food and waste products are removed from the body.

The processes of digestion, absorption, and elimination occur in the **gastrointestinal (GI) tract,** the organs of which work together to process foods. *Gastro-* refers to the stomach, and of course *intestinal* refers to the large and small intestines; however, the GI tract begins at the mouth and ends at the anus (**Focus Figure 3.3** on page 78). It is a long, continuous tube composed of several distinct organs, including the mouth, pharynx, esophagus, stomach, small intestine, and large intestine. The flow of food between these organs is controlled by **sphincters,** which are tight rings of muscle that open when a nerve signal indicates that food is ready to pass into the next section. The sphincters associated with each region of the GI tract are shown in several figures later in this chapter. Assisting the GI tract are several **accessory organs of digestion,** including the salivary glands, liver,

Do You Eat in Response to External or Internal Cues?

HIGHLIGHT

In this chapter, you learn the differences between appetite and hunger, as well as the influence of learning on food choices. So now you might be curious to investigate your own reasons for eating what and when you do. Whether you're trying to lose weight, gain weight, or maintain your current healthful weight, you'll probably find it intriguing to keep a log of the reasons behind your decisions about what, when, where, and why you eat. Are you eating in response to internal sensations telling you that your body *needs* food, or in response to your emotions, a situation, or a prescribed diet? Keeping a "cues" log for 1 full week would give you the most accurate picture of your eating habits, but even logging 2 days of meals and snacks should increase your cue awareness.

Each day, every time you eat a meal, snack, or beverage other than water, make a quick note of the following:

- **When you eat.** Many people eat at certain times (for example, 6 PM) whether they are hungry or not.

- **What you eat and how much.** A cup of yogurt and a handful of nuts? An apple? A 20-oz cola?

- **Where you eat.** This includes while sitting at the dining room table, watching television, driving in the car, and so on.

- **With whom you eat.** Are you alone or with others? If with others, are they eating as well? Have they offered you food?

- **Your emotions.** Many people overeat when they are happy, especially when celebrating with others. Some people eat excessively when they are anxious, depressed, bored, or frustrated. Still others eat as a way of denying feelings because they don't want to identify and deal with them. For some, food becomes a substitute for emotional fulfillment.

- **Your sensations: what you see, hear, or smell.** Are you eating because you walked past the kitchen and spied a batch of homemade cookies or smelled coffee roasting?

- **Any dietary restrictions.** Are you choosing a particular food because it is allowed on your current diet plan? Or are you hungry but drinking a diet soda to stay within a certain allowance of Calories? Are you restricting yourself because you feel guilty about having eaten too much at another time?

- **Your physiologic hunger.** Rate your hunger on a scale from 1 to 5 as follows:

  1 = you feel full or even stuffed
  2 = you feel satisfied but not uncomfortably full
  3 = neutral; you feel no discernible satiation nor hunger
  4 = you feel hungry and want to eat
  5 = you feel strong physiologic sensations of hunger and need to eat

After keeping a log for 2 or more days, you might become aware of patterns you'd like to change. For example, maybe you notice that you often eat when you are not actually hungry but are worried about homework or personal relationships. Or maybe you notice that you can't walk past the snack bar without going in. This self-awareness may prompt you to take positive steps to change those patterns. For instance, instead of stifling your worries with food, write down exactly what you are worried about, including steps you can take to address your concerns. And the next time you approach the snack bar, before going in, check with your gut: are you truly hungry? If so, then purchase a healthful snack, maybe a yogurt, a piece of fruit, or a bag of peanuts. If you're not really hungry, take a moment to acknowledge the strength of this visual cue—and then walk on by.

---

pancreas, and gallbladder, each of which has a specific role in the digestion and absorption of nutrients.

Imagine that you ate a turkey sandwich for lunch today. It contained two slices of bread spread with mayonnaise, some turkey, two lettuce leaves, and a slice of tomato. Let's travel along with the sandwich and see what happens as it enters your GI tract and is digested and absorbed into your body.

Digestion Begins in the Mouth

Believe it or not, the first step in the digestive process is not your first bite of that sandwich. It is your first thought about what you wanted for lunch as you stood in line at the deli. In this **cephalic phase** of digestion, hunger and appetite work together to prepare the GI tract to digest food. The nervous system stimulates the release of digestive juices in preparation

cephalic phase The earliest phase of digestion, in which the brain thinks about and prepares the digestive organs for the consumption of food.

The digestive system consists of the organs of the gastrointestinal (GI) tract and associated accessory organs. The processing of food in the GI tract involves ingestion, mechanical digestion, chemical digestion, propulsion, absorption, and elimination.

ORGANS OF THE GI TRACT

MOUTH

Ingestion Food enters the GI tract via the mouth.

Mechanical digestion Mastication tears, shreds, and mixes food with saliva.

Chemical digestion Salivary amylase and lingual lipase begin the digestion of carbohydrates and lipids.

PHARYNX AND ESOPHAGUS

Propulsion Swallowing and peristalsis move food from mouth to stomach.

STOMACH

Mechanical digestion Mixes and churns food with gastric juice into a liquid called chyme.

Chemical digestion Pepsin begins digestion of proteins, and gastric lipase continues to break lipids apart.

Absorption A few fat-soluble substances are absorbed through the stomach wall.

SMALL INTESTINE

Mechanical Digestion and **Propulsion** Segmentation mixes chyme with digestive juices; peristaltic waves move it along tract.

Chemical digestion Digestive enzymes from pancreas and brush border digest most classes of nutrients.

Absorption Nutrients are absorbed into blood and lymph through enterocytes.

LARGE INTESTINE

Chemical digestion Some remaining food residues are digested by bacteria.

Absorption Reabsorbs salts, water, and vitamins.

Propulsion Compacts waste into feces and propels it toward the rectum.

RECTUM

Elimination Temporarily stores feces before voluntary release through the anus.

ACCESSORY ORGANS

SALIVARY GLANDS

Produce saliva, a mixture of water, mucus, enzymes, and other chemicals.

LIVER

Produces bile to emulsify fats.

GALLBLADDER

Stores bile before release into the small intestine through the bile duct.

PANCREAS

Produces digestive enzymes and bicarbonate, which are released into the small intestine via the pancreatic duct.

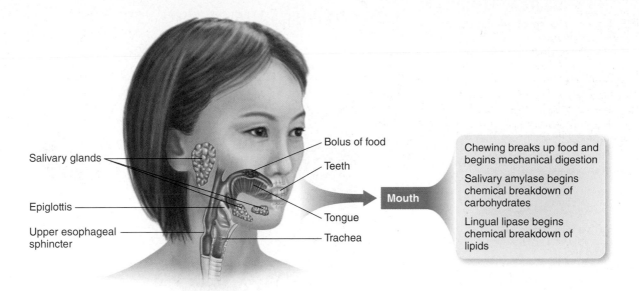

FIGURE 3.4 Where your food is now: the mouth. Chewing moistens food and mechanically breaks it down into pieces small enough to swallow, while salivary amylase begins the chemical digestion of carbohydrates and lingual lipase begins the chemical digestion of lipids.

for food entering the GI tract, and sometimes we experience some involuntary movement commonly called "hunger pangs."

Now, let's stop smelling that sandwich and take a bite and chew! Chewing moistens the food and mechanically breaks it down into pieces small enough to swallow (**Figure 3.4**). The presence of food initiates not only mechanical digestion via chewing but also chemical digestion through the secretion of hormones and other substances throughout the gastrointestinal tract. As the teeth cut and grind the different foods in the sandwich, more surface area of the foods is exposed to the digestive juices in the mouth. Foremost among these is **saliva,** which is secreted from the **salivary glands.**

Without saliva, we could not taste the foods we eat. That's because taste occurs when chemicals dissolved in saliva bind to chemoreceptors called *taste receptors* located in structures called *taste buds* on the surface of the tongue. Taste receptors are able to detect at least five distinct tastes: bitter, sweet, salty, sour, and *umami*, a savory taste due to the presence of glutamic acid, an amino acid that occurs naturally in meats and other protein-rich foods. Flavors, such as turkey or tomato, reflect complex combinations of these five basic tastes. As noted earlier, taste depends significantly on the sense of smell, called *olfaction*. To achieve olfaction, odorants dissolved in mucus bind to chemoreceptors in the nasal cavity called *olfactory receptor cells*. These cells then transmit their data to the olfactory bulb of the brain.

Saliva also initiates the chemical digestion of carbohydrates. It accomplishes this through the actions of salivary amylase, a digestive enzyme. **Enzymes** are compounds— usually proteins—that act as catalysts; that is, they induce chemical changes in other substances to speed up bodily processes (**Figure 3.5**). They can be reused because they essentially are unchanged by the chemical reactions they catalyze.

Salivary amylase is only one of many enzymes that assist the body in digesting foods. Another enzyme active in the mouth is lingual lipase, which is secreted by tongue cells during chewing and begins the breakdown of lipids. By the way, enzyme names usually end in *ase*, so they are easy to recognize as we go through the digestive process. Various *amylases* assist in the digestion of carbohydrates, *lipases* are involved with lipid digestion, and *proteases* help digest proteins.

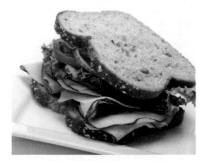

Digestion of a sandwich starts before you even take a bite.

saliva A mixture of water, mucus, enzymes, and other chemicals that moistens the mouth and food, binds food particles together, and begins the digestion of carbohydrates.

salivary glands A group of glands found under and behind the tongue and beneath the jaw that releases saliva continually as well as in response to the thought, sight, smell, or presence of food.

enzymes Small chemicals, usually proteins, that act on other chemicals to speed up bodily processes but are not changed during those processes.

FIGURE 3.5 Enzymes speed up the body's chemical reactions, including those essential to digestion and absorption as well as many other biological processes. Here, an enzyme joins two small compounds to create a larger compound; however, enzymes active in digestion typically facilitate reactions that break molecules apart. Notice that the enzyme itself is not changed in the process.

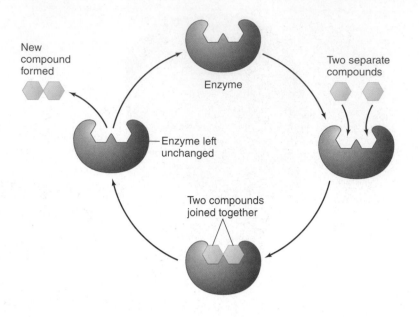

Saliva contains many other components, including the following:

- Bicarbonate, which helps neutralize acids
- Mucus, which moistens the food and the oral cavity, ensuring that food easily travels down the esophagus
- Antibodies, proteins that defend against bacteria entering the mouth
- Lysozyme, an enzyme that inhibits bacterial growth in the mouth and may assist in preventing tooth decay

In reality, very little digestion occurs in the mouth. This is because we do not hold food in our mouth for very long and because the most powerful digestive chemicals are secreted further along in the GI tract.

The Esophagus Propels Food into the Stomach

The mass of food that has been chewed and moistened in the mouth is referred to as a **bolus.** This bolus is swallowed (**Figure 3.6**) and propelled to the stomach through the esophagus. Swallowing is a very complex process involving voluntary and involuntary motion. A tiny flap of tissue called the *epiglottis* acts as a trapdoor covering the entrance to the trachea (windpipe). The epiglottis is normally open, allowing us to breathe freely even while chewing (Figure 3.6a). As our bite of sandwich moves toward the pharynx, the brain is sent a signal to temporarily raise the soft palate and close the openings to the nasal passages, preventing aspiration of food or liquid into the sinuses (Figure 3.6b). The brain also signals the epiglottis to close during swallowing, so that food and liquid cannot enter the trachea. Sometimes this protective mechanism goes awry—for instance, when we try to eat and talk at the same time. When this happens, we experience the sensation of choking and typically cough involuntarily and repeatedly until the offending food or liquid is expelled from the trachea.

As the trachea closes, the sphincter muscle at the top of the esophagus, called the *upper esophageal sphincter,* opens to allow the passage of food. The **esophagus** then transports the food to the stomach (**Figure 3.7**). A muscular tube, the esophagus propels food along its length by contracting two sets of muscles: inner sheets of circular muscle squeeze the food, while outer sheets of longitudinal muscle push food along the length of the tube. Together, these rhythmic waves of squeezing and pushing are called **peristalsis.** We will see later in this chapter that peristalsis occurs throughout the GI tract.

To view a step-by-step animation of the complex process of swallowing, visit MedlinePlus at http://www.nlm.nih.gov. Click on Medline Plus on the left hand side and click on "Videos & Cool Tools." Press on the "Anatomy Videos" button and click on "Swallowing."

bolus A mass of food that has been chewed and moistened in the mouth.

esophagus A muscular tube of the GI tract connecting the back of the mouth to the stomach.

peristalsis Waves of squeezing and pushing contractions that move food, chyme, and feces in one direction through the length of the GI tract.

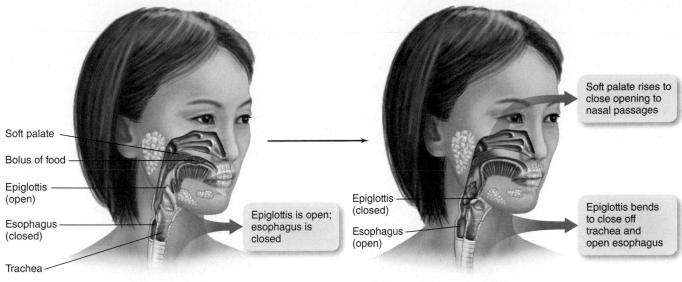

Soft palate

Bolus of food

Epiglottis (open)

Esophagus (closed)

Trachea

Soft palate rises to close opening to nasal passages

Epiglottis is open; esophagus is closed

Epiglottis (closed)

Esophagus (open)

Epiglottis bends to close off trachea and open esophagus

(a) Chewing

(b) Swallowing

FIGURE 3.6 Chewing and swallowing are complex processes. **(a)** During the process of chewing, the epiglottis is open and the esophagus is closed, so that we can continue to breathe as we chew. **(b)** During swallowing, the epiglottis closes, so that food does not enter the trachea and obstruct our breathing. Also, the soft palate rises to seal off the nasal passages to prevent the aspiration of food or liquid into the sinuses.

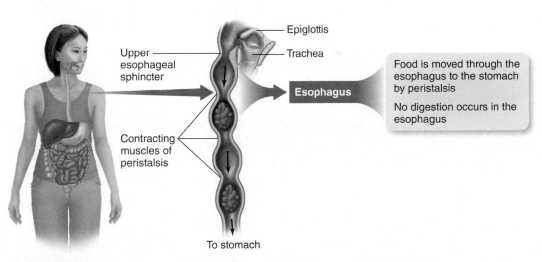

Epiglottis

Upper esophageal sphincter

Trachea

Contracting muscles of peristalsis

Esophagus

Food is moved through the esophagus to the stomach by peristalsis

No digestion occurs in the esophagus

To stomach

FIGURE 3.7 Where your food is now: the esophagus. Peristalsis, the rhythmic contraction and relaxation of both circular and longitudinal muscles in the esophagus, propels food toward the stomach. Peristalsis occurs throughout the GI tract.

Gravity also helps transport food down the esophagus, which is one reason it is wise to sit or stand upright while eating. Together, peristalsis and gravity can transport a bite of food from the mouth to the opening of the stomach in 5 to 8 seconds. At the end of the esophagus is another sphincter muscle, the *gastroesophageal sphincter,* also referred to as the *lower esophageal sphincter,* which is normally tightly closed. When food reaches the end of the esophagus, this sphincter relaxes to allow the passage of food into the stomach. In some people, this sphincter is continually somewhat relaxed. Later in the chapter, we'll discuss this disorder and the unpleasant symptoms it can prompt.

RECAP

The cephalic phase of digestion prepares the GI tract for digestion. Chewing initiates the mechanical digestion of food by breaking it into smaller components and mixing all the nutrients together. Chewing also stimulates chemical digestion through the secretion of digestive juices, such as saliva. Swallowing causes the nasal passages to close and the epiglottis to cover the trachea to prevent food from entering the sinuses and lungs. The upper esophageal sphincter opens as the trachea closes. The esophagus is a muscular tube that transports food from the mouth to the stomach via peristalsis. Once food reaches the stomach, the gastroesophageal sphincter opens to allow food into the stomach.   ■

The Stomach Mixes, Digests, and Stores Food

The **stomach** is a J-shaped organ. Its size varies with different individuals; in general, its volume is about 6 fluid ounces (¾ cup) when it is empty. The stomach wall contains four layers, the innermost of which is crinkled into large folds called *rugae*, which flatten progressively to accommodate food. This allows the stomach to expand to hold about 1 gallon of food and liquid. As food is released into the small intestine, the rugae reform, and the stomach gradually contracts in size again.

Before any food reaches the stomach, the brain sends signals to the stomach to stimulate and prepare it to receive food. For example, the hormone *gastrin*, secreted by stomach-lining cells called *G cells*, stimulates gastric glands to secrete a digestive fluid referred to as **gastric juice.** Gastric glands are lined with two important types of cells—parietal cells and chief cells—which secrete the various components of gastric juice (**Figure 3.8**).

The parietal cells secrete the following:

■ *Hydrochloric acid (HCl)*, which keeps the stomach interior very acidic. To be precise, the pH of HCl is 1.0, which means that it is ten times more acidic than pure lemon juice and a hundred times more acidic than vinegar! For a review of the negative logarithms behind the pH scale, see the ***You Do the Math*** box (page 83). The acidic environment of the stomach interior kills any bacteria and/or germs that may have entered the body with the sandwich. HCl is also extremely important for digestion because it starts to denature proteins, which means it breaks the bonds that maintain their structure. This is an essential preliminary step in protein digestion.

stomach A J-shaped organ where food is partially digested, churned, and stored until released into the small intestine.

gastric juice Acidic liquid secreted within the stomach; it contains hydrochloric acid, pepsin, and other compounds.

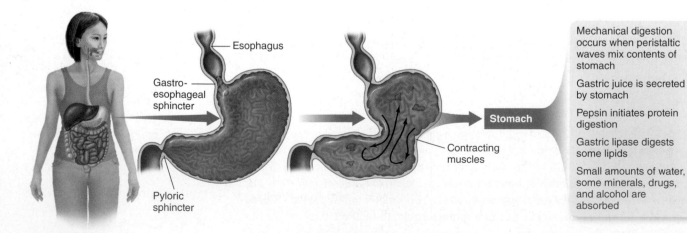

FIGURE 3.8 Where your food is now: the stomach. In the stomach, the protein in your sandwich begins to be digested and minimal digestion of lipids continues. Your meal is churned into chyme and stored until release into the small intestine.

YOU Do the Math
Negative Logarithms and the pH Scale

Have you ever been warned that the black coffee, orange juice, or cola you enjoy is corroding your stomach? If so, relax. It's a myth. How can you know for sure? Take a look at the pH scale (**Figure 3.9**). As you can see, the scale shows that hydrochloric acid (HCl) has a pH of 1.0 and gastric juice is 2.0, whereas soft drinks (including cola) are 3.0, orange juice is 4.0, and black coffee is 5.0. Not sure what all of these numbers mean?

An abbreviation for the *potential of hydrogen*, pH is a measure of the hydrogen ion concentration of a solution; that is, the potential of a substance to release to take up hydrogen ions in solution. Since an acid by definition is a compound that releases hydrogen ions, and a base is a compound that binds them, we can also say that pH is a measure of a compound's acidity or alkalinity. The precise measurements of pH range from 0 to 14, with 7.0 designated as pH neutral. Pure water is exactly neutral, and human blood is close to neutral, normally ranging from about 7.35 to 7.45.

The pH scale is a negative base-10 logarithmic scale. As you may recall from high school math classes, a base-10 logarithm ($\log_{10}$) tells you how many times you multiply by 10 to get the desired number. For example, $\log_{10}(1{,}000) = 3$ because to get 1,000 you have to multiply 10 three times ($10 \times 10 \times 10$). The pH scale is negative because an *increased* number on the scale identifies a corresponding *decrease* in concentration. These facts taken together mean that:

- For every increase of a single digit, the concentration of hydrogen ions decreases by ten-fold.
- For every decrease of a single digit, the concentration of hydrogen ions increases by ten-fold.

For example, milk has a pH of 6, which is one digit lower than 7. Milk is therefore ten times more acidic than pure water. Baking soda, at pH 9, is two digits higher than 7, and thus baking soda is 100 times less acidic than pure water: $2 = \log_{10}(100)$.

Now you do the math:

1. Is the pH of blood normally slightly acidic or slightly alkaline (basic)?

2. Identify the relative acidity of black coffee as compared to pure water and as compared to HCl.

3. Identify the relative acidity of soft drinks as compared to pure water and as compared to HCl.

If you answered correctly, you can appreciate the fact that, since the tissues lining your stomach wall are adequately protected (by mucus and bicarbonate) from the acidity of HCl, they are not likely to be damaged by coffee, cola, or any other standard beverage. On the other hand, if you were to down an entire bottle of pure lemon juice (pH 2.0), the release of all those additional hydrogen ions into the already acidic environment of your stomach would likely make you very sick. Your blood pH would drop, your breathing rate would increase, and you would almost certainly vomit. However, the juice would not corrode your stomach.

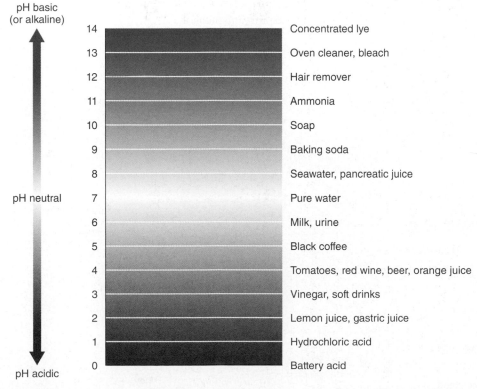

FIGURE 3.9 The pH scale identifies the levels of acidity or alkalinity of various substances. More specifically, pH is defined as the negative logarithm of the hydrogen ion concentration of any solution. Each one-unit change in pH from high to low represents a tenfold increase in the concentration of hydrogen ions. This means that gastric juice, which has a pH of 2, is 100,000 times more acidic than pure water, which has a pH of 7.

■ *Intrinsic factor,* a protein critical to the absorption of vitamin B_{12} (discussed in more detail in Chapter 8). Vitamin B_{12} is present in animal-based foods, such as the turkey in your sandwich.

The chief cells secrete the following:

■ *Pepsinogen,* an inactive enzyme, which HCl converts into the active enzyme *pepsin.* Like other protein-digesting enzymes, pepsin must be secreted in an inactive form, or it would begin to digest the cells that produced it. Once activated, pepsin begins the digestion of protein. It in turn activates many other GI enzymes that contribute to digesting your sandwich.

■ *Gastric lipase,* an enzyme active in lipid digestion. Although lingual lipase in the mouth and gastric lipase in the stomach begin to break apart the lipids in the turkey and mayonnaise in your sandwich, only minimal digestion of lipids occurs until they reach the small intestine.

The stomach also plays a role in mechanical digestion, by mixing and churning the food with the gastric juice until it becomes a liquid called **chyme.** This mechanical digestion facilitates chemical digestion, because enzymes can access the liquid chyme more easily than solid forms of food.

Despite the acidity of gastric juice, the stomach itself is not eroded because *mucous neck cells* in gastric glands and *mucous surface cells* in the stomach lining secrete a protective layer of mucus (**Figure 3.10**). Any disruption of this mucus barrier can cause gastritis (inflammation of the stomach lining) or an ulcer (a condition that is discussed later in this chapter). Other lining cells secrete bicarbonate, a base, which neutralizes acid near the surface of the stomach's lining.

Although most absorption occurs in the small intestine, some substances are absorbed through the stomach lining and into the blood. These include water, fluoride, some lipids, and some lipid-soluble drugs, including aspirin and alcohol.

chyme A semifluid mass consisting of partially digested food, water, and gastric juices.

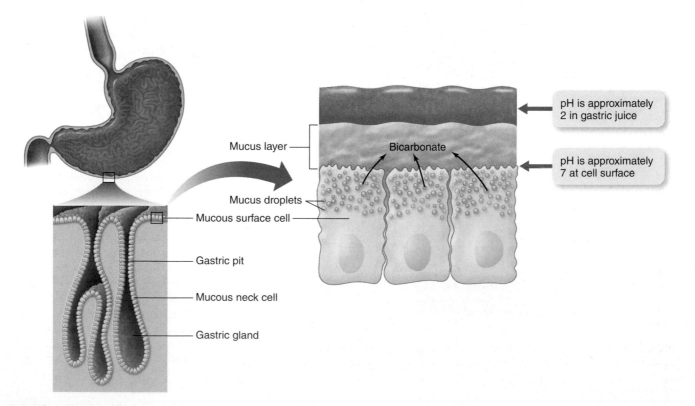

Mucus layer

Bicarbonate

pH is approximately 2 in gastric juice

pH is approximately 7 at cell surface

Mucus droplets

Mucous surface cell

Gastric pit

Mucous neck cell

Gastric gland

FIGURE 3.10 The stomach is protected from the acidity of gastric juice by a layer of mucus.

Another of the stomach's jobs is to store chyme while the next part of the digestive tract, the small intestine, gets ready for the food. Remember that the capacity of the stomach is about 1 gallon. If this amount of chyme were to move into the small intestine all at once, it would overwhelm it. Chyme stays in the stomach for about 2 hours before it is released periodically in spurts into the duodenum, which is the first part of the small intestine. Regulating this release is the *pyloric sphincter* (see Figure 3.8).

Most Digestion and Absorption Occurs in the Small Intestine

The **small intestine** is the longest portion of the GI tract, accounting for about two-thirds of its length. However, at only an inch in diameter, it is comparatively narrow.

The small intestine is composed of three sections (**Figure 3.11**). The *duodenum* is the section of the small intestine that is connected via the pyloric sphincter to the stomach. The *jejunum* is the middle portion, and the last portion is the *ileum*. It connects to the large intestine at another sphincter, called the *ileocecal valve*.

Most digestion and absorption take place in the small intestine. Here, the carbohydrates, lipids, and proteins in your turkey sandwich are broken down into their smallest components, molecules that the body can then absorb into the circulation. Digestion and absorption are achieved in the small intestine through the actions of enzymes, accessory organs (the pancreas, gallbladder, and liver), and some unique anatomical features. The details of these actions are discussed in the following sections in this chapter. Once digestion and absorption are completed in the small intestine, the residue is passed into the large intestine.

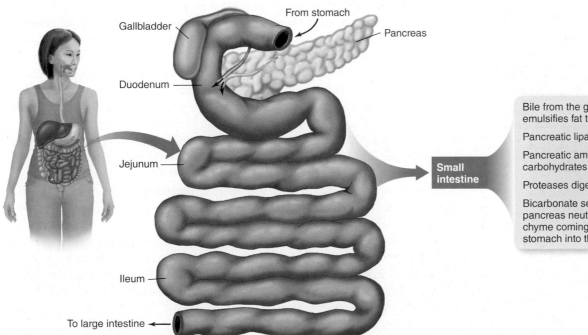

FIGURE 3.11 Where your food is now: the small intestine. Here, most of the digestion and absorption of the nutrients in your sandwich takes place.

The Large Intestine Stores Food Waste Until It Is Excreted

The **large intestine** is a thick, tubelike structure that frames the small intestine on three and one-half sides (**Figure 3.12**). It begins with a tissue sac called the *cecum*, which explains the name of the sphincter—the *ileocecal valve*—which connects it to the ileum of the small intestine. From the cecum, the large intestine continues up along the right side of the small intestine as the *ascending colon*. The *transverse colon* runs across the top of

small intestine The longest portion of the GI tract, where most digestion and absorption takes place.

large intestine The final organ of the GI tract, consisting of the cecum, colon, rectum, and anal canal and in which most water is absorbed and feces are formed.

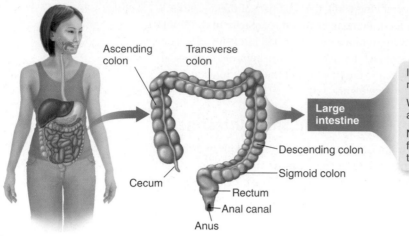

Ascending colon

Transverse colon

Large intestine

Intestinal bacteria digest any remaining food particles

Water and chemicals are absorbed into the bloodstream

Non-digestible matter forms feces, which are excreted through the rectum

Descending colon

Sigmoid colon

Cecum

Rectum

Anal canal

Anus

FIGURE 3.12 Where your food is now: the large intestine. Most water absorption occurs here, as does the formation of food wastes into semisolid feces.

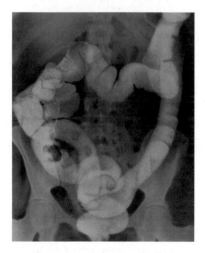

The large intestine is a thick, tubelike structure that stores the undigested mass leaving the small intestine and absorbs any remaining nutrients and water.

the small intestine, and then the *descending colon* comes down on the left. These regions of the colon are characterized by *haustra*, regular, saclike segmentations that contract to move food toward the *sigmoid colon*, which extends from the bottom left corner to the *rectum*. The last segment of the large intestine is the *anal canal*, which is about 1½ inches long.

What has happened to our turkey sandwich? The residue that finally reaches the large intestine bears little resemblance to the chyme that left the stomach several hours before. This is because a majority of the nutrients have been absorbed, leaving mostly water and indigestible food material, such as the outer husks of the tomato seeds and the fibers in the lettuce.

The GI tract hosts a population of trillions of bacterial cells, more than the number of cells making up the human body. Collectively called the *GI flora*, most of these live in the large intestine, where they perform several beneficial functions. First, they finish digesting some of the nutrients remaining in food residues. The by-products of this bacterial digestion are reabsorbed into the body, where they return to the liver and are either stored or used as needed. In addition, the GI flora ferment fibrous wastes, producing certain vitamins that are absorbed by the large intestine. The GI flora are also thought to stimulate the immune system, inhibit the growth of harmful bacteria, and reduce the risk for diarrhea. In fact, these bacteria are so helpful that they are referred to as **probiotics,** meaning "for life."[2] For more information on the role of probiotics in human health, see the ***Nutrition Myth or Fact?*** essay at the end of this chapter.

No other digestion occurs in the large intestine. Instead, it stores the digestive mass for 12 to 24 hours, absorbing water, lipid breakdown products, and electrolytes and leaving a semisolid mass called *feces*. Peristalsis occurs weakly to move the feces through the colon, except for one or more stronger waves of peristalsis each day that force the feces more powerfully toward the rectum for elimination.

RECAP

Gastric glands in the stomach secrete gastric juice, which contains hydrochloric acid, the enzymes pepsin and gastric lipase, and intrinsic factor. Bicarbonate and mucus protect the stomach lining from erosion. The stomach mixes food into a substance called chyme, which is released periodically through the pyloric sphincter into the small intestine, where most digestion and absorption occurs. Bicarbonate, bile, and a variety of digestive enzymes play important roles in the process. Small amounts of undigested food, nondigestible food material, and water enter the large intestine. Bacteria in the colon assist with the final digestion of any remaining food particles. The remaining semisolid mass, called feces, is then eliminated from the body.

probiotics Microorganisms, typically bacteria, theorized to benefit human health.

How Does the Body Accomplish Chemical Digestion?

 Identify the primary role of enzymes and of hormones in accomplishing chemical digestion.

 Discuss the roles of the gallbladder, pancreas, and liver in accomplishing chemical digestion.

Now that you have learned about the structure and functions of the GI tract, you are ready to delve more deeply into the specific activities of the various enzymes, hormones, and accessory organs involved in chemical digestion.

Enzymes and Hormones Play Roles in Digestion

Enzymes are released into the gastrointestinal tract as needed, in a process controlled by the nervous system and various hormones. Upon release, they catalyze **hydrolysis** reactions, chemical reactions that break down substances by the addition of water. In this process, which is described in detail in Chapter 7, a reactant—such as a portion of a protein—is broken down into two products.

We've introduced a few digestive enzymes produced in the mouth and stomach, but most are synthesized by the pancreas and small intestine. **Table 3.1** lists many of the enzymes that play a critical role in digestion and specifies where they are produced and their primary actions. Enzymes are usually specific to the substance they act upon, and this is true for the digestive enzymes. You can see in this table enzymes specific to the digestion of carbohydrates, lipids, and proteins, all of which are too large to be directly absorbed from the gastrointestinal tract. In contrast, subunits of the energy nutrients, as well as water, vitamins, minerals, and alcohol, do not require enzymatic digestion and can be absorbed in their original form.

TABLE 3.1 Digestive Enzymes Produced in the Gastrointestinal Tract and Their Actions

Organ Where Produced	Enzyme	Site of Action	Primary Action
Mouth	Salivary amylase Lingual lipase	Mouth	Digests carbohydrates Digests lipids
Stomach	Pepsin Gastric lipase	Stomach	Digests proteins Digests lipids
Pancreas	Proteases (trypsin, chymotrypsin, carboxypolypeptidase) Elastase Pancreatic lipase Cholesterol esterase Pancreatic amylase (amylase)	Small intestine	Digest proteins Digests fibrous proteins Digests lipids Digests cholesterol Digests carbohydrates
Small intestine	Carboxypeptidase, aminopeptidase, dipeptidase Lipase Sucrase, maltase, and lactase	Small intestine	Digest proteins Digests lipids Digest the simple carbohydrates sucrose, maltose, and lactose

Regulation of gastrointestinal function involves the action of more than 80 hormones and hormone-like substances. We identified a few of the hormones involved in hunger and satiety earlier in this chapter. **Table 3.2** identifies those important in regulating digestion. These are gastrin, secretin, CCK (which we met earlier), gastric inhibitory peptide (GIP), and somatostatin.

Accessory Organs Produce, Store, and Secrete Chemicals That Aid in Digestion

Along with the salivary glands, the gallbladder, pancreas, and liver are considered accessory organs of digestion. As you will learn in the following sections, these organs are critical to the production, storage, and secretion of enzymes and other substances involved in chemical digestion.

hydrolysis A chemical reaction that breaks down substances by the addition of water.

TABLE 3.2 Hormones Involved in the Regulation of Digestion

Hormone	Production Site	Target Organ	Actions
Gastrin	Stomach	Stomach	Stimulates secretion of HCl and pepsinogen (inactive form of pepsin) Stimulates gastric motility Promotes proliferation of gastric mucosal cells
Secretin	Small intestine (duodenum)	Pancreas Stomach	Stimulates secretion of pancreatic bicarbonate (which neutralizes acidic chyme) Decreases gastric motility
Cholecystokinin (CCK)	Small intestine (duodenum and jejunum)	Pancreas Gallbladder Stomach	Stimulates secretion of pancreatic digestive enzymes Stimulates gallbladder contraction Slows gastric emptying
Gastric inhibitory peptide (GIP)	Small intestine	Stomach Pancreas	Inhibits gastric juice secretion Slows gastric emptying Stimulates insulin release
Somatostatin	Stomach Small intestine Pancreas	Stomach Small Intestine Pancreas	Inhibits release of gastrin and slows gastric emptying Inhibits release of secretin, CCK, and GIP and reduces smooth muscle contraction in the small intestine Inhibits release of pancreatic hormones and digestive enzymes

gallbladder A pear-shaped organ beneath the liver that stores bile and secretes it into the small intestine.

bile Fluid produced by the liver and stored in the gallbladder; it emulsifies lipids in the small intestine.

pancreas A gland located behind the stomach that secretes digestive enzymes.

Nutrition
MILESTONE

Does bile act like soap? As long ago as

1767, a French pharmacist by the name of Cadet presented a chemical analysis of bile to the French Academy, in which he described bile as an "animal soap." Before the close of the century, the French chemist de Fourcroy had repeated Cadet's experiments and confirmed his results: bile caused fatty substances to combine with water in much the same way soap does! Even today, bile from oxen and other animals is mixed with other ingredients to produce bile soap, various preparations of which are marketed for laundry use and even for skin care.

The Gallbladder Stores Bile

Cholecystokinin (CCK), which is released in the small intestine in response to the presence of proteins and lipids, signals the **gallbladder** to contract. The gallbladder is located beneath the liver (see Focus Figure 3.3) and stores a greenish fluid, **bile,** produced by the liver. Contraction of the gallbladder sends bile through the *common bile duct* into the duodenum. Bile then *emulsifies* the lipids; that is, it breaks the lipids into smaller globules and disperses them, so that they are more accessible to digestive enzymes.

The Pancreas Produces Enzymes, Hormones, and Bicarbonate

The **pancreas** manufactures, holds, and secretes digestive enzymes. It is located behind the stomach (see Focus Figure 3.3). The pancreas stores these enzymes in their inactive forms, and they are activated in the small intestine; this is important because, if the enzymes were active in the pancreas, they would facilitate digestion of the pancreas. Enzymes secreted by the pancreas include *pancreatic amylase, pancreatic lipase,* and *proteases,* which catalyze the digestion of carbohydrates, lipids, and proteins.

The pancreas is also responsible for manufacturing insulin and glucagon, hormones mentioned earlier for their roles in hunger and satiety. Both hormones are important in regulating the amount of glucose in the blood.

Another essential role of the pancreas is to secrete bicarbonate into the duodenum. As noted earlier, bicarbonate is a base, whereas chyme leaving the stomach is very acidic. The pancreatic bicarbonate neutralizes this acidic chyme. This allows the pancreatic enzymes to work effectively and ensures that the lining of the duodenum is not eroded. The first portion of the duodenum is also protected by mucus produced by special glands.

The Liver Produces Bile and Regulates Blood Nutrients

The **liver** is a triangular-shaped organ of about 3 lb of tissue that rests almost entirely within the protection of the rib cage on the right side of the body (see Focus Figure 3.3). It is the largest digestive organ; it is also one of the most important organs in the body, performing more than 500 discrete functions. One important job of the liver is to synthesize many of the chemicals the body uses in carrying out metabolic processes. For example, the liver synthesizes bile, which, as we just discussed, is then stored in the gallbladder until needed for the emulsification of lipids.

Another important function of the liver is to receive the products of digestion. Lipids and fat-soluble vitamins are absorbed from the GI tract into a tissue fluid called lymph, which is drained by lymphatic vessels that eventually release into the bloodstream. Other nutrients are water-soluble and are absorbed into capillaries (microscopic blood vessels) that drain into the **portal venous system** (**Figure 3.13**). This specialized group of veins drains blood from parts of the stomach, spleen, pancreas, and small and large intestines into a large, central vein, the hepatic portal vein (*hepatic* refers to the liver). This allows absorbed nutrients to be transported to the liver for processing before the blood delivers them into the general circulation. After the liver removes the digestion products from the bloodstream, it can process them for storage or release back into the bloodstream those that are needed elsewhere in the body.

For instance, after we eat a meal, the liver picks up excess glucose from the blood and stores it as glycogen, releasing it into the bloodstream when we need energy later in the day. It also stores certain vitamins and manufactures blood proteins. The liver can even make glucose when necessary to ensure that our blood levels stay constant. Thus, the liver plays a major role in regulating the level and type of fuel circulating in our blood.

Have you ever wondered why people who abuse alcohol are at risk for liver damage? That's because another of its functions is to remove from the blood wastes and toxins such as alcohol, medications, and other drugs. When you drink, your liver works hard to replace the cells poisoned with alcohol, but over time scar tissue forms. The scar tissue blocks the free flow of blood through the liver, so any further toxins accumulate in the blood, causing confusion, coma, and, ultimately death. (Alcohol is discussed **In Depth 4.5** on pages 152–163.)

liver The largest accessory organ of the GI tract and one of the most important organs of the body. Its functions include the production of bile and processing of nutrient-rich blood from the small intestine.

portal venous system A system of blood vessels that drains blood and various products of digestion from the digestive organs and spleen and delivers them to the liver.

FIGURE 3.13 The portal venous system is a group of veins that drains regions of the digestive system and transports the blood to the liver. There, the blood is filtered through liver cells, which detoxify alcohol and other harmful agents, as well as use or store nutrients or package them before releasing them back into the general circulation for delivery to distant body cells.

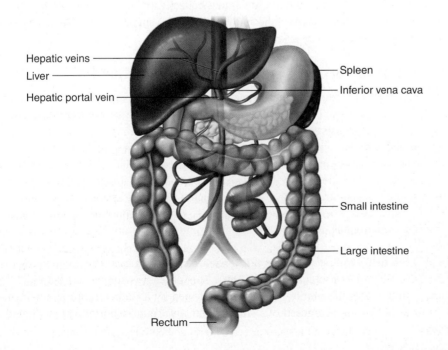

Hepatic veins
Liver
Hepatic portal vein
Spleen
Inferior vena cava
Small intestine
Large intestine
Rectum

RECAP

Enzymes speed up the digestion of food through hydrolysis. Hormones act as chemical messengers to regulate digestion. The digestive accessory organs include the gallbladder, pancreas, and liver. The gallbladder stores bile, which is produced by the liver. Bile emulsifies lipids into droplets that are more easily accessed by digestive enzymes. The pancreas synthesizes and secretes digestive enzymes, the hormones insulin and glucagon, and bicarbonate. The liver synthesizes bile, processes nutrients absorbed from the small intestine, regulates blood glucose levels, and stores glucose as glycogen. ■

LO 6 Explain how the anatomy of the small intestine's lining contributes to its absorptive function.

LO 7 List and describe the four types of absorption that occur in the small intestine.

How Does the Body Absorb and Transport Digested Nutrients?

Although some nutrient absorption occurs in the stomach and large intestine, the majority occurs in the small intestine. Its extensive surface area and specialized absorptive cells enables the small intestine to handle this responsibility.

A Specialized Lining Enables the Small Intestine to Absorb Food

The lining of the small intestine is especially well suited for absorption. If you were to examine the inside of the lining, which is also referred to as the *mucosal membrane*, you would notice that it is heavily folded (**Focus Figure 3.14**). This feature increases the surface area of the small intestine, allowing it to absorb more nutrients than if it were smooth.

Within these larger folds, you would notice even smaller, finger-like projections called *villi*, whose constant movement helps them encounter and trap nutrient molecules. The villi are composed of numerous specialized absorptive cells called **enterocytes.** Inside each villus are capillaries and a **lacteal,** which is a small lymphatic vessel. The capillaries and lacteals absorb some of the end products of digestion. Water-soluble nutrients are absorbed directly into the bloodstream, whereas fat-soluble nutrients are absorbed into lymph. Each enterocyte of each villus has hairlike projections called *microvilli.* The microvilli look like tiny brushes and are sometimes collectively referred to as the **brush border.** These intricate folds increase the surface area of the small intestine tremendously, increasing its absorptive capacity as well.

enterocytes Specialized absorptive cells in the villi of the small intestine.

lacteal A small lymphatic vessel located inside the villi of the small intestine.

brush border The microvilli of the small intestine's lining. These microvilli tremendously increase the small intestine's absorptive capacity.

passive diffusion A transport process in which ions and molecules, following their concentration gradient, cross the cell membrane without the use of a carrier protein or the requirement of energy.

facilitated diffusion A transport process in which ions and molecules are shuttled across the cell membrane with the help of a carrier protein.

Four Types of Absorption Occur in the Small Intestine

Nutrients are absorbed across the mucosal membrane and into the bloodstream or lymph via four mechanisms: passive diffusion, facilitated diffusion, active transport, and endocytosis. These are illustrated in **Figure 3.15** (page 92).

Passive diffusion is a simple process in which nutrients cross into the enterocytes without the use of a carrier protein or the requirement of energy (Figure 3.15a). Passive diffusion can occur when the wall of the intestine is permeable to the nutrient and the concentration of the nutrient in the GI tract is higher than its concentration in the enterocytes. Thus, the nutrient is moving from an area of higher concentration to an area of lower concentration. Lipids, water, vitamin C, and some minerals are absorbed via passive diffusion.

Facilitated diffusion occurs when nutrients are shuttled across the enterocytes with the help of a carrier protein (Figure 3.15b). This process is similar to passive diffusion in that it does not require energy and is driven by a concentration gradient. Fructose (a carbohydrate composed of a single sugar unit) is transported via facilitated diffusion.

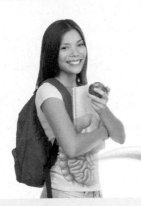

The small intestine is highly adapted for absorbing nutrients. Its length—about 20 feet—provides a huge surface area, and its wall has three structural features—circular folds, villi, and microvilli—that increase its surface area by a factor of more than 600.

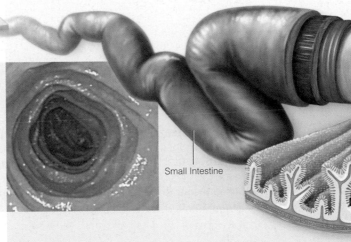

Small Intestine

CIRCULAR FOLDS

The lining of the small intestine is heavily folded, resulting in increased surface area for the absorption of nutrients.

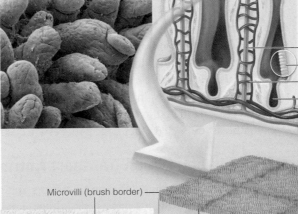

Villi

Lacteal
Enterocyte
Capillaries
Crypt

VILLI

The folds are covered with villi, thousands of finger-like projections that increase the surface area even further. Each villus contains capillaries and a lacteal for picking up nutrients absorbed through the enterocytes and transporting them throughout the

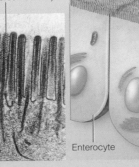

Microvilli (brush border)

MICROVILLI

The cells on the surface of the villi, enterocytes, end in hairlike projections called microvilli that together form the brush border through which nutrients are absorbed.

Enterocyte

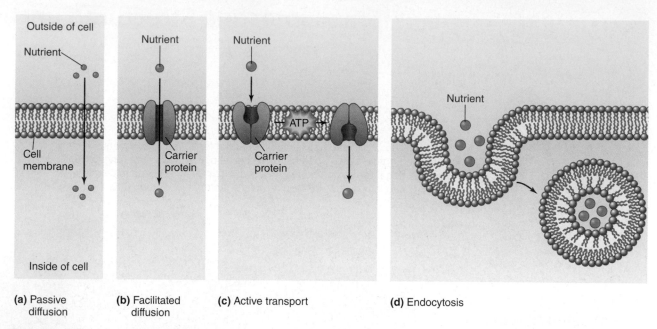

(a) Passive diffusion

(b) Facilitated diffusion

(c) Active transport

(d) Endocytosis

FIGURE 3.15 The four types of absorption that occur in the small intestine. **(a)** In passive diffusion, nutrients at a higher concentration outside the cells diffuse along their concentration gradient into the enterocytes without the use of a carrier protein or the requirement of energy. **(b)** In facilitated diffusion, nutrients are shuttled across the enterocytes with the help of a carrier protein without the use of energy. **(c)** In active transport, energy is used along with a carrier protein to transport nutrients against their concentration gradient. **(d)** In endocytosis, a small amount of the intestinal contents is engulfed by the cell membrane of the enterocyte and released into the interior of the cell.

Active transport requires the use of energy to transport nutrients in combination with a carrier protein (Figure 3.15c). The energy, which is derived from adenosine triphosphate (ATP), and the assistance of the carrier protein allow for the absorption of nutrients against their concentration gradient, meaning the nutrients can move from areas of low to high concentration. Glucose, amino acids, and certain minerals are among the nutrients absorbed via active transport. In addition to being absorbed via passive diffusion, vitamin C can be absorbed via active transport.

Endocytosis (also called pinocytosis) is a form of active transport by which a small amount of the intestinal contents is engulfed by the enterocyte's cell membrane and incorporated into the cell (Figure 3.15d). Some proteins, including the antibodies contained in breast milk, and other large particles are absorbed in this way.

Blood and Lymph Transport Nutrients and Wastes

Two circulating fluids transport nutrients and waste products throughout the body: blood travels through the cardiovascular system, and lymph travels through the lymphatic system (**Figure 3.16**). The oxygen we inhale into our lungs is carried by our red blood cells. This oxygen-rich blood then travels to the heart, where it is pumped out to the body. Blood travels to all of our tissues to deliver oxygen, nutrients, and other materials and to pick up carbon dioxide and other waste products. In the enterocytes, blood in the capillaries picks up water and water-soluble nutrients, and lymph in the lacteals picks up most lipids and fat-soluble vitamins, as well as any fluids that have escaped from the blood capillaries. Lymph nodes are clusters of immune cells that filter microbes and other harmful agents from the lymph fluid (see Figure 3.16). The lymph eventually returns to the bloodstream in an area near the heart where the lymphatic and blood vessels join together.

active transport A transport process that requires the use of energy to shuttle ions and molecules across the cell membrane in combination with a carrier protein.

endocytosis A transport process in which ions and molecules are engulfed by the cell membrane, which folds inwardly and is released in the cell interior (also called pinocytosis).

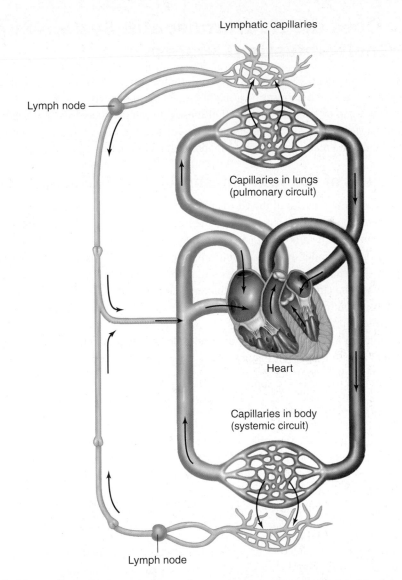

FIGURE 3.16 Blood travels through the cardiovascular system to transport nutrients and fluids and to pick up waste products. Lymph travels through the lymphatic system and transports most lipids and fat-soluble vitamins.

As discussed earlier, when blood leaves the GI system, it is transported via the portal venous system to the liver. The waste products picked up by the blood as it circulates around the body are filtered and excreted by the kidneys. In addition, much of the carbon dioxide remaining in the blood, once it reaches the lungs, is exhaled into the outside air, making room for oxygen to attach to the red blood cells and repeat this cycle of circulation again.

RECAP

The folded mucosal membrane of the small intestine contains multiple villi and microvilli that significantly increase absorptive capacity. Nutrients are absorbed through one of four mechanisms: passive diffusion, facilitated diffusion, active transport, and endocytosis. Most nutrients and waste products are absorbed into capillaries and transported throughout the body in the bloodstream, whereas lipids and fat-soluble vitamins are absorbed into lacteals and transported through lymph, which is eventually released into the cardiovascular system. ◼

LO 8 Identify three gastrointestinal tract movements and three divisions of the nervous system that contribute to gastrointestinal function.

How Does the Neuromuscular System Support the Gastrointestinal System?

Now that you can identify the organs involved in digestion and absorption and the complex tasks they each perform, you might be wondering—who's the boss? In other words, what organ or system controls all of these interrelated processes? The answer is the neuromuscular system. Its two components, nerves and muscles, partner to coordinate and regulate the digestion and absorption of food and the elimination of waste.

The Muscles of the Gastrointestinal Tract Mix and Move Food

To view an animation explaining peristalsis, visit MedlinePlus at http://www .nlm.nih.gov. Go to the Medlinline Plus link, click on the "Videos & Cool Tools" button, then the "Anatomy Videos" link and choose "Peristalsis" to begin!

The purposes of the muscles of the GI tract are to mix food, ensure efficient digestion and optimal absorption of nutrients, and move the intestinal contents from the mouth toward the anus. Once we swallow a bolus of food, peristalsis begins in the esophagus and continues throughout the remainder of the gastrointestinal tract. Peristalsis is accomplished through the actions of circular muscles and longitudinal muscles that run along the entire GI tract (**Figure 3.17a**). The circular and longitudinal muscles continuously contract and relax, causing subsequent constriction and bulging of the tract. This action pushes the contents from one area to the next.

The stomach is surrounded by its own set of longitudinal, circular, and diagonal muscles that assist in digestion (**Figure 3.18**). These muscles alternately contract and relax, churning the stomach contents and moving them toward the pyloric sphincter. The pyloric sphincter stays closed while gastric juices are secreted and the chyme is mixed. Once the chyme is completely liquefied, the pyloric sphincter is stimulated to open, and small amounts of chyme are regularly released into the small intestine.

segmentation Rhythmic contraction of the circular muscles of the small intestine, which squeezes chyme, mixes it, and enhances the digestion and absorption of nutrients from the chyme.

In the small intestine, a unique pattern of motility called **segmentation** occurs (see Figure 3.17b). Segmentation, accomplished by the rhythmic contraction of circular muscles in the intestinal wall, squeezes the chyme, mixes it, and enhances its contact with digestive enzymes and enterocytes.

haustration Involuntary, sluggish contraction of the haustra of the proximal colon, which moves wastes toward the sigmoid colon.

The colon also exhibits uncoordinated movements called **haustration.** As each haustrum fills with chyme, its distention stimulates sluggish contractions that move wastes

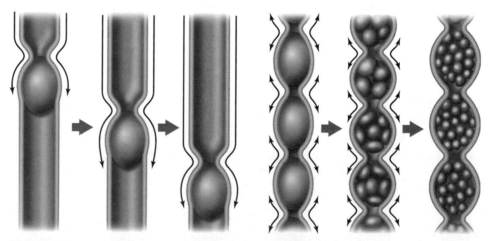

(a) Peristalsis   (b) Segmentation

FIGURE 3.17 Peristalsis and segmentation. **(a)** Peristalsis occurs through the actions of circular muscles and longitudinal muscles that run along the entire GI tract. These muscles continuously contract and relax, causing subsequent constriction and bulging of the tract, which pushes the intestinal contents from one area to the next. **(b)** Segmentation occurs through the rhythmic contraction of the circular muscles of the small intestine. This action squeezes the chyme, mixes it, and enhances its contact with digestive enzymes and enterocytes.

into the next haustrum and toward the sigmoid colon. However, two or more times each day, a much stronger and more sustained **mass movement** of the colon occurs, pushing wastes forcibly toward the rectum.

The muscles of the GI tract contract at varying rates, depending on their location and whether or not food is present. The stomach tends to contract more slowly, about three times per minute, whereas the small intestine may contract up to ten times per minute when chyme is present. The contractions of haustra are slow, occurring at a rate of about two per hour. As with an assembly line, the entire GI tract functions together, so that materials are moved in one direction, absorption of nutrients is maximized, and wastes are removed as needed.

In order to process the large amount of food we consume daily, we use both voluntary and involuntary muscles. Muscles in the mouth are primarily voluntary; that is, they are under our conscious control. Once we swallow, the involuntary muscles just described largely take over to propel food through the rest of the GI tract. This enables us to continue digesting and absorbing food while we're working, exercising, and even sleeping. We're now ready to identify the master controller behind these involuntary muscular actions.

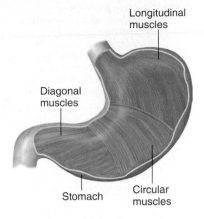

FIGURE 3.18 The stomach has longitudinal, circular, and diagonal muscles. These three sets of muscles aid digestion by alternately contracting and relaxing; these actions churn the stomach contents and move them toward the pyloric sphincter.

Nerves Control the Contractions and Secretions of the Gastrointestinal Tract

The contractions and secretions of the gastrointestinal tract are controlled by three types of nerves:

- The **enteric nervous system (ENS),** which is localized in the wall of the GI tract, and is part of the autonomic nervous system, the division of the peripheral nervous system (PNS) that regulates many internal functions
- Other branches of the autonomic nervous system outside the GI tract
- The central nervous system (CNS), which includes the brain and spinal cord

Some digestive functions are carried out entirely within the ENS. For instance, the control of peristalsis and segmentation is enteric, occurring without assistance from beyond the GI tract. In addition, enteric nerves regulate the secretions of the various digestive glands whose roles we have discussed in this chapter.

Enteric nerves also work in collaboration with the rest of the PNS and the CNS. For example, we noted earlier in this chapter that, in response to fasting, receptors in the stomach and intestinal walls (ENS receptors) stimulate peripheral nerves to signal the hypothalamus, part of the CNS. We then experience the sensation of hunger.

Finally, some functions, such as the secretion of saliva, are achieved without enteric involvement. A variety of stimuli from the smell, sight, taste, and tactile sensations from food trigger special salivary cells in the CNS; these cells then stimulate increased activity of the salivary glands.

RECAP

The coordination and regulation of digestion are directed by the neuromuscular system. Voluntary muscles assist us with chewing and swallowing. Once food is swallowed, involuntary muscles of the GI tract function together, so that materials are processed in a coordinated manner. Involuntary movements include the mixing and churning of chyme by muscles in the stomach wall, as well as peristalsis, segmentation, haustration, and mass movement. The enteric nerves of the GI tract work with the rest of the peripheral nervous system and the central nervous system to achieve the digestion, absorption, and elimination of food.

mass movement Involuntary, sustained, forceful contraction of the colon that occurs two or more times a day to push wastes toward the rectum.

enteric nervous system (ENS) The autonomic nerves in the walls of the GI tract.

LO 9 Describe the causes, symptoms, and treatments of gastroesophageal reflux disease, peptic ulcers, food allergies, celiac disease, vomiting, inflammatory bowel diseases, and functional gastrointestinal disorders.

LO 10 Compare the incidence of colorectal cancer with that of other cancers of the gastrointestinal system, and explain the role of screening in reducing colorectal cancer deaths.

What Disorders Are Related to Digestion, Absorption, and Elimination?

Considering the complexity of digestion, absorption, and elimination, it's no wonder that sometimes things go wrong. Disorders of the neuromuscular system, hormonal imbalances, infections, allergies, and a host of other disorders can disturb gastrointestinal functioning, as can merely consuming the wrong types or amounts of food for our unique needs. Whenever there is a problem with the GI tract, the absorption of nutrients can be affected. If absorption of a nutrient is less than optimal for a long period of time, malnutrition can result. Let's look more closely at some GI tract disorders and what you might be able to do if they affect you.

Belching and Flatulence Are Common

Many people complain of problems with belching (eructation) and/or flatulence (passage of intestinal gas). The primary cause of belching is swallowed air. Eating too fast, wearing improperly fitting dentures, chewing gum, sucking on hard candies or a drinking straw, and gulping food or fluid can increase the risk of swallowing air. To prevent or reduce belching, avoid these behaviors.

Although many people find *flatus* (intestinal gas) uncomfortable and embarrassing, its presence in the GI tract is completely normal, as is its expulsion. Flatus is a mixture of many gases, including nitrogen, hydrogen, oxygen, methane, and carbon dioxide. Interestingly, all of these are odorless. It is only when flatus contains sulfur that it causes the embarrassing odor associated with flatulence.

Foods most commonly reported to cause flatus include those rich in fibers, starches, and sugars, such as beans, dairy products, and some vegetables. The partially digested carbohydrates from these foods pass into the large intestine, where they are fermented by bacteria, producing gas. Other food products that may cause flatus, intestinal cramps, and diarrhea include products made with the fat substitute olestra, sugar alcohols, and quorn (a meat substitute made from fungus).

Because many of the foods that can cause flatus are healthful, it is important not to avoid them. Eating smaller portions can help reduce the amount of flatus produced and passed. In addition, products such as Beano can offer some relief. Beano is an over-the-counter supplement that contains alpha-galactosidase, an enzyme that digests the complex sugars in gas-producing foods.

Heartburn and Gastroesophageal Reflux Disease (GERD) Are Caused by Reflux of Gastric Juice

We noted earlier that, even as you're chewing your first bite of food, your stomach is beginning to secrete gastric juice to prepare for digestion. When you swallow, the food is propelled along the esophagus, and the gastroesophageal sphincter relaxes to permit it to enter the stomach. As this occurs, it's normal for a small amount of gastric juice to flow "backwards" into the lower esophagus for a moment. This phenomenon is technically known as gastroesophageal reflux, or GER.

However, in some people, peristalsis in the esophagus is weak and the food exits too slowly, or the gastroesophageal sphincter is overly relaxed and stays partially open, allowing too much gastric juice to enter the esophagus. In either case, the result is that gastric juice isn't cleared from the lower esophagus quickly and completely.

Although the stomach is protected from the highly acidic gastric juice by a thick coat of mucus, the esophagus does not have this coating. Thus, the gastric juice burns it (**Figure 3.19**). When this happens, the person experiences a painful sensation in the region of the chest behind the sternum (breastbone). This symptom is commonly called **heartburn.** Many people take over-the-counter antacids to raise the pH of the gastric juice, thereby relieving the heartburn. A nondrug approach is to repeatedly swallow: this action causes

For reliable information on dozens of common GI disorders, visit the National Institute of Diabetes and Digestive and Kidney Diseases at http://www.niddk.nih.gov. **Go to the Health Information tab, click on the "Health Topics" link, and click on "Digestive Diseases."**

heartburn The painful sensation that occurs over the sternum when gastric juice backs up into the lower esophagus.

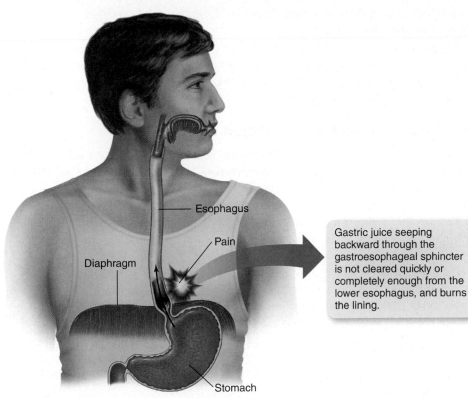

Esophagus

Pain

Diaphragm

Gastric juice seeping backward through the gastroesophageal sphincter is not cleared quickly or completely enough from the lower esophagus, and burns the lining.

Stomach

FIGURE 3.19 The mechanism of heartburn and gastroesophageal reflux disease is the same: acidic gastric juices seep backward through an open, or relaxed, sphincter into the lower portion of the esophagus and pool there, burning its lining. The pain is felt above the sternum, over the heart.

any acid pooled in the esophagus to be swept down into the stomach, eventually relieving the symptoms.

Occasional heartburn is common and not a cause for concern; however, heartburn is also the most common symptom of **gastroesophageal reflux disease (GERD),** a chronic disease in which episodes of GER cause heartburn or other symptoms more than twice per week. These other symptoms of GERD include chest pain, trouble swallowing, burning in the mouth, the feeling that food is stuck in the throat, wheezing, and hoarseness.[3]

The exact causes of GERD are unknown. However, a number of factors may contribute, including the following:[3]

- A hiatal hernia, which occurs when the upper part of the stomach lies above the diaphragm muscle. Normally, the horizontal diaphragm muscle separates the stomach from the chest cavity and helps keep gastric juice from seeping into the esophagus. Gastric juice can more easily enter the esophagus in people with a hiatal hernia.
- Cigarette smoking or inhaling secondhand smoke
- Overweight and obesity
- Pregnancy
- Certain medications, including sedatives, pain relievers, antidepressants, asthma medications, and many antihistamines

One way to reduce the symptoms of GERD is to identify the types of foods or situations that trigger episodes, and then avoid them. Eating smaller meals also helps. After a meal, stay upright for at least 3 hours. This keeps the chest area elevated and minimizes the amount of acid that can back up into the esophagus. People with GERD who smoke should stop, and, if they are overweight, they should lose weight. Taking an antacid before a meal

gastroesophageal reflux disease (GERD) A painful type of heartburn that occurs more than twice per week.

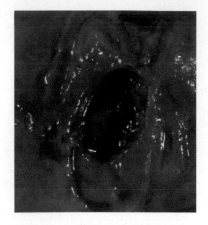

FIGURE 3.20 A peptic ulcer.

can help prevent symptoms, and many other over-the-counter and prescription medications are now available to treat GERD.

It is important to treat GERD, as it can lead to bleeding and ulcers in the esophagus. Scar tissue can develop in the esophagus, making swallowing very difficult. Some people with GERD develop a condition called Barrett's esophagus, which can lead to cancer. Asthma can also be aggravated or even caused by GERD.

A Peptic Ulcer Is an Area of Erosion in the GI Tract

A **peptic ulcer** is an area of the GI tract that has been eroded away by a combination of hydrochloric acid and the enzyme pepsin (**Figure 3.20**). In almost all cases, it is located in the stomach area (*gastric ulcer*) or the part of the duodenum closest to the stomach (*duodenal ulcer*). It causes a burning pain in the abdominal area, typically 1 to 3 hours after eating a meal. Complications include stomach obstruction, internal bleeding, or perforation of the ulcer through the GI tract wall and life-threatening infection.[4]

The bacterium *Helicobacter pylori (H. pylori)* plays a key role in the development of most peptic ulcers.[4] *H. pylori* infection is common in children, and appears to be a beneficial member of our GI flora, offering some protection against asthma and allergies, GERD, and even obesity;[5,6] moreover, the great majority of people with *H. pylori* infection do not develop ulcers. For this reason, eradication of the bacterium in children is not advised; however, in adults with *H. pylori* infection and symptoms of a peptic ulcer, treatment includes antibiotics effective against the bacterium. In addition, antacids are used to buffer the acidity of gastric juice, and the same medications used to treat GERD can be used to treat peptic ulcers. Special diets are not recommended as often as they once were because they do not reduce acid secretion. In fact, we now know that ulcers are not caused by stress or spicy foods.

Although most peptic ulcers are caused by *H. pylori* infection, some are caused by a prolonged use of nonsteroidal anti-inflammatory drugs (NSAIDs), including the pain relievers aspirin and ibuprofen. Acetaminophen use does not cause ulcers. The NSAIDs appear to cause ulcers by preventing the stomach from protecting itself from acidic gastric juices.

RECAP

Belching is commonly caused by behaviors that cause us to swallow air. Foods that may cause flatulence include those rich in fibers, starches, and sugars. Heartburn is caused by the seepage of gastric juices into the esophagus. Gastroesophageal reflux disease (GERD) is a painful type of heartburn that occurs more than twice per week. Peptic ulcers are caused by erosion of the GI tract by hydrochloric acid and pepsin. The two major causes of peptic ulcers are *Helicobacter pylori* infection and the use of nonsteroidal anti-inflammatory drugs. ■

Some People Experience Disorders Related to Specific Foods

You check out the ingredients list on your energy bar, and you notice that it says "Produced in a facility that processes peanuts." The carton of soy milk you're drinking from proclaims "Gluten free!" What's all the fuss about? To some people, consuming certain food ingredients can be dangerous, even life-threatening. To learn more about product labeling for potential food offenders, see the ***Nutrition Label Activity*** box.

Disorders related to specific foods can be clustered into three main groupings: food intolerances, food allergies, and a genetic disorder called celiac disease. We discuss these separately.

peptic ulcer An area of the GI tract that has been eroded away by the acidic gastric juice of the stomach. The two main causes of peptic ulcers are *Helicobacter pylori* infection and the use of nonsteroidal anti-inflammatory drugs.

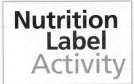

Recognizing Common Allergens in Foods

The US Food and Drug Administration (FDA) requires food labels to clearly identify any ingredients containing protein derived from the eight major allergenic foods.[1] Manufacturers must identify "in plain English" the presence of ingredients that contain protein derived from the following:

- Milk
- Eggs
- Fish
- Crustacean shellfish (crab, lobster, shrimp, and so on)
- Tree nuts (almonds, pecans, walnuts, and so on)
- Peanuts
- Wheat
- Soybeans

Although more than 160 foods have been identified as causing food allergies in sensitive individuals, the FDA requires labeling for only these eight foods because together they account for over 90% of all documented food allergies in the United States and represent the foods most likely to result in severe or life-threatening reactions.[1]

These eight allergenic foods must be indicated in the list of ingredients; alternatively, near the ingredients list, the label must say "Contains" followed by the name of the food. For example, the label of a product containing the milk-derived protein casein would have to use the term *milk* in addition to the term *casein*, so that those who have milk allergies would clearly understand the presence of an allergen they need to avoid.[1] Any food product found to contain an undeclared allergen is subject to recall by the FDA.

Look at the ingredients list from an energy bar, shown below, and answer the following questions:

- Which of the FDA's eight allergenic foods does this bar definitely contain?
- If you were allergic to peanuts, would eating this bar pose any risk to you?

  Yes or No
- If you were allergic to almonds, would eating this bar pose any risk to you?

  Yes or No

(Answers are located online in the MasteringNutrition Study Area.)

Ingredients: Soy protein isolate, rice flour, oats, milled flaxseed, brown rice syrup, evaporated cane juice, sunflower oil, soy lecithin, cocoa, nonfat milk solids, salt. **Contains soy and dairy. May contain traces of peanuts and other nuts.**

Reference

1. US Food and Drug Administration (FDA). 2014, October 23. Food Allergies: What You Need to Know. www.fda .gov/food/resourcesforyou/consumers/ucm079311.htm

---

Food Intolerance

A **food intolerance** is a cluster of GI symptoms (often gas, abdominal pain, and diarrhea) that occurs following consumption of a particular food. The immune system plays no role in intolerance, and although episodes are unpleasant, they are usually transient, resolving after the offending food has been eliminated from the body. An example is lactose intolerance. It occurs in people whose bodies do not produce sufficient quantities of the enzyme lactase, which facilitates the breakdown of the milk sugar lactose. (Lactose intolerance is discussed in more detail in Chapter 4.) People can also have an intolerance to wheat, soy, and other foods, but as with lactose intolerance, the symptoms pass once the offending food is out of the person's system.

Food Allergy

A **food allergy** is a hypersensitivity reaction of the immune system to a particular component (usually a protein) in a food. This reaction causes the immune cells to release chemicals that cause either limited or systemic (whole-body) inflammation. Although much less common than food intolerances, food allergies can be far more serious. In the United States, approximately 2% of adults and 4% to 8% of children have food allergies, and 150 to 200 Americans die each year because of allergic reactions to foods.[7]

> Watch a video explaining the problem of food allergies at http://www.fda.gov. Type "food allergies what you need to know" into the search bar, then click on the link. At the top of the page, click on the link to see the video.

food intolerance Gastrointestinal discomfort caused by certain foods that is not a result of an immune system reaction.

food allergy An allergic reaction to food, caused by a reaction of the immune system.

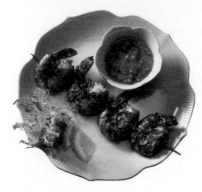

For some people, eating a meal of grilled shrimp with peanut sauce would cause a severe allergic reaction.

You may have heard stories of people being allergic to foods as common as peanuts, shellfish, or eggs. In many such people, the allergic inflammatory reaction is localized, so the damage is limited; for instance, a person's mouth and throat might itch whenever he or she eats cantaloupe. Other localized reactions include swelling of the mouth or face, a skin rash, vomiting, and wheezing. But in some cases, consumption of the offending food can cause a severe, life-threatening reaction known as *anaphylaxis*. In anaphylaxis, the airways become constricted and clogged with mucus, leading to respiratory collapse. The throat may swell and cause suffocation. At the same time, blood vessels dilate and became more permeable, so that blood pressure plummets, leading to circulatory collapse. This state, called *anaphylactic shock*, can be fatal if not treated immediately.[7] For this reason, many people with known food allergies carry with them a kit containing an injection of a powerful stimulant called epinephrine. This drug can reduce symptoms long enough to buy the victim time to get emergency medical care.

Celiac Disease

Celiac disease, also known as *celiac sprue*, is a disease that severely damages the lining of the small intestine and interferes with the absorption of nutrients.[8] As in food allergy, the body's immune system causes the disorder. There is a strong genetic predisposition to celiac disease, with the risk now linked to specific gene markers. Approximately 1 in every 133 Americans is thought to have celiac disease, but among those with a close family member with the disease, the rate is 1 in 22.[8]

Whereas many foods prompt food allergies, in celiac disease the offending food component is always *gliadin*, a fraction of a protein called *gluten* that is found in wheat, rye, and barley. When people with celiac disease eat a food made with one of these grains, their immune system triggers an inflammatory response that erodes the villi of the small intestine. If the person is unaware of the disorder and continues to eat gluten, repeated immune reactions cause the villi to become greatly decreased, so that there is less absorptive surface area. In addition, the enzymes secreted at the brush border of the small intestine become reduced. As a result, the person becomes unable to absorb certain nutrients properly—a condition known as *malabsorption*. Over time, malabsorption can lead to malnutrition (poor nutrient status). Deficiencies of fat-soluble vitamins A, D, E, and K, as well as iron, folic acid, and calcium, are common in those suffering from celiac disease, as are inadequate intakes of protein and total energy.[8]

Symptoms of celiac disease often mimic those of other intestinal disturbances, such as irritable bowel syndrome (discussed ahead), so the condition is often misdiagnosed. Some of the symptoms of celiac disease include fatty stools (due to poor fat absorption) with an odd odor; abdominal bloating and cramping; diarrhea, constipation, or vomiting; and weight loss. However, other puzzling symptoms do not appear to involve the GI tract. These include an intensely itchy rash called *dermatitis herpetiformis*, unexplained anemia, fatigue, osteoporosis (poor bone density), arthritis, infertility, seizures, anxiety, irritability, and depression, among others.[8]

Diagnostic tests for celiac disease include a variety of blood tests that screen for the presence of antigliadin antibodies or for the genetic markers of the disease. Definitive diagnosis requires a biopsy of the small intestine showing atrophy of the villi. Because long-term complications of undiagnosed celiac disease include an increased risk for intestinal cancer, early diagnosis can be life-saving.

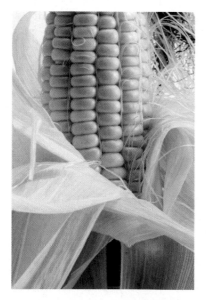

For people with celiac disease, corn is a gluten-free source of carbohydrates.

Currently, there is no cure for celiac disease. Treatment is with a special diet that excludes all forms of wheat, rye, and barley. Oats are allowed, but they are often contaminated with wheat flour from processing, and even a microscopic amount of wheat can cause an immune response. Although many gluten-free foods are now available, and the FDA now regulates the labeling of such foods, a gluten-free diet is challenging and nutritional counseling is essential. Someday, however, gluten-free foods may be unnecessary. Earlier, we discussed the beneficial functions of certain types of bacteria in the GI tract. Now, researchers have discovered that beneficial mouth bacteria are able to degrade gluten.[8,9] Thus, researchers are looking into the potential of developing probiotic breads and other gluten-containing foods that would be safe for people with celiac disease to consume.

celiac disease A disorder characterized by an immune reaction that damages the lining of the small intestine when the individual is exposed to a component of a protein called gluten.

Nonceliac Gluten Sensitivity

Recent surveys suggest that as many as 100 million Americans consume at least some foods specifically formulated to be gluten-free.[10] Many of these Americans consume gluten-free products believing that they're more healthful, or will help them lose weight. These claims are largely unfounded. However, there is "undisputable and increasing evidence" for a disorder that is related to gluten consumption but is not celiac disease.[10] This is called *nonceliac gluten sensitivity (NCGS)*. Signs and symptoms of the disorder can vary greatly, from abdominal bloating and diarrhea to bone and joint pain to depression and confusion; however, the common factor is that patients improve on a gluten-free diet.[11,12] Research into the factors contributing to NCGS is ongoing. In the meantime, if you believe that you might be "gluten sensitive," don't stop eating gluten-containing foods without consulting your doctor to determine whether or not you have celiac disease. That's because antibody tests for celiac disease are not sensitive in people who aren't currently consuming gluten.

Vomiting Can Be Acute or Chronic

Vomiting is the involuntary expulsion of the contents of the stomach and duodenum from the mouth. The reflex is triggered when substances or sensations stimulate a cluster of cells in the brain stem to signal a strong wave of contractions that begin in the small intestine and surge upward. The sphincter muscles of the GI tract relax, allowing the chyme to pass.

One or two episodes of vomiting often accompany a gastrointestinal infection, typically with the norovirus, which is often spread via contaminated water or food. Vomiting triggered by infection is classified as one of the body's innate defenses, as it removes harmful agents before they are absorbed. Certain medical procedures, medications, illicit drugs, motion sickness, and even severe pain can also trigger acute vomiting.

In contrast, *cyclic vomiting syndrome (CVS)* is a chronic condition characterized by recurring cycles of severe nausea and vomiting that can last for hours or days, alternating with symptom-free periods.[13] The number of people affected is unknown, but the condition is thought to be somewhat common, and people of all ages can be affected. The vomiting may be severe enough to cause dehydration, and the person may need to be hospitalized.

Anxiety, excitement, allergies, infections, and a variety of other disturbances may trigger CVS. These triggers are similar to those involved in migraine headaches, and the same medications used for migraines may be prescribed for CVS, along with antinausea and anti-emesis drugs.[13]

Crohn's Disease and Colitis Are Inflammatory Bowel Diseases

Two inflammatory bowel diseases are Crohn's disease and ulcerative colitis. The precise causes of these disorders are unknown, but both have been linked to an immune response to a virus or bacterium. Both also are associated with similar symptoms.

Crohn's Disease

Crohn's disease causes inflammation in the small intestine, usually the ileum, and affects the entire thickness of the wall. Experts speculate that the inflammation is caused by an inappropriate immune reaction to an otherwise harmless bacterium or virus.[14]

The symptoms of Crohn's disease include diarrhea, abdominal pain, rectal bleeding, weight loss, and fever. If allowed to progress, Crohn's disease can cause blockage of the intestine and the development of ulcers that tunnel through the tissue layers and commonly require surgical treatment. Crohn's disease also results in deficiencies in protein, energy, and vitamins and is associated with arthritis, kidney stones, gallstones, and diseases of the liver.

Because it shares many symptoms with other intestinal disorders, Crohn's disease can be difficult to diagnose. Treatment may involve a combination of medications that suppress the immune response, as well as nutritional supplements. In some cases, a period of bowel rest—that is, intravenous feeding—helps the affected tissues to heal. Up to 20% of patients eventually require surgery to treat the disease.[14]

vomiting The involuntary expulsion of the contents of the stomach and duodenum from the mouth.

Crohn's disease A chronic disease that causes inflammation in the small intestine, leading to diarrhea, abdominal pain, rectal bleeding, weight loss, and fever.

Ulcerative Colitis

Ulcerative colitis (UC) is a chronic disease characterized by inflammation and ulceration of the mucosa, or innermost lining, of the colon. Ulcers may bleed and produce pus and mucus. The disease typically develops between ages 15 and 30 or after 60 and is more common in people with a family member who has UC.[15]

The causes of UC are unknown. Researchers believe that an overactive immune system and genetics contribute. There is also some evidence that use of certain medications such as NSAIDs, antibiotics, and oral contraceptives may slightly increase the risk. The resulting signs and symptoms include diarrhea (which may be bloody), an urgent need to have a bowel movement, weight loss, anemia, nausea, fever, and fatigue. Most people have mild symptoms, but about 10% experience profuse bleeding, severe abdominal cramping, and fevers.[15] A variety of medications are used to treat symptoms, and some people require surgery.

RECAP

Food intolerances are digestive problems caused by the consumption of certain foods, but not due to an immune reaction. Food allergies are hypersensitivities to food ingredients caused by an immune reaction. Food allergies can cause localized symptoms, such as itching and swelling, or life-threatening inflammation and anaphylactic shock. In people with celiac disease, the consumption of gluten, a protein found in wheat, rye, and barley, causes an immune reaction that erodes the lining of the small intestine. Vomiting is a defensive response to the presence of harmful agents in the GI tract. Cyclic vomiting syndrome is a pattern of recurring episodes of severe vomiting that can last hours or days. Crohn's disease and ulcerative colitis are inflammatory bowel diseases. Crohn's disease usually affects the entire thickness of the ileum of the small intestine, whereas colitis is inflammation and ulceration of the innermost lining of the colon. ■

Diarrhea, Constipation, and Irritable Bowel Syndrome Are Functional Disorders

As their name implies, functional disorders affect the regular function of the gastrointestinal tract. Food may move through the small or large intestine too quickly or too slowly, prompting discomfort, bloating, or other symptoms.

Diarrhea

Diarrhea is the frequent (more than three times in one day) passage of loose, watery stools. Other symptoms may include cramping, abdominal pain, bloating, nausea, fever, and blood in the stools. Acute diarrhea is usually caused by an infection of the gastrointestinal tract, or use of medications such as antibiotics. Chronic diarrhea is more often due to an underlying disorder of the GI tract.[16]

Whatever the cause, diarrhea can be harmful if it persists for a long period of time because the person can lose large quantities of water and electrolytes and become severely dehydrated. **Table 3.3** reviews the signs and symptoms of dehydration, which is particularly dangerous in infants and young children. In fact, a child can die from dehydration in just a few days. Adults, particularly the elderly, can also become dangerously ill if severely dehydrated.

A condition referred to as *traveler's diarrhea* has become a common health concern due to the expansion in global travel. Traveler's diarrhea is discussed in the ***Highlight*** box (page 103).

Constipation

At the opposite end of the spectrum is **constipation,** which is typically defined as a condition in which no stools are passed for 2 or more days; however, it is important to recognize that some people normally experience bowel movements only every second or third day. Thus, the definition of constipation varies from one person to another. In addition to being infrequent, the stools are usually hard, small, and difficult to pass.

ulcerative colitis A chronic disease of the colon, indicated by inflammation and ulceration of the mucosa, or innermost lining, of the colon.

diarrhea A condition characterized by the frequent passage of loose, watery stools.

constipation A condition characterized by the absence of bowel movements for a period of time that is significantly longer than normal for the individual.

Traveler's Diarrhea—What Is It and How Can You Prevent It?

Diarrhea is the rapid movement of fecal matter through the large intestine, often accompanied by large volumes of water. *Traveler's diarrhea* (also called *dysentery*) is experienced by people traveling to countries outside of their own and is usually caused by a viral or bacterial infection. Diarrhea is the body's way of ridding itself of the invasive agent. The large intestine and even some of the small intestine become irritated by the microbes and the resulting immune response. This irritation leads to increased secretion of fluid and increased peristalsis of the large intestine, causing watery stools and a higher-than-normal frequency of bowel movements.

Travelers generally get diarrhea from consuming water or food that is contaminated with fecal matter. Symptoms include fatigue, lack of appetite, abdominal cramps, and watery diarrhea. In some cases, you may also experience nausea, vomiting, and low-grade fever. Usually, this diarrhea passes within 4 to 6 days, and people recover completely.

What can you do to prevent traveler's diarrhea? The National Digestive Diseases Clearinghouse advises that travelers to high-risk areas avoid the following:[1]

- Drinking tap water, using tap water to brush their teeth, and using ice made from tap water
- Drinking unpasteurized milk or milk products

- Eating raw fruits and vegetables, including lettuce and fruit salads, unless they peel the fruits or vegetables themselves
- Eating raw or rare meat and fish
- Eating meat or shellfish that is not hot when served
- Eating food from street vendors

Travelers can drink bottled water, soft drinks, and hot drinks, such as coffee or tea.

If you do suffer from traveler's diarrhea, it is important to replace the fluid and nutrients lost as a result of the illness. Specially formulated oral rehydration solutions are usually available in most countries at local pharmacies or stores. Antibiotics may also be prescribed to kill the bacteria. Once treatment is initiated, the diarrhea should cease within 2 to 3 days. If the diarrhea persists for more than 10 days after the initiation of treatment, or if there is blood in your stools, you should return to a physician immediately to avoid serious medical consequences.

Reference

1. Data from National Digestive Diseases Information Clearinghouse (NDDIC). Update 2013, November 25. Diarrhea. NIH Publication No. 11–5176. http://www.niddk.nih.gov/health-information/health-topics/digestive-diseases/diarrhea/Pages/ez.aspx.

TABLE 3.3 Signs and Symptoms of Dehydration in Adults and Children

Signs and Symptoms in Adults	Signs and Symptoms in Children
Thirst	Dry mouth and tongue
Dizziness or fainting	No tears when crying
Less frequent urination	No wet diapers for 3 hours or more
Dark-colored urine	High fever
Fatigue	Sunken eyes, cheeks, or soft spots in the skull
Dry skin	Being more cranky or drowsy than usual

Source: Data from National Digestive Diseases Information Clearinghouse (NDDIC). Update 2013, November 25. Diarrhea. NIH Publication No. 11–5176. http://www.niddk.nih.gov/health-information/health-topics/digestive-diseases/diarrhea/Pages/ez.aspx

Constipation is frequent in people who have disorders affecting the nervous system, which in turn affect the muscles of the large intestine, as they do not receive the appropriate neurologic signals needed for involuntary muscle movement to occur. For these individuals, drug therapy is often needed to maintain bowel functioning.

Many people experience temporary constipation at some point in their lives in response to a variety of factors. Often people have trouble with it when they travel, when their schedule is disrupted, if they change their diet, or if they are on certain medications. Increasing fiber and fluid in the diet is one of the mainstays of preventing constipation. Five servings of fruits and vegetables each day and six or more servings of whole grains is helpful to most people. If you eat breakfast cereal, make sure you buy one containing at least 2 to 3 g of fiber per serving.

(The dietary recommendation for fiber and the role it plays in maintaining healthy elimination is discussed in detail in Chapter 4.) Staying well hydrated by drinking lots of water is especially important when increasing fiber intake. Exercising also helps reduce the risk for constipation.

Irritable Bowel Syndrome

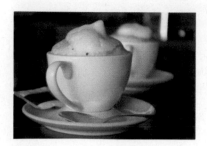

Consuming caffeinated drinks is one of several factors that have been linked with irritable bowel syndrome (IBS), a disorder that interferes with normal functioning of the colon.

Irritable bowel syndrome (IBS) is a functional GI disorder that is characterized by abdominal cramps, bloating, and either constipation or diarrhea. It is one of the most common disorders, with most studies suggesting it affects 10% to 15% of Americans. More women than men are diagnosed with IBS, which typically first appears before age 45.[17]

The causes of IBS are not well understood; however, research does suggest that, in people with IBS, the enteric nervous system responds to stress by triggering spasms of the colon.[17] Some researchers believe that the problem stems from conflicting messages between the CNS and the ENS. Whatever the cause, the normal movement of the colon appears to be disrupted. In some people with IBS, food moves too quickly through the colon and fluid cannot be absorbed fast enough, which causes diarrhea. In others, the movement of the colon is too slow and too much fluid is absorbed, leading to constipation. Large meals, meals high in fat, milk, alcohol, drinks containing caffeine or artificial sweeteners, and beans and cabbage—which may trigger intestinal gas—are thought to cause physiologic stress linked to IBS.

Treatment options include certain medications to treat diarrhea or constipation, stress management, and regular physical activity. Dietary modifications can also help. These include eating smaller meals, avoiding foods that exacerbate symptoms, eating a higher-fiber diet, and drinking at least six to eight glasses of water each day. Moreover, regular consumption of probiotic foods may help. For more information on probiotics, see the *Nutrition Myth or Fact?* at the end of this chapter.[17]

Cancer Can Develop in Any Part of the Gastrointestinal System

Cancer can develop in any region of the GI tract or in the gallbladder, liver, or pancreas; together, these sites account for over 330,000 cancers each year, and over 155,000 cancer deaths.[18] Of these, sites commonly affected include the oral cavity and pharynx, esophagus, stomach, pancreas, and the liver and bile duct. The most common GI cancer, however, is colorectal cancer—cancer affecting the colon or rectum. It is diagnosed in more than 136,000 Americans annually, making it the third most common cancer in men as well as in women. It is also the third most deadly, killing more than 50,000 Americans annually.[18]

Smoking, obesity, a diet high in red or processed meats and low in fruits and vegetables, and genetic factors are thought to increase the risk for colorectal cancer. In contrast, consumption of milk and calcium, and higher blood levels of vitamin D appear to decrease risk.[18]

Symptoms of colorectal cancer include a persistent change in bowel habits, rectal bleeding, unexplained weight loss, and abdominal pain or discomfort. Symptoms typically arise, however, only when the cancer is advanced. Thus, screening is recommended beginning at age 50, and mortality from colorectal cancer has been declining for two decades in part because of increased screening.[18] Screening options include an annual stool test that looks for occult blood (hidden blood) in a stool sample, and an internal imaging test called a *colonoscopy* that is performed every 5 to 10 years. Colonoscopy can detect both cancer and precancerous polyps—small masses of abnormal but noninvasive cells—and remove any polyps that are present. Malignant tumors require surgery, and possibly radiation and/or chemotherapy.

RECAP

irritable bowel syndrome (IBS) A stress-related disorder that interferes with normal functions of the colon. Symptoms are abdominal cramps, bloating, and constipation or diarrhea.

Diarrhea is the frequent passage of loose or watery stools, whereas constipation is the failure to have a bowel movement for 2 or more days or within a time period that is normal for the individual. Diarrhea should be treated quickly to avoid dehydration. Constipation often can be corrected by increasing your intake of fiber and water. Irritable bowel syndrome (IBS) causes abdominal cramps, bloating, and constipation or diarrhea. The most common GI cancer is colorectal cancer.

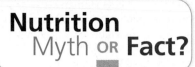

Should You Grow Your Microbiome?

We like to think of ourselves as discrete, individual organisms, but it's not true. We're actually "super-organisms." The human body is a lush microbial ecosystem containing about 100 trillion *microorganisms* (microscopic organisms such as bacteria), collectively known as the **human microbiome.** The human body is home to nearly triple the number of microbial cells as it is human cells.[1] Of course, these microorganisms have their own genes, which interact with our human cells and genes in a dizzying number of ways that affect our health. Although microorganisms live on our skin, in our urinary tract, and elsewhere in our body, here we'll focus on the *GI flora*.

Benefits of Our Resident Microbes

Researchers have identified many ways in which the GI flora benefit human health. For example, genes carried by these bacteria enable humans to digest foods and absorb nutrients that otherwise would be unavailable to us.[2] It seems likely that genes in our GI flora complement the functions of human genes required for biological pathways involved in digestion—genes that may be missing or incompletely encoded in the human genome.[3] Moreover, GI flora are thought to:[3–7]

- Manufacture enzymes that help us digest our food and absorb nutrients from food
- Supply key nutrients used to replace worn-out components of the GI tract
- Produce certain essential vitamins
- Protect against GI infections
- Provide some protection against the development of obesity and type 2 diabetes
- Degrade potential carcinogens (cancer-causing agents) in foods
- Produce anti-inflammatory chemicals, thereby providing some protection against disorders characterized by inflammation, such as certain GI cancers, esophagitis and gastritis (inflammation of the esophagus and stomach, respectively), inflammatory bowel disorders, eczema, and asthma and allergies.

Given this research, you're probably wondering how you can maintain a large and healthy population of microorganisms in your GI tract. That's where probiotics and prebiotics, two types of functional foods, come in.

Probiotic and Prebiotic Foods

You learned in Chapter 2 that *functional foods* may have biologically active ingredients with the potential to provide health benefits beyond basic nutrition.[8] These include both whole and processed foods. Here, we discuss two types of processed functional foods: probiotic and prebiotic foods. They qualify as functional foods because, in addition to the nutrients they provide, they help grow your microbiome.

Yogurt is one of a group of so-called *probiotic foods*: foods or food supplements containing microorganisms which beneficially affect consumers by improving the intestinal microbial balance.[8] Interest in probiotic foods was sparked in the early 1900s with the work of Elie Metchnikoff, a Nobel Prize–winning scientist. Dr. Metchnikoff linked the long, healthy lives of Bulgarian peasants with their consumption of fermented milk products, such as yogurt. Subsequent research identified the bacteria in fermented milk products as the factor that promoted health.

In the United States, probiotics include fortified milk, yogurt, and a creamy beverage called *kefir*, which is made from fermented milk. Probiotics are also sold in supplement form. The bacterial species most frequently used in these foods and supplements are *Lactobacillus* and *Bifidobacterium*.

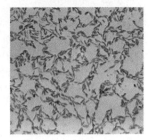

The human body is a microbial ecosystem containing about 100 trillion microscopic organisms, such as this GI bacteria.

When a person consumes probiotics, the bacteria adhere to the intestinal wall for a few days. There, they're thought to exert the beneficial actions identified with the GI flora. An enormous volume of studies now links probiotics consumption to these health benefits. For example, studies support a reduction in "transit time" of wastes through the colon in people who regularly consume yogurt, reducing their risk for constipation.[9] The probiotics in yogurt may also help regulate blood glucose: A recent observational study found that people who consume 12 ounces of yogurt daily have an 18% reduced risk for type 2 diabetes.[10] And some laboratory studies have shown that probiotics can help reduce infection and inflammation,[3] an effect that may reduce college students' susceptibility to colds! In a recent randomized, double-blind, placebo-controlled study, nearly 600 college students were given either a probiotic supplement or a placebo. Those who consumed the probiotic supplement experienced significantly fewer cold/flu symptoms and significantly more healthy days than students who received the placebo.[11]

It's important to remember that, in order to be effective, a minimum number of bacteria must be present in probiotic foods or supplements. Commercial yogurts meeting the National Yogurt Association Standards contain 100 million live and active cultures per gram. So a 1-cup serving (8 oz, or 227 grams) of yogurt contains more than 22 billion bacteria. This is considered more than the estimated effective dose.

Bacteria live only for a short time. This means that probiotic foods and supplements should be consumed on a daily basis to be most effective. They must also be properly stored and consumed within a relatively brief period of time to confer maximal benefit. In general, refrigerated foods containing probiotics have a shelf life of 3 to 6 weeks, whereas refrigerated supplements keep about 12 months. However, because the probiotic content of foods is much more stable than that of supplements, yogurt and other probiotic foods may be a better health bet.

Now that you know a little more about probiotics, you may be wondering how they're related to prebiotics. We've said that probiotics contain living and helpful bacteria that boost the population count in your GI tract. In contrast, *prebiotics* are nondigestible food ingredients (typically carbohydrates) that benefit the consumer by stimulating the growth and/or

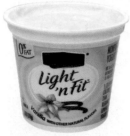

Beneficial bacteria are found in probiotic foods like yogurt or kefir.

activity of these helpful bacteria.[8] By doing so, they improve digestion and metabolism, help regulate the inflammatory response, and in general complement the action of probiotics.

An example is inulin, a carbohydrate found in a few fruits, onions and certain green vegetables, and some grains. Like other prebiotics, inulin travels through the GI tract without being digested or absorbed until it reaches the colon, where it nourishes colonies of helpful resident bacteria. In other words, prebiotics don't feed you, but they do feed your microbiome.

In addition to whole prebiotic foods, many processed foods claim to be prebiotic. For example, inulin is added to certain brands of yogurt, milk, and cottage cheese, some fruit juices, cookies, and fiber bars and supplements. Watch out, though, that your desire to feed your flora doesn't cause you to overindulge. Cookies, sweet granola bars, and other products touted as prebiotic may have just as many Calories and just as much fat as regular versions of the same foods.

Critical Thinking Questions

- Now that you've read about the benefits of a healthy population of GI flora, what do you think might be the potential downside of routinely administering broad-spectrum antibiotics to infants and toddlers with common disorders such as ear infections?
- Explain the difference between a probiotic food and a prebiotic food. Give an example of a food that might correctly be categorized as both!
- You've probably read Internet health blogs or other publications equating processed foods with junk foods. Do they deserve their bad reputation? Why or why not?

References

1. Reid, A., and S. Greene. 2013. Human Microbiome FAQ. A Report From the American Academy of Microbiology. *http://academy.asm.org/images/stories/documents/FAQ_Human_Microbiome.pdf*.

2. National Institutes of Health. 2012. NIH Human Microbiome Project defines normal bacterial makeup of the body. *NIH News*. June 13, 2012. Available at http://www.nih.gov/news/health/jun2012/nhgri-13.htm

3. Hemarajata, P. and J. Versalovic, 2013. Effects of probiotics on gut microbiota: mechanisms of intestinal immunomodulation and neuromodulation. *Therap.Adv. Gastroenterol*. 6(1):39–51. Available at http://www.ncbi.nlm.nih.gov/pmc/articles/PMC3539293/

4. Krajmalnik-Brown, R., Z. E. Ilhan, D. W. Kang, and J. K DiBaise. 2012. Effects of gut microbes on nutrient absorption and energy regulation. *Nutr. Clin. Pract*. 27(2):201–214.

5. Yoon, M. Y., K. Lee, and S. S. Yoon. 2014. Protective role of gut commensal microbes against intestinal infections. *J. Microbiol*. 52(12):983–989. doi: 10.1007/s12275-014-4655-2.

6. Munyaka, P. A. E. Khafipou, and J. E. Ghia. 2014. External influence of early childhood establishment of gut microbiota and subsequent health implications. *Front. Pediatr*. 2:109.

7. Mueller, N. T., R. Whyaat, L. Hoepner, S. Overfield, M. G. Dominquez-Bello, E. M. Widen . . . A. Rundle. 2014. Prenatal exposure to antibiotics, cesarean section and risk of childhood obesity. *Intl. J. Obes*.1–6. doi: 10.1038/ijo.2014.180.

8. United States Food and Drug Administration. 2012, April 6. Regulatory Information: Complementary and Alternative Medicine Products and Their Regulation by the Food and Drug Administration. Available at http://www.fda.gov/RegulatoryInformation/Guidances/ucm144657.htm#iv

9. Magro, D. O. 2014. Effect of yogurt containing polydextrose, *Lactobacillus acidophilus* NCFM and *Bifidobacterium lactis* HN019: a randomized, double-blind, controlled study in chronic constipation. *Nutri. J*. 13:75. doi: 10.1186/1475-2891-13-75.

10. Chen, M., Q. Sun, E. Giovannucci, D. Mozaffarain, J. E. Manson, W. C. Willet, and F. B. Hu. 2014. Dairy consumption and risk of type 2 diabetes: 3 cohorts of U.S. adults and an updated meta-analysis. *BMC Med*. 12:215. doi:10.1186/s12916-014-0215-1

11. Langkamp-Henken, B., C. C. Rowe, A. L. Ford, M. C. Christman, C. Nieves, L. Khouri,...and W. J. Dahl. 2015. *Bifidobacterium bifidum* R0071 results in a greater proportion of healthy days and a lower percentage of academically stressed students reporting a day of cold/flu: a randomised, double-blind, placebo-controlled study. *Br. J. Nutr*. 113(3):426–434.

STUDY **PLAN**   Mastering Nutrition™

Customize your study plan—and master your nutrition!—in the Study Area of MasteringNutrition.

TEST YOURSELF | *ANSWERS*

1 **T**   Sometimes you may have an appetite even though you are not hungry. These feelings are referred to as "cravings" and are associated with physical or emotional cues.

2 **F** Your brain, not your stomach, is the primary organ responsible for telling you when you are hungry.

3 **F** Even extreme food restriction, such as near-starvation, does not cause the stomach to shrink permanently. Likewise, the stomach doesn't stretch permanently. The folds in the wall of the stomach flatten as it expands to accommodate a large meal, but they re-form over the next few hours as the food empties into the small intestine. Only after gastric surgery, when a very small stomach "pouch" remains, can stomach tissue stretch permanently.

4 **T** Although there are individual variations in how we respond to food, the entire process of digestion and absorption of one meal usually takes about 24 hours.

5 **T** Most ulcers result from an infection by the bacterium *Helicobacter pylori* (*H. pylori*). Contrary to popular belief, ulcers are not caused by stress or spicy food.

summary

 Scan to hear an MP3 Chapter Review in **MasteringNutrition**.

LO 1
- Hunger is a physiologic drive that prompts us to eat. It is regulated by the hypothalamus, which contains a cluster of cells called the feeding center and a cluster called the satiety center. These work together to regulate food intake by integrating signals from three sources: nerve cells in the gastrointestinal tract, hormones, and the amount and type of food we eat.
- Foods that contain fiber, water, and large amounts of protein have the highest satiety value.
- Appetite is a psychological desire to consume specific foods; this desire is influenced by sensory data, social and cultural cues, and learning.

LO 2
- Digestion is the process of breaking down foods into molecules small enough to be transported into enterocytes. Absorption is the process of taking molecules of food out of the gastrointestinal tract and into the circulation. Elimination is the process of removing undigested food and waste products from the body.
- In the mouth, chewing starts the mechanical digestion of food. Saliva contains salivary amylase, an enzyme that initiates the chemical digestion of carbohydrates. Lingual lipase begins to digest some lipids.
- Food moves to the stomach through the esophagus via a process called peristalsis. Peristalsis involves rhythmic waves of squeezing and pushing food through the gastrointestinal tract.
- The stomach mixes and churns food together with gastric juices. Hydrochloric acid and the enzyme pepsin initiate protein digestion, and a minimal amount of fat digestion occurs through the action of gastric lipase.
- The stomach periodically releases the partially digested food, referred to as chyme, into the small intestine.

- Most of the digestion and absorption of nutrients occurs in the small intestine.
- The large intestine digests any remaining food particles, absorbs water and chemicals, and moves feces to the rectum for elimination. Microorganisms residing in the GI tract are referred to as the GI flora. These include probiotics, helpful bacteria and other microorganisms in the large intestine that perform beneficial functions.

LO 3
- At a pH of 1.0, hydrochloric acid keeps the environment of the stomach highly acidic. HCl begins to denature proteins and converts pepsinogen to pepsin, a protein-digesting enzyme.

LO 4
- Enzymes facilitate the digestion of food via the process of hydrolysis. Most digestive enzymes are synthesized by the pancreas and small intestine.
- Hormones that regulate digestion include gastrin, secretin, cholecystokinin (CCK), gastric inhibitory peptide, and somatostatin.

LO 5
- The gallbladder stores bile and secretes it into the small intestine. Bile emulsifies lipids into small droplets that are more accessible to pancreatic enzymes.
- The pancreas manufactures and secretes digestive enzymes into the small intestine. Pancreatic amylase digests carbohydrates, pancreatic lipase digests lipids, and proteases digest proteins. The pancreas also synthesizes two hormones that play a critical role in carbohydrate metabolism, insulin and glucagon.
- The liver processes, packages, and stores nutrients, detoxifies the blood, synthesizes bile, and regulates the metabolism of monosaccharides, fatty acids, and amino acids.

LO 6
- The lining of the small intestine has folds, villi, and microvilli that increase its surface area and absorptive capacity.

LO 7
- The four types of absorption that occur in the small intestine are passive diffusion, facilitated diffusion, active transport, and endocytosis.

LO 8 ■ The neuromuscular system involves coordination of the muscles of the GI tract to produce three characteristic movements: peristalsis, segmentation, and haustration. The enteric nervous system, other branches of the autonomic nervous system, and the central nervous system together act to move food along the gastrointestinal tract and to control digestion, absorption, and elimination.

LO 9 ■ Belching results from swallowed air. Flatulence is entirely normal, but may be increased by the consumption of foods rich in certain types of fiber.

■ Heartburn occurs when gastric juice pools in the esophagus and burns its lining. Gastroesophageal reflux disease (GERD) is a more painful type of heartburn that occurs more than twice per week.

■ A peptic ulcer is an area in the stomach or duodenum that has been eroded away by hydrochloric acid and pepsin. It is typically caused by infection with *Helicobacter pylori* or by use of nonsteroidal anti-inflammatory drugs.

■ A food intolerance is a cluster of GI symptoms such as gas and diarrhea that occur following consumption of a particular food, but in which the immune system is not involved. Food allergies, in contrast, are hypersensitivity immune reactions. These can be localized, such as a minor skin rash, or systemic, resulting in anaphylaxis, which can lead to respiratory and circulatory collapse.

■ People with celiac disease cannot eat gluten, a protein found in wheat, rye, and barley. A fraction of the gluten protein called gliadin prompts an immune reaction that damages intestinal villi, leading to malabsorption of nutrients and malnutrition. Nonceliac gluten sensitivity is not well understood, but appears to cause a range of symptoms due to consumption of gluten in the absence of celiac disease.

■ Acute vomiting is usually a protective response, whereas cyclic vomiting syndrome is a chronic disorder that can lead to severe dehydration.

■ Crohn's disease is a form of inflammatory bowel disorder that causes inflammation in the small intestine, whereas ulcerative colitis damages the mucosal lining of the colon. The causes of these diseases are unknown.

■ Diarrhea is the frequent (more than three times per day) elimination of loose, watery stools. Constipation is a condition in which no stools are passed for 2 or more days or for a length of time considered abnormally long for the individual. Irritable bowel syndrome is a stress-related disorder that interferes with normal functions of the colon, causing pain, diarrhea, and/or constipation.

LO 10 ■ Cancer can develop in any region of the GI tract or in the gallbladder, liver, or pancreas; however, colorectal cancer is the most common of the GI cancers, and is the third leading cause of cancer and cancer deaths in both men and women.

■ Colon cancer screening allows for the detection and removal of precancerous polyps. Increased screening has contributed to a decrease in colon cancer mortality in the last two decades.

review questions

LO 1 1. The region of brain tissue that is responsible for prompting us to seek food is the
  a. pituitary gland.
  b. satiety center.
  c. hypothalamus.
  d. thalamus.

LO 2 2. In traveling through your GI tract, chyme would encounter
  a. the esophagus, then the stomach.
  b. the duodenum, then the jejunum, and then the ileum.
  c. the liver, then the gallbladder, and then the pancreas.
  d. the jejunum, then the transverse colon, the ascending colon, and finally the anus.

LO 3 3. The parietal cells of the stomach secrete hydrochloric acid, which
  a. begins to denature proteins.
  b. accomplishes protein digestion.
  c. begins to digest carbohydrates.
  d. is more acidic than battery acid.

LO 4 4. Which of the following statements about chemical digestion is true?
  a. Enzymes are chemical messenger molecules that are important in regulating many aspects of digestion.
  b. Hormones are nearly always produced in the same organ whose activity they assist.
  c. Most hormones and enzymes involved in digestion are nonspecific, acting on a wide variety of compounds.
  d. Upon release into the GI tract, digestive enzymes typically facilitate hydrolysis reactions.

LO 5 5. Bile is a greenish fluid that
  a. is produced by the gallbladder.
  b. is stored by the pancreas.
  c. is necessary for the absorption of vitamin B_{12}.
  d. emulsifies lipids.

LO 6 6. The lining of the small intestine
  a. has muscular ridges called rugae that flatten to increase its absorptive capacity.
  b. is studded with lymph nodes that absorb nutrients from the chyme.
  c. has fingerlike projections called villi that contain capillaries and a lacteal that pick up absorbed nutrients.
  d. has absorptive cells called enterocytes that line the microvilli.

LO 7 7. A process in which nutrients are shuttled across enterocytes with the help of a carrier protein but no use of energy is
a. passive diffusion.
b. facilitated diffusion.
c. active transport.
d. endocytosis.

LO 8 8. Which of the following processes moves food along the entire GI tract?
a. mass movement
b. peristalsis
c. haustration
d. segmentation

LO 9 9. Gastroesophageal reflux disease is caused
a. by pooling of gastric juice in the lower esophagus.
b. when a hypersensitivity immune response triggers inflammation of the esophagus and stomach.
c. by ulceration of the lining of the colon.
d. by an inappropriate response of enteric nerves to stress.

LO 10 10. Colorectal cancer
a. accounts for nearly one-fourth of all cancers of the gastrointestinal system.
b. is the most common cancer in both men and women.
c. can be successfully treated during a colonoscopy.
d. can be detected with a screening test before it produces signs or symptoms.

true or false

LO 1 11. True or false? Hunger is more physiological, and appetite is more psychological.

LO 2 12. True or false? Vitamins and minerals are digested in the small intestine.

LO 5 13. The pancreas secretes inactive enzymes, hormones, and bicarbonate.

LO 8 14. True or false? The nerves in the walls of the GI tract are part of the central nervous system.

LO 9 15. True or false? Acute diarrhea is typically protective.

LO 2 16. Explain why it can be said that you are what you eat.

17. Why doesn't the acidic environment of the stomach cause it to digest itself?

LO 6 18. Imagine that the lining of your small intestine were smooth, like the inside of a rubber tube. Would this design be efficient in performing absorption? Why or why not?

LO 9 19. Create a table comparing the area of inflammation, symptoms, and treatment options for celiac disease, Crohn's disease, and ulcerative colitis.

20. After dinner, your roommate lies down to rest for a few minutes before studying. When he gets up, he complains of a sharp, burning pain in his chest. Offer a possible explanation for his pain.

math review

LO 2 21. Some people use baking soda as an antacid. The pH of baking soda is 9.0. The pH of gastric juice is 2.0. Express the alkalinity of baking soda in relation to gastric juice using a logarithmic equation.

Answers to Review Questions and Math Review are located on the MasteringNutrition Study Area and in the back of the book.

web links

www.digestive.niddk.nih.gov
National Digestive Diseases Information Clearinghouse (NDDIC)
Explore this site to learn more about the disorders covered in this chapter.

www.healthfinder.gov
Health Finder
This site has further information on the disorders related to digestion, absorption, and elimination.

www.foodallergy.org
Food Allergy & Anaphylaxis Network (FAN)
Visit this site to learn more about common food allergies.

www.csaceliacs.org
Celiac Sprue Association—National Celiac Disease Support Group
The website for this national educational organization provides information and referral services for individuals with celiac disease.

www.ccfa.org
Crohn's & Colitis Foundation of America
Search this site to learn more about the most current research, news and advocacy information on Crohn's disease and ulcerative colitis.

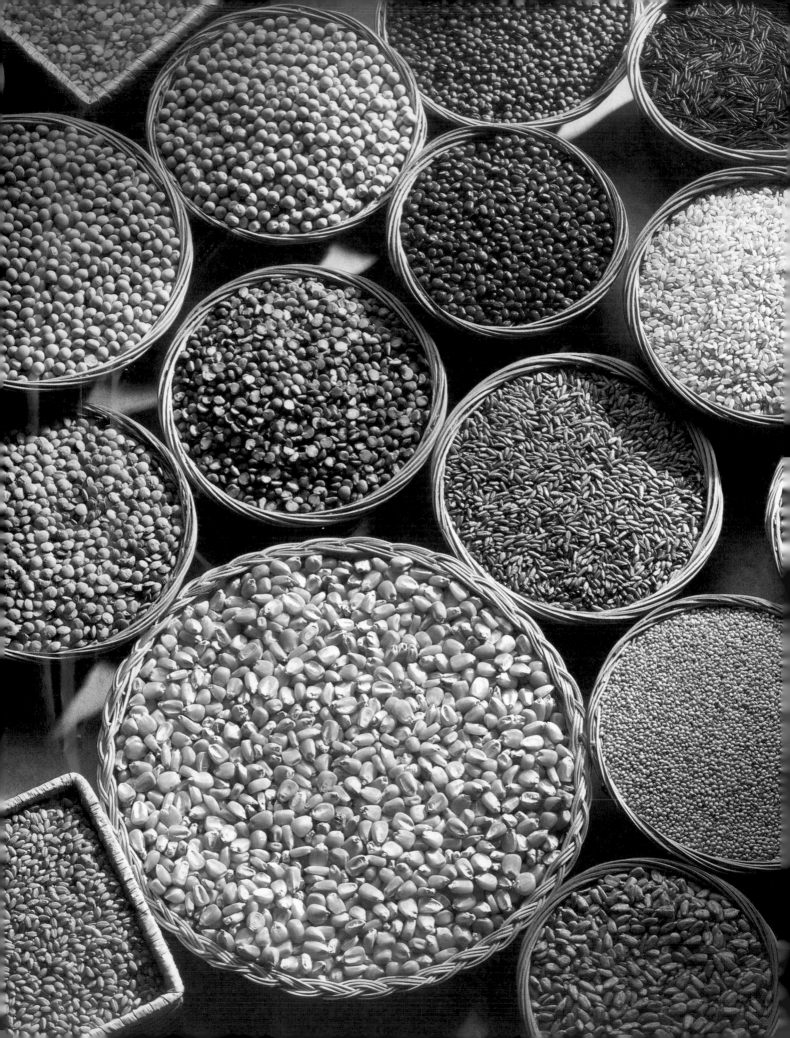

4 Carbohydrates: Plant-Derived Energy Nutrients

Learning Outcomes

After studying this chapter, you should be able to:

1 Compare and contrast simple and complex carbohydrates, *pp. 113–114*.

2 Describe the difference between alpha and beta bonds, and discuss how these bonds are related to the digestion of fiber and lactose intolerance, *pp. 114–116*.

3 Explain the properties and health benefits of the soluble and insoluble fibers found in fiber-rich carbohydrate foods, *pp. 118–119*.

4 Discuss how carbohydrates are digested and absorbed by the body, *pp. 119–121*.

5 List four functions of carbohydrates in the body, *pp. 125–126*.

6 Define the RDA and AMDR for carbohydrates and the AI for fiber, *pp. 128–129*.

7 Identify the potential health risks associated with diets high in added sugars, *pp. 129–131*.

8 List four types of foods that are generally good sources of fiber, *pp. 131–133*.

9 Identify several alternative sweeteners, and discuss their role in a healthful diet, *pp. 137–138*.

10 Describe type 1 and type 2 diabetes, and discuss how diabetes differs from hypoglycemia, *pp. 142–145*.

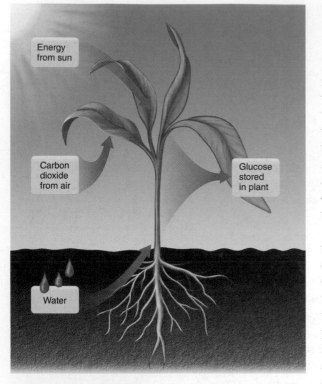

FIGURE 4.1 Plants make carbohydrates through the process of photosynthesis. Water, carbon dioxide, and energy from the sun are combined to produce glucose.

LO 1 Compare and contrast simple and complex carbohydrates.

LO 2 Describe the difference between alpha and beta bonds, and discuss how these bonds are related to the digestion of fiber and lactose intolerance.

LO 3 Explain the properties and health benefits of the soluble and insoluble fibers found in fiber-rich carbohydrate foods.

carbohydrates One of the three macronutrients, a compound made up of carbon, hydrogen, and oxygen that is derived from plants and provides energy.

glucose The most abundant sugar molecule, a monosaccharide generally found in combination with other sugars; the preferred source of energy for the brain and an important source of energy for all cells.

I t's common for college seniors to stress out about their future: Will I get into grad school? find a good job? be able to make new friends? But Sara, a 21-year-old college senior, has more critical concerns. She wonders how long her kidneys will be able to keep functioning, and whether or not she'll go blind. Sara was diagnosed with type 2 diabetes when she was 16 years old. Her doctor prescribed weight loss and oral medication, but she's been unable to keep the weight off, and recently her blood glucose soared out of control despite the drugs. As a result, she was started on insulin injections. Sara is not alone: A 2012 study found that a combination of oral medication and an intensive weight-loss program failed to control blood glucose in 47% of young participants, including those who adhered strictly to the treatment protocol.[1]

Thirty years ago, type 2 diabetes was so rare in anyone younger than middle age it was known as *adult-onset diabetes*. Now it is diagnosed in thousands of children and teens each year. The U.S. Centers for Disease Control and Prevention reports that, if current trends continue, the prevalence of diabetes among young people less than 20 years of age will increase 178% by 2050.[2] This is a major public health concern, as diabetes is the leading cause of surgical leg and foot amputations, blindness, and kidney failure among U.S. adults. As discussed in Chapter 1, it is also the seventh leading cause of death.

What is diabetes, and why are we discussing it in a chapter on carbohydrates? Does carbohydrate consumption somehow lead to diabetes—or, for that matter, to obesity or any other disorder? Several diets that have been popular for decades—including the Zone Diet,[3] Sugar Busters,[4] and Dr. Atkins' New Diet Revolution[5]—claim that carbohydrates are bad for your health and waistline. Are carbohydrates a health menace, and should we reduce our intake?

In this chapter, we explore the differences between simple and complex carbohydrates and learn why some carbohydrates are better than others. We also learn how the human body breaks down carbohydrates and uses them to maintain our health and to fuel our activity and exercise. Because carbohydrate metabolism sometimes goes wrong, we also discuss its relationship to some common health disorders, including diabetes.

What Are Carbohydrates?

As mentioned previously (in Chapter 1), **carbohydrates** are one of the three macronutrients. As such, they are an important energy source for the entire body and are the preferred energy source for nerve cells, including those of the brain. We will say more about their functions later in this chapter.

The term *carbohydrate* literally means "hydrated carbon." When something is said to be *hydrated*, it contains water, which is made up of hydrogen and oxygen (H_2O). The chemical abbreviation for carbohydrate (CHO) indicates the atoms it contains: carbon, hydrogen, and oxygen.

We obtain carbohydrates predominantly from plant foods, such as fruits, vegetables, and grains. Plants make the most abundant form of carbohydrate, called **glucose**, through a process called **photosynthesis**. During photosynthesis, the green pigment of plants, called *chlorophyll*, absorbs sunlight, which provides the energy needed to fuel the manufacture of glucose. As shown in **Figure 4.1**, water absorbed from the earth by the roots of plants combines with carbon dioxide present in the leaves to produce the carbohydrate glucose. Plants continually store glucose and use it to support their own growth. Then, when we eat plant foods, our bodies digest, absorb, and use the stored glucose.

Carbohydrates can be classified as *simple* or *complex*. Simple carbohydrates contain either one or two molecules, whereas complex carbohydrates contain hundreds to thousands of molecules.

Simple Carbohydrates Include Monosaccharides and Disaccharides

Simple carbohydrates are commonly referred to as *sugars*. Four of these sugars are called **monosaccharides** because they consist of a single sugar molecule (*mono*, meaning "one," and *saccharide*, meaning "sugar"). The other three sugars are **disaccharides**, which consist of two molecules of sugar joined together (*di*, meaning "two").

Glucose, Fructose, Galactose, and Ribose Are Monosaccharides

Glucose, fructose, and *galactose* are the three most common monosaccharides in our diet. Each of these monosaccharides contains 6 carbon atoms, 12 hydrogen atoms, and 6 oxygen atoms (**Figure 4.2**). Very slight differences in the structure of these three monosaccharides cause major differences in their level of sweetness.

Given what you've just learned about how plants manufacture glucose, it probably won't surprise you to discover that glucose is the most abundant monosaccharide found in our diet and in our bodies. Glucose does not generally occur by itself in foods but attaches to other sugars to form disaccharides and complex carbohydrates. In our bodies, glucose is the preferred source of energy for the brain, and it is a very important source of energy for all cells.

Fructose, the sweetest natural sugar, occurs in fruits and vegetables. Fructose is also called **levulose,** or *fruit sugar*. In many processed foods, it is a component of *high-fructose corn syrup*. This syrup is made from corn and is used to sweeten soft drinks, desserts, candies, and jellies.

Galactose does not occur alone in foods. It joins with glucose to create lactose, one of the three most common disaccharides.

Ribose is a five-carbon monosaccharide. Very little ribose is found in our diet; our bodies produce ribose from the foods we eat, and ribose is contained in ribonucleic acid (RNA), a component of the genetic material of our cells.

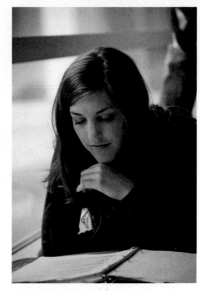

Glucose is the preferred source of energy for the brain.

photosynthesis A process by which plants use sunlight to fuel a chemical reaction that combines carbon and water into glucose, which is then stored in their cells.

simple carbohydrate A monosaccharide or disaccharide, such as glucose; commonly called *sugar*.

monosaccharide The simplest of carbohydrates; consists of one sugar molecule, the most common form of which is glucose.

disaccharide A carbohydrate compound consisting of two monosaccharide molecules joined together.

galactose A monosaccharide that joins with glucose to create lactose, one of the three most common disaccharides.

fructose The sweetest natural sugar; a monosaccharide that occurs in fruits and vegetables; also called *levulose*, or *fruit sugar*.

levulose Another term for fructose, or fruit sugar.

high-fructose corn syrup A type of corn syrup in which part of the sucrose is converted to fructose, making it sweeter than sucrose or regular corn syrup; most high-fructose corn syrup contains 42% to 55% fructose.

ribose A five-carbon monosaccharide that is located in the genetic material of cells.

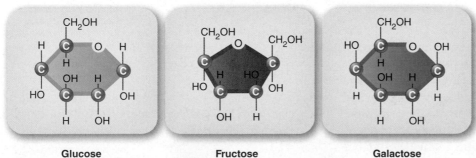

Glucose	Fructose	Galactose
Most abundant sugar molecule in our diet; good energy source	Sweetest natural sugar; found in fruit, high-fructose corn syrup	Does not occur alone in foods; binds with glucose to form lactose

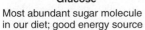

FIGURE 4.2 The three most common monosaccharides. Notice that all three monosaccharides contain identical atoms: 6 carbon, 12 hydrogen, and 6 oxygen. It is only the arrangement of these atoms that differs.

lactose Also called *milk sugar,* a disaccharide consisting of one glucose molecule and one galactose molecule; found in milk, including human breast milk.

maltose A disaccharide consisting of two molecules of glucose; does not generally occur independently in foods but results as a by-product of digestion; also called *malt sugar.*

fermentation The anaerobic process in which an agent causes an organic substance to break down into simpler substances and results in the production of ATP.

sucrose A disaccharide composed of one glucose molecule and one fructose molecule; sweeter than lactose or maltose.

alpha bond A type of chemical bond that can be digested by enzymes found in the human intestine.

beta bond A type of chemical bond that cannot be easily digested by enzymes found in the human intestine.

Lactose, Maltose, and Sucrose Are Disaccharides

The three most common disaccharides found in foods are *lactose, maltose,* and *sucrose* (**Figure 4.3**). **Lactose** (also called *milk sugar*) consists of one glucose molecule and one galactose molecule. Interestingly, human breast milk has a higher amount of lactose than cow's milk, which makes human breast milk taste sweeter.

Maltose (also called *malt sugar*) consists of two molecules of glucose. It does not generally occur by itself in foods but rather is bound together with other molecules. As our bodies break down these larger molecules, maltose results as a by-product. Maltose is also the sugar that results from *fermentation* during the production of beer and other alcoholic beverages. **Fermentation** is the anaerobic process in which an agent, such as yeast, causes an organic substance to break down into simpler substances and results in the production of adenosine triphosphate (ATP). Maltose is formed during the anaerobic breakdown of sugar in grains and other foods into alcohol. Contrary to popular belief, very little maltose remains in alcoholic beverages after the fermentation process is complete; thus, alcoholic beverages are not good sources of carbohydrate.

Sucrose is composed of one glucose molecule and one fructose molecule. Because sucrose contains fructose, it is sweeter than lactose or maltose. Sucrose provides much of the sweet taste found in honey, maple syrup, fruits, and vegetables. Table sugar, brown sugar, powdered sugar, and many other products are made by refining the sucrose found in sugarcane and sugar beets. Are honey and other naturally occurring forms of sucrose more healthful than manufactured forms? The nearby ***Highlight: Are All Forms of Sugar the Same?*** investigates this question.

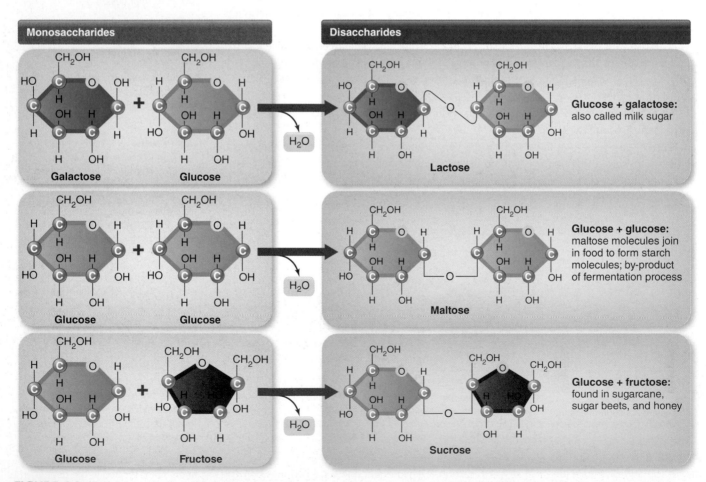

FIGURE 4.3 Galactose, glucose, and fructose join together in different combinations to make the disaccharides lactose, maltose, and sucrose.

The two monosaccharides that compose a disaccharide are attached by a bond between oxygen and one carbon on each of the monosaccharides (**Figure 4.4**). Two forms of this bond occur in nature: an **alpha bond** and a **beta bond**. As you can see in Figure 4.4a, sucrose is produced by an alpha bond joining a glucose molecule and a fructose molecule. The disaccharide maltose is also produced by an alpha bond. In contrast, lactose is produced by a beta bond joining a glucose molecule and a galactose molecule (Figure 4.4b). Alpha bonds are easily digestible by humans, whereas beta bonds are very difficult to digest and may even be nondigestible. As you will learn later in this chapter, many people do not possess enough of the enzyme lactase, needed to break the beta bond present in lactose, which causes the condition referred to as *lactose intolerance*. Beta bonds are also present in high-fiber foods, leading to our inability to digest most forms of fiber.

RECAP

Carbohydrates contain carbon, hydrogen, and oxygen. Simple carbohydrates include monosaccharides and disaccharides. Glucose, fructose, galactose, and ribose are monosaccharides; lactose, maltose, and sucrose are disaccharides. In disaccharides, two monosaccharides are linked together with either an alpha bond or a beta bond. Alpha bonds are easily digestible by humans, whereas beta bonds are not easily digestible.

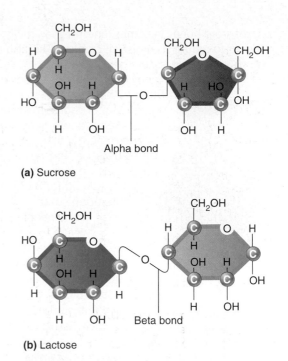

(a) Sucrose

(b) Lactose

FIGURE 4.4 The two monosaccharides that compose a disaccharide are attached by either (a) an alpha bond or (b) a beta bond between oxygen and one carbon of each monosaccharide.

HIGHLIGHT

Are All Forms of Sugar the Same?

Sucrose has become the target of a great deal of negative press. In particular, sucrose in the form of refined table sugar is commonly identified as being less healthful than sweeteners such as **honey**, **molasses**, and **raw sugar** because it is a product refined from sugarcane and sugar beets. These "natural" sweeteners are claimed to be more natural and nutritious than refined table sugar. Does the scientific evidence support this claim?

honey A sweet, sticky liquid sweetener made by bees from the nectar of flowers; contains glucose and fructose.

molasses A thick, brown syrup that is separated from raw sugar during manufacturing; it is considered the least refined form of sucrose.

white sugar Another name for sucrose, or table sugar.

raw sugar The sugar that results from the processing of sugar beets or sugarcane; it is approximately 96% to 98% sucrose; true raw sugar contains impurities and is not stable in storage; the raw sugar available to consumers has been purified to yield an edible sugar.

concentrated fruit juice sweetener A form of sweetener made with concentrated fruit juice, commonly pear juice.

confectioner's sugar A highly refined, finely ground white sugar; also referred to as powdered sugar.

corn sweeteners A general term for any sweetener made with corn starch.

Remember that sucrose consists of one glucose molecule and one fructose molecule joined together. From a chemical perspective, honey is almost identical to sucrose, because honey also contains glucose and fructose molecules in almost equal amounts. However, enzymes in bees' "honey stomachs" separate some of the glucose and fructose molecules; as a result, honey looks and tastes slightly different from sucrose. As you know,

corn syrup A syrup produced by the partial hydrolysis of corn starch.

dextrose An alternative term for glucose.

granulated sugar Another term for white sugar, or table sugar.

invert sugar A sugar created by heating a sucrose syrup with a small amount of acid; inverting sucrose results in its breakdown into glucose and fructose, which reduces the size of the sugar crystals; due to its smooth texture, it is used in making candies, such as fondant and some syrups.

maple sugar A sugar made by boiling maple syrup.

natural sweeteners A general term for any naturally occurring sweeteners, such as fructose, honey, and raw sugar.

turbinado sugar The form of raw sugar that is purified and safe for human consumption; it is sold as "Sugar in the Raw" in the United States.

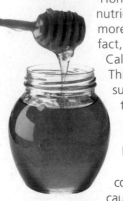

bees store honey in combs, and they fan it with their wings to reduce its moisture content. This also alters the appearance and texture of honey.

Honey does not contain any more nutrients than sucrose, so it is not a more healthful choice than sucrose. In fact, per tablespoon, honey has more Calories (energy) than table sugar. This is because the crystals in table sugar take up more space on a spoon than the liquid form of honey, so a tablespoon contains less sugar. However, some people argue that honey is sweeter, so you use less.

It is important to note that honey commonly contains bacteria that can cause fatal food poisoning in infants. The more mature digestive system of older children and adults is immune to the effects of these bacteria, but babies younger than 12 months should never be given honey.

Are raw sugar and molasses more healthful than table sugar? Actually, the "raw sugar" available in the United States is not really raw. Truly raw sugar is made up of the first crystals obtained when sugar is processed. Sugar in this form contains dirt, parts of insects, and other by-products that make it illegal to sell in the United States. The raw sugar products in American stores have actually gone through more than half of the same steps in the refining process used to make table sugar. Raw sugar has a more coarse texture than **white sugar** and is unbleached; in most markets, it is also significantly more expensive.

Molasses is the syrup that remains when sucrose is made from sugarcane. It is reddish brown in color, with a distinctive taste that is less sweet than table sugar. It does contain some iron, but this iron does not occur naturally. It is a contaminant from the machines that process the sugarcane! Incidentally, blackstrap molasses is the residue of a third boiling of the syrup. It contains less sugar than light or dark molasses but more minerals.

Table 4.1 compares the nutrient content of table sugar, raw sugar, honey, and molasses. As you can see, none of them contain many nutrients that are important

TABLE 4.1 Nutrient Comparison of Four Different Sugars

	Table Sugar	Raw Sugar	Honey	Molasses
Energy (kcal)	49	55	64	58
Carbohydrate (g)	12.6	13.8	17.3	14.95
Fat (g)	0	0	0	0
Protein (g)	0	0	0.06	0
Fiber (g)	0	0	0	0
Vitamin C (mg)	0	0	0.1	0
Vitamin A (IU)	0	0	0	0
Thiamin (mg)	0	0	0	0.008
Riboflavin (mg)	0.002	0.003	0.008	0
Folate (μg)	0	0	0	0
Calcium (mg)	0	2	1	41
Iron (mg)	0.01	0.05	0.09	0.94
Sodium (mg)	0	0	1	7
Potassium (mg)	0	4	11	293

Note: *Nutrient values are identified for 1 tablespoon of each product.*

Source: U.S. Department of Agriculture, Agricultural Research Service. 2014. USDA National Nutrient Database for Standard Reference, Release 27.

for health. This is why highly sweetened products are referred to as "empty Calories."

As introduced in Chapter 2 and discussed later in this chapter, it is added sugars in general—that is, any form of sugars and syrups added to foods during processing or preparation—that have become a concern in the American diet. Added sugars are not chemically different from naturally occurring sugars. However, foods and beverages with added sugars have lower levels of vitamins, minerals, and fiber than fruits and other foods that naturally contain simple sugars. That's why most healthcare organizations recommend that we limit our consumption of added sugars. The Nutrition Facts panel includes a list of total sugars, but a distinction is not generally made between added sugars and naturally occurring sugars. Thus, you need to check the ingredients label. Below is a list of terms for sugars. You'll find one or more of these terms on the labels of foods containing added sugars. To maintain a diet low in added sugars, limit foods in which a form of added sugar is listed as one of the first few ingredients on the label.

Oligosaccharides and Polysaccharides Are Complex Carbohydrates

complex carbohydrate A nutrient compound consisting of long chains of glucose molecules, such as starch, glycogen, and fiber.

oligosaccharides Complex carbohydrates that contain 3 to 10 monosaccharides.

Complex carbohydrates, the second major classification of carbohydrate, generally consist of long chains of glucose molecules. Technically, any carbohydrates with three or more monosaccharides are considered complex carbohydrates.

Oligosaccharides are carbohydrates that contain 3 to 10 monosaccharides (*oligo*, meaning "few"). Two of the most common oligosaccharides found in our diet are **raffinose** and **stachyose.** Raffinose is composed of galactose, glucose, and fructose. It is commonly

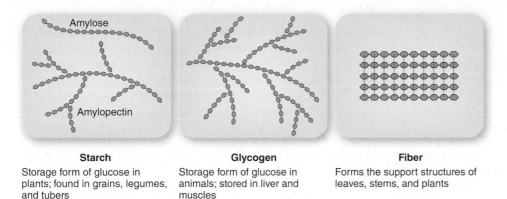

Starch	**Glycogen**	**Fiber**
Storage form of glucose in plants; found in grains, legumes, and tubers	Storage form of glucose in animals; stored in liver and muscles	Forms the support structures of leaves, stems, and plants

FIGURE 4.5 Polysaccharides, also referred to as complex carbohydrates, include starch, glycogen, and fiber.

found in beans, cabbage, brussels sprouts, broccoli, and whole grains. Stachyose is composed of two galactose molecules, a glucose molecule, and a fructose molecule. It is found in many beans and other legumes.

Raffinose and stachyose are part of the raffinose family of oligosaccharides (RFOs). Because humans do not possess the enzyme needed to break down these RFOs, they pass into the large intestine undigested. Once they reach the large intestine, they are fermented by bacteria that produce gases such as carbon dioxide, methane, and hydrogen. The product Beano® contains the enzyme alpha-galactosidase; this is the enzyme needed to break down the RFOs in the intestinal tract. Thus, this product can help to reduce the intestinal gas caused by eating beans and various vegetables.

Most **polysaccharides** consist of hundreds to thousands of glucose molecules (*poly*, meaning "many").[6] The polysaccharides include starch, glycogen, and most fibers (**Figure 4.5**).

Starch Is a Polysaccharide Stored in Plants

Plants store glucose not as single molecules but as polysaccharides in the form of **starch**. The two forms of starch are *amylose* and *amylopectin* (see Figure 4.5). Amylose is a straight chain of glucose molecules, whereas amylopectin is highly branched. Both forms of starch are found in starch-containing foods. The more open-branched structure of amylopectin increases its surface area and thus its exposure to digestive enzymes; as a result, it is more rapidly digested than amylose. In turn, amylopectin raises blood glucose more quickly than amylose.

Excellent food sources of starch include grains (wheat, rice, corn, oats, and barley), legumes (peas, beans, and lentils), and tubers (potatoes and yams). Our cells cannot use the complex starch molecules exactly as they occur in plants. Instead, the body must break them down into the monosaccharide glucose, from which we can then fuel our energy needs.

Our bodies easily digest most starches, in which alpha bonds link the numerous glucose units; however, starches linked by beta bonds are largely indigestible and are called *resistant*. Technically, resistant starch is classified as a type of fiber. When our intestinal bacteria ferment resistant starch, a short-chain fatty acid called *butyrate* is produced. Consuming resistant starch may be beneficial: some research suggests that butyrate reduces the risk for cancer.[7] Legumes contain more resistant starch than do other types of vegetables, fruits, or grains. This quality, plus their high protein and fiber content, makes legumes a healthful food.

Glycogen Is a Polysaccharide Stored by Animals

Glycogen is the storage form of glucose for animals, including humans. After an animal is slaughtered, most of the glycogen is broken down by enzymes found in animal tissues. Thus, very little glycogen exists in meat. As plants contain no glycogen, it is not a dietary source of carbohydrate. We store glycogen in our muscles and liver. We can very quickly break down the glycogen stored in the liver into glucose when we need it for energy. The storage and use of glycogen are discussed in more detail on pages 121–122.

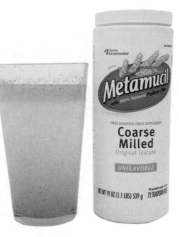

Dissolvable laxatives are examples of soluble fiber.

raffinose An oligosaccharide composed of galactose, glucose, and fructose. Also called melitose, it is found in beans, cabbage, broccoli, and other vegetables.

stachyose An oligosaccharide composed of two galactose molecules, a glucose molecule, and a fructose molecule; found in the Chinese artichoke and various beans and other legumes.

polysaccharide A complex carbohydrate consisting of long chains of glucose.

starch The storage form of glucose (as a polysaccharide) in plants.

glycogen The storage form of glucose (as a polysaccharide) in animals.

Fiber Is a Polysaccharide That Gives Plants Their Structure

Like starch, fiber is composed of long polysaccharide chains; however, the body does not easily break down the beta bonds that connect fiber molecules. This means that most fibers pass through the digestive system without being digested and absorbed, so they contribute no energy to our diet. However, fiber offers many other health benefits (see pages 126–128).

There are currently a number of definitions of fiber. The Food and Nutrition Board of the Institute of Medicine uses three distinctions: *dietary fiber, functional fiber,* and *total fiber.*[6]

- **Dietary fiber** is the nondigestible parts of plants that form the support structures of leaves, stems, and seeds (see Figure 4.5). In a sense, you can think of dietary fiber as the plant's "skeleton."
- **Functional fiber** consists of nondigestible forms of carbohydrates that are extracted from plants or manufactured in a laboratory and have known health benefits. Functional fiber is added to foods and is the form found in fiber supplements. Examples of functional fiber sources you might see on nutrition labels include cellulose, guar gum, pectin, inulin, and psyllium.
- **Total fiber** is the sum of dietary fiber and functional fiber.

Fiber can also be classified according to its chemical and physical properties as soluble or insoluble.

Soluble Fibers   **Soluble fibers** dissolve in water. They are also **viscous**, forming a gel when wet, and they are fermentable; that is, they are easily digested by bacteria in the colon. Soluble fibers are typically found in citrus fruits, berries, oat products, and beans.

Research suggests that regular consumption of soluble fibers reduces the risks for cardiovascular disease and type 2 diabetes by lowering blood cholesterol and blood glucose levels. The possible mechanisms by which fiber reduces the risk for various diseases are discussed in more detail on pages 126–128.

Soluble fibers include the following:

- *Pectins*, which contain chains of galacturonic acid and other monosaccharides. Pectins are found in the cell walls and intracellular tissues of many fruits and berries. They can be isolated and used to thicken foods, such as jams and yogurts.
- *Fructans* contain chains of fructose molecules, and serve as important storage sites for polysaccharides in the stems of many vegetables and grasses, including artichokes, asparagus, leeks, onions, garlic, and wheat. One commonly isolated fructan is inulin, which is used to alter the texture and stability of foods and can be used to replace sugar, fat and flour. As we discussed in Chapter 3, inulin is also added to foods as a prebiotic.
- *Gums* contain galactose, glucuronic acid, and other monosaccharides. Gums are a diverse group of polysaccharides that are viscous. They are typically isolated from seeds and are used as thickening, gelling, and stabilizing agents. Guar gum and gum arabic are common gums used as food additives.
- *Mucilages* are similar to gums and contain galactose, mannose, and other monosaccharides. Two examples include psyllium and carrageenan. Psyllium is the husk of psyllium seeds, which are also known as plantago or flea seeds. Carrageenan comes from seaweed. Mucilages are used as food stabilizers.

Insoluble Fibers   **Insoluble fibers** are those that do not typically dissolve in water. These fibers are usually nonviscous and cannot be fermented by bacteria in the colon. They are generally found in whole grains, such as wheat, rye, and brown rice, as well as in many vegetables and some fruits. These fibers are not associated with reducing cholesterol levels but are known for promoting regular bowel movements, alleviating constipation, and reducing the risk for a bowel disorder called diverticulosis (discussed later in this chapter). Examples of insoluble fibers include the following:

- *Lignins* are noncarbohydrate forms of fiber. Lignins are found in the woody parts of plant cell walls and in carrots and the seeds of fruits. Lignins are also found in brans (the outer husk of grains such as wheat, oats, and rye) and other whole grains.

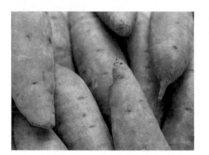

Tubers, such as these sweet potatoes, are excellent food sources of starch.

dietary fiber The nondigestible carbohydrate parts of plants that form the support structures of leaves, stems, and seeds.

functional fiber The nondigestible forms of carbohydrate that are extracted from plants or manufactured in the laboratory and have known health benefits.

total fiber The sum of dietary fiber and functional fiber.

soluble fibers Fibers that dissolve in water.

viscous Having a gel-like consistency; viscous fibers form a gel when dissolved in water.

insoluble fibers Fibers that do not dissolve in water.

- *Cellulose* is the main structural component of plant cell walls. Cellulose is a chain of glucose units similar to amylose, but unlike amylose, cellulose contains beta bonds that are not digestible by humans. Cellulose is found in whole grains, fruits, and legumes and other vegetables. It can also be extracted from wood pulp or cotton, and it is added to foods as an agent for anti-caking, thickening, and texturizing.
- *Hemicelluloses* contain glucose, mannose, galacturonic acid, and other monosaccharides. Hemicelluloses are found in plant cell walls and they surround cellulose. They are the primary component of cereal fibers and are found in whole grains and vegetables. Although many hemicelluloses are insoluble, some are also classified as soluble.

Fiber-Rich Carbohydrates   Materials written for the general public usually don't refer to the carbohydrates found in foods as complex or simple; instead, resources such as the *Dietary Guidelines for Americans 2010* emphasize eating **fiber-rich carbohydrates**, such as fruits, vegetables, and whole grains.[8] This term is important, because fiber-rich carbohydrates are known to contribute to good health, but not all complex carbohydrate foods are fiber-rich. For example, potatoes that have been processed into frozen hash browns retain very little of their original fiber. On the other hand, some foods rich in simple carbohydrates (such as fruits) are also rich in fiber. So when you're reading labels, it pays to check the grams of dietary fiber per serving. And if the food you're considering is fresh produce and there's no label to read, that almost guarantees it's fiber-rich.

RECAP

Complex carbohydrates include oligosaccharides and polysaccharides. The three types of polysaccharides are starch, glycogen, and fiber. Starch is the storage form of glucose in plants, whereas glycogen is the storage form of glucose in animals. Fiber forms the support structures of plants. Soluble fibers dissolve in water, are viscous, and can be digested by bacteria in the colon, whereas insoluble fibers do not dissolve in water, are not viscous, and cannot be digested. Fiber-rich carbohydrates are known to contribute to good health.

How Does the Body Break Down Carbohydrates?

LO 4 Discuss how carbohydrates are digested and absorbed by the body.

Glucose is the form of sugar that our bodies use for energy, and the primary goal of carbohydrate digestion is to break down polysaccharides and disaccharides into monosaccharides, which can then be converted to glucose. Chapter 3 provided an overview of gastrointestinal function. Here, we focus specifically and in more detail on the digestion and absorption of carbohydrates. **Focus Figure 4.6** (page 120) provides a visual tour of carbohydrate digestion.

Digestion Breaks Down Most Carbohydrates into Monosaccharides

Carbohydrate digestion begins in the mouth when the starch in the foods you eat mixes with your saliva during chewing (Focus Figure 4.6). Saliva contains an enzyme called **salivary amylase**, which breaks down starch into smaller particles and eventually into the disaccharide maltose. (*Amyl-* is a prefix referring to starch, and the suffix *-ase* indicates an enzyme.) The next time you eat a piece of bread, notice that you can actually taste it becoming sweeter; this indicates the breakdown of starch into maltose. Disaccharides are not digested in the mouth.

As the bolus of food leaves the mouth and enters the stomach, all digestion of carbohydrates ceases. This is because the acid in the stomach inactivates the salivary amylase enzyme (Focus Figure 4.6).

The majority of carbohydrate digestion occurs in the small intestine. As the contents of the stomach enter the small intestine, an enzyme called **pancreatic amylase** is secreted by the pancreas into the small intestine (Focus Figure 4.6). Pancreatic amylase continues to digest any remaining starch into maltose. Additional enzymes found in the microvilli

fiber-rich carbohydrates A group of foods containing either simple or complex carbohydrates that are rich in dietary fiber. These foods, which include most fruits, vegetables, and whole grains, are typically fresh or moderately processed.

salivary amylase An enzyme in saliva that breaks starch into smaller particles and eventually into the disaccharide maltose.

pancreatic amylase An enzyme secreted by the pancreas into the small intestine that digests any remaining starch into maltose.

The primary goal of carbohydrate digestion is to break down polysaccharides and disaccharides into monosaccharides that can then be converted to glucose.

ORGANS OF THE GI TRACT

ACCESSORY ORGANS

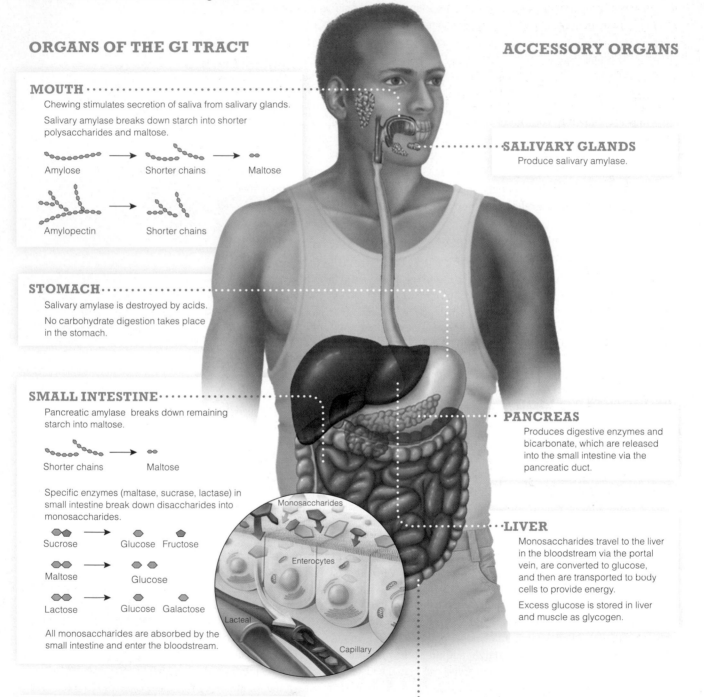

MOUTH

Chewing stimulates secretion of saliva from salivary glands.

Salivary amylase breaks down starch into shorter polysaccharides and maltose.

Amylose → Shorter chains → Maltose

Amylopectin → Shorter chains

SALIVARY GLANDS

Produce salivary amylase.

STOMACH

Salivary amylase is destroyed by acids.

No carbohydrate digestion takes place in the stomach.

SMALL INTESTINE

Pancreatic amylase breaks down remaining starch into maltose.

Shorter chains → Maltose

Specific enzymes (maltase, sucrase, lactase) in small intestine break down disaccharides into monosaccharides.

Sucrose → Glucose Fructose

Maltose → Glucose

Lactose → Glucose Galactose

All monosaccharides are absorbed by the small intestine and enter the bloodstream.

Monosaccharides

Enterocytes

Lacteal

Capillary

PANCREAS

Produces digestive enzymes and bicarbonate, which are released into the small intestine via the pancreatic duct.

LIVER

Monosaccharides travel to the liver in the bloodstream via the portal vein, are converted to glucose, and then are transported to body cells to provide energy.

Excess glucose is stored in liver and muscle as glycogen.

LARGE INTESTINE

Some carbohydrates pass into the large intestine undigested.

Bacteria ferment some undigested carbohydrate.

Remaining fiber is excreted in feces.

of the mucosal cells that line the intestinal tract work to break down disaccharides into monosaccharides (Focus Figure 4.6):

- Maltose is broken down into glucose by the enzyme **maltase**.
- Sucrose is broken down into glucose and fructose by the enzyme **sucrase**.
- Lactose is broken down into glucose and galactose by the enzyme **lactase**.

Once digestion of carbohydrates is complete, all monosaccharides are then absorbed into the mucosal cells lining the small intestine, where they pass through and enter into the bloodstream. Glucose and galactose are absorbed across the enterocytes via active transport using a carrier protein saturated with sodium. This process requires energy from the breakdown of ATP. Fructose is absorbed via facilitated diffusion and therefore requires no energy. (Refer to Chapter 3 for a description of these transport processes.) The absorption of fructose takes longer than that of glucose or galactose. This slower absorption rate means that fructose stays in the small intestine longer and draws water into the intestines via osmosis. This not only results in a smaller rise in blood glucose when consuming fructose but can also lead to diarrhea.

The Liver Converts Most Non-Glucose Monosaccharides into Glucose

Once the monosaccharides enter the bloodstream, they travel to the liver, where fructose and galactose are converted to glucose (Focus Figure 4.6). If needed immediately for energy, the glucose is released into the bloodstream, where it can travel to the cells to provide energy. If glucose is not needed immediately for energy, it is stored as glycogen in the liver and muscles. Enzymes in liver and muscle cells combine glucose molecules to form glycogen (an anabolic, or building, process) and break glycogen into glucose (a catabolic, or destructive, process), depending on the body's energy needs. On average, the liver can store 70 g (280 kcal) and the muscles can store about 120 g (480 kcal) of glycogen. Between meals, our bodies draw on liver glycogen reserves to maintain blood glucose levels and support the needs of our cells, including those of our brain, spinal cord, and red blood cells (**Figure 4.7**).

The glycogen stored in our muscles continually provides energy to the muscles, particularly during intense exercise. Endurance athletes can increase their storage of muscle glycogen from two to four times the normal amount through a process called *glycogen, or carbohydrate, loading*

maltase A digestive enzyme that breaks maltose into glucose.

sucrase A digestive enzyme that breaks sucrose into glucose and fructose.

lactase A digestive enzyme that breaks lactose into glucose and galactose.

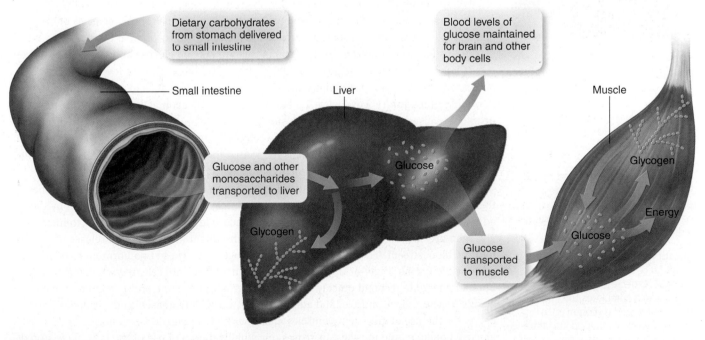

FIGURE 4.7 Glucose is stored as glycogen in both the liver and muscle. The glycogen stored in the liver maintains blood glucose between meals; muscle glycogen provides immediate energy to the muscle during exercise.

(see Chapter 14). Any excess glucose is stored as glycogen in the liver and muscles and saved for such future energy needs as exercise. Once the carbohydrate storage capacity of the liver and muscles is reached, any excess glucose can be stored as fat in adipose tissue.

Fiber Is Excreted from the Large Intestine

As previously mentioned, humans do not possess enzymes in the small intestine that can break down fiber. Thus, fiber passes through the small intestine undigested and enters the large intestine, or colon. There, bacteria ferment some previously undigested carbohydrates, causing the production of gases such as hydrogen, methane, and sulfur and a few short-chain fatty acids such as acetic acid, butyric acid, and propionic acid. The cells of the large intestine use these short-chain fatty acids for energy. It is estimated that fermented fibers yield about 1.5 to 2.5 kcal/g.[6] This is less than the 4 kcal/g provided by carbohydrates that are digested and absorbed in the small intestine; the discrepancy is due to the fact that fermentation of the fibers in the colon is an anaerobic process, which yields less energy than the aerobic digestive process of other carbohydrates. Obviously, the fibers that remain totally undigested contribute no energy to our bodies. Fiber remaining in the colon adds bulk to our stools and is excreted in feces (Focus Figure 4.6). In this way, fiber assists in maintaining bowel regularity. The health benefits of fiber are discussed later in this chapter.

A Variety of Hormones Regulate Blood Glucose Levels

Our bodies regulate blood glucose levels within a fairly narrow range to provide adequate glucose to the brain and other cells. A number of hormones, including insulin, glucagon, epinephrine, norepinephrine, cortisol, and growth hormone, assist the body with maintaining blood glucose.

When we eat a meal, our blood glucose level rises. But glucose in our blood cannot help the nerves, muscles, and other tissues function unless it can cross into their cells. Glucose molecules are too large to cross cell membranes independently. To get in, glucose needs assistance from the hormone **insulin**, which is secreted by the beta cells of the pancreas (**Focus Figure 4.8** top panel). Insulin is transported in the blood to the cells of tissues throughout the body, where it stimulates special carrier proteins, called *glucose transporters*, located in cells. The arrival of insulin at the cell membrane stimulates glucose transporters to travel to the surface of the cell, where they assist in transporting glucose across the cell membrane and into the cell. Insulin can be thought of as a key that opens the gates of the cell membrane, enabling the transport of glucose into the cell interior, where it can be used for energy. Insulin also stimulates the liver and muscles to take up glucose and store it as glycogen.

When you have not eaten for a period of time, your blood glucose level declines. This decrease in blood glucose stimulates the alpha cells of the pancreas to secrete another hormone, **glucagon** (Focus Figure 4.8 bottom panel). Glucagon acts in an opposite way to insulin: it causes the liver to convert its stored glycogen into glucose, which is then secreted into the bloodstream and transported to the cells for energy. Glucagon also assists in the breakdown of body proteins to amino acids, so that the liver can stimulate *gluconeogenesis* ("generating new glucose"), the production of glucose from amino acids.

Epinephrine, norepinephrine, cortisol, and growth hormone are additional hormones that work to increase blood glucose. Epinephrine and norepinephrine are secreted by the adrenal glands and nerve endings when blood glucose levels are low. They act to increase glycogen breakdown in the liver, resulting in a subsequent increase in the release of glucose into the bloodstream. They also increase gluconeogenesis. These two hormones are also responsible for our "fight-or-flight" reaction to danger; they are released when we need a burst of energy to respond quickly. Cortisol and growth hormone are secreted by the adrenal glands to act on liver, muscle, and adipose tissue. Cortisol increases gluconeogenesis and decreases the use of glucose by muscles and other body organs. Growth hormone decreases glucose uptake by the muscles, increases our mobilization and use of the fatty acids stored in our adipose tissue, and increases the liver's output of glucose.

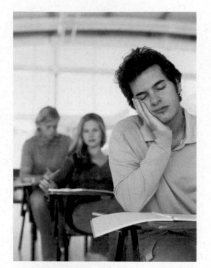

Our red blood cells, brain, and nerve cells primarily rely on glucose. This is why we get tired, irritable, and shaky when we have not eaten for a prolonged period of time.

insulin A hormone secreted by the beta cells of the pancreas in response to increased blood levels of glucose that facilitates uptake of glucose by body cells.

glucagon A hormone secreted by the alpha cells of the pancreas in response to decreased blood levels of glucose; it stimulates the liver to convert stored glycogen into glucose, which is released into the bloodstream and transported to cells for energy.

Our bodies regulate blood glucose levels within a fairly narrow range to provide adequate glucose to the brain and other cells. Insulin and glucagon are two hormones that play a key role in regulating blood glucose.

HIGH BLOOD GLUCOSE

1 **Insulin secretion:** When blood glucose levels increase after a meal, the pancreas secretes the hormone insulin from the beta cells into the bloodstream.

2 **Cellular uptake:** Insulin travels to the tissues. There, it stimulates glucose transporters within cells to travel to the cell membrane, where they facilitate glucose transport into the cell to be used for energy.

3 **Glucose storage:** Insulin also stimulates the storage of glucose in body tissues. Glucose is stored as glycogen in the liver and muscles (glycogenesis), and is stored as triglycerides in adipose tissue (lipogenesis).

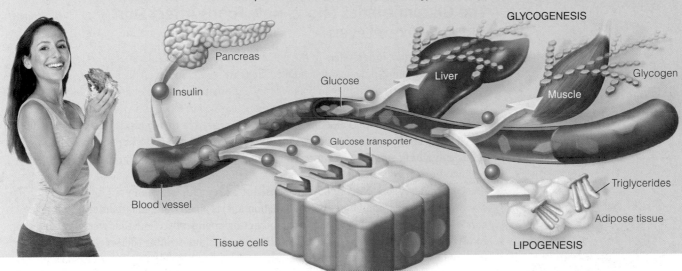

LOW BLOOD GLUCOSE

1 **Glucagon secretion:** When blood glucose levels are low, the pancreas secretes the hormone glucagon from the alpha cells into the bloodstream.

2 **Glycogenolysis:** Glucagon stimulates the liver to convert stored glycogen into glucose, which is released into the blood and transported to the cells for energy.

3 **Gluconeogenesis:** Glucagon also assists in the breakdown of proteins and the uptake of amino acids by the liver, which creates glucose from amino acids.

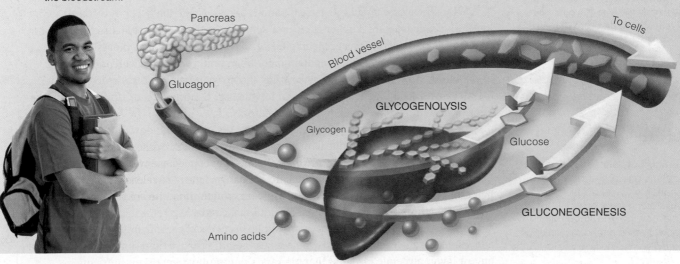

Normally, the effects of these hormones balance each other to maintain blood glucose within a healthy range. If this balance is altered, it can lead to health conditions such as diabetes (pages 140–143) or hypoglycemia (pages 144–145).

RECAP

Carbohydrate digestion starts in the mouth and continues in the small intestine. Glucose and other monosaccharides are absorbed into the bloodstream and travel to the liver, where non-glucose monosaccharides are converted to glucose. Glucose is used by the cells for energy, converted to glycogen and stored in the liver and muscles for later use, or converted to fat and stored in adipose tissue. Various hormones are involved in regulating blood glucose. Insulin lowers blood glucose levels by facilitating the entry of glucose into cells. Glucagon, epinephrine, norepinephrine, cortisol, and growth hormone raise blood glucose levels by a variety of mechanisms. ■

The Glycemic Index Shows How Foods Affect Our Blood Glucose Levels

The term **glycemic index** refers to the potential of foods to raise blood glucose levels. Foods with a high glycemic index cause a sudden surge in blood glucose. This in turn triggers a large increase in insulin, which may be followed by a dramatic drop in blood glucose. Foods with a low glycemic index cause low to moderate fluctuations in blood glucose. When foods are assigned a glycemic index value, they are often compared to the glycemic effect of pure glucose.

The glycemic index of a food is not always easy to predict. Most people assume that foods containing simple sugars have a higher glycemic index than starches, but this is not always the case. For instance, although instant potatoes are a starchy food, they have a glycemic index value of 85, while the value for an apple is only 38!

The type of carbohydrate, the way the food is prepared, and its fat and fiber content can all affect how quickly the body absorbs it. It is important to note that we eat most of our foods combined into a meal. In this case, the glycemic index of the total meal becomes more important than the ranking of each food.

For determining the effect of a food on a person's glucose response, some nutrition experts believe the **glycemic load** is more useful than the glycemic index. A food's glycemic load is the number of grams of carbohydrate it contains multiplied by the glycemic index of that carbohydrate. For instance, carrots are recognized as a vegetable having a relatively high glycemic index of about 68; however, the glycemic load of carrots is only 3. This is because there is very little total carbohydrate in a serving of carrots. The low glycemic load of carrots means that carrot consumption is unlikely to cause a significant rise in glucose and insulin.

Why do we care about the glycemic index and glycemic load? Foods or meals with a lower glycemic load are a better choice for someone with diabetes, because they will not trigger dramatic fluctuations in blood glucose. They may also reduce the risk for heart disease, because they generally contain more fiber, and fiber helps decrease fat levels in the blood. A recent systematic review has shown that eating a lower glycemic index diet decreases total blood cholesterol and low-density lipoproteins, or LDL (a blood lipid associated with increased risk for heart disease).[9]

Despite some encouraging research findings, the glycemic index and glycemic load remain controversial. Many nutrition researchers feel that the evidence supporting their health benefits is weak. In addition, many believe the concepts of the glycemic index/load are too complex for people to apply to their daily lives. Other researchers insist that helping people choose foods with a lower glycemic index/load is critical to the prevention and treatment of many chronic diseases. Until this controversy is resolved, people are encouraged to eat a variety of fiber-rich and less processed carbohydrates, such as beans and lentils, fresh vegetables, and whole-wheat bread, because these forms of carbohydrates have a lower glycemic load and they contain a multitude of important nutrients.

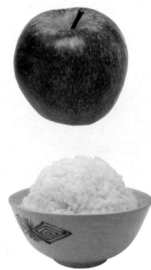

An apple has a much lower glycemic index (38) than a serving of white rice (56).

To find out the glycemic index and glycemic load of over 100 foods, visit www.health.harvard.edu. Type "Glycemic index 100 foods" in the search bar, then click on the link.

glycemic index A rating of the potential of foods to raise blood glucose and insulin levels.

glycemic load The amount of carbohydrate in a food multiplied by the glycemic index of the carbohydrate.

RECAP

The glycemic index is a value that indicates the potential of foods to raise blood glucose and insulin levels. The glycemic load is the amount of carbohydrate in a food multiplied by the glycemic index of the carbohydrate in that food. Foods with a high glycemic index/load cause sudden surges in blood glucose and insulin, whereas foods with a low glycemic index/load cause low to moderate fluctuations in blood glucose. Diets with a low glycemic index/load are associated with a reduced risk for cardiovascular disease, but some researchers feel that the evidence supporting their health benefits is weak.

Why Do We Need Carbohydrates?

LO 5 List four functions of carbohydrates in the body.

We have seen that carbohydrates are an important energy source for our bodies. Let's learn more about this and discuss other functions of carbohydrates.

Carbohydrates Provide Energy

Carbohydrates, an excellent source of energy for all of our cells, provide 4 kcal of energy per gram. Some of our cells can also use lipids and even protein for energy if necessary. However, our red blood cells can use only glucose, and the brain and other nervous tissues rely primarily on glucose. This is why you get tired, irritable, and shaky when you have not eaten carbohydrates for a prolonged period of time.

Carbohydrates Fuel Daily Activity

Many popular diets—such as Dr. Atkins' New Diet Revolution and the Sugar Busters plan—are based on the idea that our bodies actually "prefer" to use dietary fats and/or protein for energy. They claim that current carbohydrate recommendations are much higher than we really need.

In reality, the body relies mostly on both carbohydrates and fats for energy. In fact, as shown in **Figure 4.9** our bodies always use some combination of carbohydrates and fats to fuel daily activities. Fat is the predominant energy source used by our bodies at rest and during low-intensity activities, such as sitting, standing, and walking. Even during rest, however, our brain cells and red blood cells still rely on glucose.

Carbohydrates Fuel Exercise

When we exercise, whether running, briskly walking, bicycling, or performing any other activity that causes us to breathe harder and sweat, we begin to use more glucose than fat. Whereas fat breakdown is a slow process and requires oxygen, we can break down glucose very quickly either with or without oxygen. Even during very intense exercise, when less oxygen is available, we can still break down glucose very quickly for energy. That's why when you are exercising at maximal effort carbohydrates are providing almost 100% of the energy your body requires.

If you are physically active, it is important to eat enough carbohydrates to provide energy for your brain, red blood cells, and muscles. In general, if you do not eat enough carbohydrate to support regular exercise, your body will have to rely on fat and protein as alternative energy sources. One advantage of becoming highly trained for endurance-type events, such as marathons and triathlons, is that our muscles are able to store more glycogen, which provides us with additional glucose we can use during exercise. (See Chapter 14 for more information on how exercise affects intake recommendations, use, and storage of carbohydrates.)

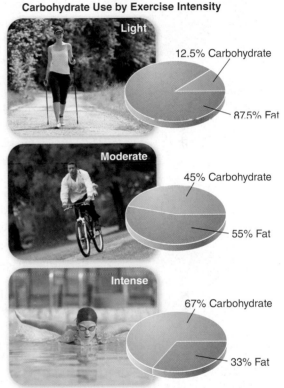

Carbohydrate Use by Exercise Intensity

Light — 12.5% Carbohydrate / 87.5% Fat

Moderate — 45% Carbohydrate / 55% Fat

Intense — 67% Carbohydrate / 33% Fat

FIGURE 4.9 Amounts of carbohydrate and fat used during light, moderate, and intense exercise. (*Source:* Figure data adapted from the "Regulation of endogenous fat and carbohydrate metabolism in relation to exercise intensity and duration" by Romijn et al., from *American Journal of Physiology*, September 1, 1993. Copyright © 1993 by The American Physiological Society. Reprinted with permission.)

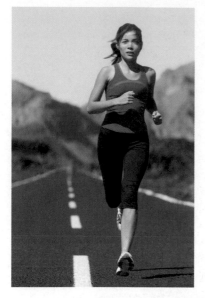

When we exercise or perform any other activity that causes us to breathe harder and sweat, we begin to use more glucose than fat.

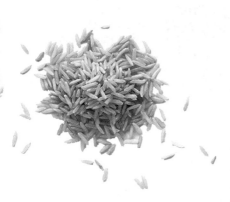

Brown rice is a good food source of dietary fiber.

ketosis The process by which the breakdown of fat during fasting states results in the production of ketones.

ketones Substances produced during the breakdown of fat when carbohydrate intake is insufficient to meet energy needs. They provide an alternative energy source for the brain when glucose levels are low.

ketoacidosis A condition in which excessive ketones are present in the blood, causing the blood to become very acidic, which alters basic body functions and damages tissues. Untreated ketoacidosis can be fatal. This condition is often found in individuals with untreated diabetes mellitus.

Low Carbohydrate Intake Can Lead to Ketoacidosis

When we do not eat enough carbohydrates, the body seeks an alternative source of fuel for the brain and begins to break down stored fat. This process, called **ketosis**, produces an alternative fuel called **ketones**. (The metabolic process of ketosis is discussed in more detail in Chapter 7.)

Ketosis is an important mechanism for providing energy to the brain during situations of fasting, low carbohydrate intake, or vigorous exercise. However, ketones also suppress appetite and cause dehydration and acetone breath (the breath smells like nail polish remover). If inadequate carbohydrate intake continues for an extended period of time, the body will produce excessive amounts of ketones. Because many ketones are acids, high ketone levels cause the blood to become very acidic, leading to a condition called **ketoacidosis**. The high acidity of the blood interferes with basic body functions, causes the loss of lean body mass, and damages many body tissues. People with untreated diabetes are at high risk for ketoacidosis, which can lead to coma and even death. (See pages 140–144 for further details about diabetes.)

Carbohydrates Spare Protein

If the diet does not provide enough carbohydrate, the body will make its own glucose from protein. As noted earlier, this process, called gluconeogenesis, involves breaking down the proteins in blood and tissues into amino acids, then converting them to glucose.

When our bodies use proteins for energy, the amino acids from these proteins cannot be used to make new cells, repair tissue damage, support the immune system, or perform any other function. During periods of starvation or when eating a diet that is very low in carbohydrate, our bodies will take amino acids from the blood first, and then from other tissues, such as muscles and the heart, liver, and kidneys. Using amino acids in this manner over a prolonged period of time can cause serious, possibly irreversible, damage to these organs. (See Chapter 6 for more details on using protein for energy.)

Fiber Helps Us Stay Healthy

The terms *simple* and *complex* can cause confusion when discussing the health effects of carbohydrates. As we explained earlier, these terms are used to designate the number of sugar molecules present in the carbohydrate. However, when distinguishing carbohydrates in terms of their effect on our health, it is more appropriate to talk about them in terms of their nutrient density and their fiber content. Although we cannot digest fiber, research indicates that it helps us stay healthy and may prevent many digestive and chronic diseases. The following are potential benefits of fiber consumption:

- Helps prevent hemorrhoids, constipation, and other intestinal problems by keeping our stools moist and soft. Fiber gives gut muscles "something to push on" and makes it easier to eliminate stools.
- Reduces the risk for *diverticulosis,* a condition that is caused in part by trying to eliminate small, hard stools. A great deal of pressure must be generated in the large intestine to pass hard stools. This increased pressure weakens intestinal walls, causing them to bulge outward and form pockets (**Figure 4.10**). Feces and fibrous materials can get trapped in these pockets, which become infected and inflamed. This painful condition is typically treated with antibiotics or surgery.
- May reduce the risk of colon cancer. Although there is some controversy surrounding this claim, many researchers believe that fiber binds cancer-causing substances and speeds their elimination from the colon. However, recent studies of colon cancer and fiber have shown that their relationship is not as strong as previously thought.
- May reduce the risk of heart disease by delaying or blocking the absorption of dietary cholesterol into the bloodstream (**Figure 4.11**, page 128). In addition, when soluble

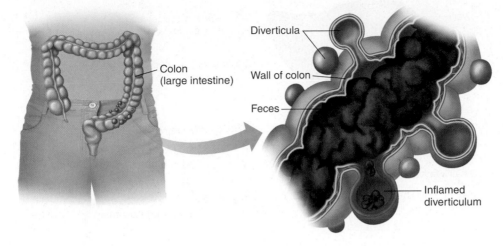

FIGURE 4.10 Diverticulosis occurs when bulging pockets form in the wall of the colon. These pockets become infected and inflamed, demanding proper treatment.

fibers are digested, bacteria in the colon produce short-chain fatty acids that may reduce the production of low-density lipoprotein (LDL) to healthful levels.

- May lower the risk for type 2 diabetes. In slowing digestion and absorption, fiber also slows the release of glucose into the blood. It thereby improves the body's regulation of insulin production and blood glucose levels.

- May enhance weight loss, as eating a high-fiber diet causes a person to feel more full. Fiber absorbs water, expands in our large intestine, and slows the movement of food through the upper part of the digestive tract. Also, people who eat a fiber-rich diet tend to eat fewer fatty and sugary foods.

RECAP

Carbohydrates are an important energy source at rest and during exercise, and they provide 4 kcal of energy per gram. Carbohydrates are necessary in the diet to spare body protein and prevent ketosis. Dietary helps prevent hemorrhoids, constipation, and diverticulosis; may reduce the risk for colon cancer, heart disease, and type 2 diabetes; and may assist with weight loss.

How Much Carbohydrate Should We Eat?

Proponents of low-carbohydrate diets claim that eating carbohydrates makes you gain weight. However, anyone who consumes more Calories than he or she expends will gain weight, whether those Calories are in the form of simple or complex carbohydrates, protein, or fat. Moreover, fat is twice as "fattening" as carbohydrate: it contains 9 kcal per gram, whereas carbohydrate contains only 4 kcal per gram. In fact, eating carbohydrate sources that are high in fiber and micronutrients has been shown to reduce the overall risk for obesity, heart disease, and diabetes. Thus, not all carbohydrates are bad, and even foods with **added sugars**—in limited amounts—can be included in a healthful diet.

The Recommended Dietary Allowance (RDA) for carbohydrate is based on the amount of glucose the brain uses.[6] The current RDA for adults 19 years of age and older is 130 g of carbohydrate per day. It is important to emphasize that this RDA does not cover the amount of carbohydrate needed to support daily activities; it covers only the amount of carbohydrate needed to supply adequate glucose to the brain.

Recall from Chapter 1 that the Acceptable Macronutrient Distribution Range (AMDR) is the range of intake for the energy-yielding nutrients associated with a decreased risk for chronic diseases. The AMDR for carbohydrates is 45% to 65% of total energy intake.

LO 6 Define the RDA and AMDR for carbohydrates and the AI for fiber.

LO 7 Identify the potential health risks associated with diets high in added sugars.

LO 8 List four types of foods that are generally good sources of fiber.

added sugars Sugars and syrups that are added to food during processing or preparation.

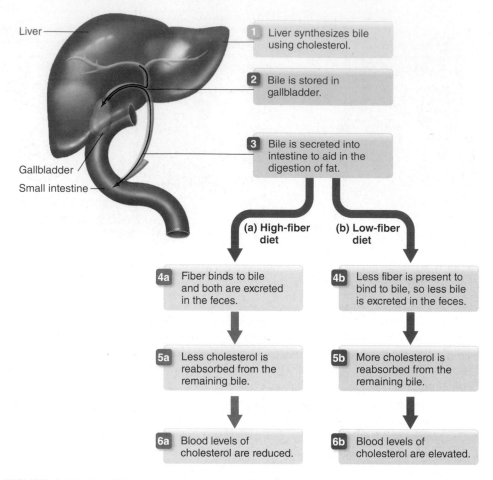

Liver

1 Liver synthesizes bile using cholesterol.

2 Bile is stored in gallbladder.

3 Bile is secreted into intestine to aid in the digestion of fat.

Gallbladder

Small intestine

(a) High-fiber diet

(b) Low-fiber diet

4a Fiber binds to bile and both are excreted in the feces.

4b Less fiber is present to bind to bile, so less bile is excreted in the feces.

5a Less cholesterol is reabsorbed from the remaining bile.

5b More cholesterol is reabsorbed from the remaining bile.

6a Blood levels of cholesterol are reduced.

6b Blood levels of cholesterol are elevated.

FIGURE 4.11 How fiber might help decrease blood cholesterol levels. **(a)** When we eat a high-fiber diet, fiber binds to the bile that is produced from cholesterol, resulting in relatively more cholesterol being excreted in the feces. **(b)** When a lower-fiber diet is consumed, less fiber (and thus cholesterol) is bound to bile and excreted in the feces.

Table 4.2 compares the carbohydrate recommendations from the Institute of Medicine with the *Dietary Guidelines for Americans* related to carbohydrate-containing foods.[6,8] As you can see, the Institute of Medicine provides specific numeric recommendations, whereas the *Dietary Guidelines for Americans* are general suggestions about eating foods high in fiber and low in added sugars. Most health agencies agree that most of the carbohydrates you eat each day should be high in fiber, whole-grain, and unprocessed. As recommended in the USDA Food Patterns, eating at least half your grains as whole grains and eating the suggested amounts of fruits and vegetables each day will ensure that you get enough fiber-rich carbohydrates in your diet. Although fruits are predominantly composed of simple sugars, they are good sources of vitamins, some minerals, and fiber.

Most Americans Eat Too Much Added Sugar

The average carbohydrate intake per person in the United States is approximately 50% of total energy intake. For some people, almost half of this amount consists of sugars. Where does all this sugar come from? Some sugar comes from healthful food sources, such as fruit and milk. Some comes from foods made with refined grains, such as soft white breads, saltine crackers, and pastries. As discussed in the ***Highlight*** on page 115, much of the rest comes from added sugars. For example, many processed foods include high-fructose corn syrup (HFCS), an added sugar.

The most common source of added sugars in the U.S. diet is sweetened soft drinks; we drink an average of 40 gallons per person each year. Consider that one 12-oz sugared cola

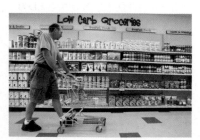

Many popular diets claim that current carbohydrate recommendations are much higher than we really need.

TABLE 4.2 Dietary Recommendations for Carbohydrates

Institute of Medicine Recommendations*	Dietary Guidelines for Americans†
Recommended Dietary Allowance (RDA) for adults 19 years of age and older is 130 g of carbohydrate per day.	Limit the consumption of foods that contain refined grains, especially refined grain foods that contain solid fats, added sugars, and sodium.
The Acceptable Macronutrient Distribution Range (AMDR) for carbohydrate is 45–65% of total daily energy intake.	Reduce the intake of Calories from solid fats and added sugars.
Added sugar intake should be 25% or less of total energy intake each day.	Increase vegetable and fruit intake.
	Eat a variety of vegetables, especially dark-green and red and orange vegetables and beans and peas.
	Consume at least half of all grains as whole grains. Increase whole-grain intake by replacing refined grains with whole grains.
	Choose foods that provide more potassium, dietary fiber, calcium, and vitamin D, which are nutrients of concern in American diets. These foods include vegetables, fruits, whole grains, and milk and milk products.

Sources: *Institute of Medicine, Food and Nutrition Board. 2005. Dietary Reference Intakes for Energy, Carbohydrates, Fiber, Fat, Fatty Acids, Cholesterol, Protein, and Amino Acids (Macronutrients).* Washington, DC: The National Academy of Sciences. Reprinted by permission.

†U.S. Department of Health and Human Services and U.S. Department of Agriculture. *2015–2020 Dietary Guidelines for Americans.* 8th Edition. December 2015. Available at http://health.gov/dietaryguidelines/2015/guidelines.

contains 38.5 g of sugar, or almost 10 teaspoons. If you drink the average amount, you are consuming more than 16,420 g of sugar (about 267 cups) each year! Other common sources of added sugars include cookies, cakes, pies, fruit drinks, fruit punches, and candy. Even many non-dessert items, such as peanut butter, yogurt, flavored rice mixes, and even salad dressing, contain added sugars.

If you want a quick way to figure out the amount of sugar in a processed food, check the Nutrition Facts panel on the box for the line that identifies "Sugars." You'll notice that the amount of sugar in a serving is identified in grams. Divide the total grams by 4 to get teaspoons. For instance, one national brand of yogurt contains 21 grams of sugar in a half-cup serving. That's more than 5 teaspoons of sugar! Doing this simple math before you buy may help you choose among different, more healthful versions of the same food.

Sugars Are Blamed for Many Health Problems

Why do sugars have such a bad reputation? First, they are known to contribute to tooth decay. Second, many people believe they cause hyperactivity in children. Third, eating a lot of sugar could increase the levels of unhealthful lipids in our blood, increasing our risk for heart disease. High intakes of sugar have also been blamed for causing diabetes and obesity. Let's learn the truth about these claims.

Sugar Causes Tooth Decay

Sugars do play a role in dental problems, because the bacteria that cause tooth decay thrive on sugar. These bacteria produce acids, which eat away at tooth enamel and can eventually cause cavities and gum disease (**Figure 4.12**). Eating sticky foods that adhere to teeth—such as caramels, crackers, sugary cereals, and licorice—and sipping sweetened beverages over a period of time are two behaviors that increase the risk for tooth decay. This means that people shouldn't suck on hard candies or caramels, slowly sip soda or juice, or put babies to bed with a bottle unless it contains water. As we have seen, even breast milk contains sugar, which can slowly drip onto the baby's gums. As a result, infants should not routinely be allowed to fall asleep at the breast.

To reduce your risk for tooth decay, brush your teeth after each meal, after drinking sugary drinks, and after snacking on sweets. Drinking fluoridated water and using a fluoride toothpaste will also help protect your teeth.

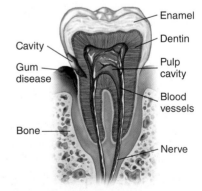

FIGURE 4.12 Eating sugar can cause an increase in cavities and gum disease. This is because bacteria in the mouth consume sugars present on the teeth and gums and produce acids, which eat away at these tissues.

There Is No Link between Sugar and Hyperactivity in Children

Although many people believe that eating sugar causes hyperactivity and other behavioral problems in children, there is little scientific evidence to support this claim. Some children actually become less active shortly after a high-sugar meal! However, it is important to emphasize that most studies of sugar and children's behavior have only looked at the effects of sugar a few hours after ingestion. We know very little about the long-term effects of sugar intake on the behavior of children. Behavioral and learning problems are complex issues, most likely caused by a multitude of factors. Because of this complexity, the Institute of Medicine has stated that, overall, there does not appear to be enough evidence that eating too much sugar causes hyperactivity or other behavioral problems in children.[6] Thus, there is no Tolerable Upper Intake Level for sugar.

High Sugar Intake Can Lead to Unhealthful Levels of Blood Lipids

Research evidence does suggest that consuming a diet high in added sugars is associated with unhealthful changes in blood lipids. For example, higher intakes of added sugars are associated with higher blood levels of low-density lipoproteins (LDL) and lower levels of high-density lipoproteins (HDL). These are risk factors for heart disease. Two recent studies have shown that people who consume sugar-sweetened beverages have an increased risk of heart disease and premature mortality from cardiovascular disease.[10,11] Although the Institute of Medicine has yet to set an upper tolerable intake limit for sugar, the growing body of evidence suggests that eating high amounts of added sugars may be harmful. As such, it is prudent to eat a diet low in added sugars. Because added sugars are a component of many processed foods and beverages, careful label reading is advised.

High Sugar Intake Is Associated with Diabetes and Obesity

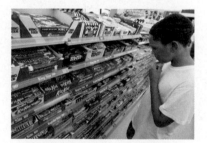

Foods with added sugars, such as candy, have lower levels of vitamins, minerals, and fiber than foods that naturally contain simple sugars.

Recent studies suggest that eating a diet high in added sugars is associated with a higher risk for diabetes; this relationship is particularly strong between higher intakes of sugar-sweetened beverages and diabetes. An observational study examined the relationship between diabetes and sugar intake across 175 countries and found that for every 150 kcal per person per day increase in availability of sugar (equivalent to about one can of soft drink per day), the prevalence of diabetes increased by 1.1%.[12] Although the exact mechanisms explaining this relationship are not clear, experts have speculated that the dramatic increase in glucose and insulin levels that occur when we consume high amounts of rapidly absorbable carbohydrates (which includes any form of sugar, including high-fructose corn syrup) may stimulate appetite, increase food intake, and promote weight gain, thereby increasing our risk for diabetes. High-fructose corn syrup in particular negatively affects how we metabolize and store body fat; this can in turn cause body cells to become more resistant to the normal actions of insulin and increase our risk for diabetes.

There is also evidence linking sugar intake with obesity. For example, a recent systematic review of randomized controlled trials and observational studies found that reducing intake of sugars in adults results in weight loss and increasing intake of sugars results in weight gain.[13] The authors stated that the increase in weight is due to the excess Calorie intake and not due to the sugars per se. This same review found that children who consume one or more servings of sugar-sweetened beverages per day had a 1.5 times higher risk of being overweight than those children consuming none or very little. Another recent study examined the effect of consuming a high protein-low glycemic index diet as compared to a normal protein-high glycemic index diet on prevention of weight regain in adults, weight loss in children, and ability of families in the study to maintain the diet.[14] Results showed that the high protein-low glycemic index diet resulted in substantially higher weight loss and prevention of weight regain, and improved blood pressure and blood lipids. Moreover, families were more likely to stay on the diet, finding it less restrictive and more acceptable.

It is important to emphasize that if you consume more energy than you expend, you will gain weight. It makes intuitive sense that people who consume extra energy from high-sugar foods are at risk for obesity, just like people who consume extra energy from fat or protein. However, more evidence is accumulating that the type of carbohydrates consumed may play a role in increasing one's risk for obesity. In addition to the increased potential for obesity, another major concern about high-sugar diets is that they tend to be low in nutrient density because the intake of high-sugar foods tends to replace that of more nutritious foods. Despite these recent findings, the relationship between added sugars and obesity is still controversial and is discussed in more detail in the end of chapter *Nutrition Myth or Fact?* (page 146).

RECAP

The RDA for carbohydrate is 130 g per day; this amount is sufficient only to supply adequate glucose to the brain. The AMDR for carbohydrate is 45% to 65% of total energy intake. Added sugars are sugars and syrups added to foods during processing or preparation. Sugar causes tooth decay but does not appear to cause hyperactivity in children. High intakes of sugars are associated with increases in unhealthful blood lipids and increased risks for heart disease, diabetes, and obesity.

Most Americans Eat Too Little Fiber-Rich Carbohydrates

Do you get enough fiber-rich carbohydrate each day? Most people in the United States eat only about two servings of fruits or vegetables each day, and most don't consistently choose whole-grain breads, pastas, and cereals. As explained earlier, fruits, vegetables, and whole-grain foods are rich in micronutrients and fiber. Whole grains also have a lower glycemic index than refined carbohydrates; thus, they prompt a more gradual release of insulin and result in less severe fluctuations in both insulin and glucose.

Table 4.3 defines the terms commonly used on nutrition labels for breads and cereals. Read the label for the bread you eat—does it list *whole-wheat* flour or just *wheat* flour? Although most labels for breads and cereals list wheat flour as the first ingredient, this term actually refers to enriched white flour, which is made when flour is processed. To gain a

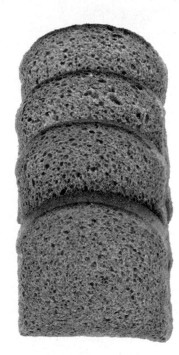

Whole-grain foods provide more nutrients and fiber than foods made with enriched flour.

TABLE 4.3 Terms Used to Describe Grains and Cereals on Nutrition Labels

Term	Definition
Brown bread	Brown bread may or may not be made using whole-grain flour. Many brown breads are made with white flour with brown (caramel) coloring added.
Enriched (or fortified) flour or grain	Enriching or fortifying grains involves adding nutrients to refined foods. In order to use this term in the United States, a minimum amount of iron, folate, niacin, thiamin, and riboflavin must be added. Other nutrients can also be added.
Refined flour or grain	Refining involves removing the coarse parts of food products; refined wheat flour is flour in which all but the internal part of the kernel has been removed.
Stone ground	This term refers to a milling process in which limestone is used to grind any grain. Stone ground does not mean that bread is made with whole grain, as refined flour can be stone ground.
Unbleached flour	Unbleached flour has been refined but not bleached; it is very similar to refined white flour in texture and nutritional value.
Wheat flour	This term means any flour made from wheat; it includes white flour, unbleached flour, and whole-wheat flour.
White flour	White flour has been bleached and refined. All-purpose flour, cake flour, and enriched baking flour are all types of white flour.
Whole-grain flour	This is flour made from grain that is not refined; whole grains are milled in their complete form, with only the husk removed.
Whole-wheat flour	Whole-wheat flour is an unrefined, whole-grain flour made from whole wheat kernels.

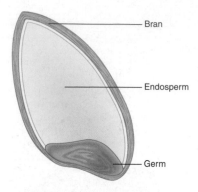

Bran

Endosperm

Germ

FIGURE 4.13 A whole grain includes the bran, endosperm, and germ.

better understanding of the difference between whole-grain and processed grain products, it's important to learn about what makes a whole grain whole, and how whole grains are processed to reduce their fiber content.

What Makes a Whole Grain Whole?

Grains are grasses that produce edible kernels. A kernel of grain is the seed of the grass. If you were to plant a kernel of barley, a blade of grass would soon shoot up. Kernels of different grains all share a similar design. As shown in **Figure 4.13**, they consist of three parts:

- The outermost covering, called the *bran*, is very high in fiber and contains most of the grain's vitamins and minerals.
- The *endosperm* is the grain's midsection and contains most of the grain's carbohydrates and protein.
- The *germ* sits deep in the base of the kernel, surrounded by the endosperm, and is rich in healthful fats and some vitamins.

Whole grains are kernels that retain all three of these parts.

The kernels of some grains also have a *husk* (hull): a thin, dry coat that is inedible. Removing the husk is always the first step in milling (grinding) these grains for human consumption.

People worldwide have milled grains for centuries, usually using heavy stones. A little milling removes only a small amount of the bran, leaving a crunchy grain suitable for cooked cereals. For example, cracked wheat and hulled barley retain much of the kernel's bran. Whole-grain flours are produced when whole grains are ground and then recombined. Because these hearty flours retain a portion of the bran, endosperm, and germ, foods such as breads made with them are rich in fiber and an array of vitamins and minerals.

With the advent of modern technology, processes for milling grains became more sophisticated, with seeds being repeatedly ground and sifted into increasingly finer flours, retaining little or no bran and therefore little fiber and few vitamins and minerals. For instance, white wheat flour, which consists almost entirely of endosperm, is high in carbohydrate but retains only about 25% of the wheat's fiber, vitamins, and minerals. In the United States, manufacturers of breads and other baked goods made with white flour are required by law to enrich their products with vitamins and minerals to replace some of those lost in processing. **Enriched foods** are foods in which nutrients that were lost during processing have been added back, so the food meets a specified standard. However, enrichment replaces only a handful of nutrients and leaves the product low in fiber. Notice that the terms *enriched* and *fortified* are not synonymous: **fortified foods** have nutrients added that did not originally exist in the food (or existed in insignificant amounts). For example, some breakfast cereals have been fortified with iron, a mineral that is not present in cereals naturally.

When choosing breads, crackers, and other baked goods, look for whole wheat, whole oats, or similar whole grains on the ingredient list. This ensures that the product contains the fiber and micronutrients that nature packed into the plant's seed.

We Need at Least 25 Grams of Fiber Daily

How much fiber do we need? The Adequate Intake for fiber is 25 g per day for women and 38 g per day for men, or 14 g of fiber for every 1,000 kcal per day that a person eats.[6] Most people in the United States eat only 12 to 18 g of fiber each day, getting only half of the fiber they need. Although fiber supplements are available, it is best to get fiber from food, because foods contain additional nutrients, such as vitamins and minerals.

It's important to drink plenty of fluid as you increase your fiber intake, as fiber binds with water to soften stools. Inadequate fluid intake with a high-fiber diet can actually result

enriched foods Foods in which nutrients that were lost during processing have been added back, so that the food meets a specified standard.

fortified foods Foods in which nutrients are added that did not originally exist in the food or existed in insignificant amounts.

in hard, dry stools that are difficult to pass through the colon. At least eight 8-oz glasses of fluid each day are commonly recommended.

Can you eat too much fiber? Excessive fiber consumption can lead to problems such as intestinal gas, bloating, and constipation. Also, because fiber causes the body to eliminate more water in the feces, a very-high-fiber diet could result in dehydration. Fiber also binds certain vitamins and minerals: a diet with too much fiber can reduce our absorption of iron, zinc, calcium, and vitamin D. In children, some elderly, the chronically ill, and other at-risk populations, extreme fiber intake can even lead to malnutrition—they feel full before they have eaten enough to provide adequate energy and nutrients. Although some societies are accustomed to a very-high-fiber diet, most people in the United States find it difficult to tolerate more than 50 g of fiber per day.

 To see a vast menu of high-fiber choices and find out how much fiber the foods you eat provide, visit the Fiber-o-Meter at www.webmd.com. Type "fiber-o-meter" in the search bar, then click on the link.

Hunting for Fiber

Eating the amounts of whole grains, legumes and other vegetables, fruits, and nuts and seeds recommended in the USDA Food Patterns will ensure that you get adequate fiber. **Figure 4.14** lists some common foods and their fiber content. You can use this information to design a diet that includes adequate fiber.

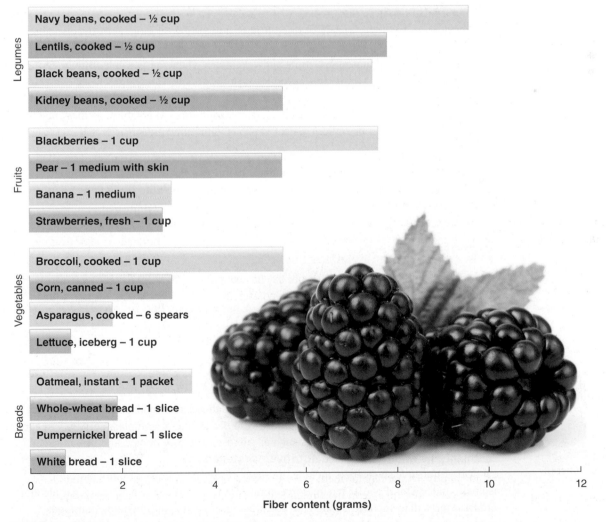

FIGURE 4.14 Fiber content of common foods.

Note: The Adequate Intake for fiber is 25 g per day for women and 38 g per day for men.
(*Source:* Data from US Department of Agriculture, Agricultural Research Service. 2014. USDA National Nutrient Database for Standard Reference, Release 27. Nutrient Data Laboratory home page. www.ars.usda.gov/ba/bhnrc/ndl.)

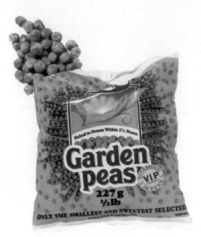

Frozen vegetables and fruits can be a healthful alternative when fresh produce is not available.

Meal Focus Figure 4.15 compares the food and fiber content of two diets, one high in fiber-rich carbohydrates and one high in refined carbohydrates. Here are some hints for selecting healthful carbohydrate sources:

- Select breads and cereals that are made with *whole* grains, such as wheat, oats, barley, and rye (make sure the label says "whole" before the word *grain*). Two slices of whole-grain bread provide 4–6 grams of fiber.
- Switch from a low-fiber breakfast cereal to one that has at least 4 grams of fiber per serving.
- For a mid-morning snack, stir 1–2 tablespoons of whole ground flaxseed meal (4 grams of fiber) into a cup of low-fat or nonfat yogurt. Or choose an apple or a pear, with the skin left on (approximately 5 grams of fiber).
- Instead of potato chips with your lunchtime sandwich, have a side of carrot sticks or celery sticks (approximately 2 grams of fiber per serving).
- Eat legumes frequently, every day if possible (approximately 6–8 grams of fiber per serving). Canned or fresh beans, peas, and lentils are excellent sources of fiber-rich carbohydrates, vitamins, and minerals. Have them as your main dish, as a side, or in soups, chili, and other dishes.
- Don't forget the greens! A cup of cooked leafy greens provides about 4 grams of fiber, and a salad is rich in fiber.
- For dessert, try fresh, frozen, or dried fruit or a high-fiber granola with sweetened soy milk.
- When shopping, choose fresh fruits and vegetables whenever possible. Buy frozen vegetables and fruits when fresh produce is not available. Check frozen selections to make sure there is no sugar or salt added.
- Be careful when buying canned fruits, legumes, and other vegetables, as they may be high in added sugar or sodium. Select versions without added sugar or salt, or rinse before serving.

Try the **Nutrition Label Activity** on page 136 to learn how to recognize various carbohydrates on food labels. Armed with this knowledge, you'll be ready to make more healthful food choices.

RECAP

The Adequate Intake for fiber is 25 g per day for women and 38 g per day for men. Most Americans eat only half of the fiber they need each day. Foods high in fiber include whole grains and cereals, fruits, and vegetables. The more processed the food, the less fiber it is likely to contain.

<table><tr><td></td></tr></table>

LO 9   Identify several alternative sweeteners, and discuss their role in a healthful diet.

What's the Story on Alternative Sweeteners?

Most of us love sweets but want to avoid the extra Calories and tooth decay that go along with them. Remember that all carbohydrates, whether simple or complex, contain 4 kcal of energy per gram. Because sweeteners such as sucrose, fructose, honey, and brown sugar contribute energy, they are called **nutritive sweeteners.**

Other nutritive sweeteners include the *sugar alcohols,* such as mannitol, sorbitol, isomalt, and xylitol. Popular in sugar-free gums, mints, and diabetic candies, sugar alcohols are less sweet than sucrose. Foods with sugar alcohols have health benefits that foods made with sugars do not have, such as a reduced glycemic response and decreased risk for dental caries. Also, because sugar alcohols are absorbed slowly and incompletely from the intestine, they provide less energy than sugar, usually 2 to 3 kcal of energy per gram. However, because they are not completely absorbed from the intestine, they can attract water into the large intestine and cause diarrhea.

nutritive sweeteners Sweeteners, such as sucrose, fructose, honey, and brown sugar, that contribute Calories (energy).

a day of meals

about 2,410 calories (kcal)

about 2,182 calories (kcal)

BREAKFAST

1 cup Froot Loops Cereal
1 cup skim milk
2 slices of white bread with
   1 tbsp of butter
8 fl. oz orange juice

1 cup Cheerios
1 cup skim milk
1 medium banana
2 slices whole-wheat toast with
   1 tbsp light margarine
8 fl. oz orange juice

LUNCH

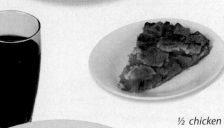

McDonald's Quarter Pounder
1 small French Fries
1 packet ketchup
16 fl oz cola beverage
15 jelly beans

Tuna Sandwich with:

2 slices of whole wheat bread
3 oz tuna packed in water,
   drained
1 tsp Dijon mustard
1 tbsp reduced-calorie
   mayonnaise
1 large carrot, sliced
1 cup raw cauliflower
2 tbsp fat-free ranch dressing
8 fl oz non-fat fruit yogurt

DINNER

½ chicken breast, roasted
1 cup mashed potatoes
½ cup sliced cooked carrots
12 fl oz cola beverage
Apple pie (1/8 of 9-inch pie)

1/2 chicken breast, roasted
1 cup brown rice
1 cup steamed broccoli

Spinach salad:

1 cup chopped spinach
1 boiled egg
2 slices turkey bacon
3 cherry tomatoes
2 tbsp cream poppyseed
   dressing
1 cup fresh blueberries with
   ½ cup whipped cream
8 fl oz cranberry juice

nutrient analysis

2,410 kcal
58.3% of energy from carbohydrates
29.2% of energy from fat
12.5% of energy from protein
15.6 grams of dietary fiber

Double the fiber intake!

nutrient analysis

2,181 kcal
58.5% of energy from carbohydrates
22.3% of energy from fat
19.2% of energy from protein
32 grams of dietary fiber

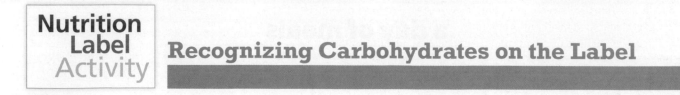

Recognizing Carbohydrates on the Label

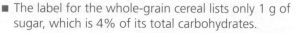

Figure 4.16 shows labels for two breakfast cereals. The cereal on the left (a) is processed and sweetened, whereas the one on the right (b) is a whole-grain product with no added sugar. Which is the better breakfast choice? Fill in the label data below to find out!

- Check the center of each label to locate the amount of total carbohydrate.

  1. For the sweetened cereal, the total carbohydrate is _____ g.

  2. For the whole-grain cereal, the total carbohydrate is _____ g for a smaller serving size.

- Look at the information listed as subgroups under Total Carbohydrate. The label for the sweetened cereal lists all types of carbohydrates in the cereal: dietary fiber, sugars, and other carbohydrate (which refers to starches). Notice that this cereal contains 13 g of sugar—half of its total carbohydrates.

  3. How many grams of dietary fiber does the sweetened cereal contain? _____

- The label for the whole-grain cereal lists only 1 g of sugar, which is 4% of its total carbohydrates.

  4. How many grams of dietary fiber does the whole-grain cereal contain? _____

- To calculate the percentage of Calories that comes from carbohydrate, do the following:

  a. Calculate the *Calories* in the cereal that come from carbohydrate. Multiply the total grams of carbohydrate per serving by the energy value of carbohydrate:

  26 g of carbohydrate × 4 kcal/g = 104 kcal from carbohydrate

  b. Calculate the *percentage of Calories* in the cereal that comes from carbohydrate. Divide the kcal from carbohydrate by the total Calories for each serving:

  (104 kcal/120 kcal) × 100 = 87% Calories from carbohydrate

Which cereal should you choose to increase your fiber intake? Check the ingredients for the sweetened cereal. Remember that they're listed in order from highest to lowest amount. The second and third ingredients listed are sugar and brown sugar, and the corn and oat flours are not whole-grain. Now look at the ingredients for the other cereal—it contains whole-grain oats. Although the sweetened product is enriched with more B vitamins, iron, and zinc, the whole-grain cereal packs 4 g of fiber per serving, not to mention 5 g of protein, and it contains no added sugars. Overall, it is a more healthful choice.

(a) Nutrition Facts

Serving Size: 3/4 cup (30g)
Servings Per Package: About 14

Amount Per Serving	Cereal	Cereal With 1/2 Cup Skim Milk
Calories	120	160
Calories from Fat	15	15
	% Daily Value**	
Total Fat 1.5g*	2%	2%
Saturated Fat 0g	0%	0%
Trans Fat 0g		
Polyunsaturated Fat 0g		
Monounsaturated Fat 0.5g		
Cholesterol 0mg	0%	1%
Sodium 220mg	9%	12%
Potassium 40mg	1%	7%
Total Carbohydrate 26g	9%	11%
Dietary Fiber 1g	3%	3%
Sugars 13g		
Other Carbohydrate 12g		
Protein 1g		

INGREDIENTS: Corn Flour, Sugar, Brown Sugar, Partially Hydrogenated Vegetable Oil (Soybean and Cottonseed), Oat Flour, Salt, Sodium Citrate (a flavoring agent), Flavor added [Natural & Artificial Flavor, Strawberry Juice Concentrate, Malic Acid (a flavoring agent)], Niacinamide (Niacin), Zinc Oxide, Reduced Iron, Red 40, Yellow 5, Red 3, Yellow 6, Pyridoxine Hydrochloride (Vitamin B6), Riboflavin (Vitamin B2), Thiamin Mononitrate (Vitamin B1), Folic Acid (Folate) and Blue 1.

(b) Nutrition Facts

Serving Size: 1/2 cup dry (40g)
Servings Per Container: 13

Amount Per Serving	
Calories	150
Calories from Fat	25
	% Daily Value*
Total Fat 3g	5%
Saturated Fat 0.5g	2%
Trans Fat 0g	
Polyunsaturated Fat 1g	
Monounsaturated Fat 1g	
Cholesterol 0mg	0%
Sodium 0mg	0%
Total Carbohydrate 27g	9%
Dietary Fiber 4g	15%
Soluble Fiber 2g	
Insoluble Fiber 2g	
Sugars 1g	
Protein 5g	

INGREDIENTS: 100% Natural Whole Grain Rolled Oats.

FIGURE 4.16 Labels for two breakfast cereals: **(a)** processed and sweetened cereal; **(b)** whole-grain cereal with no sugar added.

In addition to nutritive sweeteners, a number of other products have been developed to sweeten foods without promoting tooth decay and weight gain. Because these products provide little or no energy, they are called **non-nutritive**, or *alternative*, **sweeteners.**

Limited Use of Alternative Sweeteners Is Not Harmful

Research has shown alternative sweeteners to be safe for adults, children, and individuals with diabetes. Women who are pregnant should discuss the use of alternative sweeteners with their healthcare provider. In general, it appears safe for pregnant women to consume alternative sweeteners in amounts within the Food and Drug Administration (FDA) guidelines.[15] These amounts, known as the **Acceptable Daily Intake (ADI)**, are estimates of the amount of a sweetener that someone can consume each day over a lifetime without adverse effects. The estimates are based on studies conducted on laboratory animals, and they include a 100-fold safety factor. It is important to emphasize that actual intake by humans is typically well below the ADI.

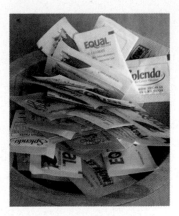

Contrary to recent media reports claiming severe health consequences related to the consumption of alternative sweeteners, major health agencies have determined that these products are safe for us to consume.

Saccharin

Discovered in the late 1800s, *saccharin* is about 300 times sweeter than sucrose. Concerns arose in the 1970s that saccharin could cause cancer; however, more than 20 years of subsequent research failed to link saccharin to cancer in humans. Based on this evidence, in May 2000 the National Toxicology Program of the U.S. government removed saccharin from its list of products that may cause cancer. No ADI has been set for saccharin, and it is used in foods and beverages and as a tabletop sweetener. It is sold as Sweet 'n Low (also known as "the pink packet") in the United States.

Acesulfame-K

Acesulfame-K (acesulfame potassium) is marketed under the names Sunette and Sweet One. It is a calorie-free sweetener that is 200 times sweeter than sugar. It is used to sweeten gums, candies, beverages, instant tea, coffee, gelatins, and puddings. The taste of acesulfame-K does not change when it is heated, so it can be used in cooking. The body does not metabolize acesulfame-K, so it is excreted unchanged by the kidneys. The ADI for acesulfame-K is 15 mg per kg body weight per day. For example, the ADI in an adult weighing 150 pounds (68 kg) would be 1,020 mg.

Aspartame

Aspartame, also called Equal ("the blue packet") and NutraSweet, is one of the most popular alternative sweeteners currently in use. Aspartame is composed of two amino acids: phenylalanine and aspartic acid. When these amino acids are separate, one is bitter and the other has no flavor—but joined together, they make a substance that is 180 times sweeter than sucrose. Although aspartame contains 4 kcal of energy per gram, it is so sweet that only small amounts are used; thus, it ends up contributing little or no energy. Heat destroys the dipeptide bonds that bind the two amino acids in aspartame (see Chapter 6), so it cannot be used in cooking because it loses its sweetness.

Although there are numerous claims that aspartame causes headaches and dizziness and can increase a person's risk for cancer and nerve disorders, studies do not support these claims.[16] A significant amount of research has been done to test the safety of aspartame.

The ADI for aspartame is 50 mg per kg body weight per day. For an adult weighing 150 pounds (68 kg), the ADI would be 3,400 mg. **Table 4.4** on page 138 shows how many servings of aspartame-sweetened foods would have to be consumed to exceed the ADI. Because the ADI is a very conservative estimate, it would be difficult for adults or children to exceed this amount of aspartame intake. However, drinks sweetened with aspartame, which are extremely popular among children and teenagers, are very low in nutritional value. They should not replace more healthful beverages, such as milk, water, and 100% fruit juice.

mannitol A type of sugar alcohol.

sorbitol A type of sugar alcohol.

xylitol A type of sugar alcohol.

non-nutritive sweeteners Also called *alternative sweeteners;* manufactured sweeteners that provide little or no energy.

Acceptable Daily Intake (ADI) An estimate made by the Food and Drug Administration of the amount of a non-nutritive sweetener that someone can consume each day over a lifetime without adverse effects.

TABLE 4.4 Foods and Beverages That a Child and an Adult Would Have to Consume Daily to Exceed the ADI for Aspartame

Foods and Beverages	50-lb Child	150-lb Adult
12 fl. oz carbonated soft drink OR	6	20
8 fl. oz powdered soft drink OR	11	33
4 fl. oz gelatin dessert OR	14	42
Packets of tabletop sweetener	32	97

Source: "Aspartame" from The Calorie Control website, 2015. http://www.caloriecontrol.org/sweeteners-and-lite /sugar-substitutes/aspartame

Some people should not consume aspartame at all: those with the disease *phenylketonuria (PKU)*. This is a genetic disorder that prevents the breakdown of the amino acid phenylalanine. Because a person with PKU cannot metabolize phenylalanine, it builds up to toxic levels in the tissues of the body and causes irreversible brain damage. In the United States, all newborn babies are tested for PKU; those who have it are placed on a phenylalanine-limited diet. Some foods that are common sources of protein and other nutrients for many growing children, such as meats and milk, contain phenylalanine. Thus, it is critical that children with PKU not waste what little phenylalanine they can consume on nutrient-poor products sweetened with aspartame.

Sucralose

Sucralose is marketed under the brand name Splenda and is known as "the yellow packet." It is made from sucrose, but chlorine atoms are substituted for the hydrogen and oxygen normally found in sucrose, and it passes through the digestive tract unchanged, without contributing any energy. It is 600 times sweeter than sucrose and is stable when heated, so it can be used in cooking. It has been approved for use in many foods, including chewing gum, salad dressings, beverages, gelatin and pudding products, canned fruits, frozen dairy desserts, and baked goods. Studies have shown sucralose to be safe. The ADI for sucralose is 5 mg per kg body weight per day. For example, the ADI of sucralose in an adult weighing 150 pounds (68 kg) would be 340 mg.

Neotame, Stevia, and Advantame

Neotame is an alternative sweetener that is 7,000 times sweeter than sugar. Manufacturers use it to sweeten a variety of products, such as beverages, dairy products, frozen desserts, and chewing gums.

Stevia was approved as an alternative sweetener by the FDA in 2008. It is produced from a purified extract of the stevia plant, native to South America. Stevia is 200 times sweeter than sugar. It is currently used commercially to sweeten beverages and is available in powder and liquid forms for tabletop use. Stevia is also called Rebiana, Reb-A, Truvia, and Purevia.

Advantame was approved as an alternative sweetener in 2014. It is Calorie-free and 20,000 times sweeter than sugar. Although derived from aspartame, it is so much sweeter that very little is used; therefore, it is considered safe for people with phenylketonuria to consume. Advantame is used to sweeten foods such as frozen desserts, beverages, and chewing gum.

The Effect of Artificial Sweeteners on Weight Management Is Unclear

Although artificial sweeteners are used to reduce the energy content of various foods, their role in weight loss and maintenance of healthy body weight is unclear. Although the popular media have recently linked drinking diet soft drinks with weight gain, a recent review concluded that there is no evidence that artificial sweeteners cause weight gain, and they may help people to lose weight.[17] In addition, a recent randomized controlled trial found that participants in a behavioral weight loss program who consumed at least 24 fluid ounces per day of an artificially sweetened beverage lost more weight after 12 weeks than participants who drank only water, suggesting that artificial sweeteners can be an effective part of a weight loss program.[18]

However, this doesn't mean that consuming artificial sweeteners will necessarily help us maintain a healthy body weight. Remember that, to prevent weight gain, you need to balance the total number of kcal you consume against the number you expend. If you're expending an average of 2,000 kcal a day and you consume about 2,000 kcal per day, then you'll neither gain nor lose weight. But if, in addition to your normal diet, you regularly indulge in "treats," you're bound to gain weight, whether they are sugar free or not. Consider the Calorie count of these artificially sweetened foods:

- One cup of nonfat chocolate frozen yogurt with artificial sweetener = 199 Calories
- One sugar-free chocolate cookie = 100 Calories
- One serving of no-sugar-added hot cocoa = 55 Calories

Does the number of Calories in these foods surprise you? *Remember, sugar free doesn't mean Calorie free.* Make it a habit to check the Nutrition Facts panel to find out how much energy is really in your food!

RECAP

Alternative sweeteners can be used in place of sugar to sweeten foods. Most of these products do not promote tooth decay and contribute little or no energy. The alternative sweeteners approved for use in the United States are considered safe when consumed in amounts less than the acceptable daily intake. The role of artificial sweeteners in weight loss and maintenance of healthy body weight is unclear. ◼

*Nutri-*Case

Hannah

"Last night, my mom called and said she'd be late getting home from work, so I made dinner. I was tired after my classes and I had a lot of homework to get to, so I kept it simple. I made us each a cheeseburger—no bun!—served with frozen french fries and some carrot sticks with guacamole on the side. We both had a cola, too. Later that night, though, when I was studying, I got a snack attack and raided a package of sugar-free cookies. I ate maybe three or four, but I didn't think it was a big deal because they're sugar-free. Then when I checked the package label this morning, I found out that each cookie has 90 Calories! It bummed me out—until those cookies, I'd been doing pretty well on my new low-carb diet!"

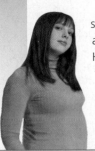

Hannah takes public transportation to the community college she attends and does not engage in regular physical activity. Without analyzing the precise grams of carbohydrate or number of Calories in Hannah's meal, would you agree that before the cookies she'd been "doing pretty well" on her low-carb diet? In other words, would you describe her meal as low carb? Would you characterize her meal as low in energy? About how many grams of dietary fiber do you think were in the meal?

LO 10 Describe type 1 and type 2 diabetes, and discuss how diabetes differs from hypoglycemia.

What Disorders Are Related to Carbohydrate Metabolism?

Health conditions that affect the body's ability to absorb and/or use carbohydrates include diabetes, hypoglycemia, and lactose intolerance.

Diabetes: Impaired Regulation of Glucose

Hyperglycemia is the term referring to higher-than-normal levels of blood glucose. **Diabetes** is a chronic disease in which the body can no longer regulate glucose within normal limits, and blood glucose levels become dangerously high. It is imperative to detect and treat the disease as soon as possible, because excessive fluctuations in glucose injure tissues throughout the body. If not controlled, diabetes can lead to blindness, seizures, stroke, kidney failure, nerve disease, and cardiovascular disease.

It is estimated that 29.1 million people in the United States—9.3% of the total population, including adults and children—have diabetes. It is speculated that of this 29.1 million, 8.1 million people have diabetes but do not know it.[19] **Figure 4.17** shows the percentage of adults with diabetes from various ethnic groups in the United States.[19] As you can see, diabetes is more common in Asian Americans, Hispanics, African Americans, and Native Americans and Native Alaskans than in Caucasians.

Diabetes Damages Blood Vessels

Diabetes causes disease when chronic exposure to elevated blood glucose levels damages the body's blood vessels, and this in turn damages other body tissues. As the concentration of glucose in the blood increases, a shift in the body's chemical balance allows glucose to attach to certain body proteins, including ones that make up blood vessels. Glucose coats these proteins like a sticky glaze, causing damage and dysfunction.

Damage to large blood vessels results in problems referred to as *macrovascular complications*. These include cardiovascular disease, which occurs because damage to artery walls allows fatty plaque to accumulate and narrow or block the vessel.

Damage to small blood vessels results in problems referred to as *microvascular complications*. For example, the kidneys' microscopic blood vessels, which filter blood and produce urine, become thickened. This impairs their function and can lead to kidney failure. Blood vessels that serve the eyes can swell and leak, leading to blindness.

When blood vessels that supply nutrients and oxygen to nerves are affected, *neuropathy*, damage to the nerves, can also occur. This condition leads to a loss of sensation, most commonly in the hands and feet. At the same time, circulation to the limbs is reduced overall. Together, these changes increase the risk of injury, infection, and tissue death (necrosis), leading to a greatly increased number of toe, foot, and lower leg amputations in people. with diabetes.

Because uncontrolled diabetes impairs carbohydrate metabolism, the body begins to break down stored fat, producing ketones for fuel. A build-up of excessive ketones can lead to ketoacidosis, a condition in which the brain cells do not get enough glucose to function properly. The person will become confused and lethargic and have trouble breathing. If left unchecked, ketoacidosis may result in coma and death. Indeed, as a result of cardiovascular disease, kidney failure, ketoacidosis, and other complications, diabetes is the seventh leading cause of death in the United States as highlighted in Chapter 1.

The two main forms of diabetes are type 1 and type 2. Some women develop a third form, *gestational diabetes,* during pregnancy (see Chapter 16). See **Focus Figure 4.18** for an overview of the processes involved in type 1 and type 2 diabetes.

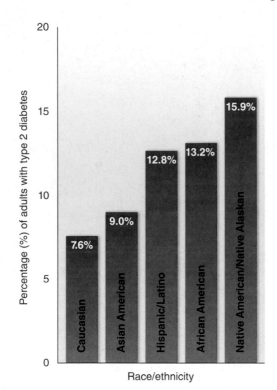

FIGURE 4.17 The percentage of adults from various ethnic and racial groups in the United States with type 2 diabetes. (*Source*: CDC National Center for Chronic Disease Prevention and Health Promotion, Division of Diabetes Translation. 2014. National Diabetes Statistics Report, 2014. http://www.cdc.gov/diabetes/pubs/statsreport14/national-diabetes-report-web.pdf.)

hyperglycemia A condition in which blood glucose levels are higher than normal.

diabetes A chronic disease in which the body can no longer regulate glucose.

Diabetes is a chronic disease in which the body can no longer regulate glucose within normal limits, and blood glucose becomes dangerously high.

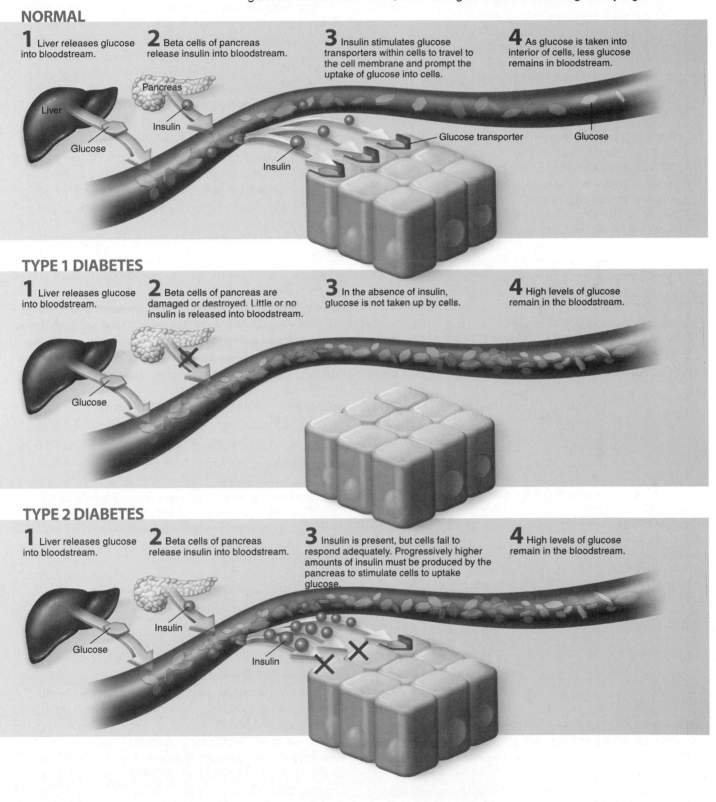

NORMAL

1 Liver releases glucose into bloodstream.

2 Beta cells of pancreas release insulin into bloodstream.

3 Insulin stimulates glucose transporters within cells to travel to the cell membrane and prompt the uptake of glucose into cells.

4 As glucose is taken into interior of cells, less glucose remains in bloodstream.

Pancreas

Liver

Insulin

Glucose

Insulin

Glucose transporter

Glucose

TYPE 1 DIABETES

1 Liver releases glucose into bloodstream.

2 Beta cells of pancreas are damaged or destroyed. Little or no insulin is released into bloodstream.

3 In the absence of insulin, glucose is not taken up by cells.

4 High levels of glucose remain in the bloodstream.

Glucose

TYPE 2 DIABETES

1 Liver releases glucose into bloodstream.

2 Beta cells of pancreas release insulin into bloodstream.

3 Insulin is present, but cells fail to respond adequately. Progressively higher amounts of insulin must be produced by the pancreas to stimulate cells to uptake glucose.

4 High levels of glucose remain in the bloodstream.

Insulin

Glucose

Insulin

Nutrition
MILESTONE

By the late 19th century, scientists had discovered a link between the pancreas and diabetes. Experiments had shown that, without a pancreas, an otherwise healthy animal would develop the disease quickly. Still, no one knew how to treat diabetes: nutritional therapies ranged from low-carbohydrate diets to starvation. For children, a diagnosis of diabetes was essentially a death sentence.

Then, in **1921**, Canadian surgeon Frederick Banting had an idea. He and his medical assistant removed the pancreas from a dog, thereby inducing diabetes. They then injected the diabetic dog with secretions extracted from a cluster of cells in the pancreas called the islets of Langerhans. They called this extraction *isletin*. A few injections of isletin a day cured the dog of diabetes. They then purified the substance—which we now call insulin—and repeated their experiment several times before trying it on a 14-year-old boy dying of diabetes. The injection reversed all signs of the disease in the boy. Banting published a paper on his research in 1922 and received a Nobel Prize the following year.

In Type 1 Diabetes, the Body Does Not Produce Enough Insulin

Approximately 5% to 10% of people with diabetes have **type 1 diabetes**, in which the body cannot produce enough insulin. When people with type 1 diabetes eat a meal and their blood glucose rises, the pancreas is unable to secrete insulin in response. Glucose therefore cannot move into body cells and remains in the bloodstream. The kidneys try to expel the excess blood glucose by excreting it in the urine. In fact, the medical term for the disease is *diabetes mellitus* (from the Greek *diabainein*, "to pass through," and Latin *mellitus*, "sweetened with honey"), and frequent urination is one of its warning signs (see **Table 4.5** for other symptoms). If blood glucose levels are not controlled, a person with type 1 diabetes will become confused and lethargic and have trouble breathing. This is because the brain cells are not getting enough glucose to function properly. As discussed earlier, uncontrolled diabetes can lead to ketoacidosis; left untreated, the ultimate result is coma and death.

Type 1 diabetes is classified as an *autoimmune disease.* This means that the body's immune system attacks and destroys its own tissues—in this case, the beta cells of the pancreas.[20]

Most cases of type 1 diabetes are diagnosed in adolescents around 10 to 14 years of age, although the disease can appear in infants, young children, and adults. It has a genetic link, so siblings and children of those with type 1 diabetes are at greater risk.[20]

The only treatment for type 1 diabetes is the administration of insulin by injection or pump several times daily. Insulin is a hormone composed of protein, so it would be digested in the intestine if taken as a pill. Individuals with type 1 diabetes must also monitor their blood glucose levels closely to ensure that they remain within a healthful range (**Figure 4.19**).

In Type 2 Diabetes, Cells Become Less Responsive to Insulin

In **type 2 diabetes**, body cells become resistant (less responsive) to insulin. This type of diabetes develops progressively, meaning that the biological changes resulting in the disease occur over a long period of time. Approximately 90% to 95% of all cases of diabetes are classified as type 2.

Obesity is the most common trigger for a cascade of changes that eventually results in the disorder. It is estimated that 80% to 90% of the people with type 2 diabetes are overweight or obese. One factor linking obesity to diabetes is the inappropriate accumulation of lipids in muscle, the liver, and beta cells, which reduces the ability of body

type 1 diabetes A disorder in which the pancreas cannot produce enough insulin.

type 2 diabetes A progressive disorder in which body cells become less responsive to insulin.

TABLE 4.5 Signs and Symptoms of Type 1 and Type 2 Diabetes

Type 1 Diabetes	Type 2 Diabetes*
Increased or frequent urination	Any of the type 1 signs and symptoms
Excessive thirst	Greater frequency of infections
Constant hunger	Sudden vision changes
Unexplained weight loss	Slow healing of wounds or sores
Extreme fatigue	Tingling or numbness in the hands or feet
Blurred vision	Very dry skin

Sources: Data adapted from U.S. Dept. of Health and Human Services, National Diabetes Information Clearinghouse (NDIC). Available online at http://diabetes.niddk.nih.gov/dm/pubs/type1and2/index.aspx#signs and from Centers for Disease Control and Prevention, Basics about Diabetes, available at http://www.cdc.gov/diabetes/basics/diabetes.html. *Some people with type 2 diabetes experience no symptoms.

cells to respond to insulin. As a result, the cells of many obese people begin to exhibit a condition called *insulin insensitivity* (insulin resistance).

The pancreas attempts to compensate for this insensitivity by secreting more insulin. At first, the increased secretion of insulin is sufficient to maintain normal blood glucose levels. However, over time, a person who is insulin insensitive will have to circulate very high levels of insulin to use glucose for energy. Eventually, this excessive production becomes insufficient for preventing a rise in fasting blood glucose. The resulting condition is referred to as **impaired fasting glucose**, meaning glucose levels are higher than normal but not high enough to indicate a diagnosis of type 2 diabetes. Some health professionals refer to this condition as **pre-diabetes**, because people with impaired fasting glucose are more likely to get type 2 diabetes than are people with normal fasting glucose levels. Ultimately, the pancreas becomes incapable of secreting these excessive amounts of insulin and stops producing the hormone altogether.

In short, in type 2 diabetes, blood glucose levels may be elevated because (1) the person has developed insulin insensitivity, (2) the pancreas can no longer secrete enough insulin, or (3) the pancreas has entirely stopped insulin production.

Diabetes is diagnosed when two or more tests of a person's fasting blood glucose indicate values in the clinically defined range. Another measure, glycosylated hemoglobin (abbreviated at HbA1c, or simply A1c) provides information about a person's average blood glucose levels over the past three months and can also be used to diagnose diabetes (see **Table 4.6**).

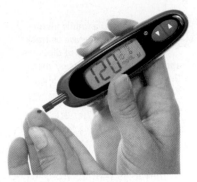

FIGURE 4.19 Monitoring blood glucose requires pricking the fingers several times each day and measuring the blood glucose level using a glucometer.

Who Is at Risk for Type 2 Diabetes?

As noted, obesity is the most common trigger for type 2 diabetes. But many other factors also play a role. For instance, relatives of people with type 2 diabetes are at increased risk, as are people with a sedentary lifestyle. A cluster of risk factors referred to as *metabolic syndrome* is also known to increase the risk for type 2 diabetes. The criteria for metabolic syndrome include a waist circumference greater than 88 cm (35 in.) for women and 102 cm (40 in.) for men, elevated blood pressure, and unhealthful levels of certain blood lipids and blood glucose.

Increased age is another risk factor for type 2 diabetes. Most cases develop after age 45, and almost 26% of Americans 65 years of age and older have diabetes. As mentioned in the chapter-opening story, type 2 diabetes in children and adolescents was virtually unheard of until about 20 years ago, but is increasing dramatically in this age group. In the United States, about 208,000 people younger than 20 years of age are estimated to have diagnosed diabetes, which is about 0.25% of that population age group.[19]

 To calculate your current level of risk for type 2 diabetes, take the National Diabetes Education Program's risk test at http://ndep.nih.gov. Type "diabetes risk test" into the search box to begin!

Lifestyle Choices Can Help Prevent or Control Diabetes

Type 2 diabetes is thought to have become an epidemic in the United States because of a combination of our poor eating habits, sedentary lifestyles, increased obesity, and an aging population. We can't control our age, but we can and do control how much and what types of foods we eat and how much physical activity we engage in—and that, in turn, influences our risk for obesity. Currently, over 34% of American college students are either overweight or obese.[21] Although adopting a healthful diet is important, moderate daily exercise may prevent the onset of type 2 diabetes more effectively than dietary changes alone.

TABLE 4.6 Values for fasting blood glucose and HbA1c indicating normal, pre-diabetes, and diabetes

Diagnosis	Fasting Blood Glucose (mg/dL)	HbA1c (%)
Normal	70-99	<5.7
Pre-diabetes	100-125	5.7-6.4
Diabetes	≥126	≥6.5

Source: American Diabetes Association. 2014. Diagnosing Diabetes and Learning About Prediabetes. http://www.diabetes.org/diabetes-basics/diagnosis/.

impaired fasting glucose Fasting blood glucose levels that are higher than normal but not high enough to lead to a diagnosis of type 2 diabetes.

prediabetes A term used synonymously with *impaired fasting glucose;* it is a condition considered to be a major risk factor for both type 2 diabetes and heart disease.

To download a family history tool that you can use to track your family history of diabetes and other chronic diseases, visit the U.S. Surgeon General's My Family Health Portrait at https://familyhistory.hhs.gov.

(See Chapter 14 for examples of moderate exercise programs.) Exercise will also assist in weight loss, and studies show that losing only 10 to 30 pounds can reduce or eliminate the symptoms of type 2 diabetes.[22] In summary, by eating a healthy diet, staying active, and maintaining a healthful body weight, you should be able to keep your risk for type 2 diabetes low.

What if you've already been diagnosed with type 2 diabetes? The Academy of Nutrition and Dietetics emphasizes that there is no *single* diet or eating plan for people with diabetes. You should follow guidelines to eat more healthfully in the same way you would to reduce your risk for heart disease, cancer, and overweight or obesity. One difference is that you may need to eat less carbohydrate and slightly more fat or protein to help regulate your blood glucose levels. Carbohydrates are still an important part of the diet, so, if you're eating less, make sure your choices are rich in nutrients and fiber. Because precise nutritional recommendations vary according to each individual's responses to foods, consulting with a registered dietitian/nutritionist is essential.

The Academy of Nutrition and Dietetics identifies the following basic strategies for eating more healthfully while living with diabetes:[23]

- Eat meals and snacks regularly and at planned times throughout the day.
- Try to eat about the same amount and types of food at each meal or snack.
- Follow the *Dietary Guidelines for Americans* or the USDA Food Patterns to guide healthy food choices to maintain a healthy weight and support heart health (see Chapter 2).
- Seek the expert advice of a registered dietitian/nutritionist to assist you with carbohydrate counting and using the exchange system.

In addition, people with diabetes should avoid alcoholic beverages, which can cause hypoglycemia, a drop in blood glucose that can cause confusion, clumsiness, and fainting. If left untreated, this can lead to seizures, coma, and death. The symptoms of alcohol intoxication and hypoglycemia are very similar. People with diabetes, their companions, and even healthcare providers may confuse these conditions; this can result in a potentially life-threatening situation.

When blood glucose levels can't be adequately controlled with lifestyle changes, oral medications may be required. These drugs work in either of two ways: they improve body cells' sensitivity to insulin or reduce the amount of glucose the liver produces. Interestingly, these drugs may not be as effective in treating young people. A 2012 study found that oral medications are not as effective in children and teens with type 2 diabetes as compared to adults.[1] Finally, if the pancreas can no longer secrete enough insulin, then people with type 2 diabetes must have daily insulin injections, just like people with type 1 diabetes.

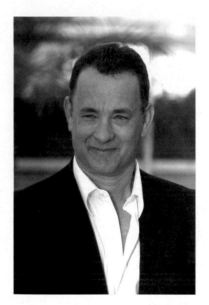

Actor Tom Hanks has type 2 diabetes.

RECAP

Diabetes is a disease that results in dangerously high levels of blood glucose. Type 1 diabetes typically appears at a young age; the pancreas cannot secrete sufficient insulin, so insulin injections are required. Type 2 diabetes develops over time and may be triggered by obesity: body cells become insensitive to the effects of insulin or the pancreas no longer secretes sufficient insulin for bodily needs. Supplemental insulin may or may not be needed to treat type 2 diabetes. Diabetes increases the risk for dangerous complications, such as heart disease, blindness, kidney disease, and amputations. Many cases of type 2 diabetes could be prevented or delayed by eating a balanced diet, getting regular exercise, and achieving and/or maintaining a healthful body weight.

Hypoglycemia: Low Blood Glucose

In **hypoglycemia**, fasting blood glucose falls to lower-than-normal levels. One cause of hypoglycemia is excessive production of insulin, which lowers blood glucose too far. People with diabetes can develop hypoglycemia if they inject too much insulin or if they exercise and fail to eat enough carbohydrates. Two types of hypoglycemia can develop in people who do not have diabetes: reactive and fasting.

hypoglycemia A condition marked by blood glucose levels that are below normal fasting levels.

Reactive hypoglycemia occurs when the pancreas secretes too much insulin after a high-carbohydrate meal. The symptoms of reactive hypoglycemia usually appear about 1 to 4 hours after the meal and include nervousness, shakiness, anxiety, sweating, irritability, headache, weakness, and rapid or irregular heartbeat. Although many people experience these symptoms from time to time, they are rarely caused by true hypoglycemia. A person diagnosed with reactive hypoglycemia must eat smaller meals more frequently to level out blood insulin and glucose levels.

Fasting hypoglycemia occurs when the body continues to produce too much insulin, even when someone has not eaten. This condition is usually secondary to another disorder, such as cancer; liver infection; alcohol-induced liver disease; or a tumor in the pancreas. Its symptoms are similar to those of reactive hypoglycemia but occur more than 4 hours after a meal.

Lactose Intolerance: Inability to Digest Lactose

Sometimes our bodies do not produce enough of the enzymes necessary to break down certain carbohydrates before they reach the colon. A common example is **lactose intolerance**, in which the body does not produce sufficient amounts of the enzyme lactase in the small intestine and therefore cannot digest foods containing lactose.

Lactose intolerance should not be confused with a milk allergy. People who are allergic to milk experience an immune reaction to the proteins found in cow's milk. Symptoms of milk allergy include skin reactions, such as hives and rashes; intestinal distress, such as nausea, vomiting, cramping, and diarrhea; and respiratory symptoms, such as wheezing, runny nose, and itchy and watery eyes. In severe cases, anaphylactic shock can occur. In contrast, symptoms of lactose intolerance are limited to the GI tract and include intestinal gas, bloating, cramping, nausea, diarrhea, and discomfort. These symptoms resolve spontaneously within a few hours.

Although some infants are born with lactose intolerance, it is more common to see lactase enzyme activity decrease after 2 years of age. In fact, it is estimated that up to 70% of the world's adult population will lose some ability to digest lactose as they age. In the United States, lactose intolerance is more common in Native American, Asian, Hispanic, and African American adults than in Caucasians.

Not everyone experiences lactose intolerance to the same extent. Some people cannot tolerate any dairy products. However, many people who are lactose intolerant can consume multiple small servings of dairy products without symptoms. This will enable them to meet their calcium requirements.[24] People with more severe lactose intolerance need to find foods that can supply enough calcium for normal growth, development, and maintenance of bones. Many can tolerate specially formulated milk products that are low in lactose, whereas others take pills or use drops that contain the lactase enzyme when they eat dairy products. Calcium-fortified soy milk and orange juice are excellent substitutes for cow's milk. Many lactose-intolerant people can also digest yogurt and aged cheese, as the bacteria or molds used to ferment these products break down the lactose during processing.

How can you tell if you are lactose intolerant? Many people discover that they have problems digesting dairy products by trial and error. But because intestinal gas, bloating, and diarrhea may indicate other health problems, you should consult a physician to determine the cause.

Tests for lactose intolerance include drinking a lactose-rich beverage and testing blood glucose levels over a 2-hour period. If you do not produce the normal amount of glucose, this means that your body is unable to digest the lactose in the beverage. A similar test involves measuring hydrogen levels in the breath, as lactose-intolerant people breathe out more hydrogen when they drink a beverage that contains lactose.

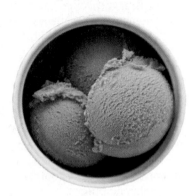

Milk products, such as ice cream, are hard to digest for people who are lactose intolerant.

lactose intolerance A disorder in which the body does not produce sufficient lactase enzyme and therefore cannot digest foods that contain lactose, such as cow's milk.

RECAP

Hypoglycemia refers to lower-than-normal blood glucose levels. It results from overproduction of insulin. Lactose intolerance is an inability to digest lactose because of insufficient production of the enzyme lactase.

Nutrition Myth OR Fact?

Are Added Sugars the Cause of the Obesity Epidemic?

Almost every day in the news we see headlines about obesity: "More Americans Overweight!" "The Fattening of America," "Obesity Is a National Epidemic!" These headlines accurately reflect the state of weight in the United States. Over the past 30 years, obesity rates have increased dramatically for both adults and children. Obesity has become public health enemy number one, as many chronic diseases, such as type 2 diabetes, heart disease, high blood pressure, and arthritis, go hand in hand with obesity.

Genetics cannot be held solely responsible for the rapid rise in obesity that has occurred in the past few decades. Our genetic makeup takes thousands of years to change; humans who lived even 100 years ago had essentially the same genetic makeup as we do. We need to look at the effect of our lifestyle changes over the same period.

One lifestyle factor that has come to the forefront of nutrition research is the contribution of added sugars to overweight and obesity. Consuming more energy than we expend causes weight gain. Consuming higher amounts of added sugars is a factor in weight gain for many people because they do not compensate for these increased Calories by increasing their energy expenditure through exercise or by reducing their energy intake from other foods.

One source of the added sugars in our diet is sugary drinks. Their role in increasing our risk for obesity has received a great deal of attention in recent years. These beverages include soft drinks, fruit drinks, energy drinks, bottled coffees and teas, and vitamin water drinks. It is estimated that U.S. children's intake of sugary drinks has increased threefold since the late 1970s, with approximately 10% of children's energy intake coming from these beverages.[1]

HFCS, in particular, has garnered a great deal of attention because it is the sole caloric sweetener in sugared soft drinks and represents more than 40% of caloric sweeteners added to other foods and beverages in the United States. More than a decade ago, researchers have linked the increased use and consumption of HFCS with the rising rates of obesity since the

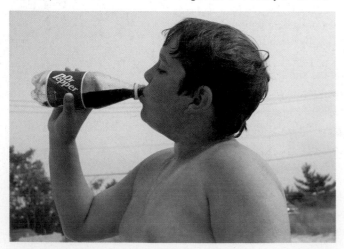

1970s, when HFCS first appeared.[2] HFCS is made by converting the starch in corn to glucose and then converting some of the glucose to fructose, which is sweeter. Fructose is metabolized differently from glucose: because it is absorbed farther down in the small intestine, it does not stimulate insulin release from the pancreas. Because insulin release inhibits food intake, this failure of fructose to stimulate insulin release could result in people consuming more total Calories in a meal than they would if they had consumed the same amount of glucose. In addition, fructose enters body cells via a transport protein not present in brain cells; thus, unlike glucose, fructose cannot enter brain cells and stimulate satiety signals. If we don't feel full, we are likely to continue eating or drinking.

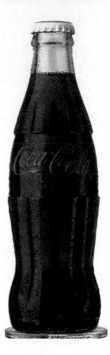

The growing evidence linking the consumption of sugar-sweetened beverages with overweight and obesity in children has led to dramatic changes in soft drink availability in schools and at school-sponsored events. In 2006, the soft drink industry agreed to a voluntary ban on sales of all sweetened soft drinks in elementary and high schools. Following on from this, the Healthy, Hunger-Free Kids Act of 2010 required the U.S. Department of Agriculture to issue new Smart Snacks in School nutrition standards for *competitive foods and beverages,* which are the foods and beverages sold outside of the school meals program during the day. The minimum standards set limits on the amount of energy, salt, sugar, and fat in foods and beverages, and also promote healthier snack foods such as whole grains, low-fat dairy, fruits, vegetables, and higher protein foods. Schools can opt to do more, and there is a wide variation in state policies regulating the availability and content of competitive foods. Thus, despite these positive changes, there is still ample availability of foods and beverages containing added sugars in the marketplace.

For this reason, the changes to the Nutrition Facts panel proposed by the FDA in 2014 include the addition of a line declaring "Added Sugars." This is due to the fact that Americans consume about 16% of their total energy from added sugars, with the primary sources being sugary drinks (soda, energy and sports drinks, and sugar-sweetened fruit drinks) and candy.[3]

Although the evidence pinpointing added sugars and HFCS as major contributors to the obesity epidemic may appear strong, some nutrition professionals disagree. It has been proposed that soft drinks would have contributed to the obesity epidemic whether the sweetener was sucrose or fructose, and that their contribution to obesity is due to increased consumption as a result of advertising, increases in serving sizes, and virtually unlimited access. It is possible that the obesity epidemic has resulted from increased consumption of energy (from sweetened soft drinks and other high-energy foods) *and* a reduction in physical activity levels, and added sugars themselves are not to blame.

This issue is extremely complex, and more research needs to be done in humans before we can fully understand how added sugars contribute to our diet and our health.

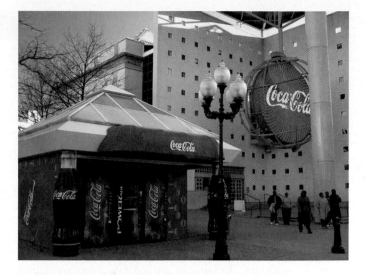

Critical Thinking Questions

1. After reading this, do you think added sugars in foods and beverages should be tightly regulated, or even banned? Why or why not?
2. Should reducing consumption of sugary drinks be up to individuals, or should it be encouraged via special taxes and/or bans on coupons, two-for-one pricing, free refills in restaurants, and other promotions that would make these drinks more expensive overall? Defend your answer.
3. Should there be an upper tolerable limit set for added sugars? Why or why not?

References

1. Te Moranga, L., S. Mallard, and J. Mann. 2013. Dietary sugars and body weight: systematic review and meta-analyses of randomized controlled trials and cohort studies. *BMJ* 346:e7492.

2. Bray G. A., S. J. Nielsen, and B. M. Popkin. 2004. Consumption of high-fructose corn syrup in beverages may play a role in the epidemic of obesity. *Am. J. Clin. Nutr.* 79:537–543.
3. U.S. Food and Drug Administration. 2014. Factsheet on the New Proposed Nutrition Facts Label. http://www.fda.gov/Food/GuidanceRegulation /GuidanceDocumentsRegulatoryInformation /LabelingNutrition/ucm387533.htm

STUDY **PLAN** MasteringNutrition™

Customize your study plan—and master your nutrition!—in the Study Plan of MasteringNutrition.

TEST YOURSELF | *ANSWERS*

1 **T** Our brains rely almost exclusively on glucose for energy, and our body tissues utilize glucose for energy both at rest and during exercise.

2 **F** At 4 kcal/g, carbohydrates have less than half the energy of a gram of fat. Eating a high-carbohydrate diet will not cause people to gain body fat unless their total diet contains more energy (kcal) than they expend. In fact, eating a diet high in complex, fiber-rich carbohydrates is associated with a lower risk for obesity.

3 **F** Although specific estimates are not yet available, significantly higher rates of type 2 diabetes are now being reported in children and adolescents; these higher rates are attributed to increasing obesity rates in young people.

4 **F** There is no evidence that diets high in sugar cause hyperactivity in children.

5 **T** Contrary to recent reports claiming harmful consequences related to the consumption of alternative sweeteners, major health agencies have determined that these products are safe for most people to consume in limited quantities.

summary

Scan to hear an MP3 Chapter Review in MasteringNutrition.

LO 1
- Carbohydrates contain carbon, hydrogen, and oxygen. Plants make the carbohydrate glucose during photosynthesis.
- Simple sugars include mono- and disaccharides. The three primary monosaccharides are glucose, fructose, and galactose.
- Two monosaccharides joined together are called disaccharides. Glucose and fructose join to make sucrose; glucose and glucose join to make maltose; and glucose and galactose join to make lactose.
- Oligosaccharides are complex carbohydrates that contain 3 to 10 monosaccharides.
- Polysaccharides are complex carbohydrates that typically contain hundreds to thousands of monosaccharides. The three types of polysaccharides are starches, glycogen, and fiber.
- Starches are the storage form of glucose in plants.
- Glycogen is the storage form of glucose in humans. Glycogen is stored in the liver and in muscles.

LO 2
- Monosaccharides are attached by a bond between oxygen and one carbon on each of the monosaccharides. There are two forms of this bond: alpha bonds are easily digestible by humans, whereas beta bonds are very difficult to digest.
- The monosaccharides in the disaccharide lactose and many forms of fiber are linked with beta bonds. Lactose is difficult to digest in people who lack adequate levels of the enzyme lactase. Many types of fiber are not digestible.

LO 3
- Dietary fiber is the nondigestible parts of plants, whereas functional fiber is a nondigestible form of carbohydrate extracted from plants or manufactured in the laboratory. Fiber may reduce the risk for certain diseases.
- Soluble fibers dissolve in water, are viscous, and are fermentable by bacteria residing in the colon. They are associated with a reduced risk for cardiovascular disease and type 2 diabetes. Insoluble fibers do not typically dissolve in water, are not viscous, and are usually not fermentable by colonic bacteria. They are associated with a reduced risk for constipation and diverticulosis.
- Fiber-rich carbohydrates are a group of foods containing either simple or complex carbohydrates that are rich in dietary fiber. These foods, which include most fruits, vegetables, and whole grains, are typically fresh or moderately processed.

LO 4
- Carbohydrate digestion starts in the mouth, where chewing and an enzyme called salivary amylase start breaking down the carbohydrates in food.
- Digestion continues in the small intestine. Specific enzymes are secreted to break starches into smaller mono- and disaccharides. As disaccharides pass through the intestinal cells, they are digested into monosaccharides.
- Glucose and other monosaccharides are absorbed into the bloodstream and travel to the liver, where all non-glucose molecules are converted to glucose.
- Glucose is transported in the bloodstream to the cells, where it is used for energy, stored in the liver or muscle as glycogen, or converted to fat and stored in adipose tissue.
- Insulin is secreted when blood glucose increases sufficiently, and it assists with the transport of glucose into cells.
- Glucagon, epinephrine, norepinephrine, cortisol, and growth hormone are secreted when blood glucose levels are low, and they assist with the conversion of glycogen to glucose, with gluconeogenesis, and with reducing the use of glucose by muscles and other organs.
- The glycemic index and the glycemic load are values that indicate how much a food increases glucose levels.

LO 5
- All cells can use glucose for energy. The red blood cells, brain, and central nervous system prefer to use glucose exclusively.
- Using glucose for energy helps spare body proteins, and glucose is an important fuel for the body during exercise.
- Fiber helps us maintain the healthy elimination of waste products. Eating adequate fiber may reduce the risk for constipation, hemorrhoids, and diverticulosis, as well as colon cancer, heart disease, and type 2 diabetes. A high-fiber diet may also prevent excessive weight gain.

LO 6
- The Acceptable Macronutrient Distribution Range for carbohydrate is 45% to 65% of total energy intake.
- The Adequate Intake for fiber is 25 g per day for women and 38 g per day for men, or 14 g of fiber for every 1,000 kcal of energy consumed.

LO 7 ■ High sugar intake can cause tooth decay, elevate triglyceride and low-density lipoprotein levels in the blood, and contribute to type 2 diabetes and obesity. It does not appear to cause hyperactivity in children.

LO 8 ■ Fiber-rich carbohydrates include whole grains and cereals, fruits, and legumes and other vegetables. Eating 6 to 11 servings of breads/grains and 5 to 9 servings of fruits and vegetables helps ensure that you meet your fiber-rich carbohydrate goals. Many nuts and seeds are also good sources of fiber.

LO 9 ■ Alternative sweeteners are added to some foods because they sweeten foods without promoting tooth decay and add little or no Calories to foods.

■ All alternative sweeteners approved for use in the United States are believed to be safe when consumed at levels at or below the Acceptable Daily Intake levels defined by the FDA.

■ Non-nutritive sweeteners provide little or no energy to the diet. They include saccharin, acesulfame-K, aspartame, and sucralose, as well as relatively newer sweeteners such as neotame, stevia, and advantame. The role of artificial sweeteners in weight loss and maintenance of healthy body weight is unclear. What is clear, however, is that many foods marketed as sugar free nevertheless contain significant Calories.

LO 10 ■ Diabetes is caused by insufficient insulin or by the cells becoming resistant or insensitive to insulin. It causes dangerously high blood glucose levels. The two primary types of diabetes are type 1 and type 2.

■ Type 1 diabetes is a disorder in which the pancreas can no longer produce sufficient insulin to meet body needs. It is classified as an autoimmune disorder and typically arises in adolescence. Type 2 diabetes is a progressive disorder in which body cells become less responsive to insulin. Obesity is a common trigger. Although the great majority of cases arise in adulthood, children are increasingly being diagnosed with type 2 diabetes.

■ A lower-than-normal blood glucose level is defined as hypoglycemia. There are two types: reactive and fasting. Reactive hypoglycemia occurs when too much insulin is secreted after a high-carbohydrate meal; fasting hypoglycemia occurs when blood glucose drops because the body continues to produce too much insulin, even though no food has been eaten.

■ Lactose intolerance results from an insufficient amount of the enzyme lactase. Symptoms include intestinal gas, bloating, cramping, diarrhea, and discomfort following consumption of dairy products.

review questions

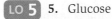

LO 1 **1.** Glucose, fructose, and galactose are
a. monosaccharides.
b. disaccharides.
c. oligosaccharides.
d. polysaccharides.

LO 2 **2.** Beta bonds are found linking monosaccharides within
a. lactose.
b. resistant starches.
c. cellulose.
d. all of the above.

LO 3 **3.** Insoluble fibers
a. are viscous, forming a gel when wet.
b. can be fermented by bacteria residing in the colon.
c. are generally found in whole grains, as well as many vegetables and some fruits.
d. include pectins, fructans, gums, and mucilages.

LO 4 **4.** The glycemic index rates
a. the potential of foods to prompt the secretion of pancreatic amylase.
b. the potential of foods to raise blood glucose and insulin levels.
c. the ratio of insulin to cortisol in the blood following a carbohydrate-rich meal.
d. the potential of a given diet for increasing the risk for diabetes.

LO 5 **5.** Glucose
a. is the predominant energy source used by our bodies at rest.
b. is obtained from the breakdown of muscle glycogen reserves maintains blood glucose levels between meals.
c. can be released from the breakdown of ketones to meet body needs when carbohydrate intake is low.
d. can be metabolized for energy very quickly either with or without oxygen.

LO 6   6. Which of the following statements about the DRIs for carbohydrates is true?

  a. The current AI for fiber adults 19 years of age and older is 130 g per day.
  b. The AMDR for carbohydrates is 45% to 65% of total energy intake.
  c. The RDA for carbohydrates covers the amount of carbohydrate needed to support daily activities.
  d. A key DRI for carbohydrates is to make half of your grain choices whole grains.

LO 7   7. Research evidence supports an association between

  a. sugar consumption and hyperactivity in children.
  b. a high-sugar diet and obesity.
  c. consumption of high-fructose corn syrup and increased sensitivity of body cells to insulin.
  d. exceeding the Institute of Medicine's upper tolerable intake limit for sugar and an increased risk for heart disease.

LO 8   8. Good sources of fiber include

  a. legumes and other vegetables, fruits, whole grains, and nuts and seeds.
  b. potatoes and other starchy vegetables, fruit juices, grains, and dairy foods.
  c. meat, fish, poultry, and tofu.
  d. rice and pasta, peanut butter, eggs, and yogurt and other fermented dairy foods.

LO 9   9. Aspartame should not be consumed by people who have

  a. phenylketonuria.
  b. type 1 diabetes.
  c. lactose intolerance.
  d. a milk allergy.

LO 10   10. Type 1 diabetes

  a. typically arises in middle and older adulthood.
  b. is a progressive disorder in which body cells become less responsive to insulin.
  c. is characterized by autoimmune destruction of the beta cells of the pancreas.
  d. can be prevented by maintaining a healthful body weight.

true or false?

LO 1   11. **True or false?** Glycogen is a polysaccharide.

LO 4   12. **True or false?** Insulin and inulin are pancreatic hormones important in carbohydrate metabolism.

LO 8   13. In the United States, manufacturers are required by law to fortify breads made with white flour, that is, to add back some of the vitamins and minerals lost in processing.

LO 9   14. **True or false?** Sugar alcohols are non-nutritive sweeteners.

LO 10   15. **True or false?** Whereas higher-than-normal blood glucose levels are characteristic of diabetes, lower-than-normal blood glucose levels characterize hypoglycemia.

Short Answer

LO 1   16. Create a table listing the molecular composition and food sources of each of the following carbohydrates: glucose, fructose, lactose, and sucrose.

LO 3   17. Your niece, Lilly, is 6 years old and is learning about MyPlate in her first-grade class. She points out the "grains" group and proudly lists her favorite food choices from this group: "saltine crackers, pancakes, and spaghetti." Explain to Lilly, in words she could understand, the difference between fiber-rich carbohydrates and refined carbohydrates and why fiber-rich carbohydrates are more healthful food choices.

LO 4   18. Describe the role of insulin in regulating blood glucose levels.

LO 5   19. Identify at least four ways in which fiber helps us maintain a healthy digestive system.

LO 10   20. Explain how obesity can trigger type 2 diabetes.

math review

LO 6 **21.** Simon is trying to determine how much carbohydrate he should consume in his diet to meet the AMDR for health. His total energy intake needed to maintain his current weight is 3,500 kcal per day. Simon has learned that the AMDR for carbohydrate is 45% to 65% of total energy intake. How many (a) kcal and (b) grams of carbohydrate should Simon consume each day?

Answers to Review Questions and Math Review can be found online in the MasteringNutrition Study Area.

web links

www.eatright.org
Academy of Nutrition and Dietetics
Visit this website to learn more about diabetes, low- and high-carbohydrate diets, and general healthful eating habits.

www.foodinsight.org
Food Insight—International Food Information Council Foundation (IFIC)
Search this site to find out more about sugars and low-calorie sweeteners.

www.ada.org
American Dental Association
Go to this site to learn more about tooth decay, as well as other oral health topics.

www.nidcr.nih.gov
National Institute of Dental and Craniofacial Research (NIDCR)

Find out more about recent oral and dental health discoveries, and obtain statistics and data on the status of dental health in the United States.

www.diabetes.org
American Diabetes Association
Find out more about the nutritional needs of people living with diabetes.

www.niddk.nih.gov
National Institute of Diabetes and Digestive and Kidney Diseases (NIDDK)
Learn more about diabetes, including treatment, complications, U.S. statistics, clinical trials, and recent research.

www.caloriecontrol.org
Calorie Control Council
This site provides information about reducing energy and fat in the diet, achieving and maintaining a healthy weight, and eating various low-calorie, reduced-fat foods and beverages.

IN DEPTH

Alcohol

After reading this In Depth, you will be able to:

1 Describe two potential benefits and two potential concerns related to "moderate drinking," pp. 153–155.

2 Explain how the body metabolizes alcohol, pp. 155–156.

3 Distinguish between alcohol abuse and alcohol dependence, p. 156.

4 List four dangerous consequences of binge drinking among young Americans, pp. 156–159.

5 Discuss the risks of maternal alcohol consumption during fetal development, pp. 160–161.

6 Identify at least three strategies for limiting your drinking and three signs of an alcohol problem, pp. 160–162.

7 Discuss how to help a loved one with an alcohol problem, p. 162.

No one should have to spend his 21st birthday in an emergency room, but that's what happened to Todd the night he turned 21. His friends took him off campus to celebrate, and, with their encouragement, he attempted to drink 21 shots before the bar closed at 2 AM. Fortunately for Todd, when he passed out and couldn't be roused, his best friend noticed his cold, clammy skin and erratic breathing and drove him to the local emergency room. There, his stomach was pumped and he was treated for alcohol poisoning. He regained consciousness but felt sick and shaky for several more hours. Not everyone is so lucky. In the United States, 2,200 people die of alcohol poisoning each year. That's about six deaths every day.[1]

What makes excessive alcohol intake so dangerous, and why is moderate alcohol consumption often considered healthful? How can you tell if someone is struggling with alcohol addiction, and what can you do to help? What if that someone is you? We explore these questions *In Depth* here.

Alcohols are chemical compounds structurally similar to carbohydrates, with one or more hydroxyl (OH) groups (**Figure 1**). **Ethanol**, the specific type of alcohol found in beer, wine, and distilled spirits such as whiskey and vodka, has one hydroxyl group. Throughout this discussion, the common term *alcohol* will be used to represent the specific compound *ethanol*.

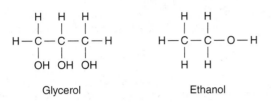

Glycerol   Ethanol

FIGURE 1 Chemical structures of glycerol and alcohol (ethanol).

What Do We Know about Moderate Alcohol Intake?

LO 1 Describe two potential benefits and two potential concerns related to "moderate drinking."

Alcohol intake is usually described as "drinks per day." A **drink** is defined as the amount of a beverage that provides ½ fluid ounce of pure alcohol. For example, 12 oz of beer, 10 oz of a wine cooler, 4 to 5 oz of wine, and 1½ oz of 80-**proof** whiskey, scotch, gin, or vodka are each equivalent to one drink (**Figure 2**). The term "proof" reflects the alcohol content of distilled spirits: 100-proof liquor is 50% alcohol whereas 80-proof liquor is 40% alcohol.

The *Dietary Guidelines for Americans* advise "If alcohol is consumed, it should be consumed in moderation—up to one

drink per day for women and two drinks per day for men—and only by adults of legal drinking age." Notice that this definition of **moderate drinking** is based on a maximal daily intake; a person who does not drink any alcohol on weekdays but downs a six-pack of beer most Saturday nights would *not* be classified as a "moderate drinker"! The *Dietary Guidelines for Americans* also identify groups of individuals who should not consume alcohol at all, including women who are or may become pregnant and women who are breastfeeding. In addition, people who cannot restrict their drinking to moderate levels and those taking medications that interact with alcohol should not drink at all, nor should individuals driving, operating machinery, or engaging in other tasks that require attention and coordination. Finally, anyone younger than the legal drinking age should not consume alcohol.

As we discuss here, both health benefits and concerns are associated with moderate alcohol intake. When deciding whether or how much alcohol to drink, you need to weigh the pros and cons of alcohol consumption against your own personal health history.

Benefits of Moderate Alcohol Intake

In most people, moderate alcohol intake offers some psychological benefits; it can reduce stress and anxiety while improving self-confidence. It can also have nutritional benefits. Moderate use of alcohol can improve appetite and dietary intake, which can be of great value to the elderly and people with a chronic disease that suppresses appetite.

In addition, moderate alcohol consumption may reduce the risk of subsequent age-related cognitive decline or dementia, including certain tests of attention, mental speed and flexibility.[2] It has also been linked to lower rates of heart disease, especially in older adults and in people already at risk for heart disease, such as those with type 2 diabetes. Consumption of a moderate amount of alcohol in any form (wine, beer, or distilled spirits) increases levels of the "good" type of cholesterol (HDL) while decreasing the concentration

alcohol Chemically, a compound characterized by the presence of a hydroxyl group; in common usage, a beverage made from fermented fruits, vegetables, or grains and containing ethanol.

ethanol A specific alcohol compound (C_2H_5OH) formed from the fermentation of dietary carbohydrates and used in a variety of alcoholic beverages.

drink The amount of an alcoholic beverage that provides approximately 0.5 fl. oz of pure ethanol.

proof A measure of the alcohol content of a liquid; 100-proof liquor is 50% alcohol by volume, 80-proof liquor is 40% alcohol by volume, and so on.

moderate drinking Alcohol consumption of up to one drink per day for women and up to two drinks per day for men.

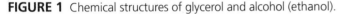

FIGURE 2 What does one drink look like? A drink is equivalent to 1½ oz of distilled spirits, 4 to 5 oz of wine, 10 oz of wine cooler, or 12 oz of beer.

of "bad" cholesterol (LDL); it also reduces the risk of abnormal clot formation in the blood vessels.[3]

Recently, there has been a great deal of interest in **resveratrol**, a chemical found in red wines, grapes, and other plant foods. Some researchers, based on experiments with mice, are proposing that resveratrol may be able to lower our risk for certain chronic diseases, such as diabetes, heart disease, and liver disease. However, the amount in red wine is too minimal to provide a health benefit.[4]

Concerns of Moderate Alcohol Intake

Not everyone responds to alcohol in the same manner. A person's age, genetic makeup, state of health, and use of medications can influence both immediate and long-term responses to alcohol intake, even at moderate levels. For example, women appear to be at increased risk for breast cancer when consuming low to moderate amounts of alcohol.[5] In some studies, moderate use of alcohol has been linked to a higher rate of bleeding in the brain, resulting in what is termed *hemorrhagic stroke;* however, other research has found that light to moderate alcohol consumption does not increase the risk for stroke.[6]

Another concern is the effect of alcohol on our waistlines! As we pointed out in Chapter 1, alcohol is not classified as a nutrient because it does not serve any unique metabolic role in humans. Although it provides virtually no nutritional value, alcohol does provide energy: at 7 kcal/g, alcohol has a relatively high Calorie content. Only fat (9 kcal/g) has more Calories per gram. As illustrated in **Figure 3**, if you're watching your weight, it makes sense to strictly limit your consumption of alcohol to stay within your daily energy needs.

Alcohol intake may also increase your *food* intake, because alcoholic beverages enhance appetite, particularly during social events, leading some people to overeat. Both current and lifelong intakes of alcohol increase the risk for obesity in both males and females, particularly for those who binge drink.[7]

> To find out how many Calories your alcoholic beverages are costing you, go to http://rethinkingdrinking.niaaa.nih.gov/, go to the "Tools" tab on the left hand side, click the "Calculators" link and select "Alcohol Calorie calculator" to begin.

The potential for drug–alcohol interactions is well known; many medications carry a warning label advising consumers to avoid alcohol while taking the drug. Alcohol magnifies the effect of certain painkillers, sleeping pills, antidepressants, and

resveratrol A chemical known to play a role in limiting cell damage from the by-products of metabolic reactions. It is found in red wine and certain other plant-based foods.

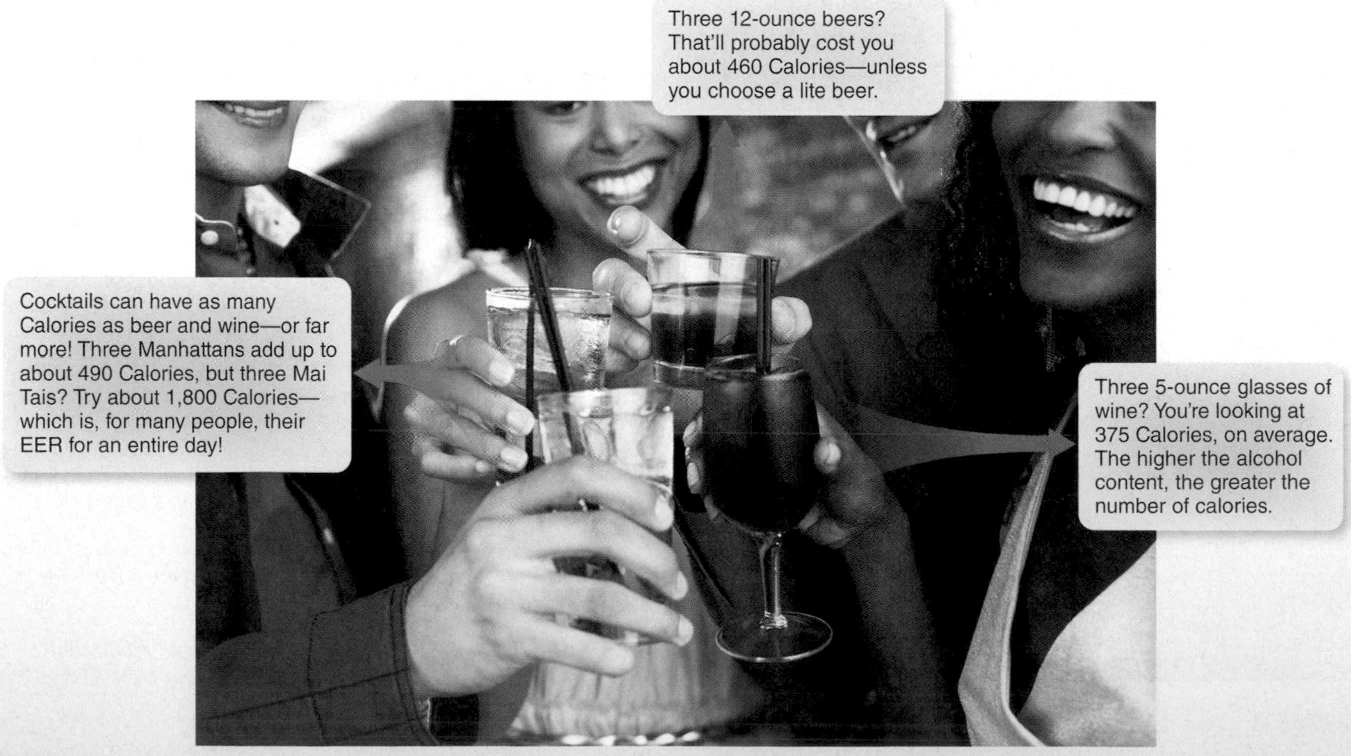

Three 12-ounce beers? That'll probably cost you about 460 Calories—unless you choose a lite beer.

Cocktails can have as many Calories as beer and wine—or far more! Three Manhattans add up to about 490 Calories, but three Mai Tais? Try about 1,800 Calories—which is, for many people, their EER for an entire day!

Three 5-ounce glasses of wine? You're looking at 375 Calories, on average. The higher the alcohol content, the greater the number of calories.

FIGURE 3 Going out for a few drinks? You might want to stick to just one—Calories in alcoholic beverages really add up!

antianxiety medications and can lead to loss of consciousness. It also increases the risk for gastrointestinal bleeding in people taking aspirin or ibuprofen, as well as the risk for stomach bleeding and liver damage in people taking acetaminophen (Tylenol). In diabetics using insulin or oral medications to lower blood glucose, alcohol can exaggerate the drug's effect, leading to an inappropriately low level of blood glucose.

As you can see, there are both benefits and risks to moderate alcohol consumption. Experts agree that people who are currently consuming alcohol in moderation and who have low or no risk for alcohol addiction or medication interaction can safely continue their current level of use. Adults who abstain from alcohol, however, should not start drinking just for the possible health benefits. Individuals who have a personal or family history of alcoholism or fall into any other risk category should consider abstaining from alcohol use, even at a moderate level.

How Is Alcohol Metabolized?

LO 2 Explain how the body metabolizes alcohol.

Alcohol is absorbed directly from both the stomach and the small intestine; it does not require digestion prior to absorption. Consuming foods with some fat, protein, and fiber slows the absorption of alcohol and can reduce *blood alcohol concentration (BAC)* by as much as 50% compared to peak BAC when drinking on an empty stomach. Carbonated alcoholic beverages are absorbed very rapidly, which explains why champagne and sparkling wines are so quick to generate an alcoholic "buzz."

The process of alcohol metabolism is discussed in detail in Chapter 7, but a brief overview will introduce you to the basics. Although most alcohol is oxidized, or broken down, in the liver, a small amount is metabolized in the stomach before it has even been absorbed. Cells in both the stomach and the liver secrete the enzyme *alcohol dehydrogenase (ADH),* which triggers the first step in alcohol degradation, while *aldehyde dehydrogenase (ALDH)* takes the breakdown process one step further (**Figure 4**). In women, ADH in the stomach is less active than in men; thus, women do not oxidize as much alcohol in their stomach, leaving up to 30% to 35% more intact alcohol to be absorbed.

Once absorbed, the alcohol moves through the bloodstream to the liver, where it is broken down at a fairly steady rate. On average, a healthy adult metabolizes the equivalent of one drink per hour. If someone drinks more than that, such as two, three or more alcoholic drinks in an hour, the excess alcohol is released back into the bloodstream, where it elevates BAC and triggers a range of behavioral and metabolic reactions. Through the blood, alcohol is quickly and completely distributed throughout all body fluids and tissues, including the brain. Anytime you consume more than one alcoholic beverage per hour, you are exposing every tissue in your body to the toxic effects of alcohol.

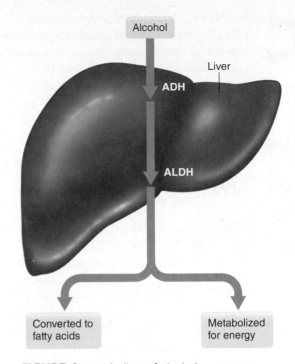

FIGURE 4 Metabolism of alcohol.

Despite what you may have heard, there is no effective intervention to speed up the breakdown of alcohol (**Table 1**). The key to keeping your BAC below the legal limit is to drink alcoholic beverages while eating a meal or large snack, to drink alcoholic beverages very slowly, to have no more than one drink per hour, and to limit your total consumption of alcohol on any one occasion.

A person who steadily increases his or her alcohol consumption over time becomes more tolerant of a given intake of alcohol. Chronic drinkers experience *metabolic tolerance,* a condition in which the liver becomes more efficient in its breakdown of alcohol. This means that the person's BAC rises more slowly after consuming a certain number of drinks.

TABLE 1 Myths about Alcohol Metabolism

The Claim	The Reality
Physical activity, such as walking around, will speed up the breakdown of alcohol.	Muscles don't metabolize alcohol; the liver does.
Drinking a lot of coffee will keep you from getting drunk.	Coffee does not cause alcohol to be excreted in the urine.
Using a sauna or steam room will force the alcohol out of your body.	Very little alcohol is lost in sweat; the alcohol will remain in your bloodstream.
Herbal and nutritional products are available that speed up the breakdown of alcohol.	There is no scientific evidence that commercial supplements will increase the rate of alcohol metabolism; they will not lower blood alcohol levels.

In addition, chronic drinkers develop what is called *functional tolerance*, meaning they show few, if any, signs of impairment or intoxication, even at high BACs. As a result, these individuals may consume twice as much alcohol as when they first started drinking before they reach the same state of euphoria.

What Are Alcohol Abuse and Dependence?

LO 3 Distinguish between alcohol abuse and alcohol dependence.

The National Institute on Alcohol Abuse and Alcoholism (NIAAA) recognizes two general types of *alcohol use disorders:* alcohol abuse and alcohol dependence, commonly known as alcoholism. In the United States, about 18 million people have an alcohol use disorder.[8]

Alcohol abuse is a pattern of alcohol consumption, whether chronic or occasional, that results in distress, danger, or harm to one's health, functioning, or interpersonal relationships. Both chronic and occasional alcohol abuse can eventually lead to alcoholism.

Binge drinking is a form of alcohol abuse defined as the consumption of five or more alcoholic drinks on one occasion by a man or four or more drinks for a woman. In a recent survey, nearly 25% of people ages 18 or older reported binge drinking within the previous month.[8] People who binge-drink report engaging in about four episodes a month.[9]

Among the many consequences of binge drinking is an increased risk for potentially fatal falls, drownings, and automobile accidents. Acts of physical violence, including vandalism and physical and sexual assault, are also associated with binge drinking. The consequences also carry over beyond a particular episode: binge drinking impairs cognition, planning, problem solving, memory, and inhibition, leading to significant social, educational, and employment problems. About 25% of college students who binge-drink report academic consequences of their drinking, from missed classes to a low GPA.[10] Finally, hangovers, which are discussed shortly, are practically inevitable, given the amount of alcohol consumed during a binge.

Alcohol dependence, commonly known as *alcoholism*, is a disease characterized by:

- *Craving:* a strong need or urge to drink alcoholic beverages
- *Loss of control:* the inability to stop once drinking has begun
- *Physical dependence:* the presence of nausea, sweating, shakiness, and other signs of withdrawal after stopping alcohol intake
- *Tolerance:* the need to drink larger and larger amounts of alcohol to get the same "high," or pleasurable sensations, associated with alcohol intake

What Are the Effects of Alcohol Abuse?

LO 4 List four dangerous consequences of binge drinking among young Americans.

LO 5 Discuss the risks of maternal alcohol consumption during fetal development.

Alcohol is a drug. It exerts a narcotic effect on virtually every part of the brain, acting as a sedative and depressant. Alcohol also has the potential to act as a direct toxin; in high concentrations, it can damage or destroy cell membranes and internal cell structures. As shown in **Figure 5**, an alcohol intake between ½ and 1 drink per day is associated with the lowest risk of mortality for both men and women. The risk of death increases sharply as alcohol intake increases above 2 drinks per day for women, and 3½ drinks per day for men. These increased mortality risks are related to alcohol's damaging effects on the brain, the liver, and other organs, as well as its role in motor vehicle accidents and other traumatic injuries.

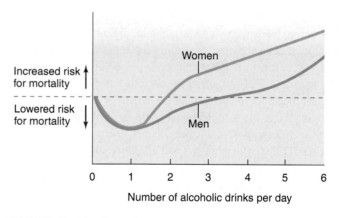

FIGURE 5 The effect of alcohol consumption on mortality risk. Consuming ½ to 1 drink per day is associated with the lowest mortality risk for all adults. The risk of death increases sharply at levels of alcohol intake above 2 drinks per day for women and about 3½ drinks per day for men.

alcohol abuse A pattern of alcohol consumption, whether chronic or occasional, that results in harm to one's health, functioning, or interpersonal relationships.

binge drinking The consumption of five or more alcoholic drinks on one occasion for a man, or four or more drinks for a woman.

alcohol dependence A disease state characterized by alcohol craving, loss of control, physical dependence, and tolerance.

alcohol hangover A consequence of drinking too much alcohol; symptoms include headache, fatigue, dizziness, muscle aches, nausea and vomiting, sensitivity to light and sound, extreme thirst, and mood disturbances.

Alcohol Hangovers

Alcohol hangover is an extremely unpleasant consequence of drinking too much alcohol. It lasts up to 24 hours, and its symptoms include headache, fatigue, dizziness, muscle aches, nausea and vomiting, sensitivity to light and sound, and extreme thirst. Some people also experience depression, anxiety, irritability, and other mood disturbances. While some of the aftereffects of a binge may be due to nonalcoholic compounds known as *congeners* (found in red wines, brandy, and whiskey, for example), most of the consequences are directly related to the alcohol itself. These include the following:

■ *Fluid and electrolyte imbalance:* Some of the symptoms occur because of alcohol's effect as a *diuretic,* a compound that increases urine output. Alcohol inhibits the release of the hormones that normally regulate urine production, prompting an excessive loss of fluid and electrolytes and contributing to dizziness and lightheadedness.

■ *Irritation and inflammation:* Alcohol irritates the lining of the stomach, causing inflammation (gastritis) and increasing gastric acid production. This may account for the abdominal pain, nausea, and vomiting seen in most hangovers.

■ *Metabolic disturbances:* Alcohol disrupts normal body metabolism, leading to low levels of blood glucose and elevated levels of lactic acid. These disturbances contribute to the characteristic fatigue, weakness, and mood changes seen after excessive alcohol intake.

■ *Biological disturbances:* Alcohol disrupts various biological rhythms, such as sleep patterns and cycles of hormone secretion, leading to an effect similar to that of jet lag.

While many folk remedies, including various herbal products, claim to prevent or reduce hangover effects, few have proven effective. Drinking water or other nonalcoholic beverages will minimize the risk for dehydration, and toast or dry cereal is effective in bringing blood glucose levels back to normal. Getting adequate sleep can counteract the fatigue, and the use of antacids can help reduce nausea and abdominal pain. While aspirin, ibuprofen, and acetaminophen might be useful for headaches, aspirin and ibuprofen can cause an upset stomach and gastrointestinal bleeding, and interactions between acetaminophen and alcohol can cause liver damage.[11]

Reduced Brain Function

Alcohol is known for its ability to alter behavior, mainly through its effects on the brain. Even at low intakes, alcohol impairs reasoning and judgment (**Figure 6**). Alcohol also interferes with normal sleep patterns, alters sight and speech, and leads to loss of both fine and gross motor skills such as handwriting, hand–eye coordination, and balance. Many people who drink experience unexpected mood swings, intense anger, or unreasonable irritation. Others react in the opposite direction, becoming sad, withdrawn, and lethargic. When teens or young adults chronically consume excessive amounts of alcohol, they may permanently alter brain structure and function.[12] Intellectual functioning and memory can be lost or compromised. In addition, early exposure to alcohol increases the risk for future alcohol addiction and may contribute to lifelong deficits in memory, motor skills, and muscle coordination.[13]

As BAC Increases, So Does Impairment

Blood Alcohol Concentration (BAC)

Life Threatening
- Loss of consciousness
- Danger of life-threatening alcohol poisoning
- Significant risk of death in most drinkers due to suppression of vital life functions

0.31–0.45%

Severe Impairment
- Speech, memory, coordination, attention, reaction time, balance significantly impaired
- All driving-related skills dangerously impaired
- Judgment and decision making dangerously impaired
- Blackouts (amnesia)
- Vomiting and other signs of alcohol poisoning common
- Loss of consciousness

0.16–0.30%

Increased Impairment
- Perceived beneficial effects of alcohol, such as relaxation, give way to increasing intoxication
- Increased risk of aggression in some people
- Speech, memory, attention, coordination, balance further impaired
- Significant impairments in all driving skills
- Increased risk of injury to self and others
- Moderate memory impairments

0.06–0.15%

Mild Impairment
- Mild speech, memory, attention, coordination, balance impairments
- Perceived beneficial effects, such as relaxation
- Sleepiness can begin

0.0–0.05%

FIGURE 6 Effects of increasing blood alcohol concentration on brain function. The first brain region affected is the cerebral cortex, which governs reasoning and judgment. At increasing levels of impairment, the cerebellum, which controls and coordinates movement, the hippocampus, which is involved in memory storage, and the brain stem, which regulates consciousness, breathing, and other essential functions, may become involved.

Alcohol Poisoning

At very high intakes of alcohol, a person is at risk for **alcohol poisoning**, a metabolic state that occurs in response to binge drinking. At high BACs, the respiratory center of the brain is depressed. This reduces the level of oxygen reaching the brain and increases the individual's risk for death by respiratory or cardiac failure. Like Todd in our opening story, many binge drinkers lose consciousness, but their blood alcohol level can still continue to rise as the alcohol in their GI tract is absorbed and released into the bloodstream. Moreover, alcohol irritates the GI tract, and vomiting—even while unconscious—is common. The person can choke on their vomit and suffocate.

For these reasons, if someone passes out after a night of hard drinking, he or she should never be left alone to "sleep it off." If the person has cold and clammy skin, a bluish tint to the skin, or slow or irregular breathing, or if the person exhibits confusion or stupor, or cannot be roused, seek emergency healthcare immediately.

Reduced Liver Function

The liver performs an astonishing number and variety of body functions, including nutrient metabolism, glycogen storage, the synthesis of many essential compounds, and the detoxification of medications and other potential poisons. As noted earlier, it is the main site of alcohol metabolism. When an individual's rate of alcohol intake exceeds the rate at which the liver can break down the alcohol, liver cells are damaged or destroyed. The longer the alcohol abuse continues, the greater the damage to the liver.

Fatty liver (also called *alcoholic steatosis*), a condition in which abnormal amounts of fat build up in the liver, is an early yet reversible sign of liver damage commonly linked to alcohol abuse. Once alcohol intake stops and a healthful diet is maintained, the liver is able to heal and resume normal function.

Alcoholic hepatitis is a more severe condition of liver inflammation, resulting in loss of appetite, nausea and vomiting, abdominal pain, and jaundice (a yellowing of the skin and eyes, reflecting reduced liver function). Mental confusion and impaired immune response often occur with alcoholic hepatitis. While avoidance of alcohol and a healthful diet often result in full recovery, many people experience lifelong complications from alcoholic hepatitis.

Cirrhosis of the liver is often the result of long-term alcohol abuse; liver cells are scarred, blood flow through the liver is impaired, and liver function declines (**FIGURE 7**). This condition almost always results in irreversible damage to the liver and can be life-threatening. Blood pressure increases dramatically, large amounts of fluid are retained in the abdominal cavity, and metabolic wastes accumulate. In some cases, liver function fails completely, resulting in the need for a liver transplant or the likelihood of death.

Nutri-Case

Theo

"I was driving home from a post-game party last night when I was pulled over by the police. The officer said I seemed to be driving 'erratically' and asked me how many drinks I'd had. I told him I'd only had three beers and explained that I was pretty tired from the game. Then, just to prove I was fine, I offered to count backward from a hundred, but I must have sounded sober, because he didn't make me do it. I can't believe he thought I was driving drunk! Still, maybe three beers after a game really is too much."

Do you think it is physiologically possible that Theo's driving had been impaired after consuming three beers? To answer, you'll need to consider both Theo's body weight and the effect of playing a long basketball game. What other factors that influence the rate of alcohol absorption or breakdown could have affected Theo's BAC? How could all of these factors influence a decision about whether "three beers after a game really is too much"?

alcohol poisoning A potentially fatal condition in which an overdose of alcohol results in cardiac and/or respiratory failure.

fatty liver An early and reversible stage of liver disease often found in people who abuse alcohol, characterized by the abnormal accumulation of fat within liver, and cells; also called alcoholic steatosis.

alcoholic hepatitis A serious condition of inflammation of the liver caused by alcohol.

cirrhosis of the liver End-stage liver disease characterized by significant abnormalities in liver structure and function; may lead to complete liver failure.

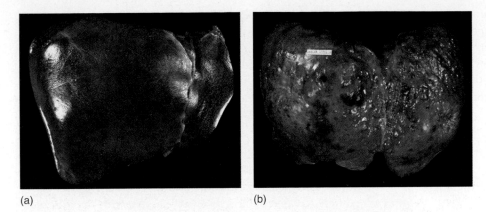

(a)   (b)

FIGURE 7 Cirrhosis of the liver is often caused by chronic alcohol abuse. **(a)** A healthy liver; **(b)** a liver damaged by cirrhosis.

Increased Risk for Chronic Disease

While moderate drinking may provide some health benefits, it is clear that chronically high intakes of alcohol damage a number of body organs and systems, increasing a person's risk for chronic disease and death:[14]

- *Bone health:* Men and women who are alcohol dependent experience an increased loss of calcium in the urine, impaired vitamin D activation, and decreased production of certain hormones that enhance bone formation with the result that up to 40% of alcoholics have osteoporosis.
- *Pancreatic injury and diabetes:* Alcohol damages the pancreas, which produces insulin, and decreases the body's ability to properly respond to insulin. The result is chronically elevated blood glucose levels and an increased risk for diabetes.
- *Cancer:* Research has most strongly linked alcohol consumption, particularly at high intakes, to increased risk for cancer of the mouth and throat, esophagus, stomach, liver, colon, and female breast.[15]

Malnutrition

As alcohol intake increases to 30% or more of total energy intake, appetite is lost and intake of healthful foods declines. Over time, the diet becomes deficient in protein, fats, carbohydrates, vitamins A and C, and minerals such as iron, zinc, and calcium (**Figure 8**). End-stage alcoholics may consume as much as 90% of their daily energy intake from alcohol, displacing virtually all foods. Even if food intake is maintained, the toxic effects of alcohol lead to impaired food digestion, nutrient absorption, and nutrient metabolism.

Long-term exposure to alcohol damages not only the liver but also the stomach, small intestine, and pancreas. Alcohol increases gastric acid production, leading to stomach ulcers, gastric bleeding, and damage to the cells that produce gastric enzymes, mucus, and other proteins. The lining of the small intestine is also damaged by chronic alcohol abuse, reducing nutrient absorption, while damage to the pancreas reduces the production of pancreatic digestive enzymes. As a result, the digestion of foods and absorption of nutrients, such as the fat-soluble vitamins (A, D, E, and K), vitamin B$_6$, folate, and zinc, become inadequate, leading to malnutrition and inappropriate weight loss.

Not only are dietary intake, food digestion, and nutrient absorption negatively affected by alcohol abuse but so, too, is the ability of body cells to utilize nutrients. For example, even if an alcoholic were to take vitamin D supplements, his or her liver would be so damaged that its cells could not activate the vitamin D. Many chronic alcoholics are unable to synthesize the liver proteins that carry vitamins and minerals to target tissues. Other vitamins and minerals are negatively affected because the

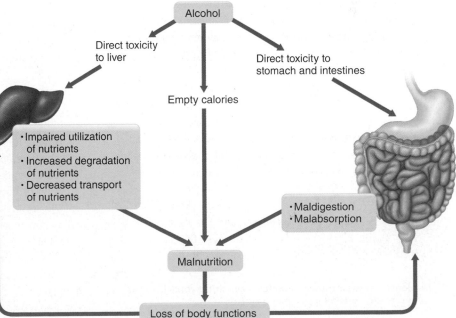

FIGURE 8 Alcohol-related malnutrition. Excess alcohol consumption contributes directly and indirectly to widespread nutrient deficiencies.

159

liver is too damaged to maintain normal nutrient storage capacity. Across the whole spectrum, from food intake to cell nutrient metabolism, alcohol abuse increases the risk for malnutrition.

Increased Risk for Traumatic Injury

Excessive alcohol intake is the third leading preventable, lifestyle-related cause of death for Americans of all ages, contributing to nearly 80,000 deaths per year. In the 4 years between 2006 and 2010, there were nearly 90,000 deaths directly attributed to alcohol among working age adults, accounting for nearly 10% of all deaths among this subset of American adults.[16] It has been estimated that as many as 6,000 young Americans die each year from alcohol-related motor vehicle accidents, suicides, and homicides and an additional 600,000 college age students are unintentionally injured while under the influence of alcohol.[17] As previously noted, rates of physical and sexual assaults, vandalism, accidental falls, and drownings also increase when people are under the influence of alcohol.

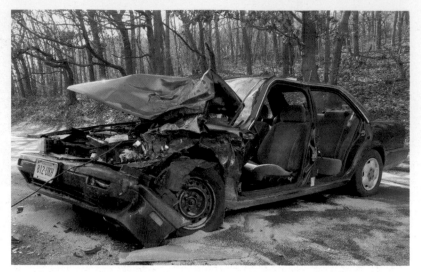

Excessive alcohol intake greatly increases the risks for car accidents and other traumatic injuries.

Fetal and Infant Health Problems

No level of alcohol consumption is considered safe for pregnant women. Women who are or think they may be pregnant should abstain from all alcoholic beverages. As discussed in the nearby *Highlight* box, fetal alcohol syndrome, which is caused by alcohol intake in a childbearing woman, is a critical problem in the United States.

Women who are breastfeeding should also abstain from alcohol because it easily passes into the breast milk at levels equal to blood alcohol concentrations. If consumed by the infant, the alcohol in breast milk can slow motor development and depress the central nervous system. Alcohol also reduces the mother's ability to produce milk, putting the infant at risk for malnutrition.

Taking Control of Your Alcohol Intake

LO 6 Identify at least three strategies for limiting your drinking and three signs of an alcohol problem.

Knowing that a moderate intake of alcohol may provide some health benefits and that excessive intake results in a wide range of problems, what can you do to control your drinking?

The following are practical strategies that can help you avoid the negative consequences of excessive alcohol consumption:[18]

■ Think about *why* you are planning to drink. Is it to relax and socialize, or are you using alcohol to release stress? If the latter, try some stress-reduction techniques that don't involve alcohol, such as exercise, yoga, meditation, or simply talking with a friend. Avoid known triggers—people, places, and events that inevitably lead to excess alcohol intake.

■ Make sure you have a protein-containing meal or snack before your first alcoholic drink; having food in the stomach delays gastric emptying, which means more of the alcohol can be broken down in the stomach before it even gets the chance to be absorbed into the bloodstream.

■ "Pace and Space" your drinks. Consume only one alcoholic beverage per hour and stop entirely after two or at most three drinks. Rotate (space) between alcoholic and nonalcoholic drinks. Start with a large glass of water, iced tea, or soda. Once your thirst has been satisfied, your rate of fluid intake will drop. Remember, a glass of pure orange juice doesn't look any different from one laced with vodka, so no one will even know what it is you are or are not drinking! Dilute hard liquor with large amounts of soda, water, juice, or iced tea. These diluted beverages are cheaper and lower in Calories, too!

■ Whether or not your drink is diluted, sip slowly to allow your liver time to keep up with your alcohol intake.

■ Know how to say "No." If your friends pressure you to drink, volunteer to be the designated driver. You'll have a "free pass" for the night in terms of saying no to alcoholic drinks.

■ Decide in advance what your alcohol intake will be, and plan some strategies for sticking to your limit. If you are going to a bar, for example, take only enough money to buy two beers and two sodas. If you are at a party, stay occupied dancing, sampling the food, or talking with friends, and stay as far away from the bar area as you can.

Fetal Alcohol Syndrome

Alcohol is a known **teratogen** (a substance that causes fetal harm) that readily crosses the placenta into the fetal bloodstream. Because the immature fetal liver cannot effectively break down the alcohol, it accumulates in the fetal blood and tissues, increasing the risk for various birth defects. The effects of maternal alcohol intake are dose-related: the more the mother drinks, the greater the potential harm to the fetus. In addition to the amount of alcohol consumed during pregnancy, the timing of the mother's alcohol intake influences the risk for fetal complications. Binge or frequent drinking during the first trimester of pregnancy is more likely to result in birth defects and other permanent abnormalities, whereas alcohol consumption in the third trimester typically results in low birth weight and growth retardation.

Fetal alcohol syndrome (FAS) is the most severe consequence of maternal alcohol consumption. The CDC reports estimates of 0.2 to 1.5 cases of FAS per 1,000 live births in the United States.[1] FAS is characterized by malformations of the face, limbs, heart, and nervous system. The facial malformations persist throughout the child's life (**Figure 9**). Exposure to alcohol while in the womb impairs fetal growth; FAS babies are often underweight at birth and rarely normalize their growth after birth. Newborn and infant death rates are abnormally high, and those who do survive suffer from emotional, behavioral, social, learning, and developmental problems throughout life. FAS is one of the most common causes of mental retardation in the United States and the only one that is completely preventable, an important fact considering the cost of FAS is nearly $4 billion per year in the United States.[1]

Conditions associated with maternal alcohol consumption are collectively known as **fetal alcohol spectrum disorders (FASD)**. In addition to FAS, they include the following:

- *Alcohol-related birth defects (ARBD):* Children with ARBD are born with heart, skeletal, kidney, ear, and eye malformations.
- *Alcohol-related neurodevelopmental disorder (ARND):* Children with ARND demonstrate a range of life-long developmental, behavioral, and mental problems, including hyperactivity and attention deficit disorder.

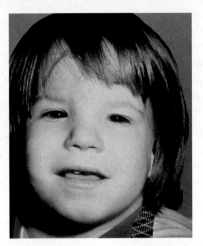

FIGURE 9 A child with fetal alcohol syndrome (FAS). The facial features typical of children with FAS include a short nose with a low, wide bridge; drooping eyes with an extra skinfold; and a flat, thin upper lip. These external traits are typically accompanied by behavioral problems and learning disorders. The effects of FAS are irreversible.

- *Fetal alcohol effects (FAE):* A more subtle set of consequences related to maternal alcohol intake, FAE is usually not identified at birth but becomes evident when the child enters preschool or kindergarten, where the child may exhibit impaired learning abilities. It is estimated that the incidence of FAE is ten times greater than that of FAS.

Can a pregnant woman safely consume any amount of alcohol? Although some pregnant women do have an occasional alcoholic drink with no apparent ill effects, there is no amount of alcohol known to be safe. In one study, researchers identified a number of subtle but long-term negative consequences, including negative impacts on child behavior and cognition, of light to moderate alcohol consumption during pregnancy.[2] The best advice regarding alcohol intake during pregnancy is to abstain if there is any chance of becoming pregnant, as well as throughout the pregnancy.

References:

1. Centers for Disease Control and Prevention. 2015. Fetal Alcohol Spectrum Disorders: Data and Statistics. http://www.cdc.gov/ncbddd/fasd/data.html.
2. Flak, A. L., S. Su, J. Bertrand, C. H. Denny, U. S. Kesmodel, and M. E. Cogswell. 2014. The association of mild, moderate, and binge prenatal alcohol exposure and child neuropsychological outcomes: a meta-analysis. *Alcoholism: Clin. Exp. Res* 38:214–226.

teratogen A substance or compound known to cause fetal harm or birth defects.

fetal alcohol syndrome (FAS) A set of serious, irreversible alcohol-related birth defects characterized by certain physical and mental abnormalities, including malformations of the face, limbs, heart, and nervous system; impaired growth; and a spectrum of mild to severe cognitive, emotional, and physical problems.

fetal alcohol spectrum disorders (FASD) An umbrella designation for a wide range of clinical outcomes that can result from prenatal exposure to alcohol. Fetal alcohol syndrome (FAS), alcohol-related neurodevelopmental disorder (ARND), and alcohol-related birth defects (ARBD) are components of FASD.

If you have trouble keeping your drinking moderate, for example by practicing the strategies just listed, then even if you're not dependent on alcohol, you should be concerned about your alcohol intake. In addition to the amount you drink, you should be concerned if you drink at inappropriate times. This includes, for example, before or while driving a car, while at work/school, or when you need to deal with negative emotions. If you answer "yes" to one or more of the following questions, provided by the NIAAA, you may have a problem with alcohol abuse:

- Have you ever felt you should cut down on your drinking?
- Have people annoyed you by criticizing your drinking?
- Have you ever felt bad or guilty about your drinking?
- Do you drink alone when you feel angry or sad?

- Has your drinking ever made you late for school or work?
- Have you ever had a drink first thing in the morning to steady your nerves or get rid of a hangover?
- Do you ever drink after promising yourself you won't?

If you think you have an alcohol problem, it is important for you to speak with a trusted friend, relative, coach, teacher, counselor, or healthcare provider. In addition, many campuses have support groups that can help. Taking control of your alcohol intake will allow you to take control of your life.

Talking to Someone about Alcohol Addiction

LO 7 Discuss how to help a loved one with an alcohol problem.

You may suspect that a close friend or relative might be one of the nearly 18 million Americans with an alcohol use disorder. If your friend or relative uses alcohol to calm down, cheer up, or relax, that may be a sign of alcohol dependency. The appearance of tremors or other signs of withdrawal as well as the initiation of secretive behaviors when consuming alcohol are other indications that alcohol has become a serious problem.

Many people become defensive or hostile when asked about their use of alcohol; denial is very common. The single hardest step toward sobriety is often the first: accepting the fact that help is needed. Some people respond well when confronted by a single person, while others benefit more from a group intervention. There should be no blaming or shaming; alcohol use disorders are medical

conditions with a genetic component. The National Institute on Alcoholism and Alcohol Abuse suggests the following approaches when trying to get a friend or relative into treatment:

- *Stop "covering" and making excuses:* Often, family and friends will make excuses to others to protect the person from the results of his or her drinking. It is important, however, to stop covering for that person so he or she can experience the full consequences of inappropriate alcohol consumption.
- *Intervene at a vulnerable time:* The best time to talk to someone about problem drinking is shortly after an alcohol-related incident, such as a DUI arrest, an alcohol-related traffic accident, or a public scene. Wait until the person is sober and everyone is relatively calm.
- *Be specific:* Tell the person exactly why you are concerned; use examples of specific problems associated with his or her drinking habits (e.g., poor school or work performance; legal problems; inappropriate behaviors). Explain what will happen if the person chooses not to get help—for example, no longer going out with the person if alcohol will be available, no longer riding with him or her in motor vehicles, moving out of a shared home, and so on.
- *Get help:* Professional help is available from community agencies, healthcare providers, online sites, school or worksite wellness centers, and some religious organizations. Several contacts and websites are listed at the end of this *In Depth*. If the person indicates a willingness to get help, call immediately for an appointment and/or immediately take him or her to a treatment center. The longer the delay, the more likely it is that the person will experience a change of heart.
- *Enlist the support of others:* Whether or not the person agrees to get help, calling upon other friends and relatives can often be effective, especially if one of these people has battled alcohol abuse. Formal support groups, such as Al-Anon and Alateen, can provide additional information and guidance.

Treatment for alcohol use disorders works for many, but not all, individuals. Success is measured in small steps, and relapses are common. Most scientists agree that people who abuse alcohol cannot just "cut down." Complete avoidance of all alcoholic beverages is the only way for most people who abuse alcohol to achieve full and ongoing recovery.

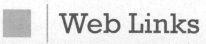 # Web Links

www.aa.org
Alcoholics Anonymous, Inc.
This site provides both links to local AA groups and information on the AA program.

www.al-anon.alateen.org
Al-Anon Family Group Headquarters, Inc.

This site provides links to local Al-Anon and Alateen groups, which offer support to spouses, children, and other loved ones of people addicted to alcohol.

www.niaaa.nih.gov
National Institute on Alcohol Abuse and Alcoholism
Visit this website for information on the prevalence, consequences, and treatments of alcohol-related disorders. Information for healthcare providers, people struggling with alcohol abuse, and family members is available free of charge.

www.collegedrinkingprevention.gov
College Drinking: Changing the Culture
The NIAAA developed this website for college students seeking information and advice on the subject of college drinking. Services include self-assessment questionnaires, answers to frequently asked questions, news articles, research, and links to support groups.

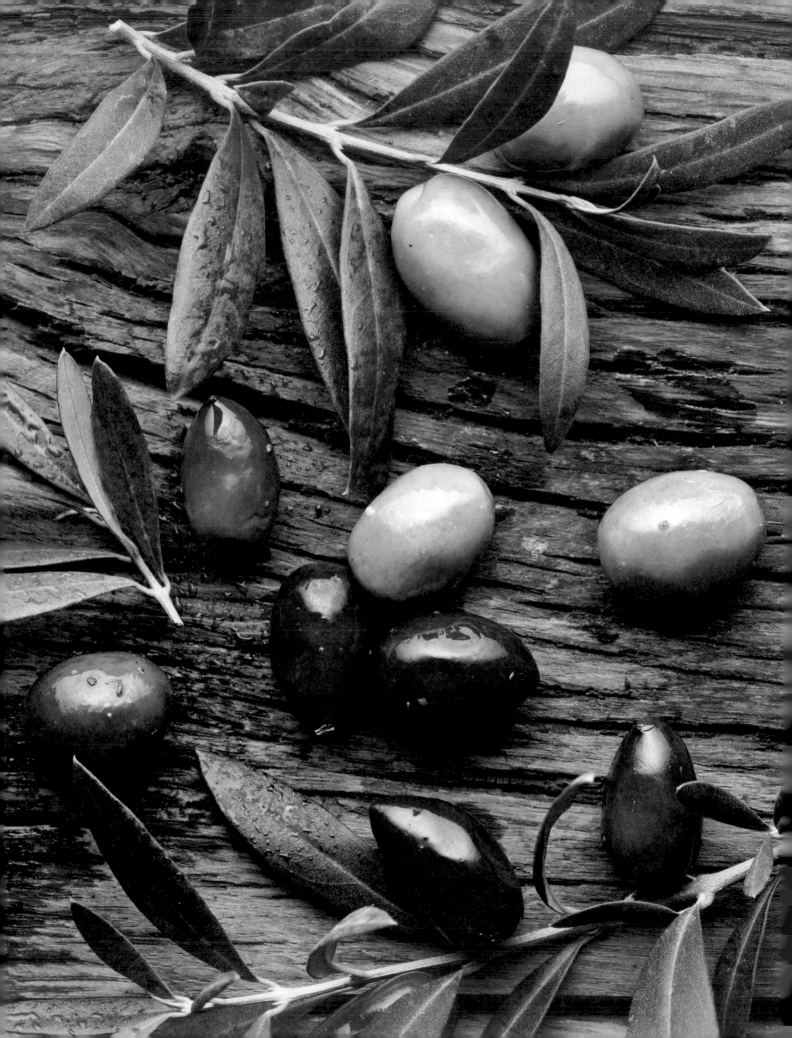

5 Lipids: Essential Energy-Supplying Nutrients

Learning Outcomes

After studying this chapter, you should be able to:

1 List and describe the three types of lipids found in foods, *pp. 166–176.*

2 Discuss how the level of saturation of a fatty acid affects its shape and the form it takes, *pp. 168–171.*

3 Explain the derivation of the term *trans* fatty acid and how *trans* fatty acids can negatively affect health, *pp. 170–171.*

4 Identify the two essential fatty acids, their chemical structure, and their beneficial functions, *pp. 171–174.*

5 Describe the steps involved in fat digestion, absorption, transport, and uptake, *pp. 176–181.*

6 List at least three physiologic functions of fat in the body, *pp. 182–185.*

7 Identify the DRIs for total fat, saturated fat, and the two essential fatty acids, *pp. 185–188.*

8 Distinguish between common food sources of fats considered beneficial and those considered less healthful, *pp. 188–194.*

9 Describe the role of blood lipids and dietary fats in the development of cardiovascular disease, *pp. 194–205.*

10 Identify lifestyle recommendations for the prevention or treatment of cardiovascular disease, *pp. 201–205.*

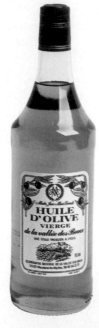

Some lipids, such as olive oil, are liquid at room temperature.

How would you feel if you purchased a bag of potato chips and were charged an extra 5% "fat tax"? What if you ordered fish and chips in your favorite restaurant only to be told that, in an effort to avoid lawsuits, fried foods were no longer being served? Sound surreal? Believe it or not, these and dozens of similar scenarios are being proposed, threatened, and defended in the current "obesity wars" raging around the globe. From Maine to California, from Iceland to New Zealand, local and national governments and healthcare policy advisors are scrambling to find effective methods for combating their rising rates of obesity. For reasons we explore in this chapter, many of their proposals focus on limiting consumption of foods high in saturated fats—for instance, requiring food vendors and manufacturers to reduce the portion size of these foods; taxing them, or increasing their purchase price; levying fines on manufacturers who produce them; removing these foods from vending machines; banning advertisements of these foods to children; and using food labels and public service announcements to warn consumers away from these foods. At the same time, "food litigation" lawsuits have been increasing, including allegations against restaurant chains and food companies for failing to warn consumers of the health dangers of eating their energy-dense, high-saturated-fat foods.

Is saturated fat really such a menace? Does a diet high in saturated fat cause obesity, heart disease, or diabetes? What exactly *is* saturated fat, anyway? Are there good and bad fats?

Although some people think that all dietary fat should be avoided, a certain amount of fat is absolutely essential for life and health. In this chapter, we'll discuss the function of fat in the human body; explain how dietary fat is digested, absorbed, transported, and stored; and help you distinguish between dietary fats that may be beneficial and those considered more harmful. You'll also assess how much fat you need in your diet and learn about the role of diet and lifestyle in the development of heart disease and other disorders.

LO 1 List and describe the three types of lipids found in foods.

LO 2 Discuss how the level of saturation of a fatty acid affects its shape and the form it takes.

LO 3 Explain the derivation of the term *trans* fatty acid and how *trans* fatty acids can negatively affect health.

LO 4 Identify the two essential fatty acids, their chemical structure, and their beneficial functions.

What Are Lipids?

Lipids are a large and diverse group of substances that are distinguished by the fact that they are insoluble in water. Think of a salad dressing made with vinegar (which is mostly water) and olive oil—a lipid. Shaking the bottle *disperses* the oil but doesn't *dissolve* it; that's why it separates back out again so quickly. Lipids are found in all sorts of living things, from bacteria to plants to human beings. In fact, their presence on your skin explains why you can't clean your face with water alone—you need some type of soap to break down the insoluble lipids before you can wash them away.

In this chapter, we focus on lipids that are synthesized within the body or found in foods. In the body, lipids are stored in adipose tissues that protect and insulate organs; are combined with phosphorus in cell membranes; and occur as steroids in bile salts, sex hormones, and other substances.[1] In foods, lipids occur as both fats and oils. These two forms are distinguished by the fact that fats, such as butter and lard, are solid at room temperature, whereas oils, such as olive oil, are liquid at room temperature. Dietary guidelines, food labels, and other nutrition information intended for the general public use the term *fats* when referring to the lipid content of diets and foods. We adopt this practice throughout this textbook, reserving the term *lipids* for discussions of chemistry and metabolism.

Three types of lipids are commonly found in foods and in the cells and tissues of the human body. These are triglycerides, phospholipids, and sterols. Let's take a look at each.

Triglycerides Are the Most Common Food-Based Lipid

Most of the fat we eat (95%) is in the form of triglycerides (also called triacylglycerols), which is the same form in which most body fat is stored. As reflected in the prefix *tri-*, a

lipids A diverse group of organic substances that are insoluble in water; lipids include triglycerides, phospholipids, and sterols.

triglyceride is a molecule consisting of a *three*-carbon glycerol backbone with *three* fatty acid chains, one attached to each carbon (**Figure 5.1**). **Glycerol** is an alcohol composed of three carbon atoms (Figure 5.1a). A **fatty acid** is a long chain of carbon atoms bound to each other as well as to hydrogen atoms (Figure 5.1b). It is an acid because it contains an acid group (carboxyl group) at the alpha (α) end of the chain.

A triglyceride forms when three fatty acids attach to glycerol via condensation reactions. Notice in Figure 5.1c the loss of an H from glycerol and an OH from the carboxyl group at each of the points at which a fatty acid has bonded to glycerol in the triglyceride compound.

Triglycerides are classified by the type of fatty acids attached to the glycerol backbone. These fatty acids can vary by their chain length (number of carbons in each fatty acid), by their level of saturation (how much hydrogen is attached to each carbon atom in the

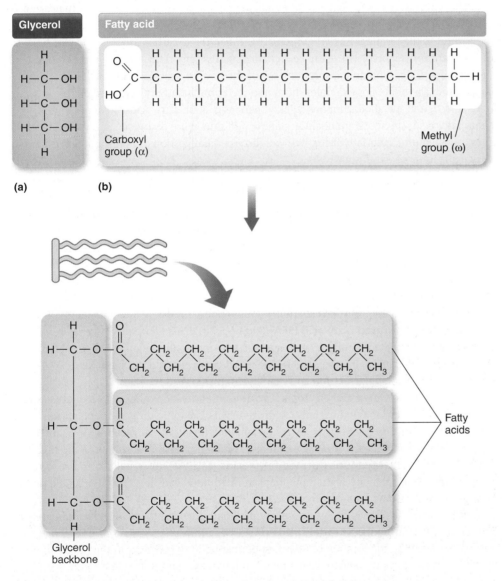

FIGURE 5.1 A triglyceride is composed of one molecule of glycerol and three fatty acids chains. **(a)** Structure of glycerol. **(b)** Structure of a fatty acid showing the carboxyl carbon (α) and the methyl carbon (ω) ends. **(c)** Via condensation reactions, the carboxyl carbon of each of three fatty acids has bonded to the glycerol's three oxygen atoms, releasing three molecules of water and forming the triglyceride.

triglyceride A molecule consisting of three fatty acids attached to a three-carbon glycerol backbone.

glycerol An alcohol composed of three carbon atoms; it is the backbone of a triglyceride molecule.

fatty acid An acid composed of a long chain of carbon atoms bound to each other as well as to hydrogen atoms, with a carboxyl group at the alpha end of the chain.

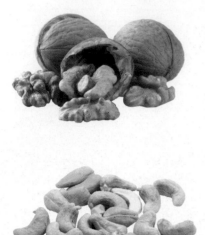

Walnuts and cashews are high in monounsaturated fatty acids.

fatty acid chain), and by their shape, which is determined in some cases by how they are commercially processed. All of these factors influence how the triglyceride is used within the body and how it affects our health.

Fatty Acids Vary in Chain Length

The fatty acids attached to the glycerol backbone can vary in the number of carbons they contain, a quality referred to as their *chain length*. In general, they contain an even number of carbons from 4 to 24; however, by far the most common fatty acids in our diet are 18 carbons in length.

- **Short-chain fatty acids** are usually fewer than 6 carbon atoms in length.
- **Medium-chain fatty acids** are 6 to 12 carbons in length.
- **Long-chain fatty acids** are 14 or more carbons in length.

The carbons of a fatty acid can be numbered beginning with the carbon of the carboxyl end (COOH), which is designated the α-carbon (that is, the *alpha*, or first, carbon), or from the carbon of the terminal methyl group (CH_3), called the ω-carbon (that is, the *omega*, or last, carbon) (Figure 5.1b). Fatty acid chain length is important because it determines the method of digestion and absorption and affects how triglycerides are metabolized and used within the body. For example, short- and medium-chain fatty acids are digested, transported, and metabolized more quickly than long-chain fatty acids. In general, long-chain fatty acids are more abundant in nature, and thus more abundant in our diet, than short- or medium-chain fatty acids. We will discuss the digestion of lipids and absorption of fatty acids in more detail shortly.

Fatty Acids Vary in Level of Saturation

The fatty acids attached to glycerol can also vary by the type of carbon bonds they contain. Within a fatty acid chain, an atom of carbon has the potential to make four bonds with other atoms, such as another carbon or hydrogen. In fatty acid chains, most carbons are bonded to two other carbons and two hydrogens; however, adjacent carbons may share a double bond that excludes hydrogen. The less hydrogen in a fatty acid chain, the less saturated that chain is considered to be.

If a fatty acid has no carbons sharing a double bond anywhere along its length, it is referred to as a **saturated fatty acid (SFA)** (**Figure 5.2a**). This is because every carbon atom in the chain is saturated with hydrogen: each has the maximum amount of hydrogen bound to it. Some foods that are high in saturated fatty acids are coconut oil, palm kernel oil, butter, cheese, whole milk, cream, lard, and beef fat.

If, within the chain of carbon atoms, two are bound to each other with a double bond, then this double carbon bond excludes hydrogen. This lack of hydrogen at *one* part of the molecule results in a fat that is referred to as *monounsaturated* (recall from Chapter 4 that the prefix *mono-* means "one"). A monounsaturated molecule is shown in the middle panel of Figure 5.2a. **Monounsaturated fatty acids (MUFAs)** are usually liquid at room temperature. Foods that are high in monounsaturated fatty acids are olive oil, canola oil, peanut oil, and cashew nuts.

If the fatty acids have *more than one* double bond, they contain even less hydrogen and are referred to as **polyunsaturated fatty acids (PUFAs)** (see Figure 5.2a). PUFAs can be further classified by the location of their first double bond. If it is next to the third carbon from the omega carbon, they are called omega-3 fatty acids and if it is next to the sixth carbon, they are called omega-6 fatty acids. These two categories of PUFAs are discussion in detail shortly. Polyunsaturated fatty acids are also liquid at room temperature and include soy, canola, corn, and safflower oils.

Foods vary in the types of fatty acids they contain. For example, animal fats provide approximately 40% to 60% of their energy from saturated fats, whereas plant fats provide 80% to 90% of their energy from monounsaturated and polyunsaturated fats (**Figure 5.3**, page 170). Notice that most oils are a good source of both MUFAs and PUFAs. Diets higher in plant foods are usually lower in saturated fats than diets high in animal products.

---

short-chain fatty acids Fatty acids fewer than six carbon atoms in length.

medium-chain fatty acids Fatty acids that are 6 to 12 carbon atoms in length.

long-chain fatty acids Fatty acids that are 14 or more carbon atoms in length.

saturated fatty acid (SFA) Fatty acids that have no carbons joined together with a double bond; these types of fatty acids are generally solid at room temperature.

monounsaturated fatty acids (MUFAs) Fatty acids that have two carbons in the chain bound to each other with one double bond; these types of fatty acids are generally liquid at room temperature.

polyunsaturated fatty acids (PUFAs) Fatty acids that have more than one double bond in the chain; these types of fatty acids are generally liquid at room temperature.

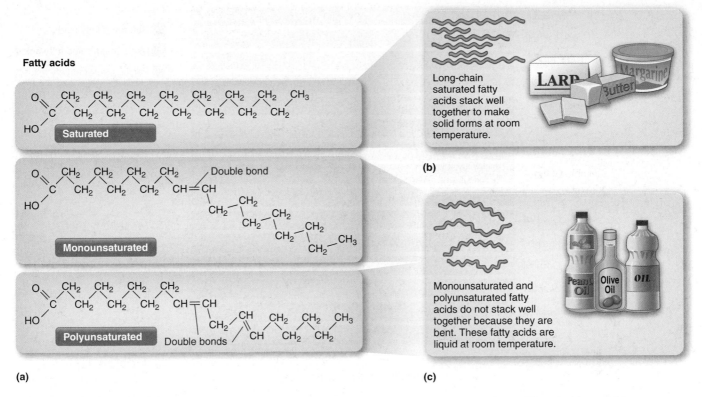

FIGURE 5.2 Examples of levels of saturation among fatty acids and how these levels of saturation affect the shape of fatty acids. **(a)** Saturated fatty acids are saturated with hydrogen, meaning they have no carbons bonded together with a double bond. Monounsaturated fatty acids contain two carbons bound by one double bond. Polyunsaturated fatty acids have more than one double bond linking carbon atoms. **(b)** Saturated fats have straight fatty acids packed tightly together and are solid at room temperature. **(c)** Unsaturated fats have "kinked" fatty acids at the area of the double bond, preventing them from packing tightly together; they are liquid at room temperature.

Fatty Acid Carbon Bonding Affects Shape

Have you ever noticed how many toothpicks are packed into a small box? Two hundred or more! But if you were to break a bunch of toothpicks into V shapes anywhere along their length, how many could you then fit into the same box? It would be very few because the bent toothpicks would jumble together, taking up much more space. Molecules of saturated fat are like straight toothpicks: they have no double carbon bonds and always form straight, rigid chains. As they have no kinks, these chains can pack together tightly (see Figure 5.2b). That is why saturated fats, such as the fat in meats, are solid at room temperature.

In contrast, each double carbon bond of unsaturated fats gives them a kink along their length (see Figure 5.2c). This means that they are unable to pack together tightly—for example, to form a stick of butter—and instead are liquid at room temperature. Monounsaturated and polyunsaturated fatty acids are fluid and flexible, qualities that are important in fatty acids that become part of cell membranes, as well as in those that transport substances in the bloodstream.

Unsaturated fatty acids can occur in either a *cis* or a *trans* shape, and only *cis* fatty acids are kinked. The prefix *cis-* indicates a location on the same side. A *cis fatty acid* has both hydrogen atoms located on the same side of the double bond (**Figure 5.4a**, page 170). This positioning gives the *cis* molecule a pronounced kink at the double carbon bond. We typically find the *cis* fatty acids in nature and thus in foods such as plant oils, fresh vegetables, and whole grains.

The prefix *trans-* denotes across or opposite. In a *trans fatty acid*, the hydrogen atoms are attached on diagonally opposite sides of the double carbon bond (Figure 5.4b). This positioning makes *trans* fatty acid fats straighter and more rigid, just like saturated fats.

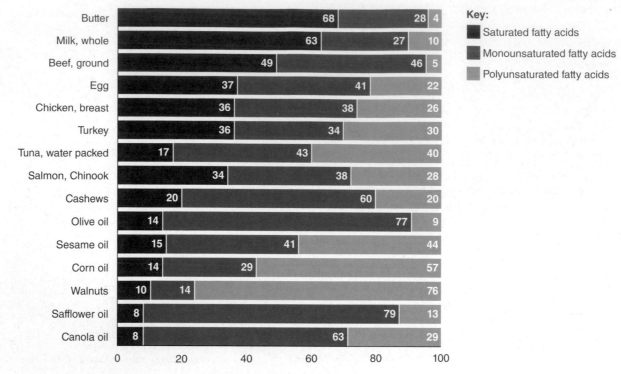

Key:
- ■ Saturated fatty acids
- ■ Monounsaturated fatty acids
- ■ Polyunsaturated fatty acids

Food	Saturated	Monounsaturated	Polyunsaturated
Butter	68	28	4
Milk, whole	63	27	10
Beef, ground	49	46	5
Egg	37	41	22
Chicken, breast	36	38	26
Turkey	36	34	30
Tuna, water packed	17	43	40
Salmon, Chinook	34	38	28
Cashews	20	60	20
Olive oil	14	77	9
Sesame oil	15	41	44
Corn oil	14	29	57
Walnuts	10	14	76
Safflower oil	8	79	13
Canola oil	8	63	29

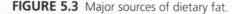

Percentage (%) of total fat kcal

FIGURE 5.3 Major sources of dietary fat.

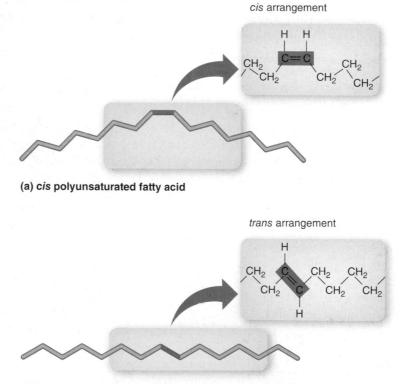

cis arrangement

(a) *cis* polyunsaturated fatty acid

trans arrangement

(b) *trans* polyunsaturated fatty acid

FIGURE 5.4 Structure of **(a)** a *cis* and **(b)** a *trans* polyunsaturated fatty acid. Notice that *cis* fatty acids have both hydrogen atoms located on the same side of the double bond. This positioning makes the molecule kinked. In *trans* fatty acids, the hydrogen atoms are attached on diagonally opposite sides of the double carbon bond. This positioning makes them straighter and more rigid.

Although small amounts of naturally occurring *trans* fatty acids are found in meats and full-fat dairy products, the majority of *trans* fatty acids are commercially produced by manipulating the fatty acid during food processing. For example, in the **hydrogenation** of oils, such as corn or safflower oil, hydrogen is added to the fatty acids. In this process, the double bonds found in the monounsaturated and polyunsaturated fatty acids in the oil are broken, and additional hydrogen is inserted at diagonally opposite sides of the double bonds. This process straightens out the molecules, making the oil more solid at room temperature—as well as more saturated. The hydrogenation of fats helps foods containing these fats, such as cakes, cookies, and crackers, resist rancidity, because the additional hydrogen reduces the tendency of the carbon atoms in the fatty acid chains to undergo oxidation.

The hydrogenation process can be controlled to make the oil more or less saturated: if only some of the double bonds are broken, the fat produced is called *partially hydrogenated,* a term you will see frequently on food labels. For example, corn oil margarine is a partially hydrogenated fat made from corn oil. Margarines that are even partially hydrogenated have more *trans* fatty acids than butter, unless the label indicates otherwise.

Does the straight, rigid shape of the saturated and *trans* fats we eat have any effect on our health? Absolutely! Research during the past two decades has shown that saturated and *trans* fatty acids raise blood cholesterol levels and appear to change cell membrane function and the way cholesterol is removed from the blood. For these reasons, diets high in saturated or *trans* fatty acids are associated with an increased risk for cardiovascular disease.

Because of these health concerns, food manufacturers are required to list the amount of saturated and *trans* fatty acids per serving on the Nutrition Facts panel of food labels. Nevertheless, the U.S. Food and Drug Administration (FDA) allows products that have less than 1 g of *trans* fat per serving to claim that they are *trans* fat free. So even if the Nutrition Facts panel states 0 g *trans* fats, the product can still have ½ g of *trans* fat per serving. If the ingredients list states that the product contains partially hydrogenated oils (PHOs), it contains *trans* fats. However, the FDA ruled in 2015 that PHOs are no longer generally recognized as safe (GRAS) and must be phased out of foods within three years. Until then, choose low-fat meats and dairy to avoid them.[2]

Given the fact that many margarines have more *trans* fatty acids than butter does, which is the more healthful choice for your morning toast? Check out the ***Highlight: Is Margarine More Healthful Than Butter?*** to find out.

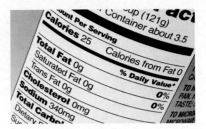

The U.S. Food and Drug Administration (FDA) requires that both saturated and *trans* fats be listed as separate line items on Nutrition Facts Panels for conventional foods and some dietary supplements. Research studies show that diets high in these fatty acids can increase the risk of cardiovascular disease.

Some Triglycerides Contain Essential Fatty Acids

The length of the fatty acid chain and the placement of the double bonds determine the function of the fatty acid within the body. As noted earlier, the carbons of a fatty acid can be numbered beginning from the α-carbon of the beginning carboxyl group (α is the first letter in the Greek alphabet) or from the ω-carbon of the terminal methyl group (ω is the last letter in the Greek alphabet). In **Figure 5.5** (page 172), we have illustrated this, numbering the carbons from the ω-carbon.[3] When synthesizing fatty acids, the body cannot insert double bonds before the ninth carbon from the ω-carbon.[3] For this reason, fatty acids with double bonds closer to the methyl end (at ω-3 and at ω-6) are considered **essential fatty acids (EFAs)**—because the body cannot synthesize them, they must be obtained from food.

There are two such EFAs: linoleic acid and alpha-linolenic acid (ALA). The body synthesizes these EFAs into longer chain fatty acids that are precursors to biological compounds called *eicosanoids* essential to growth and health.[4] Eicosanoids get their name from the Greek word *eicosa*, which means "twenty," as they are synthesized from fatty acids with 20 carbon atoms. Among the most potent regulators of cellular function

hydrogenation The process of adding hydrogen to unsaturated fatty acids, making them more saturated and thereby more solid at room temperature.

essential fatty acids (EFAs) Fatty acids that must be consumed in the diet because they cannot be made by the body. The two essential fatty acids are linoleic acid and alpha-linolenic acid (ALA).

FIGURE 5.5 The two essential fatty acids. **(a)** In linoleic acid (omega-6 fatty acid), counting from the terminal methyl group (the ω-carbon), the first double bond occurs at the sixth carbon. **(b)** In alpha-linolenic acid (omega-3 fatty acid), counting from the terminal methyl group (the ω-carbon), the first double bond occurs at the third carbon.

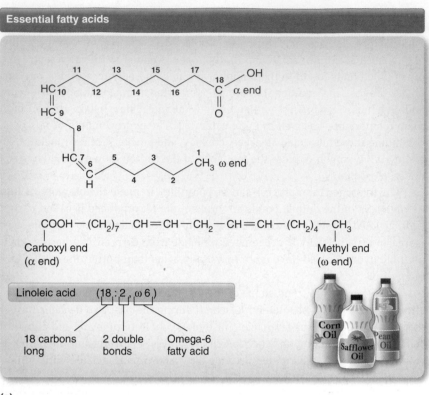

(a)

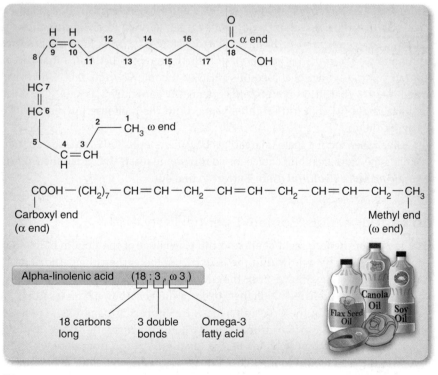

(b)

HIGHLIGHT

Is Margarine More Healthful Than Butter?

Your toast just popped up! Which will it be: butter or margarine? As you've seen in Figure 5.3, butter is 65% saturated fat. It contains 30 grams of cholesterol in 1 tablespoon. In contrast, corn oil margarine is just 2% saturated fat, with no cholesterol. But how much *trans* fat does that margarine contain? And which is better—the more natural and more saturated butter or the more processed and less saturated margarine?

You're not the only one asking this question. Until recently, vegetable-based oils were hydrogenated to make margarines. These products were filled with *trans* fats, which can increase the consumer's risk of heart disease, as well as harm cell membranes, weaken immune function, and inhibit the body's natural anti-inflammatory hormones. Some margarines also contained harmful amounts of toxic metals, such as nickel and aluminum, as by-products of the hydrogenation process. These are among some of the reasons researchers began warning consumers against these margarines several years ago.

So does that mean that butter is the better choice? A decade ago, that may have been the case, but food manufacturers now offer "*trans*-fat-free margarines and spreads" that contain no *trans* fats, no cholesterol, and low amounts of saturated fats. The American Heart Association[1] advises consumers to choose these *trans*-fat-free margarines over butter. However, some whole-food advocates point out that such manufactured products are still "non-foods" and recommend that consumers choose unprocessed nut butters (peanut, walnut, cashew, and almond butters). These natural alternatives are rich in essential fatty acids and other heart-healthy unsaturated fats.

Remember, a label claiming that a margarine has zero *trans* fatty acids doesn't guarantee that the product is *trans* fatty acid free (see the accompanying table). You have to look for margarines free of partially hydrogenated oils. That is the only way you will know your spread is entirely free of *trans* fatty acids. Check out the table to help you decide which spreads you're going to include in your diet.

Spreads for Your Bread*

Brand Name	Energy (kcal)	Sat Fat (g)	*Trans* fat (g)	Sodium (mg)
Tubs and Squeezes Made without Partially Hydrogenated Oils				
Promise Fat Free; I Can't Believe It's Not Butter (fat free)	5	0	0	90
Country Crock Omega Plus Light	50	1	0	80
Smart Balance Omega Light	50	1.5	0	80
Parkay Squeeze	70	1.5	0	110
Canola Harvest Original	100	1.5	0	100
Tubs and Sticks Made with Partially Hydrogenated Oils				
Blue Bonnet Light	50	1	1	80
Blue Bonnet (Original)	70	1.5	1.5	125
Fleischmann's Original	80	2	1.5	110
Butter				
Butter, any brand, stick	100	7.5	0.4	80
Land O'Lakes Light with Canola Oil	50	2	0	90
Shortening				
Crisco, stick or tub	100	3	0.5	0
Nut Butters				
Peanut butter	95	1.5	0	78
Almond butter	99	1	0	70

*All portion sizes are 1 tablespoon.
Source: Hurley, J., and B. Liebman. 2009. Covering the Spreads. Tracking down the butters and margarines. *Nutrition Action Health Letter*, September 13–15. Food Processor-SQL, Version 10.3, ESHA Research, Salem, OR; Websites of various margarine manufacturers.

linoleic acid An essential fatty acid found in vegetable and nut oils; an omega-6 fatty acid.

alpha-linolenic acid (ALA) An essential fatty acid found in leafy green vegetables, flaxseed oil, soy oil, fish oil, and fish products; an omega-3 fatty acid.

eicosapentaenoic acid (EPA) A metabolic derivative of alpha-linolenic acid.

docosahexaenoic acid (DHA) A metabolic derivative of alpha-linolenic acid; together with EPA, it appears to reduce the risk of heart disease.

phospholipids A type of lipid in which a fatty acid is combined with another compound that contains phosphate; unlike other lipids, phospholipids are soluble in water.

in nature, eicosanoids are produced in nearly every cell within the body.[4] They help regulate gastrointestinal tract motility, secretory activity, blood clotting, vasodilatation and vasoconstriction, vascular permeability, and inflammation. Some of the more familiar are prostaglandins, thromboxanes, and leukotrienes. There must be a balance between the various eicosanoids to assure that the appropriate amount of blood clotting or dilation/constriction of the blood vessels occurs. Now let's look more closely at the two essential fatty acids in our diet.

Linoleic Acid   An omega-6 fatty acid, **linoleic acid** is found primarily in vegetable and nut oils, such as sunflower, safflower, corn, soy, and peanut oils. If you eat lots of vegetables or use vegetable oil-based margarines or vegetable oils, you are probably getting adequate amounts of this essential fatty acid in your diet. Linoleic acid is metabolized in the body to arachidonic acid, which is a precursor to a number of eicosanoids.

Alpha-Linolenic Acid   An omega-3 fatty acid, **alpha-linolenic acid (ALA)** was only recognized to be essential in the mid-1980s. It is found primarily in dark green, leafy vegetables, flaxseeds and flaxseed oil, soybeans and soybean oil, walnuts and walnut oil, and canola oil. ALA is also a precursor of two omega-3 fatty acids now recognized for their role in protecting against cardiovascular disease: **eicosapentaenoic acid (EPA)** and **docosahexaenoic acid (DHA)**. Unfortunately, only a limited amount of dietary ALA is converted to EPA and DHA within the body; therefore, it is important to consume these key fatty acids directly.[5] They are found in fish, shellfish, and fish oils. Fish that naturally contain more oil, such as salmon and tuna, are higher in EPA and DHA than lean fish, such as cod and flounder. Research indicates that diets high in EPA and DHA stimulate the production of prostaglandins and thromboxanes that reduce inflammatory responses in the body, reduce blood clotting and plasma triglycerides, and thereby reduce an individual's risk for heart disease. For people who avoid fish or follow a vegetarian diet, intakes of EPA and DHA can be low, unless fish oil or microalgae oil supplements or marine plants such as seaweed are consumed.[6]

Nutrition
MILESTONE

In **1935**, J. A. Urquhart, a physician working among the Inuit people of the Arctic Circle in Canada, reported that in 7 years of serving this population, he had encountered no cases of heart disease, diabetes, or cancer. Over the next 50 years, studies from other researchers working among Inuit groups in Canada and Greenland continued to report similar surprising findings. How could the Inuit—whose diets were made up of as much as 75% fat—have had such extremely low rates of heart disease? The key, the researchers soon discovered, was in the *type* of fat the Inuit consumed. Cold-water fish and sea mammals, such as seal, walrus, and whales, which were staples of the Inuit diet, are very low in saturated fats, high in monounsaturated fats, and particularly rich in polyunsaturated omega-3 fatty acids—particularly EPA and DHA.

RECAP

Fat is essential for health. Triglycerides are the most common fat found in food. A triglyceride is made up of glycerol and three fatty acids. These fatty acids can be classified based on chain length, level of saturation, and shape. The essential fatty acids, linoleic acid and alpha-linolenic acid, cannot be synthesized by the body and must be consumed in the diet.   ■

Phospholipids Combine Lipids with Phosphate

Along with the triglycerides just discussed, we also find **phospholipids** in the foods we eat. They are abundant, for example, in egg yolks, peanuts, and soybeans and are present in processed foods containing emulsifiers, additives that help foods stay blended.

Phospholipids consist of a glycerol backbone with fatty acids attached at the first and second carbons and another compound that contains phosphate attached at the third carbon (**Figure 5.6a**). Because phosphates are soluble in water, phospholipids are soluble in water, a property that enables them to assist in transporting fats in the bloodstream. We discuss this concept in more detail later in this chapter (page 180).

The phospholipids are unique in that they have a hydrophobic (water-avoiding) end, which is their lipid "tail," and a hydrophilic (water-attracting) end, which is their phosphate "head." In the cell

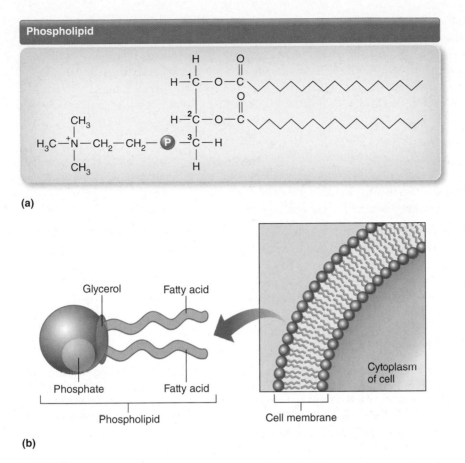

FIGURE 5.6 The structure of a phospholipid. **(a)** Detailed biochemical drawing of the phospholipid phosphatidylcholine, in which the phosphate is bound to choline and attached to the glycerol backbone at the third carbon. This phospholipid is commonly called lecithin and is found in foods such as egg yolks, as well as in the body. **(b)** Phospholipids consist of a glycerol backbone with two fatty acids and a compound that contains phosphate. This diagram illustrates the placement of the phospholipids in the cell membrane structure.

membrane, this quality helps them regulate the transport of substances into and out of the cell (Figure 5.6b). Phospholipids also help with digestion of dietary fats. In the liver, phospholipids called *lecithins* combine with bile salts and electrolytes to make bile. As you recall (from Chapter 3), bile emulsifies lipids. Note that the body manufactures phospholipids, so it is not essential to include them in the diet.

Sterols Have a Ring Structure

Sterols are a type of lipid with a multiple-ring structure quite different from that of triglycerides or phospholipids (**Figure 5.7a**, page 176). Plant foods contain some sterols, but they are not very well absorbed. However, plant sterols have a healthful function: they appear to block the absorption of dietary cholesterol, the most commonly occurring sterol in the diet and the sterol associated with an increased risk for cardiovascular disease if blood levels are abnormal (Figure 5.7b). We'll discuss plant sterols and their ability to lower blood cholesterol in more depth later in this chapter. Cholesterol is found in animal-based foods primarily as cholesterol esters, in which a fatty acid is attached to the cholesterol ring structure (Figure 5.7c). It is abundant in the fatty part of animal products, such as butter, egg yolks, whole milk, meats, and poultry. Lean meats and low- or reduced-fat milk, yogurt, and cheeses have little cholesterol.

sterols A type of lipid found in foods and the body that has a ring structure; cholesterol is the most common sterol that occurs in our diets.

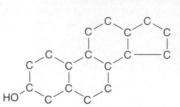
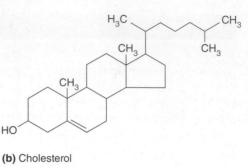

(a) Sterol ring structure   **(b)** Cholesterol

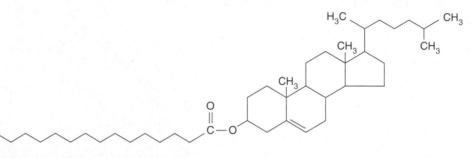

(c) Cholesterol ester

FIGURE 5.7 Sterol structure. **(a)** Sterols are lipids that contain multiple ring structures. When an OH group is added to the rings—as shown here—the compound is considered a steroid. **(b)** Cholesterol is the most commonly occurring steroid in the diet. **(c)** When a fatty acid is attached to the cholesterol molecule, it is called a cholesterol ester. Cholesterol esters are a common form of cholesterol in our diet.

It is not necessary to consume exogenous (dietary) cholesterol because the body continually synthesizes all the cholesterol it needs. Most of the body's endogenous cholesterol production occurs in the liver, which releases the cholesterol into the blood to supply other tissues. Whether exogenous or endogenous, cholesterol is used in the structure of every cell membrane, where it works in conjunction with fatty acids and phospholipids to help maintain cell membrane integrity and modulate fluidity. It is particularly plentiful in the neural cells that make up the brain, spinal cord, and nerves. The body also uses cholesterol to make several important sterol compounds, including sex hormones (estrogen, androgens such as testosterone, and progesterone), adrenal hormones, and vitamin D. In addition, cholesterol is the precursor for the bile salts that are a primary component of bile, which helps emulsify lipids in the small intestine prior to digestion. Thus, despite cholesterol's bad reputation, it is absolutely essential to human health.

RECAP

Phospholipids combine two fatty acids and a glycerol backbone with a phosphate-containing compound, making them soluble in water. Sterols have a multiple-ring structure; cholesterol is the most commonly occurring sterol in our diet.   ■

 LO 5 Describe the steps involved in fat digestion, absorption, transport, and uptake.

How Does the Body Break Down Lipids?

Because lipids are not soluble in water, they cannot enter the bloodstream easily from the digestive tract. Thus, their digestion, absorption, and transport within the body differ from those of carbohydrates and proteins, which are water-soluble substances.

The digestion and absorption of lipids were discussed in detail in Chapter 3, but we briefly review the process here (**Focus Figure 5.8**). Dietary fats are usually mixed with other

focus figure 5.8 | Lipid Digestion Overview

The majority of lipid digestion takes place in the small intestine, with the help of bile from the liver and digestive enzymes from the pancreas. Micelles transport the end products of lipid digestion to the enterocytes for absorption and eventual transport via the blood or lymph.

ORGANS OF THE GI TRACT

MOUTH

Lingual lipase secreted by tongue cells and mixed with saliva digests some triglycerides.

Little lipid digestion occurs here.

STOMACH

Most fat arrives intact at the stomach, where it is mixed and broken into droplets.

Gastric lipase digests some triglycerides.

SMALL INTESTINE

Bile from the gallbladder breaks fat into smaller droplets.

Lipid-digesting enzymes from the pancreas break triglycerides into monoacylglycerides and fatty acids.

 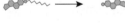

Lipid-digesting enzymes from the pancreas break dietary cholesterol esters and phospholipids into their components.

Products of fat digestion combine with bile salts to form micelles.

Micelles transport lipid digestion products to the enterocytes.

Within enterocytes, components from micelles reform triglycerides and are repackaged as chylomicrons for transport into the lymphatic system.

Shorter fatty acids can be absorbed directly into the bloodstream.

ACCESSORY ORGANS

SALIVARY GLANDS

Produce saliva.

LIVER

Produces bile, which is stored in the gallbladder.

GALLBLADDER

Contracts and releases bile into the small intestine.

PANCREAS

Produces lipid-digesting enzymes, which are released into the small intestine.

Micelles

Chylomicron

Short fatty acids

Capillary

Lacteal

foods. Lingual lipase, a salivary enzyme released during chewing, plays a minor role in the breakdown of lipids in food, so most lipids reach the stomach intact. The primary role of the stomach in lipid digestion is to mix and break up the lipid into smaller droplets. Because lipids are not soluble in water, these droplets typically float on top of the watery digestive juices in the stomach until they are passed into the small intestine.

The Gallbladder, Liver, and Pancreas Assist in Fat Digestion

Because lipids are not soluble in water, their digestion requires the help of bile from the gallbladder and digestive enzymes from the pancreas. Recall (from Chapter 3) that the gallbladder is a sac attached to the underside of the liver and the pancreas is an oblong-shaped organ sitting below the stomach. Both have a duct connecting them to the small intestine. As lipids enter the small intestine from the stomach, the gallbladder contracts and releases bile. The contraction of the gallbladder is primarily caused by the release of cholecystokinin (CCK) (also called pancreozymin) from the duodenal mucosal cells into the circulation. Secretin, another hormone released from the duodenal mucosa, also plays a role in gallbladder contraction. The same gut hormones also cause the release of the pancreatic aqueous phase (bicarbonate and water) and the pancreatic digestive enzymes into the gut.

Although bile is stored in the gallbladder, it is actually produced in the liver. It is composed primarily of bile salts made from cholesterol, lecithins and other phospholipids, and electrolytes (for example, sodium, potassium, chloride, and calcium). *Lecithins* (also called phosphatidylcholine; see Figure 5.6a) are phospholipids in which a phosphate-containing compound and choline are combined and attached at the third carbon on the glycerol backbone. They are the primary emulsifiers in bile: the hydrophobic tails of lecithin molecules attract lipid droplets, clustering them together in tiny spheres, while the hydrophilic heads form a water-attracting shell. Lecithins enable bile to act much as soap, breaking up lipids into smaller and smaller droplets with a greater surface area (**Figure 5.9a**). The more droplets there are, the greater the chance that digestive enzymes will be able to reach their target. Interestingly, lecithins are abundant in egg yolk, which is frequently used as an emulsifier in cooking—for instance, when oil and vinegar are combined to make mayonnaise.

At the same time the bile is mixing with the lipids to emulsify them, lipid-digesting enzymes produced in the pancreas travel through the pancreatic duct into the small intestine. Each lipid product requires a specific digestive enzyme or enzymes. For example, triglycerides require both pancreatic lipase and co-lipase for digestion. The co-lipase anchors the pancreatic lipase to the lipid droplet, so that it can break the fatty acids away from their glycerol backbones. Each triglyceride molecule is broken down into two free fatty acids, which are removed from the first and third carbons on the glycerol backbone, and one *monoacylglyceride*, a glycerol molecule with one fatty acid still attached at the second carbon on the glycerol backbone (Figure 5.9b).

Specific enzymes also assist in the digestion of cholesterol esters and phospholipids. As noted in Figure 5.7c, when a fatty acid is attached to cholesterol it is called a cholesterol ester. Some of the cholesterol in our diet is in this form; thus, we need *cholesterol esterase*, an enzyme released from the pancreas, to break the ester bond between cholesterol and its attached fatty acid and release a free cholesterol molecule and a free fatty acid. Phospholipase enzymes are responsible for breaking phospholipids into smaller parts. Thus, the end products of digestion are much smaller molecules, which can be more easily captured and transported to the enterocytes for absorption.

Absorption of Lipids Occurs Primarily in the Small Intestine

The majority of lipid absorption occurs in the mucosal lining of the small intestine with the help of micelles (see Figure 5.8). A **micelle** is a spherical compound made up of bile salts and biliary phospholipids that can capture the lipid digestion products, such as free fatty acids, free cholesterol, and the monoglycerides, and transport them to the enterocytes for

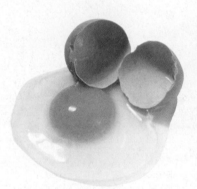

Lecithins are abundant in egg yolk, which is used as an emulsifier in products such as mayonnaise.

micelle A spherical compound made up of bile salts and biliary phospholipids that transports lipid digestion products to the intestinal mucosal cell.

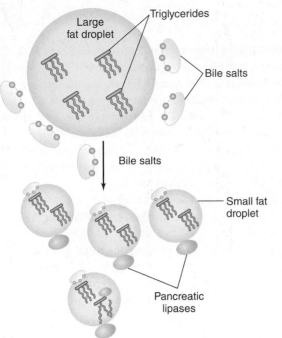

(a)

FIGURE 5.9 Action of bile salts, pancreatic lipase, and micelles in lipid digestion and absorption. **(a)** Large fat droplets filled with triglycerides are emulsified by bile into smaller and smaller droplets. Pancreatic lipase can then access the triglycerides and break them apart into free fatty acids and monoglycerides. **(b)** In the presence of pancreatic enzymes, triglycerides are broken down into fatty acids and monoacylglycerides. **(c)** These products, along with cholesterol and cholesterol esters, are trapped in the micelle, a spherical compound made up of bile salts and biliary phospholipids. The micelle then transports these lipid digestion products to the intestinal mucosal cell, and these products are then absorbed into the cell.

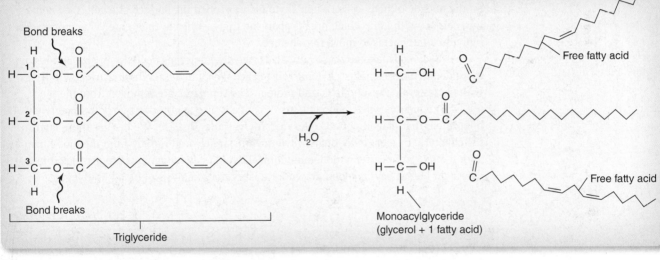

(b)

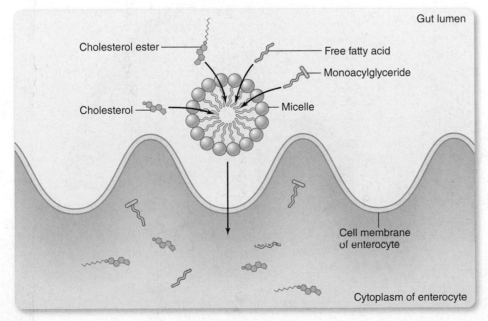

(c)

absorption (Figure 5.9c). The micelle has a hydrophobic core and a hydrophilic surface, which is excellent for transporting lipids in the watery environment of the gut.

How do the absorbed lipids—which do not mix with water—get into the bloodstream? Within the enterocytes, the fatty acids and monoglycerides are reformulated back into triglycerides and then packaged into lipoproteins before they're released into the bloodstream. A **lipoprotein** is a spherical compound with triglycerides clustered in the center along with cholesterol esters, free cholesterol, and other hydrophobic lipids and phospholipids and proteins forming the outside of the sphere (**Figure 5.10**). The specific lipoprotein produced in the enterocytes to transport lipids from a meal is called a **chylomicron**.

The process of forming a chylomicron begins with the re-creation of the triglycerides and the cholesterol esters in the endoplasmic reticulum of the enterocytes (**Figure 5.11**). These products are then loosely enclosed within an outer shell made of phospholipids and proteins. The chylomicron is now soluble in water because phospholipids and proteins are water soluble. Once chylomicrons are formed, they are transported out of the enterocytes to the lymphatic system, which empties into the bloodstream through the thoracic duct at the left subclavian vein in the neck. In this way, the dietary fat consumed in a meal is transported into the blood. This is why, soon after a meal containing fat, there is an increase of chylomicrons in the blood.

The triglycerides within chylomicrons are used by cells throughout the body. They are released with the help of an enzyme called **lipoprotein lipase**, or LPL, which is found on the outside of body cells. When chylomicrons touch the surface of a cell, they come into contact with LPL, which breaks apart the triglycerides in their core. This process frees individual fatty acids to move into the cell.

As body cells take up these fatty acids, the chylomicrons decrease in size and become more dense. These smaller chylomicrons, called *chylomicron remnants,* are now filled with cholesterol, phospholipid, and protein. The remnants are removed from the blood by the liver, which recycles their contents. Liver cells also synthesize two additional types of lipoprotein that play important roles in cardiovascular disease. We discuss these later in the chapter. For most individuals, chylomicrons are cleared rapidly from the blood, usually within 6 to 8 hours after a moderate-fat meal, which is why patients are instructed to fast overnight before having blood drawn for a laboratory analysis of blood lipid levels.

lipoprotein A spherical compound in which fat clusters in the center and phospholipids and proteins form the outside of the sphere.

chylomicron A lipoprotein produced in the mucosal cell of the intestine; transports dietary fat out of the intestinal tract.

lipoprotein lipase An enzyme that sits on the outside of cells and breaks apart triglycerides, so that their fatty acids can be removed and taken up by the cell.

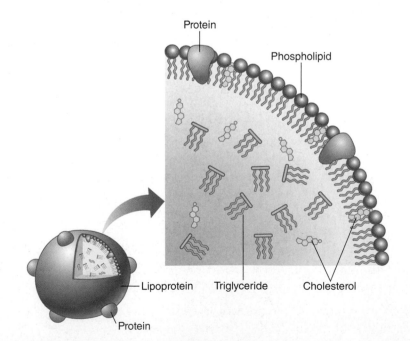

FIGURE 5.10 Structure of a lipoprotein. Notice that the fat clusters in the center of the molecule and the phospholipids and proteins, which are water soluble, form the outside of the sphere. This enables lipoproteins to transport fats in the bloodstream.

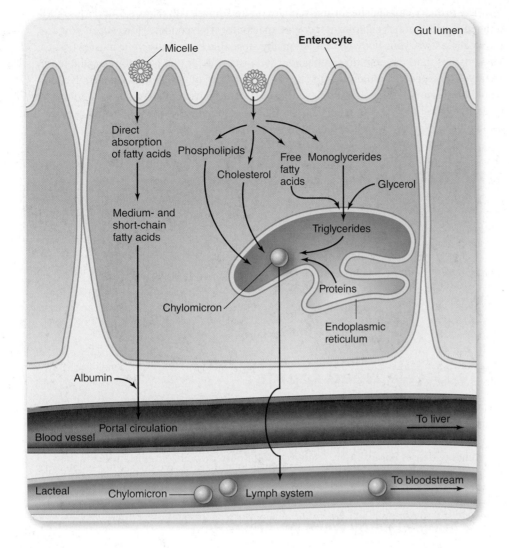

FIGURE 5.11 The reassembly of the lipid components (for example, triglycerides) into a chylomicron, which is then released into the lymphatic circulation and then into the bloodstream at the thoracic duct. Short- and medium-chain fatty acids are transported directly into the portal circulation (for example, the blood going to the liver).

As mentioned earlier, short- and medium-chain fatty acids (those less than 14 carbons in length) can be transported in the body more readily than long-chain fatty acids. This is because short- and medium-chain fatty acids transported to the mucosal cells do not have to be re-formed into triglycerides and incorporated into chylomicrons (see Figure 5.11). Instead, they can travel in the portal bloodstream bound to either the transport protein albumin or a phospholipid. In general, our diet is low in short- and medium-chain fatty acids; however, they can be extracted from certain oils for clinical use in feeding patients who cannot digest long-chain fatty acids.

Fat Is Stored in Adipose Tissues for Later Use

We've said that, after a meal, the chylomicrons begin to circulate through the blood. There are three primary fates of the fatty acids in their core:

1. Body cells, especially muscle cells, can take them up and use them as a source of energy.
2. Cells can use them to make lipid-containing compounds needed by the body.
3. If the body doesn't need the fatty acids for immediate energy, muscle and adipose cells can re-create the triglycerides (using glucose for the glycerol backbone) and store them for later use.

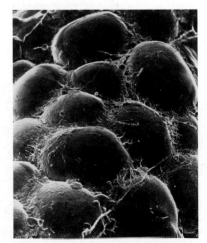

Adipose tissue. During times of weight gain, excess fat consumed in the diet is stored in the adipose tissue.

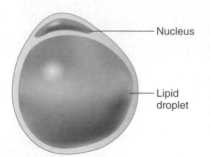

FIGURE 5.12 Diagram of an adipose cell.

The primary storage site for triglycerides is the adipose cell (**Figure 5.12**). This is the only body cell that has significant storage capacity for triglycerides. However, if you are physically active, your body will preferentially store this extra fat in your muscle tissues. This ensures that, the next time you go out for a run, the fat will be readily available for energy. Thus, people who engage in physical activity are more likely to have triglyceride stored in the muscle tissue and to have less body fat—something many of us would prefer. Of course, fat stored in your adipose tissues can also be used for energy during exercise, but it must be broken down first and then transported to your muscle cells.

RECAP

Fat digestion begins when fats are emulsified by bile. Lipid-digesting enzymes from the pancreas subsequently digest the triglycerides into two free fatty acids and one monoglyceride. These are transported into the intestinal mucosal cells with the help of micelles. Once inside the mucosal cells, triglycerides are re-formed and packaged into lipoproteins called chylomicrons. Dietary fat, in the form of triglycerides, is transported by the chylomicrons to cells within the body that need energy. Triglycerides stored in the muscle tissue are used as a source of energy during physical activity. Excess triglycerides are stored in the adipose tissue and can be used whenever the body needs energy. ■

LO 6 List at least three physiologic functions of fat in the body.

Why Do We Need Lipids?

Dietary fat is a primary source of energy because fat has more than twice the energy per gram as carbohydrate or protein. Fat provides 9 kilocalories (kcal) per gram, whereas carbohydrate and protein provide only 4 kcal per gram. This means that fat is much more energy dense. For example, 1 tablespoon of butter or oil contains approximately 100 kcal, whereas it takes 2.5 cups of steamed broccoli or 1 slice of whole-wheat bread to provide 100 kcal.

Lipids Supply Energy When We Are at Rest

At rest, we are able to deliver plenty of oxygen to our cells, so that metabolic functions can occur. Just as a candle needs oxygen for the flame to continue burning, our cells need oxygen to use fat for energy. Thus, approximately 30% to 70% of the energy used at rest by the muscles and organs comes from lipids.[5] The exact amount of energy coming from lipids at rest will depend on how much fat you are eating in your diet, how physically active you are, and whether you are gaining or losing weight. If you are dieting, more lipid will be used for energy than if you are gaining weight. During times of weight gain, more of the fat consumed in the diet is stored in the adipose tissue, and the body uses more dietary protein and carbohydrate as fuel sources at rest.

Lipids Fuel Physical Activity

Lipids are the major energy source during physical activity, especially those lasting 30 minutes or more, and one of the best ways to lose body fat is to exercise and moderately reduce energy intake. During aerobic exercise, such as running or cycling, lipids can be mobilized from muscle tissue, adipose tissue, and blood lipoproteins. A number of hormonal changes signal the body to break down stored energy to fuel the working muscles. The hormonal responses, and the amount and source of the lipids used, depend on your level of fitness; the type, intensity, and duration of the exercise; and how well fed you are before you exercise.

For example, adrenaline (that is, epinephrine) strongly stimulates the breakdown of stored fat. Within minutes of beginning exercise, blood levels of epinephrine rise dramatically. Through a cascade of events, this surge of epinephrine activates an enzyme

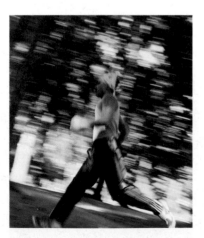

Lipids, in the form of dietary fat, provide energy and help our body perform essential physiologic functions.

within adipose cells called *hormone-sensitive lipase.* This enzyme works to remove single fatty acids from the stored triglycerides. When all three free fatty acids on the glycerol backbone have been removed, the free fatty acids and the glycerol are released into the blood.

Epinephrine also signals the pancreas to *decrease* insulin production. This is important, because insulin inhibits fat breakdown. Thus, when the need for fat as an energy source is high, blood insulin levels are typically low. As you might guess, blood insulin levels are high when we are eating, because during this time our need for energy from stored fat is low and the need for fat storage is high.

Once fatty acids are released from the adipose cells, they travel in the blood attached to the transport protein albumin, to the muscle cells. There, they enter the mitochondria, the cell's energy-generating structures, and use oxygen to produce ATP, which is the cell's energy source. Becoming more physically fit means you can deliver more oxygen to the muscle cells to use the fatty acids delivered there. In addition, you can exercise longer when you are fit. Because the body has only a limited supply of stored carbohydrate as glycogen in muscle tissue, the longer you exercise, the more fatty acids you use for energy. This point is illustrated in **Figure 5.13**. In this example, an individual is running for 4 hours at a moderate intensity. As the muscle glycogen levels become depleted, the body relies on fatty acids from the adipose tissue as a fuel source.

Under normal circumstances, fatty acids cannot be used to produce glucose[7]; however, recall that the breakdown of triglycerides also frees molecules of glycerol into the bloodstream. Some of this free glycerol travels to the liver, where it can be used for the production of modest amounts of glucose (in the process of gluconeogenesis).

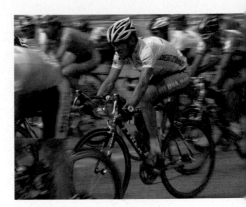

The longer you exercise, the more fat you use for energy. Cyclists in a long-distance race make greater use of fat stores as the race progresses.

Lipids Stored in Body Fat Provide Energy for Later Use

The body stores extra energy in the form of body fat, which then can be used for energy at rest, during exercise, or during periods of low energy intake. Having a readily available energy source in the form of fat allows the body to always have access to energy even

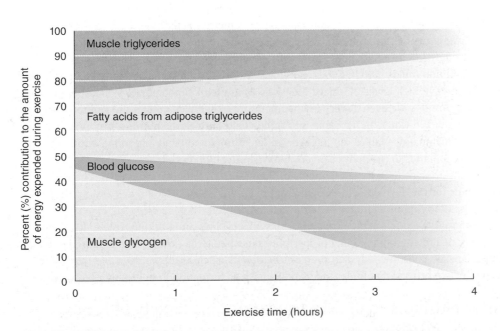

FIGURE 5.13 Various sources of energy used during exercise. As a person exercises for a prolonged period of time, fatty acids from adipose cells contribute relatively more energy than do carbohydrates stored in the muscle or circulating in the blood. (*Source:* Data from Coyle, E. F. 1995. Substrate utilization during exercise in active people. *Am. J. Clin. Nutr.* 61[Suppl.]:968S–979S. Used with permission.)

when we choose not to eat (or are unable to eat), when we are exercising, and while we are sleeping. The body has small amounts of stored carbohydrate in the form of glycogen—only enough to last about 1 to 2 days—and there is no place that the body can store extra protein. We cannot consider our muscles and organs as a place where "extra" protein is stored! For these reasons, the fat stored in adipose and muscle tissues is necessary to fuel the body between meals. Although too much stored adipose tissue can harm our health, some fat storage is essential.

Essential Fatty Acids Contribute to Important Biological Compounds

As discussed earlier, EFAs are needed to make a number of important biological compounds. They also are important constituents of cell membranes, help prevent DNA damage, and help fight infection. In the fetus, EFAs are essential for normal growth and development, especially for the development of the brain and visual centers.

Dietary Fat Enables the Transport of Fat-Soluble Vitamins

Dietary fat enables the absorption and transport of the fat-soluble vitamins (A, D, E, and K) needed by the body for many essential metabolic functions. The fat-soluble vitamins are transported in the gut to the intestinal cells for absorption as part of micelles, and they are transported in the blood to the body cells as part of chylomicrons.[7] Vitamin A is important for normal vision and night vision. Vitamin D helps regulate blood calcium and phosphorus concentrations within normal ranges, which indirectly helps maintain bone health. Vitamin E keeps cell membranes healthy throughout the body, and vitamin K is important for the proteins involved in blood clotting and bone health. We discuss these vitamins in detail in later chapters.

Lipids Help Maintain Cell Function and Provide Protection to the Body

Lipids, especially PUFAs, phospholipids, and cholesterol, are a critical part of every cell membrane, where they help maintain membrane integrity, determine what substances are transported into and out of the cell, and regulate what substances can bind to the cell. Thus, lipids strongly influence the function of cells.

In addition, lipids help maintain cell fluidity. For example, wild salmon live in very cold water and have high levels of omega-3 fatty acids in their cell membranes. These fatty acids stay fluid and flexible even at very low temperatures, thereby enabling the fish to swim in extremely cold water. In the same way, lipids help our cell membranes stay fluid and flexible. This quality enables red blood cells, for example, to bend and move through the smallest capillaries in the body, delivering oxygen to all body cells.

Lipids are also primary components of the tissues of the nervous system. The body uses lipids for the development, growth, and maintenance of these tissues and for the transmission of impulses from one nerve cell to another.

Although we often think of body fat as "bad," it plays an important role in keeping the body healthy and functioning properly. Besides being the primary site of stored energy, adipose tissue pads the body and protects the organs, such as the kidneys and liver, when we fall or are bruised. Fat under the skin also acts as insulation to help retain body heat.

Fats Contribute to the Flavor, Texture, and Satiety of Foods

Dietary fat adds flavor and texture to foods. Fat makes salad dressings smooth and ice cream "creamy," and it gives cakes and cookies their moist, tender texture. Frying foods in melted fat or oil, as with doughnuts or french fries, gives them a crisp, flavorful coating; however, eating such foods regularly can be unhealthful because they are high in saturated and/or *trans* fatty acids.

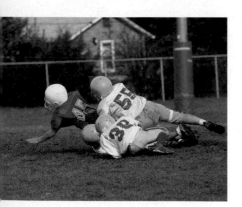

Adipose tissue pads the body and protects the organs when we fall or are bruised.

We often hear that fats contribute to satiation and satiety. First, what does this mean? A food or nutrient is said to contribute to *satiation* if that food makes you feel full and causes you to stop eating. A food or nutrient is said to contribute to *satiety* if it contributes to a feeling of fullness that subsequently reduces the amount of food you eat at the next meal or lengthens the time between meals.[8,9]

A number of research studies have compared the effects of fat and carbohydrate on both satiation and satiety. In general, this research has found little difference between these two macronutrients when energy intake has been controlled.[8] However, research also indicates that the energy density of a food contributes significantly to both satiety and satiation.[10] For every gram of fat you consume, you get more than twice the energy; thus, foods that contain a high proportion of fat are higher in energy density. Foods high in fat also stimulate the release of satiety factors in the small intestine, but our response to these satiety factors becomes blunted with chronic fat ingestion. This may explain why it is so easy to overeat high-fat, palatable foods and end up consuming more Calories than we would if we selected foods with lower energy densities. Satiety is also affected by the level of gastric distention produced by the food consumed, and by how quickly food empties from the stomach, which can also be affected by the energy density of food.[11]

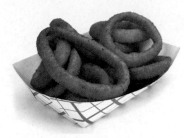

Fat adds texture and flavor to foods.

RECAP

Dietary fats provide the majority of energy required at rest and are a major fuel source during exercise, especially endurance exercise. They also provide essential fatty acids. Dietary fats help transport the fat-soluble vitamins into the body, help regulate cell function, and maintain cell membrane integrity. Stored body fat in the adipose tissue helps protect vital organs and pads the body. Fats contribute to the flavor and texture of foods, and because fats are energy dense, they are one factor that contributes to the satiety we feel after a meal. ■

How Much Dietary Fat Should We Eat?

The latest research comparing low-carbohydrate to low-fat diets has made Americans wonder what, exactly, is a healthful level of dietary fat and what foods contain the most beneficial fats. We'll explore these issues here.

Dietary Reference Intake (DRI) for Total Fat

The Acceptable Macronutrient Distribution Range (AMDR) for fat is 20% to 35% of total energy.[12] This recommendation is based on evidence indicating that higher intakes of fat increase the risk for obesity and its complications, especially heart disease and diabetes, but that diets too low in fat and too high in processed carbohydrate can also increase the risk for heart disease if they cause an unhealthful shift in blood lipids.[12] Within this range of fat intake, we're also advised to limit intake of saturated fat and minimize our intake of *trans* fatty acids as much as possible; these changes will lower our risk for heart disease.

Because carbohydrate is essential in replenishing glycogen, athletes and other physically active people are advised to consume less fat and more carbohydrate, especially if they participate in endurance activities. Specifically, it is recommended that athletes consume 20% to 25% of their total energy from fat, 55% to 60% of energy from carbohydrate, and 12% to 15% of energy from protein.[13] This percentage of fat intake is still within the AMDR and represents approximately 45 to 55 g of fat per day for an athlete consuming 2,000 kcal per day, and 78 to 97 g of fat per day for an athlete consuming 3,500 kcal per day.

Although many people trying to lose weight consume less than 20% of their energy from fat, this practice may do more harm than good, especially if they are also limiting their energy intake (eating fewer than 1,500 kcal per day). Research suggests that very-low-fat diets, or those with less than 15% of energy from fat, do not provide additional health or

LO 7 Identify the DRIs for total fat, saturated fat, and the two essential fatty acids.

LO 8 Distinguish between common food sources of fats considered beneficial and those considered less healthful.

Exactly how much fat should you eat per day? Find out with the fat intake calculator at **www.healthcalculators.org**. Click on the "Fat Intake" link to begin!

performance benefits over moderate-fat diets and are usually very difficult to follow.[14] In fact, most people find that they feel better, are more successful in weight maintenance, and are less preoccupied with food if they keep their fat intakes at 20% to 25% of energy intake. Additionally, people attempting to reduce their dietary fat frequently eliminate protein-rich foods, such as meat, dairy, eggs, and nuts. These foods are also potential sources of many essential vitamins and minerals important for good health and for maintaining an active lifestyle. Diets extremely low in fat may also be deficient in essential fatty acids.

Dietary Reference Intakes for Essential Fatty Acids

Dietary Reference Intakes (DRIs) for the two essential fatty acids are[12]

- *Linoleic acid.* The Adequate Intake (AI) for linoleic acid is 14 to 17 g per day for men and 11 to 12 g per day for women 19 years and older. Using the typical energy intakes for adult men and women, this translates into an AMDR of 5% to 10% of energy.
- *Alpha-linolenic acid.* The AI for ALA is 1.6 g per day for adult men and 1.1 g per day for adult women. This translates into an AMDR of 0.6% to 1.2% of energy.

For example, an individual consuming 2,000 kcal per day should consume about 11–22 g per day of linoleic acid and about 1.3–2.6 g per day of ALA. This level of intake would keep one within the 5:1 to 10:1 ratio of linoleic acid to ALA recommended by the World Health Organization and supported by the Institute of Medicine.[12] Because these fatty acids compete for the same enzymes to produce various eicosanoids that regulate body functions, this ratio helps keep the eicosanoids produced in balance; that is, one isn't overproduced at the expense of another.

Most Americans appear to get adequate amounts of linoleic acid, probably because of the high amount of salad dressings, vegetable oils, margarine, and mayonnaise we eat. In contrast, our consumption of ALA, as well as EPA and DHA, is more variable and can be low in the diet of people who do not eat dark green, leafy vegetables; fish or fish oil; walnuts; soy products; canola oil; or flaxseeds or their oil. So rather than attempting to monitor your linoleic acid to ALA ratio, focus on consuming healthful amounts of the foods listed in **Table 5.1**.

Limit Saturated and *Trans* Fat

Research over the last two decades has shown that diets high in saturated and *trans* fatty acids negatively influence blood lipid levels, change cell membrane function, and alter the way cholesterol is removed from the blood. For these reasons, researchers believe that diets high in saturated and *trans* fatty acids can increase the risk for cardiovascular disease.

Reduce Your Intake of Saturated Fats

The recommended intake of saturated fats is less than 7% to 10% of our total energy; our average intake is between 11% and 12% of energy.[15] According to data from the National Health and Nutrition Examination Survey (NHANES), about 64% of adults in the United States exceed the dietary recommendation for saturated fats.[16] Let's look at the primary sources of saturated fats in the American diet.

- **Animal products.** Meats and dairy contain a mixture of fatty acids, including saturated fats. However, these foods are rich in a variety of nutrients, and are a regular part of the diet of many people. If you consume animal products, instead of trying to avoid them entirely, choose them wisely. For meats, the precise amount of saturated fat will depend on the cut and how it is prepared. For example, red meats, such as beef, pork, and lamb, typically have more fat than skinless chicken or fish. Thus, lean meats are lower in saturated fat than regular cuts. In addition, broiled, grilled, or baked meats have less saturated fat than fried meats. Dairy products may also be high in saturated fat. Whole-fat milk has three times the saturated fat of low-fat milk, and nearly twice the energy.

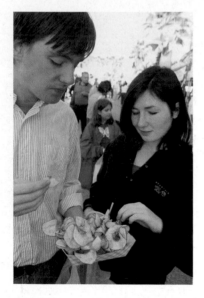

Americans consume more saturated fat than recommended; *trans* fat intake should be as low as possible.

TABLE 5.1 Omega-3 Fatty Acid Content of Selected Foods

Food Item	Total Omega-3	DHA	EPA
	g/Serving		
Flaxseed oil, 1 tbsp.	7.25	0.00	0.00
Salmon oil (fish oil), 1 tbsp.	4.39	2.48	1.77
Sardine oil, 1 tbsp.	3.01	1.45	1.38
Flaxseed, whole, 1 tbsp.	2.50	0.00	0.00
Herring, Atlantic, broiled, 3 oz	1.83	0.94	0.77
Salmon, Coho, steamed, 3 oz	1.34	0.71	0.46
Canola oil, 1 tbsp.	1.28	0.00	0.00
Sardines, Atlantic, w/ bones, oil, 3 oz	1.26	0.43	0.40
Trout, rainbow fillet, baked, 3 oz	1.05	0.70	0.28
Walnuts, English, 1 tbsp.	0.66	0.00	0.00
Halibut, fillet, baked, 3 oz	0.53	0.31	0.21
Shrimp, canned, 3 oz	0.47	0.21	0.25
Tuna, white, in oil, 3 oz	0.38	0.19	0.04
Crab, Alaska King, steamed, 3 oz	0.36	0.10	0.25
Scallops, broiled, 3 oz	0.31	0.14	0.17
Smart Balance Omega-3 Buttery Spread (1 tbsp.)	0.32	0.01	0.01
Tuna, light, in water, 3 oz	0.23	0.19	0.04
Avocado, California, fresh, whole	0.22	0.00	0.00
Haddock, baked (3oz)	0.14	0.09	0.04
Spinach, cooked, 1 cup	0.17	0.00	0.00
Eggland's Best, 1 large egg, with omega-3	0.12	0.06	0.03

EPA = eicosapentaenoic acid; DHA = docosahexaenoic acid
Source: Data from Food Processor SQL, Version 10.3, ESHA Research, Salem, OR, and manufacturer labels.

- **Grain products.** Baked goods and snack foods, including pastries, cookies, and muffins, may be rich in saturated fats. Tortilla chips, microwave and movie-theater popcorn, snack crackers, and packaged rice and pasta mixes may also be high in saturated fat.
- **Vegetables and vegetable spreads/dressings.** We often don't think of plant foods as having high amounts of saturated fats, but if these foods are fried, breaded, or drenched in sauces they can become a source of saturated fat. For example, a small baked potato (138 g) has no fat and 134 kcal, whereas a medium serving (134 g) of french fries cooked in vegetable oil has 427 kcal, 23 g of fat, and 5.3 g of saturated fat. This is one-third of the saturated fat recommended for an entire day for a person on a 2,000-kcal/day diet.

As you can see, it's easy to reduce your intake of saturated fats by making smart choices when you shop, prepare, and cook foods.

Avoid *Trans* Fatty Acids

The Institute of Medicine recommends that we keep our intake of *trans* fatty acids to an absolute minimum.[12] The majority of our *trans* fat intake comes from deep-fried fast or frozen foods, some tub margarines, and bakery products, such as cookies and crackers.[12, 17-19]

Currently, the average American's consumption of industrially produced *trans* fatty acids is only about 2% to 3% of total energy intake; however, the negative health effect of this *trans* fat intake appears to be dramatic. Many health professionals feel that diets high in *trans* fatty acids increase the risk for cardiovascular disease even more than diets high in saturated fats.[20,21] A research review that involved over 140,000 individuals showed that for every 2% increase in energy intake from *trans* fatty acids, there was a 23% increase in incidence of cardiovascular disease.[20] A 2012 review of current U.S. top-selling packaged foods showed that 9% of these foods contained partially hydrogenated oils, yet 84% of these products reported they had no *trans* fatty acids.[19] How can you limit the level of *trans* fats in the foods you buy? The next time you are in the grocery store, read the labels and look for foods made with partially hydrogenated oils (PHOs). These foods *do* contain *trans* fatty acids even if the label says they have zero *trans* fats.[19]

What about Dietary Cholesterol?

Consumers are confused about whether they should avoid dietary cholesterol. This confusion is understandable given that health experts have changed their message over the years as they have learned more about saturated fat and cholesterol metabolism and their relationship to cardiovascular disease.[22,23] Here are three points to keep in mind:

- First, our body can make cholesterol. The majority is produced in the liver and intestine. Thus, we never have to worry about getting enough cholesterol in our diet. When we consume cholesterol, our body typically reduces its internal production, which keeps our total cholesterol pool constant.
- Second, we absorb only about 40% to 60% of the cholesterol we consume.[23] The exact amount absorbed depends on a number of factors, including genetics, body size, health status and the types of foods we consume.[22,24] The cholesterol not absorbed is lost in the feces.
- Third, our body recycles cholesterol, so again, we always have enough.

A diet high in saturated fats can impair cholesterol metabolism in the liver as well as cholesterol uptake by body cells.[25] Thus, by keeping our intake of saturated fats within the recommended ranges, we in turn can avoid excessive levels of cholesterol in our blood. Because saturated fat and cholesterol are typically found in the same foods, namely, fatty animal products, following the recommendation from the Institute of Medicine to limit your intake of dietary cholesterol to less than 300 mg/day will also help keep your intake of saturated fats low.[12] However, there appears to be no direct link between dietary cholesterol and cardiovascular disease and no other countries give a dietary cholesterol recommendation.[26] The new 2015 Dietary Guidelines for Americans will not recommend a specific limit on dietary cholesterol. USDA and DHHS. Scientific Report of the 2015 Dietary Guidelines Advisory Committee. February 2015. Web link: http://health.gov /dietaryguidelines/2015-scientific-report/PDFs/Scientific-Report-of-the-2015-Dietary- Guidelines-Advisory-Committee.pdf.

Select Beneficial Fats

As we have explored in this chapter, some high-fat diets, especially those high in saturated and *trans* fatty acids, can contribute to chronic diseases, including heart disease and cancer. However, unsaturated fatty acids do not have this negative effect and are absolutely essential to good health. Thus, a sensible health goal would be to eat the appropriate amounts and types of fat.

In general, it is prudent to switch to more healthful sources of fats without increasing your total fat intake. For example, use olive oil and canola oil for cooking and a nut butter on your toast. Dairy products can be high in saturated fats, so select low- and reduced-fat versions when possible.

Eat More Sustainable Fish

To keep our oceans healthy, make sure you select fish from the sustainable fish list at www.seafoodwatch.org/. Or download a guide to the best seafood choices for your region at by clicking on the "Seafood Recommendations" tab and going to "Consumer Guides."

Table 5.1 identified the omega-3 fatty acid content of various foods. As you can see, the best source of DHA and EPA is fish. Moreover, fish is low in saturated fats. So select fish at least twice a week instead of meat sources of protein. Especially look for wild-caught salmon, line-caught tuna, line-caught cod and rock fish, and Pacific sardines.

It is important to recognize that there can be some risk associated with eating large amounts of fish on a regular basis. Depending on the species of fish and the level of pollution in the water in which it is caught, the fish may contain high levels of toxins, such as mercury, polychlorinated biphenyls (PCBs), and other environmental contaminants. Types of fish that are currently considered safe to consume include salmon (except from the Great Lakes region), farmed trout, flounder, sole, mahi mahi, and cooked shellfish. Line-caught tuna, either fresh or canned, is low in mercury. These tuna are smaller, usually less than 20 pounds, and have had less exposure to mercury in their lifetime. Fish more likely to be contaminated are shark, swordfish, golden bass, golden snapper, marlin, bluefish, and largemouth and smallmouth bass. (For more information on seafood safety, see Chapter 15.)

Pick Plants

Of course, healthful fats include not only the essential fatty acids but also polyunsaturated and monounsaturated fats in general. An easy way to shift your diet toward these healthful fats—without increasing your total fat intake—is to replace animal-based foods with versions derived from plants. For example, drink soy milk or almond milk instead of cow's milk. Order your Chinese take-out with tofu instead of beef. Use thin slices of avocado in a sandwich in place of cheese, or serve tortilla chips with guacamole instead of nachos. Use beans, peas, and lentils more frequently as the main source of protein in your meal, or add them to your meat-based dish, so that you use less meat overall.

> Concerned about the saturated fat in the meat you eat? For a guide on leanest cuts of beef, go to www.mayoclinic.org and search for "cuts of beef."

Plant oils are excellent sources of healthful unsaturated fatty acids, so cook with naturally occurring plant oils, such as olive, canola, soybean, or walnut oil in place of butter or lard. Naturally occurring oils have not been hydrogenated and contain no *trans* fatty acids. You can also use these oils to dress your salad.

Nuts and seeds provide another way to increase the healthful fats in your diet. They are rich in unsaturated fats and provide protein, minerals, vitamins, and fiber. They are high in energy: a 1 oz serving of nuts (about 4 tablespoons) contains 160–180 kcal. So eat them in moderation, for instance by sprinkling a few on your salad, yogurt, or breakfast cereal. Spread a nut butter on your morning toast, or pack a peanut butter and jelly sandwich instead of a meat sandwich for lunch. Or add some nuts or seeds to raisins and pretzel sticks for a quick trail mix.

Three popular seeds high in EFAs are pumpkin seeds, flaxseeds, and chia seeds:

- Pumpkin seeds are a delicious source of omega-3 fatty acids and plant sterols, which reduce the body's absorption of cholesterol. They're also very high in several minerals, including magnesium and zinc.
- Flaxseeds are from flax, a flowering plant grown in many parts of the world. Ground flaxseeds and their oil provide both omega-6 and omega-3 fatty acids. They can be mixed into yogurt and other creamy foods, and you can sprinkle ground flaxseeds on breakfast cereal or mix them into the batter of pancakes, breads, and other baked goods.
- Chia seeds are from a desert plant grown in Mexico. They have a nutty taste and are high in omega-3 fatty acids, protein, and fiber. Sprinkle some on cereal, in yogurt, or on stir-fried vegetables, or toss some into the batter of muffins or other baked goods.

Shop for Lower-Fat Options

When shopping, look for lower-fat versions of the processed foods you buy. Read food labels and do the math! Most importantly, look for foods with no hydrogenated oils and lower amounts of saturated fat per serving.

Here are a few more tips to help you choose and cook foods low in saturated and *trans* fats:

- Select liquid or tub margarines/butters over hard stick forms. Fats that are solid at room temperature are usually high in *trans* or saturated fats. Read the label to make sure the margarine does not contain any partially hydrogenated oils, even if the label says no *trans* fatty acids. Also, select margarines made from healthful fats, such as canola oil.

- Buy reduced-fat salad dressings and mayonnaise or those made with healthful fats, such as olive oil and vinegar blends. Remember, a tablespoon of full-fat salad dressing or mayonnaise contains 100 kcal. Salad dressings can also contain partially hydrogenated oils, so read the labels.
- Select low-fat or nonfat milk, yogurt, cheese, and cheese spreads. If you can't imagine life without "real" cheese, then buy sharp cheddar and hard, dry cheeses, such as Parmesan. These have less fat than mild, creamy cheeses, and they provide more flavor.
- When purchasing meat and poultry, choose cuts lower in fat. When preparing these foods at home, trim any visible fat before cooking, and remove the skin from poultry. Bake or broil instead of frying.

Putting these tips into practice can make a big reduction in your intake of saturated and *trans* fats as well as total energy. Need more convincing? Compare the two sets of meals in **Meal Focus Figure 5.14**.

Don't Let the Fats Fool You!

Americans commonly add fat to foods to improve their taste. Added fats, such as oils, butter, cream, shortening, margarine, mayonnaise, and salad dressings, are called **visible fats** because we can easily see what type of fat we're adding, and how much.

In contrast, when fat is added in the preparation of a frozen entrée or a fast-food burger and fries, we may not know how much or what type of fat is actually there. In fact, we might not realize that a food contains any fat at all. We call fats in prepared and processed foods **invisible fats** because they are hidden within the food. In fact, their invisibility often tricks us into choosing them over more healthful foods. For example, a slice of yellow cake is much higher in fat (40% of total energy) than a slice of angel food cake (1% of total energy), yet many consumers assume that the fat content of these foods is the same, because they are both cake.

The majority of the fat in the average American diet is invisible. Foods that can be high in invisible fats are baked goods, regular-fat dairy products, processed meats or meats that are highly marbled or not trimmed, and most convenience and fast foods, such as hamburgers, hot dogs, chips, ice cream, french fries, and other fried foods.

Because high-fat diets have been associated with obesity, many Americans have tried to reduce their total fat intake. Food manufacturers have been more than happy to provide consumers with low-fat alternatives to their favorite foods. However, these foods may not always have fewer Calories, and many replace the fat with processed carbohydrates, which negatively impact blood lipids. Turn to the ***Nutrition Label Activity: How Much Fat Is in This Food?*** (on page 192) to learn how to avoid being fooled by the fats in the foods you buy.

Watch Out When You're Eating Out!

Many college students eat most of their meals in dining halls, fast-food restaurants, and other food establishments. If that describes you, watch out! The menu items you choose each day may be increasing the amount of fat in your diet, including your intake of saturated and *trans* fats. A high fat intake is especially difficult to avoid if you regularly eat fast food. According to national data, fast-food consumers have higher total energy, total fat, and saturated fat intakes than those who eat fast food infrequently.[27] And although many fast food restaurants have eliminated *trans* fatty acids from their menus, some still have items, such as desserts and shakes, that contain *trans* fatty acids. The following are a few tips and strategies you can use to improve the amount and type of fat in your menu choices.

- When dining out, select a fish high in omega-3 fatty acid, such as wild-caught salmon, or try a vegetarian entrée made with tofu or tempeh. If you do choose meat, ask that it be trimmed of fat and broiled rather than fried.
- Cut back on packaged or bakery pastries, such as Danish, croissants, doughnuts, cakes, tarts, pies, and brownies. These baked goods are typically high in saturated and *trans* fatty acids.

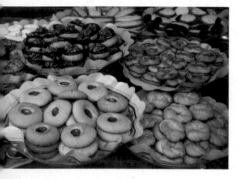

Baked goods are often high in invisible fats.

visible fats Fats we can see in our foods or see added to foods, such as butter, margarine, cream, shortening, salad dressings, chicken skin, and untrimmed fat on meat.

invisible fats Fats that are hidden in foods, such as the fats found in baked goods, regular-fat dairy products, marbling in meat, and fried foods.

a day of meals

HIGH in saturated fat
calories (kcal)

LOW in saturated fat
calories (kcal)

BREAKFAST

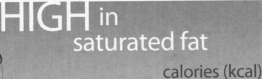

1 egg, fried
2 slices bacon
2 slices white toast with
   2 tsp. butter
8 fl. oz whole milk

2 egg whites, scrambled
2 slices whole-wheat toast
   with 2 tsp. olive oil spread
1 grapefruit
8 fl. oz skim milk

LUNCH

McDonald's Quarter Pounder
with cheese
McDonald's French fries, small
12 fl. oz cola beverage

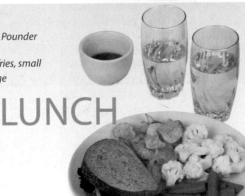

Tuna Sandwich

3 oz tuna (packed in water)
2 tsp. reduced fat mayonnaise
2 leaves red leaf lettuce
2 slices rye bread
1 large carrot, sliced with
   1 cup raw cauliflower with
   2 tbsp. low-fat Italian salad
   dressing
1 1-oz bag of salted potato chips
24 fl. oz water

DINNER

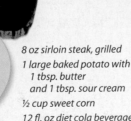

8 oz sirloin steak, grilled
1 large baked potato with
   1 tbsp. butter
   and 1 tbsp. sour cream
½ cup sweet corn
12 fl. oz diet cola beverage

1 cup minestrone soup
4 oz grilled salmon
1 cup brown rice with 2 tsp.
   slivered almonds
1 cup steamed broccoli
1 dinner roll with 1 tsp. butter
12 fl. oz iced tea

nutrient analysis

2,316 kcal
36.6% of energy from carbohydrates
39.1% of energy from fat
16% of energy from saturated fat
15.3% of energy from unsaturated fat
23% of energy from protein
15.3 grams of dietary fiber
2,713 milligrams of sodium

11% LESS saturated fat

nutrient analysis

2,392 kcal
46.6% of energy from carbohydrates
28.1% of energy from fat
5% of energy from saturated fat
18.8% of energy from unsaturated fat
17.5% of energy from protein
28 grams of dietary fiber
2,713 milligrams of sodium

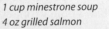

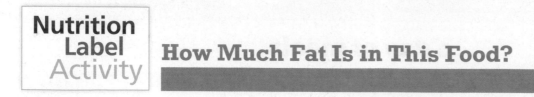

Nutrition Label Activity

How Much Fat Is in This Food?

Since high-fat diets have been associated with obesity, many Americans are trying to reduce their total fat intake. Because of this concern, food manufacturers have been more than happy to provide consumers with low-fat alternatives to their favorite foods—so you can have your cake and eat it, too! The FDA and the USDA have set specific regulations on allowable label claims for reduced-fat products. The following claims are defined for one serving:

- Fat-free = less than 0.5 g of fat
- Low-fat = 3 g or less of fat
- Reduced or less fat: at least 25% less fat as compared to a standard serving
- Light: one-third fewer Calories or 50% less fat as compared with a standard serving amount

There are now thousands of fat-modified foods in the market. However, if you're choosing such foods because of a concern about your weight, beware! Lower-fat versions of foods may not always be lower in Calories. The reduced fat is often replaced with added sugars, resulting in a very similar total energy intake.

You can see this for yourself by studying **Table 5.2**, where we list a number of full-fat foods with their lower-fat alternatives. If you were to incorporate such foods into your diet on a regular basis, you could significantly reduce the amount of fat you consume. Still, your choices may or may not reduce the amount of energy you consume. For example, as you can see in the table, drinking nonfat milk instead of whole milk would dramatically reduce both your fat and your energy intake. However, eating fat-free instead of regular Fig Newton cookies would not significantly reduce your energy intake. Thus, if you're looking for foods lower in both fat and energy, read the Nutrition Facts panel of modified-fat foods carefully before you buy.

Two cracker labels are shown in **Figure 5.15**; one cracker is higher in fat than the other. Let's review how you can determine the percentage of energy coming from fat in each product.

1. Divide the total kcal from fat by the total kcal per serving, and multiply the answer by 100.

   - For the regular wheat crackers: 50 kcal/150 kcal = 0.33 × 100 = 33%.

     Thus, for the regular crackers, the total energy coming from fat is 33%.

   - For the reduced-fat wheat crackers: 35 kcal/130 kcal = 0.269 × 100 = 27%.

     Thus, for the reduced-fat crackers, the total energy coming from fat is 27%.

     You can see that, although the total amounts of energy per serving are not very different between these two crackers, the levels of fat are quite different.

TABLE 5.2 Comparison of Full-Fat, Reduced-Fat, and Low-Fat Foods

Product and Serving Size	Version	Energy (kcal)	Protein (g)	Carbohydrate (g)	Fat (g)
Milk, 8 oz	Whole, 3.3% fat	150	8.0	11.4	8.2
	2% fat	121	8.1	11.7	4.7
	Skim (nonfat)	86	8.4	11.9	0.5
Mayonnaise, 1 tbsp.	Regular	100	0.0	0.0	11.0
	Light	50	0.0	1.0	5.0
Margarine, corn oil, 1 tbsp.	Regular	100	0.0	0.0	11.0
	Reduced-fat	60	0.0	0.0	7.0
Peanut butter, 1 tbsp.	Regular	95	4.1	3.1	8.2
	Reduced-fat	81	4.4	5.2	5.4
Wheat Thins, 18 crackers	Regular	158	2.3	21.4	6.8
	Reduced-fat	120	2.0	21.0	4.0
Cookies, Oreo, 3 cookies	Regular	160	2.0	23.0	7.0
	Reduced-fat	130	2.0	25.0	3.5
Cookies, Fig Newton, 3 cookies	Regular	210	3.0	30.0	4.5
	Fat-free	204	2.4	26.8	0.0

Source: Data from Food Processor-SQL, Version 9.9, ESHA Research, Salem, OR.

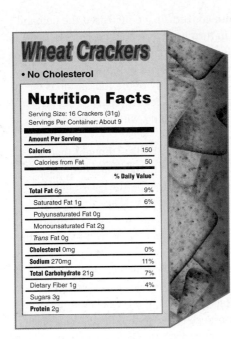

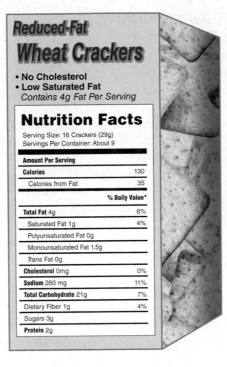

(a)   **(b)**

FIGURE 5.15 Labels for two types of wheat crackers. **(a)** Regular wheat crackers.
(b) Reduced-fat wheat crackers.

2. If the total kcal per serving from fat is not indicated on the label, you can quickly calculate this value by multiplying the grams of total fat per serving by 9 (as there are 9 kcal per gram of fat):

- For the regular wheat crackers: 6 g fat × 9 kcal g = 54 kcal of fat.

  To calculate percentage of kcal from fat, divide the kcal from fat by the total kcal per serving, then multiply by 100:

- 54 kcal/150 kcal = 0.36 × 100 = 36%.

  You can see that this value is not exactly the same as the 50 kcal reported on the label or the 33% of kcal

from fat calculated in example 1. The values on food labels are rounded off, so your estimations may not be identical when you do this second calculation.

Referring again to Table 5.2, compare regular cheddar cheese to low-fat cheddar cheese; then answer the following questions:

1. What is the percentage of energy from fat in the regular-fat cheddar cheese vs. the low-fat cheese?
2. How much does the percentage of fat decrease by selecting the low-fat cheese?
3. If you select the low-fat cheese, how many kcal do you save? How many grams of fat do you save?

- Consider splitting an entrée with your dinner companion and have a dinner salad or broth-based soup as a first course.
- On your salad, choose olive oil and vinegar instead of a high-fat dressing. Always order the dressing on the side, so that you can monitor the amount you use. Instead of buttering your bread, dip it in olive oil.
- Order a baked potato or brown rice instead of french fries or potatoes au gratin. At fast-food restaurants, either skip the french fries or order the smallest serving for portion control. Some fast-food restaurants allow you to replace the french fries in a meal order with fruit.
- Order pizza with vegetable toppings instead of pepperoni or sausage. Try the whole-wheat crust if it is available.
- Share or skip dessert or choose fruit, a yogurt parfait, or angel-food cake.
- Order coffee drinks with skim or reduced fat milk instead of cream or whole milk, and accompany them with a biscotti instead of a brownie.

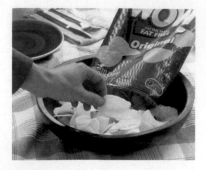

Snack foods have been the primary target for fat replacers, such as Olean, because it is more difficult to significantly reduce the fat in these types of foods without dramatically changing the taste.

Be Aware of Fat Replacers

The rising rates of obesity and its associated health concerns have increased the demand for low-fat versions of our favorite foods, which in turn has created a booming industry for *fat replacers*, substances that mimic the palate-pleasing and flavor-enhancing properties of fats with fewer Calories. Fat replacers can be either carbohydrate-, protein- or fat-based, but all types share the goal of mimicking the palatability of the full-fat foods we like.[28] Snack foods and desserts have been the primary target for fat replacers because it is difficult to simply reduce or eliminate the fat in these products without dramatically changing their taste.

In the mid-1990s, both food industry executives and nutritionists thought that fat replacers would be the answer to our growing obesity problem. They reasoned that, if we replace some of the fats in snack and fast foods with these products, we might be able to reduce both energy and fat intake and help Americans manage their weight better. Unfortunately, this has not proven to be true. It is evident from our growing obesity problem that fat replacers don't help Americans lose weight or even maintain their current weight.

Products such as olestra (brand name Olean) hit the market in 1996 with a lot of fanfare, but the hype was short-lived. Initially, foods containing olestra had to bear a label warning of potential gastrointestinal side effects. In 2003, the U.S. FDA announced that this warning was no longer necessary, as more recent research indicated that olestra caused only mild, infrequent discomfort. However, even with the new labeling, only limited foods in the marketplace now contain olestra.

More recently, a new group of fat replacers has been developed using proteins, such as the whey protein found in milk. Like their predecessors, these new fat replacers lower the fat content of food, but in addition they improve the food's total nutrient profile and decrease its Calorie content. This means we can have a low-fat ice cream with the mouth-feel, finish, and texture of a full-fat ice cream that is also higher in protein and lower in Calories than traditional ice cream. So don't be surprised if you see more products containing protein-based fat replacers on your supermarket shelves in the next few years.

RECAP

The AMDR for total fat is 20% to 35% of total energy. The AI for linoleic acid is 14–17 g per day for adult men and 11–12 g per day for adult women. The AI for alpha-linolenic acid is 1.6 g per day for adult men and 1.1 g per day for adult women. Health professionals recommend that we reduce our intake of saturated fat to less than 10% of our total energy intake and our intake of *trans* fatty acids to the absolute minimum. A healthful dietary strategy is to switch from saturated and *trans* fats to unsaturated fats. We can do this by choosing fish and plant-based foods more often, when shopping, cooking at home, and eating out. Visible fats can be easily recognized, but invisible fats are added to our food during manufacturing or cooking, so we are not aware of how much we are consuming.

 LO 9 Describe the role of blood lipids and dietary fats in the development of cardiovascular disease.

LO 10 Identify lifestyle recommendations for the prevention or treatment of cardiovascular disease.

What Role Do Lipids Play in Cardiovascular Disease and Cancer?

According to the Centers for Disease Control and Prevention, diseases of the heart are the leading cause of death in the United States, accounting for more than 611,000 deaths in 2013.[29,30] Cancer is a close second, with over 584,000 deaths, and stroke is the fifth, causing over 128,000 deaths.[30] Combined, these three disease categories accounted for nearly 51% of all deaths in 2013.[30] So it's important to take a look at these diseases and the dietary and lifestyle factors that can influence their development. Let's start with a look at cardiovascular disease, since it is projected that, by the year 2030, 40% of the U.S. population will have some form of cardiovascular disease.[31]

Cardiovascular Disease Involves the Heart or Blood Vessels

Cardiovascular disease is a general term used to refer to any abnormal condition involving dysfunction of the heart (*cardio-* means "heart") or blood vessels (*vasculature*). There are many forms of this disease, but the three most common are the following:

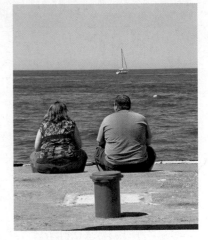

Being overweight is associated with higher rates of death from cardiovascular disease.

■ *Coronary heart disease* (also called *coronary artery disease*) occurs when blood vessels supplying the heart (the *coronary arteries*) become blocked or constricted; such blockage reduces the flow of blood—and the oxygen and nutrients it carries—to the heart. This can result in chest pain, called *angina pectoris*, and lead to a heart attack. It is also a key risk factor for sudden cardiac arrest, which is routinely fatal unless the heart is restarted within minutes.

■ *Stroke* is caused by blockage or rupture of one of the blood vessels supplying the brain (the *cerebral arteries*). When this occurs, the region of the brain depending on that artery for oxygen and nutrients cannot function. As a result, the movement, speech, or other body functions controlled by that part of the brain suddenly stop.

■ *Hypertension*, also called *high blood pressure*, is a condition that may not cause any symptoms, but it increases your risk for a heart attack or stroke. If your blood pressure is high, that means that the force of the blood flowing through your arteries is above normal. (We will discuss hypertension and the dietary and lifestyle factors that affect it in Chapter 9.)

To understand cardiovascular disease, we need to look at an underlying condition called *atherosclerosis*.

Atherosclerosis Is Narrowing of Arteries

Atherosclerosis is a condition in which arterial walls accumulate deposits of lipids and scar tissue, which build up to such a degree that they impair blood flow (**Focus Figure 5.16**, page 196). It's a complex process that begins with injury to the cells that line the insides of all arteries. Factors that commonly promote such injury are the forceful pounding of blood under high pressure and blood-vessel damage from irritants, such as the nicotine in tobacco or the excessive blood glucose in people with poorly controlled diabetes. Whatever the cause, the injury attracts immune cells, which trigger vessel inflammation, which is increasingly being recognized as an important marker of cardiovascular disease.[32] Inflamed vessels become weakened, allowing lipids, mainly cholesterol, to seep through the layers of the vessel wall and become oxidized. Immune cells engulf the oxidized lipids and accumulate as foam cells. These are joined by calcium, protein fibers, and other debris that eventually becomes trapped in thick, grainy deposits called *plaque*. The term *atherosclerosis* reflects the presence of these deposits: *athere* is a Greek word meaning "a thick porridge."

As plaque forms, the interior of the blood vessel narrows and slowly diminishes the blood supply to any tissues "downstream," including the heart muscle or the brain. As a result, these tissues—including heart muscle—wither and gradually lose their ability to function. Alternatively, the blockage may occur suddenly because a plaque ruptures and *platelets*, substances in blood that promote clotting, stick to the damaged area. This quickly obstructs the artery, causing the death of the tissue it supplies. The clot can also detach and travel in the bloodstream until it completely occludes a narrow vessel in the heart or brain. Any of these processes can lead to a heart attack, sudden cardiac arrest, or stroke.

Risk Factors for Cardiovascular Disease

During the past two decades, researchers have identified a number of factors that increase the risk for cardiovascular disease. Some of these risk factors are nonmodifiable, meaning they are beyond your control. These include age (the older you are, the higher your risk), male gender, and family history. For example, you have an increased risk for cardiovascular disease if one of your parents has suffered a heart attack, especially at a young age.

cardiovascular disease A general term that refers to abnormal conditions involving dysfunction of the heart or blood vessels, including coronary heart disease, stroke, and hypertension.

atherosclerosis A disease in which arterial walls accumulate deposits of lipids and scar tissue, which build up to a point at which they impair blood flow.

focus figure 5.16 | Atherosclerosis

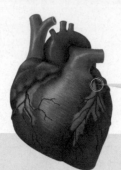

Plaque accumulation within coronary arteries narrows their interior and impedes the flow of oxygen-rich blood to the heart.

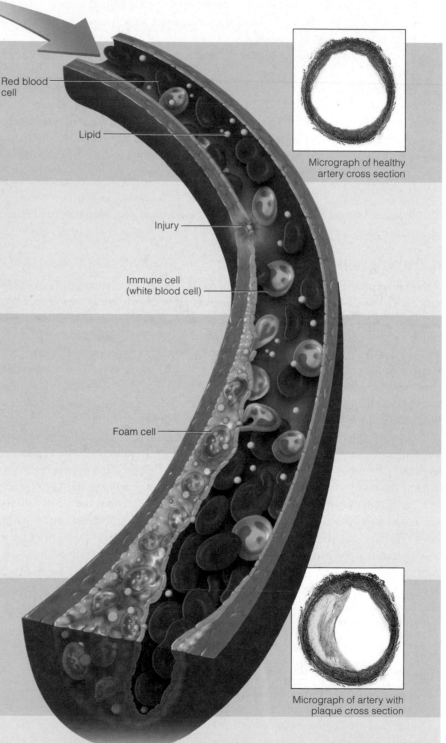

Red blood cell

Lipid

Injury

Immune cell (white blood cell)

Foam cell

Micrograph of healthy artery cross section

Micrograph of artery with plaque cross section

HEALTHY ARTERY

Blood flows unobstructed through normal, healthy artery.

ARTERIAL INJURY

The artery's lining is injured, attracting immune cells, and prompting inflammation.

LIPIDS ACCUMULATE IN WALL

Lipids, particularly cholesterol-containing LDLs, seep beneath the wall lining. The LDLs become oxidized. Immune cells, attracted to the site, engulf the oxidized LDLs and are transformed into foam cells.

FATTY STREAK

The foam cells accumulate to form a fatty streak, which releases more toxic and inflammatory chemicals.

PLAQUE FORMATION

The foam cells, along with platelets, calcium, protein fibers, and other substances, form thick deposits of plaque, stiffening and narrowing the artery. Blood flow through the artery is reduced or obstructed.

Other risk factors are modifiable, meaning they are at least partly within your control. Following is a brief description of each of these modifiable risk factors. Notice that many of them have a dietary component.[33-36]

- *Obesity:* Being obese is associated with higher rates of cardiovascular disease and higher rates of death from cardiovascular disease. The risk is due primarily to a greater occurrence of hypertension, inflammation, abnormal blood lipids (discussed in more detail shortly), and type 2 diabetes in individuals who are overweight. Chapter 13 explores the influence of body weight on an individual's overall cardiometabolic risk.

- *Physical inactivity:* Numerous research studies have shown that physical activity can reduce your risk for cardiovascular disease by improving several risk factors associated with the disease. Regular physical activity can reduce body fat and weight, improve blood lipids, lower resting blood pressure, and reduce blood glucose levels both at rest and after eating. Physical activity can also significantly reduce the risk for type 2 diabetes, a major cardiovascular disease risk factor.[34] According to the 2008 US Physical Activity Guidelines, physical activity can reduce your risk for heart disease by 20% to 30%, stroke by 25% to 30%, and type 2 diabetes by 25% to 35%.[37]

- *Smoking:* There is strong evidence that smoking increases your risk for blood-vessel injury and cardiovascular disease. Research indicates that smokers have a two- to six-fold greater chance of developing cardiovascular disease than nonsmokers, depending on age and gender.[38] If you smoke, quitting is one of the best ways to reduce your risk for cardiovascular disease. People who stop smoking live longer than those who continue to smoke, and smokers who quit by age 30 reduce their chances of dying from a smoking-related disease by more than 90%.[39]

- *Type 2 diabetes:* As discussed (in Chapter 4), for many individuals with type 2 diabetes, the condition is directly related to being overweight or obese. The risk for cardiovascular disease is three times higher in women with diabetes and two times higher in men with diabetes compared to individuals without diabetes.

- *Inflammation:* Earlier, we explained the role of blood-vessel inflammation in the development of atherosclerosis. C-reactive protein (CRP) is a nonspecific marker of inflammation that is associated with cardiovascular disease. Risk for cardiovascular disease appears to be higher in individuals who have high blood inflammatory markers, such as CRP, in addition to other risk factors, such as abnormal blood lipids.[36,40] Thus, reducing the factors that promote inflammation, such as obesity and a diet low in omega-3 fatty acids and high in saturated fats, can reduce the risk for cardiovascular disease.

- *Abnormal blood lipids:* As we explain next, levels of certain blood lipids are associated with an increased or decreased risk for cardiovascular disease. Making lifestyle changes, such as lowering your intake of saturated and *trans* fat, increasing your physical activity and soluble fiber intake, and achieving a healthful body weight, can help improve your blood lipid profile.

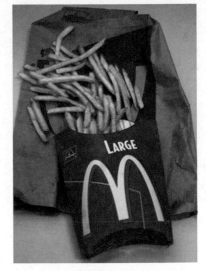

Lowering your intake of saturated fats and avoiding all *trans* fats—such as those found in french fries—can help improve your blood lipid profile, especially when accompanied by increasing your physical activity and soluble fiber intake.

The Role of Blood Lipids in Cardiovascular Disease

Recall that lipids are transported in the blood by lipoproteins made up of a lipid center and a protein outer coat. Because lipoproteins are soluble in blood, they are commonly called *blood lipids.*

The names of lipoproteins reflect their proportion of lipid, which is less dense, to protein, which is very dense (**Figure 5.17**, page 198). For example, very-low-density lipoproteins (VLDLs) have a high ratio of lipid to protein. Let's look at each of these blood lipids in more detail to determine how they are linked to heart disease risk.

Chylomicrons At 85% triglyceride, chylomicrons have the lowest density. As you learned earlier, the blood contains chylomicrons only after a meal. They are produced in the enterocytes to transport dietary fat into the lymph system and from there into

Use this online risk assessment tool to estimate your 10-year risk of having a heart attack: http://cvdrisk.nhlbi.nih.gov

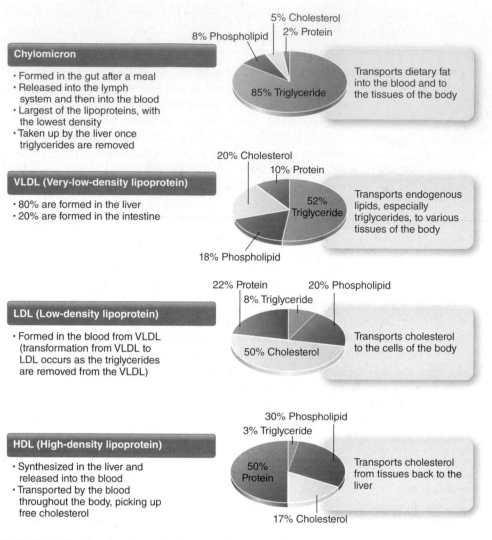

Chylomicron

- Formed in the gut after a meal
- Released into the lymph system and then into the blood
- Largest of the lipoproteins, with the lowest density
- Taken up by the liver once triglycerides are removed

5% Cholesterol
2% Protein
8% Phospholipid
85% Triglyceride

Transports dietary fat into the blood and to the tissues of the body

VLDL (Very-low-density lipoprotein)

- 80% are formed in the liver
- 20% are formed in the intestine

20% Cholesterol
10% Protein
52% Triglyceride
18% Phospholipid

Transports endogenous lipids, especially triglycerides, to various tissues of the body

LDL (Low-density lipoprotein)

- Formed in the blood from VLDL (transformation from VLDL to LDL occurs as the triglycerides are removed from the VLDL)

22% Protein
8% Triglyceride
20% Phospholipid
50% Cholesterol

Transports cholesterol to the cells of the body

HDL (High-density lipoprotein)

- Synthesized in the liver and released into the blood
- Transported by the blood throughout the body, picking up free cholesterol

30% Phospholipid
3% Triglyceride
50% Protein
17% Cholesterol

Transports cholesterol from tissues back to the liver

FIGURE 5.17 The chemical components of various lipoproteins. Notice that chylomicrons contain the highest proportion of triglycerides, making them the least dense, and high-density lipoproteins (HDLs) have the highest proportion of protein, making them the most dense.

the bloodstream. **Focus Figure 5.18** illustrates the transport and distribution of chylomicrons and the other lipoproteins.

Very-Low-Density Lipoproteins More than half of the substance of **very-low-density lipoproteins (VLDLs)** is triglyceride. The liver is the primary source of VLDLs, but they are also produced in the intestines. VLDLs are primarily transport vehicles ferrying triglycerides from their source to the body's cells, including to adipose tissues for storage. The enzyme lipoprotein lipase (LPL) frees most of the triglyceride from the VLDL molecules, resulting in its uptake by the body's cells.

Diets high in fat, simple sugars, and extra Calories can increase the production of endogenous VLDLs, whereas diets high in omega-3 fatty acids can help reduce their production. In addition, exercise can reduce VLDLs, because the fat produced in the body is quickly used for energy instead of remaining to circulate in the blood.

Low-Density Lipoproteins The molecules resulting when VLDLs release their triglyceride load are much higher in cholesterol, phospholipids, and protein and therefore somewhat more dense. These **low-density lipoproteins (LDLs)** circulate in the blood, delivering their cholesterol to cells with specialized LDL receptors. Diets high in saturated and *trans* fat *decrease* the removal of LDLs by body cells, apparently by blocking these receptor sites.

very-low-density lipoprotein (VLDL) A lipoprotein made in the liver and intestine that functions to transport endogenous lipids, especially triglycerides, to the tissues of the body.

low-density lipoprotein (LDL) A lipoprotein formed in the blood from VLDLs that transports cholesterol to the cells of the body; often called "bad cholesterol."

Dietary and endogenous lipids are transported in the body via several different lipoprotein compounds, such as chylomicrons, VLDLs, LDLs, and HDLs.

CHYLOMICRONS

Chylomicrons are produced in the enterocytes to transport dietary lipids. The enzyme lipoprotein lipase (LPL), found on the endothelial cells in the capillaries, hydrolyzes the triglycerides in the chylomicrons into fatty acids and glycerol, which enter body cells (such as muscle and adipose cells), leaving a chylomicron remnant. Chylomicron remnants are dismantled in the liver.

VLDLs

VLDLs (very-low-density lipoproteins) are produced primarily in the liver to transport endogenous fat in the form of triglycerides into the bloodstream. Lipoprotein lipase hydrolyzes the triglycerides in the VLDLs, allowing the fatty acids to enter body cells, especially muscle and adipose cells. Glycerol is also released and is transported back to the liver.

LDLs

LDLs (low-density lipoproteins) are created with the removal of most of the VLDLs' triglyceride load. LDLs are rich in cholesterol, which they deliver to body cells with LDL receptors. LDLs not taken up by the cells are primarily taken up by the liver for degradation.

HDLs

HDLs (high-density lipoproteins) are produced in the liver and circulate in the blood, picking up cholesterol from dying cells, other lipoproteins, and arterial plaques. They return this cholesterol to the liver, where it can be recycled or eliminated from the body through bile.

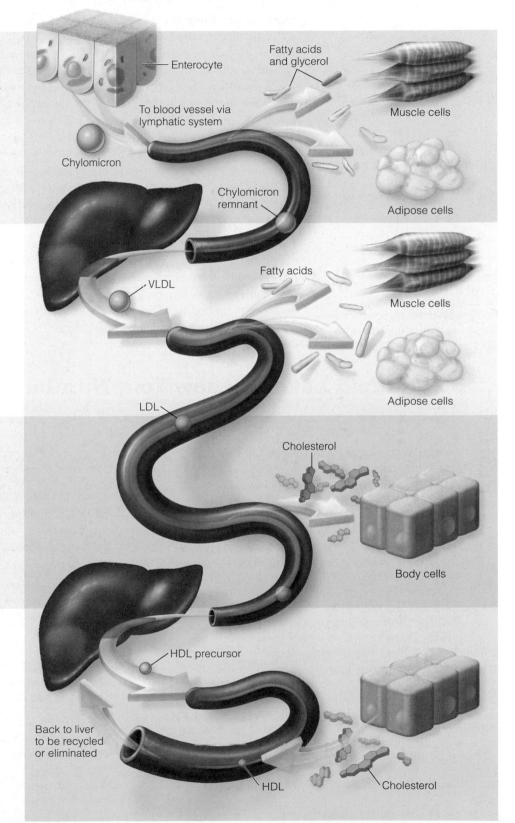

Enterocyte

Fatty acids and glycerol

To blood vessel via lymphatic system

Chylomicron

Muscle cells

Chylomicron remnant

Adipose cells

VLDL

Fatty acids

Muscle cells

Adipose cells

LDL

Cholesterol

Body cells

HDL precursor

Back to liver to be recycled or eliminated

HDL

Cholesterol

What happens to LDLs not taken up by body cells? As shown in Figure 5.18, they are primarily taken up by the liver for degradation. As they degrade over time, they release their cholesterol; thus, failure to remove LDLs from the bloodstream results in an increased load of cholesterol in the blood. The more cholesterol circulating in the blood, the greater the risk that some of the LDLs will be oxidized and contribute to atherosclerosis (see Figure 5.16). Because high blood levels of LDL-cholesterol increase the risk for cardiovascular disease, it is commonly called "bad cholesterol."

High-Density Lipoproteins   As their name indicates, **high-density lipoproteins (HDLs)** are small, dense lipoproteins with a very low cholesterol content and a high protein content. They are released from the liver and intestines to circulate in the blood, picking up cholesterol from dying cells and arterial plaques and transferring it to other lipoproteins, which return it to the liver. This process is called reverse cholesterol transport.[41] The liver takes up the cholesterol and uses it to synthesize bile, thereby removing it from the circulatory system. HDLs also have anti-inflammatory properties, which also help keep LDLs from oxidation.[41] High blood levels of HDL-cholesterol are therefore associated with a low risk for cardiovascular disease. That's why HDL-cholesterol is often referred to as "good cholesterol." There is some evidence that diets high in omega-3 fatty acids and participation in regular physical exercise can modestly increase HDL-cholesterol levels. Refer to the *Highlight: Blood Lipid Levels: Know Your Numbers!* to gain more insight into your own blood lipid levels.

high-density lipoprotein (HDL) A lipoprotein made in the liver and released into the blood. HDLs function to transport cholesterol from the tissues back to the liver; often called "good cholesterol."

Total Serum Cholesterol   Normally, as the dietary level of cholesterol increases, the body decreases the amount of cholesterol it makes, which keeps the body's level of cholesterol constant. Unfortunately, this feedback mechanism does not work well in everyone. For some individuals, eating dietary cholesterol doesn't decrease the amount of cholesterol produced in the body, and their total body cholesterol level rises. This also increases the level of cholesterol in the blood. These individuals may benefit from reducing their intake of dietary cholesterol and saturated fat.

Blood Lipid Levels: Know Your Numbers!

One of the most important steps you can take to reduce your own risk for heart disease is to know your "numbers"—that is, your blood lipid values. In addition, if you are considering a career in nutrition or healthcare, you'll need to be able to work with your clients to track their blood lipid levels as they change their diet and lifestyle to decrease their risk for cardiovascular disease. So it's important to keep a record of blood lipid values and have them checked every 1 to 2 years.

How are blood lipids, such as LDL-cholesterol or HDL-cholesterol, actually measured? First, a blood sample is taken and the lipoproteins in the blood are extracted. Total cholesterol is determined by breaking apart all the lipoproteins and measuring their combined cholesterol content. You can see from Figure 5.17 that each of the lipoproteins contains some cholesterol and some triglycerides. The same process is used to determine total blood triglyceride level. The next step is to measure the amount of cholesterol in the LDLs and HDLs, because these two lipoproteins can either raise or lower an individual's risk for heart disease. These lipoproteins are separated and the amount of cholesterol in each one is determined to give an LDL-cholesterol and an HDL-cholesterol value. Once these values are determined, you can compare them to the following "target" levels, which identify healthful ranges for each blood lipid, and see how you measure up.

The target lipid values are as follows:[1]

Total cholesterol (mg/d): <200 mg/dL
LDL-cholesterol (mg/d): <130 mg/dL
HDL-cholesterol (mg/d): >40 mg/dL
Triglycerides (mg/d): <150 mg/dL

Reference

1. National Institutes of Health. 2002. *Third Report of the National Cholesterol Education Program: Detection, Evaluation and Treatment of High Blood Cholesterol in Adults (ATP III).* Bethesda, MD: National Cholesterol Education Program, National Heart, Lung, and Blood Institute, NIH. Available at www.nhlbi.nih.gov /guidelines/cholesterol/atp3xsum.pdf.

Both dietary cholesterol and saturated fats are found in animal foods; thus, by limiting their intake of animal products or selecting low-fat animal products, people reduce their intake of both saturated fat and cholesterol. According to the 2010 Dietary Guidelines, Americans get the majority of their dietary cholesterol from eggs and egg mixed dishes (25%), chicken and chicken mixed dishes (12%), beef and beef mixed dishes (6%), and all types of beef burgers (5%). Selecting fish, poultry without the skin, lean cuts of meat, plant sources of protein, and low-fat dairy products, as well as consuming egg whites without yolks, can dramatically reduce the amount of cholesterol in the diet.

The Role of Dietary Fats in Cardiovascular Disease

Research indicates that high intakes of saturated and *trans* fatty acids increase the blood's level of the lipids associated with cardiovascular disease—namely, total blood cholesterol and the cholesterol found in VLDLs and LDLs. It has also been shown that *trans* fatty acids can raise blood LDL-cholesterol, and lower HDL-cholesterol levels, more than saturated fatty acids.[16] Moreover, in vegetable oils converted to solids (for example, corn oil to corn oil margarine), the level of saturated fat dramatically increases, along with the level of *trans* fatty acids. Hence, to reduce the risk for heart disease, we must reduce our intake of high-fat animal products, hydrogenated vegetable products, and commercially prepared foods high in *trans* fatty acids. But if you already avoid *trans* fats, then is limiting saturated fat also necessary? News headlines in the past few years have pointed to studies suggesting that saturated fat isn't harmful after all. Who's right? Are saturated fats bad or benign? See the **Nutrition Myth or Fact?** at the end of this chapter to find out.

The FDA requires that both saturated fat and *trans* fatty acid content be listed on labels for conventional foods and some dietary supplements. Restaurants are required to provide nutrition facts—including saturated and *trans* fat content—for their menu items at the consumer's request, and some local ordinances require restaurants to post this information. Use the healthy eating strategies listed earlier in this chapter whenever you're eating out.

Conversely, omega-3 fatty acids decrease our risk for heart disease by reducing inflammation and blood triglycerides and increasing HDLs.[42,43] Moreover, replacing saturated fats with monounsaturated and polyunsaturated fatty acids lowers both total and LDL-cholesterol levels.[35,44]

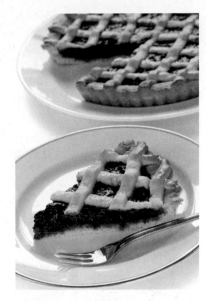

Saturated and *trans* fats are often hidden in processed and prepared foods, such as pies. Without a label, it is impossible to know the amount of fat in each serving of these types of foods, so their intake should be limited.

Lifestyle Changes Can Prevent or Reduce Cardiovascular Disease

The Centers for Disease Control and Prevention,[45] the American Heart Association, and American College of Cardiology have made the following dietary and lifestyle recommendations to improve blood lipid levels and reduce the risk for cardiovascular disease:[42,46,47,49]

- Follow the DRIs for total fat, saturated fat, and *trans* fat. Increase intake of dietary omega-3 fatty acids from dark green, leafy vegetables; fatty fish; soybeans or soybean oil; walnuts or walnut oil; flaxseed meal or oil; or canola oil.
- Increase dietary intakes of whole grains, fruits, and vegetables, so that total dietary fiber is 20–30 g per day, with 10–25 g per day coming from fiber sources such as oat bran, beans, and fruits. This type of fiber reduces LDL-cholesterol.[15,22]
- Make sure to consume the RDA of vitamin B6, B12, and folate to help maintain low blood levels of the amino acid homocysteine. High homocysteine levels in the blood are associated with increased risk for cardiovascular disease. (In Depth 7.5 lists the DRIs for all vitamins.)
- Select and prepare foods with less salt to help keep your blood pressure normal (< 120/80 mm Hg). (See Chapter 9.)
- Eat smaller meals and snacks throughout the day instead of eating most of your Calories in the evening before bed. This approach decreases the load of fat entering the body at any one time. Exercising after a meal also helps keep blood lipids and glucose within normal range.
- Add plant sterols to your diet. There is strong clinical research evidence that the consumption of 2–3 g/day of plant sterols can reduce blood LDLs.[15] Plant sterols are isolated from plant oils and then mixed into commercial margarines, salad dressings, milk, yogurt, or pills. Researchers do not know exactly how plant sterols reduce LDL-cholesterol, but one suggested mechanism is that they block the absorption of dietary cholesterol but are not absorbed themselves.[50]

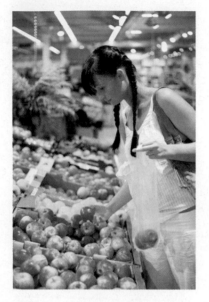

Watch Dr. Penny Kris-Etherton from Pennsylvania State University talk about the AHA's food-based approach at www.heart.org by searching for "Saturated Fats" and clicking on the first article.

Consuming whole fruits and vegetables can reduce your risk for cardiovascular disease.

- Maintain blood glucose and insulin concentrations within normal ranges. High blood glucose levels are associated with high blood triglycerides, which can eventually translate into higher LDLs in the blood. (See Chapter 4.)
- Maintain a healthy body weight. Obesity promotes inflammation; thus, keeping body weight within a healthy range helps keep inflammation low.[51,52] In addition, blood pressure values have been shown to decrease three to four points in people who have lost 10 pounds of body weight.[53]
- Maintain an active lifestyle. Exercise most days of the week for 30–60 minutes whenever possible. Exercise helps maintain a healthful blood lipid profile, body weight, and blood pressure and reduces your risk for diabetes.
- Consume no more than two alcoholic drinks per day for men and one drink per day for women. People diagnosed with hypertension should abstain from drinking alcohol entirely. (See In Depth 4.5.)
- If you smoke, stop. As noted earlier, smoking significantly increases the risk for cardiovascular disease.

The impact of diet on reducing the risk for cardiovascular disease was clearly demonstrated in the Dietary Approaches to Stop Hypertension (DASH) study, which is discussed in detail in Chapter 9. Although this study focused on dietary interventions to reduce hypertension, the results showed that eating the DASH way can also dramatically improve blood lipids. The DASH diet includes high intakes of fruits, vegetables, whole grains, low-fat dairy products, poultry, fish, and nuts and low intakes of fats, red meat, sweets, and sugar-containing beverages. Combining the DASH dietary approach with an active lifestyle significantly reduces the risk for cardiovascular disease.

Prescription Medications Can Reduce Cardiovascular Disease Risk

Sometimes medications are needed in addition to lifestyle changes to reduce cardiovascular risk. A number of medications on the market help lower LDL-cholesterol. The following are some of the most common:

- *Endogenous cholesterol synthesis inhibitors:* These types of drugs, typically called *statins,* block an enzyme in the cholesterol synthesis pathway. Thus, these drugs lower blood levels of LDL-cholesterol and VLDL-cholesterol. Statins also have an important anti-inflammatory effect that contributes to the reduction in cardiovascular disease risk independent of their effect on blood lipids.[32]
- *Bile acid sequestrants:* These types of drugs bind the bile acids, preventing them from being reabsorbed by the intestinal tract. Because bile acids are made from cholesterol, blocking their reabsorption means the liver must use cholesterol already in the body to make new bile acids. Continually eliminating bile acids from the body reduces the total cholesterol pool.

*Nutri-*Case

Gustavo

"Sometimes I wonder where doctors get their funny ideas. Yesterday I had my annual checkup and my doctor says, 'You're doing great! Your weight is fine, your blood sugar's good. . . . The only thing that concerns me is that your blood pressure is a little high. So I want you to watch your diet. Don't sprinkle salt on your food. Eat fish more often. When you eat meat, trim off all the fat. Use one of the new heart-healthy margarines instead of butter, and cook with olive oil instead of lard. And when you have eggs, don't eat the yolks.'

I know he means well, but my wife's just starting to get around again after breaking her hip. How am I supposed to go home and tell her that now she has to learn a whole new way to cook too?"

Do you think Gustavo's objection to his physician's advice is valid? Why or why not? Identify at least two interventions or resources that might help Gustavo and his wife.

- *Nicotinic acid:* Therapeutic doses of nicotinic acid, a form of niacin, favorably affect all blood lipids when given pharmacologically. (The form of niacin found in multivitamin supplements does not affect lipids.) Unfortunately, this drug has a number of side effects, such as flushing of the skin, gastrointestinal distress, and liver problems.[16] Because of this, it is used less frequently than the other two drugs.

The Role of Dietary Fat in Cancer

Cancer develops as a result of a poorly understood interaction between the environment and genetic factors. In addition, most cancers take years to develop, so examining the impact of dietary fat on cancer development can be a long and difficult process. Currently, research shows that obesity, poor nutrition, and physical inactivity may account for 25% to 30% of several major cancers, including colon cancer and postmenopausal breast cancer.[54] Of course, a diet high in fat can contribute to obesity, but there is no strong evidence that a certain type or amount of fat causes cancer.

Three types of cancer that have been studied extensively for their possible relationship to dietary fat intake are breast cancer, colon cancer, and prostate cancer:

- *Breast cancer:* Currently, no clinical trials show a link between the amount or type of fat consumed and increased risk for breast cancer.[55,56] One confounding factor is that the influence of diet on breast cancer is difficult to separate from the influence of body weight.[56]
- *Colon cancer:* Recent research shows that a Western diet high in red meat, fat, refined grains, and desserts is associated with a greater occurrence of colon cancer compared to a diet high in fruits, vegetables, poultry, and fish.[57,58] Because we now know that physical activity can reduce the risk for colon cancer, earlier diet and colon cancer studies that did not control for this factor are now being questioned.
- *Prostate cancer:* As with other cancers, the exact link between dietary fat intake and prostate cancer is not clear.[59,60] Research shows that there is a consistent link between prostate cancer risk and consumption of animal fats, but not other types of fats. The exact mechanism by which animal fats may contribute to prostate cancer has not yet been identified. Men who consume diets high in animal fat also have lower intakes of fruits and vegetables.

Until we know more about the link between diet, especially fat, and cancer, the American Institute for Cancer Research recommends the following diet and lifestyle changes to reduce your risk:[61]

- Maintain a healthy body weight. Avoid weight gain and increases in waist circumference throughout adulthood.
- Engage in moderate physical activity, the equivalent of brisk walking, for at least 30 minutes a day. For improved fitness, aim for 60 minutes or more of moderate activity, or 30 minutes of vigorous activity every day. Limit nonessential sedentary behaviors, such as watching television and playing video games.
- Limit consumption of sugary drinks and other sources of empty Calories.
- Eat a variety of fruits, legumes and other vegetables, and whole unprocessed grains.
- Limit consumption of red meats, such as beef, pork, and lamb, and avoid processed meats.
- If you drink alcohol, limit intake to two drinks/day for men and one drink/day for women.
- Limit consumption of salty foods and foods processed with salt.
- Don't use supplements to protect against cancer.

RECAP

The types of fats we eat can significantly influence our health and risk for disease. Saturated and *trans* fatty acids increase our risk for heart disease, whereas omega-3 fatty acids can reduce our risk. Other risk factors for heart disease include being overweight, being physically inactive, smoking, having high blood pressure, and having diabetes. High levels of LDL-cholesterol and low levels of HDL-cholesterol increase your risk for heart disease. Making appropriate changes in diet and lifestyle behaviors may reduce your risk for some types of cancer. ■

Nutrition Myth OR Fact?   Are Saturated Fats Bad or Benign?

Saturated fats are in the news. As you read in Chapter 5, decades of research has suggested that diets high in saturated fatty acids (SFA) are associated with increased risk of coronary heart disease (CHD), the most common form of cardiovascular disease (CVD). However, the headlines in 2014 trumpeted the conclusions of new research indicating that saturated fats don't deserve their bad rap. How is it that the scientific community could be so divided on what appears to be a simple question of physiology? Let's look at the studies involved and why they brought about such controversy.

In 2014, researchers from the United Kingdom published a meta-analysis of 32 observational studies examining the relationship between saturated fat intake and the risk of coronary disease.[1] Their conclusion stated that there is no clear evidence that supports the current cardiovascular guidelines that encourage "high consumption of polyunsaturated fatty acids and low consumption of total saturated fats." Immediately upon the publication of this article, researchers from the American Heart Association (AHA) and other public health organizations around the world began reviewing the analysis' methodology, data, and conclusions. The following key criticisms emerged from these reviews:

- Two-thirds of the research studies included in the analysis were observational in nature and relied on self-reported diets. This means the researchers, using questionnaires or diet records, had asked people what they typically ate, and then looked at coronary outcomes 5–23 years later. These types of studies do not provide information about cause and effect. To answer the question of whether or not a high-SFA diet increases the risk for CHD, researchers need to feed diets lower in SFAs and then look to see whether there is a decreased occurrence of CHD or cardiac death in subsequent years and if these coronary events can be predicted based on changes in blood lipids over the same time period. They then compare these results to individuals consuming a control or typical diet. In fact, an earlier meta-analysis of eight randomized clinical trials (RCTs) comparing diets in this way found that when polyunsaturated fats (PUFA) replaced SFAs in the diet, coronary events were reduced by 19%.[2] This corresponded to a 10% reduction in CHD risk based on changes in blood lipids. They also found that for each decrease in total cholesterol of 40 mg/dL there was a 24% decrease in CHD events. Overall, 13,614 people, the majority male, were followed for an average of 4.5 years. Half had begun the study already having CHD. Those individuals who were on the diet longer had a great positive outcome with dietary change.

- They included research studies other scientists thought were inappropriate or misinterpreted or studies in which *trans* fatty acids were fed as margarine as part of the intervention.[3,4] Given that the link between *trans* fatty acid

consumption and CVD is well-established, such studies should have been excluded.

- The researchers made some minor calculation errors, which required them to rerun their data after the original article was published.[5] They also made assumptions about their results that other researchers could not agree with, such as saying the outcomes for a few people in a study could be generalized to the whole population.[3] For any one individual, the risk of developing CVD based on diet will depend on that individual's CVD risk factors at baseline. Thus, how much benefit is derived from a dietary change may depend on whether an individual started the study with high or low risk factors for CVD (e.g. normal or poor blood lipid profile; family history of CVD) or having already experienced a cardiovascular event.

This controversy surrounding SFA and CHD has emphasized the importance of carefully evaluating the quality of the nutrition-related research you read. When reviewing the literature about diet and CVD risk, considering the issues bulleted below will help you apply the findings to yourself or a client:

- What are your current CVD risk factors? These are listed on page 197 and including, smoking, obesity, physical activity level, family history, and blood lipids. If your CVD risks are high you may respond differently to a dietary and lifestyle change compared to an individual who has low risks. In addition, there are always confounding factors to consider. For example, the number of individuals classified as overweight or obese has increased dramatically in most developed countries over the last 20 years. This in turn has dramatically increased the prevalence of chronic disease. We also know that people who lose weight and become more fit decrease their CVD risk even if their SFA intake doesn't change dramatically. In short, energy balance makes a critical contribution to the diet-CVD discussion (see Chapter 13).

- If you reduce your dietary intake of SFAs, with what do you replace them? In the past, many people replaced fat in their diet with refined carbohydrates. We now know that this approach to reducing CVD doesn't work: when SFAs are replaced with refined carbohydrates and sugars, CVD risk factors—including LDL-cholesterol, small-particle LDLs (spLDLs, discussed below), inflammation, insulin resistance and body weight—increase.

- We don't eat fatty acids: we eat whole foods. Using a food-based approach for lowering your risk of CVD should make dietary recommendations easier to follow. The AHA, for example, encourages consumers to eat more whole fruits and vegetables, including legumes, as well as whole grains, low-fat dairy, poultry, fish, and nuts, and to limit your intake of red meat and added sugars, including sugary beverages.

These are important considerations, but keep in mind that the current recommendation to limit dietary SFA intake in order to reduce CVD risk is based on two key assumptions:[6,7]

1. Higher intakes of SFAs increase blood total cholesterol and LDL-cholesterol, lipids associated with increased risk for CVD.

2. Lowering LDL-cholesterol will reduce the risk of CVD.

The relationship between diet and CVD is complex, and as our understanding of this relationship grows, these simple assumptions are being challenged. For example, researchers are beginning to identify new markers in the blood that might predict CVD risk more precisely than total or LDL-cholesterol.[6,7] These include spLDLs, which are commonly referred to as "atherogenic" because they are able to easily penetrate the arterial wall and become oxidized, the first step in the atherosclerosis process (see Figure 5.16).[8] Lifestyle changes associated with increased spLDLs are obesity and diets high in refined sugars, whereas exercise is associated with improvements in the cardioprotective HDLs.[9] Unfortunately, assessment of LDL-cholesterol doesn't tell you if you have spLDLs, which is why your total-cholesterol/HDL-cholesterol ratio or non-HDL-cholesterol is considered by some researchers to be a better predictor of your CVD risk.[10,11] Also, tests for spLDLs are not yet widely available to the public.

In addition, new markers for tracking dietary intake are being identified. For example, if you eat dairy products, certain fatty acids unique to dairy products will show up in your blood. Researchers can now design studies that can allow them to determine how much dairy is in participants' diets without having to rely on diet records. These studies should avoid some of the design pitfalls of our current observational studies.

As always, it's helpful also to bear in mind that we eat foods, not single nutrients. Any given food containing SFAs might also contain other important nutrients, fiber, phytochemicals, or probiotics. For example, dairy contains saturated fat, but also contains protein, calcium, riboflavin, other micronutrients, and may contain probiotics.[6,7] Increasing low-fat dairy intake will increase the dietary calcium intake, which increases fecal fat excretion.[12] The calcium binds some of the fat in the diet and reduces the fat absorption, which might be one reason why diets high in dairy might contribute to weight loss. This example illustrates the importance of a looking at whole foods, not just single nutrients in foods, when considering human physiology and health.

So what's the bottom line? Governments, public health organizations, and registered dietitians don't base dietary recommendations on one study, but on a body of research evidence. This doesn't mean the current SFA recommendations won't change, but only that more research would be needed before the scientific community could responsibly conclude that saturated fats are not related to CVD risk. Until then, eating a variety of whole foods while limiting red meat and sugars is our best recommendation for lowering your risk of CVD.

Critical-Thinking Questions

- What is a meta-analysis? Why might a meta-analysis of eight randomized clinical trials provide more valid, reliable evidence about SFAs and CVD risk than a meta-analysis of 32 mostly observational studies?

- You want dessert. You avoid the ice cream in your freezer—too much saturated fat!—and go for the fat-free mango sorbet, which has no saturated fat, *trans* fat, or cholesterol, but does have 36 grams of sugar in a half-cup serving. Why do researchers suggest that such trade-offs aren't as smart as you might think?

- Look at your own diet. What whole-food dietary changes are you willing to make to help lower your lifetime risk of CVD? How much effort and cost would it take to make these changes?

References

1. Chowdhury, R., S. Warnakula, S. Kunutsor, F. Crowe, H. A. Ward, L. Johnson, O. H. Franco, A. S. Butterworth, N. G. Forouhi, S. G. Thompson, K. T. Khaw, D. Mozaffarian, J. Danesh, and E. Di Angelantonio (2014). Association of Dietary, Circulating, and Supplement Fatty Acids With Coronary Risk: a systematic review and meta-analysis. *Ann. Intr. Med.* 160:6.

2. Mozaffarian, D., R. Micha, and S. Wallace (2010). Effects on coronary heart disease of increasing polyunsaturated fat in place of saturated fat: a systematic review and meta-analysis of randomized controlled trials. *PLoS Med.* 7(3).

3. Dawczynski, C., M. E. Kleber, W. März, G. Jahreis, and S. Lorkowski (2014). Association of dietary, circulating, and supplement fatty acids with coronary risk. *Ann. Intr. Med.*161(6):453–454.

4. Liebman, B. F., M. B. Katan, and M. F. Jacobson (2014). Association of dietary, circulating, and supplement fatty acids with coronary risk. *Ann. Intr. Med.*161(6):454–455.

5. Willett, W. C., M. J. Stampfer, and F. M. Sacks (2014). Association of dietary, circulating, and supplement fatty acids with coronary risk. *Ann. Intr. Med.* 161(6):453.

6. Astrup, A. 2014. A changing view on saturated fatty acids and dairy: from enemy to friend. *Am. J. Clin. Nutri.* 100(6): 1407–1408.

7. Astrup, A. 2014. Yogurt and dairy product consumption to prevent cardiometabolic diseases: epidemiologic and experimental studies. *Am J. Clin. Nutri.* 99(5):1235S–1242S.

8. Barona, J., and M. L. Fernandez. 2012. Dietary cholesterol affects plasma lipid levels, the intravascular processing of lipoproteins and reverse cholesterol transport without increasing the risk for heart disease. *Nutrients* 4(8):1015–1025.

9. Chandra, A., and A. Rohatgi. 2014. The role of advanced lipid testing in the prediction of cardiovascular disease. *Curr. Atheroscl. Rep.* 16(3):394.

10. Lewington, S., G. Whitlock, R. Clarke, P. Sherliker, J. Emberson, J. Halsey, N. Qizilbash, R. Peto, and R. Collins. 2007. Blood cholesterol and vascular mortality by age, sex, and blood pressure: a meta-analysis of individual data from 61 prospective studies with 55,000 vascular deaths. *Lancet* 370(9602):1829–1839.

11. Robinson, J. G., S. Wang, B. J. Smith, and T. A. Jacobson. 2009. "Meta-analysis of the relationship between non-high-density lipoprotein cholesterol reduction and coronary heart disease risk." *J. Am. Coll. Cardiol.* 53(4):316–322.

12. Bendsen, N. T., A. L. Hother, S. K. Jensen, J. K. Lorenzen, and A. Astrup. 2008. Effect of dairy calcium on fecal fat excretion: a randomized crossover trial. *Int. J. Obes. (Lond.)* 32(12): 1816–1824.

STUDY PLAN   MasteringNutrition™

Customize your study plan—and master your nutrition!—in the Study Plan of MasteringNutrition.

summary

Scan to hear an MP3 Chapter Review in MasteringNutrition.

LO 1
- Fats and oils are forms of a larger and more diverse group of substances called lipids; most lipids are insoluble in water.
- The three types of lipids commonly found in foods are triglycerides, phospholipids, and sterols.

LO 2
- Most of the fat we eat is in the form of triglycerides; a triglyceride is a molecule that contains three fatty acids attached to a glycerol backbone.
- Short-chain fatty acids are usually less than 6 carbon atoms in length; medium-chain fatty acids are 6 to 12 carbons in length; and long-chain fatty acids are 14 or more carbons in length.

- Saturated fatty acids have no carbons attached together with a double bond, which means that every carbon atom in the fatty acid chain is saturated with hydrogen. They are straight in shape and solid at room temperature.
- Monounsaturated fatty acids contain one double bond between two carbon atoms. Polyunsaturated fatty acids contain more than one double bond between carbon atoms. Unsaturated fatty acids are usually liquid at room temperature.

LO 3
- A *cis* fatty acid has hydrogen atoms located on the same side of the double bond in an unsaturated fatty acid. This *cis* positioning produces a kink in the unsaturated fatty acid and is the shape found in naturally occurring unsaturated fatty acids.
- A *trans* fatty acid has hydrogen atoms located on opposite sides of the double carbon bond.

This positioning causes *trans* fatty acids to be straighter and more rigid, like saturated fats. This *trans* positioning results when oils are hydrogenated during food processing.

LO 4 ■ The essential fatty acids (linoleic acid and alpha-linolenic acid) must be obtained from food. These fatty acids are precursors to important biological compounds called eicosanoids, which are essential for growth and health.

■ Linoleic acid is found primarily in vegetable and nut oils. Alpha-linolenic acid (ALA) is found in dark green, leafy vegetables; flaxseeds and oil; walnuts and walnut oil; soybean oil and soy foods; canola oil; and fish products and fish oil. EPA and DHA are metabolic derivatives of ALA that appear to reduce the risk of heart disease.

LO 5 ■ The majority of fat digestion and absorption occurs in the small intestine. Fat is emulsified by bile, which is produced by the liver and stored in the gallbladder. The emulsified fat is then acted on by pancreatic enzymes, which break it into even smaller particles that are taken up by the micelles.

■ Lipid digestion products are transported to enterocytes by micelles.

■ Because fats are not soluble in water, triglycerides are packaged into lipoproteins before being released into the bloodstream for transport to the cells.

■ Phospholipids consist of a glycerol backbone and two fatty acids with a phosphate group; phospholipids are soluble in water and assist with transporting fats in the bloodstream.

■ Sterols have a ring structure; cholesterol is the most common sterol in our diet.

■ Dietary fat is primarily used either as an energy source for the cells or to make lipid-containing compounds in the body, or it is stored in the muscle and adipose tissue as triglyceride for later use.

LO 6 ■ Fats are a primary energy source during rest and exercise; are our major source of stored energy; provide essential fatty acids; enable the transport of fat-soluble vitamins; help maintain cell function; provide protection for body organs; and contribute to the flavor, texture, and satiety of foods.

LO 7 ■ The AMDR for fat is 20% to 35% of total energy intake. Our intake of saturated fats and *trans* fatty acids should be kept to a minimum. Individuals who limit fat intake to less than 15% of energy intake need to make sure that essential fatty acid needs are met, as well as protein and energy needs.

■ For the essential fatty acids, 5% to 10% of energy intake should be in the form of linoleic acid and 0.6% to 1.2% as alpha-linolenic acid.

LO 8 ■ Limit consumption of saturated and trans fats by choosing lower-fat versions of animal-based foods, limiting pastries and other high-fat baked goods, and avoiding fried and breaded vegetables and heavy sauces. Check food labels for partially hydrogenated oils, which indicate that the product contains *trans* fats.

■ Select beneficial unsaturated fats by eating more sustainable fish, and choosing plant oils, tofu, legumes, nuts, and seeds more often, including when eating out. Watch for invisible fats found in cakes, cookies, marbling in meat, regular-fat dairy products, and fried foods.

■ Fat replacers are substances that mimic the palate-pleasing and flavor-enhancing properties of fats with fewer Calories. They can be carbohydrate-, protein- or fat-based, but all types share the goal of mimicking the palatability of the full-fat foods.

LO 9 ■ Cardiovascular disease is characterized by dysfunction of the heart (*cardio-* means "heart") or blood vessels (*vasculature*). An underlying condition contributing to cardiovascular disease is atherosclerosis, the accumulation of deposits of lipids and other debris in arteries.

■ Diets high in saturated fat and *trans* fatty acids can increase our risk for cardiovascular disease.

■ High levels of circulating low-density lipoproteins, or LDLs, increase total blood cholesterol concentrations and contribute to the formation of plaque on arterial walls, leading to an increased risk for cardiovascular disease. This is why LDL-cholesterol is sometimes called the "bad cholesterol."

■ High-density lipoproteins, or HDLs, function to return cholesterol to the liver, reducing our blood cholesterol levels and our risk for cardiovascular disease. This is why HDL-cholesterol is sometimes called the "good cholesterol."

LO 10 ■ In addition to diet, other risk factors for cardiovascular disease are overweight or obesity, physical inactivity, smoking, high blood pressure, and diabetes.

■ Research shows that obesity increases the risk for certain cancers. A diet high in fat can contribute to obesity, but there is no strong evidence that a certain type or amount of fat causes cancer.

review questions

LO 1 1. The type of lipid found most abundantly in foods is
a. triglycerides.
b. *trans* fatty acids.
c. phospholipids.
d. sterols.

LO 2 2. Fatty acids with one double bond between two of their carbon atoms are referred to as
a. saturated.
b. monounsaturated.
c. polyunsaturated.
d. steroids.

LO 3 3. *Trans* fatty acids
a. have no double carbon bonds.
b. have double carbon bonds in which both hydrogen atoms are located on the same side of the double bond.
c. are synthesized in the liver and intestine, and therefore do not need to be consumed in the diet.
d. increase the blood's level of the lipids associated with cardiovascular disease.

LO 4 4. Alpha-linolenic acid (ALA) is
a. a precursor to linoleic acid.
b. a metabolic derivative of EPA and DHA.
c. also known as arachidonic acid.
d. found in leafy green vegetables, flaxseed oil, and fatty fish.

LO 5 5. Triglycerides within chylomicrons are taken up by body cells with the help of
a. lipoprotein lipase.
b. gastric lipase.
c. pancreatic lipase.
d. bile.

LO 6 6. Fats
a. provide less energy, gram for gram, than carbohydrates, but are metabolized more efficiently.
b. are a major source of fuel for the body both during physical activity and at rest.
c. enable the digestion of fat-soluble vitamins.
d. keep foods from turning rancid.

LO 7 7. The AMDR for fat is
a. 10% to 25% of total energy.
b. 15% to 30% of total energy.
c. 20% to 35% of total energy.
d. There is no AMDR for fat.

LO 8 8. Three healthful sources of beneficial fats are
a. skim milk, lamb, and fruits.
b. oats, broth-based soups, and red wine.
c. vegetables, fish, and seeds.
d. whole milk, egg whites, and stick margarine.

LO 9 9. The risk for cardiovascular disease is reduced in people who have high blood levels of
a. triglycerides.
b. very-low-density lipoproteins.
c. low-density lipoproteins.
d. high-density lipoproteins.

LO 10 10. The risk for heart disease is reduced in people who
a. smoke.
b. strictly limit their intake of cholesterol.
c. drink at least two glasses of red wine a day.
d. engage in regular physical activity.

true or false?

LO 1 11. **True or false?** Lecithin is a sterol found in egg yolks and is emulsified by bile.

LO 3 12. **True or false?** *Trans* fatty acids are produced by food manufacturers; they do not occur in nature.

LO 6 13. **True or false?** During a long bike ride, lipids are mobilized from adipose tissue for use as energy.

LO 8 14. **True or false?** A serving of food labeled *reduced fat* has at least 25% fewer Calories than a full-fat version of the same food.

LO 10 15. **True or false?** To reduce your risk for cardiovascular disease, avoid eating most of your Calories in the evening before bed.

short answer

LO 6 16. Explain the link between dietary fat and bone health.

LO 6 17. You have volunteered to participate in a 20-mile walk-a-thon to raise money for a local charity. You have been training for several weeks, and the event is now 2 days away. An athlete friend of yours advises you to "load up on carbohydrates" today and tomorrow and says you should avoid eating any foods that contain fat during the day of the walk-a-thon. Do you take this advice? Why or why not?

LO 10 18. Caleb's father is feeling down after an appointment with his doctor. He tells Caleb that his "blood test didn't turn out so good." He then adds, "My doctor told me I can't eat any of my favorite foods anymore. He says red meat and butter have too much fat. I guess I'll have to switch to cottage cheese and margarine!" What type of blood test do you think Caleb's father had? How should Caleb respond to his father's intention to switch to cottage cheese and margarine? Finally, suggest a nondietary lifestyle choice that might improve his health.

math review

LO 7 19. Your friend Maria has determined that she needs to consume about 2,000 kcal per day to maintain her healthful weight. Create a chart for Maria showing the recommended maximum number of Calories she should consume in each of the following forms: unsaturated fat, saturated fat, linoleic acid, alpha-linolenic acid, and *trans* fatty acids.

LO 8 20. Hannah believes that if she limits her fat intake, she will lose weight. After classes, she treats herself to a cup (8 ounces) of nonfat frozen yogurt topped with 4 tablespoons of fat-free chocolate syrup. The yogurt contains 35 grams of carbohydrate, 0.5 gram of fat, and 6 grams of protein. The chocolate syrup contains 48 grams of carbohydrate and 2 grams of protein. First, what do you think of Hannah's approach to weight loss? Second, approximately how many kcal are in her after-class snack? Third, propose a nutrient-dense snack with approximately the same number of kcal and a healthful level of unsaturated fat.

Answers to Review Questions and Math Review can be found online in the MasteringNutrition Study Area.

web links

www.heart.org/HEARTORG
American Heart Association
Learn the best ways to lower and manage your blood cholesterol levels.

www.nhlbi.nih.gov/chd
National Cholesterol Education Program
Check out this site for information on how a healthful diet can lower your cholesterol levels.

www.nhlbi.nih.gov
National Heart, Lung, and Blood Institute
Use the online risk assessment tool to estimate your personal risks for having a heart attack.

www.nlm.nih.gov/medlineplus
Medline Plus Health Information
Search for "fats" or "lipids" to locate resources and learn the latest news on dietary lipids, heart disease, and cholesterol.

www.nih.gov
National Institutes of Health
Go to this clearinghouse site for a wide range of resources, reports, and other useful tools on the subjects we cover in this chapter.

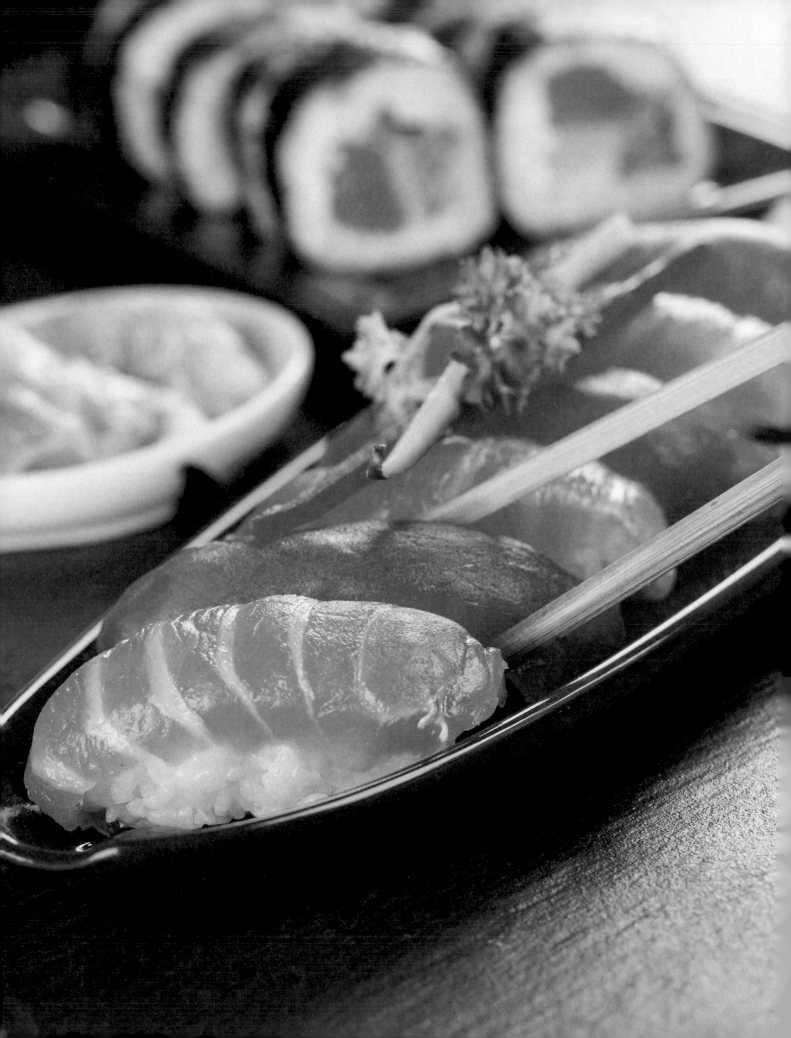

6 Proteins: Crucial Components of All Body Tissues

Learning Outcomes

After studying this chapter, you should be able to:

1 Illustrate the structure of an amino acid molecule including its five essential components, *p. 212*.

2 Differentiate among essential amino acids, nonessential amino acids, and conditionally essential amino acids, *pp. 212–214*.

3 Explain how amino acids are assembled to form proteins and the relationship between protein shape and function, *pp. 214–221*.

4 Discuss how proteins are digested and absorbed by the body, *pp. 221–223*.

5 Describe at least four functions of proteins in the body, *pp. 223–227*.

6 Calculate an individual's Recommended Dietary Allowance for protein, *p. 230*.

7 Discuss the relationship between a high-protein diet and heart disease, bone loss, and kidney disease, *pp. 231–233*.

8 Identify both animal and plant foods that are excellent sources of dietary protein, *pp. 233–237*.

9 Discuss the health benefits, challenges, and nutritional quality of a balanced and adequate vegetarian diet, *pp. 238–241*.

10 Describe two disorders related to inadequate protein intake or genetic abnormalities, *pp. 241–243*.

W hat do tennis pro Venus Williams, ultramarathon runner Scott Jurek, Olympic gold medalist skier Bode Miller, and dozens of other winning athletes have in common? They're vegetarians! Although statistics on the prevalence of vegetarianism among athletes aren't available, national surveys have found that 4% of all Americans age 8 and up report that they are vegetarian (never eat meat, poultry, or fish), and another 14% say that more than half of their meals are vegetarian.[1]

What exactly is a vegetarian? Do you qualify? If so, how do you plan your diet to include sufficient protein, especially if you play competitive sports? Are there real advantages to eating meat, or is plant protein just as good?

It seems as if everybody has an opinion about protein, both how much you should consume and from what sources. In this chapter, we address these and other questions to clarify the importance of protein in the diet and dispel common myths about this crucial nutrient.

What Are Proteins?

Proteins are large, complex molecules found in all living things. Although best known as a part of our muscle mass, proteins are critical components of all tissues of the human body, including bones, blood, and skin. They also function in metabolism, immunity, fluid balance, and nutrient transport, and they can provide energy in certain circumstances.

Like carbohydrates and lipids, proteins are made up of carbon, hydrogen, and oxygen. They also contain a special form of nitrogen that the body can readily use. Carbohydrates and lipids do not provide nitrogen. Proteins are available from a wide variety of both animal and plant foods. In addition, the human body is able to synthesize them according to instructions provided by our genetic material, or DNA. We'll explore how DNA dictates the structure of proteins shortly.

The Building Blocks of Proteins Are Amino Acids

The proteins in our body are made from a combination of building blocks called **amino acids,** molecules composed of a central carbon atom connected to four other groups: an amine group, an acid group, a hydrogen atom, and a side chain (**Figure 6.1a**). The word *amine* means "nitrogen-containing," and nitrogen is indeed the essential component of the amine portion of the molecule.

As shown in Figure 6.1b, the portion of the amino acid that makes each unique is its side chain. The amine group, acid group, and carbon and hydrogen atoms do not vary. Variations in the structure of the side chain give each amino acid its distinct properties.

The singular term *protein* is misleading, as there are potentially an infinite number of unique types of proteins in living organisms. Most of the body's proteins are made from combinations of just 20 amino acids, identified in **Table 6.1** (page 214). Two of the 20 amino acids listed in Table 6.1, cysteine and methionine, are unique in that their side chains contain sulfur. This property affects the types of chemical bonds they form. By combining a few dozen to more than 300 of these 20 amino acids in various sequences, our body synthesizes an estimated 10,000 to 50,000 unique proteins. **Figure 6.2** illustrates how the components of a protein differ from those of a carbohydrate, such as starch. As you can see, starch is composed of a chain of glucose molecules. In contrast, the protein insulin is composed of 51 amino acids connected in a specific order, or sequence. Notice that different regions of the molecule are connected by unique disulfide bridges linking the sulfur-containing cysteine amino acids. We'll discuss the structure of proteins in more detail shortly.

The Body Can Synthesize Only Some Amino Acids

Of the 20 amino acids in the body, nine are classified as essential. This does not mean that they are more important than the others. Instead, an **essential amino acid** is one that the

LO 1 Illustrate the structure of an amino acid molecule including its five essential components.

LO 2 Differentiate among essential amino acids, nonessential amino acids, and conditionally essential amino acids.

proteins Large, complex molecules made up of amino acids and found as essential components of all living cells.

amino acids Nitrogen-containing molecules that combine to form proteins.

essential amino acids Amino acids not produced by the body, or not produced in sufficient amounts, so they must be obtained from food.

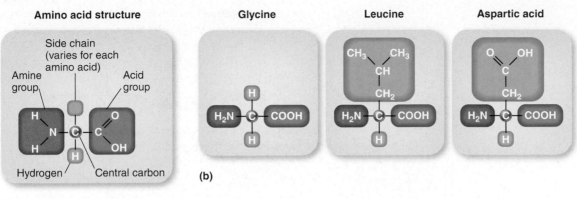

FIGURE 6.1 Structure of an amino acid. **(a)** All amino acids contain five parts: a central carbon atom, an amine group that contains nitrogen, an acid group, a hydrogen atom, and a side chain. **(b)** Only the side chain differs for each of the 20 amino acids, giving each its unique properties.

body cannot produce at all or cannot produce in sufficient quantities to meet its physiologic needs. Thus, essential amino acids must be obtained from food. Without the proper amount of essential amino acids in our bodies, we lose our ability to make the proteins and other nitrogen-containing compounds we need.

Nonessential amino acids are just as important to the body as essential amino acids, but the body can synthesize them in sufficient quantities, so we do not need to consume them in our diet. We make nonessential amino acids by transferring the amine group from other amino acids to a different acid group and side chain. This process is called **transamination** and it is shown in **Figure 6.3** (page 214). The acid groups and side chains can be donated by amino acids, or they can be made from the breakdown products of

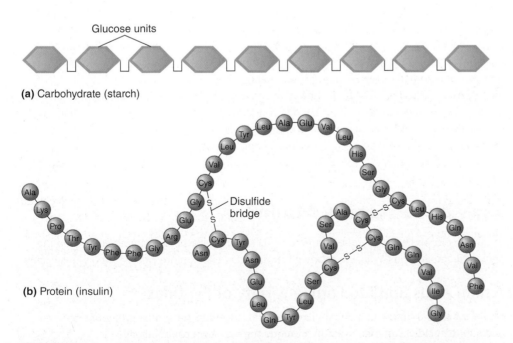

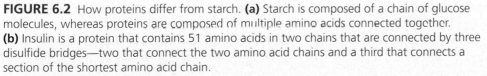

FIGURE 6.2 How proteins differ from starch. **(a)** Starch is composed of a chain of glucose molecules, whereas proteins are composed of multiple amino acids connected together. **(b)** Insulin is a protein that contains 51 amino acids in two chains that are connected by three disulfide bridges—two that connect the two amino acid chains and a third that connects a section of the shortest amino acid chain.

nonessential amino acids Amino acids that can be manufactured by the body in sufficient quantities and therefore do not need to be consumed regularly in our diet.

transamination The process of transferring the amine group from one amino acid to another in order to manufacture a new amino acid.

Transamination

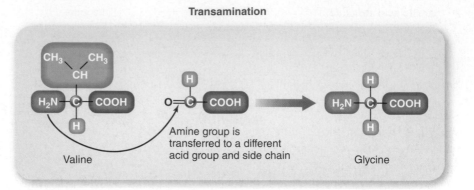

FIGURE 6.3 Transamination. Our bodies can make nonessential amino acids by transferring the amine group from an essential amino acid to a different acid group and side chain.

TABLE 6.1 Amino Acids of the Human Body

Essential Amino Acids	Nonessential Amino Acids
These amino acids must be consumed in the diet.	These amino acids can be manufactured by the body.
Histidine	Alanine
Isoleucine	Arginine
Leucine	Asparagine
Lysine	Aspartic acid
Methionine	Cysteine
Phenylalanine	Glutamic acid
Threonine	Glutamine
Tryptophan	Glycine
Valine	Proline
	Serine
	Tyrosine

carbohydrates and fats. Thus, by combining parts of different amino acids, the necessary nonessential amino acid can be made.

Under some conditions, a nonessential amino acid can become an essential amino acid. In this case, the amino acid is called a **conditionally essential amino acid.** Consider what occurs in the disease known as phenylketonuria (PKU). As previously discussed (in Chapter 4), someone with PKU cannot metabolize phenylalanine (an essential amino acid). Normally, the body uses phenylalanine to produce the nonessential amino acid tyrosine, so the inability to metabolize phenylalanine results in failure to make tyrosine. In this situation, tyrosine becomes a conditionally essential amino acid that must be provided by the diet. Other conditionally essential amino acids include arginine, cysteine, and glutamine.

RECAP

Proteins are critical components of all the tissues of the human body. Like carbohydrates and lipids, they contain carbon, hydrogen, and oxygen. Unlike the other macronutrients, they also contain nitrogen and some contain sulfur, and their structure is dictated by DNA. The building blocks of proteins are amino acids. The amine group of the amino acid contains nitrogen. The portion of the amino acid that changes, giving each amino acid its distinct identity, is the side chain. The body uses 20 amino acids. It cannot make nine essential amino acids, so we must obtain them from our diet. The body can make 11 nonessential amino acids from parts of other amino acids, carbohydrates, and fats. When the body's need to synthesize a nonessential amino acid exceeds its ability to do so, that amino acid is classified as conditionally essential.

 Explain how amino acids are assembled to form proteins and the relationship between protein shape and function.

conditionally essential amino acids Amino acids that are normally considered nonessential but become essential under certain circumstances when the body's need for them exceeds the ability to produce them.

peptide bond Unique types of chemical bond in which the amine group of one amino acid binds to the acid group of another in order to manufacture dipeptides and all larger peptide molecules.

How Are Proteins Made?

As stated, our bodies can synthesize proteins by selecting the needed amino acids from the pool of all amino acids available at any given time. Let's look more closely at how this occurs.

Amino Acids Bond to Form a Variety of Peptides

Figure 6.4 shows that, when two amino acids join together, the amine group of one binds to the acid group of another in a unique type of chemical bond called a **peptide bond.** In this dehydration synthesis reaction, a molecule of water is released as a by-product.

Two amino acids joined together form a *dipeptide,* and three amino acids joined together are called a *tripeptide.* The term *oligopeptide* is used to identify a string of four to nine amino acids, and a *polypeptide* is 10 or more amino acids bonded together.

As a polypeptide chain grows longer, it begins to fold into any of a variety of complex shapes that give proteins their sophisticated structure.

Genes Regulate Amino Acid Binding

Each of us is unique because we inherited a specific "code" that integrates the code from each of our parents. Each person's genetic code dictates minor differences in amino acid sequences, which in turn lead to differences in our bodies' individual proteins. These differences in proteins result in the unique physical and physiologic characteristics each one of us possesses.

The Structure of Genes

A *gene* is a segment of deoxyribonucleic acid (DNA) that serves as a template for the synthesis of a particular protein. All body cells (except mature red blood cells) contain a full set of that person's genes; however, individual cells *use* only some of their genes. **Gene expression** is the process by which cells use genes to make proteins.

The building blocks of DNA are **nucleotides,** molecules composed of a "backbone" made up of a phosphate group and a pentose sugar called deoxyribose, to which is attached one of four nitrogenous bases: adenine (A), guanine (G), cytosine (C), or thymine (T). Within DNA molecules, these nucleotides occur in two long, parallel chains coiled into the shape of a double helix (**Figure 6.5**, page 216). Because nucleotides vary only in their nitrogenous bases, the astonishing variability of DNA arises from the precise sequencing of nucleotides along these chains.

Chains of nucleotides are held together by hydrogen bonds that link their nitrogenous bases. Each base can bond only to its *complementary base:* A always bonds to T, and G always bonds to C. The complementary nature of bases guides the transfer of genetic instructions from DNA into the resulting protein.

Transcription and Translation

Proteins are actually manufactured at the site of ribosomes in the cell's cytoplasm. But DNA never leaves the nucleus. So for gene expression to occur, a gene's DNA has to replicate itself—that is, it must make an exact copy of itself, which can then be carried out to the cytoplasm. DNA replication ensures that the genetic information in the original gene is identical to the genetic information used to build the protein. Through the process of replication, DNA provides the instructions for building every protein in the body.

Nutrition
MILESTONE

In **1934**, Dr. Asbjøn Følling, a Norwegian physician and biochemist, examined children with mental retardation who were excreting urine that smelled unusually strong. He found that the urine contained a substance called phenylpyruvic acid, which is a by-product of the breakdown of the amino acid phenylalanine. Although a small amount of this by-product in the urine is normal, a large amount indicates an inability to completely break down phenylalanine. Initially named Følling's disease, this condition is now known as phenylketonuria, or PKU. It is a genetic disorder that causes a deficiency in the enzyme that breaks down phenylalanine.

In people with PKU, phenylalanine can build up in the body, causing brain damage, seizures, and psychiatric disorders. As a result of Følling's discovery, United States healthcare providers now screen the blood of all newborns for PKU. Those newborns found to have PKU are prescribed a diet low in phenylalanine, and they can develop into healthy children and adults.

gene expression The process of using a gene to make a protein.

nucleotide A molecule composed of a phosphate group, a pentose sugar called deoxyribose, and one of four nitrogenous bases: adenine (A), guanine (G), cytosine (C), or thymine (T).

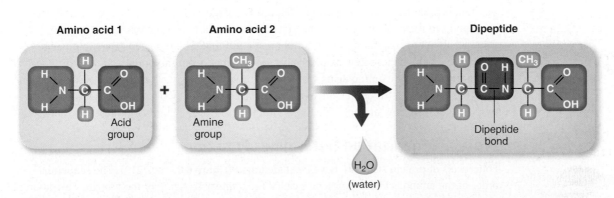

FIGURE 6.4 Amino acid bonding. Two amino acids join together to form a dipeptide. By combining multiple amino acids, proteins are made.

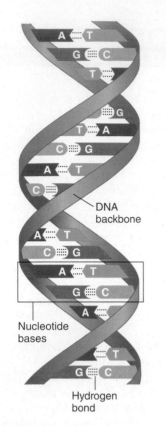

FIGURE 6.5 The double helix of DNA. DNA is a complex compound made up of molecules called nucleotides, each of which consists of a deoxyribose sugar and phosphate backbone and a nitrogenous base. Hydrogen bonding of complementary bases holds the two strands of DNA together.

transcription The process through which messenger RNA copies genetic information from DNA in the nucleus.

translation The process that occurs when the genetic information carried by messenger RNA is translated into a chain of amino acids at the ribosome.

Cells use a special molecule to copy, or transcribe, the information from DNA and carry it to the ribosomes. This molecule is *messenger RNA* (*messenger ribonucleic acid*, or *mRNA*). In contrast with DNA, RNA is a single strand of nucleotides, and its four nitrogenous bases are A, G, C, and U ("U" stands for uracil, which takes the place of the thymine found in DNA). Also, as its name suggests, it contains the pentose sugar ribose instead of deoxyribose. During **transcription**, mRNA copies to its own base sequence the genetic information from DNA's base sequence (**Focus Figure 6.6,** no. 1). The mRNA then detaches from the DNA and leaves the nucleus, carrying its genetic "message" to the ribosomes in the cytoplasm (Focus Figure 6.6, no. 2).

Once the genetic information reaches the ribosomes, **translation** occurs; that is, the language of the mRNA nucleotide sequences is translated into the language of amino acid sequences, or proteins. At the ribosomes, mRNA binds with ribosomal RNA (rRNA) and its nucleotide sequences are distributed, somewhat like orders for parts in an assembly plant, to molecules of transfer RNA (tRNA) (Focus Figure 6.6, no. 3). Now the tRNA molecules roam the cytoplasm until they succeed in binding with the specific amino acid that matches their "order." They then transfer their amino acid to the ribosome, which assembles the amino acids into proteins (Focus Figure 6.6, no. 4). Once the amino acids are loaded onto the ribosome, tRNA works to maneuver each amino acid into its proper position (Focus Figure 6.6, no. 5). When synthesis of the new protein is completed, it is released from the ribosome and can either go through further modification in the cell or can be functional in its current state (Focus Figure 6.6, no. 6).

The proper sequencing of amino acids determines both the shape and function of a particular protein. Genetic abnormalities can occur when the DNA contains errors in proper nucleotide sequencing or when mistakes occur in the translation of this sequencing. Two examples of the consequences of these types of genetic abnormalities, sickle cell anemia and cystic fibrosis, are discussed later in this chapter.

Again, although the genes for making every protein in our bodies are contained within each cell nucleus, not all genes are expressed and each cell does not make every type of protein. For example, each cell contains the DNA to manufacture the hormone insulin. However, only the beta cells of the pancreas *express* the insulin gene to produce insulin. As we explored (in the ***Nutrition Myth or Fact?*** in Chapter 1), our physiologic needs alter gene expression, as do various nutrients. For instance, a cut in the skin that causes bleeding will prompt the production of various proteins that clot the blood. Or if we consume more dietary iron than we need, the gene for ferritin (a protein that stores iron) will be expressed, so that we can store this excess iron. Our genetic makeup and how appropriately we express our genes are important factors in our health.

Protein Turnover Involves Synthesis and Degradation

Our bodies constantly require new proteins to function properly. *Protein turnover* involves both the synthesis of new proteins and the degradation of existing proteins to provide the building blocks for those new proteins (**Figure 6.7**, page 218). This process allows the cells to respond to the constantly changing demands of physiologic functions. For instance, skin cells live only for about 30 days and must continually be replaced. The amino acids needed to produce these new skin cells can be obtained from the body's *amino acid pool*, which includes those amino acids we consume in our diet as well as those that are released from the breakdown of other cells in our bodies. The body's pool of amino acids is used to produce not only new amino acids but also other products, including glucose, fat, and urea.

Protein Organization Determines Function

Four levels of protein structure have been identified (**Figure 6.8**, page 219). The sequential order of the amino acids in a protein is called the *primary structure* of the protein. The different amino acids in a polypeptide chain possess unique chemical attributes that cause the chain to twist and turn into a characteristic spiral shape, or to fold into a so-called pleated sheet.

focus figure 6.6 | Protein Synthesis

Cell ——
Nucleus ——

In the nucleus, genetic information from DNA is transcribed by messenger RNA (mRNA), which then carries it to ribosomes in the cytoplasm, where this genetic information is translated into a chain of amino acids that eventually make a protein.

1 Part of the DNA unwinds, and a section of its genetic code is transcribed to the mRNA inside the nucleus.

2 The mRNA leaves the nucleus via a nuclear pore and travels to the cytoplasm.

3 Once the mRNA reaches the cytoplasm, it binds to a ribosome via ribosomal RNA (rRNA). The code on the mRNA is translated into the instructions for a specific order of amino acids.

4 The transfer RNA (tRNA) binds with specific amino acids in the cytoplasm and transfers the amino acids to the ribosome as dictated by the mRNA code.

5 The amino acid is added to the growing amino acid chain, and the tRNA returns to the cytoplasm.

6 Once the synthesis of the new protein is complete, the protein is released from the ribosome. The protein may go through further modifications in the cell or can be functional in its current state.

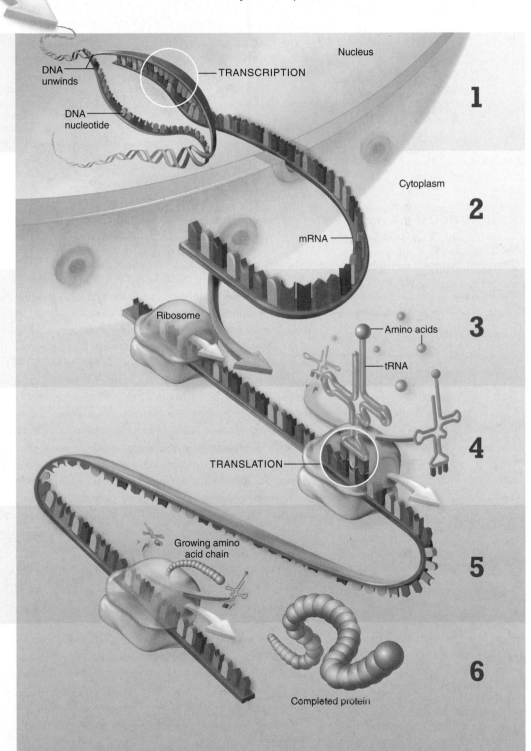

Nucleus

DNA unwinds

DNA nucleotide

TRANSCRIPTION

Cytoplasm

mRNA

Ribosome

Amino acids

tRNA

TRANSLATION

Growing amino acid chain

Completed protein

1

2

3

4

5

6

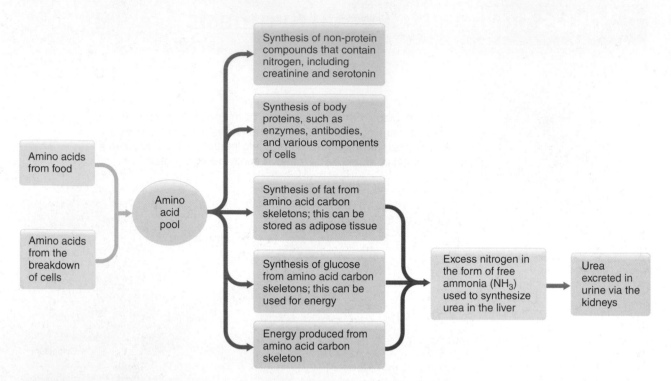

FIGURE 6.7 Protein turnover involves the synthesis of new proteins and the breakdown of existing proteins to provide building blocks for new proteins. Amino acids are drawn from the body's amino acid pool and can be used to build proteins, fat, glucose, and non-protein nitrogen-containing compounds. Urea is produced as a waste product from any excess nitrogen, which is then excreted by the kidneys.

These shapes are also referred to as the protein's *secondary structure*. The stability of the secondary structure is achieved by hydrogen bonds that create a bridge between two protein strands or two parts of the same strand of protein (see Figure 6.2). The spiral or pleated sheet of the secondary structure further folds into a unique three-dimensional shape, referred to as the protein's *tertiary structure*. Both hydrogen bonds and disulfide bridges between sulfur atoms maintain the tertiary shape, which is critically important because it determines each protein's function in the body. Often, two or more identical or different polypeptides bond to form an even larger protein with a *quaternary structure*, which may be *globular* or *fibrous*.

The importance of the shape of a protein to its function cannot be overemphasized. For example, the protein strands in muscle fibers are much longer than they are wide (Figure 6.8d). This structure plays an essential role in enabling muscle contraction and relaxation. In contrast, the proteins that form red blood cells are globular in shape, and they result in the red blood cells being shaped like flattened discs with depressed centers, similar to a miniature doughnut (**Figure 6.9,** page 219). This structure and the flexibility of the proteins in the red blood cells permit them to change shape and flow freely through even the tiniest capillaries to deliver oxygen and still return to their original shape.

Protein Denaturation Affects Shape and Function

Proteins can uncoil and lose their shape when they are exposed to heat, acids, bases, heavy metals, alcohol, and other damaging substances. The term used to describe this change in the shape of proteins is **denaturation.** Everyday examples of protein denaturation that we can see are the stiffening of egg whites when they are whipped, the curdling of milk when lemon juice or another acid is added, and the solidifying of eggs as they cook.

Denaturation does not affect the primary structure of proteins. However, when a protein is denatured, its function is also lost. For instance, denaturation of critical body proteins on exposure to heat or acidity is harmful, because it prevents them from performing their functions. This type of denaturation can occur during times of high fever or when blood pH is out of the normal range. In some cases, however, denaturation is helpful. For instance,

denaturation The process by which proteins uncoil and lose their shape and function when they are exposed to heat, acids, bases, heavy metals, alcohol, and other damaging substances.

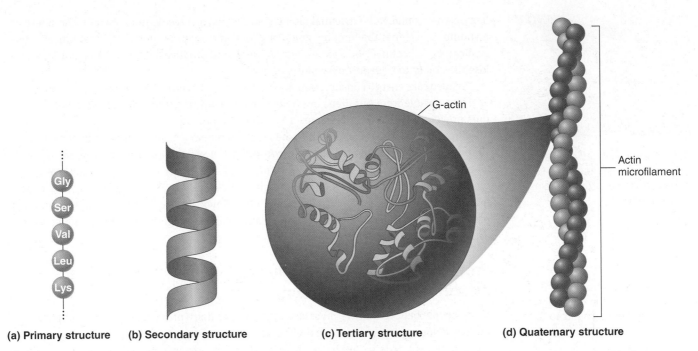

(a) Primary structure   **(b) Secondary structure**   **(c) Tertiary structure**   **(d) Quaternary structure**

FIGURE 6.8 Levels of protein structure. **(a)** The primary structure of a protein is the sequential order of amino acids. **(b)** The secondary structure of a protein is the twisting or folding of the amino acid chain. **(c)** The tertiary structure is a further folding that results in the three-dimensional shape of the protein. **(d)** In proteins with a quaternary structure, two or more polypeptides interact, forming a larger protein, such as the actin molecule illustrated here. In this figure, strands of actin molecules intertwine to form contractile elements involved in generating muscle contractions.

denaturation of proteins during the digestive process allows for their breakdown into amino acids and the absorption of these amino acids from the digestive tract into the bloodstream.

Protein Synthesis Can Be Limited by Missing Amino Acids

For protein synthesis to occur, all essential amino acids must be available to the cell. If this is not the case, the amino acid that is missing or in the smallest supply is called the **limiting amino acid.** Without the proper combination and quantity of essential amino acids, protein synthesis slows to the point at which proteins cannot be generated. For instance, the protein

limiting amino acid The essential amino acid that is missing or in the smallest supply in the amino acid pool and is thus responsible for slowing or halting protein synthesis.

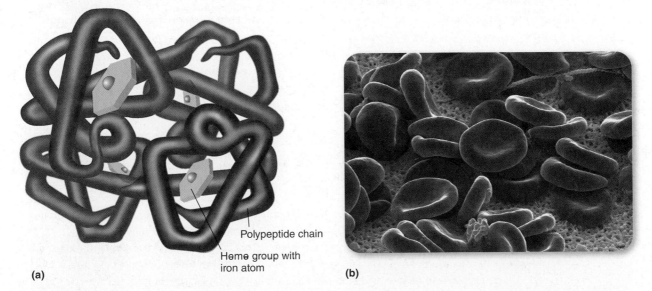

Polypeptide chain

Heme group with iron atom

(a)

(b)

FIGURE 6.9 Protein shape determines function. **(a)** Hemoglobin, the protein that forms red blood cells, is globular in shape. **(b)** The globular shape of hemoglobin results in red blood cells being shaped like flattened discs.

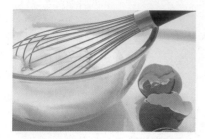

Stiffening egg whites adds air through the beating action, which denatures some of the proteins within them.

incomplete proteins Foods that do not contain all of the essential amino acids in sufficient amounts to support growth and health.

complete proteins Foods that contain sufficient amounts of all nine essential amino acids.

mutual supplementation The process of combining two or more incomplete protein sources to make a complete protein.

hemoglobin contains the essential amino acid histidine. If we do not consume enough histidine, it becomes the limiting amino acid in hemoglobin production. As no other amino acid can be substituted, our bodies become unable to produce adequate hemoglobin, and we lose the ability to transport oxygen to our cells.

Inadequate energy consumption also limits protein synthesis. If there is not enough energy available from our diets, our bodies will use any accessible amino acids for energy, thus preventing them from being used to build new proteins.

Protein that do not contain all of the essential amino acids in sufficient quantities to support growth and health are called **incomplete** (*low-quality*) **proteins.** Proteins that have all nine of the essential amino acids in sufficient quantities are considered **complete** (*high-quality*) **proteins.** The most complete protein sources are foods derived from animals and include egg whites, meat, poultry, fish, and milk. Soybeans are the most complete source of plant protein. In general, the typical American diet is very high in complete proteins, as we eat proteins from a variety of food sources.

Protein Synthesis Can Be Enhanced by Mutual Supplementation

Many people believe that we must consume meat or dairy products to obtain complete proteins. Not true! Consider a meal of beans and rice. Beans are low in the amino acids methionine and cysteine but have adequate amounts of isoleucine and lysine. Rice is low in isoleucine and lysine but contains sufficient methionine and cysteine. By combining beans and rice, a complete protein source is created.

Mutual supplementation is the process of combining two or more incomplete protein sources to make a complete protein. The two foods involved are called complementary foods; these foods provide **complementary proteins** (**Figure 6.10**) which, when combined, provide all nine essential amino acids.

Combining Complementary Foods

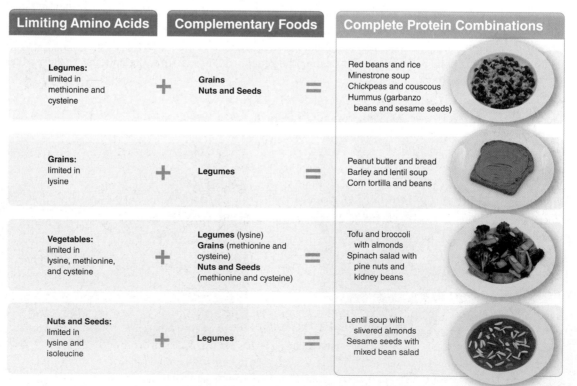

Limiting Amino Acids	Complementary Foods	Complete Protein Combinations
Legumes: limited in methionine and cysteine	**+** **Grains** **Nuts and Seeds**	**=** Red beans and rice Minestrone soup Chickpeas and couscous Hummus (garbanzo beans and sesame seeds)
Grains: limited in lysine	**+** **Legumes**	**=** Peanut butter and bread Barley and lentil soup Corn tortilla and beans
Vegetables: limited in lysine, methionine, and cysteine	**+** **Legumes** (lysine) **Grains** (methionine and cysteine) **Nuts and Seeds** (methionine and cysteine)	**=** Tofu and broccoli with almonds Spinach salad with pine nuts and kidney beans
Nuts and Seeds: limited in lysine and isoleucine	**+** **Legumes**	**=** Lentil soup with slivered almonds Sesame seeds with mixed bean salad

FIGURE 6.10 Complementary food combinations.

It is not necessary to eat complementary proteins at the same meal. Recall that we maintain a free pool of amino acids in the blood; these amino acids come from food and sloughed-off cells. When we eat one complementary protein, its amino acids join those in the free amino acid pool. These free amino acids can then combine to synthesize complete proteins. However, it is wise to eat complementary-protein foods during the same day, as partially completed proteins cannot be stored and saved for a later time. Mutual supplementation is important for people eating a vegetarian diet, particularly if they consume no animal products whatsoever.

RECAP

Amino acids bind via peptide bonds to form proteins. Genes regulate the amino acid sequence, and thus the structure, of all proteins. During transcription, mRNA copies to its own base sequence the genetic information from DNA. mRNA carries this information from the cell nucleus to the ribosomes in the cytoplasm, where translation into proteins occurs. Protein turnover involves the synthesis and degradation of proteins, so that the body can constantly adapt to a changing environment. The shape of a protein determines its function. When a protein is denatured by heat or damaging substances, such as acids, it loses its shape and its function. When a particular amino acid is limiting, protein synthesis cannot occur. A complete protein provides all nine essential amino acids. Mutual supplementation combines two or more complementary-protein sources to make a complete protein. ∎

How Does the Body Break Down Proteins?

LO 4 Discuss how proteins are digested and absorbed by the body.

In this section, we will review how proteins are digested and absorbed. As you review each step in this process, refer to **Focus Figure 6.11** (page 222) for a visual overview of the process of protein digestion.

Stomach Acids and Enzymes Break Proteins into Short Polypeptides

Virtually no enzymatic digestion of proteins occurs in the mouth. As shown in Focus Figure 6.11, proteins in food are chewed, crushed, and moistened with saliva to ease swallowing and to increase the surface area of the protein for more efficient digestion. There is no further digestive action on proteins in the mouth.

When proteins reach the stomach, hydrochloric acid denatures the protein strands. It also converts the inactive enzyme, *pepsinogen*, into its active form, **pepsin,** which is a protein-digesting enzyme. Although pepsin is itself a protein, it is not denatured by the acid in the stomach because it has evolved to work optimally in an acidic environment. The hormone *gastrin* controls both the production of hydrochloric acid and the release of pepsin; thinking about food or actually chewing food stimulates the gastrin-producing cells located in the stomach. Pepsin begins breaking proteins into single amino acids and shorter polypeptides via hydrolysis; these amino acids and polypeptides then travel to the small intestine for further digestion and absorption.

Enzymes in the Small Intestine Break Polypeptides into Single Amino Acids

As the polypeptides reach the small intestine, the pancreas and the small intestine secrete enzymes that digest them into oligopeptides, tripeptides, dipeptides, and single amino acids (see Focus Figure 6.11). The enzymes that digest polypeptides are called **proteases;** proteases found in the small intestine include trypsin, chymotrypsin, and carboxypeptidase.

The cells in the wall of the small intestine then absorb the single amino acids, dipeptides, and tripeptides. Peptidases, enzymes located in the intestinal cells, break the

complementary proteins Proteins contained in two or more foods that together contain all nine essential amino acids necessary for a complete protein. It is not necessary to eat complementary proteins at the same meal.

pepsin An enzyme in the stomach that begins the breakdown of proteins into shorter polypeptide chains and single amino acids.

proteases Enzymes that continue the breakdown of polypeptides in the small intestine.

focus figure 6.11 | Protein Digestion Overview

Digestion of dietary proteins into single amino acids occurs primarily in the stomach and small intestine. The single amino acids are then transported to the liver, where they may be converted to glucose or fat, used for energy or to build new proteins, or transported to cells as needed.

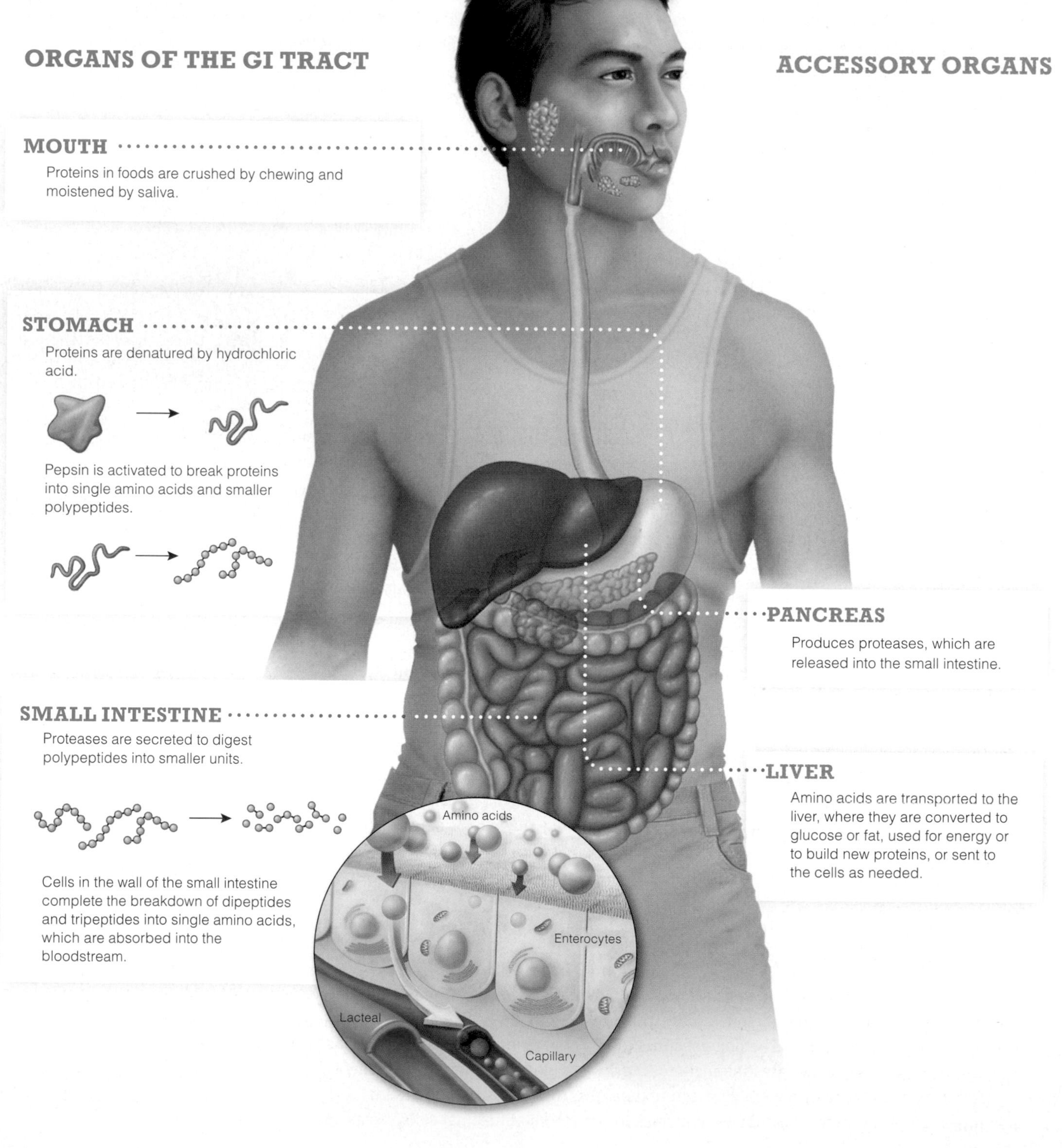

ORGANS OF THE GI TRACT
ACCESSORY ORGANS
MOUTH
Proteins in foods are crushed by chewing and moistened by saliva.
STOMACH
Proteins are denatured by hydrochloric acid.
Pepsin is activated to break proteins into single amino acids and smaller polypeptides.
SMALL INTESTINE
Proteases are secreted to digest polypeptides into smaller units.
Cells in the wall of the small intestine complete the breakdown of dipeptides and tripeptides into single amino acids, which are absorbed into the bloodstream.
Amino acids
Enterocytes
Lacteal
Capillary
PANCREAS
Produces proteases, which are released into the small intestine.
LIVER
Amino acids are transported to the liver, where they are converted to glucose or fat, used for energy or to build new proteins, or sent to the cells as needed.

dipeptides and tripeptides into single amino acids. Dipeptidases break dipeptide bonds, whereas tripeptidases break tripeptide bonds. The amino acids are then transported via the portal vein to the liver. Once in the liver, amino acids may be converted to glucose or fat, combined to build new proteins, used for energy, or released into the bloodstream and transported to other cells as needed (see Focus Figure 6.11).

The cells of the small intestine have different sites that specialize in transporting certain types of amino acids, dipeptides, and tripeptides. This fact has implications for users of amino acid supplements. When very large doses of supplements containing single amino acids are taken on an empty stomach, they typically compete for the same absorption sites. This competition can block the absorption of other amino acids and could in theory lead to deficiencies. In reality, people rarely take very large doses of single amino acids on an empty stomach. We discuss the use of amino acid supplements in more detail later in this chapter.

Protein Digestibility Affects Protein Quality

Earlier in this chapter, we discussed how various protein sources differ in quality of protein. The quantity of essential amino acids in a protein determines its quality: higher-protein-quality foods are those that contain more of the essential amino acids in sufficient quantities needed to build proteins, and lower-protein-quality foods contain fewer essential amino acids.

A number of methods are used to estimate a food's protein quality. One method is to calculate a *chemical score*. A **chemical score** is a comparison of the amount of the limiting amino acid in a food to the amount of the same amino acid in a reference food. The amino acid that is found to have the lowest proportion in the test food as compared to the reference food is defined as the limiting amino acid. Thus, the chemical score of a protein gives an indication of the lowest amino acid ratio calculated for any amino acid in a particular food.

Another factor in protein quality is *digestibility*, or how well our bodies can digest a protein. The **protein digestibility corrected amino acid score (PDCAAS)** uses the chemical score and a correction factor for digestibility to calculate a value for protein quality. Proteins with higher digestibility are more complete. Animal protein sources, such as meat and dairy products, are highly digestible, as are many soy products; we can absorb more than 90% of these protein sources. Legumes are also highly digestible (about 70% to 80%). Grains and many vegetable proteins are less digestible, with PDCAAS values ranging from 60% to 90%.

These measures of protein quality are useful when determining the quality of protein available to populations of people. However, these measures are impractical and are not used for individual diet planning.

chemical score A method used to estimate a food's protein quality; it is a comparison of the amount of the limiting amino acid in a food to the amount of the same amino acid in a reference food.

protein digestibility corrected amino acid score (PDCAAS) A measurement of protein quality that considers the balance of amino acids as well as the digestibility of the protein in the food.

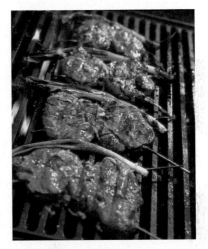

Meats are highly digestible sources of dietary protein.

RECAP

In the stomach, hydrochloric acid denatures proteins and converts pepsinogen to pepsin; pepsin breaks proteins into smaller polypeptides and individual amino acids. In the small intestine, proteases break polypeptides into smaller fragments and single amino acids. Enzymes in the cells in the wall of the small intestine break the smaller peptide fragments into single amino acids, which are then transported to the liver for distribution to our cells. Taking high doses of individual amino acid supplements can lead to deficiencies of other amino acids. Protein digestibility and the provision of essential amino acids influence protein quality.

Why Do We Need Proteins?

LO 5 Describe at least four functions of proteins in the body.

The functions of proteins in the body are so numerous that only a few can be described in detail in this chapter. Note that proteins function most effectively when we also consume adequate amounts of energy as carbohydrates and fat. When there is not enough energy available, the body uses proteins as an energy source, limiting their availability for the functions described in this section.

Proteins Contribute to Cell Growth, Repair, and Maintenance

The proteins in the body are dynamic, meaning that they are constantly being broken down, repaired, and replaced. When proteins are broken down, many amino acids are recycled into new proteins. Think about all of the new proteins that are needed to allow an embryo to develop and grow. In this case, an entirely new human body is being made! In fact, a newborn baby has more than 10 trillion body cells.

Even in adulthood, all cells are constantly turning over, as damaged or worn-out cells are broken down and their components are used to create new cells. Red blood cells live for only about 4 months and then are replaced by new cells that are produced in bone marrow. The cells lining the intestinal tract are replaced every 3 to 6 days. The "old" intestinal cells are treated just like the proteins in food; they are digested and the amino acids absorbed back into the body. The constant turnover of proteins from our diet is essential for such cell growth, repair, and maintenance.

Proteins Act as Enzymes and Hormones

Recall that enzymes are compounds—usually proteins—that speed up chemical reactions, without being changed by the chemical reaction themselves. Enzymes can increase the rate at which reactants bond, break apart, or exchange components. Each cell contains thousands of enzymes that facilitate specific cellular reactions. For example, the enzyme phosphofructokinase (PFK) is critical to driving the rate at which we break down glucose and use it for energy during exercise. Without PFK, we would be unable to generate energy at a fast enough rate to allow us to be physically active.

Although some hormones are made from lipids, many are made from amino acids or from peptides. For example, thyroid hormone, which regulates many aspects of metabolism, is an amino acid hormone, and insulin, which acts on cell membranes to facilitate the transport of glucose into cells, is a peptide hormone (see Figure 6.2b).

Proteins Help Maintain Fluid and Electrolyte Balance

Electrolytes are electrically charged atoms (ions) that assist in maintaining fluid balance. For our bodies to function properly, fluids and electrolytes must be maintained at healthy levels inside and outside cells and within blood vessels. Proteins attract fluids, and the proteins that are in the bloodstream, in the cells, and in the spaces surrounding the cells work together to keep fluids moving across these spaces in the proper quantities to maintain fluid balance and blood pressure. When protein intake is deficient, the concentration of proteins in the bloodstream is insufficient to draw fluid from the tissues and across the blood vessel walls; fluid then collects in the tissues, causing **edema** (**Figure 6.12**). In addition to being uncomfortable, edema can lead to serious medical problems.

Sodium (Na^+) and potassium (K^+) are examples of common electrolytes. Under normal conditions, Na^+ is more concentrated outside the cell, and K^+ is more concentrated inside the cell. This proper balance of Na^+ and K^+ is accomplished by the action of **transport proteins** located within the cell membrane. **Figure 6.13** (page 226) shows how these transport proteins work to pump Na^+ outside and K^+ inside of the cell. The conduction of nerve signals and contraction of muscles depend on a proper balance of electrolytes. If protein intake is deficient, we lose our ability to maintain these functions, resulting in potentially fatal changes in the rhythm of the heart. Other consequences of chronically low protein intakes include muscle weakness and spasms, kidney failure, and, if conditions are severe enough, death.

Proteins Help Maintain Acid–Base Balance

The body's cellular processes result in the constant production of acids and bases. These substances are transported in the blood to be excreted through the kidneys and the lungs. The human body maintains very tight control over the pH, or the acid–base balance, of the blood (see Chapter 3). The body goes into a state called **acidosis** when the blood becomes

edema A potentially serious disorder in which fluids build up in the tissue spaces of the body, causing fluid imbalances and a swollen appearance.

transport proteins Protein molecules that help transport substances throughout the body and across cell membranes.

acidosis A disorder in which the blood becomes acidic; that is, the level of hydrogen in the blood is excessive. It can be caused by respiratory or metabolic problems.

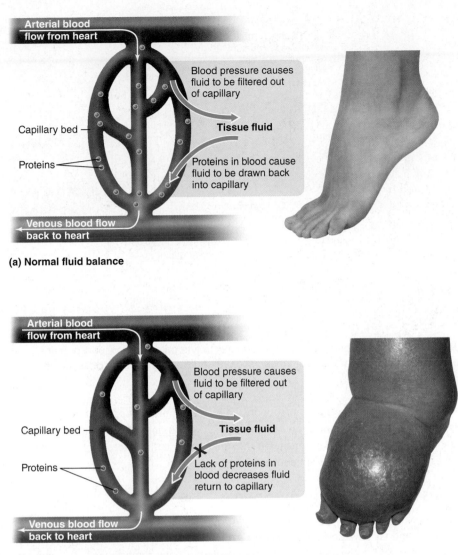

(a) Normal fluid balance

Arterial blood flow from heart

Blood pressure causes fluid to be filtered out of capillary

Capillary bed

Tissue fluid

Proteins

Proteins in blood cause fluid to be drawn back into capillary

Venous blood flow back to heart

(b) Edema caused by insufficient protein in bloodstream

Arterial blood flow from heart

Blood pressure causes fluid to be filtered out of capillary

Capillary bed

Tissue fluid

Proteins

Lack of proteins in blood decreases fluid return to capillary

Venous blood flow back to heart

FIGURE 6.12 The role of proteins in maintaining fluid balance. The heartbeat exerts pressure that continually pushes fluids in the bloodstream through the arterial walls and out into the tissue spaces. By the time blood reaches the veins, the pressure of the heartbeat has greatly decreased. In this environment, proteins in the blood are able to draw fluids out of the tissues and back into the bloodstream. **(a)** This healthy (non-swollen) tissue suggests that body fluids in the bloodstream and in the tissue spaces are in balance. **(b)** When the level of proteins in the blood is insufficient to draw fluids out of the tissues, edema can result. This foot with edema is swollen due to fluid imbalance.

too acidic. **Alkalosis** results if the blood becomes too basic. Both acidosis and alkalosis can be caused by respiratory or metabolic problems. Acidosis and alkalosis can cause coma and death by denaturing body proteins.

Proteins are excellent **buffers,** meaning they help maintain proper acid–base balance. Acids contain hydrogen ions, which are positively charged. The side chains of proteins have negative charges that attract the hydrogen ions and neutralize their detrimental effects on the body. Proteins can release the hydrogen ions when the blood becomes too basic. By buffering acids and bases, proteins maintain acid–base balance and blood pH.

Proteins Help Maintain a Strong Immune System

Antibodies are special proteins that are critical components of the immune system. When a foreign substance attacks the body, the immune system produces antibodies to defend against it. Bacteria, viruses, toxins, and allergens (substances that cause allergic reactions) are examples of *antigens;* that is, substances that generate antibody production.

Each antibody is designed to target one specific antigen. When that substance invades the body, antibodies are produced to neutralize it or tag it for destruction by immune cells. Once antibodies have been made, the body "remembers" this process and can respond more quickly the next time that invader appears. *Immunity* refers to the development of the molecular memory to produce antibodies quickly upon subsequent invasions.

alkalosis A disorder in which the blood becomes basic; that is, the level of hydrogen in the blood is deficient. It can be caused by respiratory or metabolic problems.

buffers Proteins that help maintain proper acid–base balance by attaching to, or releasing, hydrogen ions as conditions change in the body.

antibodies Defensive proteins of the immune system. Their production is prompted by the presence of bacteria, viruses, toxins, and allergens.

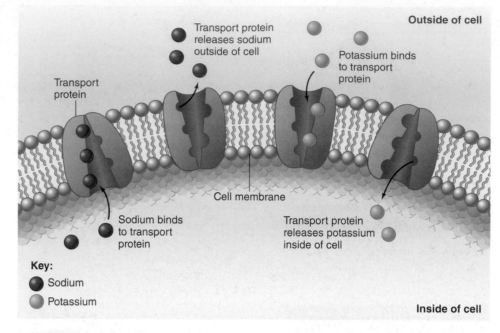

FIGURE 6.13 Transport proteins help maintain electrolyte balance. Transport proteins in the cell membrane pick up potassium and sodium and transport them across the cell membrane.

Adequate protein is necessary to support the increased production of antibodies that occurs in response to a cold, flu, or other infection. If we do not consume enough protein, our resistance to infection is weakened. On the other hand, eating more protein than we need does not improve immune function.

Proteins Serve as an Energy Source

The body's primary energy sources are carbohydrate and fat. Remember that both carbohydrate and fat have specialized storage forms that can be used for energy—glycogen for carbohydrate and triglycerides for fat. Proteins do not have a specialized storage form for energy. This means that, when proteins need to be used for energy, they are taken from the blood and body tissues, such as the liver and skeletal muscle. In healthy people, proteins contribute very little to energy needs. Because we are efficient at recycling amino acids, protein needs are relatively low compared to needs for carbohydrate and fat.

To use proteins for energy, the liver removes the amine group from the amino acids in a process called **deamination.** The nitrogen bonds with hydrogen, creating ammonia, which is a toxic compound that can upset acid–base balance. To avoid this, the liver quickly combines ammonia with carbon dioxide to make *urea*, which is much less toxic. The urea is then transported via the bloodstream to the kidneys, where the urea is filtered out of the blood and is subsequently excreted in the urine (**Figure 6.14**). The remaining fragments of the amino acid contain carbon, hydrogen, and oxygen. The body can use these fragments to generate energy or to build carbohydrates. Certain amino acids can be converted into glucose via gluconeogenesis. This is a critical process during times of low carbohydrate intake or starvation. Fat cannot be converted into glucose, but body proteins can be broken down and converted into glucose to provide needed energy to the brain.

To protect the proteins in our body tissues, it is important that we regularly eat an adequate amount of carbohydrate and fat to provide energy. We also need to consume enough dietary protein to meet our needs without drawing on the proteins that already are playing an active role in our bodies. Unfortunately, the body cannot store excess dietary protein. As a consequence, eating too much protein results in the removal and excretion of the nitrogen in the urine and the use of the remaining components for energy. Any remaining components not used for energy can be converted and stored as body fat.

deamination The process by which an amine group is removed from an amino acid. The nitrogen is then transported to the kidneys for excretion in the urine, and the carbon and other components are metabolized for energy or used to make other compounds.

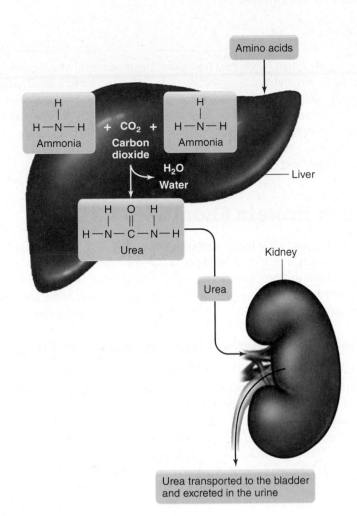

FIGURE 6.14 Urea excretion. The process of deamination leads to the creation of ammonia, which the liver quickly combines with carbon dioxide to make urea. The urea is then transported via the bloodstream to the kidneys, where the urea is filtered out of the blood and is subsequently excreted in the urine.

Proteins Assist in the Transport and Storage of Nutrients

Proteins act as carriers for many important nutrients in the body. As previously discussed (in Chapter 5), lipoproteins contain lipids bound to proteins, which allows the transport of hydrophobic lipids through the watery medium of blood. Another example of a transport protein is transferrin, which carries iron in the blood. Ferritin, in contrast, is an example of a storage protein: it is the compound in which iron is stored in the liver.

As discussed on page 226, transport proteins are located in cell membranes and allow for the proper transport of many nutrients across the cell membrane. These transport proteins also help in the maintenance of fluid and electrolyte balance and conduction of nerve impulses.

Other Roles of Proteins

The amino acids from proteins can also be used to make compounds such as **neurotransmitters,** which are chemical messengers that transmit messages from one nerve cell to another. Examples of neurotransmitters include epinephrine and norepinephrine, both of which stimulate the sympathetic nervous system, and *melatonin*, which plays a critical role in the regulation of sleep. Proteins also assist in blood clotting via a mass of protein fibers called *fibrin;* fibrin is developed from the protein *fibrinogen.* Connective tissue, the most abundant type of tissue in the body, is composed mainly of another protein, *collagen.*

 To learn more about how blood clots and wounds heal, go to www.medlineplus.gov, click on "Videos and Cool Tools," then click on "Anatomy Videos," and then click "blood clotting."

neurotransmitters Chemical messengers that transmit messages from one nerve cell to another.

RECAP

Proteins serve many important functions: (1) enabling the production, growth, repair, and maintenance of body cells and tissues; (2) acting as enzymes and hormones; (3) maintaining fluid and electrolyte balance; (4) maintaining acid–base balance; (5) making antibodies, important proteins of the immune system; (6) providing energy when carbohydrate and fat intake are inadequate; (7) transporting and storing nutrients; and (8) producing compounds such as neurotransmitters, fibrin, and collagen. Proteins function best when adequate amounts of energy, carbohydrate, and fat are consumed. ■

 LO 6 Calculate an individual's Recommended Dietary Allowance for protein.

LO 7 Discuss the relationship between a high-protein diet and heart disease, bone loss, and kidney disease.

LO 8 Identify both animal and plant foods that are excellent sources of dietary protein.

How Much Protein Should We Eat?

Consuming adequate protein is a major concern of many people. In fact, one of the most common concerns of active people and athletes is that their diets are deficient in protein (see the *Nutrition Myth or Fact?* essay at the end of this chapter for a discussion of this topic). This concern about dietary protein is generally unnecessary, as we can easily consume the protein our bodies need by eating an adequate and varied diet.

Nitrogen Balance Is a Method Used to Determine Protein Needs

A highly specialized procedure referred to as *nitrogen balance* is used to determine a person's protein needs. Nitrogen is excreted through the body's processes of recycling or using proteins; thus, the balance can be used to estimate if protein intake is adequate to meet protein needs.

Typically performed only in experimental laboratories, the nitrogen-balance procedure involves measuring both nitrogen intake and nitrogen excretion over a 2-week period. A standardized diet, the nitrogen content of which has been measured and recorded, is fed to the study participant. The person is required to consume all of the foods provided. Because the majority of nitrogen is excreted in the urine and feces, laboratory technicians directly measure the nitrogen content of the subject's urine and fecal samples. Small amounts of nitrogen are excreted in the skin, hair, and body fluids such as mucus and semen, but because of the complexity of collecting nitrogen excreted via these routes, the measurements are estimated. Then, technicians add the estimated nitrogen losses to the nitrogen measured in the subject's urine and feces. Nitrogen balance is then calculated as the difference between nitrogen intake and nitrogen excretion.

People who consume more nitrogen than is excreted are considered to be in positive nitrogen balance (**Figure 6.15**). This state indicates that the body is retaining or adding protein, and it occurs during periods of growth, pregnancy, or recovery from illness or a protein deficiency. People who excrete more nitrogen than is consumed are in negative nitrogen balance. This situation indicates that the body is losing protein, and it occurs during starvation or when people are consuming very-low-energy diets. This is because, when energy intake is too low to meet energy demands over a prolonged period of time, the body metabolizes body proteins for energy. The nitrogen from these proteins is excreted in the urine and feces. Negative nitrogen balance also occurs during severe illness, infections, high fever, serious burns, or injuries that cause significant blood loss. People in these situations require increased dietary protein. A person is in nitrogen balance when nitrogen intake equals nitrogen excretion. This indicates that protein intake is sufficient to cover protein needs. Healthy adults who are not pregnant are in nitrogen balance.

Although nitrogen balance has been used for many years as a method to estimate protein needs in humans, it has been criticized because it is so time and labor-intensive for both research participants and scientists. In addition, because it is not possible to collect and measure all of the nitrogen excreted each day, this method is recognized as underestimating protein needs.[2]

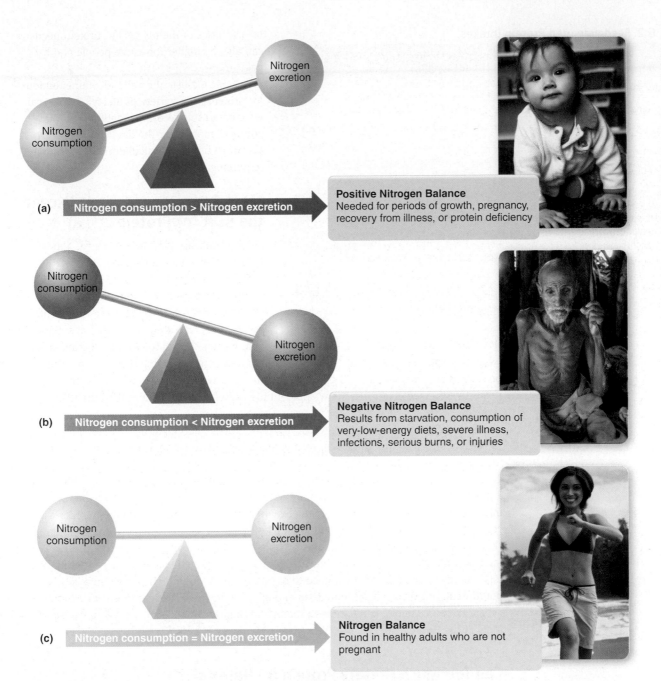

FIGURE 6.15 *Nitrogen balance* describes the relationship between how much nitrogen (protein) we consume and how much we excrete each day. **(a)** Positive nitrogen balance occurs when nitrogen consumption is greater than excretion. **(b)** Negative nitrogen balance occurs when nitrogen consumption is less than excretion. **(c)** Nitrogen balance is maintained when nitrogen consumption equals excretion.

Recommended Dietary Allowance for Protein

How much protein should we eat? The RDA for sedentary people is 0.8 g per kilogram of body weight per day. The recommended percentage of energy that should come from protein is 10% to 35% of total energy intake. Protein needs are higher for children, adolescents, and pregnant/lactating women because more protein is needed during times of growth and development (refer to Chapters 17 and 18 for details on protein needs during

TABLE 6.2 Recommended Protein Intakes

Group	Protein Intake (grams per kilogram* body weight)
Sedentary adults[1]	0.8
Nonvegetarian endurance athletes[2]	1.2 to 1.4
Nonvegetarian strength athletes[2]	1.2 to 1.7
Vegetarian endurance athletes[2]	1.3 to 1.5
Vegetarian strength athletes[2]	1.3 to 1.8

*To convert body weight to kilograms, divide weight in pounds by 2.2.
Weight (lb)/2.2 Weight (kg)
Weight (kg) × protein recommendation (g/kg body weight per day) = protein intake (g/day)

[1]Data from Food and Nutrition Board, Institute of Medicine. 2005. Dietary Reference Intakes for Energy, Carbohydrate, Fiber, Fat, Fatty Acids, Cholesterol, Protein, and Amino Acids (Macronutrients). Washington, DC: National Academies Press. Available at http://www.nap.edu/openbook.php?isbn=0309085373.

[2]Data American College of Sports Medicine, American Dietetic Association, and Dietitians of Canada. 2009. Joint position statement. Nutrition and athletic performance. *Med. Sci. Sports Exerc.* 41(3): 709–731.

these phases of the life cycle). Protein needs can also be higher for active people and for vegetarians.

Table 6.2 lists the daily recommendations for protein for a variety of lifestyles. How can we convert this recommendation into total grams of protein for the day? In the **You Do the Math** box, let's calculate Theo's protein requirements.

Most Americans Meet or Exceed the RDA for Protein

Surveys indicate that Americans eat almost 16% of their total daily energy intake as protein.[3] Men report eating about 73 to 104 g of protein each day, and women consume 59 to 72 g per day. Putting these values into perspective, let's assume that the average man weighs 75 kg (165 lb) and the average woman weighs 65 kg (143 lb). Their protein requirements (assuming they are not athletes or vegetarians) are 60 g and 52 g per day for men and women at this average weight, respectively. As you can see, many adults in the United States eat more than the RDA for protein.

Research indicates that the protein intake of athletes participating in a variety of sports can also well exceed current recommendations.[4] For instance, the protein intake for some female distance runners is 1.2 g per kg body weight per day, accounting for 15% of their total daily energy intake. In addition, some male bodybuilders consume 3 g per kg body weight per day, accounting for almost 38% of their total daily energy intake! However, certain groups of athletes are at risk for low protein intakes. Athletes who consume inadequate energy and limit food choices, such as some distance runners, figure skaters, female gymnasts, and wrestlers who are dieting, are all at risk for low protein intakes. Unlike people who consume adequate energy, individuals who are restricting their total energy intake (kilocalories) need to pay close attention to their protein intake. It's not difficult, however, to get more than enough protein without exceeding your energy needs. For an example, compare the protein and Calorie counts in two days' meals in **Meal Focus Figure 6.16**.

Can Too Much Dietary Protein Be Harmful?

High protein intakes have been identified with increased health risks. Three health conditions that have received particular attention are heart disease, bone loss, and kidney disease.

High Protein Intake and Heart Disease

High-protein diets composed of predominantly animal sources are associated with higher blood cholesterol levels. Until recently, this was assumed to be due to the saturated fat in animal products, which has been shown to increase blood cholesterol levels and the risk for heart disease. Interestingly, a recent review draws into question these widely held assumptions, as it found that eating more saturated fat was *not* associated with an increased risk for heart disease.[5] The authors of this study suggest that this may be due to two reasons: (1) the LDL cholesterol linked with saturated fat intake is of a sub-type that is not associated with increasing a person's risk for heart disease, and (2) saturated fat also increases a person's HDL cholesterol, which is protective again heart disease. This topic is

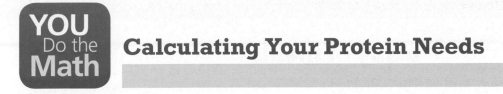

YOU Do the Math

Calculating Your Protein Needs

Theo wants to know how much protein he needs each day. During the off-season, he works out three times a week at a gym and practices basketball with friends every Friday night. He is not a vegetarian. Although Theo exercises regularly, he would not be considered an endurance athlete or as a strength athlete during the off-season. At this level of physical activity, Theo's requirement for protein probably ranges from the RDA of 0.8 up to 1.0 g per kilogram of body weight per day. To calculate the total number of grams of protein Theo should eat each day,

1. Convert Theo's weight from pounds to kilograms. Theo presently weighs 200 lb. To convert this value to kilograms, divide by 2.2:

$$(200 \text{ lb})/(2.2 \text{ lb/kg}) = 91 \text{ kg}$$

2. Multiply Theo's weight in kilograms by his RDA for protein, like so:

$$(91 \text{ kg}) \times (0.8 \text{ g/kg}) = 72.8 \text{ g of protein per day}$$

$$(91 \text{ kg}) \times (1.0 \text{ g/kg}) = 91 \text{ g of protein per day}$$

What happens during basketball season, when Theo practices, lifts weight, and has games 5 or 6 days a week? This will probably raise his protein needs to approximately 1.2 to 1.7 g per kilogram of body weight per day. How much more protein should he eat? See below:

$$91 \text{ kg} \times 1.2 \text{ g/kg} = 109.2 \text{ g of protein per day}$$

$$91 \text{ kg} \times 1.7 \text{ g/kg} = 154.7 \text{ g of protein per day}$$

Now calculate your own recommended protein intake based on your activity level.

Answers will vary depending on body weight and individual activity levels.

---

still highly contentious, and as discussed in Chapter 5, nutrition experts stress that eating less saturated fat, and replacing it with more healthful foods higher in polyunsaturated fats, such as nuts, avocados, fish, whole grains, and olive oil, is the best approach to reducing one's risk for heart disease. A recent study found that consuming a diet high in fish and fewer high-fat dairy products and meats is associated with lowering inflammation and endothelial function, which are recognized risk factors for cardiovascular disease.[6] Although we do not yet know the optimal AMDR of protein to reduce the risk for cardiovascular disease within a population, it appears that consuming protein sources low in saturated fat may help.

High Protein Intake and Bone Loss

How might a high-protein diet lead to bone loss? Until recently, nutritionists have been concerned about high-protein diets because they increase calcium excretion. This may be because animal products contain more of the sulfur amino acids (methionine and cysteine). Metabolizing these amino acids makes the blood more acidic, and calcium is pulled from the bone to buffer these acids. Although eating more protein can cause an increased excretion of calcium, it is very controversial whether high protein intakes actually cause bone loss. In fact, we do know that eating too little protein causes bone loss, which increases the risk for fractures and osteoporosis. Higher intakes of animal and soy protein have been shown to protect bone in middle-aged and older women. A recent systematic review of the literature concluded that there is no evidence to support the contention that high-protein diets lead to bone loss, except in people consuming inadequate calcium.[7]

High Protein Intake and Kidney Disease

A high-protein diet can increase the risk of acquiring kidney disease in people who are susceptible. Because people with diabetes have higher rates of kidney disease, it was

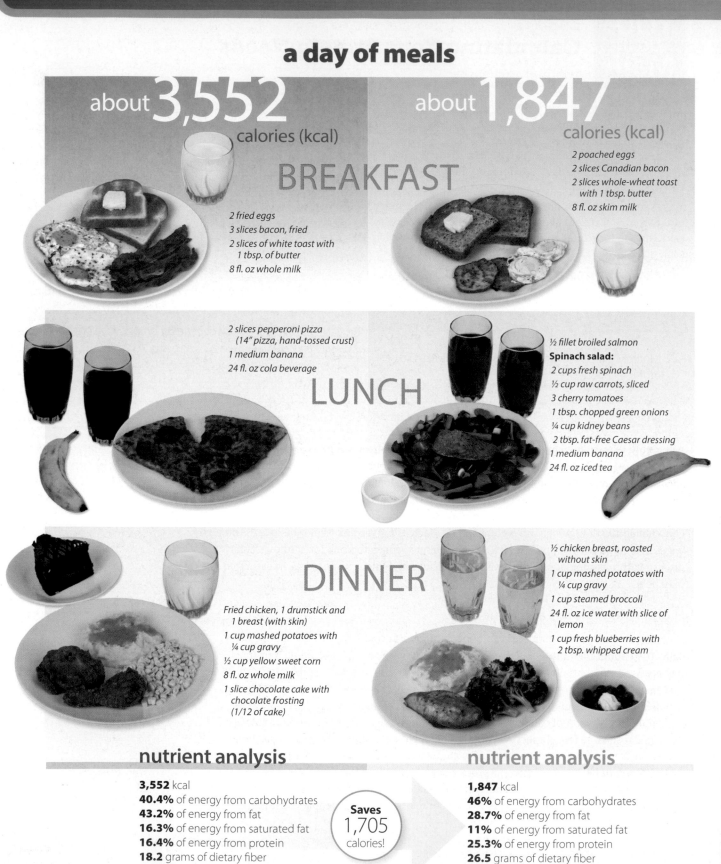

meal focus figure 6.16 | Maximizing Healthy Protein Intake

a day of meals

about 3,552 calories (kcal)

BREAKFAST

2 fried eggs
3 slices bacon, fried
2 slices of white toast with
  1 tbsp. of butter
8 fl. oz whole milk

LUNCH

2 slices pepperoni pizza
  (14" pizza, hand-tossed crust)
1 medium banana
24 fl. oz cola beverage

DINNER

Fried chicken, 1 drumstick and
  1 breast (with skin)
1 cup mashed potatoes with
  ¼ cup gravy
½ cup yellow sweet corn
8 fl. oz whole milk
1 slice chocolate cake with
  chocolate frosting
  (1/12 of cake)

about 1,847 calories (kcal)

2 poached eggs
2 slices Canadian bacon
2 slices whole-wheat toast
  with 1 tbsp. butter
8 fl. oz skim milk

½ fillet broiled salmon
Spinach salad:
  2 cups fresh spinach
  ½ cup raw carrots, sliced
  3 cherry tomatoes
  1 tbsp. chopped green onions
  ¼ cup kidney beans
  2 tbsp. fat-free Caesar dressing
1 medium banana
24 fl. oz iced tea

½ chicken breast, roasted
  without skin
1 cup mashed potatoes with
  ¼ cup gravy
1 cup steamed broccoli
24 fl. oz ice water with slice of
  lemon
1 cup fresh blueberries with
  2 tbsp. whipped cream

nutrient analysis

3,552 kcal
40.4% of energy from carbohydrates
43.2% of energy from fat
16.3% of energy from saturated fat
16.4% of energy from protein
18.2 grams of dietary fiber
6,246 milligrams of sodium

Saves 1,705 calories!

nutrient analysis

1,847 kcal
46% of energy from carbohydrates
28.7% of energy from fat
11% of energy from saturated fat
25.3% of energy from protein
26.5 grams of dietary fiber
3,280 milligrams of sodium

previously assumed that they would benefit from a lower-protein diet. However, the evidence is inconclusive regarding the optimal amount of protein that people with diabetes should consume. The American Diabetes Association does not recommend a reduction in protein intake even in people with diabetes-related kidney disease, as it does not improve kidney function or reduce cardiovascular disease risk.[8]

In addition, there is no evidence that eating more protein causes kidney disease in healthy people who are not susceptible to this condition. In fact, a review of studies assessing the effect of high protein intakes on renal function in athletes has found that regularly consuming over 2 g of protein per kilogram of body weight per day does not appear to cause unhealthy changes in kidney function.[9] Thus, experts agree that eating no more than 2 g of protein per kilogram of body weight each day is safe for healthy people.

It is important for people who consume a lot of protein to drink more water. This is because eating more protein increases protein metabolism and urea production. As mentioned earlier, urea is a waste product that forms when nitrogen is removed during amino acid metabolism. Adequate fluid is needed to flush excess urea from the kidneys. This is particularly important for athletes, who need more fluid due to higher sweat losses.

Protein: Much More Than Meat!

Table 6.3 compares the protein content of a variety of foods. Although some people think that the only good sources of protein are beef, pork, poultry, and seafood, many other foods are rich in proteins. These include dairy products (milk, cheese, yogurt, and so on), eggs, legumes (including soy products), whole grains, and nuts. Fruits and many vegetables are not particularly high in protein; however, these foods provide fiber and many vitamins and minerals and are excellent sources of carbohydrates. Thus, eating them can help provide the carbohydrates and energy you need, so that your body can use proteins for building and maintaining tissues.

After reviewing Table 6.3, you might be wondering how much protein you typically eat. See the **Nutrition Label Activity** box (page 235) to find out.

Legumes

Legumes include soybeans, kidney beans, pinto beans, black beans, garbanzo beans (chickpeas), lima beans, green peas, black-eyed peas, and lentils. Would you be surprised to learn that the quality of the protein in some of these legumes is almost equal to that of meat? It's true! The quality of soybean protein is almost identical to that of meat and is available as soy milk, tofu, textured vegetable protein, and tempeh, a firm cake made by cooking and fermenting whole soybeans. For more information about the nutrients in soy, claims regarding its health benefits, and ways to enjoy soy, check out the **Highlight** box (page 236).

The protein quality of other legumes is also relatively high. In addition to being excellent sources of protein, legumes are high in fiber, iron, calcium, and many of the B-vitamins. They are also low in saturated fat. Eating legumes regularly, including foods made from soybeans, may help reduce the risk for heart disease by lowering LDL cholesterol levels. Diets high in legumes and soy products are also associated with lower rates of some cancers. Legumes are not nutritionally complete, however, as they do not contain vitamins B_{12}, C, or A. They're also deficient in methionine, an essential amino acid; however, combining them with grains, nuts, or seeds gives you a complete protein.

How can you add more legumes to your daily diet? Try these suggestions:

- Instead of cereal, eggs, or a doughnut, microwave a frozen bean burrito for a quick, portable breakfast.

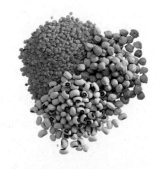

The quality of the protein in some legumes, such as these black-eyed peas, lentils, and garbanzo beans, is almost equal to that of meat.

TABLE 6.3 Protein Content of Commonly Consumed Foods

Food	Serving Size	Protein (g)
Beef		
Ground, lean, baked (15% fat)	3 oz	22
Beef tenderloin steak, broiled (1/8-in. fat)	3 oz	21.5
Top sirloin, broiled (1/8-in. fat)	3 oz	23
Poultry		
Chicken breast, broiled, no skin (bone removed)	½ breast	27
Chicken thigh, bone and skin removed	1 thigh	20
Turkey breast, roasted, Louis Rich	3 oz	15
Seafood		
Salmon, Chinook, baked	3 oz	22
Shrimp, steamed	3 oz	19
Tuna, light, in water, drained	3 oz	22
Pork		
Pork loin chop, broiled	3 oz	21
Ham, roasted, extra lean (5% fat)	3 oz	18
Dairy		
Whole milk (3.3% fat)	8 fl. oz	7.7
Skim milk	8 fl. oz	8.3
Low-fat, plain yogurt	8 fl. oz	12
Cottage cheese, low-fat (2%)	1 cup	27
Soy Products		
Tofu	½ cup	10
Tempeh, cooked	3 oz	15.5
Soy milk	1 cup	8
Beans		
Refried	½ cup	6
Kidney, red	½ cup	8
Black	½ cup	7.6
Nuts		
Peanuts, dry roasted	1 oz	6.7
Peanut butter, creamy	2 tbsp.	8
Almonds, blanched	1 oz	6

Sources: Values obtained from U.S. Department of Agriculture, Agricultural Research Service. 2013. USDA National Nutrient Database for Standard Reference, Release 26. Available online at http://ndb.nal.usda.gov/.

- If you normally have a side of bacon, ham, or sausage with your eggs for breakfast, have a side of black beans instead.
- Make your pancakes with soy milk or pour soy milk on your cereal.
- For lunch, try a sandwich made with hummus (a garbanzo bean spread), cucumbers, tomato, avocado, and/or lettuce on whole-wheat bread or in a whole-wheat pocket.
- Add garbanzo beans, kidney beans, or fresh peas to tossed salads, or make a three-bean salad with kidney beans, green beans, and garbanzo beans.
- Make a side dish using legumes, such as peas with pearl onions; succotash (lima beans, corn, and tomatoes); or homemade chili with kidney beans and tofu instead of meat.
- Make black bean soup, lentil soup, pea soup, minestrone soup, or a batch of dal (a type of yellow lentil used in Indian cuisine) and serve over brown rice. Top with plain yogurt, a traditional accompaniment in many Asian cuisines.
- Make tacos or burritos with black or pinto beans instead of shredded meat.
- Make a "meatloaf" using cooked, mashed lentils instead of ground beef.
- For fast food at home, keep canned beans on hand. Serve over rice with a salad for a complete and hearty meal.

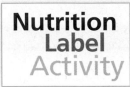

Nutrition Label Activity

How Much Protein Do You Eat?

Theo wants to know if his diet contains enough protein. To calculate his protein intake, he records all the foods he eats for 3 days in a food diary. The foods Theo consumed for 1 of his 3 days are listed on the left in the following table, and the protein content of those foods is listed on the right. Theo recorded the protein content listed on the Nutrition Facts Panel for those foods with labels. For products without labels, he used the nutrient analysis program that came with this book. There is also a U.S. Department of Agriculture website that lists the energy and nutrient content of thousands of foods (http://ndb.nal.usda.gov/).

Foods Consumed	Protein Content (g)
Breakfast	
Brewed coffee (2 cups) with 2 tbsp. half and half	1.4
1 large bagel (5-in. diameter)	13
Low-fat cream cheese (2 tbsp.)	1.6
Mid-Morning Snack	
Cola beverage (32 fl. oz)	0
Low-fat strawberry yogurt (1 cup)	10
Fruit and nut granola bar (2; 37 g each)	5.7
Lunch	
Ham and cheese sandwich:	
Whole-wheat bread (2 slices)	4
Mayonnaise (1.5 tbsp.)	0.2
Extra-lean ham (4 oz)	24
Swiss cheese (2 oz)	15
Iceberg lettuce (2 leaves)	0.3
Sliced tomato (3 slices)	0.5
Banana (1 large)	1.5
Wheat Thin crackers (20)	3.6
Bottled water (20 fl. oz)	0.0

Foods Consumed	Protein Content (g)
Dinner	
Cheeseburger:	
Broiled ground beef (1/2 lb, cooked)	52
American cheese (1 oz)	5
Seeded bun (1 large)	8
Ketchup (2 tbsp.)	0.5
Mustard (1 tbsp.)	0.7
Shredded lettuce (1/2 cup)	0.3
Sliced tomato (3 slices)	0.5
French fries (30; 2- to 3-in. strips)	5
Baked beans (2 cups)	24
2% low-fat milk (2 cups)	16
Evening Snack	
Chocolate chip cookies (4; 3-in.-diameter)	3
2% low-fat milk (1 cup)	8
Total protein intake for the day:	**203.8 g**

As calculated in the **You Do the Math** box (page 231), Theo's RDA during the off-season is 72.8 to 91 g of protein. He is consuming 2.3 to 2.8 times that amount! You can see that he does not need to use amino acid or protein supplements, because he has more than adequate amounts of protein to build lean tissue. Now calculate your own protein intake using food labels and a diet analysis program. Do you obtain more protein from animal or non-animal sources? If you consume mostly non-animal sources, are you eating soy products and complementary foods throughout the day? If you eat animal-based products on a regular basis, notice how much protein you consume from even small servings of meat and dairy products.

- Use soy nut butter (similar to peanut butter), soy deli meats, or soy cheese in sandwiches.
- Try soy sausages, bacon, hot dogs, burgers, ground "beef," and "chicken" patties.
- Toss cubes of prepackaged flavored, baked tofu or tempeh or a handful of edamame into stir-fried vegetables and serve over Chinese noodles or rice.
- Order soy-based dishes, such as spicy bean curd and miso soup, at Asian restaurants.
- Instead of potato chips or pretzels for snacks, try one of the new bean chips.
- Dip fresh vegetables in bean dip.
- Have hummus on wedges of pita bread.
- Add roast soy "nuts" to your trail mix.
- Keep frozen tofu desserts, such as tofu ice cream, in your freezer.

HIGHLIGHT

What's So Great about Soy?

Twenty years ago, if you were able to find a soy-based food in a traditional grocery store in the United States or Canada, it was probably soy milk. Now, it seems there are soy products in almost every aisle, from miso soup to soy-based hot dogs and burgers, and even tofu ice cream. Why the explosion? What's so great about soy, and should you give it a try?

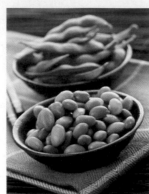

What Is Soy?

Before we explore the health claims tied to soy-based foods, let's define some terms. First, all soy-based foods start with soybeans, a staple in many Asian countries. Soybeans provide all essential amino acids and have almost twice as much protein as any other legume (7–10 grams of protein in 1 cup of soy milk). Although they also pack three to ten times as much fat as other beans, almost all of it is unsaturated. Soy also contains antioxidants. Here are some common varieties of soy-based foods you might find in your local supermarket:

- *Soy milk* is a beverage produced when soybeans are ground with water. Flavorings are added to make the drink palatable, and many brands of soy milk are fortified with calcium and vitamins D and B_{12}.

- *Tofu* is made from soy milk coagulated to form curds. If the coagulant used is calcium sulfate, the resulting product is high in calcium. Tofu is usually sold in blocks, like cheese, and is used as a meat substitute. Although many people object to its bland taste and mushy texture, tofu adapts well to many seasonings, and when drained and frozen before cooking it develops a chewy texture similar to meat.

- *Tempeh* is a more flavorful and firmer-textured meat substitute made from soybeans fermented with grains. It is often used in stir-fried dishes.

- *Miso* is a paste made from fermented soybeans and grains. It is used sparingly as a base for soups and sauces, as it is high in sodium.

- *Edamame* are precooked, frozen soybeans eaten as a snack or in salads and other dishes.

Soy May Reduce Your Risk for Chronic Disease

Proponents say that a diet high in soy protein can reduce your risk for heart disease and certain types of cancer. Let's review the research behind these claims.

The U.S. Food and Drug Administration (FDA) allows food manufacturers to put labels on products high in soy protein stating that a daily diet containing 25 grams of soy protein and low in saturated fat and cholesterol may reduce the risk for heart disease.[1] The FDA reviewed 27 relevant clinical studies before concluding that diets providing four servings a day of soy-based foods (not supplements) can provoke a modest reduction in blood levels of LDL-cholesterol. The American Heart Association therefore recommends consuming soy milk and tofu as part of a heart-healthy diet.[2]

Many studies suggest that soy protects against prostate cancer, which is the most common cancer in men.[3] It is unclear, however, whether or not soy reduces a woman's risk for breast cancer. The American Cancer Society (ACS) states that "a number of laboratory and animal experiments and human observational studies suggest that soy may reduce the risk for several types of cancer, including breast, prostate, ovarian, and uterine cancer," and recommends consuming soy foods as part of a balanced, plant-based diet.[4]

Adding Soy to Your Diet

If you decide that you want to try soy, how do you go about it? A first step for many people is to substitute soy milk for cow's milk on its own, on cereal, in smoothies, or in recipes for baked goods. Different brands of soy milk can have very different flavors, so try a few before you decide you don't like the taste. Refer to the list of tips (pages 234–235) for more ways to add soy—and other legumes—to your diet.

References

1. Department of Health and Human Services. U.S. Food and Drug Administration. 2013. Food. Guidance for Industry: A Food Labeling Guide (11. Appendix C: Health Claims). http://www.fda.gov/food/guidanceregulation/guidancedocumentsregulatoryinformation/labelingnutrition/ucm064919.htm

2. American Heart Association. 2014. Getting Healthy. Nutrition Center. Try These Tips for Heart-health Grocery Shopping. http://www.heart.org/HEARTORG/GettingHealthy/NutritionCenter/HeartSmartShopping/Try-These-Tips-for-Heart-Healthy-Grocery-Shopping_UCM_001884_Article.jsp.

3. Centers for Disease Control and Prevention. 2013. Cancer Prevention and Control. Cancer Among Men. http://www.cdc.gov/cancer/dcpc/data/men.htm.

4. American Cancer Society. 2013. Soybean. http://www.cancer.org/treatment/treatmentsandsideeffects/complementaryandalternativemedicine/dietandnutrition/soybean.

Nuts

Nuts are another healthful high-protein food. In fact, the USDA Food Patterns counts one-third cup of nuts or two tablespoons of peanut butter as equivalent to 1 ounce—about one-third of a serving—of meat! Moreover, studies show that consuming about 2 to 5 oz of nuts per week, in particular walnuts and peanuts, significantly reduces people's risk for cardiovascular disease and premature mortality from a range of causes.[10-12] Although the exact mechanism behind this is not known, nuts contain many nutrients and other substances that are associated with health benefits, including fiber, unsaturated fats, potassium, folate, plant sterols, and *antioxidants*, substances that can protect our cells from damage (see Chapter 10).

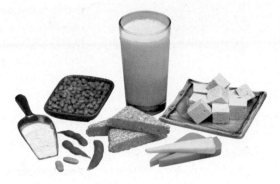

Soy products are also a good source of dietary protein.

"New" Foods

A new source of non-meat protein that is available on the market is *quorn*, a protein product derived from fermented fungus. It is mixed with a variety of other foods to produce various types of meat substitutes. Other "new" foods high in protein include some very ancient grains! For instance, you may have heard of pastas and other products made with quinoa (pronounced keen-wah), a plant so essential to the diet of the ancient Incas that they considered it sacred. No wonder: quinoa, which is cooked much like rice, provides 8 g of protein in a 1-cup serving. It's highly digestible and, unlike many more familiar grains, provides all nine essential amino acids. A similar grain called amaranth also provides complete protein. Teff, millet, and sorghum are grains long cultivated in Africa as rich sources of protein. They are now widely available in the United States. Although these three grains are low in the essential amino acid lysine, combining them with legumes produces a complete-protein meal.

Protein and Amino Acid Supplements—Any Truth to the Hype?

"Amino acid supplements—you can't gain without them!" This is just one of the headlines found in bodybuilding magazines and Internet sites touting amino acid supplements as the key to achieving increased power, strength, and performance "perfection." Many athletes who read these claims believe that taking amino acid supplements will boost their energy during performance, replace proteins metabolized for energy during exercise, enhance muscle growth and strength, and hasten recovery from intense training or injury. Should you believe the hype?

As noted earlier in this chapter, we use very little protein for energy during exercise, and most Americans already consume more than they need. A diet providing adequate energy and meeting or exceeding the athlete's RDA for protein (refer to Table 6.2) will support either strength or endurance training and performance without the need for amino acid supplements. What about the claims related to muscle-building? Although some research has shown that intravenous infusions of various amino acids in the laboratory can stimulate certain hormones that enhance the building of muscle, there is little evidence that taking amino acid supplements orally can build muscle or improve strength. Because these supplements are relatively expensive, there is no need to put in a dent in your wallet by taking expensive amino acid supplements, as the benefits can be derived by consuming a glass of milk after exercise![4]

RECAP

The RDA for protein for most nonpregnant, nonlactating, nonvegetarian sedentary adults is 0.8 g per kg body weight. Children, pregnant women, nursing mothers, vegetarians, and active people need slightly more. Most people, including athletes, who eat enough kilocalories and carbohydrates have no problem meeting their RDA for protein. Eating too much protein may increase a susceptible person's risk for kidney disease. Good sources of protein include beef pork, poultry, and fish, eggs, dairy products, soy and other legumes, nuts, quorn, quinoa, and other ancient grains. Amino acid supplements are not necessary to support muscle growth or exercise performance, assuming energy and protein intakes are adequate. ■

LO 9 Discuss the health benefits, challenges, and nutritional quality of a balanced and adequate vegetarian diet.

Can a Vegetarian Diet Provide Adequate Protein?

Vegetarianism is the practice of restricting the diet mostly or entirely to foods of plant origin, including vegetables, fruits, grains, and nuts. Many vegetarians are college students; moving away from home and taking responsibility for one's eating habits appears to influence some young adults to try vegetarianism as a lifestyle choice.

Types of Vegetarian Diets

There are almost as many types of vegetarian diets as there are vegetarians. Some people who consider themselves vegetarians regularly eat poultry and fish. Others avoid the flesh of animals but consume eggs, milk, and cheese liberally. Still others strictly avoid all products of animal origin, including milk and eggs, and even by-products such as candies and puddings made with gelatin. A type of "vegetarian" diet receiving significant media attention recently is the plant-based diet: it consists mostly of plant foods, as well as eggs, dairy, and occasionally red meat, poultry, and/or fish.

Table 6.4 identifies the various types of vegetarian diets, ranging from the most inclusive to the most restrictive. Notice that the more restrictive the diet, the more challenging it becomes to achieve an adequate protein intake.

TABLE 6.4 Terms and Definitions of a Vegetarian Diet

Type of Diet	Foods Consumed	Comments
Plant-based (also called semivegetarian, partial vegetarian, or flexitarian)	Vegetables, grains, nuts, fruits, legumes; sometimes seafood, poultry, eggs, dairy products	Typically exclude or limit red meat; may also avoid or limit other meats
Pescovegetarian	Similar to semivegetarian but excludes all red meat and poultry	*Pesco* means "fish," which is included
Lacto-ovo-vegetarian	Vegetables, grains, nuts, fruits, legumes, dairy products (*lacto*), eggs (*ovo*)	Excludes red meat, poultry, and seafood; relies on dairy products and eggs for animal sources of protein
Lactovegetarian	Similar to lacto-ovo-vegetarian but excludes eggs	Relies on milk and cheese for animal sources of protein
Ovovegetarian	Similar to lacto-ovo-vegetarian but excludes dairy products	Relies on eggs as an animal source of protein
Vegan (also called strict vegetarian)	Only plant-based foods (vegetables, grains, nuts, seeds, fruits, legumes)	May not provide adequate vitamin B_{12}, zinc, iron, or calcium
Macrobiotic diet	Vegan type of diet; becomes progressively more strict until almost all foods are eliminated; at the extreme, only brown rice and small amounts of water or herbal tea	Taken to the extreme, can cause malnutrition and death
Fruitarian	Only raw or dried fruit, seeds, nuts, honey, vegetable oil	Very restrictive diet; deficient in protein, calcium, zinc, iron, vitamin B_{12}, riboflavin, other nutrients

vegetarianism The practice of restricting the diet mostly or entirely to foods of plant origin, including vegetables, fruits, grains, and nuts.

Why Do People Become Vegetarians?

When discussing vegetarianism, one of the most often asked questions is why people would make this food choice. The most common responses are included here.

Religious, Ethical, and Food-Safety Reasons

Some make the choice for religious or spiritual reasons. Several religions prohibit or restrict the consumption of animal flesh; however, generalizations can be misleading. For example, whereas certain sects within Hinduism forbid the consumption of meat, perusing the menu at any Indian restaurant will reveal that many other Hindus regularly consume small quantities of meat, poultry, and fish. Many Buddhists are vegetarians, as are some Christians, including Seventh Day Adventists.

Many vegetarians are guided by their personal philosophy to choose vegetarianism. These people feel that it is morally and ethically wrong to consume animals and, in some cases, any products from animals (such as dairy products or eggs). They may consume milk and eggs but choose to purchase them only from family farms where they feel animals are treated humanely.

There is also a great deal of concern about meat-handling practices, because contaminated meat has occasionally made its way into our food supply. For example, several outbreaks of severe illness, sometimes resulting in permanent disability and even death, have been traced to hamburgers served at fast-food restaurants, as well as ground beef sold in markets and consumed at home.

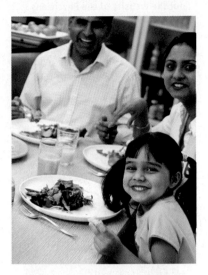

People who follow certain sects of Hinduism refrain from eating meat.

Ecological Benefits

Many people choose vegetarianism because of their concerns about the effect of meat production on the global environment. Due to the high demand for meat in developed nations, meat production has evolved from small family farming operations into the larger system of agribusiness. Critics point to the environmental costs of agribusiness, including massive uses of natural resources to support animals, and methane and other greenhouse-gas emissions produced by animals themselves. For an in-depth discussion of this complex and emotionally charged topic, refer to the ***Nutrition Myth or Fact?*** essay at the end of Chapter 16.

Health Benefits

Still others practice vegetarianism because of its health benefits. Research over several years has consistently shown that a varied and balanced vegetarian diet can reduce the risk for many chronic diseases. Its health benefits include the following:

- Reduced intake of fat and total energy, which reduces the risk for obesity. This may in turn lower a person's risk for type 2 diabetes.
- Lower blood pressure, which may be due to a higher intake of fruits and vegetables. People who eat vegetarian diets tend to be nonsmokers, to drink alcohol in moderation if at all, and to exercise more regularly, which are also factors known to reduce blood pressure and help maintain a healthy body weight.
- Reduced risk for heart disease, which may be due to lower saturated fat intake and a higher consumption of *antioxidants*, which are found in plant-based foods. As noted earlier, antioxidants (discussed in detail in Chapter 10) help protect our cells. They are abundant in fruits and vegetables.
- Fewer digestive problems, such as constipation and diverticular disease, perhaps due to the higher fiber content of vegetarian diets. Diverticular disease (discussed in Chapter 4) occurs when the wall of the bowel (large intestine) pouches and becomes inflamed.
- Reduced risk for some cancers. Research shows that vegetarians may have lower rates of cancer, particularly colorectal cancer. Many components of a vegetarian diet

If you're interested in trying a vegetarian diet but don't know where to begin, check out the website of the Physicians Committee for Responsible Medicine at www.pcrm.org. Click on the Health and Nutrition button, then scroll down to the left-side margin until you see "Free Vegetarian Starter Kit." Open it up and get started!

could contribute to reducing cancer risks, including antioxidants, fiber, no intake of red meats and processed meats (which increase the risk for colorectal cancer), and lower consumption of *carcinogens* (cancer-causing agents) that are formed when cooking meat.[13]

■ Reduced risk for kidney disease, kidney stones, and gallstones. The lower protein contents of vegetarian diets, plus the higher intake of legumes and vegetable proteins such as soy, may be protective against these conditions.

What Are the Challenges of a Vegetarian Diet?

Although a vegetarian diet can be healthful, it also presents some challenges. Limiting the consumption of animal products introduces the potential for inadequate intakes of certain nutrients, especially for people consuming a vegan, macrobiotic, or fruitarian diet. **Table 6.5** lists the nutrients that can be deficient in a vegan type of diet plan and describes good non-animal sources that can provide these nutrients. Vegetarians who consume dairy and/or egg products obtain these nutrients more easily.

Research indicates that individuals with a history of disordered eating are more likely to switch to a vegetarian diet.[14] Instead of eating a healthful variety of non-animal foods, people with disordered eating problems may use vegetarianism as an excuse to restrict many foods from their diet. Experts suggest that the possibility of disordered eating should be considered if the switch to a vegetarian diet is accompanied by unnecessary weight loss.[14]

Can a vegetarian diet provide enough protein? Because high-quality non-meat protein sources are quite easy to obtain in developed countries, a well-balanced vegetarian diet can provide adequate protein. In fact, the American Dietetic Association endorses an appropriately planned vegetarian diet as healthful, nutritionally adequate, and beneficial in reducing and preventing various diseases. As you can see, the emphasis is on a *balanced* and *adequate* vegetarian diet; thus, it is important for vegetarians to eat complementary proteins and obtain enough energy from other macronutrients to spare protein from being used as an energy source. Although the digestibility of a vegetarian diet is potentially lower than that of an animal-based diet, there is no separate protein recommendation for vegetarians who consume complementary plant proteins.[15]

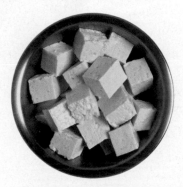

Vegetarians should eat two to three servings of beans, nuts, seeds, eggs, or meat substitutes (such as tofu) daily.

TABLE 6.5 Nutrients of Concern in a Vegan Diet

Nutrient	Functions	Non-Meat/Nondairy Food Sources
Vitamin B_{12}	Assists with DNA synthesis; protection and growth of nerve fibers	Vitamin B_{12}–fortified cereals, yeast, soy products, and other meat analogues; vitamin B_{12} supplements
Vitamin D	Promotes bone growth	Vitamin D–fortified cereals, margarines, and soy products; adequate exposure to sunlight; supplementation may be necessary for those who do not get adequate exposure to sunlight
Riboflavin (vitamin B_2)	Promotes release of energy; supports normal vision and skin health	Whole and enriched grains, green leafy vegetables, mushrooms, beans, nuts, seeds
Iron	Assists with oxygen transport; involved in making amino acids and hormones	Whole-grain products, prune juice, dried fruits, beans, nuts, seeds, leafy vegetables such as spinach
Calcium	Maintains bone health; assists with muscle contraction, blood pressure, and nerve transmission	Fortified soy milk and tofu, almonds, dry beans, leafy vegetables, calcium-fortified juices, fortified breakfast cereals
Zinc	Assists with DNA and RNA synthesis, immune function, and growth	Whole-grain products, wheat germ, beans, nuts, seeds

Theo

Nutri-Case

"No way would I ever become a vegetarian! The only way to build up your muscles is to eat meat. I was reading in a bodybuilding magazine last week about a new diet called the *Protein Path to Power* that says if you eat a diet really high in lean meats and cut out the junk foods, you'll gain muscle but not fat because 'protein makes protein, but fat and sugar make fat.' That makes sense to me. Besides, after a game I just crave meat. If I don't have it, I feel sort of like my batteries don't get recharged. Competitive athletes just can't perform without meat."

What specific claims does Theo make here about the role of meat in the diet? Do you think these claims are valid? Why or why not?

Using MyPlate

Although the USDA has not designed a version of MyPlate specifically for people following a vegetarian diet, healthy eating tips for vegetarians are available at MyPlate online (see the Web Links section at the end of this chapter). For example, to meet their needs for protein and calcium, lacto-vegetarians can consume low-fat or nonfat dairy products. Vegans and ovovegetarians can consume calcium-fortified soy milk or one of the many protein bars fortified with calcium.

In addition to protein and calcium, vegans need to pay special attention to consuming foods high in vitamins D, B_{12}, and riboflavin (B_2) and the minerals zinc and iron. Supplementation of these micronutrients may be necessary for certain individuals if they cannot consume adequate amounts in their diet.

The Vegetarian Resource Group offers a colorful, downloadable vegan MyPlate poster. Go to www.vrg.org, then click on "Guides and Handouts" on the left-side margin, then click on "My Vegan Plate Color Handout."

RECAP

People who consider themselves vegetarians may limit their consumption of animal products or avoid them entirely. Some people choose vegetarianism for religious or ethical reasons, or because of concerns about food safety, the environment, or their health. A balanced vegetarian diet may reduce the risk for obesity, type 2 diabetes, heart disease, digestive problems, some cancers, kidney disease, kidney stones, and gallstones. Whereas varied vegetarian diets can provide enough protein, vegetarians who consume no animal products need to make sure they consume adequate plant sources of protein and supplement their diet with good sources of vitamin D, vitamin B_{12}, riboflavin, calcium, iron, and zinc. ■

What Disorders Are Related to Protein Intake or Metabolism?

LO 10 Describe two disorders related to inadequate protein intake or genetic abnormalities.

Consuming inadequate protein can result in severe illness and death. Typically, this occurs when people do not consume enough total energy, but a diet deficient specifically in protein can have similar effects.

Protein–Energy Malnutrition Can Lead to Debility and Death

When a person consumes too little protein and energy, the result is **protein–energy malnutrition** (also called *protein–Calorie malnutrition*). Two diseases that can follow are marasmus and kwashiorkor (**Figure 6.17**, page 242).

protein–energy malnutrition
A disorder caused by inadequate consumption of protein. It is characterized by severe wasting.

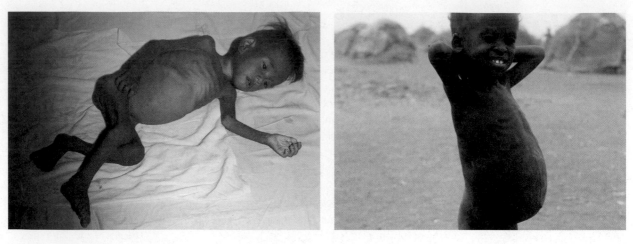

(a)   (b)

FIGURE 6.17 Two forms of protein–energy malnutrition: **(a)** marasmus and **(b)** kwashiorkor.

Marasmus Results from Grossly Inadequate Energy Intakes

Marasmus is a disease that results from grossly inadequate intakes of protein, energy, and other nutrients. Essentially, people with marasmus slowly starve to death. It is most common in young children (6 to 18 months of age) living in impoverished conditions who are severely undernourished. For example, the children may be fed diluted cereal drinks that are inadequate in energy, protein, and most nutrients. People suffering from marasmus have the look of "skin and bones," as their body fat and tissues are wasting. The consequences of marasmus include the following:

- Wasting and weakening of muscles, including the heart muscle
- Stunted brain development and learning impairment
- Depressed metabolism and little insulation from body fat, causing a dangerously low body temperature
- Stunted physical growth and development
- Deterioration of the intestinal lining, which further inhibits absorption of nutrients
- *Anemia* (abnormally low levels of hemoglobin in the blood)
- Severely weakened immune system
- Fluid and electrolyte imbalances

If marasmus is left untreated, death from dehydration, heart failure, or infection will result. Treating marasmus involves carefully correcting fluid and electrolyte imbalances. Protein and carbohydrates are provided once the body's condition has stabilized. Fat is introduced much later, as the protein levels in the blood must improve to the point at which the body can use them to carry fat, so that it can be safely metabolized by the body.

Kwashiorkor Results from a Low-Protein Diet

Kwashiorkor often occurs in developing countries when infants are weaned early due to the arrival of a subsequent baby. This deficiency disease is typically seen in young children (1 to 3 years of age) who no longer drink breast milk. Instead, they often are fed a low-protein, starchy cereal. Recent research suggests that dysfunctional GI bacteria combined with a low-protein diet interact to contribute to the development of kwashiorkor.[16] Unlike marasmus, kwashiorkor often develops quickly and causes the person to look swollen, particularly in the belly. This is because the low protein content of the blood is inadequate to keep fluids from seeping into the tissue spaces. These are other symptoms of kwashiorkor:

- Some weight loss and muscle wasting, with some retention of body fat
- Retarded growth and development but less severe than that seen with marasmus
- Edema, which results over time in extreme distension of the belly and is caused by fluid and electrolyte imbalances

marasmus A form of protein–energy malnutrition that results from grossly inadequate intakes of protein, energy, and other nutrients.

kwashiorkor A form of protein–energy malnutrition that is typically seen in developing countries in infants and toddlers who are weaned early. Denied breast milk, they are fed a cereal diet that provides adequate energy but inadequate protein.

- Fatty degeneration of the liver
- Loss of appetite, sadness, irritability, and apathy
- Development of sores and other skin problems; skin pigmentation changes
- Dry, brittle hair that changes color, straightens, and falls out easily

Kwashiorkor can be reversed if adequate protein and energy are given in time. Because of their severely weakened immune systems, many individuals with kwashiorkor die from infectious diseases they contract in their weakened state. Of those who are treated, many return home to the same impoverished conditions, only to develop this deficiency once again.

Many people think that only children in developing countries suffer from these diseases. However, protein–energy malnutrition occurs in all countries and affects both children and adults. In the United States, poor people living in inner cities and isolated rural areas are especially affected. Others at risk include the elderly, the homeless, people with eating disorders, those addicted to alcohol and other drugs, and individuals with wasting diseases, such as AIDS or cancer. (Chapter 16 provides more information on malnutrition and hunger.)

Disorders Related to Genetic Abnormalities

Numerous disorders are caused by defective DNA. These genetic disorders include phenylketonuria (PKU), sickle cell anemia, and cystic fibrosis.

As previously discussed (in Chapter 4), *phenylketonuria* is an inherited disease in which a person does not have the ability to break down the amino acid phenylalanine. As a result, phenylalanine and its metabolic by-products build up in tissues and can cause brain damage. Individuals with PKU must eat a diet that is severely limited in phenylalanine.

Sickle cell anemia is an inherited disorder of the red blood cells in which a single amino acid present in hemoglobin is changed. As shown in Figure 6.9, normal hemoglobin is globular, giving red blood cells a round, doughnut-like shape. The genetic alteration that occurs with sickle cell anemia causes the red blood cells to be shaped like a sickle or a crescent (**Figure 6.18**). Because sickled red blood cells are stiff and sticky, they cannot flow smoothly through the smallest blood vessels. Instead, they block the vessels, depriving nearby tissues of their oxygen supply and eventually damaging vulnerable organs, particularly the spleen. Sickled cells also have a life span of only about 10 to 20 days, as opposed to the 120-day average for globular red blood cells. The body's greatly increased demand for new red blood cells leads to severe anemia. Other signs and symptoms of sickle cell anemia include impaired vision, headaches, convulsions, bone degeneration, and decreased function of various organs. This disease occurs in any person who inherits the sickle cell gene from both parents.

Cystic fibrosis is an inherited disease that primarily affects the respiratory system and digestive tract. It is caused by a defective gene that causes cells to build and then reject an abnormal version of a protein that normally allows the passage of chloride into and out of certain cells. This alteration in chloride transport causes cells to secrete thick, sticky mucus. The linings of the lungs and pancreas are particularly affected, causing breathing difficulties, lung infections, and digestion problems that lead to nutrient deficiencies. Symptoms include wheezing, coughing, and stunted growth. The severity of this disease varies greatly; some individuals with cystic fibrosis live relatively normal lives, whereas others are seriously debilitated and die in childhood.

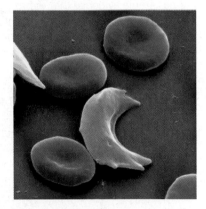

FIGURE 6.18 A sickled red blood cell.

sickle cell anemia A genetic disorder that causes red blood cells to be shaped like a sickle or crescent. These cells cannot travel smoothly through blood vessels, causing cell breakage and anemia.

cystic fibrosis A genetic disorder that causes an alteration in chloride transport, leading to the production of thick, sticky mucus that causes life-threatening respiratory and digestive problems.

RECAP

Protein–energy malnutrition can lead to marasmus and kwashiorkor. These diseases primarily affect impoverished children in developing nations. However, residents of developed countries are also at risk, especially the elderly, the homeless, people who abuse alcohol or other drugs, and people with AIDS, cancer, and other wasting diseases. Genetic disorders involving abnormal proteins include phenylketonuria, sickle cell anemia, and cystic fibrosis.

Nutrition Myth OR Fact?

Are Current Protein Recommendations High Enough?

In 2005, the Institute of Medicine concluded that a protein intake of 0.8 gram per kilogram body weight is sufficient to maintain nitrogen balance in healthy adults no matter what their activity level.[1] However, as discussed in the chapter and illustrated in Table 6.2 (page 230), there is now increasing evidence that the current RDA may not be sufficient to support optimal health and function for various groups, and experts are calling for a critical examination of the RDA to determine if it should be increased.[2]

The adequacy of the current RDA to meet the needs of active people and athletes has been questioned for a number of years. Although the Institute of Medicine states there is insufficient evidence to support the contention that these populations need increased protein intakes,[1] experts working with athletes and highly active people argue that there is ample evidence that the protein needs of these groups are higher and the current RDA cannot meet their needs.[3] They contend that athletes need more protein for several reasons:

- Regular exercise increases the transport of oxygen to body tissues, requiring changes in the oxygen-carrying capacity of the blood. To carry more oxygen, we need to produce more of the protein that carries oxygen in the blood (that is, hemoglobin, which is a protein).
- During intense exercise, we use a small amount of protein directly for energy.
- We also use protein to make glucose to prevent hypoglycemia (low blood sugar) during exercise.
- Regular exercise stimulates tissue growth and causes tissue damage, which must be repaired by additional proteins.

As a result of these increased demands for protein, the American College of Sports Medicine has concluded that strength athletes (such as weightlifters) need 1.2 to 1.7 grams of protein per kilogram body weight per day, which is equivalent to 1.8 to 2 times more protein than the current RDA (refer to Table 6.2). Similarly, endurance athletes (such as distance runners) need 1.2 to 1.4 grams of protein per kilogram body weight per day, which is equivalent to 1.5 to 1.75 times more protein.[4] More recent research suggests that optimal protein needs for both these types of athletes could as high as 1.6 to 2.25 times the current RDA, or 1.3 to 1.8 grams per kilogram body weight per day.[3]

Research examining protein needs in adults older than 65 years of age, young men, and children suggests that the protein needs for these populations—to meet optimal growth, tissue repair, and regeneration, function, and health—also are higher than the current RDA.[5–8] For instance, some researchers suggest that, to preserve lean body tissue

and physical function, older adults may need 1.29 grams of protein per kilogram of body weight, which is 1.6 times the current RDA.

What could be contributing to this discrepancy between recent research findings and the evidence used to set the RDAs for protein? One factor may be inaccuracy in the method used to determine protein needs. The current RDAs are based on evidence determined by the nitrogen-balance method. As discussed in this chapter, this method is expensive and time- and labor-intensive for both researchers and research participants; moreover, because it cannot capture all of the nitrogen excreted from the body, it underestimates protein needs. A relatively new method, referred to as the *indicator amino acid technique* (IAAO), is much less invasive and time-consuming than nitrogen balance.[1] However, this method appears to overestimate protein needs. A second factor in the discrepancy may be a lack of correspondence between nitrogen balance and health; that is, we don't currently know whether or not consuming enough protein to meet nitrogen balance optimizes health and functioning. As such, there is clearly a need to conduct research that critically examines the methods used to measure protein needs, and the amounts needed to support health-related outcomes.[1]

Does this mean that you should add more protein to your diet? Not necessarily. Contrary to popular belief, most Americans, no matter what their activity level, already consume more than twice the RDA for protein. Thus, even if the RDA were increased, it is highly likely that you are already meeting or exceeding it. As discussed in this chapter, consuming adequate protein and engaging in regular physical activity that includes resistance training will promote optimal health and function. By eating a balanced diet and consuming a variety of foods, adults can easily meet their protein requirements without the need for amino acid supplements or protein powders.

Critical Thinking Questions

- Before taking this course, did you feel you would benefit from consuming more protein? Why or why not?
- Based on the outcome of estimating your current protein intake in the Nutrition Label Activity, would you meet or exceed the suggested increase in protein intakes for active people?
- What are some adverse effects to people's health or the environment that could result from increasing the current RDA for protein?

References

1. Institute of Medicine, Food and Nutrition Board. 2005. *Dietary Reference Intakes for Energy, Carbohydrate, Fiber, Fat, Fatty Acids, Cholesterol, Protein, and Amino Acids (Macronutrients)*. Washington, DC: National Academies Press.
2. Marini, J. C. 2015. Protein recommendations: are we ready for new recommendations? *J. Nutr.* 145(1):5–6.
3. Phillips, S. M., and L. J. van Loon. 2011. Dietary protein for athletes: from requirements to optimum adaptation. *J. Sports Sci.* 29 Suppl 1:S29–S38.
4. American College of Sports Medicine, American Dietetics Association, and Dietitians of Canada. 2009. Joint position statement: nutrition and athletic performance. *Med. Sci. Sports Exerc.* 41(3):709–731.
5. Rafii, M., M. Chapman, J. Owens, R. Elango, W. W. Campbell, R. O. Ball, P. B. Pencharz, and G. Courtney-Martin. 2015. Dietary protein requirement of female adults >65 years determined by the indicator amino acid oxidation technique is higher than current recommendations. *J. Nutr.* 145(1):18–24.
6. Tang, M., G. P. McCabe, R. Elango, P. B. Pencharz, R. O. Ball, and W. W. Campbell. 2014. Assessment of protein requirements in octogenarian women with use of the indicator amino acid oxidation technique. *Am. J. Clin. Nutr.* 99:891–898.
7. Humayun, M. A., R. Elango, R. O. Ball, and P. B. Pencharz. 2007. Reevaluation of the protein requirement in young men with the indicator amino acid oxidation technique. *Am. J. Clin. Nutr.* 86:995–1002.
8. Elango, R., M. A. Humayun, R. O. Ball, and P. B. Pencharz. 2011. Protein requirement of healthy school-aged children determined by the indicator amino acid oxidation method. *Am. J. Clin. Nutr.* 94:1545–1552.

STUDY **PLAN**   MasteringNutrition™

Customize your study plan—and master your nutrition!—in the Study Area of MasteringNutrition.

TEST YOURSELF | *ANSWERS*

1 **F** Although protein can be used for energy in certain circumstances, fats and carbohydrates are the primary sources of energy for our bodies.

2 **F** There is no evidence that consuming amino acid supplements assists in building muscle tissue. Consuming adequate energy and exercising muscles, specifically using weight training, build muscle tissue.

3 **F** Excess protein is broken down and its component parts are either stored as fat or used for energy or tissue building and repair. Only the nitrogen component of protein is excreted in the urine.

4 **F** Vegetarian diets can meet and even exceed an individual's protein needs, assuming that adequate energy-yielding macronutrients, a variety of protein sources, and complementary-protein sources are consumed.

5 **T** Most people in the United States consume 1.5 to 2 times more protein than they need.

Summary

Scan to hear an MP3 Chapter Review in **MasteringNutrition**.

LO 1 ■ Unlike carbohydrates and fat, the structure of proteins is dictated by DNA; moreover, proteins contain nitrogen and some contain sulfur.

■ Amino acids are the building blocks of proteins; they are composed of a nitrogen-containing amine group, an acid group, a hydrogen atom, and a unique side chain, all bonded to a central carbon atom.

LO 2 ■ There are 20 different amino acids in our bodies: nine are essential amino acids, meaning that our bodies cannot produce them, and we must obtain them from food; 11 are nonessential, meaning our bodies can make them, so they do not need to be consumed in the diet. Conditionally essential amino acids are those that can become essential when the body's need for them exceeds its ability to produce them.

LO 3 ■ Amino acids form peptide bonds with other amino acids to produce dipeptides, tripeptides, oligopeptides, and polypeptides.

■ Our genetic makeup determines the sequence of amino acids in our proteins. *Gene expression* refers to the use of a gene in a cell to make a protein. All genes are present in cells, but not all genes are expressed.

■ Deoxyribonucleic acid (DNA) is the genetic template for gene expression and protein synthesis. The building blocks of DNA are nucleotides, molecules composed of a phosphate group, a pentose sugar called deoxyribose, and one of four nitrogenous bases.

■ Cells use various types of RNA to transcribe DNA and translate it into the sequence of amino acids unique to the given protein.

■ Protein turnover involves the synthesis of new proteins and the degradation of existing proteins.

■ The precise sequence of amino acids determines a protein's three-dimensional shape, which in turn determines its function in the body. When proteins are exposed to damaging substances, such as heat, acids, bases, and alcohol, they are denatured, meaning they lose their shape and function.

■ A limiting amino acid is one that is missing or in limited supply, preventing the synthesis of adequate proteins.

■ Mutual supplementation is the process of combining two incomplete protein sources to make a complete protein. The two foods involved in this process are called complementary proteins.

LO 4 ■ In the stomach, hydrochloric acid denatures proteins and converts pepsinogen into pepsin, an enzyme that breaks proteins strands into shorter polypeptides and single amino acids.

■ Most of the digestion of proteins occurs in the small intestine with the help of proteases secreted by the pancreas and intestinal cells. Single amino acids are absorbed into the bloodstream and transported via the portal vein to the liver.

■ Taking high doses of individual amino acid supplements on an empty stomach could in theory lead to deficiencies of other amino acids competing for the same intestinal absorption sites.

■ Protein quality is determined by its amino acid content and digestibility. Higher-quality proteins contain more essential amino acids and are more digestible. Animal sources, soy protein, and legumes are highly digestible forms of protein.

LO 5 ■ Proteins are needed to promote cell growth, repair, and maintenance. They act as enzymes and hormones; help maintain the balance of fluids, electrolytes, acids, and bases; and support healthy immune function. They are also critical for nutrient transport and storage.

LO 6 ■ The RDA for protein for sedentary adults is 0.8 g of protein per kilogram of body weight per day; protein should comprise 10% to 35% of total energy intake. Pregnant women, athletes, and certain other individuals need slightly more protein; however, most people in the United States routinely eat much more than their RDA.

LO 7 ■ Research evidence suggests that high-protein diets do not lead to increased LDL cholesterol levels if protein sources low in saturated fat are consumed. Bone health should not be compromised with high protein intakes if adequate calcium is consumed. There is no evidence that eating more protein causes kidney disease in healthy people who are not susceptible to this condition; however, high protein intakes may increase the risk of kidney disease in susceptible people.

LO 8 ■ Beef, pork, poultry, seafood, dairy foods, eggs, soy and other legumes, nuts, quorn, quinoa, and certain other "ancient grains" are excellent sources of dietary protein.

LO 9 ■ There are many forms of vegetarianism; for example, a plant-based diet may limit but not entirely exclude meat, poultry, and fish; pescovegetarians consume fish and may consume dairy products and eggs; lacto-ovo vegetarians eat only plant foods plus dairy products and eggs; vegans consume only plant foods.

■ Some people consume a vegetarian diet as a religious practice. Others choose vegetarianism because of ethical, food-safety, environmental, or health concerns.

■ Consuming a well-planned vegetarian diet may reduce the risk for obesity, heart disease, type 2 diabetes, and some forms of cancer.

■ Vegans may need to supplement their diet with vitamins B_{12} and D, riboflavin, iron, calcium, and zinc.

LO 10 ■ Marasmus and kwashiorkor are two forms of protein–energy malnutrition that results from grossly inadequate energy and protein intake.

■ Phenylketonuria is a genetic disease in which the person cannot break down the amino acid phenylalanine. The buildup of phenylalanine and its by-products leads to brain damage.

■ Sickle cell anemia is a genetic disorder of the red blood cells. Because of an alteration of one amino acid in hemoglobin, the red blood cells become sickle-shaped and cannot travel smoothly through blood vessels. This blocks the vessels, causing inadequate oxygenation of nearby tissues, organ damage, and anemia.

■ Cystic fibrosis is a genetic disease that causes an alteration in chloride transport, leading to the production of thick, sticky mucus. This mucus causes serious respiratory and digestive problems, which lead to variable levels of debilitation and, in some cases, premature death.

review questions

LO 1 1. The portion of an amino acid that contains nitrogen is called the
a. side chain.
b. amine group.
c. acid group.
d. nitrate cluster.

LO 2 2. Nonessential amino acids are
a. amino acids that the body does not need for normal functioning.
b. amino acids that the body is unable to synthesize.
c. amino acids that the body is able to synthesize in sufficient quantities to meet its needs.
d. amino acids such as phenylalanine that the body cannot metabolize.

LO 3 3. The process of combining peanut butter and whole-wheat bread to make a complete protein is called
a. deamination.
b. vegetarianism.
c. transamination.
d. mutual supplementation.

LO 4 4. Polypeptides in the small intestine are broken down by
a. hydrochloric acid.
b. pepsin.
c. proteases.
d. phosphofructokinase.

LO 5 5. Proteins
a. and carbohydrates are the body's two primary sources of energy.
b. are taken from the blood and body tissues when needed for energy.
c. are converted by the liver to urea, which is transported to the kidneys for excretion in urine.
d. contribute about 28% of an average adult's energy needs.

LO 6 6. Alyson is a 22-year-old vegetarian athlete training to compete in the New York City marathon. Her daily recommended protein intake is about
a. 1.3 to 1.5 grams per kilogram of body weight.
b. 1.2 to 1.4 grams per kilogram of body weight.
c. 0.9 to 1.0 grams per kilogram of body weight.
d. 0.8 grams per kilogram of body weight.

LO 7 7. Which of the following statements about high-protein diets is true?
a. Research evidence linking high-protein diets to an increased risk for heart attacks and strokes is conclusive.
b. Research evidence linking high-protein diets to an increased risk for bone fractures is conclusive.
c. Research suggests that higher intakes of animal and soy protein protect bone in older women.
d. Both a and b are true.

LO 8   8. Which of the following is a good source of protein, fiber, and healthful, unsaturated fats?

a. red meat
b. skim milk
c. green, leafy vegetables
d. walnuts

LO 9   9. Which of the following meals would be appropriate in a balanced and adequate vegan diet?

a. rice, pinto beans, acorn squash, soy butter, and almond milk
b. veggie dog, bun, and a banana–yogurt milkshake
c. brown rice and green tea
d. egg salad on whole-wheat toast, broccoli, carrot sticks, and soy milk

LO 10   10. In sickle cell anemia,

a. a single amino acid in hemoglobin is changed.
b. red blood cells lose their characteristic doughnut-like shape.
c. normal blood flow is disrupted.
d. all of the above are true.

true or false?

LO 3   11. **True or false?** When a protein is denatured, its shape is lost but its function is retained.

LO 4   12. **True or false?** After leaving the small intestine, amino acids are transported to the liver for distribution throughout the body.

LO 5   13. **True or false?** All hormones are proteins.

14. **True or false?** Buffers help the body maintain acid–base balance.

LO 6   15. **True or false?** Athletes typically require about three times as much protein as nonactive people.

short answer

LO 6   16. Draw a sketch showing how amino acids bond to form proteins.

17. Differentiate between the roles of mRNA and tRNA in DNA replication.

LO 7   18. Explain the relationship between excessive protein intake and an increased risk for kidney disease.

LO 9   19. You've always thought of your dad as a bit of a "health nut," so you're not surprised when you come home on spring break and he offers you

a dinner of stir-fried vegetables and something called *quorn*. Over dinner, he announces that he has joined an online vegetarian chat group. "But, Dad," you protest, "you still eat meat, don't you?" "Sure I do," he answers, "but only once or twice a week. Lots of the other people in my chat group occasionally eat meat, too!" In your opinion, is vegetarianism an identity, a lifestyle choice, or a fad? Defend your position.

LO 10   20. Explain the relationship between inadequate protein intake and the swollen bellies of children with kwashiorkor.

math review

LO 6   21. Barry is concerned he is not eating enough protein. After reading this chapter, he recorded his diet each day for 1 week to calculate how much protein he is eating. Barry's average protein intake for the week is equal to 190 g, and his daily energy intake averages 3,000 kcal. Barry weighs 182 lb. Based on your calculations, is Barry (a) meeting or exceeding the AMDR for protein and (b) meeting or exceeding the RDA for protein?

Answers to Review Questions and Math Review can be found online in the MasteringNutrition Study Area.

web links

www.eatright.org
Academy of Nutrition and Dietetics
Search for "vegetarian diets" to learn how to plan healthful meat-free meals.

fnic.nal.usda.gov
USDA Food and Nutrition Information Center
Click on "food consumption" in the left navigation bar to find a searchable database of the nutrient values of foods.

www.cdc.gov
Centers for Disease Control and Prevention
Click on "CDC A-Z Index" to learn more about E. coli and mad cow disease.

www.who.int/nutrition/en/
World Health Organization Nutrition Site
Click on "Nutrition Topics" to learn more about the worldwide scope of protein-deficiency diseases and related topics.

www.nlm.nih.gov/medlineplus
Medline Plus Health Information
Search for "sickle cell anemia" and "cystic fibrosis" to obtain additional information and resources, and the latest developments for these diseases.

www.vrg.org
Vegetarian Resource Group
Visit this site for additional information on how to build a balanced vegetarian diet.

www.choosemyplate.gov/healthy-eating-tips /tips-for-vegetarian.html
MyPlate.gov
This section of the MyPlate website contains useful, healthy eating tips for vegetarians.

www.meatlessmonday.com
Meatless Monday Campaign
Find out how to start going meatless one day a week with this innovative campaign's website.

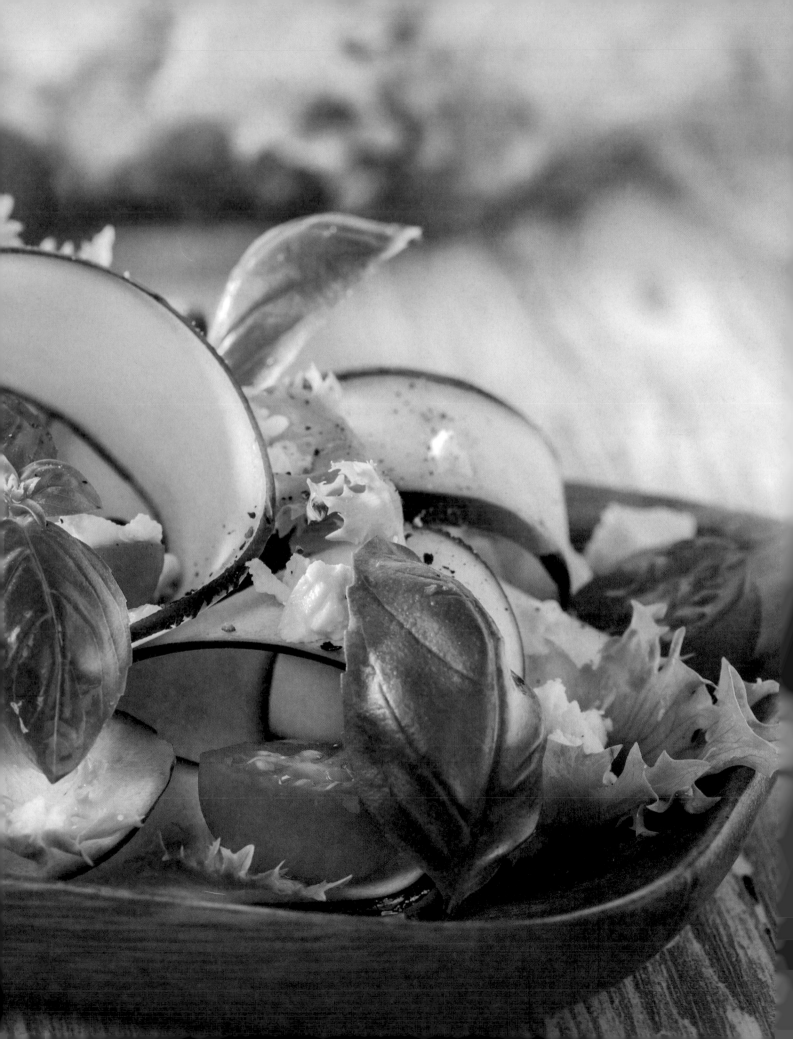

7 Metabolism: From Food to Life

Learning Outcomes

After studying this chapter, you should be able to:

1 Describe the properties of metabolism, catabolism, and anabolism, including the roles of ATP, ADP, and AMP, *pp. 252–254.*

2 Illustrate the following types of metabolic reactions: hydrolysis, dehydration synthesis, phosphorylation, and oxidation–reduction, *pp. 254–258.*

3 Identify the metabolic processes and stages involved in extracting energy from carbohydrates, *pp. 258–264.*

4 Identify the metabolic processes and stages involved in extracting energy from fats, *pp. 264–269.*

5 Explain how the catabolism of proteins differs from the catabolism of carbohydrates and lipids, *pp. 270–272.*

6 Delineate the process by which alcohol is metabolized, *pp. 272–274.*

7 Identify the body's mechanisms for storing excess glucose, triglycerides, and proteins, *pp. 275–276.*

8 Describe the processes by which glucose, fatty acids, cholesterol, and nonessential amino acids are synthesized, *pp. 276–278.*

9 Explain the role of insulin, glucagon, epinephrine, and cortisol in regulating metabolism, *pp. 279–280.*

10 Explain how the states of feasting and fasting affect metabolism, *pp. 280–284.*

TEST YOURSELF

True or False?

1 Every cell of the body is metabolically active. **T** *or* **F**

2 Certain vitamins are essential for producing energy in the body. **T** *or* **F**

3 Body fat is the only option for storing energy consumed in excess of short-term energy needs. **T** *or* **F**

4 You can increase your body's breakdown of alcohol by drinking a beverage containing caffeine. **T** *or* **F**

5 During a period of extreme starvation, the body will use heart muscle for energy and to help maintain blood glucose levels. **T** *or* **F**

Test Yourself answers are located in the Study Plan.

MasteringNutrition™

Go online for chapter quizzes, pre-tests, interactive activities, and more!

While grocery shopping, Olivia notices a new type of cereal on the shelf. A bright green banner on the label promises that the cereal is "A delicious way to boost your metabolism!" She notices other products claiming to be "High in Protein!" and to increase your metabolism and help you lose weight. Olivia has been trying to lose a few pounds so she can improve her performance on the softball team. She remembers reading an article on the Web describing a high-protein weight-loss shake. Over the next few weeks, Olivia invests over $100 on high-protein bars, shakes, and cereals, convinced they will rev up her metabolism. Yet, after 4 weeks, she is dismayed to find out she has actually gained 4 pounds.

What is "metabolism" anyway? Why is this technical term now at the center of dozens of ad campaigns? How does the body metabolize the energy-yielding nutrients, and is there anything special about protein? Just how does metabolism influence our health and body weight? We explore these and other questions in this chapter.

LO 1 Describe the properties of metabolism, catabolism, and anabolism, including the roles of ATP, ADP, and AMP.

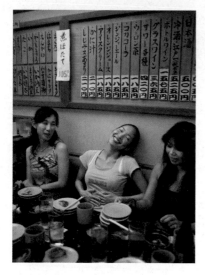

The food we eat is converted to fuel and other necessary substances through metabolism.

metabolism The sum of all the chemical and physical processes by which the body breaks down and builds up molecules.

calorimeter A special instrument in which food can be burned and the amount of heat that is released can be measured; this process demonstrates the energy (caloric) content of the food.

anabolism The process of synthesizing larger molecules from smaller ones.

catabolism The breakdown, or degradation, of larger molecules to smaller molecules.

Why Is Metabolism Essential for Life?

Although some people say they live to eat, we all have to eat to live. The food we eat each day provides the energy and nutrients the body needs to sustain life. **Metabolism** is the sum of all the chemical and physical processes by which the body breaks down and builds up molecules. When nutrition researchers burn food in a **calorimeter** to determine how much energy the food contains, carbon dioxide, water, and thermal energy (heat) are released. In a similar way, when the body uses food for fuel, carbon dioxide, water, and energy, both chemical and thermal energy, are released. Cells throughout the body require chemical energy to grow, reproduce, repair themselves, and maintain their functions. Indeed, every chemical reaction in the body either requires or releases energy. In addition, energy released as heat helps keep us warm. When cell metabolism functions properly, so, too, does the body.

Anabolism and Catabolism Require or Release Energy

As you learned in previous chapters, the end products of digestion are absorbed from the small intestine and then circulated to the body's cells. There, they may be broken down even further for energy. Alternatively, the cells may use these small, basic molecules as building blocks to synthesize compounds, such as glycogen, cholesterol, hormones, enzymes, or cell membranes, according to the body's needs. The process of making larger, chemically complex molecules from smaller, more basic ones is called **anabolism** (**Figure 7.1**). Because the process of anabolism supports the building of compounds, it is critical for growth, repair, and maintenance of the body's tissues and synthesis of the chemical products essential for human functioning. From a small subset of metabolic "building blocks," including glucose, amino acids, and fatty acids, the body is able to use anabolism to synthesize thousands of chemically complex substances.

Anabolic reactions require energy. If you've studied physics, you know that *energy* can be broadly defined as the capacity to perform work. Mechanical energy is necessary for movement, electrical energy sparks nerve impulses, and thermal energy maintains body temperature. The energy that fuels anabolic reactions is chemical energy. How exactly does the body generate this chemical energy?

Catabolism is the breakdown, or degradation, of larger, more complex molecules to smaller, more basic molecules (see Figure 7.1). The opposite of anabolism, it releases chemical energy. Catabolism of food begins with digestion, when chemical reactions break down the thousands of different proteins, lipids, and carbohydrates in the human diet into the same small group of end products: amino acids, fatty acids, glycerol, and monosaccharides (usually glucose). After absorption, these basic components are transported to body cells. When a cell needs energy, it can catabolize these components into even smaller molecules. Energy is released as a by-product of this intracellular catabolism.

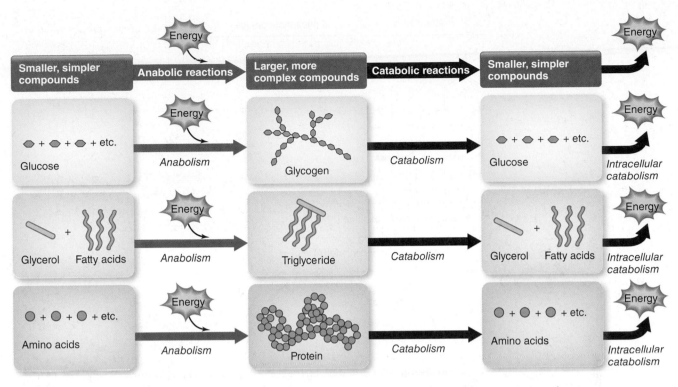

FIGURE 7.1 Anabolic reactions use energy to convert simple chemical compounds into larger, more complex structures. Catabolic reactions degrade complex compounds and produce energy.

Catabolism is also used to break down old cells or tissues that need to be repaired or replaced. The energy gained via catabolic reactions is used not only to fuel the body's work but also to build new compounds, cells, and tissues through anabolism. Thus, in response to our earlier question, the energy to fuel anabolic reactions comes from the body's catabolic reactions.

Overall, a balance between anabolism and catabolism maintains health and function. However, there are times when one of these two processes dominates. For example, fetal and childhood growth represents a net anabolic state, because more tissue is formed than broken down. However, disease is often dominated by catabolism, with more tissue being broken down than repaired. Of course, one goal of treatment is to stop or minimize these catabolic processes and allow the anabolic phase of recovery to begin.

Energy Stored in Adenosine Triphosphate Fuels the Work of All Body Cells

When cells catabolize nutrients such as glucose, they package the energy that is released during the reaction in a compound called **adenosine triphosphate (ATP)**. As you might guess from its name, a molecule of ATP includes an organic compound called adenosine and three phosphate groups (**Figure 7.2a**, page 254). The bonds between the phosphate groups store a significant amount of potential energy and are sometimes termed *high-energy phosphate bonds*. When these bonds are broken, their energy is released and can be used to do the work of the cell. This explains why ATP is often called the molecular "currency" of the cell: its phosphate bonds store energy to build new molecules, break down old molecules, and keep the cell functioning optimally.

When one high-energy phosphate bond is broken and a single phosphate group released, **adenosine diphosphate (ADP)** is produced (Figure 7.2b). When two phosphates are removed, **adenosine monophosphate (AMP)** is produced. ATP can be regenerated by adding phosphate groups back to these molecules (Figure 7.2c).

adenosine triphosphate (ATP)
A high-energy compound made up of the purine adenine, the simple sugar ribose, and three phosphate units; it is used by cells as a source of metabolic energy.

adenosine diphosphate (ADP)
A metabolic intermediate that results from the removal of one phosphate group from ATP.

adenosine monophosphate (AMP)
A low-energy compound that results from the removal of two phosphate groups from ATP.

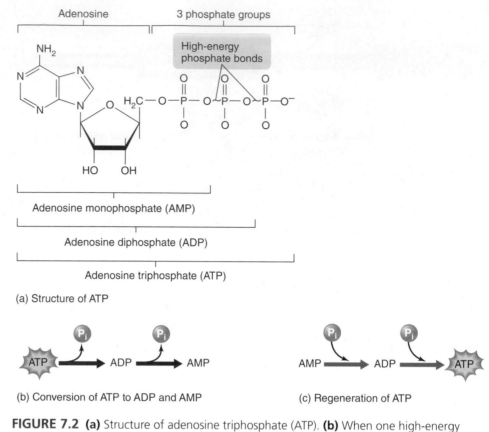

(a) Structure of ATP

(b) Conversion of ATP to ADP and AMP

(c) Regeneration of ATP

FIGURE 7.2 (a) Structure of adenosine triphosphate (ATP). **(b)** When one high-energy phosphate group is removed, adenosine diphosphate (ADP) is formed. When two high-energy phosphate groups are removed, adenosine monophosphate (AMP) is formed. **(c)** ATP can be regenerated by adding phosphate groups back to AMP and ADP through the process of phosphorylation.

A small amount of ATP is stored in every cell for immediate use. When cells need more ATP, they can generate it through the catabolism of glucose, glycerol, fatty acids, and amino acids. Thus, the food we eat each day helps the body regenerate the ATP required by our cells.

RECAP

Metabolism is sum of all the chemical and physical processes by which the body breaks down and builds up molecules. All forms of life are dependent upon metabolism for survival. A balance between anabolic and catabolic reactions helps the body achieve growth and repair and maintain health and functioning. The body uses, produces, and stores energy in the form of ATP. ■

LO 2 Illustrate the following types of metabolic reactions: hydrolysis, dehydration synthesis, phosphorylation, and oxidation–reduction.

What Chemical Reactions Are Fundamental to Metabolism?

Metabolic pathways are clusters of chemical reactions that occur sequentially and achieve a particular goal, such as the breakdown of glucose for energy. Cells use different, yet related, metabolic pathways to release the energy in each of the major energy-containing nutrients—glucose, fatty acids, and amino acids. These pathways typically occur within a specific part of a cell. This is because many metabolic enzymes are restricted to one or a few locations within the cell. As an example, the process of glycolysis, to be discussed shortly, occurs in the cytosol, the liquid portion of the cytoplasm, because all of the enzymes needed for that process can be found in the cytosol. **Figure 7.3** shows the general structure of a cell and its components.

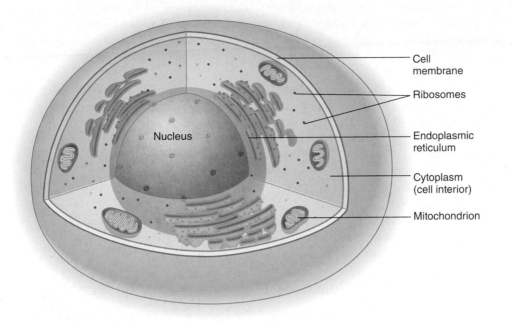

FIGURE 7.3 Structure of a typical cell. The cell membrane separates the cell from the extracellular fluid. The nucleus contains the genetic information. The cytoplasm contains the organelles, surrounded by a fluid called cytosol. Organelles include mitochondria, endoplasmic reticulum, and ribosomes.

Many other metabolic reactions take place in the cell's mitochondria, which might be compared to the furnace in your house. The mitochondria contain large numbers of metabolic enzymes and are the primary sites where chemical energy, in the form of ATP, is produced. Cells that lack mitochondria, such as red blood cells, are limited in their ability to produce energy. These cells must rely on less efficient energy-producing processes that can occur in their cytoplasm.

Metabolic pathways are limited not only to certain types of cells and certain cell structures, but they may also be limited to specific body organs or tissues. Glycogen stored in the liver can be catabolized and the resulting glucose released into the bloodstream, yet the catabolism of glycogen stored in skeletal muscle does not allow for the release of glucose into the blood. Why the difference? Muscle lacks one enzyme that catalyzes one simple step in the metabolic pathway that is found in the liver; thus, the glucose released from the catabolism of muscle glycogen is not able to pass through the muscle cell membrane into the blood.

Although all cells are metabolically active, many nutritionists view liver, muscle, and adipose cells as key locations for the integration of metabolic pathways. As this chapter unfolds, it will be possible to visualize the "networking" of metabolic pathways that occurs between these and other body cells.

Before describing each of the unique metabolic pathways involving carbohydrates, fats, and proteins, we will review a few simple chemical reactions common to all of them.

In Dehydration Synthesis and Hydrolysis Reactions, Water Reacts with Molecules

Dehydration synthesis and **hydrolysis** are chemical reactions involving water. Dehydration synthesis, also called *condensation*, is an anabolic process. It occurs when small, chemically simple units combine to produce a larger, more complex compound. In the process, water is released as a by-product. The general formula for these reactions is written as follows:

$$A\text{—}OH + H\text{—}B \rightarrow A\text{—}B + H_2O$$

For a brief introduction to mitochondria, check out www.youtube.com and enter the phrase "Mitochondria ATP Synthesis" in the Search box to locate this short video.

dehydration synthesis An anabolic process by which smaller, chemically simple compounds are joined and a molecule of water is released; also called *condensation*.

hydrolysis A catabolic process by which a large, chemically complex compound is broken apart with the addition of water.

One example is the synthesis of disaccharides from individual monosaccharides. As discussed in Chapter 4, the formation of a chemical bond between two simple sugars occurs when one monosaccharide donates a hydroxyl (OH) group and the other donates a hydrogen (H) atom. The dehydration synthesis of glucose and fructose to yield sucrose is shown in **Figure 7.4a**.

Again, dehydration synthesis is typically an anabolic process. Its opposite, termed *hydrolysis*, is usually catabolic. Recall that *hydro-* refers to water, whereas *lysis* is from a Greek word meaning to separate. In hydrolysis, a large, chemically complex compound is broken apart with the addition of water. Because the original compound becomes hydrated, this reaction is also called a *hydration* reaction. Notice that the general formula for hydrolysis reactions is opposite that of dehydration synthesis reactions:

$$A—B + H_2O \rightarrow A—OH + H—B$$

One example of hydrolysis is the catabolism or breakdown of the disaccharide sucrose to its smaller and chemically simpler monosaccharides (glucose and fructose). This process is illustrated in Figure 7.4b.

In Phosphorylation Reactions, Molecules Exchange Phosphate

The process by which one or more phosphate groups are added to a chemical compound is called **phosphorylation**. For example, glucose undergoes phosphorylation when it first enters a cell:

$C_6H_{12}O_6$	+	A—P—P—P	$\rightarrow$	$C_6H_{12}O_6$—P	+	A—P—P
Glucose		ATP		Phosphorylated glucose		ADP

phosphorylation The addition of one or more phosphate groups to a chemical compound.

The newly phosphorylated glucose can either be stored as glycogen or be oxidized for immediate energy (discussed shortly). Another example of phosphorylation is the synthesis

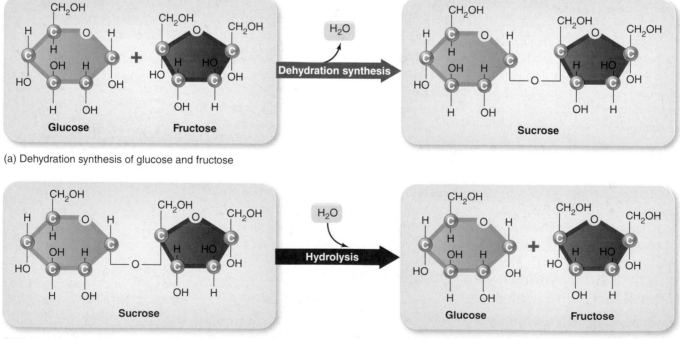

(a) Dehydration synthesis of glucose and fructose

(b) Hydrolysis of sucrose

FIGURE 7.4 (a) Dehydration synthesis of glucose and fructose. Glucose and fructose react and, with the release of water, combine to form sucrose. **(b)** Hydrolysis of sucrose. Sucrose undergoes hydrolysis, with the addition of water, to form glucose and fructose.

of ATP from ADP plus a free phosphate group (see Figure 7.2c). As you may have guessed, removal of phosphate groups, as in the breakdown of ATP (see Figure 7.2b), is called *dephosphorylation*.

In Oxidation–Reduction Reactions, Molecules Exchange Electrons

In **oxidation–reduction reactions**, the molecules involved exchange electrons, often in the form of hydrogen (which has just one electron). These reactions always occur together, as electrons gained by one molecule must be donated by another. The molecule that gives up an electron is said to be *oxidized*, because typically its electron has been removed by an oxygen atom. The molecule that has acquired an electron is said to be reduced, because, in gaining an electron (e^-), it becomes more negatively charged. In the human body, the oxygen needed for oxidation reactions is obtained from the air we breathe. Because they involve the exchange of electrons, oxidation–reduction (*redox*) reactions are classified as *exchange reactions*.

One example of a redox reaction important to metabolism involves **flavin adenine dinucleotide (FAD)** and $FADH_2$, two forms of riboflavin, one of the B-vitamins involved in energy metabolism. These compounds are required by several of the enzymes active in the electron transport chain, a key step in the production of energy. $FADH_2$ is easily oxidized, losing electrons as hydrogen, and forming FAD (**Figure 7.5**). In addition, FAD is easily reduced back to $FADH_2$ by the simple addition of hydrogen.

The production of energy from the energy-containing nutrients occurs through a series of oxidation–reduction reactions that ultimately yield carbon dioxide (CO_2) and water (H_2O). The oxidation of glucose and of fatty acids through this process is illustrated later in this chapter.

Enzymes Mediate Metabolic Reactions

During energy metabolism, one function of enzymes is to channel the energy-containing nutrients into useful metabolic pathways. For example, by increasing or decreasing the activity of one particular enzyme, the body can channel fatty acids either toward breakdown for energy or, if energy needs have already been met, toward storage as adipose tissue. Thus, enzymes help regulate metabolism.

In order to function, enzymes generally require substances called **cofactors**. These small, nonprotein substances (**Figure 7.6**, page 258) either enhance or are essential for the action of the enzyme. Many cofactors are minerals, such as iron or zinc, which may help bind different parts of an enzyme together, thereby speeding up the reaction. If the cofactor is organic (contains carbon), it is termed a **coenzyme**. Many coenzymes are derived from vitamins, particularly B-vitamins. For example, FAD and $FADH_2$, derivatives of the B-vitamin riboflavin, function as coenzymes. In short, minerals and vitamins functioning as cofactors or coenzymes are essential to ensure that metabolic pathways are as efficient as possible.

oxidation–reduction reactions Reactions in which electrons are lost by one compound (it is oxidized) and simultaneously gained by another compound (it is reduced).

flavin adenine dinucleotide (FAD) A coenzyme derived from the B-vitamin riboflavin; FAD readily accepts electrons (hydrogen) from various donors.

cofactor A small, nonprotein substance that enhances or is essential for enzyme action; trace minerals such as iron, zinc, and copper function as cofactors.

coenzyme Organic (carbon-containing) cofactor; many coenzymes are derived from B-vitamins.

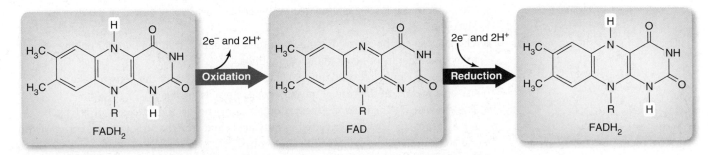

FIGURE 7.5 Oxidation and reduction of FAD and $FADH_2$. $FADH_2$ is easily oxidized to FAD, which can easily be reduced back to $FADH_2$.

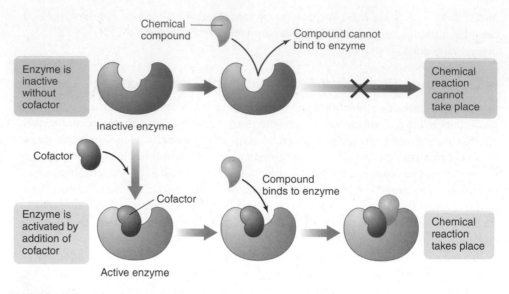

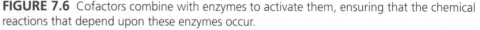

FIGURE 7.6 Cofactors combine with enzymes to activate them, ensuring that the chemical reactions that depend upon these enzymes occur.

An example of an enzyme-driven metabolic reaction is the phosphorylation of glucose, mentioned earlier. The enzyme that activates this process is **glucokinase**. When glucose concentrations in the liver rise after a meal, the activity of this enzyme increases to handle the increased load, allowing for efficient metabolism of the glucose. Not every metabolic enzyme is as responsive, however. As discussed shortly, the liver enzyme ADH that typically oxidizes alcohol does not increase in response to a sudden increase in alcohol consumption.

RECAP

Dehydration synthesis, also called condensation, is an anabolic reaction that releases water. Hydrolysis is a catabolic reaction that requires the addition of water (hydration). The reaction in which phosphate is transferred is called phosphorylation. In oxidation–reduction reactions, the molecules involved exchange electrons. Enzymes and cofactors facilitate and help regulate metabolism. Coenzymes are organic cofactors. ▪

LO 3 Identify the metabolic processes and stages involved in extracting energy from carbohydrates.

How Is Energy Extracted from Carbohydrates?

As you learned in Chapter 4, most dietary carbohydrate is digested and absorbed as glucose. The glucose is then transported to the liver, where it has a number of metabolic fates:

- The glucose can be phosphorylated, as described earlier, and stored in the liver as glycogen.
- The glucose can be phosphorylated and then metabolized in the liver for energy or used to make other glucose-containing compounds.
- The glucose can be released into circulation for other cells of the body to take up and use as a fuel or, in the case of muscle tissue, store as glycogen.
- The glucose, if consumed in excess of total energy needs and in excess of glycogen storage capacity, can be converted to fatty acids and stored as triglycerides, primarily in the adipose tissue.

glucokinase An enzyme that adds a phosphate group to a molecule of glucose.

What happens to fructose and galactose, the other dietary monosaccharides? Although there are many other metabolic options for each, both can be (a) converted into glucose through a series of reactions or (b) channeled into the glycolysis pathway (discussed shortly) for energy production. For that reason, and because glucose is the dominant monosaccharide in the human diet, this discussion will explore how the body uses glucose as an energy source.

The oxidation of glucose for the production of energy progresses through three distinct stages, each of which takes place in a different part of the cell. The three stages are

1. Glycolysis
2. The tricarboxylic acid (TCA) cycle (also known as the Krebs cycle or citric acid cycle)
3. The electron transport chain, which is where the process of oxidative phosphorylation occurs

Step by step, we will review these metabolic pathways.

In Glycolysis, Glucose Is Broken Down into Pyruvate

The metabolic pathway used by cells to produce energy from glucose begins with a sequence of reactions known as **glycolysis** (**Figure 7.7**). Because glycolysis occurs in the cytosol, even cells without mitochondria, such as red blood cells, can produce energy from

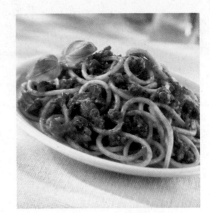

Most dietary carbohydrate is digested and absorbed as glucose.

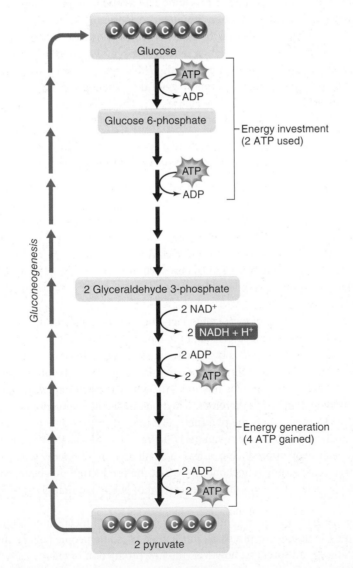

FIGURE 7.7 Overview of glycolysis. In the first stage of glucose oxidation, glucose is converted to pyruvate. A separate pathway provides for the regeneration of glucose via gluconeogenesis, which requires the input of ATP. Net production from glycolysis: two pyruvate molecules, two ATP, and two NADH 1 H+.

glycolysis A sequence of chemical reactions that converts glucose to pyruvate.

Watch a video lecture illustrating the detailed steps in glycolysis at www .youtube.com and enter the phrase "Glycolysis The Reactions" in the Search box to locate this brief animation by Virtual Cell Productions.

this pathway. Also, because the reactions of glycolysis are anaerobic (that is, do not require oxygen), this short pathway can be completed even when tissues are in an oxygen-deprived state such as during high-intensity exercise.

During glycolysis, six-carbon glucose is converted into two molecules of three-carbon pyruvate. The first step of glycolysis is the phosphorylation of glucose, which, as described earlier, yields glucose 6-phosphate and ADP. The ATP that fuels this reaction is stored in the cell. Then, several enzyme-driven reactions result in the formation of pyruvate. (These reactions are omitted from Figure 7.7 but included in the complete figure in Appendix A.) Initially, the process of glycolysis requires two ATP for the phosphorylation of glucose, but eventually this pathway produces a small amount (four molecules) of ATP, thus yielding a net of two ATP to be used as energy for the cell.

As shown in Figure 7.7, glycolysis is an oxidative pathway, because two hydrogen atoms (with their electrons) are released. These hydrogen atoms are picked up by two molecules of the coenzyme **nicotinamide adenine dinucleotide (NAD)**, derived from the B-vitamin niacin, forming two molecules of NADH, the reduced form of NAD. The metabolic fate of the newly formed NADH will be explained shortly.

If the pyruvate molecules generated by glycolysis are to be used for the production of energy, they must go through a number of additional metabolic steps, which vary depending on whether oxygen is present (*aerobic* environment) or absent (*anaerobic* environment). If energy is not immediately needed by the cell, pyruvate can be used to resynthesize glucose, which can be stored as glycogen or used in the synthesis of other carbohydrate-containing substances (which will then be stored). The resynthesis of glucose from pyruvate can be thought of as "moving back up" this stage of the metabolic pathway, which occurs through a separate series of reactions (see Figure 7.7). This reverse process is known as gluconeogenesis and will be discussed later in this chapter.

In the Absence of Oxygen, Pyruvate Is Converted to Lactate

In the absence of oxygen, the pyruvate produced through glycolysis is anaerobically converted to **lactate**. This one-step reaction involves a simple transfer of hydrogen. Both pyruvate and lactate are three-carbon compounds, so there is no loss or gain of carbon atoms. In a reversal of the hydrogen transfer that occurred in glycolysis (when NAD^+ accepted $2H^+ + 2e^-$ to form $NADH + H^+$), the conversion of pyruvate to lactate involves the transfer of $2e^- + 2H^+$ from NADH to lactate, forming NAD^+ (**Figure 7.8a**). The production of lactate therefore regenerates the NAD^+ required for the continued functioning of the glycolysis pathway.

The anaerobic conversion of pyruvate to lactate occurs in cells with few or no mitochondria, such as the red blood cells and the lens and cornea of the eye. It also occurs in the muscle cells during high-intensity exercise, when oxygen delivery to the muscle is limited. Compared with the entire three-stage oxidation of glucose, the production of energy in this phase of anaerobic glycolysis is not very efficient. The short pathway from pyruvate to lactate does not yield any ATP; therefore, when one molecule of glucose is converted to lactate, the only ATP produced is the two (net) ATP units that were generated when the glucose was initially converted to pyruvate (see Figure 7.8). The anaerobic production of lactate is, however, a way of producing at least a small amount of energy when oxygen is absent or in those cells lacking mitochondria. Again, the production of lactate, sometimes referred to as lactic acid, also allows the regeneration of NAD^+, so that glycolysis can continue.

During intense exercise, lactate and other metabolic by-products can build up in tissues, especially the muscle tissues. As discussed in Chapter 14, some people believe this build-up contributes to fatigue and soreness; however, the low production of energy as ATP through the anaerobic production of lactate is one of the many reasons individuals cannot sustain high-intensity exercise for long periods of time. After exercise, lactate can diffuse from the muscle cells into the blood, which transports it to the liver. Then, when oxygen is

nicotinamide adenine dinucleotide (NAD) A coenzyme form of the B-vitamin niacin; NAD readily accepts electrons (hydrogen) from various donors.

lactate (lactic acid) A three-carbon compound produced from pyruvate in oxygen-deprived conditions.

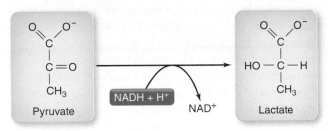

(a) Anaerobic conversion of pyruvate to lactate

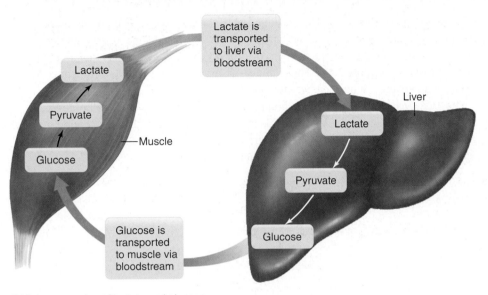

(b) Interconversion of lactate and glucose

FIGURE 7.8 (a) Anaerobic conversion of pyruvate to lactate. In the absence of oxygen, the body converts pyruvate to lactate. **(b)** Interconversion of lactate and glucose. After the anaerobic production and release of lactate by the muscle, when oxygen becomes available, the liver converts lactate back to glucose. (This process, known as the Cori cycle, is discussed in more detail in Chapter 14.)

readily available during the rest or recovery phase, it is reconverted to pyruvate, which can be used to synthesize glucose (Figure 7.8b). This process illustrates the integration of metabolism between muscle tissues and the liver, as was mentioned earlier. This cycle of glucose-to-lactate (during oxygen deprivation) followed by lactate-to-glucose (during oxygen availability) will be discussed in more detail in Chapter 14.

In the Presence of Oxygen, Pyruvate Is Converted to Acetyl CoA

In an aerobic environment where oxygen is plentiful, pyruvate is converted to a two-carbon compound known as **acetyl CoA** (**Figure 7.9**). This reaction occurs in the mitochondria and therefore does not occur in red blood cells or other cells that lack mitochondria. *CoA* is shorthand for *coenzyme A*, a coenzyme derived from the B-vitamin pantothenic acid. As with the conversion of glucose to pyruvate, the metabolic pathway taking pyruvate to acetyl CoA generates NADH + H$^+$ from the niacin-derived coenzyme NAD$^+$. Pyruvate is a three-carbon compound, whereas acetyl CoA is a two-carbon metabolite. What happens to the other carbon? It ends up within the gas carbon dioxide (CO_2), which the lungs exhale as a waste product.

Unlike the metabolic option to convert lactate to glucose, once pyruvate is metabolized to acetyl CoA, there is no "going back" to glucose synthesis. In other words, there is no metabolic option for the conversion of acetyl CoA to glucose. Once acetyl CoA is produced, it can be further metabolized to produce energy (ATP) or, when the body has adequate ATP, redirected into fatty acid synthesis (discussed shortly).

The conversion of pyruvate to acetyl CoA is a critical step in the oxidation of glucose, because it links stage 1 (glycolysis) to stage 2 (the TCA cycle). This reaction also marks the transition of cytosol-based pathways to mitochondria-based pathways. To begin this step, pyruvate moves from the cytosol into the mitochondria, where it is converted to acetyl CoA.

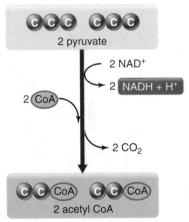

FIGURE 7.9 Aerobic conversion of pyruvate to acetyl CoA. In the presence of oxygen, the body converts pyruvate to acetyl CoA. This reaction links the first and second stages of glucose oxidation. The two pyruvate molecules were generated from glucose through glycolysis.

acetyl CoA Coenzyme A (CoA) is derived from the B-vitamin pantothenic acid; it readily reacts with two-carbon acetate to form the metabolic intermediate acetyl CoA; sometimes referred to as *acetyl coenzyme A.*

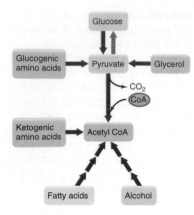

FIGURE 7.10 Metabolic crossroads. Acetyl CoA is generated as a result of carbohydrate, fatty acid, amino acid, and alcohol metabolism.

Once acetyl CoA is produced in the mitochondria, it cannot be transferred back across the mitochondrial membrane without conversion to another compound, called citrate. Thus, acetyl CoA is committed to the TCA cycle for energy production or the conversion to citrate, in which form it can move back out of the mitochondria for fatty acid synthesis.

As this chapter proceeds, it will become clear that acetyl CoA is generated not only from glucose oxidation but also from fatty acid and amino acid catabolism (**Figure 7.10**). You may be familiar with the phrase "All roads lead to Rome." In metabolism, most "roads" (metabolic pathways) lead to acetyl CoA!

The TCA Cycle Begins with the Entry of Acetyl CoA

The process of glycolysis has a clear starting point (glucose) and a clear ending point (pyruvate). The linking step (pyruvate to acetyl CoA) also has distinct start and end points. In contrast, stage 2 of glucose metabolism, the **TCA cycle**, is a continuous loop of eight metabolic reactions (**Figure 7.11**). The complete TCA cycle is illustrated in Appendix A, and a condensed version will be used here for simplicity.

The TCA cycle occurs in the mitochondria of the cell, which is where all of the necessary metabolic enzymes can be found. The mitochondria are also the location of stage 3 of glucose oxidation (involving the electron transport chain) and ATP synthesis; thus, the transition between stages 2 and 3 is highly efficient.

TCA cycle The tricarboxylic acid (TCA) cycle is a repetitive series of eight metabolic reactions, located in cell mitochondria, that metabolizes acetyl CoA for the production of carbon dioxide, high-energy GTP, and reduced coenzymes NADH and FADH$_2$.

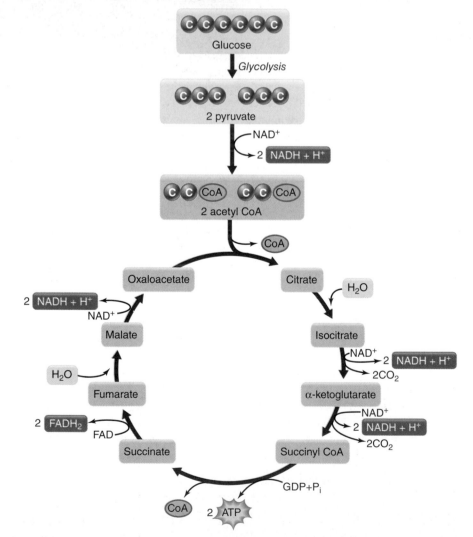

FIGURE 7.11 Overview of the TCA cycle. In the second stage of glucose oxidation, acetyl CoA enters the TCA cycle, resulting in the release of carbon dioxide, GTP (ATP), and reduced coenzymes NADH and FADH$_2$.

We think of cycles as self-regenerative, but the acetyl CoA within the TCA cycle does not regenerate. As will be seen, the two carbons that form acetyl CoA end up within two molecules of carbon dioxide. In contrast, the fate of the four-carbon compound oxaloacetate, a metabolic intermediate within the TCA cycle, does illustrate the cyclical nature of this stage of glucose oxidation: as shown in Figure 7.11, it is "used up" in the first step of the cycle, where it is converted into citrate, and is regenerated from malate in the final step of the cycle.

Oxaloacetate and other metabolic intermediates within the TCA cycle are necessary for its continued functioning; when these compounds are limited, the TCA cycle decreases in activity, and energy production sharply declines. There are several situations in which lack of oxaloacetate causes a significant decrease in energy production. One is consumption of a diet very low in carbohydrates. Although oxaloacetate can be made from some amino acids, dietary carbohydrate is the primary source. The glucose that is derived from dietary carbohydrate can be converted to acetyl CoA (stage 1, Figure 7.11), which can enter the TCA cycle and be converted to oxaloacetate. In contrast, oxaloacetate cannot be synthesized from fatty acids. If a person is following a very-low-carbohydrate diet, such as the Atkins Diet, he or she will have limited ability to produce oxaloacetate, resulting in a slowdown of the TCA cycle.

The first step of the TCA cycle begins with the entry of acetyl CoA into the cycle. As previously explained, pyruvate crosses from the cytosol into the mitochondria, where it is converted into acetyl CoA. The two-carbon acetyl CoA reacts with four-carbon oxaloacetate to form six-carbon citrate (hence the term *citric acid cycle*), and the metabolic cycle begins. By the time all eight metabolic steps are completed, the cycle has produced two molecules of carbon dioxide; this is in addition to the one carbon dioxide produced in the earlier "linking" step.

In addition to the release of carbon dioxide, a high-energy compound known as guanosine triphosphate (GTP), equivalent to one ATP, is produced. Finally, a total of eight hydrogens, with their electrons, are transferred to two coenzymes—NAD$^+$ and FAD—-producing NADH and FADH$_2$. These newly formed, hydrogen-rich coenzymes serve as the transition to stage 3, transporting the hydrogen atoms, with their electrons, to the electron transport chain.

For every molecule of glucose that goes through glycolysis, two pyruvate molecules are generated, leading to two molecules of acetyl CoA. Thus, the TCA cycle must complete two "rotations" for each molecule of glucose. From glycolysis through the TCA cycle, one molecule of glucose produces the following: six molecules of carbon dioxide (including those produced in the "linking step"), two ATP, two GTP, and 10 reduced coenzymes (including the NADH from the linking step) as sources of hydrogen and electrons. Note, however, the low energy output: this small amount of ATP and GTP will not do much to fuel the activities of the body. It is not until the final stage of glucose oxidation that energy production as ATP is significantly increased.

Oxidative Phosphorylation Captures Energy as ATP

The third and final stage of glucose oxidation, termed *oxidative phosphorylation*, occurs in the **electron transport chain** and takes place in the inner membrane of the mitochondria (**Figure 7.12**). The electron transport chain is a series of enzyme-driven reactions or couplings; various proteins, called electron carriers, alternately accept, then donate, electrons. The electrons come from the NADH and FADH$_2$ generated during glycolysis, the linking step, and the TCA cycle.

electron transport chain A series of metabolic reactions that transports electrons from NAHD or FADH$_2$ through a series of carriers, resulting in ATP production.

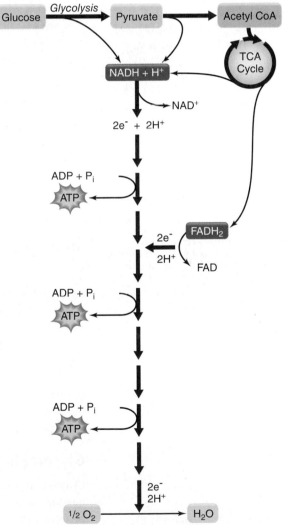

FIGURE 7.12 Overview of the electron transport chain. In the third and final stage of glucose oxidation, called *oxidative phosphorylation*, additional ATP and water are produced as electrons from NADH and FADH$_2$ and are passed from one carrier to the next along the electron transport chain.

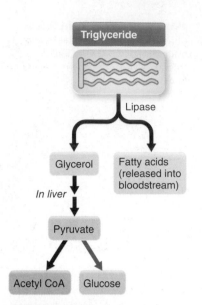

FIGURE 7.13 Conversion of glycerol to pyruvate. The glycerol derived from the catabolism of triglycerides is readily converted to pyruvate, which can be used for glucose synthesis or be converted to acetyl CoA.

As summarized in Figure 7.12, as the electrons are passed from one carrier to the next, energy is released as ATP. In this process, NADH and $FADH_2$ are oxidized (lose electrons) and their electrons are eventually donated to O_2, which is reduced to H_2O (water). The energy released from the reduction of O_2 to water is used to phosphorylate mitochondrial ADP to ATP, thereby capturing the metabolic energy in ATP's high-energy phosphate bonds. Once formed, the ATP can exit the mitochondria for use by all components of the cell.

As mentioned, the final step in the electron transport chain occurs when oxygen accepts the low-energy electrons, reacts with hydrogen, and forms water. If the cell lacks adequate oxygen for this final step, the entire electron transport chain comes to a halt. Oxygen is essential for cellular energy production; without oxygen, cell metabolism stops.

This brings the process of glucose oxidation to a close. The complete process started with glucose and resulted in the production of carbon dioxide, water, and ATP. The carbon dioxide was produced in the linking step (pyruvate to acetyl CoA) and the TCA cycle. The water was produced in the final step of the electron transport chain. ATP was produced in varying amounts during the three stages. It might surprise you to know that the amount of ATP produced by NADH and $FADH_2$ is not exact (about two to three ATP per NADH and one to two for $FADH_2$); thus, different researchers calculate different values for ATP production. Many biochemistry textbooks report a net of 30 to 32 ATP produced by the complete oxidation of one glucose molecule. Other references (including Appendix A of this textbook) use the range of 36 to 38 ATP per glucose molecule. This may seem confusing, but the study of nutrient metabolism is rarely an exact science.

RECAP

Glucose oxidation occurs in three well-defined stages: glycolysis, the TCA cycle, and oxidative phosphorylation. The conversion of pyruvate to acetyl CoA is a critical link between glycolysis and the TCA cycle. In the absence of oxygen, the pyruvate is converted to lactate, which can then be "recycled" by liver cells back into glucose. The end products of glucose oxidation are carbon dioxide, water, and ATP. ∎

LO 4 Identify the metabolic processes and stages involved in extracting energy from fats.

How Is Energy Extracted from Fats?

The fatty acids used for cellular energy can come from the triglycerides circulating in serum lipoproteins, including the dietary fat in chylomicrons, or from the triglycerides stored in body tissues, including adipose tissue. Because the triglyceride molecule is more complex than that of glucose, there are more steps involved in converting it into energy. Of course, the first step requires that each fatty acid be removed from the glycerol backbone. Through a process called **lipolysis**, dietary and adipocyte triglycerides are broken down by lipases to yield glycerol and three free fatty acids. Triglycerides in lipoproteins are broken down through the action of *lipoprotein lipase*, whereas triglycerides in adipose cells are catabolized by the enzyme *hormone-sensitive lipase*. Whether the glycerol and three free fatty acids have come from dietary fat or stored body fat, they feed into the same metabolic pathways.

Glycerol Is Converted to Pyruvate

Glycerol, the small, three-carbon backbone of triglycerides, does not produce much energy but does serve other important metabolic functions. The liver easily converts glycerol into pyruvate, another three-carbon compound (**Figure 7.13**). As previously discussed, pyruvate can be converted into acetyl CoA for entry into the TCA cycle (see Figure 7.9), or it can be used for the regeneration of glucose (see Figure 7.7). Thus, in times of low-energy or low-carbohydrate intake, the body can use the glycerol component of triglycerides as a source of glucose.

Fatty Acids Are Converted to Acetyl CoA

In yet another example of the integration of metabolism across different body organs, fatty acids released from adipose cells are attached to **albumin**, a blood protein, and transported

lipolysis The enzyme-driven catabolism of triglycerides into free fatty acids and glycerol.

albumin A serum protein, made in the liver, that transports free fatty acids from one body tissue to another.

to working cells in need of energy, such as muscle or liver cells. They are catabolized for energy through a process known as **β-oxidation**, or **fatty acid oxidation**. This metabolic pathway takes place in the mitochondria, which means that fatty acids must move from the cytosol across the mitochondrial membrane. Before the fatty acids can be transported into the mitochondria, however, they must be activated by the addition of coenzyme A (CoA), the same coenzyme used in the synthesis of acetyl CoA from pyruvate. This reaction requires an "investment" of energy from ATP. The activated fatty acids are then shuttled across the mitochondrial membrane by a compound known as **carnitine**. You might have heard that carnitine supplements can help your body burn fat. Is it true? Read the nearby *Highlight* to find out.

β-oxidation (fatty acid oxidation) A series of metabolic reactions that oxidize free fatty acids, leading to the end products of water, carbon dioxide, and ATP.

carnitine A small, organic compound that transports free fatty acids from the cytosol into the mitochondria for oxidation.

HIGHLIGHT

Are Carnitine Supplements Fat Burners?

Product labels, Internet advertisements, and TV infomercials practically shout the term "fat burner" when trying to convince consumers of the value of carnitine supplements; for years, carnitine has been included in many so-called weight-loss, fat-burning supplements. The appeal of their claim is undeniable: use this product, and body fat will "melt" away.

Carnitine shuttles fatty acids across the mitochondrial membrane. Fatty acids are oxidized along the inside of the mitochondrial membrane, because that is where the enzymes of the β-oxidation pathway are found. If fatty acids can't get across the mitochondrial membrane, they will not be oxidized as a fuel and will accumulate. It seems logical, then, that carnitine supplements will increase fat oxidation and decrease body fat stores. But do they? There are two arguments often used in marketing carnitine supplements: (1) many people are low in carnitine and so would benefit from carnitine supplements, and (2) even healthy people with normal carnitine levels could lower their body fat by taking extra carnitine. How do these arguments hold up?

Looking at the first issue, are many people low in carnitine? Two important pieces of information are often left out of advertisements for carnitine supplements: (1) carnitine is widely available from a large number of foods, and (2) humans synthesize carnitine in amounts that fully meet the needs of healthy people. Food sources of carnitine include meat, poultry, fish, and dairy products; healthy children and adults on a mixed diet get all the carnitine needed from their normal diet. What about vegetarians and vegans? It is true that they *eat* much less dietary carnitine than nonvegetarians, but the body can easily synthesize it from the amino acids lysine and methionine. Lysine is found in legumes, including soybeans, whereas methionine is plentiful in grains, nuts, and seeds. Vegetarians commonly consume these foods in abundant amounts. As long as their diet provides enough of these foods, as well as the iron, niacin, vitamin B_6, and vitamin C used as cofactors, healthy vegetarians and vegans can meet their need for carnitine through endogenous (internal) synthesis. So, well-nourished, healthy people—vegetarians and vegans included—are rarely, if ever, low in carnitine.

What about the second claim? Do high doses of carnitine supplements benefit overweight or obese people? Manufacturers promote carnitine supplements as "fat burners" by implying that high intakes will increase blood levels, then muscle levels, of carnitine. Once in the muscle, the advertisements suggest, the carnitine would trigger fat oxidation and "burn up" body fat. Most studies have shown that taking large doses of carnitine, for up to 2 weeks, does not increase muscle carnitine levels and, so, would have no effect on body fat oxidation. However, a recent small study with 12 men did show that 3 months of carnitine supplementation led to an increase in gene activity related to fat oxidation.[1] Despite this genetic change, however, none of the carnitine-supplemented men lost body fat or body weight. In addition, a review of "fat-burning" supplements concluded that there was a lack of strong scientific evidence to support the proposed role of carnitine in fat metabolism.[2] Thus, well-controlled research has failed to support either of these claims.

Are there any situations when carnitine supplements are useful? Yes, but they are rare. People with certain genetic metabolic defects must be provided with supplementary carnitine, because they are unable to synthesize or utilize it; patients with chronic kidney failure and those on dialysis treatment for kidney failure are often supplemented with carnitine as well. In general, however, there is no evidence to support the claims that carnitine supplements increase the body's rate of fat oxidation or reduce body fat. The only "burning" you might experience when buying carnitine supplements is that of the money in your wallet!

References

1. Stephens, F. B., B. T. Wall, K. Marimuthu, C. E. Shannon, D. Constantin-Teodosiu, I. A. Macdonald, and P. L. Greenhaff. 2013. Skeletal muscle carnitine loading increases energy expenditure, modulates fuel metabolism gene networks and prevents body fat accumulation in humans. *J. Physiol.* 591:4655–4666.
2. Jeukendrup, A. E., and R. Randell. 2011. Fat burners: nutrition supplements that increase fat metabolism. *Obesity Rev.* 12:841–851.

Once in the mitochondria, β-oxidation proceeds, systematically breaking down long-chain fatty acids into two-carbon segments that lead to the formation of acetyl-CoA units (**Figure 7.14**). Thus, a 16-carbon fatty acid is converted to eight acetyl-CoA units. As the two-carbon segments are cleaved off the fatty acid, high-energy electrons are transferred to the coenzymes NAD⁺ and FAD, forming NADH + H⁺ and FADH₂, which feed into the electron transport chain. As with glucose oxidation, the acetyl CoA generated from fatty acid oxidation feeds into the TCA cycle for the production of ATP. The electron-rich coenzymes produced in the TCA cycle also feed into the electron transport chain and produce additional ATP. (See Appendix A for a more detailed view of β-oxidation.)

In summary, the process of extracting energy from triglycerides starts with fatty acids and glycerol and ends with the production of carbon dioxide, water, and ATP (**Figure 7.15**). These are the same three compounds produced during the oxidation of glucose.

As noted, because fatty acids almost always have more carbons than the six found in glucose, more acetyl CoA and more ATP are produced during β-oxidation of one long-chain fatty acid than during oxidation of glucose. A single 18-carbon fatty acid yields

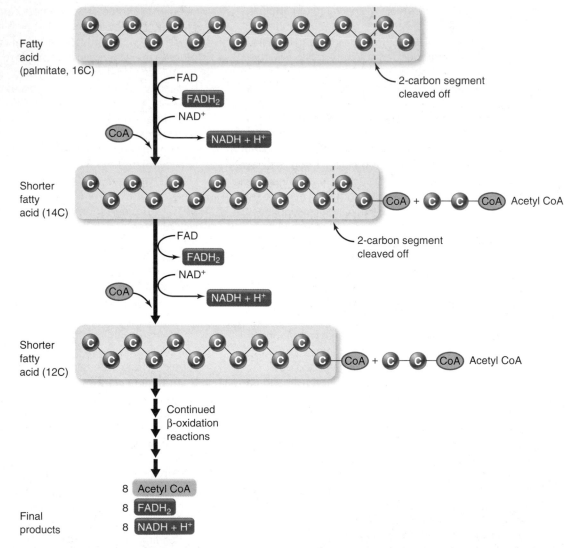

FIGURE 7.14 Overview of β-oxidation of fatty acids. Fatty acids are sequentially broken down into two-carbon segments that result in the formation of one additional acetyl CoA during each step of the process. A 16-carbon fatty acid yields eight acetyl CoA units.

nearly 3.5 times more ATP than that derived from one six-carbon molecule of glucose. More importantly, fatty acids have relatively few oxygen atoms compared with oxygen-rich glucose (**Figure 7.16**). Fatty acids thus offer numerous opportunities for oxidation, which results in a higher output of NADH and $FADH_2$ and a higher number of electrons, leading to greater production of ATP through the electron transport chain. The result is that, on a per gram basis, fatty acids have a much higher energy potential compared with carbohydrates, approximately 9 kcal/g versus approximately 4 kcal/g for carbohydrates.

Fatty Acids Cannot Be Converted to Glucose

Earlier, we noted that glycerol can be converted to pyruvate, which the liver is then able to convert to glucose. In contrast, there is no metabolic pathway to convert fatty acid–derived acetyl CoA into pyruvate for glucose synthesis. Because cells cannot convert acetyl CoA into glucose, it is impossible for fatty acids to feed into glucose production. Again, there is no metabolic pathway that allows for the conversion of fatty acids to glucose.

Ketones Are a By-Product of Fat Catabolism

Recall that the acetyl CoA that enters the TCA cycle can come from glucose or fatty acid catabolism. But the TCA cycle functions only when there is adequate oxaloacetate, a carbohydrate derivative (see Figure 7.11). In another science class, you may have heard the statement "Fat burns in the flame of carbohydrate": this need for oxaloacetate is what "the flame" refers to. Thus, if a person is following a very-low-carbohydrate diet or has too little functioning insulin to allow glucose to enter cells, oxaloacetate production falls and TCA cycle activity decreases. As fat catabolism continues during this carbohydrate-depleted state, acetyl CoA builds up, exceeding the ability of the TCA cycle to metabolize it, and accumulates in the liver cells.

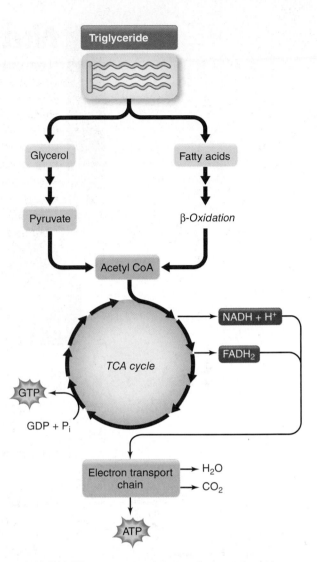

FIGURE 7.15 Extraction of energy from triglycerides. Glycerol and fatty acids can be metabolized to yield energy as ATP.

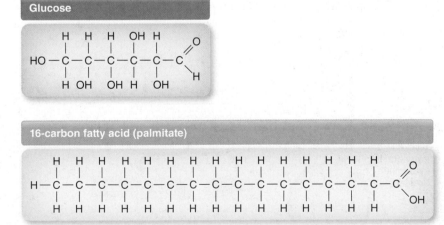

FIGURE 7.16 A comparison of glucose and fatty acid structures. In contrast with glucose, where each carbon is attached to an oxygen, there are many opportunities for oxidation of the carbon-to-hydrogen bonds of a fatty acid.

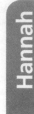

Nutri-Case

"I was walking through the Student Union this morning, minding my own business, when this really attractive guy from biology class comes up to me all friendly, like I'm his long-lost sister or something. 'Hannah! Can I walk with you to class?' Now, I hardly know this guy, so I just shrugged, 'Sure, whatever . . .' Well, before you know it, he's trying to sell me this 'awesome'—that's what he kept calling it—weight-loss supplement. He tells me it's full of pyruvate, some kind of chemical that we need to burn fat. He says that, if I take it, my body will burn a lot more fat, so I'll use up my fat stores and lose weight. By the time we got to class, he had me half-convinced, but the supplements cost $30 a bottle, and I didn't even have that much on me. So I said I'd think about it and maybe buy some next week. But I'm not sure. My mom always says if it sounds too good to be true, it is."

Should Hannah buy the pyruvate supplements? Review the metabolic pathway of β-oxidation and consider whether or not it seems logical that consuming pyruvate supplements would increase the burning of the body's fat stores. Why or why not?

As the acetyl CoA builds up, liver cells divert it into an alternative metabolic pathway leading to the synthesis of one or more **ketone bodies** (acetoacetate, acetone, and β-hydroxybutyrate or 3-hydroxybutyrate) (**Figure 7.17**). The liver constantly produces low levels of ketone bodies; however, production increases dramatically during times of very-low-carbohydrate intake, whether from prolonged fasting, starvation, or very-low-carbohydrate diets, as well as in people with type 1 diabetes who require external insulin for glucose transport into the cell. If someone with type 1 diabetes cannot obtain insulin, the body will be unable to maintain oxaloacetate production, the TCA cycle will shut down, and ketone production will increase. Ketone bodies are released from the liver into the bloodstream, where they can be taken up and used as an alternative fuel by the brain, certain kidney cells, and other body cells when their normal fuel source (glucose) is not available.

The production of energy from ketones is metabolically inefficient, because the total amount of ATP produced will be lower than what would have been produced through β-oxidation of fatty acids. A little energy, however, is better than none; thus, ketone synthesis provides a backup source of energy for carbohydrate-deprived cells.

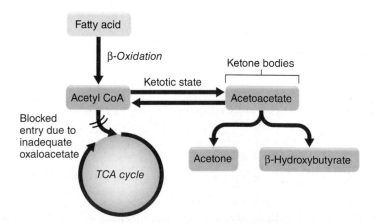

ketone bodies Three- and four-carbon compounds (acetoacetate, acetone, and β- or 3-hydroxybutyrate) derived when acetyl CoA levels become elevated.

FIGURE 7.17 Overview of ketone synthesis. Ketones are produced when acetyl CoA is blocked from entering the TCA cycle. Two molecules of acetyl CoA combine to form acetoacetate, which can be converted to acetone or β-hydroxybutyrate. These three compounds are collectively called ketone bodies. Energy is later extracted from ketones when acetoacetate is reconverted back to acetyl CoA for entry into the TCA cycle.

When the rate of ketone production increases above its use by cells, blood and urine ketone levels rise, a condition known as *ketosis*. Typical blood levels of ketones are 3 mg/dL in a healthy individual eating a mixed diet but can rise to 90 mg/dL in severe ketosis, as seen in a person with type 1 diabetes without insulin. Ketones are acidic and inappropriately lower blood pH (increasing its acidity); thus, the body attempts to eliminate them by excreting them in the urine. This process, however, also causes dehydration, as fluid is lost in the urine. As the pH of the blood falls further and dehydration becomes more severe, *ketoacidosis* occurs. If allowed to persist, ketoacidosis can result in coma or death. A classic symptom of diabetic ketoacidosis is a fruity odor on the breath, which results from increased production of the specific ketone body acetone.

Although high levels of ketone bodies are normally harmful to the body, some medical conditions are treated with ketogenic diets. These medically supervised diets are moderate in protein, high in fat and extremely low in carbohydrates (10–20 g/d). See the **You Do the Math** box to get a better idea of the strict limitations of this medical ketogenic diet. One medical condition that seems to respond to a ketogenic diet is epilepsy. The diet is sometimes prescribed when childhood epilepsy has not responded to other treatments, although it may also be effective in adolescents and adults. The ketones produced on this diet appear to reduce the number of severe seizures experienced. The exact mechanism by which the ketogenic diet exerts its antiseizure action is not yet fully understood.

 Read a father's story about the "miraculous" effect of a ketogenic diet on his son's epilepsy at www.nytimes.com; click on the "Search" button and enter the phrase "Epilepsy's Big Fat Miracle" in the for this November 21, 2010 piece.

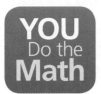
YOU Do the Math

Designing a Ketogenic Menu

As noted in our discussion on ketosis, some children with epilepsy are prescribed a ketogenic diet, in addition to their medication, to reduce the number or severity of their seizures. The benefits of the ketogenic diet for the reduction of epileptic seizures have been known for centuries; accounts of the beneficial effect of fasting on epilepsy are long-standing. American physicians have been using ketogenic diets to treat epilepsy for the past 80 years; however, we still do not know the specific mechanism by which ketones alter brain chemistry to reduce seizures.[1,2] A medical ketogenic diet is very high in fat and low in both protein and carbohydrate. Although the diet should always be developed and monitored by a registered dietitian/nutritionist (RDN) and/or physician, you can work through the calculations here to get a general idea of what a typical ketogenic menu might look like.

Most children are prescribed a diet providing 4 g of fat (36 kcal) for every 1 g of protein/carbohydrate (4 kcal). A child needing 1,500 kcal/day would be fed 150 g of fat and about 38 g of protein/carbohydrate combined. Estimating the protein requirement at about 20 g per day, that means the child could eat 18 g of carbohydrates each day. In summary, the child's daily menu would provide:

Using the nutrient data from the food composition tables, develop a 1-day menu for this child. High-fat, low-protein/carbohydrate foods include cream, butter, bacon, oils, and so forth. Small amounts of fried chicken or fish would provide fat plus protein, as would nuts and peanut butter.

Obviously, children on a medical ketogenic diet eat very few fruits and vegetables, very little milk/dairy, and few grains/cereals. An RDN would develop a strict dietary prescription identifying exactly how much of which foods are allowed; a nutrient supplement would also be prescribed. Usually, the diet is tried for about 3 months to see how well it works. If there is little or no improvement, the dietitian would then recommend a return to the normal diet.

References

1. Nei, M., J. I. Sirvenand, and M. R. Sperling. 2014. Ketogenic diet in adolescents and adults with epilepsy. *Seizure* 23:439–442.
2. O"Connor, S. E., C. Richardson, W. H. Trescher, D. L. Byler, J. D. Sather, E. H. Michael,…, and B. Zupec-Kania. 2014. The ketogenic diet for the treatment of pediatric status epilepticus. *Ped. Neurol.* 50:101–103.

1,500 kcal/day	
150 g of fat	1,350 fat kcal
20 g of protein	80 protein kcal
18 g of carbohydrate	72 carbohydrate kcal

RECAP

Triglycerides are broken down into glycerol and free fatty acids. Glycerol can be (a) converted to glucose via pyruvate or (b) oxidized for energy. Free fatty acids are oxidized to produce acetyl CoA and electron-rich coenzymes, which can enter the TCA cycle and electron transport chain. The end products of fatty acid oxidation are carbon dioxide, water, and ATP. Fatty acids cannot be converted into glucose. When cells face an inadequate supply of carbohydrate, fat catabolism increases and the excess acetyl CoA is diverted to ketone formation. ■

LO 5 Explain how the catabolism of proteins differs from the catabolism of carbohydrates and lipids.

How Is Energy Extracted from Proteins?

As you read in Chapter 6, the body's first priority in the use of protein is for the building and repair of body tissues. The body preferentially uses fat and carbohydrate as fuel sources; however, small amounts of protein are used for energy, primarily when total energy or carbohydrate intake is low. The exact amount of protein used for energy, therefore, will depend on the total energy in the diet and the amount of fat and carbohydrate consumed.

In Proteolysis, Proteins Are Broken Down to Amino Acids

During protein breakdown, called **proteolysis**, dietary proteins are digested into single amino acids or small peptides that are absorbed into the body; eventually, the small peptides are further catabolized into single amino acids. These amino acids are absorbed, then transported to the liver, where they can be made into various proteins or released into the bloodstream for uptake by other cells for their unique building and repair functions. If protein is consumed in excess of what is needed by the cells, some of this protein can be used for energy or converted into fatty acids for storage as triglycerides. Additionally, if we don't eat enough total energy or carbohydrate, the tissues can break down some of the proteins in their cells for energy. This process is explained shortly.

In Oxidative Deamination, the Amino Group Is Removed

Under conditions of starvation or extreme dieting, the body must turn to its own tissues for energy, including protein. Amino acids are unique from other energy-containing nutrients in that they contain nitrogen, which must be removed, so that the remaining carbon skeleton can be used for energy. Thus, the utilization of amino acids for energy begins with oxidative *deamination* of the amino acids, which removes their amine (NH_2), or nitrogen, group and leaves a **carbon skeleton** (**Figure 7.18**). The end products of deamination are ammonia (NH_3), derived from the amine group, and the remaining carbon skeleton, often classified as a **keto acid**. (*Note:* Even though the terms *ketone* and *keto acid* appear very similar, they are produced from completely different metabolic pathways and have very different metabolic roles. Be careful not to get the two terms confused!)

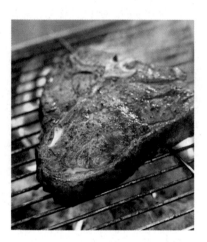

Dietary proteins are broken down into single amino acids or small peptides.

proteolysis The breakdown of dietary proteins into single amino acids or small peptides that are absorbed by the body.

carbon skeleton The unique "side group" that remains after deamination of an amino acid; also referred to as a *keto acid*.

keto acid The chemical structure that remains after deamination of an amino acid.

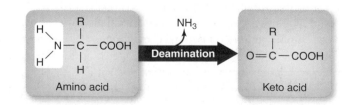

FIGURE 7.18 The process of oxidative deamination. Amino acids are deaminated when the amine group is removed; the remaining structure is known as a keto acid or carbon skeleton.

After Oxidative Deamination, the Carbon Skeleton Feeds into Energy Production

The carbon skeleton produced through oxidative deamination can be channeled into glycolysis or the TCA pathway to produce energy (**Figure 7.19**). Each of the 20 amino acids (identified in Chapter 6) has a different carbon skeleton and is classified into a number of different groups, many of which overlap. For this discussion, there are two groups of interest:

- The carbon skeletons of **glucogenic amino acids** are converted to pyruvate, which can then be used to synthesize glucose or converted to acetyl CoA for entry into the TCA cycle. The primary glucogenic amino acids are alanine, glycine, serine, cysteine, and tryptophan.
- The carbon skeletons of **ketogenic amino acids** are converted directly to acetyl CoA for entry into the TCA cycle or for use in synthesizing fatty acids. The only totally ketogenic amino acids are leucine and lysine.

Many of the amino acids can feed into the TCA cycle at different entry points. For example, some amino acids can have both ketogenic and gluconeogenic functions. These include tyrosine, phenylalanine, tryptophan, lysine, and leucine. Because amino acids can have multiple functions, it is difficult to fit them into groups. Appendix A shows how the carbon skeletons of the various amino acids can contribute to TCA cycle intermediates, glucose production, fatty acid production, and/or ketone body production.

The amount of energy, or ATP, produced from the catabolism of amino acids depends on where in the metabolic pathway the carbon skeleton enters. The "higher up" the point of entry, such as conversion to pyruvate, the greater the ATP production. No amino acid, however, generates as much ATP as one molecule of glucose or one free fatty acid.

If Consumed in Excess, the Carbon Skeleton Feeds into Fatty Acid Synthesis

When proteins are consumed in excess of cells' immediate needs for protein and energy, both glucogenic and ketogenic amino acids feed into the production of acetyl CoA, which is then used to synthesize fatty acids for storage as triglycerides. Although many bodybuilders believe that high-protein intakes lead to an increase in the synthesis of muscle mass, the reality is that the consumption of dietary protein in excess of short-term requirements for protein synthesis and cell energy leads to the same outcome as the consumption of excess dietary carbohydrate or fat: an increase in the synthesis of fatty acids and an increased deposition of triglycerides in adipose tissue.

Ammonia Is a By-Product of Protein Catabolism

Whereas some ammonia is useful as a nitrogen source for the synthesis of nonessential amino acids, high levels of ammonia are toxic to the body. Thus, the ammonia generated as a result of the deamination of amino acids must be quickly eliminated. To protect against ammonia toxicity, liver cells combine two molecules of ammonia together with carbon dioxide to form urea, which is much less toxic. **Figure 7.20** (page 272) illustrates a simplified pathway for urea synthesis; the complete metabolic pathway can be found in Appendix A. The urea produced from amino acid catabolism is released from the liver into the bloodstream, then filtered out by the kidneys and excreted in the urine. When the body has to make and excrete a large amount of urea, as occurs with a very high protein intake, the kidney excretes a large volume of urine. This in turn increases the risk for dehydration unless the individual drinks a large amount of fluid.

The processes by which energy is extracted from carbohydrates, triglycerides, and proteins are summarized in **Table 7.1** (page 272).

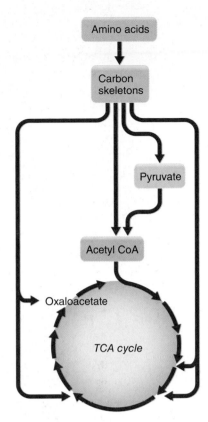

FIGURE 7.19 Extraction of energy from amino acids. The carbon skeletons of amino acids can be converted into pyruvate or acetyl CoA or can feed into the TCA cycle at various entry points. The point of entry into the catabolic pathway determines how much energy is extracted from that particular carbon skeleton.

glucogenic amino acid An amino acid that can be converted to glucose via gluconeogenesis.

ketogenic amino acid An amino acid that can be converted to acetyl CoA for the synthesis of free fatty acids.

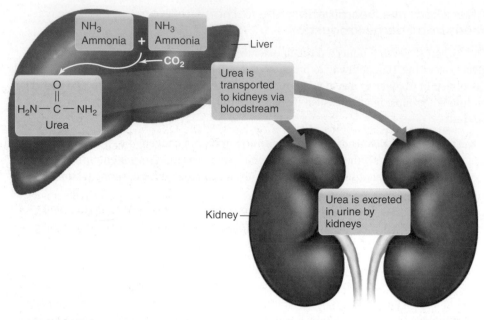

FIGURE 7.20 Overview of urea synthesis. The liver converts highly toxic ammonia, derived from deamination of amino acids, into urea. The urea is then released into the bloodstream for urinary excretion by the kidney.

RECAP

After deamination, the carbon skeletons of amino acids can be used as sources of energy. Glucogenic amino acids are converted into pyruvate, whereas ketogenic amino acids are converted into acetyl CoA. Some amino acids feed into the TCA cycle as various metabolic intermediates. The amine group released as a result of deamination can be transferred onto a keto acid for the synthesis of nonessential amino acids or, via ammonia, converted to and excreted as urea. ■

LO 6 Delineate the process by which alcohol is metabolized.

How Is Alcohol Metabolized?

We already took an *In Depth* look at alcohol (pages 152–163). Now we're ready to explore how the body metabolizes alcohol.

Alcohol Is Metabolized through Oxidation

As with glucose and fatty acids, alcohol is metabolized in a stepwise fashion through a series of oxidation reactions. These reactions may differ according to a person's alcohol intake.

TABLE 7.1 Extraction of Energy from Carbohydrate, Triglycerides, Protein, and Alcohol

Nutrient	Yields Energy as ATP?	Oxidative End Products?	Feeds into Glucose Production?	Feeds into Nonessential Amino Acid Production?	Feeds into Fatty Acid Production and Storage as Triglycerides?
Carbohydrate (glucose)	Yes	CO_2, H_2O	Yes	Yes, if source of nitrogen is available	Yes, although process is inefficient
Triglycerides: fatty acids	Yes	CO_2, H_2O	No	No	Yes
Triglycerides: glycerol	Yes	CO_2, H_2O	Yes, if carbohydrate is unavailable to cells	Yes, if source of nitrogen is available	Yes
Protein (amino acids)	Yes	CO_2, H_2O, N as urea	Yes, if carbohydrate is unavailable to cells	Yes	Yes
Alcohol	Yes	CO_2, H_2O	No	No	Yes

In people with low to moderate intakes, alcohol is oxidized first into acetaldehyde by the action of **alcohol dehydrogenase (ADH)**; then the acetaldehyde is oxidized by **aldehyde dehydrogenase (ALDH)** into acetate (**Figure 7.21**). Finally, acetate is readily converted into acetyl CoA.

In people who chronically abuse alcohol, an alternative pathway, the **microsomal ethanol oxidizing system (MEOS)**, becomes important for oxidizing the increased levels of alcohol. The name reflects the fact that this enzyme system operates in microsomes, which are fragments of the membrane of endoplasmic reticulum. Ethanol oxidizing enzymes are inducible, which means the higher the intake of alcohol, the greater their activity. As alcohol abuse increases, the MEOS increases in response.

Like the ADH pathway, the MEOS pathway results in the formation of acetyl CoA, the primary "fuel" for the TCA cycle. The oxidation of alcohol into acetaldehyde creates imbalances in two key pairs of coenzymes, $NAD^+/NADH$ and $NADP^+/NADPH$, which contribute to some of the metabolic and health problems associated with chronic alcohol abuse.

The Oxidation of Alcohol Begins in the Stomach

Although the oxidation of alcohol occurs primarily in the liver, a small but important amount of alcohol is actually oxidized in the stomach, before it is even absorbed into the bloodstream. This is known as *first-pass metabolism* and occurs via the ADH pathway. The action of gastric (stomach) ADH reduces, rather than simply delaying, the absorption of alcohol by as much as 20%. This enzyme is less active in young women than men; thus, women do not oxidize as much alcohol in their stomach, leaving more alcohol to be absorbed. As a result of this biological difference, women absorb an average of 30% to 35% more alcohol than a similar-sized man consuming the same size and type of alcoholic beverage. Gastric ADH activity decreases with age in men but apparently not in women, and there appear to be genetic differences in the amount or activity of this enzyme. Fasting for as little as 1 day prior to alcohol consumption lowers gastric ADH activity, increasing the percentage of alcohol absorbed into the bloodstream for a given intake. Women with a long history of alcohol abuse have virtually no gastric ADH activity.[3]

The Oxidation of Alcohol Continues in the Liver

Although a small amount is oxidized in the stomach, most of the alcohol consumed by an individual is rapidly absorbed into the bloodstream and transported to the liver, the primary site of alcohol oxidation. In the liver, the ADH pathway dominates at low to moderate intakes of alcohol, whereas the MEOS pathway becomes more important as the amount of alcohol consumed increases. The liver typically oxidizes alcohol at a fairly constant rate, equivalent to approximately one drink per hour, as explained in the alcohol *In Depth*. This rate varies somewhat with the individual's genetic profile, state of health, body size, use of medication, and nutritional status. If a person drinks more alcohol than the liver can oxidize over the same period of time, the excess is released back into the bloodstream. The greater the difference between rate of alcohol intake and rate of alcohol oxidation, the higher the blood alcohol concentration (BAC) (**Figure 7.22**, page 274).

Despite popular theories, there isn't much that can be done to speed up the breakdown of alcohol: it doesn't help to walk around (skeletal muscles don't oxidize alcohol), consume coffee or caffeinated beverages (caffeine doesn't increase rates of ADH or ALDH activity), or use commercial herbal or nutrient supplements (they have no impact on rates of ADH or ALDH activity). The key to avoiding the unwanted behavioral and physiologic consequences of alcohol is to consume alcohol at the rate of about one drink per hour, which then allows the liver to metabolize the alcohol at the same rate as it is consumed.

Although alcohol itself is a cellular toxin, acetaldehyde also produces specific and damaging effects. The amount of acetaldehyde that accumulates depends on the relative rates of activity for ADH and ALDH. In some ethnic groups, including certain Asian populations, the rate of ADH activity is normal or high and the activity of ALDH

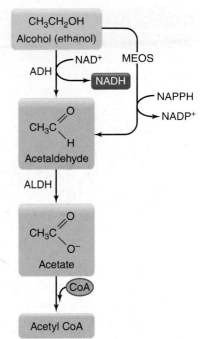

FIGURE 7.21 Pathways of alcohol metabolism. The primary metabolic by-product of alcohol oxidation is acetyl CoA.

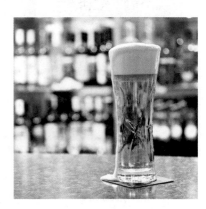

Alcohol is metabolized in the stomach and liver.

alcohol dehydrogenase (ADH) An enzyme that converts ethanol to acetaldehyde in the first step of alcohol oxidation.

aldehyde dehydrogenase (ALDH) An enzyme that oxidizes acetaldehyde to acetate.

microsomal ethanol oxidizing system (MEOS) A liver enzyme system that oxidizes ethanol to acetaldehyde; its activity predominates at higher levels of alcohol intake.

ALCOHOL IMPAIRMENT CHART

FEMALE										MALE									
Approximate blood alcohol concentration											Approximate blood alcohol concentration								
Drinks	Body Weight in Pounds									Drinks	Body Weight in Pounds								
	90	100	120	140	160	180	200	220	240			100	120	140	160	180	200	220	240
0	.00	.00	.00	.00	.00	.00	.00	.00	.00	ONLY SAFE DRIVING LIMIT	0	.00	.00	.00	.00	.00	.00	.00	.00	ONLY SAFE DRIVING LIMIT
1	.05	.05	.04	.03	.03	.03	.02	.02	.02	Impairment Begins	1	.04	.03	.03	.02	.02	.02	.02	.02	Impairment Begins
2	.10	.09	.08	.07	.06	.05	.05	.04	.04	Driving Skills Affected	2	.08	.06	.05	.05	.04	.04	.03	.03	Driving Skills Affected
3	.15	.14	.11	.10	.09	.08	.07	.06	.06	Possible Criminal Penalties	3	.11	.09	.08	.07	.06	.06	.05	.05	Possible Criminal Penalties
4	.20	.18	.15	.13	.11	.10	.09	.08	.08		4	.15	.12	.11	.09	.08	.08	.07	.06	
5	.25	.23	.19	.16	.14	.13	.11	.10	.09		5	.19	.16	.13	.12	.11	.09	.09	.08	
6	.30	.27	.23	.19	.17	.15	.14	.12	.11	Legally Intoxicated Criminal Penalties	6	.23	.19	.16	.14	.13	.11	.10	.09	Legally Intoxicated Criminal Penalties
7	.35	.32	.27	.23	.20	.18	.16	.14	.13		7	.26	.22	.19	.16	.15	.13	.12	.11	
8	.40	.36	.30	.26	.23	.20	.18	.17	.15		8	.30	.25	.21	.19	.17	.15	.14	.13	
9	.45	.41	.34	.29	.26	.23	.20	.19	.17		9	.34	.28	.24	.21	.19	.17	.15	.14	
10	.51	.45	.38	.32	.28	.25	.23	.21†	.19		10	.38	.31	.27	.23	.21	.19	.17	.16	

Your body can get rid of one drink per hour. Each 1.5 oz of 80 proof liquor, 12 oz of beer or 5 oz of table wine = 1 drink.

FIGURE 7.22 Effect of alcohol intake on blood alcohol concentration (BAC) and driving behavior. A 180-lb male will experience a BAC of .08 and a significant decline in driving skills after only three drinks. (*Sources:* Female figure adapted from "BAC Chart Female" from Pennsylvania Liquor Control Board Website, Copyright © 2012 by Pennsylvania Liquor Control Board. Reprinted with permission. Male figure adapted from "BAC Chart Male" from Pennsylvania Liquor Control Board Website, Copyright © 2012 by Pennsylvania Liquor Control Board. Reprinted with permission.)

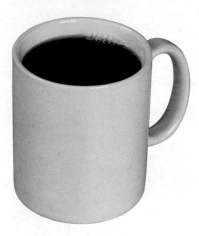

Black coffee will not speed the breakdown of alcohol.

is relatively low. When a person with this genetic profile drinks alcohol, acetaldehyde accumulates. This typically leads to facial flushing, headaches, nausea, tachycardia (rapid heartbeat), and hyperventilation (rapid breathing), which are often unpleasant enough to inhibit future intake of alcohol. Researchers have long known that people with this type of enzyme imbalance are at low risk for alcohol abuse because the downside of alcohol intake typically outweighs any pleasurable effect, even at low levels of consumption.

As an individual's alcohol intake increases over time, the liver's ADH pathway for alcohol oxidation becomes less efficient, and the MEOS pathway becomes more active. As a result of increased MEOS activity, the liver metabolizes alcohol more efficiently, and blood alcohol levels rise more slowly for a given intake of alcohol. In other words, a heavy drinker who used to reach a blood alcohol concentration (BAC) of 0.05 after only two drinks may not reach the same BAC until he has consumed four drinks. This condition reflects a metabolic tolerance to alcohol. Compared with light or moderate drinkers, people who chronically abuse alcohol must consume increasingly larger amounts before reaching a state of intoxication.

People who chronically consume alcohol in more-than-moderate amounts are at significant risk of dangerous drug–alcohol interactions. Thus, a number of pain relievers, antidepressants, and other drugs are clearly labeled "not to be consumed with alcohol." What accounts for this risk? The liver's MEOS system is used to metabolize not only alcohol but also many prescription and over-the-counter drugs, as well as illegal or street drugs. When an individual is consuming alcohol, however, the MEOS enzymes prioritize alcohol metabolism, leaving the drugs to accumulate. This "metabolic diversion" away from drug detoxification means the drug remains intact, continues to circulate in the blood, and leads to an exaggerated or intensified drug effect. The combination of drugs and alcohol can be fatal, and drug label warnings must be taken very seriously.

Although the majority of ingested alcohol is oxidized by enzymatic pathways in the stomach and liver, a small amount, typically less than 10% of intake, is excreted through the urine, breath, and sweat. Alcohol is distributed throughout all body fluids and water-based tissue spaces in roughly equivalent concentrations. Increases in blood alcohol concentration are paralleled by increases in breath vapor alcohol levels; this relationship forms the basis of the common Breathalyzer testing done by law enforcement agencies. Some people try to rid themselves of alcohol through saunas and steam rooms, but the amount of alcohol lost through the increased sweat is negligible.

RECAP

The majority of ingested alcohol is oxidized in the stomach and liver by pathways involving ADH and ALDH. As an individual's alcohol intake increases over time, these pathways for alcohol oxidation become less efficient and the MEOS pathway becomes more active. The liver oxidizes alcohol at a steady rate of approximately one drink per hour; there is no effective way to speed up the liver's oxidation of alcohol. ■

How Is Energy Stored?

The body needs stored energy it can use during times of sleep, fasting, or exercise, when energy demands persist but food is not being consumed. The body typically stores extra energy as either fat, in the form of triglycerides, or carbohydrate, in the form of glycogen. Although humans appear to have an unlimited ability to store fat, only a limited amount of carbohydrate can be stored as glycogen (**Table 7.2**). The body has no storage mechanism for amino acids or nitrogen, and the pool of free amino acids in the blood is small. Thus, most of the body's amino acids are bound up in protein molecules. These factors make triglycerides the most useful form of stored energy.

LO 7 Identify the body's mechanisms for storing excess glucose, triglycerides, and proteins.

The Energy of Dietary Glucose Is Stored as Muscle and Liver Glycogen

Recall from Chapter 4 that limited amounts of carbohydrate are stored in the body as glycogen, the storage form of glucose synthesized primarily in the liver and muscles. Glucose can easily be stored as glycogen within these tissues and, after an overnight fast, much of the carbohydrate consumed at breakfast is used to replenish the liver glycogen depleted during the night to maintain blood glucose levels.

The amount of stored glycogen will depend on the adequacy of dietary carbohydrate and the size of the individual: people on a low-carbohydrate diet store very little glycogen, and larger individuals, assuming an adequate dietary carbohydrate intake, can store more glycogen because of the larger size of their muscle tissues and livers. But even in larger individuals, typical body stores of glycogen can be quickly depleted if dietary intake of carbohydrate is low and utilization of glucose as fuel is high. The total amount of glycogen in the muscle is nearly always 2 to 3 times greater than the amount in the liver. Whereas the "average" male might store only 800 g of glycogen, a larger male athlete on a high-carbohydrate diet may store as much as 1,200 g of glycogen. Individuals who participate in endurance exercise are heavy glycogen users; therefore, they need to make sure their glycogen stores are replenished after each workout or competitive event. (Chapter 14 explores the process of carbohydrate loading for endurance athletes in detail.)

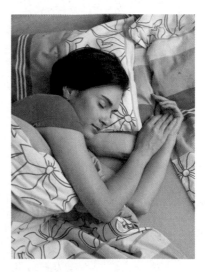

The body needs stored energy during sleep.

The Energy of Dietary Triglycerides Is Stored as Adipose Tissue

Whenever we eat in excess of energy needs, the body uses the dietary carbohydrate for energy and preferentially stores the dietary fat as body fat. A number of factors contribute to this preference:

■ The conversion of dietary fat to body fat is very efficient and requires little energy.
■ Dietary fatty acids can be taken up by adipose tissue cells and converted into stored triglycerides without dramatic changes to the fatty acid structures from their original (dietary) form.

TABLE 7.2 Body Energy Reserves of a Well-Nourished 70-kg* Male

	Triglycerides	Glycogen	Protein
Weight	15 kg	0.2 kg	6 kg
Kilocalories	135,000	800	24,000

*70 kg equals about 154 lb.

- The conversion of dietary carbohydrates to fatty acids that can be stored within the adipose cells requires a greater number of metabolic steps and is energy inefficient.
- When dietary carbohydrate is consumed in excess of the body's need, there is an increase in the oxidation of carbohydrate (glucose) over fat for energy, leaving more of the dietary fat available for storage in the adipose tissue.

Thus, when you overeat and consume a large meal, the fat within that meal will probably be converted to body fat and stored, whereas the carbohydrate in the meal will be used preferentially to fuel your body for the next 4 to 5 hours and to replenish glycogen stores.

The Energy of Dietary Proteins Is Found as Circulating Amino Acids

Although the body has no designated storage place for extra protein, some free amino acids circulating within the blood can be quickly broken down for energy if necessary. These free amino acids are either derived from dietary protein or are produced when tissue proteins are broken down. During protein catabolism, cells recycle as many of the amino acids as possible, using them to make new proteins or releasing them into the blood for uptake by other tissues. This process efficiently recycles many of the amino acids within the body, reducing the amount of protein required from food.

RECAP

The body is able to convert glucose into muscle and liver glycogen, the body's storage form of carbohydrate. Free fatty acids and glycerol are readily reassembled into triglycerides for storage in the adipose tissue, the body's largest energy depot. Technically, there are no protein stores in the human body; a small circulating pool of free amino acids can be used for energy if needed.

LO 8 Describe the processes by which glucose, fatty acids, cholesterol, and nonessential amino acids are synthesized.

How Are Key Nutrient Compounds Synthesized?

During the process of anabolism, a relatively small number of chemically simple components, including glucose, fatty acids, and amino acids, is used to synthesize a very large number of more complex body proteins, lipids, carbohydrates, and other compounds (recall Figure 7.1). The body also has the ability to synthesize glucose, fatty acids, and some amino acids. The following discussion will explore some of these common anabolic pathways.

Gluconeogenesis Is the Synthesis of Glucose

Glucose is the preferred source of energy for most body tissues, the primary energy source for the brain and other nerve cells, and the sole source for red blood cells. If the supply of glucose is interrupted, loss of consciousness and even death may occur. In the absence of adequate dietary carbohydrate, liver glycogen can sustain blood glucose levels for several hours. Beyond that time, however, if dietary carbohydrate intake is not restored, the body must synthesize glucose from noncarbohydrate substances.

The process of making new glucose from noncarbohydrate substrates is called **gluconeogenesis** (**Figure 7.23**). The primary substrates for gluconeogenesis are the glucogenic amino acids derived from the catabolism of body proteins or free glucogenic amino acids circulating in the blood. Although the body cannot make glucose from free fatty acids, a small amount of glucose can be produced from the glycerol found in triglycerides.

gluconeogenesis The synthesis of glucose from noncarbohydrate precursors, such as glucogenic amino acids and glycerol.

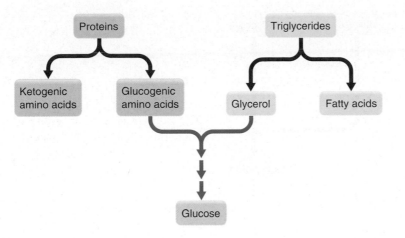

FIGURE 7.23 Overview of gluconeogenesis. In the absence of dietary carbohydrate and adequate glycogen stores, the body is able to convert glycerol and glucogenic amino acids into glucose.

The body relies on gluconeogenesis to maintain blood glucose levels at night when we are sleeping and during times of fasting as well as when rates of glucose oxidation are high, such as during trauma and exercise. Normally, the amount of body protein used for gluconeogenesis is low, but it increases dramatically during times of prolonged or severe illness, long-term fasting, or starvation. Protein catabolism for glucose production can lead to the destruction of vital tissue proteins, such as skeletal and heart muscles and organ proteins. The deadly consequences of this metabolic pathway are described in more detail in the section on starvation.

Lipogenesis Is the Synthesis of Fatty Acids

Lipogenesis is the production of fat from nonfat substances, such as carbohydrates, ketogenic amino acids, and alcohol. This process is also called *de novo* **synthesis** of fatty acids, because it is the synthesis of new fatty acids from nonfat compounds. Lipogenesis typically occurs when individuals consume any energy-producing nutrient in excess of energy needs: excess dietary carbohydrate, protein, and alcohol all contribute to lipogenesis.

Most lipogenesis occurs in liver cells. How does the liver convert the six-carbon ring of glucose or the carbon skeleton of an amino acid to a long-chain fatty acid with many carbons? Not surprisingly, the process involves many steps. As shown in **Figure 7.24** (page 278), the two-carbon acetyl CoA units derived from glucose, amino acid, and alcohol metabolism are converted into fatty acid chains. The newly synthesized fatty acids are then combined with glycerol to form triglycerides. The liver releases these triglycerides as VLDLs, which then circulate in the bloodstream. Eventually, the fatty acids are removed from the VLDLs, taken up into adipose tissue cells, and reassembled into triglycerides for storage as body fat. This is another example of the integration of metabolism that occurs between the liver and the adipose tissue.

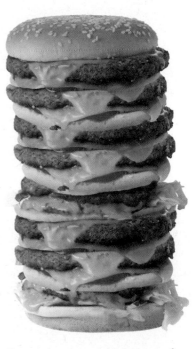

Consuming an excess amount of carbohydrate, protein, or alcohol will contribute to lipogenesis.

The Synthesis of Cholesterol

Although all cells can synthesize cholesterol, the liver and intestine synthesize as much, if not more, cholesterol than most people consume from their diet. For example, whereas healthy adults synthesize about 800 to 1,000 mg of cholesterol per day, the average American adult male consumes 300 mg per day and adult females just over 200 mg/day. The body regulates endogenous synthesis of cholesterol tightly in most healthy adults; that is, as the level of cholesterol in cells increases, the rate of endogenous cholesterol synthesis declines. This mechanism prevents hypercholesterolemia (high blood cholesterol), a known risk factor for cardiovascular disease.

lipogenesis The synthesis of free fatty acids from nonlipid precursors, such as ketogenic amino acids or ethanol.

***de novo* synthesis** The process of synthesizing a compound "from scratch."

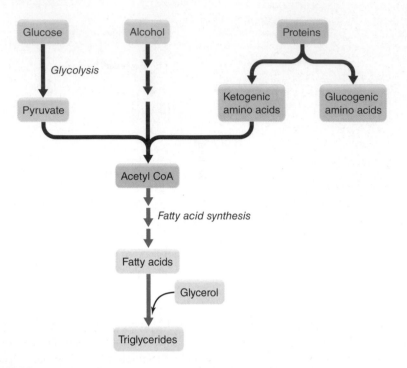

FIGURE 7.24 Overview of lipogenesis. Acetyl CoA, derived from glucose, ketogenic amino acids, or alcohol, can be converted into fatty acids for eventual storage as adipocyte triglycerides.

Cholesterol is synthesized from acetyl CoA, which is produced during the metabolism of fatty acids, alcohol, ketogenic amino acids and, through pyruvate, glucose. It is a multistep process that is closely regulated by key enzymes. Once synthesized, the cholesterol can be used in the production of bile acids, steroid hormones, and vitamin D. Cholesterol is also an essential component of cell membranes, helping to maintain their structure and function.

The Synthesis of Nonessential Amino Acids

When synthesizing any of the 11 nonessential amino acids (NEAAs), the body typically makes the carbon skeleton from carbohydrate- or fat-derived metabolites. The amine group can be provided through the process of transamination, where it is donated by one amino acid and accepted by a keto acid (**Figure 7.25**). When the keto acid accepts the donated amine group, it becomes a newly formed amino acid. The synthesis of nonessential amino acids occurs only when the body has enough energy and nitrogen to complete the necessary anabolic steps. During starvation, for example, energy intake is so low that the body stops the production of NEAAs.

Essential amino acids (EAAs) are distinguished from NEAAs by their carbon skeletons. The carbon skeletons of EAAs cannot be derived from carbohydrate or fat metabolic intermediates; therefore, EAAs must be consumed in their existing form from dietary proteins. Essential amino acids can be degraded or catabolized through several metabolic reactions, but they cannot be synthesized by cellular pathways.

RECAP

The dietary intake of carbohydrates, fats, and protein supplies the body with glucose, fatty acids, and amino acids. If nutrient intake is interrupted or inadequate, the body has the ability to endogenously synthesize glucose, almost all fatty acids, cholesterol, and 11 nonessential amino acids from readily available metabolic intermediates, including pyruvate and acetyl CoA.

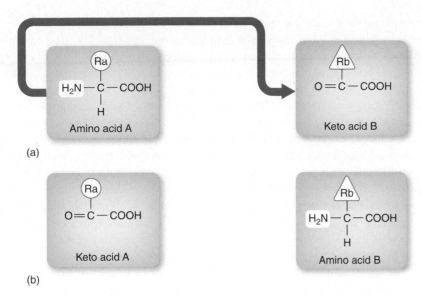

(a)

(b)

FIGURE 7.25 Transamination and the synthesis of nonessential amino acids. **(a)** Amino acid A transfers its amine group to keto acid B. **(b)** This transfer results in the formation of keto acid A and nonessential amino acid B.

What Hormones Regulate Metabolism?

LO 9 Explain the role of insulin, glucagon, epinephrine, and cortisol in regulating metabolism.

To maintain homeostasis (balanced internal conditions), the body must regulate energy storage and breakdown as needed. Several anabolic and catabolic hormones work to regulate metabolism (**Table 7.3**).

The primary anabolic hormone is insulin, which increases in the blood after a meal, especially when protein and carbohydrate are consumed. Insulin activates enzymes that promote the storage of nutrients in the body and enables cells to take up glucose (in addition to fatty acids and amino acids). These compounds are then converted into glycogen, triglycerides, and body protein. Thus, insulin increases the uptake of substrates into cells, emphasizes macronutrient storage, and turns off catabolic processes within the body (see Table 7.3). If endogenous insulin production is inhibited in any way, then exogenous insulin must be provided through insulin injections or an insulin pump. If body cells are not correctly responding to the insulin, as in people with type 2 diabetes, other medications may be required.

Conversely, glucagon, epinephrine, and cortisol are catabolic hormones that trigger the breakdown of stored triglycerides, glycogen, and body proteins for energy. They also turn off the anabolic pathways that store energy (see Table 7.3). As blood glucose drops,

TABLE 7.3 Hormonal Regulation of Metabolism

Metabolic State	Hormone	Site of Secretion	Role in Carbohydrate Metabolism	Role in Lipid Metabolism	Role in Protein Metabolism	Overall Metabolic Effect
Fed	Insulin	Pancreatic beta cells	Increases cell uptake of glucose Increases glycogen synthesis	Increases synthesis and storage of triglycerides	Increases cell uptake of amino acids and protein synthesis	Anabolic
Fasted	Glucagon	Pancreatic alpha cells	Increases glycogen degradation Increases gluconeogenesis	Increases lipolysis	Increases degradation of proteins	Catabolic
Exercise	Epinephrine	Adrenal medulla	Increases glycogen degradation	Increases lipolysis	No significant effect	Catabolic
Stress	Cortisol	Adrenal cortex	Decreases cell uptake of glucose Increases gluconeogenesis	Increases lipolysis	Decreases cell uptake of amino acids Increases degradation of proteins	Catabolic

glucagon concentrations increase, prompting the body to release glucose from stored glycogen. During exercise, blood levels of epinephrine increase quickly, stimulating the breakdown of stored energy reserves. Cortisol, which rises during times of energy deprivation and physical stress, such as injury or exercise, also triggers the catabolism of stored energy.

A rise in blood cortisol levels also occurs during times of emotional stress and is considered a hallmark of the primitive "fight-or-flight" response. Catabolism of stored energy prepares the body to either fight or flee from an enemy, two situations that typically demand high energy. In today's world, however, we do not typically physically fight or flee from our enemies, so the fatty acids and glucose that are dumped into the bloodstream in response to stress are not utilized as physiologically intended. When day-to-day stresses chronically trigger elevations in blood cortisol levels during physically inactive periods, these metabolically inappropriate responses can increase a person's risk for excessive abdominal fat storage and/or glucose intolerance.

As you can see, a number of catabolic hormones regulate substrate breakdown, and insulin is the major anabolic hormone. Homeostasis requires a balance among these hormones. If one or more of them ceases to regulate properly, normal metabolic controls fail. For example, most people with type 2 diabetes make plenty of insulin, sometimes too much. As described in Chapter 4, however, when the cells of people with type 2 diabetes don't properly respond to insulin, they fail to take up glucose for fuel and must turn to glucogenic amino acids. Normally, insulin promotes amino acid uptake and protein synthesis; in people with type 2 diabetes, however, the ineffective insulin response triggers protein catabolism. Thus, normal metabolic controls are lost, and the balance between anabolism and catabolism is disrupted.

RECAP

To maintain homeostasis, the body must regulate energy storage and breakdown as needed. The primary anabolic hormone is insulin, whereas glucagon, epinephrine, and cortisol are catabolic hormones. ∎

LO 10 Explain how the states of feasting and fasting affect metabolism.

How Do Feeding and Fasting Affect Metabolism?

Although the need for energy is constant, most people eat or fuel their body on an intermittent basis. Every night, while we sleep, the body continues its metabolic processes, drawing upon stored energy. In the morning, when we "break our fast," the body receives an infusion of new energy sources. How does the body take advantage of energy when it is available, even if not needed at that moment? And how does it remain metabolically active even in the absence of food intake? The metabolic responses to the cycles of feeding and fasting are explored here.

Metabolic Responses to Feeding

For several hours after the consumption of a meal, food is digested and nutrients are absorbed. The bloodstream is enriched with glucose, fatty acids, and amino acids. Most cells are able to meet their immediate energy needs through glucose oxidation. Only if the meal was very low in carbohydrate would body cells break down fatty acids or amino acids for fuel.

The fed state (**Focus Figure 7.26a**) is generally an anabolic state; after absorption, the end products of digestion are converted into larger, more chemically complex compounds.

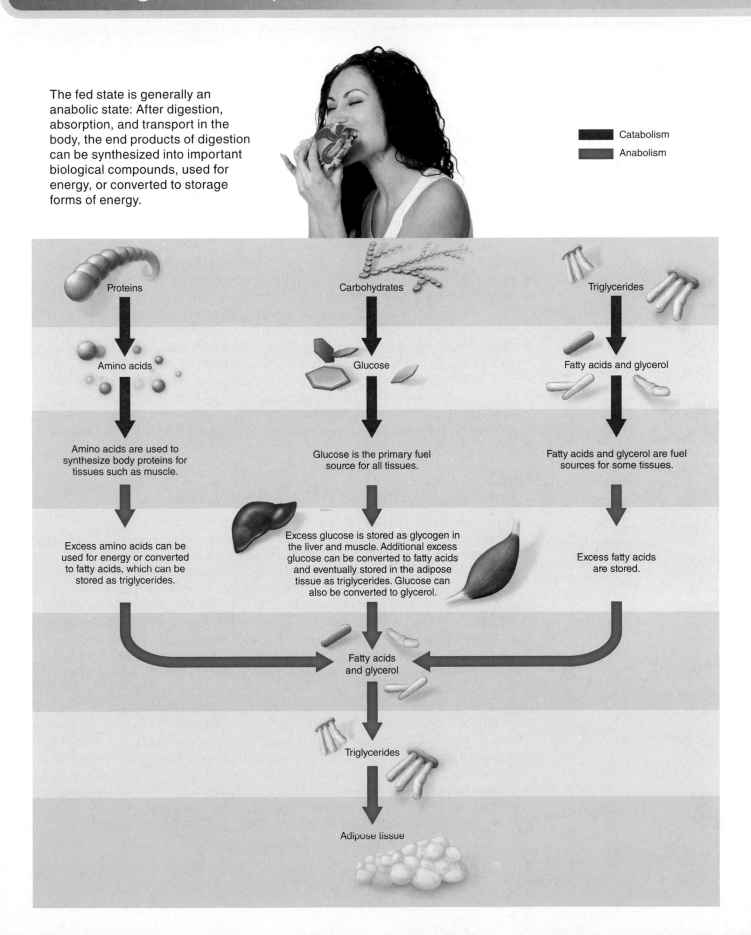

The fed state is generally an anabolic state: After digestion, absorption, and transport in the body, the end products of digestion can be synthesized into important biological compounds, used for energy, or converted to storage forms of energy.

Catabolism

Anabolism

Proteins

Amino acids

Amino acids are used to synthesize body proteins for tissues such as muscle.

Excess amino acids can be used for energy or converted to fatty acids, which can be stored as triglycerides.

Carbohydrates

Glucose

Glucose is the primary fuel source for all tissues.

Excess glucose is stored as glycogen in the liver and muscle. Additional excess glucose can be converted to fatty acids and eventually stored in the adipose tissue as triglycerides. Glucose can also be converted to glycerol.

Triglycerides

Fatty acids and glycerol

Fatty acids and glycerol are fuel sources for some tissues.

Excess fatty acids are stored.

Fatty acids and glycerol

Triglycerides

Adipose tissue

Glucose in excess of energy needs is converted to and stored as liver and muscle glycogen. Once glycogen stores are saturated, any remaining glucose is converted to fatty acids and eventually stored as triglycerides. Dietary fatty acids are combined with glycerol to form and be stored as triglycerides, largely in the adipose tissue. The liver takes up newly absorbed amino acids and converts some of them to needed proteins. The remaining amino acids are deaminated, and the carbon skeletons are converted to fatty acids for eventual storage as triglycerides.

Metabolic Responses to Short-Term Fasting

As the gap between meals lengthens beyond 3 hours or so, the body shifts from its previous anabolic state to a catabolic profile. Without a readily available supply of dietary carbohydrate, the body must turn inward in order to maintain normal blood glucose levels. **Focus Figure 7.26b** summarizes the interrelated metabolic responses to both short- and long-term fasting.

Recall that muscle glycogen is reserved for use by muscle tissue alone and is not available for normalization of blood glucose levels. Liver glycogen is broken down and glucose is released into the bloodstream; however, the supply of liver glycogen is limited. Most body cells, including muscle cells, are able to switch to the use of fatty acids as fuel, conserving the remaining blood glucose for brain and other cells that rely very heavily on glucose as fuel. As the carbohydrate-deprived state continues, ketone bodies accumulate as fatty acid–derived acetyl CoA is blocked from entering the TCA cycle. The longer a person remains in a fasting state, the greater the rate of gluconeogenesis. Glucose is synthesized from glucogenic amino acids (drawn initially from free amino acids in the blood, then largely from the breakdown of muscle protein) and glycerol (derived from the catabolism of triglycerides). These short-term adaptations will provide the glucose and energy needed to meet the body's needs for a few days.

Metabolic Responses to Prolonged Starvation

After 2 to 3 days of fasting, the body senses an approaching crisis and responds with dramatic changes in its metabolic profile. Whether the starvation is the result of a voluntary action (for example, political protest, religious ritual, or self-defined act) or involuntary circumstances (such as a severe illness, famine, war, or extreme poverty), the body shifts into survival mode. There are two overriding problems to be solved: the problem of meeting the body's need for energy and the problem of maintaining blood glucose levels in support of glucose-dependent cells, such as brain and red blood cells. The body must solve these problems while maintaining the integrity of its essential functions, including preservation of skeletal and cardiac muscle, maintenance of the immune system, and continuation of brain function for as long as possible. How, then, does the body meet these challenges?

Prolonged energy deprivation prompts the body to initiate several energy-conserving tactics. Fatigue sets in, and there is a sharp decline in voluntary physical activity. Core body temperature drops, and resting metabolic rate declines. Overall, the energy needs of the body drop dramatically. At the same time, most cells further increase their use of fatty acids as primary fuel, conserving the limited supply of glucose. Plasma levels of free fatty acids increase sharply as they move from adipose stores to the tissues and cells in need of energy. Plasma ketone levels increase to an even greater extent as they are released from the liver and circulate throughout the

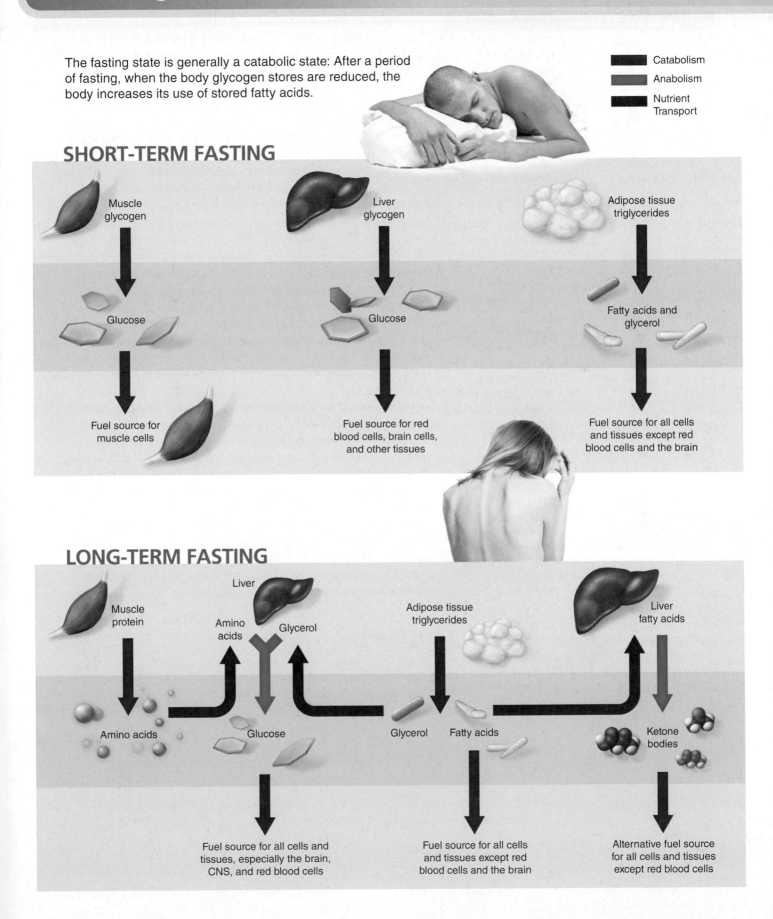

The fasting state is generally a catabolic state: After a period of fasting, when the body glycogen stores are reduced, the body increases its use of stored fatty acids.

Catabolism
Anabolism
Nutrient Transport

SHORT-TERM FASTING

Muscle glycogen → Glucose → Fuel source for muscle cells

Liver glycogen → Glucose → Fuel source for red blood cells, brain cells, and other tissues

Adipose tissue triglycerides → Fatty acids and glycerol → Fuel source for all cells and tissues except red blood cells and the brain

LONG-TERM FASTING

Muscle protein → Amino acids

Liver → Amino acids → Glycerol → Glucose → Fuel source for all cells and tissues, especially the brain, CNS, and red blood cells

Adipose tissue triglycerides → Glycerol   Fatty acids → Fuel source for all cells and tissues except red blood cells and the brain

Liver fatty acids → Ketone bodies → Alternative fuel source for all cells and tissues except red blood cells

Nutrition
MILESTONE

It would seem obvious that the solution to prolonged starvation is simply to provide food—any food. However, over 70 years ago, a severe and often fatal condition called *refeeding syndrome* was identified among newly freed prisoners of war (POWs).

During World War II, more than 140,000 Allied POWs were held under conditions of extreme deprivation. In **1945**, the war ended, and POWs returned home to comprehensive medical care and plentiful American food. Shortly thereafter, researchers began describing the onset of heart failure following refeeding of previously starved POWs, often within 4 days of the reintroduction of food.

We now understand that rapid refeeding of a previously starved individual severely disrupts the metabolic equilibrium that had allowed the person to survive during starvation. Loss of muscle and fat stores leads to a loss of intracellular electrolytes, particularly phosphate, while serum electrolyte levels remain relatively stable. Rapid reintroduction of foods high in carbohydrate forces serum phosphate into cells to support the metabolism of glucose. As serum phosphate levels plunge (often along with magnesium and potassium), the person can experience respiratory failure, heart failure, seizures, and sudden death.

Clinicians now recognize the need to gradually reintroduce food to a starved person and to carefully monitor serum electrolytes, supplementing as needed. But even today, the risk for refeeding syndrome still exists among severe anorexics, chronic alcoholics, and patients with late-stage cancer, AIDS, or severe gastrointestinal disease.

body. Yet, even with these adaptations, the need by brain cells for a certain amount of glucose remains.

There are very few options available for solving the body's "glucose problem." As stored triglycerides are broken down to provide fatty acids for fuel, the glycerol component is used to provide small amounts of glucose. Glucogenic amino acids, however, remain the major source of glucose for use by the brain. Although the brain does shift away from its normal reliance on glucose and adapts to the use of ketone bodies for fuel, day after day, the body sacrifices muscle, serum, and organ proteins in order to maintain a small but essential supply of glucose.

Over time, after weeks to even months of starvation, a new crisis arises: adipose stores become depleted, depriving the body of its most efficient source of fuel. Now, not only the brain but the entire body must survive on protein. With no other option available, the body begins to rapidly break down skeletal muscle, cardiac muscle, protein in organs such as the liver and kidney, and serum proteins, such as immune factors and transport proteins. As discussed in Chapter 6, children with marasmus illustrate this final stage of depletion. They have no visible fat stores, their muscles are atrophied, and they lack the reserves to sustain the synthesis of immune, hair, skin, and other proteins. During this advanced stage of starvation, many die of heart failure as the cardiac muscle becomes too wasted to function properly. Others die of infections due to their inability to mount normal immune responses.

How long can a person survive complete starvation? Obviously, the need for water is critical; a person will die of dehydration long before reaching these final stages of prolonged starvation. Prior health and nutritional status play an important role: if a person enters starvation with large stores of body fat, his or her survival will be prolonged. If a person has good muscle mass and adequate nutrient stores, he or she is also at a slight advantage. The elderly and young children are more susceptible to the effects of starvation. Most previously healthy adults can survive without food for 1 to 3 months, assuming no illness or trauma and an adequate supply of water. Extreme environmental conditions and increased physical activity shorten survival time.

RECAP

In the fed state, the body assumes an anabolic profile, converting newly absorbed glucose, fatty acids, and amino acids into stored glycogen and triglycerides and synthesizing some proteins. During short-term fasts, the body mobilizes stored glycogen and triglycerides to meet its need for glucose and energy. If the fasting state persists, more extreme adaptations to glucose and energy deficits occur. The body relies heavily on fatty acids and ketones as fuel sources and catabolizes proteins for gluconeogenesis. Over time, body fat and protein stores are so depleted that death occurs.

Nutrition Myth OR Fact?

"Speed Up Your Metabolism!" Is It Just a Dream?

The claims sound like a dream come true—consuming a particular food, supplement, or diet will rev up your metabolism and cause the pounds to melt away! Is there any truth to such claims? Are the recommendations safe? Let's examine the research evidence.

Claims for Single Foods or Food Components

A number of single foods or food components have been promoted as *thermogenic*, having the ability to increase our metabolic rate through the production of heat. Calories expended as heat are not available for storage as body fat or additional body weight; thus, the theory is that so-called thermogenic foods, ingredients, or supplements promote weight loss (or at least reduce the individual's rate of weight gain). What foods are promoted as thermogenic, and what are their effects on metabolism and body weight?

Caffeine

One of the most researched and highly promoted thermogenic food components is caffeine. About 90% of U.S. adults consume caffeine every day from coffee, tea, soft drinks, and, to an increasing extent, energy drinks. A recent review of the research confirmed that caffeine increases metabolism, sometimes in a dose–response manner, where higher intakes of caffeine led to greater increases in energy expenditure. Caffeine is also known to specifically increase rates of fat oxidation and, when consumed around the same time as a bout of exercise, reduces the perception of difficulty of that exercise.[1]

The effect of caffeine on metabolic rate seems to be influenced by typical or habitual caffeine intake. Individuals who usually maintain high caffeine intakes will see less of a bump in metabolic rate with additional caffeine compared to those with lower typical intakes. High caffeine intakes may also increase blood pressure, interfere with normal sleep patterns, or lead to an irregular heartbeat. It has also been shown that caffeine and caffeinated energy drinks can lead to insulin resistance and increased blood glucose levels; thus, some caution must be taken at high levels of caffeine intake.[2]

Green Tea and Green Tea Extract

One increasingly popular thermogenic agent is green tea or green tea extract. In addition to caffeine, green tea contains high levels of physiologically active polyphenols, including several catechins, which have been shown to increase energy expenditure in a number of short- and long-term studies,

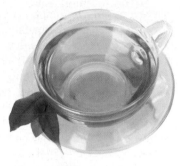

even with the removal of caffeine from green tea extract.[3] Most researchers agree that the caffeine and catechins in green tea act in a synergistic manner (their combined effect on metabolic rate is greater than simply adding their individual effects together). In agreement with other research, the beneficial effect of green tea on metabolic rate is greater when one's usual intake of caffeine is relatively low. It is important to remember, however, that increases in metabolic rate are generally very modest and don't always lead to loss of weight or body fat. As a beverage, green tea is safe, widely available, widely consumed, and inexpensive. Some, but not all, researchers express concerns about the use of green tea as a dietary supplement because it is not known what a safe and appropriate dose is.[4] The bottom line? Green tea is a great Calorie-free source of fluid and antioxidant-rich polyphenols. It may temporarily increase metabolic rate by a small amount, but its effect on body weight is minimal at best. The long-term effect of consuming concentrated green tea extract remains unknown.

Capsaicin

A compound found in hot (chili) peppers, capsaicin has been shown to increase energy expenditure in several human studies.[5] It has been estimated that an additional 15 Calories are burned for every teaspoon of cayenne pepper added to a meal. Serving meals with whole chili or hot peppers of any color will lead to a similar increase in metabolic rate and energy expenditure. While some people have a low tolerance for spicy foods, those who enjoy the taste of hot peppers can slightly increase their metabolic rate with little or no risk. Even better, additional research suggests that milder sweet peppers can also increase energy expenditure, although, again, only to a small extent. Finally, consumption of capsaicin-related compounds has been shown to decrease the caloric intake of the meal by about 75 Calories.[6] Either way,

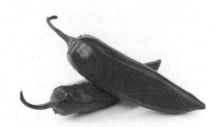

adding hot or sweet peppers to your regular diet is safe and nutritious (peppers are rich in vitamin C, as well as beta-carotene and many other phytochemicals) and may provide a short-term boost in energy expenditure and/or a slight decrease in energy intake.

Cold Water

Believe it or not, consumption of cold water has also been shown to speed up your metabolism through a process known as *water-induced thermogenesis*.[7] Studies in young adults have shown that drinking 500 mL (about 2 cups) of cold water increased energy expenditure by about 3% over 90 minutes.

Let's do some math to see how this might translate into weight loss. Many people consume a portion of their daily fluids as sweetened soft drinks. If they were to replace one 12-ounce soft drink per day with cold water, they would decrease their Calorie intake by about 180 kcal/day, which translates into the potential loss of about 19 pounds per year (at about 3,500 kcal per pound):

$$180 \text{ kcal/day} \times 365 \text{ days} = 65{,}700 \text{ kcal}/3{,}500 \text{ kcal per pound}$$
$$= \text{about 19 pounds}$$

In addition, the increased energy expenditure from drinking 12 ounces of cold water per day could theoretically amount to about 50 to 60 Calories per day, translating to a potential weight loss of just over 5 additional pounds per year:

$$50 \text{ kcal/day} \times 365 \text{ days} = \text{about } 18{,}250 \text{ kcal}/3{,}500 \text{ kcal per pound}$$
$$= \text{about 5 pounds}$$

From this simple calculation, you can see that replacing a beverage high in empty Calories with a Calorie-free beverage is a smart strategy for anyone trying to lose weight. Choosing cold water specifically is a healthful, cost-free, risk-free approach to boost one's metabolic rate and energy expenditure just a bit higher.

Dried Ginger Root

In Japanese and other cultures, ginger consumption is often associated with a "warm sensation" typically due to increased skin blood flow and/or an increase in core body temperature, both of which would increase energy expenditure or metabolic rate. Although a recent study found that ginger intake did increase fat oxidation by more than 10%, researchers failed to demonstrate any measurable increase in metabolic rate or energy expenditure at the dose given.[8]

Medium Chain Triglycerides

Coconut oil is being promoted as a "fat-burning miracle" due to its high content of medium chain triglycerides (MCT). MCT have been shown to increase rates of dietary induced thermogenesis (DIT), also known as the thermic effect of food (TEF). Normally DIT/TEF accounts for about 10% of your total energy expenditure over the course of a day. One study found that consumption of a meal with both chili powder and MCT

increased DIT/TEF by 50%.[9] Other studies, however, have failed to suggest that the impact of MCT on DIT/TEF is actually large enough to contribute to weight loss and/or decreases in body fat.[10]

Claims for Dietary Patterns

In addition to these single food or food component claims, many diet programs advertise that consumption of a high-protein diet (in which protein accounts for approximately 25% to 30% of total Calories) revs up metabolism. Research has consistently shown that this is true. When compared to diets of the same caloric intake but with lower levels of protein, high-protein diets have been shown to increase metabolic rate and energy expenditure through thermogenesis.[11] This is thought to be due to several factors:

- The thermic effect of dietary protein is about 20% to 30%, a level much higher than that of carbohydrate (5% to 15%) or fat (0% to 3%).

- High-protein diets are associated with higher levels of satiety, so people following such diets may stop eating sooner or wait longer before eating again.

- Consumption of a high-protein diet conserves lean body mass, which burns energy at a higher rate than adipose tissue. This conservation of lean body mass is important during times of energy restriction, such as when an individual is eating less to lose weight, and it's also an important consideration for athletes.[12]

In total, these metabolic responses help explain why adopting a high-protein diet increases metabolic rate and has the ability to support weight-loss efforts.

Claims for Physical Activity

If there is a single "magic bullet" for increasing metabolic rate, most researchers would agree it is physical activity. Many research studies have reported that purposeful physical activity not only increases metabolic rate during the period of activity but also increases resting metabolic rate afterwards, a phenomenon known as excessive post-exercise oxygen consumption (EPOC). The precise duration of the increased post-exercise metabolic rate varies:

- Short bouts (15–30 minutes) of moderate physical activity may increase metabolic rate for only 30 minutes or so, burning an extra 10–15 kcal.

- Longer and more intense exercise can increase metabolic rate for up to 14 hours, burning an extra 200–300 kcal. Brief sessions of low intensity exercise may produce less than .5 kg in body fat loss, whereas regular (3 times/week) vigorous activity, more than an hour in duration, can lead to as much as 3 kg of fat loss in a year, all from the increase in metabolic rate following exercise.[13]

- Endurance exercise (such as running, cycling, rowing, or swimming), interval training (cycling or running at a high rate of speed for several minutes, followed by a recovery period at a lower intensity or rate) and very-high-intensity resistance training (such as lifting extremely heavy weights at a rapid rate) has also been shown to increase post-exercise metabolic rate above baseline measures.

In addition to post-exercise increases in metabolic rate, physical activity of adequate duration and intensity increases lean body mass, which itself speeds up metabolic rate. In healthy people, increased physical activity carries virtually no risks but offers multiple benefits.

If you are looking to boost your metabolism and lose weight and/or body fat, adding single foods or food components won't hurt if the foods are readily available and part of a healthful diet, but it probably won't make much of a difference, either. Consuming a lower proportion of your Calories from carbohydrates and fats, and a higher proportion from protein, may help if you also reduce your total Calorie intake. Overall, however, regular, purposeful physical activity appears to be the most effective method for speeding up your metabolic rate and supporting weight loss.

Critical Thinking Questions

■ What would you say to your roommate if he told you he has decided to add hot chili powder to each meal? Are there any negative side effects he would need to be aware of? Are there other lifestyle changes he could make that would be more effective?

■ Why do you think that Olivia, in our chapter-opening scenario, didn't lose weight when she increased her consumption of high-protein foods, and instead, gained 4 pounds in 4 weeks? Propose at least two reasons.

■ Would you be willing and able to modify your lifestyle using any of the approaches described? Pick three of the changes reviewed and describe the impact it would have on your day-to-day activities. How realistic would it be for you to make all three changes at once?

References

1. Schubert, M. M., S. Hall, M. Leveritt, G. Grant, S. Sabapathy, and B. Desbrow. 2014. Caffeine consumption around an exercise bout: effects of energy expenditure, energy intake, and exercise enjoyment. *J. Appl. Physiol.* 117:745–754.
2. Shearer, J., and T. E. Graham. 2013. Performance effects and metabolic consequences of caffeine and caffeinated energy drink consumption on glucose disposal. *Nutr. Rev.* doi.org/10.1111/nure.12124.
3. Roberts, J. D., M. G. Roberts, M. D. Tarpey, J. C. Weekes, and C. H. Thomas. 2015. The effect of a decaffeinated green tea extract formula on fat oxidation, body composition and exercise performance. *J. Int. Soc. Sports Nutr.* 12:1. Doi:10.1186/s12970-014-0062-7.
4. Hutcheon, D. A., and J. Ziegler. 2014. Green tea: should it be used as a dietary aid? *Top. Clin. Nutr.* 29:268–277.
5. Ludy, M. J., G. E. Moore, and R. D. Mattes. 2012. The effects of capsaicin and capsiate on energy balance: critical review and meta-analysis of studies in human. *Chem Senses* 37:103–121.
6. Whiting, S., E. J. Derbyshire, and B. Tiwari. 2014. Could capsaicinoids help to support weight management? A systematic review and meta-analysis of energy intake data. *Appetite* 73:183-188.
7. Girona, M., E. K. Grasser, A. G. Dulloo, and J. P. Montani. 2014. Cardiovascular and metabolic responses to tap water ingestion in young humans: does the water temperature matter? *Acta Physiologica* 211:358–370.
8. Miyamoto, M., K. Matsuzaki, M. Katakura, T. Hara, Y. Tanabe, and O. Shido. 2015. Oral intake of encapsulated dried ginger root powder hardly affects human thermoregulatory function, but appears to facilitate fat utilization. *Int. J. Biometeorol.* doi:10.1007/soo484-015-0957-2.
9. Clegg, M. E., M. Golsorkhi, and C. J. Henry. 2013. Combined medium-chain triglyceride and chilli [sic] feeding increases diet-induced thermogenesis in normal-weight humans. *Eur. J. Nutr.* 52:1579–1585.
10. Bueno, N. B, I. V. de Melo, T. T. Florencio, and A. L. Sawaya. 2015. Dietary medium-chain triacylglycerols versus long-chain triacylglycerols for body composition in adults: systematic review and meta-analysis of randomized controlled trials. *J. Am. Coll. Nutr.* doi: 10.1080/07315724.2013.879844.
11. Bray, G. A., S. R. Smith, L. De Jonge, H. Xie, J. Rood, C. K. Martin, M. Most, C. Brock, S. Mancuso, and L. M. Redman. 2012. Effect of dietary protein content on weight gain, energy expenditure, and body composition during overeating: a randomized trial. *JAMA* 307:47–55.
12. Phillips, S. M. 2014. A brief review of higher dietary protein diets in weight loss: a focus on athletes. *Sports Med.* 44 (Suppl 2):S149–S153.
13. Shalev-Goldman, E., T. O'Neill, and R. Ross. 2014. Energy cost of exercise, post exercise metabolic rates and obesity. In: G. A. Bray and C. Bouchard, eds., *Handbook of Obesity: Epidemiology, Etiology, and Physiopathology.* 3rd Edn. Boca Raton, FL: CRC Press.

STUDY **PLAN** MasteringNutrition™

Customize your studies—and master your nutrition!—in the Study Area of MasteringNutrition.

TEST YOURSELF | ANSWERS

1 **T** All cells are metabolically active, but liver, muscle, and adipose cells are key locations for integration of metabolic pathways.

2 **T** Two vitamins that help produce energy from the macronutrients are riboflavin and niacin.

3 **F** The excess energy from dietary carbohydrate is also stored in the liver and in muscle as glycogen.

4 **F** There is no effective way to speed up the liver's breakdown of alcohol.

5 **T** During periods of starvation, body proteins are catabolized and their glucogenic amino acids are used in gluconeogenesis.

summary

Scan to hear an MP3 Chapter Review in **MasteringNutrition**.

LO 1 ■ Metabolism is the sum of all the chemical and physical processes by which the body breaks down and builds up molecules.

■ All forms of life maintain a balance between anabolic and catabolic reactions, which determines if the body achieves growth and repair or if it persists in a state of loss.

■ Cells store energy in the high-energy phosphate bonds of adenosine triphosphate (ATP). Release of a single phosphate group leaves adenosine diphosphate (ADP) and release of two leaves adenosine monophosphate (AMP). Adding phosphate groups back to these compounds regenerates ATP.

LO 2 ■ Metabolic pathways are clusters of chemical reactions that occur sequentially and achieve a particular goal, such as the breakdown of glucose for energy. These pathways are carefully controlled, either turned on or off, by hormones released within the body.

■ Dehydration synthesis is an anabolic reaction in which water is released. Hydrolysis is a catabolic reaction in which water breaks the

bonds between molecules. Phosphorylation is a chemical reaction in which phosphate is transferred. In oxidation–reduction reactions, the molecules involved exchange electrons.

■ Enzymes, cofactors, and coenzymes increase the efficiency of metabolism.

LO 3 ■ Glucose oxidation occurs in three well-defined stages: glycolysis, the TCA cycle, and oxidative phosphorylation via the electron transport chain. The end products of glucose oxidation are carbon dioxide, water, and ATP.

■ During glycolysis, six-carbon glucose is converted into two molecules of three-carbon pyruvate. If glycolysis is anaerobic, pyruvate is converted to lactate. If glycolysis is aerobic, pyruvate is converted to acetyl CoA, which then enters the TCA cycle.

■ During the TCA cycle, acetyl CoA, produced during carbohydrate, fat, or protein catabolism, results in the production of GTP or ATP, NADH, and FADH$_2$. The two final electron-rich compounds go through oxidative phosphorylation (as part of the electron transport chain) to produce energy as ATP.

■ During oxidative phosphorylation, NADH and FADH$_2$ enter the electron transport chain, where, through a series of reactions, ATP is produced.

LO 4 ■ Triglycerides are broken down into glycerol and free fatty acids.

■ Glycerol can be (a) converted to glucose or (b) oxidized for energy.

■ Free fatty acids are oxidized for energy but cannot be converted into glucose. In a carbohydrate-depleted state, fatty acids are diverted to ketone formation. The end products of fatty acid oxidation are carbon dioxide, water, and ATP.

LO 5 ■ After deamination, the carbon skeletons of amino acids can be oxidized for energy. The carbon skeletons of glucogenic amino acids are converted into pyruvate, whereas those of ketogenic amino acids are converted into acetyl CoA. Some amino acids feed into the TCA cycle as various metabolic intermediates. The end products of amino acid oxidation are carbon dioxide, water, ATP, and urea.

■ The amine group released as a result of deamination can be transferred onto a keto acid for the synthesis of nonessential amino acids or, through the production of ammonia, converted to and excreted as urea.

LO 6 ■ Alcohol metabolism begins in the stomach, where up to 20% of the alcohol consumed is oxidized. The remainder is oxidized in the liver. At high intakes, some alcohol continues to circulate in the blood, because the liver oxidizes alcohol at a steady rate of approximately one drink per hour.

■ In people with low or moderate alcohol intake, alcohol is oxidized first into acetaldehyde by ADH; then the acetaldehyde is oxidized by ALDH into acetate. In people who chronically abuse alcohol, the body uses the microsomal ethanol oxidizing system. Both pathways result in the formation of acetyl CoA.

LO 7 ■ The body extracts energy from glucose, fatty acids, glycerol, and amino acids. Glycogen is the body's storage form of carbohydrate. Triglycerides in the adipose tissue form the body's largest energy depot. Technically, there are no protein stores in the human body.

LO 8 ■ The dietary intake of carbohydrates, fats, and protein supplies the body with glucose, fatty acids, and amino acids. If intake is inadequate, the body synthesizes glucose, almost all fatty acids, cholesterol, and 11 nonessential amino acids from readily available metabolic intermediates.

■ The primary substrates for gluconeogenesis are the glucogenic amino acids. A small amount of glucose can be produced from glycerol, but the body cannot make glucose from fatty acids.

■ Excess dietary carbohydrate, protein, and alcohol all contribute to lipogenesis and triglyceride storage; excess dietary fat further increases triglyceride storage.

■ The body can make the carbon skeletons of NEAAs from carbohydrate- or fat-derived metabolites. The amine group can be provided through the process of transamination. The carbon skeletons of EAAs cannot be derived from carbohydrate or fat metabolic intermediates; therefore, EAAs must be consumed in their existing form from dietary proteins.

LO 9 ■ To maintain homeostasis, the body must regulate energy storage and breakdown as needed. The primary anabolic hormone is insulin, whereas glucagon, epinephrine, and cortisol are catabolic hormones.

LO 10 ■ In the fed state, the body converts newly absorbed glucose, fatty acids, and amino acids into stored glycogen and triglycerides.

■ During short-term fasts, the body uses stored glycogen and triglycerides to meet its need for glucose and energy. If the fast persists, the body relies heavily on fatty acids and ketones for fuel and initiates gluconeogenesis from glycerol and glucogenic amino acids to meet its glucose requirements. Over time, body fat and protein stores are so depleted that death occurs.

review questions

LO 1 1. Adenosine monophosphate
   a. can be regenerated by adding two phosphate groups to ATP.
   b. is produced when one phosphate group is released from ATP.
   c. has one high-energy phosphate bond.
   d. is composed of one molecule of adenosine bonded to one phosphate group.

LO 2 2. In which of the following types of chemical reactions is a compound catabolized by the addition of a molecule of water?
   a. hydrolysis
   b. dehydration synthesis
   c. oxidation
   d. phosphorylation

LO 3 3. In the absence of oxygen, the pyruvate produced through glycolysis is converted to

    a. lactate.
    b. acetyl CoA.
    c. oxaloacetate.
    d. NADH.

LO 4 4. Ketones are produced when

    a. people follow a high-carbohydrate, low-fat diet.
    b. oxaloacetate builds up and TCA cycle activity increases.
    c. acetyl CoA is blocked from entering the TCA cycle.
    d. All of the above can prompt the production of ketones.

LO 5 5. Amino acids are unique from other energy-yielding compounds in that

    a. they cannot be converted to glucose (gluconeogenesis).
    b. they contain nitrogen, which must be removed before the remaining compound can be used for energy.
    c. they contain ammonia, which the kidneys convert to urea and excrete from the body in urine.
    d. even when consumed to excess, they will not increase the synthesis of fatty acids.

LO 6 6. Anya skipped breakfast this morning. It is now midafternoon, and she has joined a friend for a late lunch. Although she rarely drinks alcohol, while waiting for her food to arrive, she enjoys a glass of wine. Which of the following statements best describes Anya's body's response to the alcohol?

    a. Gastric ADH oxidizes about 30% to 35% of the alcohol Anya consumes; the rest is absorbed into her bloodstream.
    b. When the alcohol enters Anya's bloodstream, her muscles quickly take it up for oxidation before her blood alcohol level increases.

    c. The microsomal ethanol oxidizing system (MEOS) breaks down about 20% of the alcohol Anya consumes before it is absorbed into her bloodstream.
    d. None of the above statements is true.

LO 7 7. Of the approximately 160,000 kcal reserves in the body of a well-nourished 70-kg male,

    a. triglycerides account for about 50%, and glycogen and protein each about 25%.
    b. about 85% is from triglycerides, and most of the remaining 15% is from protein.
    c. triglycerides, glycogen, and protein each account for about 33%.
    d. triglycerides, glycogen, protein, and water each account for about 25%.

LO 8 8. Most lipogenesis

    a. occurs when individuals consume an excess of glucogenic amino acids.
    b. occurs when acetyl CoA is converted into glycerol, which is in turn attached to fatty acid chains.
    c. occurs in liver cells.
    d. occurs in adipose cells.

LO 9 9. Glucagon, epinephrine, and cortisol are

    a. coenzymes.
    b. cofactors.
    c. anabolic hormones.
    d. catabolic hormones.

LO 10 During short-term fasts, the body uses

    a. muscle and liver glycogen for glucose for red blood cells, brain cells, and other body cells.
    b. liver glycogen for glucose for red blood cells, brain cells, and other body cells.
    c. glycerol from adipose tissue for ketone bodies.
    d. amino acids from the breakdown of body proteins for gluconeogenesis.

true or false?

LO 1 11. **True or false?** When cells engage in catabolism, chemical energy is released.

LO 3 12. **True or false?** Glycolysis yields a net of four ATP that can be used as energy for the cell.

LO 5 13. **True or false?** Liver synthesis of urea increases as dietary protein intake increases.

LO 7 14. **True or false?** The body stores enough glycogen to last about 5 to 7 days.

LO 10 15. **True or false?** Glucogenic amino acids can be converted into glucose during prolonged starvation.

short answer

LO 3 16. Explain the statement that, within the electron transport chain, energy is captured in ATP.

LO 4 17. Describe the process of fatty acid oxidation.

18. An elderly patient who has type 1 diabetes is admitted to the hospital in a state of severe ketoacidosis. The patient is comatose, but an elderly friend tells the admitting staff that he

thinks his companion is sick because recently she has not had enough money to buy insulin. Describe a possible series of physiologic events that might have led to her ketoacidosis.

day at school and eats whatever his friends are eating.

LO 5 19. Review the information you learned about phenylketonuria (PKU) in Chapters 4 and 6; then describe the physiologic events likely to occur in a child with phenylketonuria who, unknown to his parents, goes off his diet every

LO 10 20. Your aunt Winifred has been overweight her entire life. Recently, she began a very strict semistarvation diet because it promises that "all the weight you lose will be fat." What information could you share with her that would explain why her weight loss will include loss of body protein, not just body fat?

math review

LO 5 21. Your close friend Chris has just started using a "high-protein" supplement. Each serving provides a total of 1,800 mg of mixed amino acids, and the directions say to use three servings per day. If Chris weighs 170 lb, calculate (a) how much protein Chris needs, using the standard 0.8 g/kg body weight

guideline, and (b) what percentage of Chris's total protein needs is met by the three servings. If three servings of this product costs $1.50, calculate how many eggs you could buy for $1.50 and how many grams of protein those eggs would provide. How would Chris feel if you shared your results?

Answers to Review Questions and Math Review are located in the MasteringNutrition Study Area.

web links

www.nutritionandmetabolism.com
Nutrition and Metabolism
An online, peer-reviewed journal with articles concerning the integration of nutrition, exercise physiology, clinical investigations, and metabolism.

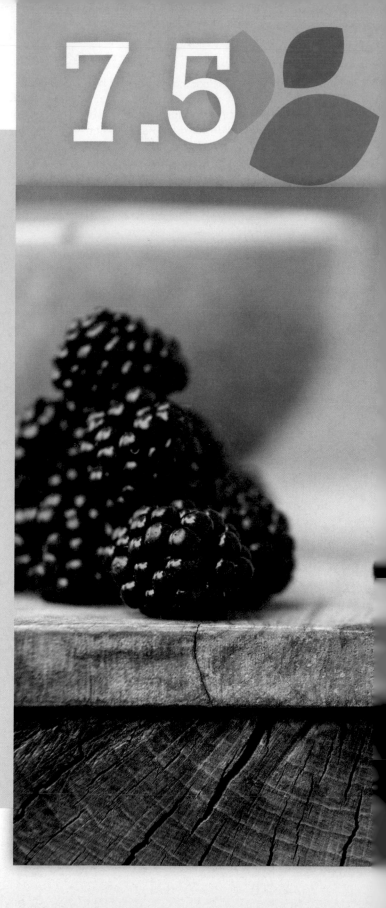

Vitamins and Minerals: Micronutrients with Macro Powers

After studying this In Depth, you should be able to:

1 Describe some incidents that led to the discovery of micronutrients, p. 293.

2 Distinguish between fat-soluble and water-soluble vitamins, pp. 293–296.

3 Describe the differences between major, trace, and ultra-trace minerals, pp. 296–299.

4 Explain why the amount of a micronutrient we consume may differ significantly from the amount our bodies absorb and use, pp. 299–301.

5 Discuss the role of micronutrient supplements in supporting or threatening our health, pp. 301–303.

Have you ever heard about the college student on a junk-food diet who developed scurvy, a disease caused by inadequate intake of vitamin C? This urban legend seems to circulate on many college campuses every year, but that might be because there's some truth behind it. Away from their families, many college students adopt diets that are deficient in one or more micronutrients. For instance, some students adopt a vegan diet with insufficient iron, while others neglect foods rich in calcium and vitamin D. Why is it important to consume adequate levels of the micronutrients, and exactly what constitutes a micronutrient, anyway? This In Depth explores the discovery of micronutrients, their classification and naming, and their impact on our health.

How Were the Micronutrients Discovered?

 Describe some incidents that led to the discovery of micronutrients.

As you recall from the previous chapters in this text, the macronutrients carbohydrates, lipids, and proteins provide energy; thus, we need to consume them in relatively large amounts. In contrast, the **micronutrients,** vitamins and minerals, are needed in much smaller amounts. They are nevertheless essential to our survival, assisting critical body functions such as energy metabolism and the formation and maintenance of healthy cells and tissues.

Much of our knowledge of vitamins and minerals comes from accidental observations of animals and humans. For instance, in the 1890s, a Dutch physician named C. Eijkman noticed that chickens fed polished rice developed paralysis, which could be reversed by feeding them whole-grain rice. Noting the high incidence of *beriberi*—a disease that results in extensive nerve damage—among hospital patients fed polished rice, Eijkman hypothesized that a highly refined diet was the primary cause of beriberi. We now know that whole-grain rice, with its nutrient rich bran layer, contains the vitamin thiamin and that thiamin deficiency results in beriberi.

Similarly, in the early 1900s, it was observed that Japanese children living in fishing villages rarely developed a type of blindness that was common among Japanese children who did not eat fish. Experiments soon showed that cod liver oil, chicken liver, and eel fat prevented the disorder. We now know that each of these foods contains vitamin A, which is essential for healthy vision.

Such observations were followed by years of laboratory research before nutritionists came to fully accept the idea that very small amounts of substances present in food are critical to good health. In 1906, English scientist F. G. Hopkins coined the term *accessory factors* for those substances; we now call them vitamins and minerals.

Avocados are a source of fat-soluble vitamins.

How Are Vitamins Classified?

 Distinguish between fat-soluble and water-soluble vitamins.

Vitamins are organic compounds that regulate a wide range of body processes. Of the 13 vitamins recognized as essential, humans can synthesize only small amounts of vitamins D and K and niacin (a B vitamin), so we must consume virtually all of the vitamins in our diet. Most people who eat a varied and healthful diet can readily meet their vitamin needs from foods alone. The exceptions to this will be discussed shortly.

Fat-Soluble Vitamins

Vitamins A, D, E, and K are **fat-soluble vitamins** (Table 1, page 294). They are found in the fatty portions of foods (butterfat, cod liver oil, corn oil, and so on) and are absorbed along with dietary fat. Fat-containing meats, dairy products, nuts, seeds, vegetable oils, and avocados are all sources of one or more fat-soluble vitamins.

In general, the fat-soluble vitamins are readily stored in the body's adipose tissue; thus, we don't need to consume them every day. While this may simplify day-to-day menu planning, there is also a disadvantage to our ability to store these nutrients. When we consume more of them than we can use, they build up in the adipose tissue, liver, and other tissues and can reach toxic levels. Symptoms of fat-soluble vitamin toxicity, described in Table 1, include damage to our hair, skin, bones, eyes, and nervous system. Overconsumption of vitamin supplements is the most common cause of vitamin toxicity in the United States; rarely do our dietary choices lead to toxicity. Of the four fat-soluble vitamins, vitamins A and D are the most toxic; **megadosing** with 10 or more times the recommended intake of either can result in irreversible organ damage and even death.

Even though we can store the fat-soluble vitamins, deficiencies can occur, especially in people who have a malabsorption disorder, such as celiac disease, that reduces their ability to absorb dietary fat. In addition, people who are "fat phobic," or eat very small amounts of dietary fat, are at risk for a deficiency due to low intake and poor absorption.

micronutrients Nutrients needed in relatively small amounts to support normal health and body functions. Vitamins and minerals are micronutrients.

Vitamins Micronutrient compounds that contain carbon and assist us in regulating our body's processes; classified as water soluble or fat soluble.

fat-soluble vitamins Vitamins that are not soluble in water but are soluble in fat; these include vitamins A, D, E, and K.

megadosing Taking a dose of a nutrient that is ten or more times greater than the recommended amount.

TABLE 1 Fat-Soluble Vitamins

Vitamin Name	Primary Functions	Recommended Intake*	Reliable Food Sources	Toxicity/Deficiency Symptoms
A (retinol, retinal, retinoic acid)	Required for ability of eyes to adjust to changes in light Protects color vision Assists cell differentiation Required for sperm production in men and fertilization in women Contributes to healthy bone Contributes to healthy immune system	RDA: Men: 900 µg/day Women: 700 µg/day UL: 3,000 µg/day	Preformed retinol: beef and chicken liver, egg yolks, milk Carotenoid precursors: spinach, carrots, mango, apricots, cantaloupe, pumpkin, yams	*Toxicity:* Fatigue, bone and joint pain, spontaneous abortion and birth defects of fetuses in pregnant women, nausea and diarrhea, liver damage, nervous system damage, blurred vision, hair loss, skin disorders *Deficiency:* Night blindness and xerophthalmia; impaired growth, immunity, and reproductive function
D (cholecalciferol)	Regulates blood calcium levels Maintains bone health Assists cell differentiation	RDA: Adults aged 19 to 70: 15µg/day Adults aged >70: 20 µg/day UL 100 µg/day	Canned salmon and mackerel, milk, fortified cereals	*Toxicity:* Hypercalcemia *Deficiency:* Rickets in children, osteomalacia and/or osteoporosis in adults
E (tocopherol)	As a powerful antioxidant, protects cell membranes, polyunsaturated fatty acids, and vitamin A from oxidation Protects white blood cells Enhances immune function Improves absorption of vitamin A	RDA: Men: 15 mg/day Women: 15 mg/day UL: 1,000 mg/day	Sunflower seeds, almonds, vegetable oils, fortified cereals	*Toxicity:* Rare *Deficiency:* Hemolytic anemia; impairment of nerve, muscle, and immune function
K (phylloquinone, menaquinone, menadione)	Serves as a coenzyme during production of specific proteins that assist in blood coagulation and bone metabolism	AI: Men: 120 µg/day Women: 90 µg/day	Kale, spinach, turnip greens, brussels sprouts	*Toxicity:* None known *Deficiency:* Impaired blood clotting, possible effect on bone health

*RDA: Recommended Dietary Allowance; UL: upper limit; AI: Adequate Intake.

The consequences of fat-soluble vitamin deficiencies, described in Table 1, include osteoporosis, the loss of night vision, and even death in the most severe cases.

Water-Soluble Vitamins

Vitamin C (ascorbic acid) and the B-vitamins (thiamin, riboflavin, niacin, vitamin B_6, vitamin B_{12}, folate, pantothenic acid, and biotin) are all **water-soluble vitamins** (Table 2). They are found in a wide variety of foods, including whole grains, fruits, vegetables, meats, and dairy products. In general, they are easily absorbed through the intestinal tract directly into the bloodstream, where they then travel to target cells.

With the exception of vitamin B_{12}, we do not store large amounts of water-soluble vitamins. Instead, our kidneys filter from our bloodstream any excess, which is excreted in urine. Because we do not maintain stores of these vitamins in our tissues, toxicity is rare. When it does occur, however, it is often from the overuse of high-potency vitamin supplements. Toxicity can cause nerve damage and skin lesions.

Because most water-soluble vitamins are not stored in large amounts, they need to be consumed on a daily or weekly

water-soluble vitamins Vitamins that are soluble in water; these include vitamin C and the B-vitamins.

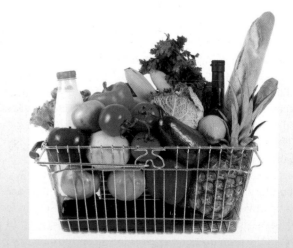

Water-soluble vitamins can be found in a variety of foods.

TABLE 2 Water-Soluble Vitamins

Vitamin Name	Primary Functions	Recommended Intake*	Reliable Food Sources	Toxicity/Deficiency Symptoms
Thiamin (vitamin B$_1$)	Required as enzyme cofactor for carbohydrate and amino acid metabolism	RDA: Men: 1.2 mg/day Women: 1.1 mg/day	Pork, fortified cereals, enriched rice and pasta, peas, tuna, legumes	*Toxicity:* None known *Deficiency:* Beriberi; fatigue, apathy, decreased memory, confusion, irritability, muscle weakness
Riboflavin (vitamin B$_2$)	Required as enzyme cofactor for carbohydrate and fat metabolism	RDA: Men: 1.3 mg/day Women: 1.1 mg/day	Beef liver, shrimp, milk and other dairy foods, fortified cereals, enriched breads and grains	*Toxicity:* None known *Deficiency:* Ariboflavinosis; swollen mouth and throat; seborrheic dermatitis; anemia
Niacin, nicotinamide, nicotinic acid	Required for carbohydrate and fat metabolism Plays role in DNA replication and repair and cell differentiation	RDA: Men: 16 mg/day Women: 14 mg/day UL: 35 mg/day	Beef liver, most cuts of meat/fish/poultry, fortified cereals, enriched breads and grains, canned tomato products	*Toxicity:* Flushing, liver damage, glucose intolerance, blurred vision *Deficiency:* Pellagra; vomiting, constipation, or diarrhea; apathy
Pyridoxine, pyridoxal, pyridoxamine (vitamin B$_6$)	Required as enzyme cofactor for carbohydrate and amino acid metabolism Assists synthesis of blood cells	RDA: Men and women aged 19 to 50: 1.3 mg/day Men aged >50: 1.7 mg/day Women aged >50: 1.5 mg/day UL: 100 mg/day	Chickpeas (garbanzo beans), most cuts of meat/fish/poultry, fortified cereals, white potatoes	*Toxicity:* Nerve damage, skin lesions *Deficiency:* Anemia; seborrheic dermatitis; depression, confusion, and convulsions
Folate (folic acid)	Required as enzyme cofactor for amino acid metabolism Required for DNA synthesis Involved in metabolism of homocysteine	RDA: Men: 400 µg/day Women: 400 µg/day UL: 1,000 µg/day	Fortified cereals, enriched breads and grains, spinach, legumes (lentils, chickpeas, pinto beans), greens (spinach, romaine lettuce), liver	*Toxicity:* Masks symptoms of vitamin B$_{12}$ deficiency, specifically signs of nerve damage *Deficiency:* Macrocytic anemia, neural tube defects in a developing fetus, elevated homocysteine levels
Cobalamin (vitamin B$_{12}$)	Assists with formation of blood cells Required for healthy nervous system function Involved as enzyme cofactor in metabolism of homocysteine	RDA: Men: 2.4 µg/day Women: 2.4 µg/day	Shellfish, all cuts of meat/fish/poultry, milk and other dairy foods, fortified cereals	*Toxicity:* None known *Deficiency:* Pernicious anemia; tingling and numbness of extremities; nerve damage; memory loss, disorientation, and dementia
Pantothenic acid	Assists with fat metabolism	AI: Men: 5 mg/day Women: 5 mg/day	Meat/fish/poultry, shiitake mushrooms, fortified cereals, egg yolk	*Toxicity:* None known *Deficiency:* Rare
Biotin	Involved as enzyme cofactor in carbohydrate, fat, and protein metabolism	RDA: Men: 30 µg/day Women: 30 µg/day	Nuts, egg yolk	*Toxicity:* None known *Deficiency:* Rare
Ascorbic acid (vitamin C)	Antioxidant in extracellular fluid and lungs Regenerates oxidized vitamin E Assists with collagen synthesis Enhances immune function Assists in synthesis of hormones, neurotransmitters, and DNA Enhances iron absorption	RDA: Men: 90 mg/day Women: 75 mg/day Smokers: 35 mg more per day than RDA UL: 2,000 mg	Sweet peppers, citrus fruits and juices, broccoli, strawberries, kiwi	*Toxicity:* Nausea and diarrhea, nosebleeds, increased oxidative damage, increased formation of kidney stones in people with kidney disease *Deficiency:* Scurvy, bone pain and fractures, depression, anemia

*RDA: Recommended Dietary Allowance; UL: upper limit; AI: Adequate Intake.

basis. Deficiency symptoms, including diseases or syndromes, can arise fairly quickly, especially during fetal development and in growing infants and children. The signs of water-soluble vitamin deficiency vary widely and are identified in Table 2.

Same Vitamin, Different Names and Forms

Food and supplement labels, magazine articles, and even nutrition textbooks often use simple, alphabetic (A, D, E, K, and so on) names for the fat-soluble vitamins. The letters reflect their order of discovery: vitamin A was discovered in 1916, whereas vitamin K was not isolated until 1939. These lay terms, however, are more appropriately viewed as "umbrellas" that unify a small cluster of chemically related compounds. For example, the term *vitamin A* refers to the specific compounds retinol, retinal, and retinoic acid. Similarly, *vitamin E* occurs naturally in eight forms, known as tocopherols, of which the primary form is alpha-tocopherol. Compounds with *vitamin D* activity include cholecalciferol and ergocalciferol, and the *vitamin K* "umbrella" includes phylloquinone and menaquinone. As you can see, most of the individual compounds making up a fat-soluble

What's the Best Way to Retain the Vitamins in Foods?

After selecting foods for their micronutrient value, it is important to store and prepare the foods properly. Minerals such as iron, calcium, and zinc are less affected by food-storage and preparation techniques, but losses of both fat- and water-soluble vitamins can be very high if food is not properly handled. Here are a few tips:

- Use as little water as possible when rinsing, storing, or cooking foods to minimize the loss of water-soluble vitamins. For maximal retention of these vitamins, steam or microwave vegetables.
- Avoid high temperatures for long periods of time to maximize retention of vitamin C, thiamin, and riboflavin.

- Store foods in tightly sealed containers. Exposure to air dramatically reduces the amount of vitamins A, C, E, and K, as well as B-vitamins. Whenever possible, eat raw fruits and vegetables as soon as they are prepared.
- Keep milk and other dairy foods out of direct light. When exposed to light, the riboflavin in these and other foods is rapidly destroyed. Using coated cardboard cartons or opaque plastic bottles will protect the riboflavin in milk.
- Don't sacrifice nutrient value for appearance. Although the addition of baking soda to certain vegetables enhances their color, it also increases the pH of the cooking water (makes it more alkaline), destroying thiamin, riboflavin, vitamin K, and vitamin C.

---

vitamin cluster have similar chemical designations (tocopherols, calciferols, and so on). Table 1 lists both the alphabetic and the chemical terms for the fat-soluble vitamins.

Similarly, there are both alphabetic and chemical designations for water-soluble vitamins. In some cases, such as *vitamin C* and *ascorbic acid*, you may be familiar with both terms. But few people would recognize *cobalamin* as *vitamin B_{12}*. Some of the water-soluble vitamins, such as niacin and vitamin B_6, mimic the "umbrella" clustering seen with vitamins A, E, D, and K: the term *vitamin B_6* includes pyridoxal, pyridoxine, and pyridoxamine. If you read any of these three terms on a supplement label, you'll know it refers to vitamin B_6.

The vitamins pantothenic acid and biotin exist in only one form. There are no other related chemical compounds linked to either vitamin. Table 2 lists both the alphabetic and chemical terms for the water-soluble vitamins.

Since all vitamins are organic compounds, they are all more or less vulnerable to degradation from exposure to heat, oxygen, or other factors. For tips on preserving the vitamins in the foods you eat, see the nearby *Highlight* for details.

How Are Minerals Classified?

LO 3 Describe the differences between major, trace, and ultra-trace minerals.

Minerals—such as calcium, iron, and zinc—are crystalline elements; that is, you'll find them on the periodic table. Because they are already in the simplest chemical form possible, the body does not digest or break them down prior to absorption. For the same reason, they cannot be degraded on exposure to heat

or any other natural process, so the minerals in foods remain intact during storage and cooking. Furthermore, unlike vitamins, they cannot be synthesized in the laboratory or by any plant or animal, including humans. Minerals are the same wherever they are found—in soil, a car part, or the human body. The minerals in our foods ultimately come from the environment; for example, the selenium in soil and water is taken up into plants and then incorporated into the animals that eat the plants. Whether humans eat the plant foods directly or eat the animal products, all of the minerals in our food supply originate from Mother Earth!

Most minerals are present in the foods and beverages we consume in the form of salts, which dissolve in the watery chyme in the GI tract, leaving their component mineral ions to be absorbed. Minerals therefore are not classified according to solubility, but according to the intake required and the amount present in the body. They are thereby classified into three groups as major, trace, or ultra-trace minerals.

Major Minerals

Major minerals are those the body requires in amounts of at least 100 mg per day. In addition, these minerals are found in the body in amounts of 5 g (5,000 mg) or higher. There are seven major minerals: sodium, potassium, phosphorus, chloride, calcium, magnesium, and sulfur. **Table 3** summarizes

Minerals Naturally occurring elements essential for the formation of blood, bone, many enzymes, and other critical compounds; classified as major, trace, or ultra-trace.

Major minerals Minerals we need to consume in amounts of at least 100 mg per day and of which the total amount present in the body is at least 5 g (5,000 mg).

TABLE 3 Major Minerals

Mineral Name	Primary Functions	Recommended Intake*	Reliable Food Sources	Toxicity/Deficiency Symptoms
Sodium	Fluid balance Acid–base balance Transmission of nerve impulses Muscle contraction	AI: Adults: 1.5 g/day (1,500 mg/day)	Table salt, pickles, most canned soups, snack foods, cured luncheon meats, canned tomato products	*Toxicity:* Water retention, high blood pressure, loss of calcium in urine *Deficiency:* Muscle cramps, dizziness, fatigue, nausea, vomiting, mental confusion
Potassium	Fluid balance Transmission of nerve impulses Muscle contraction	AI: Adults: 4.7 g/day (4,700 mg/day)	Most fresh fruits and vegetables: potatoes, bananas, tomato juice, orange juice, melons	*Toxicity:* Muscle weakness, vomiting, irregular heartbeat *Deficiency:* Muscle weakness, paralysis, mental confusion, irregular heartbeat
Phosphorus	Fluid balance Bone formation Component of ATP, which provides energy for our bodies	RDA: Adults: 700 mg/day	Milk/cheese/yogurt, soy milk and tofu, legumes (lentils, black beans), nuts (almonds, peanuts and peanut butter), poultry	*Toxicity:* Muscle spasms, convulsions, low blood calcium *Deficiency:* Muscle weakness, muscle damage, bone pain, dizziness
Chloride	Fluid balance Transmission of nerve impulses Component of stomach acid (HCl) Antibacterial	AI: Adults: 2.3 g/day (2,300 mg/day)	Table salt	*Toxicity:* None known *Deficiency:* dangerous blood acid–base imbalances, irregular heartbeat
Calcium	Primary component of bone Acid–base balance Transmission of nerve impulses Muscle contraction	RDA: Adults aged 19 to 50 and men aged 51–70: 1,000 mg/day Women aged 51–70 and adults aged >70: 1,200 mg/day UL for adults 19–50: 2,500 mg/day UL for adults aged 51 and above: 2,000 mg/day	Milk/yogurt/cheese (best-absorbed form of calcium), sardines, collard greens and spinach, calcium-fortified juices	*Toxicity:* Mineral imbalances, shock, kidney failure, fatigue, mental confusion *Deficiency:* Osteoporosis, convulsions, heart failure
Magnesium	Component of bone Muscle contraction Assists more than 300 enzyme systems	RDA: Men aged 19 to 30: 400 mg/day Men aged > 30: 420 mg/day Women aged 19 to 30: 310 mg/day Women aged >30: 320 mg/day UL: 350 mg/day	Greens (spinach, kale, collard greens), whole grains, seeds, nuts, legumes (navy and black beans)	*Toxicity:* None known *Deficiency:* Low blood calcium, muscle spasms or seizures, nausea, weakness, increased risk for chronic diseases (such as heart disease, hypertension, osteoporosis, and type 2 diabetes)
Sulfur	Component of certain B-vitamins and amino acids Acid–base balance Detoxification in liver	No DRI	Protein-rich foods	*Toxicity:* None known *Deficiency:* None known

*RDA: Recommended Dietary Allowance; UL: upper limit; AI: Adequate Intake; DRI: Dietary Reference Intake.

the primary functions, recommended intakes, food sources, and toxicity/deficiency symptoms of these minerals.

Trace and Ultra-Trace Minerals

Trace minerals are those we need to consume in amounts of less than 100 mg per day. They are found in the human body in amounts of less than 5 g (5,000 mg). Four trace minerals have an established RDA or AI: fluoride, iron, manganese, and zinc.[1] **Table 4** (page 298) identifies the primary functions, recommended intakes, food sources, and toxicity/deficiency symptoms of these minerals.

Ultra-trace minerals are those that are required in amounts less than 1 mg per day. The DRI Committee has established an RDA or AI guideline for five ultra-trace minerals: chromium, copper, iodine, molybdenum, and selenium.[1] These are included in Table 4. Other ultra-trace

minerals such as arsenic, nickel, and vanadium are thought to be important or essential for human health, but there is not yet enough research to establish an RDA or AI guideline.[1] As research into these ultra-trace minerals continue, scientists may soon be able to define a DRI value.

Same Mineral, Different Forms

Unlike vitamins, most of which can be identified by either alphabetic designations or their chemical name, minerals

Trace minerals Minerals we need to consume in amounts less than 100 mg per day and of which the total amount present in the body is less than 5 g (5,000 mg).

ultra-trace minerals Minerals we need to consume in amounts less than 1 mg per day.

TABLE 4 Trace and Ultra-Trace Minerals

Mineral Name	Primary Functions	Recommended Intake*	Reliable Food Sources	Toxicity/Deficiency Symptoms
Trace	**Minerals**			
Fluoride	Development and maintenance of healthy teeth and bones	RDA: Men: 4 mg/day Women: 3 mg/day UL: 2.2 mg/day for children aged 4 to 8; 10 mg/day for children aged > 8	Fish, seafood, legumes, whole grains, drinking water (variable)	*Toxicity:* Fluorosis of teeth and bones *Deficiency:* Dental caries, low bone density
Iron	Component of hemoglobin in blood cells Component of myoglobin in muscle cells Assists many enzyme systems	RDA: Adult men: 8 mg/day Women aged 19 to 50: 18 mg/day Women aged >50: 8 mg/day	Meat/fish/poultry (best-absorbed form of iron), fortified cereals, legumes, spinach	*Toxicity:* Nausea, vomiting, and diarrhea; dizziness and confusion; rapid heartbeat; organ damage; death *Deficiency:* Iron-deficiency microcytic anemia (small red blood cells), hypochromic anemia
Manganese	Assists many enzyme systems Synthesis of protein found in bone and cartilage	AI: Men: 2.3 mg/day Women: 1.8 mg/day UL: 11 mg/day for adults	Whole grains, nuts, leafy vegetables, tea	*Toxicity:* impairment of neuromuscular system *Deficiency:* Impaired growth and reproductive function, reduced bone density, impaired glucose and lipid metabolism, skin rash
Zinc	Assists more than 100 enzyme systems Immune system function Growth and sexual maturation Gene regulation	RDA: Men: 11 mg/day Women: 8 mg/day UL: 40 mg/day	Meat/fish/poultry (best-absorbed form of zinc), fortified cereals, legumes	*Toxicity:* Nausea, vomiting, and diarrhea; headaches; depressed immune function; reduced absorption of copper *Deficiency:* Growth retardation, delayed sexual maturation, eye and skin lesions, hair loss, increased incidence of illness and infection
Ultra-	**Trace Minerals**			
Chromium	Glucose transport Metabolism of DNA and RNA Immune function and growth	AI: Men aged 19 to 50: 35 µg/day Men aged >50: 30 µg/day Women aged 19 to 50: 25 µg/day Women aged >50: 20 µg/day	Whole grains, brewers yeast	*Toxicity:* None known *Deficiency:* Elevated blood glucose and blood lipids, damage to brain and nervous system
Copper	Assists many enzyme systems Iron transport	RDA: Adults: 900 µg/day UL: 10 mg/day	Shellfish, organ meats, nuts, legumes	*Toxicity:* Nausea, vomiting, and diarrhea; liver damage *Deficiency:* Anemia, reduced levels of white blood cells, osteoporosis in infants and growing children
Iodine	Synthesis of thyroid hormones Temperature regulation Reproduction and growth	RDA: Adults: 150 µg/day UL: 1,100 µg/day	Iodized salt, saltwater seafood	*Toxicity:* Goiter *Deficiency:* Goiter, hypothyroidism, cretinism in infant of mother who is iodine deficient
Molybdenum	Assists many enzyme systems	RDA: Adults: 45 µg/day UL: 2 mg/day	Legumes, nuts, grains	*Toxicity:* Symptoms not well defined in humans *Deficiency:* Abnormal metabolism of sulfur containing compounds
Selenium	Required for carbohydrate and fat metabolism	RDA: Adults: 55 µg/day UL: 400 µg/day	Nuts, shellfish, meat/fish/poultry, whole grains	*Toxicity:* Brittle hair and nails, skin rashes, nausea and vomiting, weakness, liver disease *Deficiency:* Specific forms of heart disease and arthritis, impaired immune function, muscle pain and wasting, depression, hostility

*RDA: Recommended Dietary Allowance; UL: upper limit; AI: Adequate Intake.

are simply referred to by their chemical name. Again, minerals in foods and supplements are often found as different salts; for example, a supplement label might identify calcium as calcium lactate, calcium gluconate, or calcium citrate. As we will discuss shortly, these different salts, while all containing the same elemental mineral, may differ in their ability to be absorbed by the body.

How Do Our Bodies Use Micronutrients?

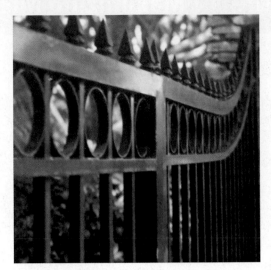

The iron in foods is chemically identical to that in a wrought iron fence.

LO 4 Explain why the amount of a micronutrient we consume may differ significantly from the amount our bodies absorb and use.

The micronutrients found in foods and supplements are not always in a chemical form that our cells can use. This discussion will highlight some of the ways in which our bodies modify the food forms of vitamins and minerals to maximize their absorption and utilization.

What We Eat Differs from What We Absorb

The most healthful diet is of no value to our bodies unless the nutrients can be absorbed and transported to the cells that need them. Unlike carbohydrates, fats, and proteins, which are efficiently absorbed (85–99% of what is eaten makes it into the blood), some micronutrients are so poorly absorbed

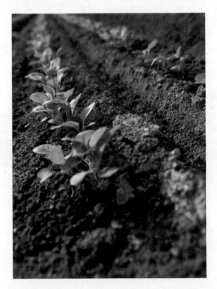

Plants absorb minerals from soil and water.

that only 3–10% of what is eaten ever enters the bloodstream.

The absorption of many vitamins and minerals depends on their chemical form. Dietary iron, for example, can be in the form of *heme iron* (found only in meats, fish, and poultry) or *non-heme iron* (found in plant and animal foods, as well as iron-fortified foods and supplements). Healthy adults absorb about 25% of the heme iron in foods, but non-heme iron absorption is lower, and varies greatly. (You will learn more about the absorption of dietary iron in Chapter 12.)

In addition, the presence of other factors within the same food influences mineral absorption. For example, approximately 30% to 45% of the calcium found in milk and dairy products is absorbed, but the calcium in spinach, Swiss chard, seeds, and nuts is absorbed at a much lower rate because factors in these foods bind the calcium and prevent its absorption. Non-heme iron, zinc, vitamin E, and vitamin B_6 are other micronutrients whose absorption can be reduced by various binding factors in foods.

Some micronutrients actually compete with one another for absorption. Several minerals, for example, use the same protein carriers to move across the mucosal cell for release into the bloodstream. Iron and zinc compete for intestinal absorption, as do iron and copper. Thus, a woman taking a high potency iron supplement will probably absorb a lower percent of dietary zinc compared to a woman who is not using iron supplements. This doesn't mean, however, that you should avoid taking an iron supplement when prescribed by your health care provider. In cases of iron deficiency, for example, you could take the iron supplement in the morning then later in the day, eat zinc-rich foods such as meats, legumes, and, as an afternoon snack, zinc-fortified cereal.

The absorption of many vitamins and minerals is also influenced by other foods within the meal. For example, the fat-soluble vitamins are much better absorbed when the meal contains some dietary fat. Calcium absorption is increased by the presence of lactose, found in milk, and non-heme iron absorption can be doubled if the meal includes vitamin C–rich foods, such as red peppers, oranges, or tomatoes. On the other hand, high-fiber foods, such as whole grains, and foods high in oxalic acid, such as tea, spinach, and rhubarb, can decrease the absorption of zinc and iron. It may seem an impossible task to correctly balance your food choices to optimize micronutrient absorption, but the best approach, as always, is to eat a variety of healthful foods every day. See an example in **Meal Focus Figure 1** (page 300), which compares a day's meals high and low in micronutrients.

meal focus figure 1 | Maximizing Micronutrients

a day of meals

low in MICRONUTRIENTS

high in MICRONUTRIENTS

BREAKFAST

1 large butter croissant
1 tbsp. strawberry jam
1 16 fl. oz latte with whole milk

1 cup All-Bran cereal
1 cup skim milk
1 grapefruit
8 fl. oz low-fat plain yogurt
2 slices rye toast with 2 tsp. butter and 1 tbsp. blackberry preserves

LUNCH

3 slices pepperoni pizza (14-inch pizza)
1.5 oz potato chips
24 fl. oz cola beverage

1 chicken breast, boneless, skinless, grilled

Spinach salad
2 cups spinach leaves
1 boiled egg
1 tbsp. chopped green onions
4 cherry tomatoes
½ medium carrot, chopped
1 tbsp. pine nuts
2 tbsp. Ranch dressing (reduced fat)
2 falafels (2-¼ inch diameter) with 2 tbsp. hummus

DINNER

6 fried chicken tenders
1 cup mashed potatoes with ½ cup chicken gravy
24 fl. oz diet cola beverage
1 yogurt and fruit parfait

2 cups minestrone soup, reduced sodium
2 whole-grain dinner rolls with 2 tsp. margarine
2 pork loin chops, roasted
1 cup mixed vegetables, cooked
8 fl. oz skim milk
1 cup fresh strawberries (sliced) with 1 tbsp. low-fat whipped cream

nutrient analysis

2,789 kcal	
46 milligrams of vitamin C	
28.6 milligrams of niacin	
929 milligrams of calcium	
13.4 milligrams of iron	
490 mcg of folate	
1,300 milligrams of sodium	

Provides more nutrients!

nutrient analysis

2,528 kcal
255 milligrams of vitamin C
42.8 milligrams of niacin
1,780 milligrams of calcium
27.5 milligrams of iron
1,335 mcg of folate
3,368 milligrams of sodium

What We Eat Differs from What Our Cells Use

Many vitamins undergo one or more chemical transformations after they are eaten and absorbed into our bodies. For example, before they can go to work for our bodies, the B vitamins must combine with other substances. For thiamin and vitamin B_6, phosphate groups are added. Vitamin D is another example: before cells can use it, the food form of vitamin D must have two hydroxyl (OH) groups added to its structure. These transformations activate the vitamin; because the reactions don't occur randomly, but only when the active vitamin is needed, they help the body maintain control over its metabolic pathways.

While the basic nature of minerals does not change, they can undergo minor modifications that change their atomic structure. Iron (Fe) may alternate between Fe^{2+} (ferrous) and Fe^{3+} (ferric); copper (Cu) may exist as Cu^{1+} or Cu^{2+}. These are just two examples of how micronutrients can be modified from one form to another to help the body make the best use of dietary nutrients.

Controversies in Micronutrient Metabolism

LO 5 Discuss the role of micronutrient supplements in supporting or threatening our health.

The science of nutrition continues to evolve, and our current understanding of vitamins and minerals will no doubt change over the next several years or decades. While some people interpret the term *controversy* as negative, nutrition controversies are exciting developments, proof of new information, and a sign of continued growth in the field.

Are Supplements Healthful Sources of Micronutrients?

For millions of years, humans relied solely on natural foodstuffs as their source of nutrients. Only within the past 75 years or so has a second option become available: purified supplemental nutrients, including those added to fortified foods. Are the micronutrients in supplements any better or worse than those in foods? Do our bodies use the nutrients from these two sources any differently?

As previously noted, the availability, or "usefulness," of micronutrients in foods depends in part on the food itself. The iron and calcium in spinach are poorly absorbed, whereas the iron in beef and the calcium in milk are absorbed efficiently. Because of these and other differences in the availability of micronutrients from different sources, it is difficult to generalize about the usefulness of supplements. Nevertheless, we can say a few things about this issue:

■ In general, it is much easier to develop a toxic overload of nutrients from supplements than it is from foods. It is very difficult, if not impossible, to develop a vitamin or mineral toxicity through diet (food) alone.

■ Some micronutrients consumed as supplements appear to be harmful to the health of certain subgroups of consumers. For example, recent research has shown that the use of common supplements, particularly iron, may actually increase the rates of death in older women.[2] Earlier, it was shown that high-potency beta-carotene supplements increase death rates among male smokers. Alcoholics are more susceptible to the potentially toxic effects of vitamin A supplements and should avoid their use unless prescribed by a healthcare provider. There is also some evidence that a high intake of vitamin A, including supplement use, increases the risk for osteoporosis and bone fractures in older women with low intakes of vitamin D.[3]

■ Most minerals are better absorbed from animal food sources than they are from supplements. The one exception might be calcium citrate-malate, used in calcium-fortified juices. The body uses this form as effectively as the calcium from milk or yogurt.

■ Enriching a low-nutrient food with a few vitamins and/or minerals does not turn it into a healthful food. For example, soda that has been fortified with selected micronutrients is still basically soda.

■ Eating a variety of healthful foods provides you with many more nutrients, phytochemicals, and other dietary factors than supplements alone. Nutritionists are not even sure they have identified all the essential nutrients; it is possible that the list of essential micronutrients will expand in the future. Supplements provide only those nutrients that the manufacturer puts in; foods provide the nutrients that have been identified as well as yet-unknown factors, which likely work in concert with one another to maintain health and functioning.

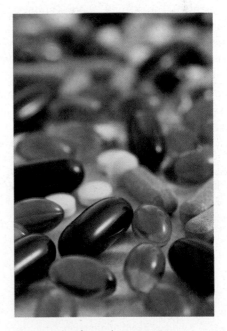

Thousands of supplements are marketed to consumers.

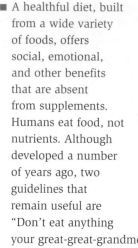
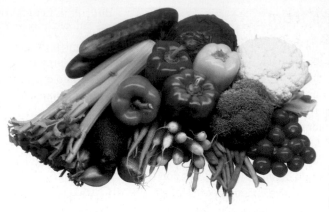

■ A healthful diet, built from a wide variety of foods, offers social, emotional, and other benefits that are absent from supplements. Humans eat food, not nutrients. Although developed a number of years ago, two guidelines that remain useful are "Don't eat anything your great-great-grandmother wouldn't recognize as food"[4] and "Eat food, not too much, mostly plants."[5]

On the other hand, micronutrient supplements can play an important role in promoting good health in some populations, such as pregnant women, children with poor eating habits, and people with certain illnesses. The risks and benefits of specific supplements versus whole foods are discussed later in this text (see Chapters 8 through 12 for specific micronutrient details).

Can Micronutrients Prevent or Treat Chronic Disease?

Researchers continue to investigate the links between macronutrients such as dietary fat and carbohydrate and the prevention and/or treatment of chronic diseases such as heart disease and diabetes. For example, there is strong agreement that *trans* fats increase risk of heart disease and high fiber diets help regulate blood glucose levels. Less clear, however, are the links between individual vitamins and minerals and certain chronic diseases.

A number of research studies have suggested, but not proven, links between the following micronutrients and disease states. In each case, adequate intake of the nutrient has been associated with lower disease risk.

■ Vitamin D and colon cancer
■ Vitamin E and complications of diabetes
■ Vitamin K and osteoporosis
■ Calcium and pregnancy-induced hypertension

> **Thinking of taking a dietary supplement?** Before you do, check out this one-minute video from the Office of Dietary Supplements at http://ods.od .nih.gov/HealthInformation /makingdecisions.sec.aspx

■ Chromium and blood glucose control in persons with diabetes
■ Magnesium and muscle wasting (sarcopenia) in older adults
■ Potassium and high blood pressure

The DRIs identify intake recommendations for large population groups; however, another subject of controversy is the question, "What is the optimal intake of each micronutrient for any given individual?" Contemporary research suggests that the answer to this question should take into account aspects of the individual's genetic profile. As you've learned (in Chapter 1), the science of *nutrigenomics* blends the study of human nutrition with that of genetics. It is becoming clear that some individuals require much higher or lower intakes of micronutrients to achieve health and prevent disease. For example, researchers have identified genetic variations in certain populations that increase their need for dietary folate.[6] Future studies may identify other examples of how our genetic profile may influence our need for vitamins and minerals.

Again, it's important to critically evaluate any claim about the protective or disease-preventing ability of a specific vitamin or mineral. Supplements that provide megadoses of

Liz **Nutri-**Case

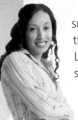

"I used to have dinner in the campus dining hall, but not anymore. It's too tempting to see everyone eating all that fattening food and then topping it off with a big dessert. My weight would balloon up in a week if I ate like that! So instead I stay in my dorm room and have a bowl of cereal with nonfat milk. The cereal box says it provides a full day's supply of all the vitamins and minerals, so I know it's nutritious. And when I eat cereal for dinner, it doesn't matter if I didn't eat all the right things earlier in the day!"

What do you think of Liz's "cereal suppers"? If the cereal provides 100% of the DV for all vitamins and minerals, then is Liz correct that it doesn't matter what else she eats during the day? If not, why not? What factors besides the percentage of DV does Liz need to consider?

micronutrients are potentially harmful, and exclusive use of vitamin/mineral therapies should never replace more traditional, proven methods of disease treatment. Current, reputable information can provide updates as the research into micronutrients continues.

Do More Essential Micronutrients Exist?

Nutrition researchers continue to explore the potential of a variety of substances to qualify as essential micronutrients. Vitamin-like factors such as carnitine and trace minerals such as boron, nickel, and silicon seem to have beneficial roles in human health, yet additional information is needed to fully define their metabolic roles. Until more research is done, such substances can't be classified as essential micronutrients.

As the science of nutrition continues to evolve, the next 50 years will be an exciting time for micronutrient research. Who knows? Within a few decades, we all might have personalized micronutrient prescriptions matched to our gender, age, and DNA!

Web Links

www.fda.gov/food/dietarysupplements/default.htm
US Food and Drug Administration
Select "Using Dietary Supplements" for information about the advantages and potential risks of supplement use.

fnic.nal.usda.gov/dietary-supplements
Food and Nutrition Information Center
Click on "General Information and Resources" to obtain information on vitamin and mineral supplements.

www.ods.od.nih.gov
Office of Dietary Supplements
This site provides summaries of current research results and helpful information about the use of dietary supplements.

lpi.oregonstate.edu
Linus Pauling Institute of Oregon State University
This site provides information on vitamins and minerals that promote health and lower disease risk. You can search for individual nutrients (for example, vitamin C) as well as types of nutrients (for example, antioxidants).

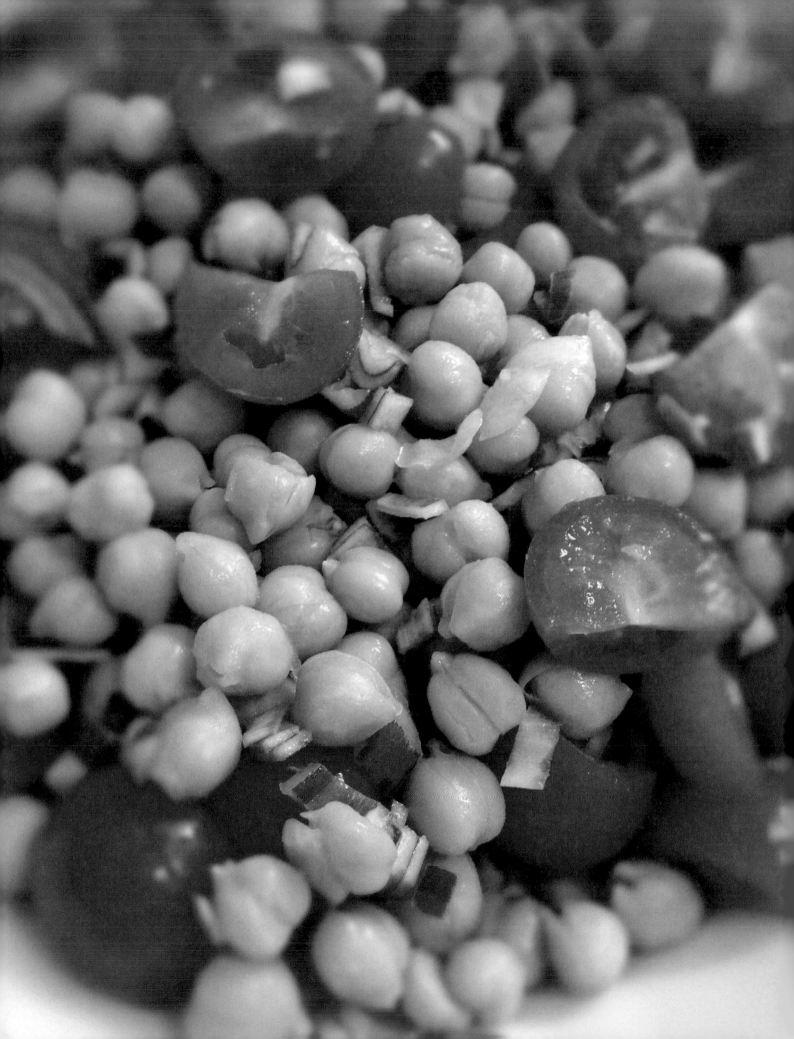

8 Nutrients Involved in Energy Metabolism

Learning Outcomes

After studying this chapter, you should be able to:

1. Describe how B-vitamins act as coenzymes to enhance the activities of enzymes involved in energy metabolism, *pp. 306–307*.
2. Identify the primary roles of thiamin, riboflavin, and niacin in energy metabolism, *pp. 308–313*.
3. Identify the deficiency disorders associated with thiamin, riboflavin, and niacin, *pp. 310–314*.
4. Explain how vitamin B_6, folate, and vitamin B_{12} function in energy metabolism and other body functions, *pp. 314–323*.
5. Discuss the roles of vitamin B_6, folate, and vitamin B_{12} in homocysteine metabolism and their association with cardiovascular disease, *pp. 315–316*.
6. Explain why adequate folate intake is especially critical during the first several weeks of pregnancy, *p. 318*.
7. Describe the roles of pantothenic acid, biotin, and choline in energy metabolism, *pp. 323–326*.
8. Discuss the roles of iodine, chromium, manganese, and sulfur in energy metabolism, *pp. 326–331*.
9. Identify the deficiency disorders associated with poor iodine intake, *pp. 327–328*.
10. Discuss the effect of poor B-vitamin intake on the ability to perform physical activity, *pp. 331–333*.

TEST YOURSELF

True or False?

1. The B-vitamins are an important source of energy for our body. **T** *or* **F**
2. A severe deficiency of certain B-vitamins active in energy metabolism can be fatal. **T** *or* **F**
3. B-vitamins are water soluble, so there is no risk of toxicity. **T** *or* **F**
4. Chromium supplementation reduces body fat and enhances muscle mass. **T** *or* **F**
5. In the United States, if we use table salt, we consume adequate iodine. **T** *or* **F**

Test Yourself answers are located in the Study Plan.

MasteringNutrition™

Go online for chapter quizzes, pre-tests, interactive activities, and more!

D r. Leslie Bernstein looked in astonishment at the 80-year-old man in his office. A leading gastroenterologist and professor of medicine at Albert Einstein College of Medicine in New York City, he had admired Pop Katz for years as one of his most healthy patients, a strict vegan and athlete who just weeks before had been accomplishing 3-mile runs as if he were 40 years younger. Now he could barely stand. He was confused, cried easily, was wandering away from the house partially clothed, and had lost control of his bladder. Tests showed that he was not suffering from Alzheimer's disease, had not had a stroke, did not have a tumor or an infection, and had no evidence of exposure to pesticides, metals, drugs, or other toxins. Blood tests were normal, except that his red blood cells were slightly enlarged. Bernstein consulted with a neurologist, who diagnosed "rapidly progressive dementia of unknown origin."

Bernstein was unconvinced: How could such a healthy man deteriorate so quickly? Then he had a flash of insight. For decades, Katz had followed a vegan diet. No animal foods, including dairy and eggs. Thus, no vitamin B_{12}. Bernstein immediately tested Katz's blood, then gave him an injection of B_{12}. The blood test confirmed Bernstein's hunch: the level of B_{12} in Katz's blood was too low to measure. The morning after his injection, Katz could sit up without help. Within a week of ongoing treatment, he could read, play card games, and hold his own in conversations. Unfortunately, the period of severe B_{12} deficiency did leave some permanent neurologic damage.[1]

In this chapter, we explore the reasons certain B-vitamins, including vitamin B_{12}, are essential to the body's breakdown and use of the macronutrients, and why severe deficiency of these vitamins is incompatible with life. We also discuss the role of the minerals iodine, chromium, manganese, and sulfur in energy metabolism; and we conclude the chapter with a look at the impact of low B-vitamin intake on our ability to work, play, and exercise.

How Does the Body Regulate Energy Metabolism?

 Describe how B-vitamins act as coenzymes to enhance the activities of enzymes involved in energy metabolism.

We've explored the digestion and metabolism of carbohydrates, lipids, proteins, and alcohol (in Chapters 3 through 7). In those chapters, you learned that the regulation of energy metabolism is a complex process involving numerous biological substances and chemical pathways. Here, we describe how certain micronutrients we consume in our diet assist us in generating energy from the carbohydrates, lipids, and proteins we eat along with them.

The Body Requires Vitamins and Minerals to Produce Energy

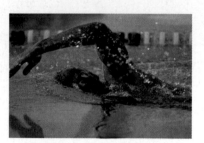

Vitamins do not provide energy directly, but the B-vitamins help the body create the energy that it needs from the foods we eat.

Although vitamins and minerals do not contain Calories and thus do not directly provide energy, the body is unable to generate energy from the macronutrients without them. The B-vitamins are particularly important in assisting energy metabolism. They include thiamin, riboflavin, vitamin B_6, niacin, folate, vitamin B_{12}, pantothenic acid, and biotin. Except for vitamin B_{12}, these water-soluble vitamins need to be consumed regularly, because the body has no storage reservoir for them. Conversely, excess amounts of these vitamins, either from food or supplementation, are easily lost in the urine.

The primary role of six of the B-vitamins (thiamin, riboflavin, niacin, vitamin B_6, pantothenic acid, and biotin) is to act as coenzymes in a number of metabolic processes. The other two B-vitamins (folate and vitamin B_{12}) function secondarily in energy metabolism, and primarily in cell regeneration and the synthesis of red blood cells. We discuss their roles as blood nutrients later in this text (in Chapter 12).

Figure 8.1 provides a simple overview of how some of the B-vitamins act as coenzymes to promote energy metabolism, and **Figure 8.2** (on page 308) shows how these coenzymes participate in the energy metabolism pathways. For instance, thiamin is part of the

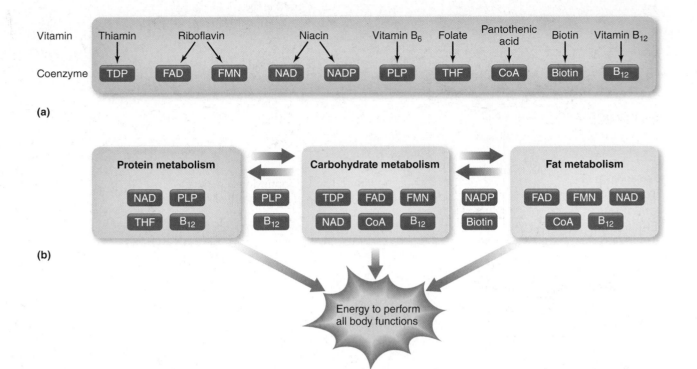

(a)

(b)

FIGURE 8.1 The B-vitamins play many important roles in the reactions involved in energy metabolism. **(a)** B-vitamins and the coenzymes they are a part of. **(b)** This chart illustrates many of the coenzymes essential for various metabolic functions; however, this is only a small sample of the thousands of roles that the B-vitamins play in our body. TPP, thiamin pyrophosphate; FAD, flavin adenine dinucleotide; FMN, flavin mononucleotide; NAD, nicotinamide adenine dinucleotide; NADP, nicotinamide adenine dinucleotide phosphate; PLP, pyridoxal phosphate; CoA, coenzyme A.

coenzyme thiamin pyrophosphate, or TPP, which is required for the breakdown of glucose. Riboflavin is a part of two coenzymes, flavin mononucleotide (FMN) and flavin adenine dinucleotide (FAD), which help break down glucose and fatty acids.

Four minerals also function in energy metabolism: the trace minerals iodine, chromium, and manganese, and the major mineral sulfur. A brief overview of the nutrients involved in energy metabolism is provided in **Table 8.1**. The specific functions of each B-vitamin and mineral involved in energy metabolism are described in this chapter.

Some Micronutrients Assist with Nutrient Transport and Hormone Production

Some micronutrients promote energy metabolism by facilitating the transport of nutrients into the cells. For instance, the mineral chromium helps improve glucose uptake into cells. Other micronutrients assist in the production of hormones that regulate metabolic processes; the mineral iodine, for example, is necessary for the synthesis of thyroid hormones, which regulate our metabolic rate and promote growth and development. These processes and their related nutrients are discussed ahead.

TABLE 8.1 Overview of Nutrients Involved in Energy Metabolism

To see the full profile of nutrients involved in energy metabolism, turn to Chapter 7.5, In Depth: Vitamins and Minerals, pages 292–303.	

Nutrient	Recommended Intake
Thiamin (vitamin B$_1$)	RDA for 19 years and older: Women = 1.1 mg/day Men = 1.2 mg/day
Riboflavin (vitamin B$_2$)	RDA for 19 years and older: Women = 1.1 mg/day Men = 1.3 mg/day
Niacin (nicotinamide and nicotinic acid)	RDA for 19 years and older: Women = 14 mg/day Men = 16 mg/day

Nutrient	Recommended Intake
Vitamin B$_6$ (pyridoxine)	RDA for 19 to 50 years of age: Women and men = 1.3 mg/day RDA for 51 years and older: Women = 1.5 mg/day Men = 1.7 mg/day
Folate (folic acid)	RDA for 19 years and older: Women and men = 400 µg/day
Vitamin B$_{12}$ (cobalamin)	RDA for 19 years and older: Women and men = 2.4 µg/day
Pantothenic acid	AI for 19 years and older: Women and men = 5 mg/day
Biotin	AI for 19 years and older: Women and men = 30 µg/day
Choline	AI for 19 years and older: Women = 425 mg/day Men = 550 mg/day

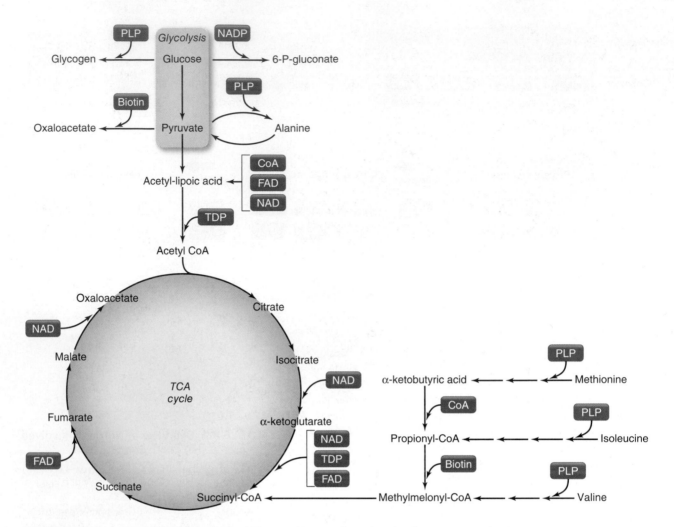

FIGURE 8.2 Example of some metabolic pathways that require B-vitamins for energy production.

RECAP

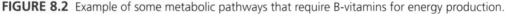

Vitamins and minerals are not direct sources of energy, but they help generate energy from carbohydrates, fats, proteins, and alcohol. Acting as coenzymes, micronutrients such as the B-vitamins assist enzymes in metabolizing macronutrients to produce energy. Minerals such as chromium and iodine assist with nutrient uptake into the cells and with regulating energy production and cell growth.

LO 2 Identify the primary roles of thiamin, riboflavin, and niacin in energy metabolism.

LO 3 Identify the deficiency disorders associated with thiamin, riboflavin, and niacin.

How Do Thiamin, Riboflavin, and Niacin Assist in Energy Metabolism?

Thiamin and riboflavin were the first B-vitamins to be discovered in the early 1900s, and therefore were initially designated vitamin B_1 and B_2. Although niacin was discovered later (1936), it is sometimes referred to as B_3. All three play critical roles in energy metabolism.

Thiamin (Vitamin B_1)

Thiamin was the first B-vitamin discovered, hence its designation as vitamin B_1. Because this compound was recognized as vital to health and has a functional amine group, it was initially called "vitamine."[2] Later, this term was applied to several other nonmineral compounds that are essential for health, and the spelling was changed to *vitamin*. Thiamin was given a new name reflecting both its thiazole and amine groups. The body converts dietary thiamin to its coenzyme thiamin diphosphate (TDP) ester, which was previously referred to as thiamin pyrophosphate, or TPP. The structures of thiamin and TDP are shown in **Figure 8.3**.

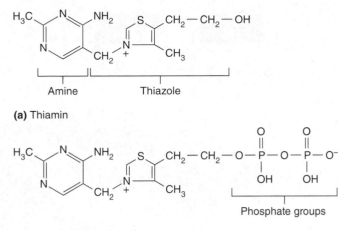

(a) Thiamin

(b) Thiamin pyrophosphate

FIGURE 8.3 Structure of **(a)** thiamin and **(b)** thiamin diphosphate (TDP) formally called thiamin pyrophosphate (TPP).

Functions of Thiamin

Thiamin is important in a number of energy-producing metabolic pathways within the body. As a part of TDP, thiamin plays a critical role in the breakdown of glucose for energy. For example, TDP is required for pyruvate dehydrogenase, the enzyme responsible for the conversion of pyruvate to acetyl-CoA (see Figure 8.2). This is a critical step in the conversion of glucose into a smaller molecule that can enter the TCA cycle. Thus, when dietary thiamin is inadequate, the body's ability to metabolize carbohydrate is diminished.

Another primary role of TDP is to act as a coenzyme in the metabolism of the branched-chain amino acids, which include leucine, isoleucine, and valine. TDP is a coenzyme for two α-keto acid dehydrogenase complexes. One of these enzyme complexes helps convert the carbon skeletons of the branched-chain amino acids into products that can enter the TCA cycle, whereas the other converts α-ketoglutarate to succinate in the TCA cycle (see Figure 8.2). The highest concentrations of the branched-chain amino acids are found in the muscle, where they make up approximately 25% of the content of the average protein. Thus, these amino acids play a significant role in providing fuel for the working muscle, especially during high-intensity exercise.[3]

TDP also assists in the production of DNA and RNA, making it important for cell regeneration and protein synthesis. Finally, it plays a role in the synthesis of neurotransmitters—chemicals that transmit messages throughout the central nervous system.

How Much Thiamin Should We Consume?

The RDA for thiamin for adults aged 19 years and older is 1.2 mg/day for men and 1.1 mg/day for women. According to NHANES III data, the average dietary intake of thiamin for men and women between the ages of 19 and 70 years is approximately 2 mg/day and approximately 1.5 mg/day, respectively.[4] Thus, it appears that the average adult in the United States gets adequate amounts of thiamin in the diet.

Those at greatest risk for poor thiamin status are the elderly, who typically have reduced total energy intakes; anyone with malabsorption syndrome; and patients on renal dialysis, since thiamin is easily cleared from the blood during dialysis. Also, people who eat a diet high in unenriched processed grains and simple sugars may be at risk for poor thiamin status.

Physically active individuals may be at risk for poor B-vitamin status, including thiamin, if their diet is made up primarily of high amounts of simple carbohydrates such as candy, soda, chips, and sport drinks and gels. Research indicates that depletion of the B-vitamins can reduce the ability to perform physical activity.[5] This is discussed in more detail at the end of the chapter.

Food Sources of Thiamin

Thiamin is found abundantly in ham and other pork products (**Figure 8.4**, on page 310). Sunflower seeds, beans, oat bran, mixed dishes that contain whole or enriched grains and meat, tuna fish,

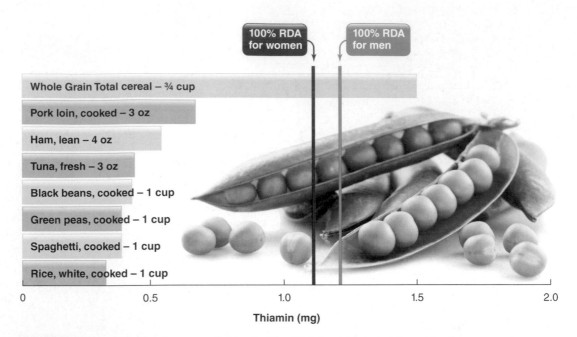

FIGURE 8.4 Common food sources of thiamin. The RDA for thiamin is 1.2 mg/day for men and 1.1 mg/day for women 19 years and older. (*Source*: Data from US Department of Agriculture, Agricultural Research Service. 2009. USDA Nutrient Database for Standard Reference, Release 22. Nutrient Data Laboratory Home Page. www.ars.usda.gov.)

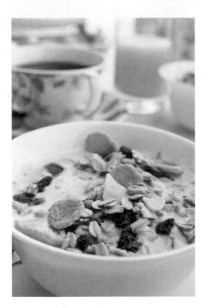

Ready-to-eat cereals are a good source of thiamin and other B-vitamins.

soy milk, and soy-based meat substitutes are also good sources. Enriched and whole-grain foods, including fortified ready-to-eat cereals, are rich in several B-vitamins, including thiamin.

What Happens If We Consume Too Much Thiamin?

Excess thiamin is readily cleared by the kidneys, and to date there have been no reports of adverse effects from consuming high amounts of thiamin from either food or supplements. Thus, the Institute of Medicine (IOM) has not been able to set a tolerable upper intake level (UL) for thiamin.[4]

What Happens If We Don't Consume Enough Thiamin?

As the B-vitamins are involved in most energy-generating processes, the deficiency symptoms include a combination of fatigue, apathy, muscle weakness, and reduced cognitive function. Thiamin-deficiency disease is called **beriberi.** In this disease, the body's inability to metabolize energy leads to muscle wasting and nerve damage; in later stages, patients may be unable to move at all. The heart muscle may also be affected, and the patient may die of heart failure. Beriberi is seen in countries in which unenriched, processed grains are a primary food source; for instance, beriberi was widespread in Asia when rice was processed and refined, and it still occurs in refugee camps and other settlements dependent on poor-quality food supplies.

Thiamin deficiency is also seen in industrialized countries in people with chronic heavy alcohol consumption and limited food intake. This alcohol-related thiamin deficiency is called Wernicke–Korsakoff syndrome. High alcohol intake contributes to thiamin deficiency in three ways: it is generally accompanied by low thiamin intake; at the same time, it increases the need for thiamin to metabolize the alcohol; and it reduces thiamin absorption. Together, these factors contribute to thiamin deficiency.[2] The symptoms of Wernicke–Korsakoff syndrome are muscle weakness, tremors, confusion, and memory impairment.[2]

Riboflavin (Vitamin B₂)

beriberi A disease caused by thiamin deficiency, characterized by muscle wasting and nerve damage.

In 1917, riboflavin became the second B-vitamin discovered; thus, it was designated vitamin B₂. The term *riboflavin* reflects its structure and color; *ribo* refers to the carbon-rich ribityl side chain, and *flavin*, which is associated with the multiring portion of the vitamin, refers

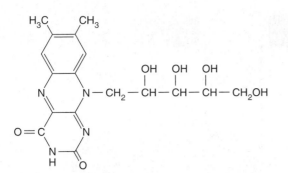

(a) Riboflavin

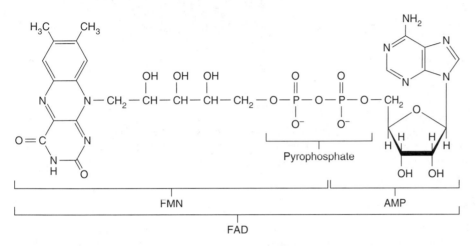

(b) Flavin mononucleotide (FMN) and flavin adenine dinucleotide (FAD) (coenzyme)

FIGURE 8.5 Structure of **(a)** riboflavin and **(b)** its coenzyme forms flavin mononucleotide (FMN) and flavin adenine dinucleotide (FAD).

to the yellow color this vitamin produces when dissolved in water (*flavus* means "yellow" in Latin) (**Figure 8.5a**). Riboflavin is relatively heat stable but sensitive to light: when exposed to light, the ribityl side chain is cleaved off and the vitamin loses its activity.

Functions of Riboflavin

Riboflavin is an important component of two coenzymes that are involved in oxidation–reduction reactions occurring within the energy-producing metabolic pathways, including the electron transport chain. These coenzymes, FMN and FAD, are involved in the metabolism of carbohydrates, fatty acids, and amino acids for energy. The structures of FMN and FAD are shown in Figure 8.5b: notice that FMN combines with adenosine monophosphate to produce FAD. For example, you will recall (from Chapter 7) that FAD and FMN function as electron acceptors in the electron transport chain, which eventually results in the production of ATP.

FAD is also a part of the α-ketoglutarate dehydrogenase complex, which converts α-ketoglutarate to succinate in one step of the TCA cycle (see Figure 8.2). It is also a coenzyme for succinate dehydrogenase, the enzyme involved in the conversion of succinate to fumarate in the next step of the TCA cycle. Finally, riboflavin is a part of the coenzyme required by glutathione peroxidase, which assists in the fight against oxidative damage. (Antioxidants are discussed in detail in Chapter 10, pages 380–417.)

Nutrition MILESTONE

Thiamin deficiency results in a disease called *beriberi*, which causes paralysis of the lower limbs. Although beriberi has been known throughout recorded history, it was not until the 19th century, when steam-powered mills began removing the outer shell of rice and other grains, that the disease became widespread, especially in Southeast Asia. At the time, it was not known that the outer layer of the grain contains the highest concentrations of B-vitamins, including thiamin.

In **1906**, Drs. Christiaan Eijkman and Gerrit Grijns, Dutch physicians living in Java, described how they could produce beriberi in chickens or pigeons by feeding them polished rice and could cure them by feeding back the rice bran that had been removed during polishing. In 1911, Polish chemist Casimir Funk was able to isolate the water-soluble, nitrogen-containing compound in rice bran that was responsible for the cure. He referred to this compound as a "vital amine" and called it thiamin.

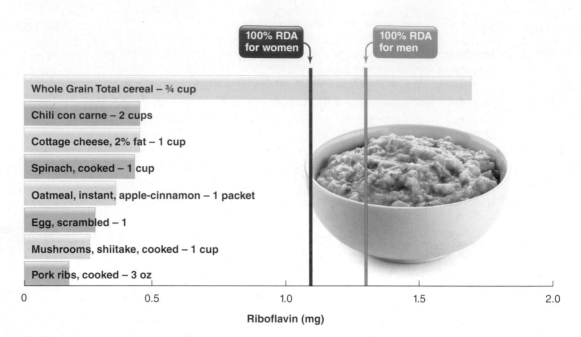

FIGURE 8.6 Common food sources of riboflavin. The RDA for riboflavin is 1.3 mg/day for men and 1.1 mg/day for women. (*Source*: Data from US Department of Agriculture, Agricultural Research Service. 2009. Nutrient Data Laboratory Home Page. www.ars.usda.gov.)

How Much Riboflavin Should We Consume?

The RDA for riboflavin for adults aged 19 years and older is 1.3 mg/day for men and 1.1 mg/day for women, respectively. Based on NHANES III data, the dietary intake of riboflavin from food for men between the ages of 19 and 70 years averages 2.0 to 2.3 mg/day (median = 2 mg/day) and for women of the same age 1.7 to 1.9 mg/day (median = 1.5 mg/day).[4] Thus, it appears that most adults in the United States get adequate amounts of riboflavin in their diet.

As with thiamin, those at greatest risk for low riboflavin intakes are the elderly, who may have reduced total energy intake; individuals who make poor food selections; those with malabsorption problems; and patients on renal dialysis.[6] Approximately one-third of the RDA for riboflavin is supplied in the American diet by milk and milk products; thus, it is easy to see how people who eliminate milk and milk products from their diet may also be at risk.[7]

Riboflavin is destroyed when it is exposed to light; thus, milk is generally stored in opaque containers. In addition to milk and other dairy products, good sources of riboflavin include eggs, meats (including organ meats), broccoli, enriched bread and grain products, and ready-to-eat cereals (**Figure 8.6**).

As with thiamin, there are no reports of adverse effects from consuming high amounts of riboflavin from either food or supplements; thus, the IOM has not been able to set a UL for riboflavin.[4]

Riboflavin deficiency is referred to as **ariboflavinosis.** Symptoms of ariboflavinosis include sore throat; swelling of the mucous membranes in the mouth and throat; lips that are dry and scaly; a purple-colored tongue; and inflamed, irritated patches on the skin. Severe riboflavin deficiency can impair the metabolism of vitamin B_6 (pyridoxine) and niacin.[4]

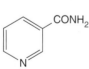

(a) Nicotinic acid   **(b)** Nicotinamide

FIGURE 8.7 Forms of niacin.
(a) Structure of nicotinic acid.
(b) Structure of nicotinamide. The generic term *niacin* is used to refer to these two compounds.

ariboflavinosis A condition caused by riboflavin deficiency.

pellagra A disease that results from severe niacin deficiency.

Niacin

Niacin is a generic name for two specific vitamin compounds, nicotinic acid and nicotinamide, which are shown in **Figure 8.7**. This B-vitamin was previously designated as vitamin B_3, a name you will sometimes still see on vitamin supplement labels. Niacin was first established as an essential nutrient in the treatment of pellagra in 1937. **Pellagra,** the deficiency of niacin, was first described in the 1700s and was common in the United States until the early 20th century. (For more information on the history of pellagra, see the *Highlight* box in Chapter 1, page 5.)

Functions of Niacin

The two forms of niacin, nicotinic acid and nicotinamide, are essential for the formation of the two coenzymes nicotinamide adenine dinucleotide (NAD) and nicotinamide adenine dinucleotide phosphate (NADP). These coenzymes, like those formed from riboflavin and thiamin, are required for the oxidation–reduction reactions involved in the catabolism of carbohydrate, fat, and protein for energy. For example, NAD- and NADP-dependent enzymes catalyze steps in the β-oxidation and synthesis of fatty acids, the oxidation of ketone bodies and ethanol, the degradation of carbohydrates, and the catabolism of amino acids.[8] Some metabolic pathways in which niacin functions are illustrated in Figure 8.2. Niacin is also an important coenzyme in DNA replication and repair and in the process of cell differentiation. Pharmaceutical preparations of niacin are sometimes prescribed for the treatment of abnormal blood lipids.[9]

How Much Niacin Should We Consume?

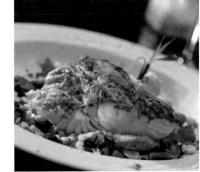

Niacin is a unique vitamin in that the body can synthesize a limited amount from the amino acid tryptophan. However, the ratio reflecting the conversion of tryptophan to niacin is 60:1; thus, the body relies on the diet to provide the majority of niacin necessary for functioning. The term *niacin equivalents (NE)* is used to express niacin intake recommendations, and it reflects the amount of niacin in our diet and the amount synthesized from tryptophan within the body. Recall that people consuming limited, corn-based diets are at significant risk for pellagra. This is not surprising, since corn is low in both niacin and the amino acid tryptophan.

Halibut is a good source of niacin.

The RDA for niacin for adults aged 19 and older is 16 mg/day of NE for men and 14 mg/day of NE for women. Based on NHANES III data, the average dietary intake of niacin from food for men and women between the ages of 19 and 70 years is approximately 27 mg/day and 21 mg/day, respectively.[4]

Good food sources of niacin include meat, fish, poultry, enriched bread products, and ready-to-eat cereals; however, the availability of this niacin for absorption varies. For example, the niacin in cereal grains is bound to other substances and is only 30% available for absorption, whereas the niacin found in meats is much more available.[4] To calculate the NE in your own diet, see **You Do the Math** (page 314). See **Figure 8.8** for the niacin content of commonly consumed foods.

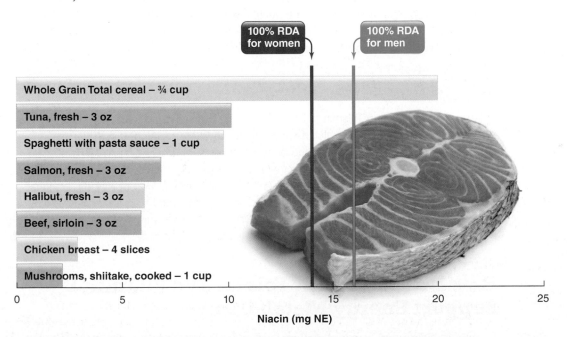

FIGURE 8.8 Common food sources of niacin. The RDA for niacin is 16 mg NE/day for men and 14 mg NE/day for women. (*Source*: Data from US Department of Agriculture, Agricultural Research Service. 2009. USDA Nutrient Database for Standard Reference, Release 22. Nutrient Data Laboratory Home Page. www.ars.usda.gov.)

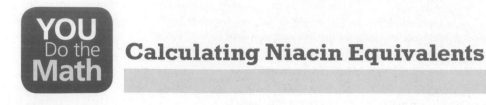

Calculating Niacin Equivalents

When you analyze your diet using the nutrient analysis program provided with this book, you will notice that the program calculates your total niacin equivalents (NE). How is this calculation done? How would you calculate your own intake of NE if the computer program was not doing this for you?

To calculate NE, you first need to determine the amount of two components of your diet: (1) total niacin intake from food in mg/day and (2) total intake of tryptophan in mg/day.

Now you are ready to do the calculation, using the following formula. Just keep in mind that 1 NE = either 60 mg of tryptophan or 1 mg of niacin.

Total NE = niacin intake from food + (tryptophan intake/60)

Now calculate the NE intake of an adult male who consumes 18.9 mg/day of niacin and 630 mg/day of tryptophan. What percentage of his total NE intake is coming from tryptophan? Is this person meeting his RDA?

There seem to be no adverse effects from the consumption of naturally occurring niacin in foods; however, niacin can cause toxicity symptoms when taken in supplement form.[4] These symptoms include *flushing*, which is burning, tingling, and itching sensations accompanied by a reddened flush, primarily on the face, arms, and chest. Liver damage, glucose intolerance, blurred vision, and edema of the eyes can be seen with very large doses of niacin taken over long periods of time. The UL for niacin is 35 mg/day and was determined based on the level of niacin below which flushing is typically not observed.

As mentioned, severe niacin deficiency causes pellagra, which is rarely seen in industrialized countries, except in cases of chronic alcoholism. Initial symptoms of pellagra include functional changes in the gastrointestinal tract, which decrease the amount of hydrochloric acid (HCl) produced and the absorption of nutrients, and lesions in the central nervous system, causing weakness, fatigue, and anorexia. These initial symptoms are followed by what have been identified as the "three Ds"—dermatitis, diarrhea, and dementia.[8] The word *pellagra* literally means "rough skin": dermatitis occurs on the parts of the body more exposed to the elements, such as the face, neck, hands, and feet. The diarrhea and dementia develop as the disease worsens, and they further affect the gastrointestinal tract and central nervous system.

RECAP

The body converts dietary thiamin to its coenzyme thiamin diphosphate, or TDP, which is important in the metabolism of glucose and the branched-chain amino acids. Thiamin-deficiency disease is called beriberi. Riboflavin is a component of two coenzymes involved in carbohydrate, fatty acid, and amino acid metabolism: flavin mononucleotide (FMN) and flavin adenine dinucleotide (FAD). Riboflavin-deficiency disease is ariboflavinosis. Niacin is essential for the formation of two coenzymes involved in carbohydrate, fatty acid, and amino acid metabolism: nicotinamide adenine dinucleotide (NAD) and nicotinamide adenine dinucleotide phosphate (NADP). Niacin-deficiency disease is pellagra.

LO 4 Explain how vitamin B_6, folate, and vitamin B_{12} function in energy metabolism and other body functions.

LO 5 Discuss the roles of vitamin B_6, folate, and vitamin B_{12} in homocysteine metabolism and their association with cardiovascular disease.

LO 6 Explain why adequate folate intake is especially critical during the first several weeks of pregnancy.

How Do Vitamin B_6, Folate, and Vitamin B_{12} Support Energy Metabolism?

Vitamin B_6, folate, and vitamin B_{12} all perform multiple roles in human functioning in addition to their roles in energy metabolism. One shared role important in cardiovascular health is in the metabolism of the amino acid homocysteine. Let's take a closer look.

Vitamin B$_6$ (Pyridoxine)

Vitamin B$_6$ is actually a group of three related compounds—pyridoxine (PN), pyridoxal (PL), and pyridoxamine (PM)—and their phosphate forms, which include pyridoxine phosphate (PNP), pyridoxal phosphate (PLP), and pyridoxamine phosphate (PMP), respectively. The structures of these compounds are shown in **Figure 8.9**.

Functions of Vitamin B$_6$

Some of the metabolic pathways in which vitamin-B$_6$ functions are illustrated in Figure 8.2. In the form of PLP, vitamin B$_6$ is a coenzyme for more than 100 enzymes involved in the metabolism of amino acids. Some of the critical roles of vitamin B$_6$ are listed here:

- *Amino acid metabolism.* Vitamin B$_6$ plays a critical role in transamination, which is a key process in making nonessential amino acids (see Chapter 6). Without adequate vitamin B$_6$, all amino acids become essential, as our body cannot make them in sufficient quantities.
- *Neurotransmitter synthesis.* Vitamin B$_6$ is a coenzyme involved in the synthesis of several neurotransmitters, a process that involves transamination. Neurotransmitters are chemicals necessary for the transmission of nerve impulses across synapses. Because of this, vitamin B$_6$ is important in cognitive function and normal brain activity. Abnormal brain waves have been observed in both infants and adults in vitamin B$_6$– deficient states.[10]
- *Carbohydrate metabolism.* Vitamin B$_6$ is a coenzyme assisting in the breakdown of stored glycogen into glucose. Thus, vitamin B$_6$ plays an important role in maintaining blood glucose during exercise. It is also important for the conversion of amino acids to glucose.
- *Heme synthesis.* The synthesis of heme, required for the production of hemoglobin and thus the transport of oxygen in red blood cells, requires vitamin B$_6$. Chronic vitamin B$_6$ deficiency can lead to small red blood cells with inadequate amounts of hemoglobin, which is called *microcytic, hypochromic anemia.*[10] (This is discussed in more detail in Chapter 12.)
- *Immune function.* Vitamin B$_6$ plays a role in maintaining the health and activity of lymphocytes and in producing adequate levels of antibodies in response to an immune challenge. The depression of immune function seen in vitamin B$_6$ deficiency may also be due to a reduction in vitamin B$_6$–dependent enzymes involved in DNA synthesis.
- *Metabolism of other nutrients.* Vitamin B$_6$ also plays a role in the metabolism of other nutrients, including niacin, folate, and carnitine.[10]
- *Reduction in cardiovascular disease (CVD) risk.* Vitamin B$_6$, folate, and vitamin B$_{12}$ are closely interrelated in some metabolic functions, including the metabolism of

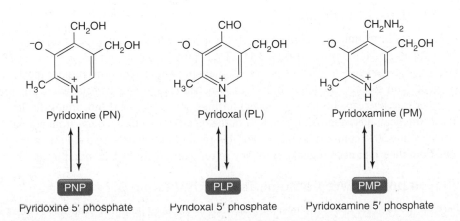

FIGURE 8.9 Structure of the vitamin B$_6$ compounds and their interconversions to the phosphorylated forms.

methionine, an essential amino acid. The body metabolizes methionine to another amino acid, called **homocysteine.** In the presence of sufficient levels of vitamin B_6, homocysteine can then be converted to the nonessential amino acid cysteine (**Figure 8.10**). In the presence of sufficient levels of folate and vitamin B_{12}, homocysteine can also be converted back to methionine if the body's level of methionine becomes deficient. If these nutrients are not available, these conversion reactions cannot occur and homocysteine will accumulate in the blood. High levels of homocysteine have been associated with an increased risk for cardiovascular disease and as a measure of poor dietary intakes of vitamin B_6, folate, and vitamin B_{12}.

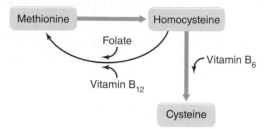

FIGURE 8.10 The body metabolizes methionine, an essential amino acid, to homocysteine. Notice, however, that homocysteine can then be converted back to methionine through a vitamin B_{12}– and folate–dependent reaction, or to cysteine through a vitamin B_6–dependent reaction. Cysteine is a nonessential amino acid important for making other biological compounds. Without these B-vitamins, blood levels of homocysteine can increase. High levels of homocysteine are a risk factor for cardiovascular disease.

How Much Vitamin B_6 Should We Consume?

The RDA for vitamin B_6 for adult men and women aged 19 to 50 years is 1.3 mg/day. For adults 51 years of age and older, the RDA increases to 1.7 mg/day for men and 1.5 mg/day for women. The increased requirement with aging is based on data indicating that more vitamin B_6 is required to maintain normal vitamin B_6 status, using blood PLP concentrations as a status indicator, in older individuals. Based on NHANES III data, the average dietary intake of vitamin B_6 from food for men and women between the ages of 19 and 70 years averages 2 mg/day and 1.5 to 1.6 mg/day, respectively.[4]

Because of the role vitamin B_6 plays in protein metabolism, it has been proposed that the requirement for vitamin B_6 be based on protein intake. Although the RDAs did not define vitamin B_6 intake in terms of protein intake, we do know that as protein intake increases more vitamin B_6 is required.[4] Fortunately, nature has combined vitamin B_6 with protein in many foods, so food sources high in protein are also typically high in vitamin B_6.

Food Sources of Vitamin B_6

Good sources of vitamin B_6 include meat, fish (especially tuna), poultry, and organ meats, which are also high in protein (**Figure 8.11**). Thus, protein and vitamin B_6 are provided together in the same food, which ensures adequate protein metabolism. Besides meat and fish, good food sources of vitamin B_6 include enriched ready-to-eat cereals, white potatoes and other starchy vegetables, bananas, and fortified soy-based meat substitutes. In the typical American diet, approximately 40% of the dietary vitamin B_6 comes from animal sources, while 60% comes from plants. For this reason, individuals who eliminate animal foods from their diet need to make sure they select plant foods high in vitamin B_6.

What Happens If We Consume Too Much Vitamin B_6?

There are no adverse effects associated with high intakes of vitamin B_6 from food sources. Vitamin B_6 supplements have been used to treat conditions such as premenstrual syndrome and carpal tunnel syndrome. Caution is required, however, when using such supplements.

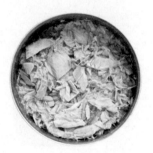

Tuna is a very good source of vitamin B_6.

homocysteine An amino acid that requires adequate levels of folate, vitamin B_6 and vitamin B_{12} for its metabolism. High levels of homocysteine in the blood are associated with an increased risk for cardiovascular disease.

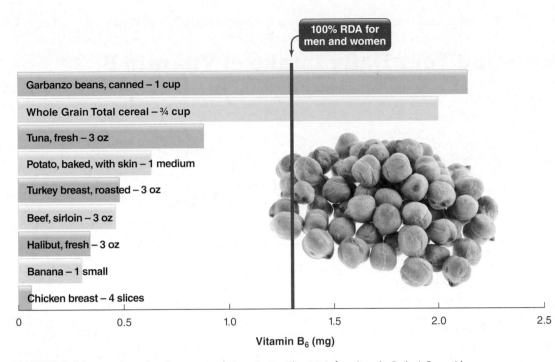

100% RDA for men and women

Garbanzo beans, canned – 1 cup

Whole Grain Total cereal – ¾ cup

Tuna, fresh – 3 oz

Potato, baked, with skin – 1 medium

Turkey breast, roasted – 3 oz

Beef, sirloin – 3 oz

Halibut, fresh – 3 oz

Banana – 1 small

Chicken breast – 4 slices

| 0 | 0.5 | 1.0 | 1.5 | 2.0 | 2.5 |

Vitamin B$_6$ (mg)

FIGURE 8.11 Common food sources of vitamin B$_6$. The RDA for vitamin B$_6$ is 1.3 mg/day for men and women aged 19 to 50 years. (*Sources:* Data from US Department of Agriculture, Agricultural Research Service. 2009. USDA Nutrient Database for Standard Reference, Release 22. Nutrient Data Laboratory Home Page. www.ars.usda.gov.)

High doses of supplemental vitamin B$_6$ have been associated with sensory neuropathy and dermatological lesions.[4] Thus, the UL for vitamin B$_6$ is set at 100 mg/day. See the ***Nutrition Myth or Fact?*** essay at the end of this chapter for more discussion of the potential relationship between high intakes of vitamin B$_6$ and premenstrual syndrome.

What Happens If We Don't Consume Enough Vitamin B$_6$?

A number of conditions appear to increase the need for vitamin B$_6$: alcoholism, certain prescription medications, intense physical activity, and chronic diseases, such as arthritis and vascular disease.[3,4,11] If we don't get enough vitamin B$_6$ in the diet, the symptoms of vitamin B$_6$ deficiency can develop. These include anemia, convulsions, depression, confusion, and inflamed, irritated patches on the skin. Notice that the symptoms associated with vitamin B$_6$ deficiency involve three tissues: skin, blood, and the nervous system. This fact reflects the role of vitamin B$_6$ in protein metabolism, red blood cell development, and the synthesis of neurotransmitters.

No specific disease is solely attributed to vitamin B$_6$ deficiency. However, recall that, if intakes of vitamin B$_6$, folate, and vitamin B$_{12}$ are low, blood levels of homocysteine increase. High blood homocysteine concentrations are an independent risk factor for cardiovascular disease.

If you're wondering whether you're getting enough vitamin B$_6$—or too much!—see the ***You Do the Math*** box (page 318) and calculate your daily intake.

Folate

Folate was originally identified as a growth factor in green, leafy vegetables (foliage), hence the name.[12] The generic term *folate* is used for all the various forms of food folate that demonstrate biological activity. Folic acid (pteroylglutamate; see **Figure 8.12**) is the form of folate found in most supplements and used in the enrichment and fortification of foods.

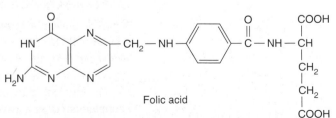

Folic acid

FIGURE 8.12 Structure of folate.

YOU Do the Math

Calculating Your Daily Intake of Vitamin B$_6$

Open up your cupboard and take a look inside. How many processed foods providing B-vitamins do you consume on a typical day? Pull out all such foods, including breads, ready-to-eat cereals, pasta, energy bars, meal replacement drinks, and so forth. Then, if you take any supplements, including vitamins, protein powders, weight-loss supplements, and so forth, line those up too.

Now, let's see if we can determine whether you are meeting or exceeding your RDA for vitamin B$_6$. We'll limit our analysis to B$_6$ because it is one of the B-vitamins with a UL. Use the template provided in the following table to document your vitamin B$_6$ intake for a typical day. On food labels, the amount of the vitamin will be given as a percentage of the daily value (%DV). Thus, you will first have to write down the %DV for each serving. Be sure to look at the serving size! If you eat two servings, you will need to multiply this value by 2, and so on. Finally, convert the %DV to the amount that you ate. For vitamin B$_6$, 100% of the DV is 2 mg. Notice that we have filled in one line of the template as an example; now you fill in the rest.

Meal	Food	%DV for B$_6$	Servings	%DV per Serving	B$_6$ Consumed (mg)
Breakfast	Wheaties	50%	2	100%	2 mg
Lunch					
Snack					
Dinner					
Supplements					
Total mg B$_6$/day:					

How much vitamin B$_6$ did you get each day from processed foods and supplements alone? How much additional vitamin B$_6$ would you estimate you get in whole foods, such as meat, fish, poultry, starchy vegetables, and bananas? Are you close to the UL for vitamin B$_6$ (100 mg for adults aged 19–70)? Although this assignment was designed to look at vitamin B$_6$, you can look at other micronutrients in your diet that have a UL.

Functions of Folate and Folic Acid

Within the body, folate functions primarily in association with folate-dependent coenzymes that act as acceptors and donors of one-carbon units. These enzymes are critical for DNA synthesis, cell differentiation, and amino acid metabolism, which occur within the cytosol, nucleus, and mitochondria of the cells. Folate's role in assisting with cell division makes it a critical nutrient during the first few weeks of pregnancy, when the combined sperm–egg cell multiplies rapidly to form the primitive tissues and structures of the human body. Without adequate folate, the embryo cannot develop properly. In particular, a group of nervous system malformations called *neural tube defects* are associated with low maternal folate intake. Folate is also essential in the synthesis of new cells, such as the red blood cells, and for the repair of damaged cells. (We will discuss the role of folate in red blood cell development more in Chapter 12.)

As already discussed, folate and vitamin B$_{12}$ are needed for the regeneration of methionine from homocysteine. High levels of homocysteine have been associated with an increased risk for cardiovascular disease.

What Factors Alter Folate Digestion, Absorption, and Balance?

Dietary folates are hydrolyzed by the brush border of the lumen and then absorbed into the enterocytes. This process is typically achieved through a carrier-mediated process, but some folates can cross the mucosal cell membrane by diffusion. Folates are then released from the enterocytes into the portal circulation, in which they are transported to the liver.[8]

The bioavailability of folate varies, depending on its source. When folic acid is taken as a supplement or in a fortified food, such as breakfast cereal, the amount absorbed is high—nearly 85% to 100%.[4] However, the bioavailability of food folate is approximately 50%.[8] When large doses of folic acid are taken as supplements, they are well absorbed, but the body has no mechanism for retaining this folate, so it is easily lost in the urine.

Because dietary folate is only half as bioavailable as synthetic folic acid, the amount of food folate in the diet is expressed as dietary folate equivalents, or DFE. In order to calculate the amount of DFE, you need to know that 1 µg of food folate is equal to 0.5 µg of folic acid taken on an empty stomach or 0.6 µg of folic acid taken with a meal.[4] Thus, to calculate the total DFE in an individual's diet, use the following equation:

µg of DFE provided in diet = µg of food folate per day + (1.7 × µg of synthetic folic acid/day)

Because this calculation can be time consuming, most nutrient databases calculate the DFE automatically, so that the total micrograms per day of folate provided in the nutrient analysis printout has already taken into account the bioavailability of the different types of folate in the diet.

Much of the folate circulating in the blood is attached to transport proteins, especially albumin, for delivery to the cells of the body. The red blood cells also contain folate attached to hemoglobin. Because this folate is not transferred out of the red blood cells to other tissues, it may be a good measure of folate status over the past 3 months—the life of red blood cells.[13] If red blood cell folate levels begin to drop, this indicates that, when the red blood cells were being formed, folate was inadequate in the body.

How Much Folate Should We Consume?

Folate is so important for good health and the prevention of birth defects that in 1998 the U.S. Department of Agriculture (USDA) mandated the fortification with folic acid of enriched breads, flours, corn meals, rice, pastas, and other grain products. Because folic acid is highly available for absorption, the goal of this fortification was to increase folate intake among all Americans and thus decrease the risk for birth defects and chronic diseases associated with low folate intakes.

The RDA for folate for adult men and women aged 19 years and older is 400 µg/day, with 600 µg/day required for pregnant women.[4] These higher levels of folate were set to minimize the risk for birth defects. The UL for folate is 1,000 µg/day.

Ready-to-eat cereals, bread, and other grain products are among the primary sources of folate in the United States; however, you need to read the label of processed grain products to make sure they contain folate. Other good food sources include liver, spinach, lentils, oatmeal, asparagus, and romaine lettuce. **Figure 8.13** shows some foods relatively high in

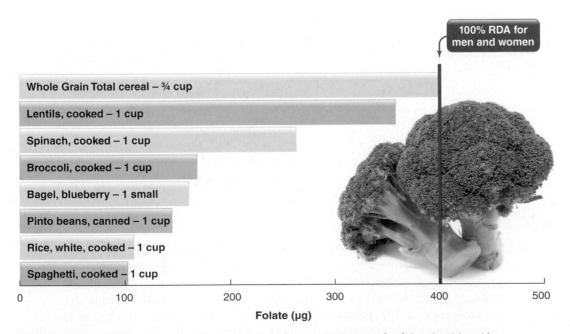

FIGURE 8.13 Common food sources of folate and folic acid. The RDA for folate is 400 µg/day for men and women. (*Sources*: Data from US Dept. of Agriculture, Agriculture Research Services. 2009. USDA Nutrient Database for Standard Reference, Release 22. Nutrient Data Laboratory Home Page. www.ars.usda.gov.)

folate. Losses of folate can occur when food is heated or when folate leaches out of cooked foods and the liquid from these foods is discarded. For this reason, cook green vegetables in a minimal amount of water and limit the time foods are exposed to high temperatures. These actions will help preserve the folate in the food.

What Happens If We Consume Too Much Folate?

There have been no studies suggesting toxic effects of consuming high amounts of folate in food; however, toxicity can occur with high amounts of supplemental folate.[8] One especially frustrating problem with folate toxicity is that it can mask a simultaneous vitamin B_{12} deficiency. This often results in a failure to detect the B_{12} deficiency and, as described in the chapter-opening case, a delay in diagnosis of B_{12} deficiency can contribute to severe damage to the nervous system. There do not appear to be any clear symptoms of folate toxicity independent from its interaction with vitamin B_{12} deficiency. However, as discussed in the **Nutrition Myth or Fact?** at the end of this chapter, researchers are becoming concerned about some possible health risks, such as increased risk for cancer and allergies, now being associated with high supplemental doses of folic acid.

What Happens If We Consume Too Little Folate?

A folate deficiency can cause many adverse health effects, including *macrocytic anemia* (discussed in Chapter 12). Again, deficiencies in folate, vitamin B_6, and vitamin B_{12} can cause elevated levels of homocysteine in the blood, a condition that is associated with heart disease. When folate intake is inadequate in pregnant women, neural tube defects can occur. (Neural tube defects are discussed in more detail in Chapter 16.)

Vitamin B_{12} (Cobalamin)

As with folate, the generic terms *vitamin B_{12}* and *cobalamin* are used to describe a number of compounds that exhibit vitamin B_{12} biological activity. These compounds have cobalt in their center and are surrounded by ring structures. See **Figure 8.14** for a diagram of the structure of cyanocobalamin, one of the forms of vitamin B_{12}. As you can see, vitamin B_{12} is a complex molecule, and the Nobel Prize was awarded for the delineation of its structure.

FIGURE 8.14 Structure of vitamin B_{12} (cyanocobalamin). As you can see, this is a highly complex molecule, and the Nobel Prize was awarded for the delineation of its structure.

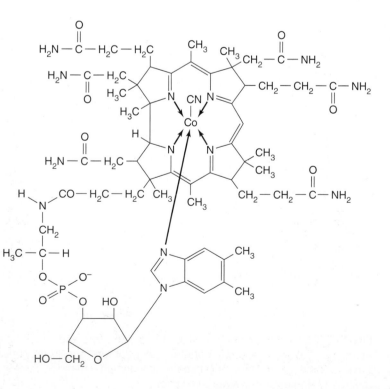

Functions of Vitamin B$_{12}$

Vitamin B$_{12}$ is part of coenzymes that assist with DNA synthesis, which is necessary for the proper formation of red blood cells.[8] As described in the chapter-opening scenario, vitamin B$_{12}$ is essential for healthy functioning of the nervous system, because it helps maintain the myelin sheath that coats nerve fibers. When this sheath is damaged or absent, the conduction of nerve signals is altered, causing numerous neurologic problems.

Adequate levels of vitamin B$_{12}$ and folate, as well as B$_6$, are also necessary for the metabolism of the amino acid homocysteine, which we discussed earlier.

What Factors Alter Vitamin B$_{12}$ Absorption, Metabolism, and Balance?

Vitamin B$_{12}$ is synthesized almost entirely by bacteria in animals. For this reason, the vitamin B$_{12}$ in our diet comes almost exclusively from meat, eggs, dairy products, and some seafood and is approximately 50% bioavailable in a typical meal.[14] Fortified plant foods such as soy milks and cereals are also good sources of vitamin B$_{12}$.

The absorption of vitamin B$_{12}$ is complex (**Figure 8.15**). In food, vitamin B$_{12}$ is bound to protein. It is released from this protein in the acidic environment of the stomach, where it is then attached to another group of proteins called R-binders. The stomach also secretes **intrinsic factor,** a protein necessary for vitamin B$_{12}$ absorption in the small intestine. The intrinsic factor and vitamin B$_{12}$–R-binder complexes formed in the stomach pass into the small intestine, where the R-binder protein is hydrolyzed by pancreatic proteolytic enzymes, after which free vitamin B$_{12}$ binds to the intrinsic factor. The vitamin B$_{12}$-intrinsic factor complexes are then recognized by receptors on the enterocytes and internalized. These receptors do not recognize vitamin B$_{12}$ alone but only when it is bound to intrinsic factor. Within the enterocytes, vitamin B$_{12}$ is released into the cytosol. The vitamin B$_{12}$ is then released from the enterocyte, bound to a protein called transcobalamin II, and then

intrinsic factor A protein secreted by cells of the stomach that binds to vitamin B$_{12}$ and aids its absorption in the small intestine.

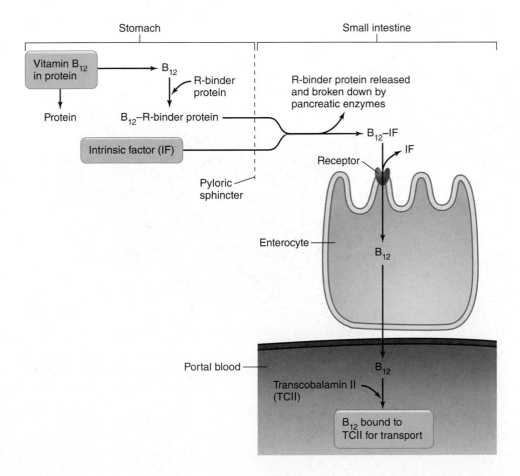

FIGURE 8.15 Digestion and absorption of vitamin B$_{12}$. (*Source:* "Advanced Nutrition and Human Metabolism (with InfoTrac®) 4e," by Gropper; Smith; Groff, 2005. Copyright © 2005 by Brooks/Cole, a part of Cengage Learning, Inc. Reproduced by permission.)

transported to the cells of the body. The body stores vitamin B_{12} in the liver, approximately 2 to 3 mg, which means we can probably survive for months without vitamin B_{12} in our diet.[4] Vitamin B_{12} is lost from the system in the urine and bile.

How Much Vitamin B_{12} Should We Consume?

The RDA for vitamin B_{12} for adult men and women aged 19 and older is 2.4 µg/day. Vitamin B_{12} is found primarily in dairy products, eggs, meats, and poultry. **Figure 8.16** displays some foods relatively high in vitamin B_{12}. Individuals consuming a vegan diet need to eat plant-based foods that are fortified with vitamin B_{12} or take vitamin B_{12} supplements or injections to ensure that they maintain adequate blood levels of this nutrient.

As we age, our sources of vitamin B_{12} may need to change. Nonvegans younger than 51 years of age are generally able to meet the RDA for vitamin B_{12} by consuming it in foods. However, it is estimated that about 10% to 30% of adults older than 50 years have a chronic inflammatory condition referred to as **atrophic gastritis,** which results in low secretion of HCl. Because HCl separates foodbound vitamin B_{12} from dietary proteins, if the acid content of the stomach is inadequate, then we cannot free up enough vitamin B_{12} from food sources alone.[4] Because atrophic gastritis can affect almost one-third of the older adult population, it is recommended that people older than 50 years of age consume foods fortified with vitamin B_{12}, take a vitamin B_{12}–containing supplement, or have periodic vitamin B_{12} injections.

There are no known adverse effects from consuming excess amounts of vitamin B_{12} from food. However, data are not available on the effects of excess amounts of vitamin B_{12} from supplements.

Vitamin B_{12} deficiency is rare but is generally associated with either dietary insufficiency or reduced absorption. Deficiency symptoms generally include those associated with

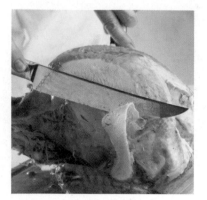

Turkey contains vitamin B_{12}.

atrophic gastritis A condition, frequently seen in people over the age of 50, in which stomach-acid secretions are low.

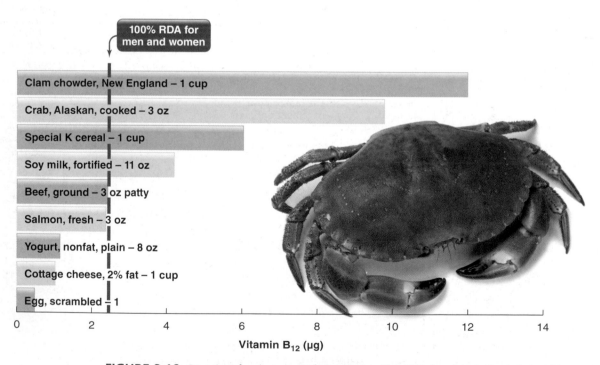

FIGURE 8.16 Common food sources of vitamin B_{12}. The RDA for vitamin B_{12} is 2.4 µg/day for men and women. (*Source:* Data from US Department of Agriculture, Agriculture Research Services. 2009. USDA Nutrient Data Base for Standard Reference, Release 22. Nutrient Data Laboratory Home Page. www.ars.usda.gov.)

anemia, as well as gastrointestinal and neurologic effects.[8,14] The symptoms of anemia include pale skin, diminished energy and exercise tolerance, fatigue, and shortness of breath. Gastrointestinal symptoms include loss of appetite, constipation, excessive gas, and changes in skin pigment.[14] Neurologic symptoms include tingling and numbness of extremities, abnormal gait, memory loss, dementia, disorientation, visual disturbances, insomnia, and impaired bladder and bowel control.[14] A deficiency of vitamin B_{12}, as with vitamin B_6 and folate, has been linked to cardiovascular disease due to high levels of homocysteine.

As noted, an important cause of vitamin B_{12} deficiency is reduced absorption. A common culprit in reduced absorption is a condition called pernicious anemia, which is caused by inadequate secretion of intrinsic factor by parietal cells of the stomach. (Pernicious anemia is discussed in more detail in Chapter 12.)

RECAP

Some of the important functions of vitamin B_6 are in amino acid and carbohydrate metabolism, neurotransmitter and heme synthesis, and maintenance of immune cells and antibodies. Without adequate intake of vitamin B_6, which plays a critical role in transamination, all amino acids become essential. Folate is critical for amino acid metabolism, as well as DNA synthesis and cell division. Inadequate intake of folate in the first several weeks of pregnancy is a risk factor for neural tube defects. Vitamin B_{12} is part of enzymes important in DNA synthesis and is essential for maintenance of the myelin sheath that coats nerve fibers. Adequate levels of vitamins B_6, B_{12}, and folate are necessary for metabolism of the amino acid homocysteine. ■

What Are the Roles of Pantothenic Acid, Biotin, and Choline in Energy Metabolism?

LO 7 Describe the roles of pantothenic acid, biotin, and choline in energy metabolism.

Pantothenic acid, biotin, and choline all play roles in lipid metabolism and other body functions. They are widely available in foods and deficiencies are rare.

Pantothenic Acid

Pantothenic acid is an essential vitamin that is metabolized into two major coenzymes: coenzyme A (CoA) and acyl carrier protein (ACP), which are shown in **Figure 8.17** (page 324). Both are essential in the synthesis of fatty acids, while CoA is essential for fatty acid oxidation, ketone metabolism, and the metabolism of carbohydrate and protein.[8] For example, in the conversion of pyruvate to acetyl-CoA, the enzyme pyruvate dehydrogenase requires CoA. Many of the metabolic reactions that require pantothenic acid for energy production are illustrated in Figure 8.2. Besides its role in energy metabolism, pantothenic acid is required in the synthesis of cholesterol and steroids and in the detoxification of drugs.

The AI for pantothenic acid for adult men and women aged 19 years and older is 5 mg/day. Pantothenic acid is widely distributed in foods, with the average daily intake at approximately 5 mg/day and usual intakes ranging from 4 to 7 mg/day.[4,8] Thus, the AI for pantothenic acid and the average dietary intake are similar. As mentioned, pantothenic acid is available from a variety of foods, including chicken, beef, egg yolk, potatoes, oat cereals, tomato products, whole grains, certain mushrooms, and organ meats (**Figure 8.18**, page 325). There are no known adverse effects from consuming excess amounts of pantothenic acid, and deficiencies of pantothenic acid are very rare.

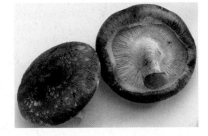

Shiitake mushrooms contain ten to twenty times more pantothenic acid than other types of mushrooms.

FIGURE 8.17 Structure of coenzymes containing pantothenic acid. **(a)** Coenzyme A (CoA). **(b)** Acyl carrier protein (ACP).

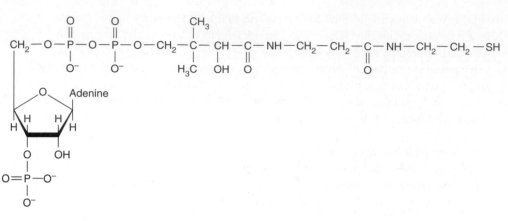

(a) Coenzyme A (CoA)

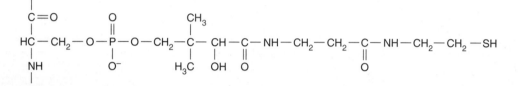

(b) Acyl carrier protein (ACP)

Biotin

Biotin is a component of four carboxylase enzymes that are present in humans. These enzymes serve as the carbon dioxide (CO_2) carrier and the carboxyl donor for substrates.[8] **Figure 8.19** shows the structure of biotin.

The enzymes that require biotin as a coenzyme are involved in fatty acid synthesis (for example, lipogenesis), gluconeogenesis, and carbohydrate, fat, and protein metabolism. For example, pyruvate carboxylase catalyzes the synthesis of oxaloacetate from pyruvate in the TCA cycle. Many of the enzyme reactions that require biotin for energy production are illustrated in Figure 8.2.

The AI for biotin for adult men and women aged 19 and older is 30 µg/day. The biotin content has been determined for very few foods, and these values are not reported in food composition tables or dietary analysis programs. In food, biotin exists as free biotin or bound to protein as biocytin, both of which appear to be widespread in foods. The free form of biotin is shown in Figure 8.19; the structure of biocytin is similar to that of free biotin but has an amino acid attached to the carboxyl end.

There are no known adverse effects from consuming excess amounts of biotin. Biotin deficiencies are typically seen only in people who consume a large number of raw egg whites over long periods of time. This is because raw egg whites contain a protein that binds with biotin and prevents its absorption. Biotin deficiencies are also seen in people fed total parenteral nutrition (nutrients administered by a route other than the GI tract) that is not supplemented with biotin. Symptoms include thinning of hair; loss of hair color; development of a red, scaly rash around the eyes, nose, and mouth; depression; lethargy; and hallucinations.

Choline

Choline is a vitamin-like substance that is important for metabolism, the structural integrity of cell membranes, and neurotransmission. It is typically grouped with the B-vitamins because of its role in fat digestion and transport and homocysteine metabolism.

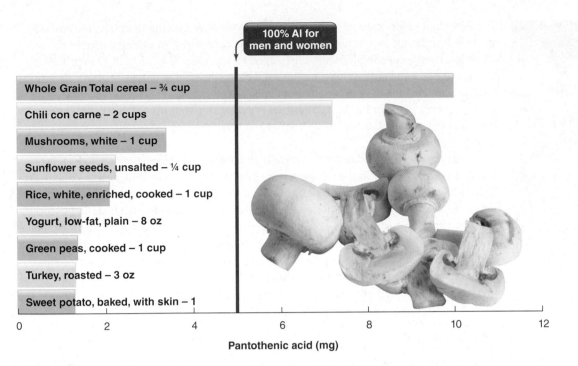

FIGURE 8.18 Common food sources of pantothenic acid. The AI for pantothenic acid is 5 mg/day for men and women. (*Source*: Data from US Dept. of Agriculture, Agriculture Research Services. 2009. USDA Nutrient Data Base for Standard Reference, Release 22. Nutrient Data Laboratory Home Page. www.ars.usda.gov.)

Specifically, choline plays an important role in the metabolism and transport of fats and cholesterol. High amounts of the choline-containing compound phosphatidylcholine are found in bile, which aids fat digestion, and in the formation of lipoproteins, which transport endogenous and dietary fat and cholesterol in the blood to the cells. Choline is also necessary for the synthesis of phospholipids and other components of cell membranes; thus, choline plays a critical role in the structural integrity of cell membranes. Finally, choline accelerates the synthesis and release of **acetylcholine,** a neurotransmitter that is involved in many functions, including muscle movement and memory storage.

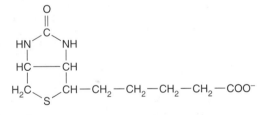

FIGURE 8.19 Structure of biotin.

Nutri-Case

Judy

"Ever since my doctor put me on this crazy diet, I've been feeling hungry and exhausted. This morning I'm sitting in the lunch room on my break, and I actually doze off and start dreaming about food! Maureen, one of the girls I work with, comes in and has to wake me up! I told her what's been going on with me, and she thinks I should start taking some B-vitamins so I stay healthy while I'm on the diet. She says B-vitamins are the most important because they give you energy. Maybe after work I'll stop off at the mall and buy some. If they give you energy, maybe they'll make it easier to stick to my diet too."

Is Judy's coworker correct when she asserts that B-vitamins "give you energy"? Either way, do you think it's likely that Judy needs to take B-vitamin supplements to ensure that she "stays healthy" while she is on her prescribed diet? Why or why not? Finally, could taking B-vitamins help Judy stick to her diet?

acetylcholine A neurotransmitter that is involved in many functions, including muscle movement and memory storage.

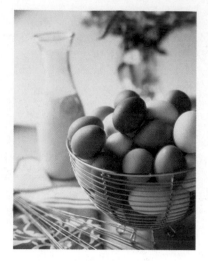

Choline is widespread in foods and can be found in eggs and milk.

Although small amounts of choline can be synthesized within the body, the amount made is insufficient for our needs; thus, choline is considered an essential dietary nutrient. Choline has an AI of 550 mg/day for men aged 19 and older and an AI of 425 mg/day for women aged 19 and older. There are limited data on the choline intake of North Americans, because choline intake is not reported in the NHANES or other large surveys. In addition, it is not reported in major nutrient databases. However, it is estimated that choline intakes in the United States and Canada range from 730 to 1,040 mg/day[4] based on the typical choline content of foods.

Choline is widespread in foods, typically in the form of phosphatidylcholine (see Figure 5.6 on page 175) in the cell membranes of the food. The food highest in choline are eggs, while other good sources are milk, liver, soybean oil, salmon, and mushrooms.[4,15] Lecithin (a more common term for phosphatidylcholine) is added to foods during processing as an emulsifying agent, which also increases choline intakes in the diet. Inadequate intakes of choline can lead to increased fat accumulation in the liver, which eventually leads to liver damage. Excessive intake of supplemental choline results in various toxicity symptoms, including a fishy body odor, vomiting, excess salivation, sweating, diarrhea, and low blood pressure. The UL for choline for adults 19 years of age and older is 3.5 g/day.

RECAP

The B-vitamins pantothenic acid and biotin assist in the metabolism of carbohydrates, fats, and protein. Both are widely available in foods. Choline is a vitamin-like substance that is required for the production of phosphatidylcholine, a compound found in bile, and for the synthesis and release of the neurotransmitter acetycholine. ∎

 LO 8 Discuss the roles of iodine, chromium, manganese, and sulfur in energy metabolism.

LO 9 Identify the deficiency disorders associated with poor iodine intake.

How Do Minerals Help Regulate Energy Metabolism?

In addition to the B-vitamins and choline, several minerals facilitate energy metabolism. These include iodine, chromium, manganese, and sulfur.

Iodine

Iodine is the heaviest trace element required for human health and a necessary component of the thyroid hormones, which help regulate human metabolism. In nature, this element is found primarily as inorganic salts in rocks, soil, plants, animals, and water as either iodine or iodide, but once it enters the GI tract, it is broken down to iodide, which is the negative ion of iodine, designated I−. Upon absorption, the majority of this iodide is taken up by the thyroid gland.[15]

Functions of Iodine

As just noted, iodine is responsible for a single function within the body: the synthesis of thyroid hormones.[16] Although iodine's function is singular, the multiple actions of thyroid hormones mean that it affects the whole body. Thyroid hormones regulate key metabolic reactions associated with body temperature, resting metabolic rate, macronutrient metabolism, and reproduction and growth.

The structure of the thyroid hormones, thyroxine (T_4) and 3, 5, 39-triiodothyronine (T_3), illustrates the placement of iodine (I) in these two hormones (**Figure 8.20**). Both are derived from the iodination of the amino acid tyrosine, shown in Figure 8.20c. Notice that thyroxine has four iodine molecules as part of its structure, whereas triiodothyronine has three—thus, the abbreviated designations T_4 and T_3. Thyroxine (T_4) is the primary circulating thyroid hormone. The removal of one iodine group is required to generate the active form of T_3.[8]

How Much Iodine Should We Consume?

The body needs relatively little iodine to maintain health. The RDA for adults 19 years of age and older is 150 µg/day. It is estimated that the iodine intake from food in the United States is approximately 200 to 300 µg/day for men and 190 to 210 µg/day for women.[17]

Very few foods are reliable sources of iodine, because the amount of iodine in foods varies according to the soil, irrigation, and fertilizers used. Saltwater foods, both fish and plants, tend to have higher amounts, because marine species concentrate iodine from seawater. Good food sources include saltwater fish, shrimp, seaweed, iodized salt, and white and whole-wheat breads made with iodized salt and bread conditioners. In addition, iodine is added to dairy cattle feed and used in sanitizing solutions in the dairy industry, making dairy foods an important source of iodine.

Iodine has been voluntarily added to salt in the United States since 1924 to combat iodine deficiency resulting from the poor iodine content of soils in this country. For many people, iodized salt is their primary source of iodine, and approximately ½ teaspoon of iodized salt meets the entire adult RDA for iodine. When you buy salt, look carefully at the package label, because stores carry both iodized and noniodized salt. Most specialty salts, such as kosher salt or sea salt, do not have iodine added. If iodine has been added to the salt, it will be clearly marked on the label.

Excess iodine intakes can cause a number of health-related problems, especially related to thyroid gland function. Too much iodine blocks the synthesis of thyroid hormones. As the thyroid gland attempts to produce more hormones, it may enlarge, a condition known as **goiter** (**Figure 8.21**, page 328). (Goiter refers to the enlargement of the thyroid gland, regardless of its cause.) Iodine toxicity generally occurs as a result of excessive supplementation. Thus, the UL for iodine is 1,100 µg/day.[17]

Paradoxically, goiter is also the most classic disorder of iodine deficiency. An insufficient supply of iodine means there is less iodine for the production of thyroid hormones. The body responds by stimulating the thyroid gland, including increasing the size of the gland, in an attempt to capture more iodine from the blood.

The development of a goiter is only one of many problems that result when iodine is insufficient in the diet. A broader term applied to the disorders associated with poor iodine intakes is *iodine deficiency disorders,* or *IDDs,* which include cretinism, growth and developmental disorders, mental deficiencies, neurologic disorders, decreased fertility, congenital abnormalities, and prenatal and infant death.[17,18,19] The World Health Organization (WHO) considers iodine deficiency to be the "greatest single cause of preventable brain damage and mental retardation" in the world.[18] If a woman experiences iodine deficiency during pregnancy, her infant has a high risk of being born with a unique form of mental impairment referred to as **cretinism.** In addition to mental impairment, the infant may suffer from stunted growth, deafness, and muteness. Among pregnant women, iodine deficiency may also increase the occurrence of spontaneous abortion, stillbirths and congenital abnormalities, and infant mortality.[19,20] The impact of mild iodine deficiency on the development of the brain and neurologic system of a child is more difficult to determine. Iodine deficiency can also cause **hypothyroidism** (low blood levels of thyroid hormone), which is characterized by decreased body temperature, an inability to tolerate cold environmental temperatures, weight gain, fatigue, and sluggishness.

According to the World Health Organization,[21] 1.88 billion people live in areas subject to iodine deficiency and are at increased risk for its health complications and consequences. A recent global assessment of iodine status showed that 30% of the world's 241 million school-age children remain iodine deficient.[22] In the United States, large areas of crop-producing lands are low in iodine, and thus foods grown on these lands are low in iodine. As recently as the beginning of the 20th century, IDDs and goiter were considered endemic

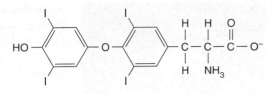

(a) Thyroxine (T$_4$)

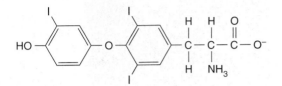

(b) 3, 5, 3′–Triiodothyronine (T$_3$)

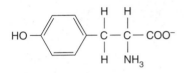

(c) Tyrosine

FIGURE 8.20 Thyroid hormones contain iodine (I). **(a)** Structure of the thyroid hormone T$_4$. **(b)** Structure of the thyroid hormone T$_3$. Both are derived from the iodination of **(c)** tyrosine, an amino acid.

Visit the Iodine Global Network to learn more about the worldwide campaign to iodize salt and prevent IDDs, at http://www.ign.org. Look for Quick Links and Resources, and click on Iodine Videos to watch the videos on iodine supplementation around the world.

goiter Enlargement of the thyroid gland; can be caused by iodine toxicity or deficiency.

cretinism A unique form of mental retardation that occurs in infants when the mother experiences iodine deficiency during pregnancy.

hypothyroidism A condition characterized by low blood levels of thyroid hormone.

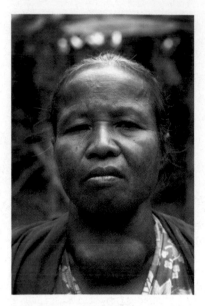

FIGURE 8.21 Goiter, or enlargement of the thyroid gland, occurs with both iodine toxicity and deficiency.

hyperthyroidism A condition characterized by high blood levels of thyroid hormone.

in the United States. However, the problem was not fully addressed until World War I, when many conscripted men were barred from military service because they had goiters. At that time, the treatment of goiters with sodium iodine was shown to be effective, and the search was on for a method of increasing iodine in the food supply by fortifying processed foods, increasing the level of iodine in the soil through fertilizers, or adding iodine to the feed of animals. After much debate, it was determined that the fortification of salt with iodine was the best solution. This action significantly reduces the risk of goiter, cretinism, low cognitive function, and iodine deficiency.[23] The World Health Organization now has a worldwide campaign to increase salt fortification with iodine,[18] especially as health organizations recommend reductions in sodium intake.

Hyperthyroidism (high blood levels of thyroid hormone) is most commonly caused by Graves' disease, which is an autoimmune disease that causes an overproduction of thyroid hormones. The symptoms include weight loss, increased heat production, muscular tremors, nervousness, a racing heartbeat, and protrusion of the eyes.

Chromium

Chromium is a trace mineral that plays an important role in carbohydrate metabolism. You may be surprised to learn that the chromium in your body is the same metal used in the chrome plating for cars. Chromium enhances the ability of insulin to transport glucose from the bloodstream into cells.[17,24] Chromium also plays important roles in the metabolism of RNA and DNA, in immune function, and in growth.

Chromium supplements are marketed to reduce body fat and enhance muscle mass and have become popular with bodybuilders and other athletes interested in improving their body composition. The *Highlight* box investigates whether taking supplemental chromium is effective in improving body composition.

HIGHLIGHT

Can Chromium Supplements Enhance Body Composition?

Chromium supplements, predominantly in the form of chromium picolinate, are popular with bodybuilders, weight lifters, and overweight individuals who want to lose body fat. This popularity stems from claims

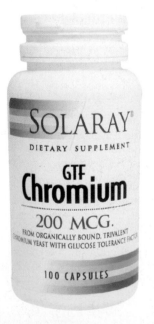

that chromium increases muscle mass and muscle strength and decreases body fat. What does the research say?

An early study of chromium supplementation was promising, in that chromium use in both untrained men and football players was found to decrease body fat and increase muscle mass.[1] These findings caused a surge in the popularity of chromium supplements and motivated many scientists across the United States to test their reproducibility. The next study of chromium supplementation found no

effects of chromium on muscle mass, body fat, or muscle strength.[2]

These contradictory reports led experts to closely examine the two studies. When they did so, they found a number of flaws in the methodology of both. One major concern with the first study was that the chromium status of the research participants prior to the study was not measured or controlled.[1] Since participants who had started the study deficient in chromium would have a more positive reaction than would be expected in people with normal chromium status, subsequent studies were designed to control for pre-study chromium status. A second major concern was that body composition was measured in both studies using calipers that measure the thickness of skinfolds at various sites on the body. Although this method can give a general estimate of body fat, it is not sensitive to small changes in muscle mass. Subsequent studies of chromium used more sophisticated methods of measuring body composition.

The results of research studies conducted since 1995 consistently show that chromium supplementation has no effect on muscle mass, body fat, or muscle strength in a variety of groups, including untrained college males and females, overweight and obese males and females, collegiate wrestlers, and older men and women.[3–10]

Neither have scientists found an effect of chromium on body composition when different types of experimental designs have been used, with varying energy intakes and exercise expenditure.[11,12] To finally put this issue at rest and provide evidence to refute supplement-company claims, three recent reviews of the chromium weight loss literature have been done.[13–15] One review examined randomized clinical trials (RCT, n=9 studies) using only overweight or obese participants (n=622) that were community based, administered by a health professional, and followed participants for up to 24 weeks past the diet.[15] Another meta-analysis used placebo-controlled, double-blind studies (n=11) where 80% compliance was reported in overweight or obese individuals.[13] All three reviews concluded that the level of weight change between treatment and placebo was small (–0.5–1.1 kilogram) and had little clinical relevance. Adverse side effects from treatment were reported in at least three studies and included watery stools, vertigo, weakness, nausea, vomiting, and dizziness.[13]

Despite these studies, many supplement companies still claim that chromium supplements enhance strength and muscle mass and reduce body fat. These claims result in millions of dollars of sales of supplements to consumers each year. Before you decide to purchase chromium supplements, read some of the studies cited here. The information they provide may help you avoid being one of the many consumers fooled by this costly nutrition myth.

References

1. Evans, G. W. 1989. The effect of chromium picolinate on insulin controlled parameters in humans. *Int. J. Biosoc. Med. Res.* 11:163–180.
2. Hasten, D. L., E. P. Rome, D. B. Franks, and M. Hegsted. 1992. Effects of chromium picolinate on beginning weight training students. *Int. J. Sports Nutr.* 2:343–350.
3. Lukaski, H. C., W. A. Siders, and J. G. Penland. 2007. Chromium picolinate supplementation in women: effects on body weight, composition and iron status. *Nutr.* 23:187–195.
4. Hallmark, M. A., T. H. Reynolds, C. A. DeSouza, C. O. Dotson, R. A. Anderson, and M. A. Rogers. 1996. Effects of chromium and resistive training on muscle strength and body composition. *Med. Sci. Sports. Exerc.* 28:139–144.
5. Pasman, W. J., M. S. Westerterp-Plantenga, and W. H. Saris. 1997. The effectiveness of long-term supplementation of carbohydrate, chromium, fiber and caffeine on weight maintenance. *Int. J. Obes. Relat. Metab. Disord.* 21:1143–1151.
6. Walker, L. S., M. G. Bemben, D. A. Bemben, and A. W. Knehans. 1998. Chromium picolinate effects on body composition and muscular performance in wrestlers. *Med. Sci. Sports Exerc.* 30:1730–1737.
7. Campbell, W. W., L. J. Joseph, S. L. Davey, D. Cyr-Campbell, R. A. Anderson, and W. J. Evans. 1999. Effects of resistance training and chromium picolinate on body composition and skeletal muscle in older men. *J. Appl. Physiol.* 86:29–39.
8. Campbell, W. W., L. J. O. Joseph, R. A. Anderson, S. L. Davey, J. Hinton, and W. J. Evans. 2002. Effects of resistive training and chromium picolinate on body composition and skeletal muscle size in older women. *Int. J. Sports Nutr. Exerc. Metab.* 12:125–135.
9. Volpe, S. L., H. W. Huang, K. Larpadisorn, and I. I. Lesser. 2001. Effect of chromium supplementation and exercise on body composition, resting metabolic rate and selected biochemical parameters in moderately obese women following an exercise program. *J. Am. Coll. Nutr.* 20:293–306.
10. Yazaki, Y., Z. Faridi, Y. Ma, A. Ali, V. Northrup, V. Y. Njike,…, and D. L. Katz. 2010. A pilot study of chromium picolinate for weight loss. *J. Altern. Complement Med.* 16(3):291–299.
11. Diaz, L. D., B. A. Watkin, Y. Li, R. A. Anderson, and W. W. Campbell. 2008. Chromium picolinate and conjugated linoleic acid do not synergistically influence diet- and exercise-induced changes in body composition and health indexes in overweight women. *J. Nutr. Biochem.* 19(1):61–68.
12. Lukaski, H. C., W. W. Bolonchuk, W. A. Siders, and D. B. Milne. 1996. Chromium supplementation and resistance training: effects on body composition, strength, and trace element status of men. *Am. J. Clin. Nutr.* 63:954–965.
13. Onakpoya, I., P. Posadzki, and E. Ernst. 2013. Chromium supplementation in overweight and obesity: a systematic review and meta-analysis of randomized clinical trials. *Obes. Rev.* 14(6), 496–507. doi: http://dx.doi.org/10.1111/obr.12026
14. Manore, M. M. 2012. Dietary Supplements for improving body composition and reducing body weight: where is the evidence? *Int. J. Sport. Nutr. Exerc. Metab.* 22(2):139–154.
15. Tian, H., X. Guo, X. Wang, Z. He, R. Sun, S. Ge, and Z. Zhang. 2013. Chromium picolinate supplementation for overweight or obese adults. *Cochrane Database Syst. Rev.* 11. doi: http://dx.doi.org/10.1002/14651858.CD010063.pub2

The body needs only small amounts of chromium. The AI for adults aged 19 to 50 years is 35 µg/day for men and 25 µg/day for women. For adults 51 years of age and older, the AI decreases to 30 µg/day and 20 µg/day for men and women, respectively.[17] The AI for individuals over 50 years was based on the energy intake of older adults, which is typically lower than that of younger individuals.

The question of whether the average diet provides adequate chromium is controversial. Chromium is widely distributed in foods, but concentrations in any particular food are not typically high. In addition, determining the chromium content of food is difficult because contamination can easily occur during laboratory analysis. Thus, we cannot determine average chromium intake from any currently existing nutrient database.

Foods identified as good sources of chromium include mushrooms, prunes, dark chocolate, nuts, whole grains, cereals, asparagus, brewer's yeast, some beers, red wine, and

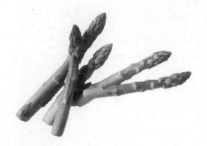

Our body contains very little chromium. Asparagus is a good dietary source of this trace mineral.

meats, especially processed meats. Dairy products are typically poor sources of chromium. Food-processing methods can also add chromium to foods, especially if the food is processed in stainless steel containers. For example, it is assumed that wine and beer derive some of their chromium content from processing.[17]

There appears to be no toxicity related to consuming chromium in the diet, but there are insufficient data to establish a UL for chromium. Because chromium supplements are widely used in the United States, the IOM has recommended more research to determine the safety of high-dose chromium supplements. Until this research is available, supplementation with high amounts of chromium is discouraged. Chromium deficiency appears to be uncommon in the United States. When chromium deficiency is induced in a research setting, glucose uptake into the cells is inhibited, causing a rise in blood glucose and insulin levels. Chromium deficiency can also result in elevated blood lipid levels and in damage to the brain and nervous system.[17]

Manganese

A trace mineral, manganese is a cofactor involved in protein, fat, and carbohydrate metabolism, gluconeogenesis, cholesterol synthesis, and the formation of urea, the primary component of urine. It also assists in the synthesis of the protein matrix found in bone tissue and in building cartilage, a tissue supporting joints. Manganese is also an integral component of superoxide dismutase, an antioxidant enzyme. Thus, it assists in the conversion of free radicals to less damaging substances, protecting the body from oxidative damage (see Chapter 10).

The AI for manganese for adults 19 years of age and older is 2.3 mg/day for men and 1.8 mg/day for women. Manganese requirements are easily met, as this mineral is widespread in foods and is readily available in a varied diet. Whole-grain foods, such as oat bran, wheat flour, whole-wheat spaghetti, and brown rice, are good sources of manganese (**Figure 8.22**). Other sources include pineapple, pine nuts, okra, spinach, and raspberries. Overall, grain products contribute approximately 37% of dietary manganese, and vegetables and beverages, primarily tea, contribute another 18% to 20%.[17]

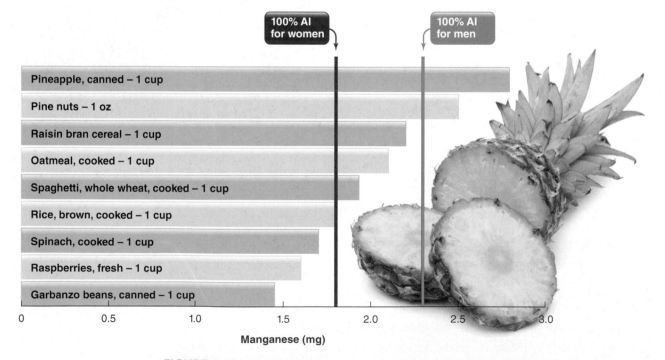

FIGURE 8.22 Common food sources of manganese. The AI for manganese is 2.3 mg/day for men and 1.8 mg/day for women. (*Source*: Data from US Department of Agriculture, Agriculture Research Service. 2009. USDA Nutrient Data Base for Standard Reference, Release 22. Nutrient Data Laboratory Home Page. www.ars.usda.gov.)

Manganese toxicity can occur in occupational environments, such as mines, in which workers inhale manganese dust. It can also result from drinking water high in manganese. Toxicity results in impairment of the neuromuscular system, causing symptoms similar to those seen in Parkinson's disease, such as muscle spasms and tremors. Elevated blood manganese concentrations and neurotoxicity were the criteria used to determine the UL for manganese, which is 11 mg/day for adults 19 years of age and older.[17]

Manganese deficiency is rare in humans. Symptoms include impaired growth and reproductive function, reduced bone density and impaired skeletal growth, impaired glucose and lipid metabolism, and skin rash.

Sulfur

Sulfur is a major mineral and a component of the B-vitamins thiamin and biotin. As such, it is essential for macronutrient metabolism. In addition, as part of the amino acids methionine and cysteine, sulfur helps stabilize the three-dimensional shapes of proteins in the body. The liver requires sulfur to assist in the detoxification of alcohol and various drugs, and sulfur helps to maintain acid–base balance.

The body is able to obtain ample amounts of sulfur from our consumption of protein-containing foods; as a result, there is no DRI specifically for sulfur. There are no known toxicity or deficiency symptoms associated with sulfur.

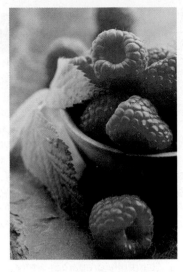

Raspberries are one of the many foods that contain manganese.

RECAP

Iodine is necessary for the synthesis of thyroid hormones, which regulate metabolic rate and body temperature. Iodine-deficiency disorders (IDDs) include cretinism, growth and developmental disorders, hypothyroidism, and many others. Both toxicity and deficiency can lead to development of a goiter. The fortification of salt with iodine has decreased the incidence of goiter and IDDs. Chromium assists the transport of glucose into the cell, the metabolism of RNA and DNA, and immune function and growth. Manganese is involved in energy metabolism, the formation of urea, the synthesis of bone and cartilage, and protection against free radicals. Sulfur is part of the B-vitamins thiamin and biotin and the amino acids methionine and cysteine. ▪

Does B-Vitamin Intake Influence the Body's Capacity for Physical Activity?

LO 10 Discuss the effect of poor B-vitamin intake on the ability to perform physical activity.

We have already discussed the classic deficiency diseases that can result when intake of selected B-vitamins is significantly inadequate, such as beriberi with thiamin deficiency and pellagra with niacin deficiency. However, what happens when intake of the B-vitamins is low, but not low enough to cause one of these deficiency diseases? In other words, what happens when the diet provides a minimum level of B-vitamins, but not enough to fully supply the metabolic pathways of the body with the coenzymes they need to support regular physical activity? Moreover, do individuals who engage in regular physical activity have higher needs for B-vitamins than sedentary adults? Researchers have attempted to answer these questions in a number of ways.

First, researchers have designed studies in which they identify individuals with poor B-vitamin status and then determine the impact of the low status on the individuals' ability to perform exercise. They can then compare the average performance of low-status individuals to the average performance of those with good B-vitamin status.

Second, they have performed controlled metabolic diet studies to determine if athletes need higher levels of B-vitamins than sedentary adults to maintain their vitamin status. For more information on this type of study, see the *Highlight: How Do Scientists Determine Vitamin Requirements?* (page 332).

HIGHLIGHT

How Do Scientists Determine Vitamin Requirements?

Throughout this book, we identify the precise amounts of the different vitamins you need to consume each day to maintain good health. But have you ever wondered how researchers determine these recommendations? Of the several methods used, one of the most rigorous is the metabolic diet study.

The goal of a metabolic diet study is to determine how vitamin assessment parameters in the blood, urine, and feces change as the dietary intake of a nutrient, such as vitamin B_6, is closely controlled. In a metabolic diet study, which may last for weeks or months, all foods eaten by study participants are carefully prepared, weighed to within 0.1 g, and recorded. Subjects are usually required to either live at the research facility (where all physical activity is monitored) or go to the research facility for all their meals. Depending on the nutrient being studied, all fluids, even water, may also be provided to the participant. Throughout the study, each participant's body weight is measured daily to prevent any increase or decrease in weight. If weight does change, energy intake is altered so that the subject returns to the baseline weight. This must be done without altering the intake of the vitamin being studied. Because many of the vitamins we talked about in this chapter help metabolize protein, fat, and/ or carbohydrate, it is important that the body stores of these macronutrients do not change during the metabolic study. This is why monitoring weight and physical activity is so important. At different times during the study, vitamin assessment parameters are measured in the blood, urine, and feces. This may require that the subject collect all urine and feces throughout the study.

For example, let's say you want to determine whether active and sedentary men have different requirements for vitamin B_6. You know that, during physical activity, carbohydrate is burned for fuel and that protein is necessary for the building and repair of muscle tissue. You also know that vitamin B_6 is very important for glucose and protein metabolism; thus, physical activity might increase the body's need for this B-vitamin.

To compare vitamin B_6 requirements, you might design a study as follows. First, you would recruit active young men between the ages of 20 and 35 years (all of equal

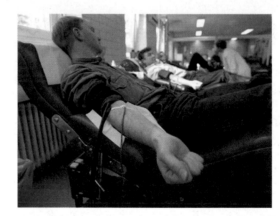

fitness levels and exercising the same number of hours/ week), as well as sedentary males of the same age. You would then feed the participants a succession of three different diets, each lasting 3 weeks, and each providing a different level of vitamin B_6. The diets would consist of the following:

1. Vitamin B_6 below the RDA (1.0 mg/day)
2. Vitamin B_6 at the level of the RDA (1.3 mg/day)
3. Vitamin B_6 above the RDA (1.6 mg/day)

Ideally, you would randomly assign these diets, so that one individual might be fed diet number 1 while another individual is on diet number 2 and another is on diet number 3. By randomly assigning the diets, you ensure that you do not dictate the order in which they are fed. Because you don't want the effect of one diet to carry over to the next diet you are feeding, you would need to include a "washout" period between diets. How long this washout period lasted would depend on the vitamin you were researching, but for our example, 6 weeks should be long enough, because vitamin B_6 is a water-soluble vitamin. During the washout period, all participants would be fed a diet providing the RDA for vitamin B_6 for normal, healthy men.

During the study period, you would need to ensure that the subjects did not eat any foods except what you fed them. In addition, study participants must be monitored to *make sure they eat all the food.* Throughout the study, the amount of vitamin B_6 in the foods would need to be determined via chemical analysis in a lab, as would the amount of vitamin B_6 in the participants' blood, urine, and fecal samples. You would also need to make sure all subjects maintained baseline body weights.

You would then determine the nutritional status of the men when they were on each of the three test diets to determine which diet was able to keep assessment parameters within normal range. You would also compare vitamin status between groups for each of the diets. If the active men had poor status on 1.3 mg/day of vitamin B_6, while the sedentary subjects had adequate status on this level, you would conclude that the RDA was not adequate for the active individuals and they would need more vitamin B_6 to maintain good status.

Third, researchers have conducted cross-sectional studies that compare the nutritional status of trained athletes to sedentary individuals to determine the frequency of poor B-vitamin status in each group. A drawback of cross-sectional studies is that the two groups of people they compare may have other differences besides their fitness level that contribute to their differences in nutritional status. Cross-sectional studies help determine whether differences exist between two groups, but more detailed studies are needed to determine if those differences are due to level of physical activity alone.

Perhaps the ideal study of the effect of physical activity on B-vitamin status would be longitudinal, controlling B-vitamin intake over several months in a study group of athletes, while varying their activity level from low to high. Researchers would then be able to monitor any changes in nutritional status and determine whether these changes affect an individual's ability to perform physical activity. Unfortunately, such studies are difficult and expensive to conduct.

Because of the role B-vitamins play in energy production during exercise, researchers generally assume that individuals with poor B-vitamin status will have a reduced ability to perform physical activity. This hypothesis has been supported in classic studies examining the effect of thiamin, riboflavin, and vitamin B_6 deficiency on work performance.[25,26] For example, a team of Dutch researchers depleted 24 healthy, active men of thiamin, riboflavin, and vitamin B_6 over an 11-week period by feeding them a diet high in unenriched processed foods, such as white bread, white rice, margarine, and soft drinks.[25] This diet provided only 50% of the RDA for thiamin, riboflavin, and vitamin B_6. When they examined the effect of this B-vitamin deficiency on the men's ability to perform physical activity, the researchers found that B-vitamin depletion decreased the ability to perform maximal work by 7% to 12%. Thus, it took only 11 weeks of eating a low-B-vitamin diet before these men were unable to exercise at the same intensity and duration as they had when they were consuming adequate amounts of these vitamins.

Notice that, in the Dutch study, the diet the participants ate was high in unenriched processed foods. In the United States, the Food and Drug Administration mandated the enrichment of foods made with refined grains, such as wheat, corn, and rice, in the 1940s. The micronutrients added back include thiamin, riboflavin, niacin, and iron. Thus, some of the nutrients lost in the milling process are replaced by the enrichment process. Moreover, as mentioned earlier, the enrichment of breads and cereals with folic acid began in 1996.

In addition to a diet high in processed foods, a poor-quality diet overall may fail to provide levels of B-vitamins high enough to support optimal physical activity. In a recent study, researchers observed that providing school children in India with a multivitamin supplement containing B-vitamins improved overall micronutrient status and also significantly improved their aerobic and endurance capacity compared to controls.[27]

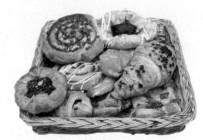

Diets high in processed foods and simple carbohydrates are low in B-vitamins.

RECAP

The hypothesis that individuals with poor B-vitamin status will have a reduced ability to perform physical activity has been supported in studies examining the effect of thiamin, riboflavin, and vitamin B_6 deficiency on work performance. Consuming a diet high in whole grains, fruits, vegetables, and lean meats and dairy will ensure that your body has adequate B-vitamins to fuel physical activity. ∎

Treating Premenstrual Syndrome with Vitamin B$_6$ and Folic Acid: Does It Work? Is It Risky?

Perform an Internet search for treatments for premenstrual syndrome (PMS) and you are likely to find many recommendations for supplementing with magnesium, calcium, vitamin E, folic acid, vitamin B$_6$, and various herbal remedies. Many PMS supplements sold in pharmacy or health food stores contain 50 to 200 mg of vitamin B$_6$ per capsule or tablet and/or 400 µg of folate, with the recommendation that the consumer take at least two capsules per day. As you learned in this chapter, the UL of vitamin B$_6$ is 100 mg/day, and high doses of vitamin B$_6$ over an extended period of time can cause neurologic disorders. The UL for folate is 1,000 µg per day. There is concern that higher doses can mask B$_{12}$ deficiency and contribute to cancer, allergies, and other diseases.[1,2] Is there research to support recommending high levels of folic acid and vitamin B$_6$ for PMS? Do the benefits of supplementing outweigh the risks for adverse effects or toxicity?

What Is PMS?

- PMS is a disorder characterized by a cluster of symptoms triggered by hormonal changes that occur 1 to 2 weeks prior to the start of menstruation. These symptoms typically fall into the two general categories in the following lists, which the American College of Obstetricians and Gynecologists uses in the diagnosis of PMS.[3]

- *Emotional symptoms:* depression, angry outbursts, irritability, crying spells, anxiety, confusion, social withdrawal, poor concentration, insomnia, increased napping, and changes in sexual desire

- *Physical symptoms:* thirst and appetite changes (food cravings), breast tenderness, bloating and weight gain, swelling of hands and feet, abdominal pain, headache, aches and pain, fatigue, skin problems, and gastrointestinal distress

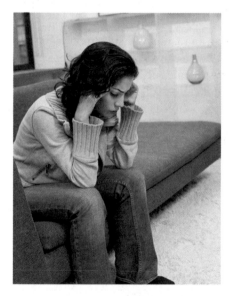

For a woman to be diagnosed with PMS, she typically has to report a pattern of symptoms meeting the following criteria.[3] The pattern must

- be present in the 5 days before her period for at least three menstrual cycles in a row.

- end within 4 days after her period starts.

- interfere with some of her normal activities.

Currently, there is no universally accepted medical treatment for PMS. Not surprisingly, given the diversity of its associated symptoms, a wide variety of clinical and alternative therapies are used:

- *Antidepressants* to help relieve the emotional symptoms of PMS

- *Hormonal contraceptives,* which can stabilize shifts in reproductive hormones

- *Diuretics* to help ease the fluid retention associated with PMS in some women

- *Nonsteroidal anti-inflammatory drugs,* such as ibuprofen or naproxen, to relieve cramping and aches and pain

- *Vitamins,* especially folic acid, vitamin B$_6$, and vitamin E

- *Minerals,* especially calcium and magnesium

- *Amino acid supplements,* such as L-tryptophan

- *Various herbs,* including ginkgo biloba, St. John's wort, ginger, evening primrose oil, and chaste tree fruit[3,4,5,6]

Unfortunately, some of these remedies have the potential for negative health consequences if taken in excess. Here, we discuss vitamin B$_6$ and folic acid.

Adverse Effects of Vitamin B$_6$ Toxicity

The *New England Journal of Medicine* first reported concerns about the use of vitamin B$_6$ for PMS in 1983. Researchers described the development of sensory neuropathy (a disorder affecting the sensory nerves) in seven women, 20 to 43 years of age, taking high doses of pyridoxine, the most common form of vitamin B$_6$ in supplements.[7]

Five of the women began with 50 to 100 mg/day of vitamin B$_6$ before steadily increasing their dose in an attempt to derive a benefit. In one case, a 27-year-old woman began taking 500 mg/day of vitamin B$_6$ to treat premenstrual edema. Over the course of a year, she gradually increased her dose to 5,000 mg/day (5 g/day), which is 50 times higher than the UL for vitamin B$_6$. She reported a tingling sensation in her neck, legs, and feet; numbness in her hands and feet; impaired walking; and impairment in handling small objects. She also noticed changes in the feeling in her lips and tongue. Within 2 months of stopping her supplement, she began to see improvement in her gait and sensation, but it was 7 months before she could walk without a cane. At the time the report was written, the numbness in her legs and hands had still not improved.

A total of four of the seven women became so severely disabled they could not walk or could walk only with a cane. The others experienced less severe symptoms, including "lightning-like" pains in their calves and shins, especially after exercise. Unfortunately, none of the women reported that the supplements had improved their premenstrual edema, made them feel better, or improved their mood, the reasons they gave for taking the supplement in the first place.

In summary, four of the seven women began feeling better within 6 months after stopping supplementation but still had diminished sensory perception. Two of them did not experience recovery until 2 to 3 years after supplementation had stopped.

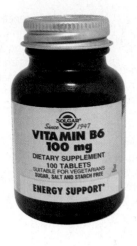

Adverse Effects of High Folic Acid Intake

It has long been recognized that high doses of folic acid can mask vitamin B_{12} deficiency and contribute to neurologic complications; however, there is now evidence that high doses of supplemental folic acid over a period of time may have other adverse health outcomes.[1,2] The amount of folic acid associated with these adverse outcomes varies greatly, ranging from 400 to over 1,000 µg/day. The following are a few of these adverse effects:

- Predisposition to allergies.[8]
- Interference with zinc absorption.
- Promotion of cancer; adequate amounts of folate might protect against cancer, but high doses of supplemental folic acid might stimulate the growth of precancerous or cancerous cells.[9]

Since commercial breads and cereals are fortified with folic acid, some researchers are concerned that women might be getting too much if they take folic acid supplements and consume significant amounts of these fortified foods daily.

Does Research Support the Treatment of PMS with Vitamin B_6 and Folic Acid?

Does a review of the research literature support the use of high doses of folic acid and vitamin B_6 for the treatment of PMS? To date, there have been nine randomized clinical trials testing whether vitamin B_6 supplementation improves PMS symptoms. These nine trials, including 940 subjects, were systematically reviewed by researchers in the United Kingdom to determine if there was enough evidence to recommend using vitamin B_6 as a treatment for PMS.[10,11] Unfortunately, none of the clinical trials met the highest criteria set for research quality. The results show that about half of the studies reported some positive effects of vitamin B_6 supplements on PMS symptoms when compared to the placebo group, but frequently the improvement was only for some of the symptoms. The authors concluded that "there was insufficient evidence of high enough quality to give a confident recommendation for using vitamin B_6 in the treatment of PMS … but results suggest that vitamin B-6 up to 100 mg/d

are likely to be of benefit in treating PMS."[11] A more recent research trial with 94 women found that 80 mg of vitamin B_6 daily for 3 months was associated with a statistically significant reduction in some PMS symptoms.[12] If vitamin B_6 is to have a positive effect on PMS, it needs to be taken daily, not just when symptoms appear.[2]

Research has reported an association between folic acid deficiency and depression,[13] but the research supporting a recommendation of folic acid for PMS treatment is weak. The Office of Women's Health has listed folic acid supplementation (400 µg) as an alternative treatment for PMS,[14] but the American College of Obstetricians and Gynecologists does not make the same recommendation.[3] Currently, there are no studies that have specifically examined the use of folic acid supplementation for the reduction of PMS symptoms.

Researchers have, however, examined whether dietary B-vitamin intake in general is associated with increased or decreased PMS diagnosis.[15] In the Nurses' Health Study II Cohort, at baseline in 1991, all women were PMS free. After 10 years, 1,057 women were confirmed with PMS and 1,968 were confirmed as PMS free. Researchers then examined their B-vitamin intake over this decade to determine if those with higher B-vitamin intake were more or less likely to be diagnosed with PMS. They found no significant associations between the incidence of PMS and dietary intakes of B-vitamins, including vitamin B_6 and folate; neither did they see an association between supplemental B_6 and PMS.

At this time, there does not appear to be strong enough evidence to recommend vitamin B_6 or folic acid supplements for the treatment of PMS, especially in the high doses typically found in PMS supplements. Some of the problems observed when reviewing these studies reveal why the authors could not give definitive recommendations. For example, one study showed that 58% of the individuals taking vitamin B_6 felt better, but so did 59% of the individuals taking the placebo; thus, there were no differences between the groups. Many of the studies showed improvement in only some of the symptoms of PMS, such as anxiety and food cravings but not headaches and depression. Finally, the level of treatment in the studies varied greatly, from 50 to 600 mg/day of vitamin B_6. Thus, although some studies suggest a benefit, the evidence for the efficacy of treating PMS with vitamin B_6 is not convincing and further research is needed.[16,10,11]

Critical Thinking Questions

- Do you think the limited benefits of treating PMS with vitamin B_6 or folic acid outweigh the risks of toxicity or negative health effects?
- What would you do if a friend told you she was taking 100 mg/day of vitamin B_6 for PMS?
- What if she told you she was taking twice that amount and had been doing so for several months?

For more information on the use of vitamins and minerals for PMS, see the National Institutes of Health (NIH) Office of Dietary Supplements in Web Links (page 339).

References

1. Arbor Clinical Nutrition Updates. 2010, December. Can folate supplements be dangerous? Part 2. 327:1–5.
2. Institute of Medicine (IOM), Food and Nutrition Board. 1998. *Dietary reference intakes for thiamin, riboflavin, niacin, vitamin B₆, folate, vitamin B₁₂, pantothenic acid, biotin, and choline*. Washington, DC: National Academy Press.
3. American College of Obstetricians and Gynecologists. 2011. Premenstrual Syndrome Fact Sheet. www.acog.org /Search?Keyword=premenstrual+syndrome (accessed Feb 2015).
4. Mayo Clinic. 2014. Premenstrual Syndrome (PMS). http://www. mayoclinic.org/diseases-conditions/premenstrual-syndrome/basics /alternative-medicine/con-20020003?p=1 (accessed, Feb 2015).
5. Lloyd, K. B., and L. B. Hornsby. 2009. Complementary and alternative medications for women's health issues. *Nutr. Clin. Prac.* 24(5): 589–608. doi: http://dx.doi. org/10.1177/0884533609343001
6. Whalen, A. M., T. M. Jurgen, and H. Naylor. 2009. Herbs, vitamins and minerals in the treatment of premenstrual syndrome: a systemic review. *Can. J. Clin. Pharmacol.* 16(3):e407–429.
7. Schaumburg, H., J. Kaplan, A. Winderbank, N. Vick, S. Rasmus, D. Pleasure, and M. J. Brown. 1983. Sensory neuropathy from pyridoxine abuse: a new megavitamin syndrome. *N. Engl. J. Med.* 309:445–448.
8. Withrow, M. J., V. M. Moore, A. R. Rumbold, and M. J. Davies. 2009. Effect of supplemental folic acid in pregnancy on childhood asthma: a prospective birth cohort study. *Am. J. Epidemiol.* 170(12):1486–1493.
9. Ebbing, M., K. H. Bønaa, O. Nygård, E. Arnesen, P. M. Ueland, Nordrehaug JE,…, and S. E. Vollset. 2009. Cancer incidence and mortality after treatment with folic acid and vitamin B₁₂. *JAMA* 203(19):2119–20026.
10. Canning S., M. Waterman, L. Dye. 2006. Dietary supplements and herbal remedies for premenstrual syndrome (PMS): a systematic research review of the evidence for their efficacy. *J. Reprod. Infant Psychol.* 24(4):363–378.
11. Wyatt, K. M., P. W. Dimmock, P. W. Jones, P. M. Shaughn O'Brien. 1999. Efficacy of vitamin b-6 in the treatment of premenstrual syndrome: systemic review. *Brit. Med. J.* 318 (May 22), 1375–1381.
12. Kashanian, M., R. Mazinani, and S. Jalalmanesh. 2007. Pyridoxine (vitamin B₆) therapy for premenstrual syndrome. *Int. J. Gynaecol. Obstet.* 96:43–44.
13. Cho, Y. J., J. Y. Han, J. S. Choi, H. K. Ahn, H. M. Ryu, M. M. Y. Kim, J. H. Yang, A. A. Nava-Ocampo, and G. Koren. 2008. Prenatal multivitamins containing folic acid do not decrease prevalence of depression among pregnant women. *J. Obstet. Gynaecol.* 28(5):482–484.
14. Department of Health and Human Services (DHHS), Office of Women's Health. 2014. Premenstrual syndrome fact sheet. http://www.womenshealth.gov/publications/our-publications /fact-sheet/premenstrual-syndrome.html (accessed Feb 2015).
15. Chocano-Bedoya, P. O., J. E. Manson, S. E. Hankinson, W. C. Willett, S. R. Johnson, L. Chasan-Taber, A. G. Ronnenberg, C. Bigelow, and E. R. Berthone-Johnson. 2011. Dietary B-vitamin intake and incident premenstrual syndrome. *Am. J. Clin. Nutri.* 93(5):1080–1086.
16. Rapkin, A. 2003. The review of treatment of premenstrual syndrome & premenstrual dysphoric disorder. *Psychoneuroendocrinology* 28:39–53.

STUDY **PLAN**   MasteringNutrition™

Customize your study plan—and master your nutrition!—the Study Area of MasteringNutrition.

TEST YOURSELF | ANSWERS

1 **F** B-vitamins do not directly provide energy. However, they play critical roles in ensuring that the body is able to generate energy from carbohydrates, fats, and proteins.

2 **T** A severe niacin deficiency can cause pellagra, which once killed thousands of people in the United States alone each year; and thiamin deficiency causes beriberi, which can result in heart failure.

3 **F** The IOM has set ULs for both niacin and vitamin B₆. High intakes of these nutrients can cause adverse effects.

4 **F** Research studies have failed to show any consistent effects of chromium supplements on reducing body fat or enhancing muscle mass.

5 **F** Not necessarily! Although much of the salt sold in the United States is iodized, you need to read the label carefully. Some brands of table salt, kosher salt, sea salt, and other specialty salts do not provide iodine.

summary

Scan to hear an MP3 Chapter Review in **MasteringNutrition**.

LO 1
- The B-vitamins include thiamin, riboflavin, vitamin B$_6$, niacin, folate, vitamin B$_{12}$, pantothenic acid, and biotin.
- The B-vitamins act as coenzymes. In this role, they activate enzymes and assist them in the metabolism of carbohydrates, fats, amino acids, and alcohol for energy; the synthesis of fatty acids and cholesterol; and gluconeogenesis.
- Food sources of the B-vitamins include whole grains, enriched breads, ready-to-eat cereals, meats, dairy products, and some fruits and vegetables.

LO 2
- The body converts dietary thiamin to its coenzyme thiamin pyrophosphate, or TPP, which is important in the metabolism of glucose and the branched-chain amino acids.
- Riboflavin is a component of two coenzymes involved in carbohydrate, fatty acid, and amino acid metabolism: flavin mononucleotide (FMN) and flavin adenine dinucleotide (FAD).
- Niacin is essential for the formation of two coenzymes involved in carbohydrate, fatty acid, and amino acid metabolism: nicotinamide adenine dinucleotide (NAD) and nicotinamide adenine dinucleotide phosphate (NADP).

LO 3
- A deficiency of thiamin can cause beriberi, riboflavin deficiency can cause ariboflavinosis, and a deficiency of niacin can cause pellagra.

LO 4
- Vitamin B$_6$ plays a critical role in transamination; without adequate B$_6$, all amino acids become essential. It is also important for carbohydrate metabolism, neurotransmitter and heme synthesis, and immune function.
- Folate is important for amino acid metabolism, DNA synthesis, and cell division as well as blood health.
- Vitamin B$_{12}$ is important for homocysteine metabolism, blood health and maintenance of the myelin sheath that coats nerve fibers. Its intestinal absorption requires adequate secretion of intrinsic factor in the stomach. It is found exclusively in animal-based foods and fortified foods.

LO 5
- Inadequate intakes of vitamin B$_6$, folate, and vitamin B$_{12}$ are associated with elevated blood levels of the amino acid homocysteine. This, in turn, is associated with an increased risk for cardiovascular disease.

LO 6
- Folate assists in cell division, and deficiency in the early weeks of pregnancy significantly increases the risk of having a baby with a neural tube defect, a central nervous system malformation.

LO 7
- The B-vitamins pantothenic acid and biotin assist in the metabolism of carbohydrates, fats and protein. Both are widely available in foods.
- Choline is a vitamin-like substance that assists with homocysteine metabolism and is a component of phosphatidylcholine found in bile. Choline also accelerates the synthesis and release of acetylcholine, a neurotransmitter.

LO 8
- Iodine is a trace mineral needed for the synthesis of thyroid hormones. Thyroid hormones are integral to the regulation of body temperature, the maintenance of resting metabolic rate, and healthy reproduction and growth.
- Chromium is a trace mineral that enhances the ability of insulin to transport glucose from the bloodstream into the cell. Chromium is also necessary for the metabolism of RNA and DNA, and it supports normal growth and immune function.
- Manganese is a trace mineral that acts as a cofactor in energy metabolism and the formation of urea.
- Sulfur is a major mineral that is a component of thiamin and biotin and the amino acids methionine and cysteine.

LO 9
- Iodine deficiency or toxicity can lead to the development of a goiter. Iodine-deficiency disorders include a form of mental impairment called cretinism, decreased fertility, hypothyroidism, growth and developmental disorders, and others.

LO 10
- Inadequate levels of the B-vitamins can reduce an individual's ability to perform physical activity. A diet high in whole grains, fruits and vegetables, lean meats, and dairy typically provides adequate levels of the B-vitamins.

review questions

LO 1 **1.** The B-vitamins

    a. act as enzymes essential for energy metabolism.

    b. act as coenzymes to promote energy metabolism.

    c. act as energy-yielding micronutrients.

    d. are essential to the synthesis of thyroid hormones and the regulation of metabolic rate.

LO 2 **2.** Vitamins required for the oxidation-reduction reactions involved in the catabolism of carbohydrates, fats, and proteins for energy include

    a. thiamin and riboflavin, but not niacin.

    b. thiamin and niacin, but not riboflavin.

    c. riboflavin and niacin, but not thiamin.

    d. thiamin, riboflavin, and niacin.

LO 3 **3.** Niacin-deficiency disease is called

    a. flushing.

    b. marasmus.

    c. pellagra.

    d. beriberi.

LO 4 **4.** A coenzyme assisting in the breakdown of stored glycogen to glucose and in the conversion of amino acids to glucose is

    a. vitamin B_6.

    b. folate.

    c. vitamin B_{12}.

    d. vitamin B_6, folate, and vitamin B_{12}.

LO 5 **5.** High blood levels of the amino acid homocysteine are associated with

    a. high blood levels of the amino acid methionine.

    b. vitamin B_6, folate, and vitamin B_{12} toxicity.

    c. an increased risk for cardiovascular disease.

    d. an increased risk for neural tube defects.

LO 6 **6.** Adequate folate intake is essential during early pregnancy because

    a. folate deficiency masks a simultaneous vitamin B_{12} deficiency.

    b. folate is critical for cell division.

    c. maternal folate deficiency increases the risk of cretinism.

    d. folate helps maintain the myelin sheath coating nerve fibers.

LO 7 **7.** Which of the following statements about choline is true?

    a. Choline is found exclusively in foods of animal origin.

    b. Choline is a B-vitamin that assists in carbohydrate metabolism.

    c. Choline is a neurotransmitter that is involved in muscle movement and memory storage.

    d. Choline is a vitamin-like compound necessary for homocysteine metabolism and the synthesis of bile.

LO 8 **8.** A trace mineral that plays an important role in carbohydrate metabolism, glucose transport into cells, RNA and DNA metabolism, immune function, and growth is

    a. iodine.

    b. chromium.

    c. manganese.

    d. sulfur.

LO 9 **9.** According to the World Health Organization (WHO), the greatest single cause of preventable brain damage and mental retardation in the world is

    a. iodine deficiency.

    b. chromium deficiency.

    c. manganese deficiency.

    d. sulfur deficiency.

LO 10 **10.** Research has consistently shown that individuals with poor B-vitamin status

    a. have a reduced ability to perform physical activity involving intense bursts of energy, such as sprinting, but not endurance activity, such as running.

    b. have a reduced ability to perform endurance activity, such as running, but not physical activity involving intense bursts of energy, such as sprinting.

    c. have a reduced ability to perform most types of physical activity.

    d. have a greatly increased risk of musculoskeletal injury with physical activity.

true or false?

LO 3 **11. True or false?** Wernicke–Korsakoff syndrome is a thiamin deficiency related to chronic alcohol abuse.

    12. True or false? In the United States, milk is fortified with riboflavin to prevent macrocytic anemia.

LO 7 **13. True or false?** Biotin is a B-vitamin involved in carbohydrate, fat, and protein metabolism.

LO 8 **14. True or false?** Iodine is necessary for the synthesis of reproductive hormones.

    15. True or false? There is no DRI for sulfur.

short answer

LO 3 **16.** Your great-aunt is on renal dialysis. Explain the implications, if any, for her B-vitamin status.

LO 4 **17.** Explain the statement that, without vitamin B_6, all amino acids become essential.

18. In the chapter-opening story, Mr. Katz was given an injection of vitamin B_{12}. Why didn't his physician simply give him the vitamin in pill form?

LO 9 **19.** Would you expect goiter to be more common in coastal regions or inland? Explain your answer.

LO 10 **20.** Identify three types of studies researchers have performed to explore the effect of B-vitamin intake on physical activity.

math review

LO 4 **21.** Calculate the DFE in the diet of an individual who consumes the following:

- Food folate = 70 μg/day; synthetic folic acid from fortified foods = 224 μg/day

How many DFE is this person getting per day? What percentage of this person's total DFE is coming from synthetic versus food folate?

Answers to Review Questions and Math Review can be found online in the MasteringNutrition Study Area and in the back of the book.

web links

www.ars.usda.gov
Nutrient Data Laboratory Home Page
Click on "Reports for Single Nutrients" to find reports listing food sources for selected nutrients.

www.unicef.org/nutrition/
UNICEF: Nutrition
This site provides information about micronutrient deficiencies in developing countries and UNICEF's efforts and programs to combat them.

www.euro.who.int/en/home
World Health Organization (WHO)
This site provides information on nutrient deficiencies throughout the world, including iodine-deficiency disorders (IDDs).

www.ods.od.nih.gov
National Institutes of Health (NIH) Office of Dietary Supplements
This site provides information on vitamins and minerals, the safe use of supplements, and the research available on the treatment of health problems and disease with various supplements.

www.lpi.oregonstate.edu
Linus Pauling Institute at Oregon State University
This site provides accurate and current information on vitamins, minerals, and phytochemicals that promote health and prevent disease. Search for information on a micronutrient using the micronutrient information center.

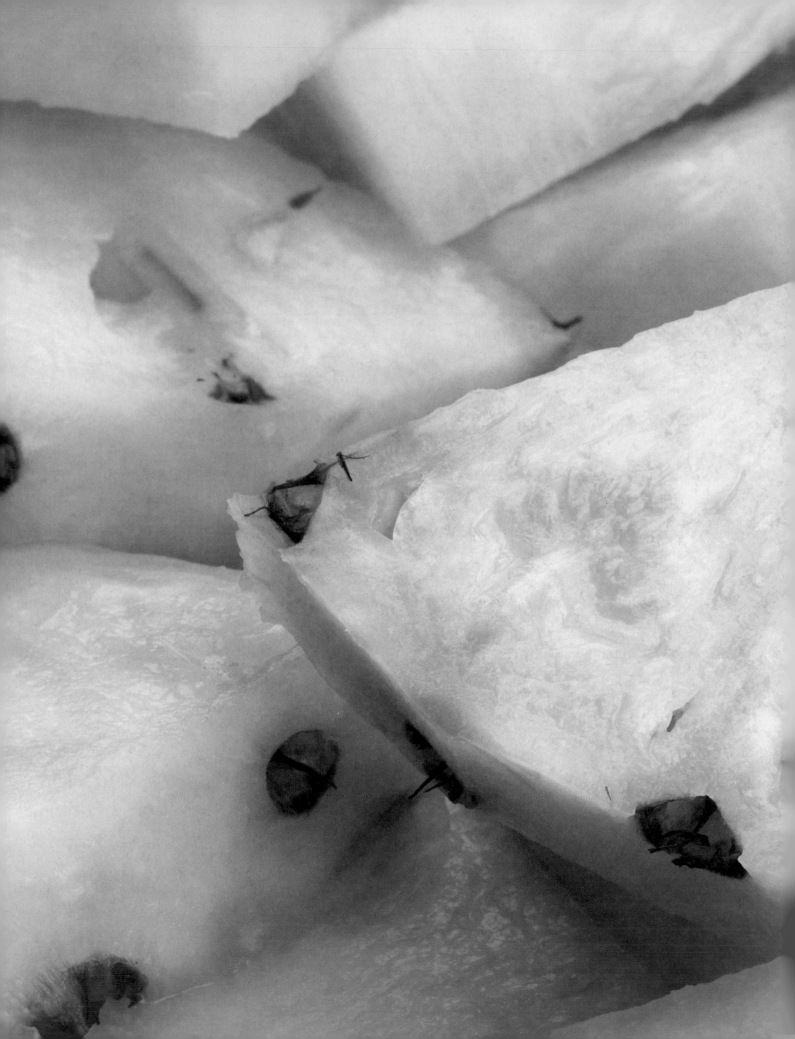

9 Nutrients Involved in Fluid and Electrolyte Balance

Learning Outcomes

After studying this chapter, you should be able to:

1 Distinguish among extracellular fluid, intracellular fluid, interstitial fluid, and intravascular fluid, *pp. 342–344.*

2 Identify the critical contributions of water and electrolytes to human functioning, *pp. 344–349.*

3 Explain how the kidneys regulate blood pressure and blood volume, *pp. 344–345.*

4 Discuss the avenues of fluid intake and excretion in the body, *pp. 350–352.*

5 Explain how the body maintains acid–base balance, *pp. 352–353.*

6 Identify the DRIs for water and compare the nutritional quality of several common beverages, *pp. 354–358.*

7 Identify the functions, DRIs, and common dietary sources of sodium, potassium, chloride, and phosphorus, *pp. 359–365.*

8 Distinguish between *hypernatremia* and *hyponatremia* and identify factors that can cause these conditions, *pp. 360–361.*

9 Describe several disorders related to fluid and electrolyte imbalance and identify their signs and symptoms, *pp. 365–371.*

10 Define *hypertension* and list three lifestyle changes that can reduce it, *pp. 367–368.*

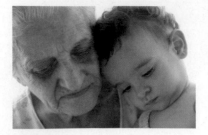

As we age, our body water content decreases: approximately 75% of an infant's body weight is composed of water, whereas an elderly adult's is only 50% or less.

I n 2011, a 14-year-old died of cardiac arrest after consuming a 24-ounce can of a popular energy drink. An autopsy revealed that caffeine toxicity had caused the death. In 2012, a 19-year-old went into cardiac arrest and died after consuming 32 ounces of the same energy drink. In 2013, the U.S. Food and Drug Administration (FDA) released records of nearly 150 adverse events between 2004 and 2012 that were linked to energy drinks. The reports included incidents of vomiting, difficulty breathing, seizures, cardiac arrests, miscarriages, and at least 18 deaths.[1]

All beverages provide water, the body's most basic nutrient. But some beverages provide other healthful nutrients, such as protein, vitamin C, or calcium, whereas still others, like drinks loaded with caffeine and added sugars, can be harmful. In this chapter, we explore the role of water and four major minerals—sodium, potassium, chloride, and phosphorus—known as electrolytes in maintaining the body's fluid balance and neuromuscular function. We also review the health benefits and drawbacks of some popular beverages, including energy drinks. Finally, we explain how blood pressure is maintained and take a look at some disorders that occur when fluids and electrolytes are out of balance.

LO 1 Distinguish among extracellular fluid, intracellular fluid, interstitial fluid, and intravascular fluid.

What Is Body Fluid?

You know, of course, that orange juice, blood, and shampoo are all fluids, but what makes them so? A **fluid** is a substance characterized by its ability to move freely and changeably, adapting to the shape of the container that holds it. This may not seem very important, but as you'll learn in this chapter, the fluid composition of cells and tissues is critical to the body's ability to function.

Body Fluid Is the Liquid Portion of Cells and Tissues

Between about 50% and 70% of a healthy adult's body weight is fluid. When we cut a finger, we can see some of this fluid dripping out as blood, but the fluid in the bloodstream can't account for such a large percentage of one's total body weight. So where is all this fluid hiding?

About two-thirds of the body's fluid is held within the walls of cells and is therefore called **intracellular fluid** (**Figure 9.1a**). Every cell in the body contains fluid. When cells lose their fluid, they quickly shrink and die. On the other hand, when cells take in too much fluid, they swell and burst apart. This is why appropriate fluid balance—which we'll discuss throughout this chapter—is so critical to life.

The remaining third of the body's fluid is referred to as **extracellular fluid** because it flows outside of the cells (see Figure 9.1a). There are two types of extracellular fluid:

1. **Interstitial fluid** flows between the cells that make up a particular tissue or organ, such as muscle fibers or the liver (Figure 9.1b).
2. **Intravascular fluid** is the fluid in the bloodstream and lymph. *Plasma* is specifically the extracellular fluid portion of blood that transports blood cells within the body's arteries, veins, and capillaries (Figure 9.1c).

Not every tissue in the body contains the same amount of fluid. Lean tissues, such as muscle, are more than 70% fluid, whereas fat tissue is between only 10% and 20% fluid. This is not surprising, considering the hydrophobic nature of lipid cells.

Body fluid levels also vary according to gender and age. Males have more lean tissue than females and thus a higher percentage of body weight as fluid. The amount of body fluid as a percentage of total weight decreases with age. About 75% of an infant's body weight is fluid, whereas the total body fluid of an elderly person is generally less than 50% of body weight. This decrease in total body fluid is, in part, a result of the loss of lean tissue that commonly occurs as people age.

fluid A substance composed of molecules that move past one another freely. Fluids are characterized by their ability to conform to the shape of whatever container holds them.

intracellular fluid The fluid held at any given time within the walls of the body's cells.

extracellular fluid The fluid outside of the body's cells, either in the body's tissues (interstitial fluid) or as the liquid portion of the blood or lymph (intravascular fluid).

interstitial fluid The fluid that flows between the cells that make up a particular tissue or organ, such as muscle fibers or the liver.

intravascular fluid The fluid in the bloodstream and lymph.

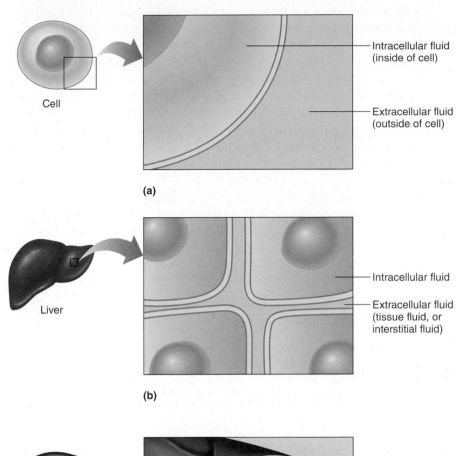

(a)

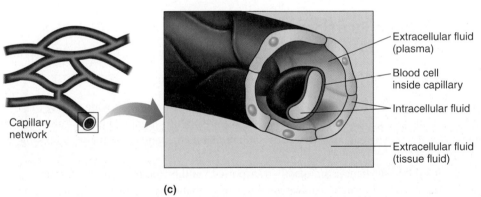

(b)

(c)

FIGURE 9.1 The components of body fluid. **(a)** Intracellular fluid is contained within the cells that make up our body tissues. Extracellular fluid is external to cells. **(b)** Interstitial fluid is external to tissue cells, and **(c)** plasma is external to blood cells.

Body Fluid Is Composed of Water and Dissolved Substances Called Electrolytes

Water is made up of molecules consisting of two hydrogen atoms bound to one oxygen atom (H_2O). Although water is essential to maintain life, we would quickly die if our cell and tissue fluids contained only water. Instead, within the body fluids are a variety of dissolved substances (called *solutes*) critical to life. These include six major minerals: sodium, potassium, chloride, phosphorus, calcium, and magnesium. We consume these minerals in compounds called *salts*, including table salt, which is made of sodium and chloride.

Mineral salts are called **electrolytes,** because when they dissolve in water, the two component minerals separate into electrically charged **ions,** which are themselves commonly referred to as electrolytes. An ion's electrical charge, which can be positive or negative, is the "spark" that stimulates nerves and causes muscles to contract, making electrolytes critical to body function.

electrolyte A compound that disassociates in solution into positively and negatively charged ions and is thus capable of conducting an electrical current; the ions in such a solution.

ion Any electrically charged particle, either positively or negatively charged.

Of the six major minerals just mentioned, four will be discussed in this chapter: sodium, potassium, chloride, and phosphorus. Because they play critical roles in bone health, calcium and magnesium will be discussed in Chapter 11. The ionic forms of sodium (Na^+) and potassium (K^+) are positively charged; that is, they are cations. In contrast, chloride (Cl^-) and phosphorus (in the form of hydrogen phosphate, or HPO_4^{2-}) are negatively charged; they are anions. In the intracellular fluid, potassium and phosphate are the predominant ions. In the extracellular fluid, sodium and chloride predominate. There is a slight difference in electrical charge on either side of the cell's membrane that is needed in order for the cell to perform its normal functions.

RECAP

Between 50% and 70% of an average healthy adult's weight is body fluid, the liquid portion of our cells and tissues. Body fluid consists of intracellular fluid—the fluid within cells—and extracellular fluid, which is beyond cell membranes. Extracellular fluid includes interstitial fluid, also called tissue fluid, and intravascular fluid flowing within blood and lymphatic vessels. Body fluid consists of water and many dissolved solutes, including ions of sodium, potassium, chloride, and phosphorus, which are called electrolytes. ■

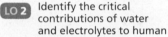

LO 2 Identify the critical contributions of water and electrolytes to human functioning.

LO 3 Explain how the kidneys regulate blood pressure and blood volume.

What Are the Functions of Water and Electrolytes?

The functions of water and electrolytes are interrelated and their levels in the body delicately balanced.

Water Performs Functions Critical to Life

Water not only quenches our thirst; it performs a number of functions that are critical to life.

Solubility and Transport

Water is an excellent **solvent,** which means it is capable of dissolving a wide variety of substances, including amino acids, glucose, the water-soluble vitamins, mineral salts, and some medications. The chemical reactions upon which life depends would not be possible without water.

Water-soluble substances are readily transported via the bloodstream. In contrast, lipids do not dissolve in water. To overcome this incompatibility, lipids and the fat-soluble vitamins are either attached to or surrounded by water-soluble proteins, so that they, too, can be transported in the blood to the cells.

Blood Volume and Blood Pressure

Blood volume is the amount of fluid in blood; thus, appropriate body fluid levels are essential to maintaining healthful blood volume. When blood volume rises inappropriately, blood pressure increases; when blood volume decreases inappropriately, blood pressure decreases. As you know, hypertension (high blood pressure) is an important risk factor for heart disease and stroke, whereas low blood pressure can cause people to feel tired, confused, or dizzy. We discuss hypertension later in this chapter.

The kidneys play a central role in the regulation of blood volume and blood pressure. While filtering the blood, they reabsorb (retain) water and other nutrients that the body needs and excrete waste products and excess water in the urine. Changes in blood volume, blood pressure, and concentration of solutes in the blood signal the kidneys to adjust the volume and concentration of urine.

Imagine that you have just finished working out for an hour, during which time you did not drink any fluids but you lost fluid through sweat. In response to the increased concentration of solutes in your blood, **antidiuretic hormone (ADH)** is released from the

For an informative video on blood pressure, visit www .nlm.nih.gov and type in "blood pressure" into the search box to begin!

solvent A substance that is capable of mixing with and breaking apart a variety of compounds. Water is an excellent solvent.

blood volume The amount of fluid in blood.

antidiuretic hormone (ADH) A hormone released from the pituitary gland in response to an increase in blood solute concentration. ADH stimulates the kidneys to reabsorb water and to reduce the production of urine.

pituitary gland (**Figure 9.2**). The action of ADH is appropriately described by its name: a **diuretic** is a substance that increases fluid loss via the urine. ADH has an antidiuretic effect, stimulating the kidneys to reabsorb water and to reduce the production of urine.

Simultaneously, your loss of fluids has reduced your blood volume. As shown on the right side of Figure 9.2, this drop in blood volume has resulted in a decrease in blood pressure. Pressure receptors in the kidney sense this reduced blood pressure, and signal the kidney to secrete the enzyme **renin.** Renin then catalyzes the conversion of a blood protein called angiotensinogen, which is produced in the liver, to another blood protein, angiotensin. Angiotensinogen is the precursor of Angiotensin I. Angiotensin I is converted to **angiotensin II,** which is a powerful vasoconstrictor; this means it works to constrict the diameter of blood vessels, which results in an increase in blood pressure.

Angiotensin II also signals the release of the hormone **aldosterone** from the adrenal glands located on top of the kidneys. Aldosterone signals the kidneys to retain sodium and chloride. Because water travels with the ionic form of these two minerals, this results in water retention, which increases blood pressure and decreases urine output. These responses help regulate fluid balance and blood pressure.

diuretic A substance that increases fluid loss via the urine. Common diuretics include alcohol and prescription medications for high blood pressure and other disorders.

renin An enzyme secreted by the kidneys in response to a decrease in blood pressure. Renin converts the blood protein angiotensinogen to angiotensin I, which eventually results in an increase in sodium reabsorption.

angiotensin II A potent vasoconstrictor that constricts the diameter of blood vessels and increases blood pressure; it also signals the release of the hormone aldosterone from the adrenal glands.

aldosterone A hormone released from the adrenal glands that signals the kidneys to retain sodium and chloride, which in turn results in the retention of water.

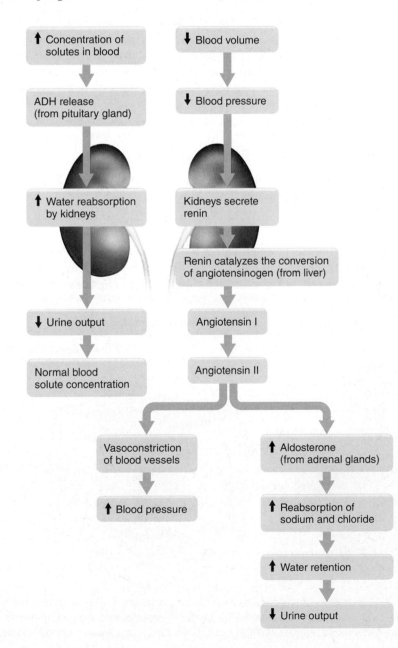

FIGURE 9.2 Regulation of blood volume and blood pressure by the kidneys.

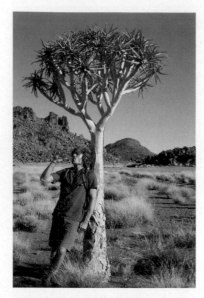

To prevent heat-related illness, a hiker needs to adjust his or her fluid intake according to the humidity level and temperature of the environment.

Would the proteins in your body tissues "cook" at the same temperature that would fry an egg? For a short, fun video from NPR on the experiment that answered this question, go to **www.npr.org**, and type in the search box **"How Much Heat Can You Take."**

Body Temperature

Just as overheating is disastrous to a car engine, a high internal temperature can cause the body to stop functioning. Fluids are vital to the body's ability to maintain its temperature within a safe range. Two factors account for the cooling power of fluids. First, water has a high capacity for heat: it takes a lot of energy to raise its temperature. Because the body contains a lot of water, only sustained high heat can increase body temperature.

Second, body fluids are our primary coolant. When heat needs to be released from the body, there is an increase in the flow of blood from the warm body core to the vessels lying just under the skin. This action transports heat out to the body periphery, where it can be released from the skin. When we are hot, the sweat glands secrete more sweat from the skin. As this sweat evaporates off of the skin's surface, heat is released into the environment. As a result, the skin and underlying blood are cooled. This process, called *evaporative cooling*, is illustrated in **Figure 9.3**. This cooler blood flows back to the body's core and reduces internal body temperature.

Tissue Protection and Lubrication

Water is a major part of the fluids that protect and lubricate tissues. The cerebrospinal fluid that surrounds the brain and spinal column protects these vital tissues from damage, and a fetus in a mother's womb is protected by amniotic fluid. Synovial fluid lubricates joints, and tears cleanse and lubricate the eyes. Saliva moistens the food we eat, the water in gastric juice dilutes the food to make chyme, and the mucus lining the walls of the intestine helps the chyme move smoothly along. Finally, the pleural fluid covering the lungs allows their friction-free expansion and retraction behind the chest wall.

Electrolytes Support Many Body Functions

Now that you know why fluid is essential to the body's functioning, we're ready to explore three critical roles of the minerals within it.

Osmotic Pressure

Cell membranes are *permeable* to water. This means that water flows easily through them. Cells cannot voluntarily regulate this flow of water and thus have no active control over the balance of fluid between the intracellular and extracellular compartments. In contrast,

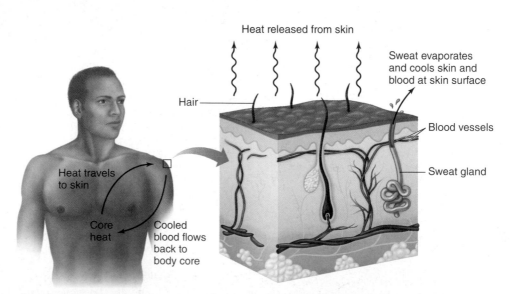

FIGURE 9.3 Evaporative cooling occurs when heat is transported from the body core through the bloodstream to the surface of the skin. The water evaporates into the air and carries away heat. This cools the blood, which circulates back to the body core, reducing body temperature.

cell membranes are *not* freely permeable to electrolytes. Sodium, potassium, and the other electrolytes stay where they are, either inside or outside of a cell, unless they are actively transported elsewhere by special proteins. So how do electrolytes help the cells maintain their fluid balance? To answer this question, we need to review a bit of chemistry.

Imagine that you have a special filter that has the same properties as cell membranes; in other words, this filter is freely permeable to water but not permeable to electrolytes. Now imagine that you insert this filter into a glass of dilute salt water to divide the glass into two chambers (**Figure 9.4a**). The water levels on both sides of the filter would, of course, be identical, because it is freely permeable to water. Now imagine that you add a full teaspoon of salt to the water on one side of the filter only (Figure 9.4b). In solution, the salt would immediately dissociate into sodium and chloride ions. You would therefore see the water on the "dilute salt water" side of the glass suddenly begin to flow through the filter to the "concentrated salt water" side of the glass (Figure 9.4c). Why would this mysterious movement of water occur? The answer is that water always moves from areas where solutes, such as sodium and chloride, are in low concentrations to areas where they are highly concentrated. This movement is referred to as **osmosis.** To put it another way, electrolytes attract water toward areas where they are concentrated. This movement of water toward solutes continues until the concentration of solutes is equal on both sides of the cell membrane.

Water follows the movement of electrolytes; this action provides a means to control movement of water into and out of the cells. The pressure that is needed to keep the particles in a solution from drawing liquid toward them across a semipermeable membrane is referred to as **osmotic pressure.** Cells can regulate the osmotic pressure, and thus the balance of fluids between their internal and extracellular environments, by using special transport proteins to actively pump electrolytes across their membranes. (For an example of how transport proteins pump sodium and potassium across the cell membrane, see Chapter 6, Figure 6.13.)

By maintaining the appropriate movement of electrolytes into and out of the cell, the body maintains a healthful balance of fluid and electrolytes between the intracellular and

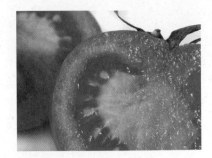

By sprinkling salt on a slice of tomato, you can see for yourself the effects of osmotic pressure.

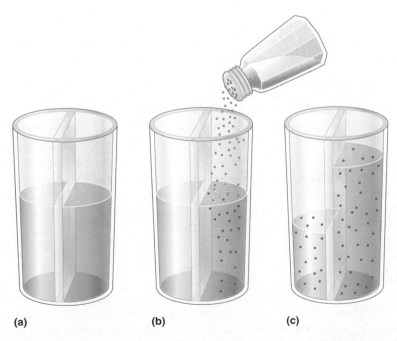

(a)   (b)   (c)

FIGURE 9.4 Osmosis. **(a)** A filter that is freely permeable to water only is placed in a glass of dilute salt water. **(b)** Additional salt is added to only one side of the glass. **(c)** Drawn by the high concentration of electrolytes, water flows to the "concentrated salt water" side of the filter. This flow of water into the concentrated solution will continue until the concentration of electrolytes on both sides of the membrane is equal.

osmosis The movement of water (or any solvent) through a semipermeable membrane from an area where solutes are less concentrated to areas where they are highly concentrated.

osmotic pressure The pressure that is needed to keep the particles in a solution from drawing liquid toward them across a semipermeable membrane.

extracellular compartments. If the concentration of electrolytes is much higher inside of the cells as compared with outside, water will flow into the cells in such large amounts that the cells can burst. On the other hand, if the extracellular environment contains too high a concentration of electrolytes, water flows out of the cells, and they can dry up. **Focus Figure 9.5** provides an illustration of how an imbalance between fluids and electrolyte intake during strenuous exercise affects the body. When you exercise, what and how much you should drink depend on multiple factors, including how strenuous your session is, how long it lasts, and how warm or humid the environment is.

Certain illnesses can threaten the delicate balance of fluid inside and outside of the cells. You may have heard of someone being hospitalized because of excessive diarrhea or vomiting. When this happens, the body loses a great deal of fluid from the intestinal tract and extracellular compartment. This causes the loss of both water and electrolytes. In some cases, the relative loss of water is greater than the loss of electrolytes, and the body's extracellular electrolyte concentration then becomes very high. In response, a great deal of intracellular fluid leaves the cells to try to balance the high electrolyte concentration in the extracellular fluid. These imbalances in fluid and electrolytes change the flow of electrical impulses through the heart, causing an irregular heart rate that can be fatal if left untreated. Food poisoning and eating disorders involving repeated vomiting and diarrhea can also result in death from life-threatening fluid and electrolyte imbalances, including disorders that create an excessive loss of electrolytes versus an excessive loss of fluid.

Nerve Impulse Conduction

In addition to their role in maintaining fluid balance, electrolytes are critical in enabling nerves to respond to stimuli. Nerve impulses are initiated at the membrane of a nerve cell in response to a change in the degree of electrical charge across the membrane. An influx of sodium into a nerve cell causes the cell to become slightly less negatively charged. This is called *depolarization* (**Figure 9.6**, page 350). If enough sodium enters the cell, the change in electrical charge triggers an *action potential,* an electrical signal that is then propagated along the length of the cell. Once the signal is transmitted, that portion of cell membrane returns to its normal electrical state through the release of potassium to the outside of the cell. This return of the cell to its initial electrical state is termed *repolarization.* Thus, both sodium and potassium play critical roles in ensuring that nerve impulses are generated, transmitted, and completed.

Muscle Contraction

Muscles contract because of a series of complex physiologic changes that we will not describe in detail here. Simply stated, muscles are stimulated to contract in response to stimulation of nerve cells. As described earlier, sodium and potassium play a key role in the generation of nerve impulses, or electrical signals. When a muscle fiber is stimulated by an electrical signal, changes occur that lead to an increased flow of calcium ions from their storage site in the sarcoplasmic reticulum. This release of calcium ions stimulates muscle contraction. The muscles can relax after a contraction once the electrical signal is complete and calcium has been pumped back into its storage site.

RECAP

Water serves many important functions, including dissolving and transporting substances, and contributing to blood volume and blood pressure. The kidneys help regulate blood volume and blood pressure by altering their excretion in urine or their reabsorption into blood of water and solutes, including electrolytes. Water also plays a key role in maintaining body temperature, and in cushioning and lubricating body tissues. Electrolytes help regulate fluid balance by controlling the movement of fluid into and out of cells. Electrolytes, specifically sodium and potassium, play a key role in generating nerve impulses in response to stimuli. Calcium is an electrolyte important in muscle contraction.

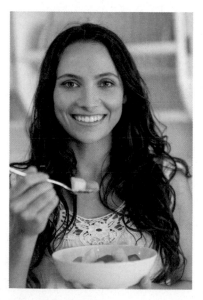

Fruits and vegetables are delicious sources of dietary water.

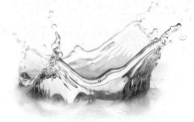

The health of our body's cells depends on maintaining the proper balance of fluids and electrolytes on both sides of the cell membrane, both at rest and during exercise. Let's examine how this balance can be altered under various conditions of exercise and fluid intake.

MODERATE EXERCISE

When you are appropriately hydrated, engaged in moderate exercise, and not too hot, the concentration of electrolytes is likely to be the same on both sides of cell membranes. You will be in fluid balance.

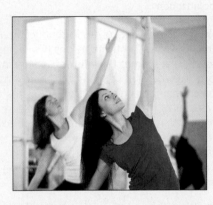

Concentration of electrolytes about equal inside and outside cell

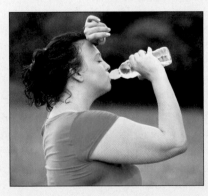

STRENUOUS EXERCISE WITH RAPID AND HIGH WATER INTAKE

If a person drinks a great deal of water quickly during intense, prolonged exercise, the extracellular fluid becomes diluted. This results in the concentration of electrolytes being greater inside the cells, which causes water to enter the cells, making them swell. Drinking moderate amounts of water or sports drinks more slowly will replace lost fluids and restore fluid balance.

Lower concentration of electrolytes outside

H_2O

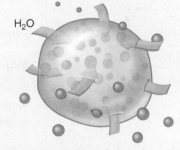

Higher concentration of electrolytes inside

STRENUOUS EXERCISE WITH INADEQUATE FLUID INTAKE

If a person does not consume adequate amounts of fluid during strenuous exercise of long duration, the concentration of electrolytes becomes greater outside the cells, drawing water away from the inside of the cells and making them shrink. Consuming sports drinks will replace lost fluids and electrolytes.

Higher concentration of electrolytes outside

H_2O

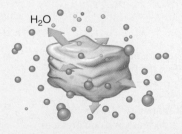

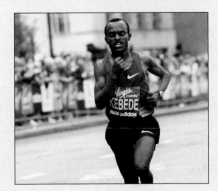

Lower concentration of electrolytes inside

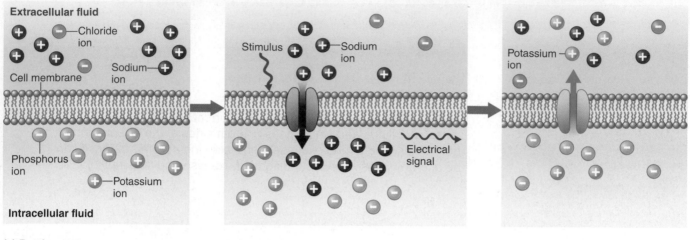

(a) Resting state

(b) Depolarization

(c) Repolarization

FIGURE 9.6 The role of electrolytes in conduction of a nerve impulse. **(a)** In the resting state, the intracellular fluid has slightly more ions with a negative charge. **(b)** A stimulus causes changes to occur that prompt the influx of sodium into the interior of the cell. Sodium has a positive charge, so when this happens, the charge inside the cell becomes slightly positive. This is called depolarization. If enough sodium enters the cell, an action potential is transmitted to adjacent regions of the cell membrane. **(c)** Release of potassium to the exterior of the cell allows the first portion of the membrane to return to the resting state almost immediately. This is called repolarization.

LO 4 Discuss the avenues of fluid intake and excretion in the body.

How Does the Body Maintain Fluid Balance?

The proper balance of fluid is maintained in the body by a series of mechanisms that prompt us to drink and retain fluid when we are dehydrated and to excrete fluid as urine when we consume more than we need.

We Gain Fluids through Consumption and Metabolism

You obtain the fluid you need each day from two primary sources. As much as 90% of your body's requirement for fluid must be obtained from the consumption of beverages and foods. The remainder is metabolic water produced by body cells.

Imagine that, at lunch, you ate a ham sandwich and a bag of salted potato chips. Now it's almost time for your afternoon seminar to end and you are very thirsty. When the instructor dismisses class, you dash to the nearest drinking fountain. What prompted you to suddenly feel so thirsty?

The body's command center for fluid intake is a cluster of nerve cells in the same part of the brain we studied in relation to food intake; that is, the *hypothalamus*. Within the hypothalamus is a group of cells, collectively referred to as the **thirst mechanism,** that causes us to consciously desire fluids. The thirst mechanism prompts us to feel thirsty when it is stimulated by the following:

thirst mechanism A cluster of nerve cells in the hypothalamus that stimulates our conscious desire to drink fluids in response to an increase in the concentration of salt in our blood or a decrease in blood pressure and blood volume.

- Increased concentration of salt and other dissolved substances in the blood. Remember that ham sandwich and those potato chips? Both of these foods are salty, and eating them increased the blood's sodium concentration.
- A reduction in blood volume and blood pressure. This can occur when fluids are lost through profuse sweating, blood loss, vomiting, diarrhea, or simply when fluid intake is too low.

■ Dryness in the tissues of the mouth and throat. Tissue dryness reflects a lower amount of fluid in the bloodstream, which causes a reduced production of saliva.

Once the hypothalamus detects such changes, it stimulates the release of ADH to signal the kidneys to reduce urine flow and return more water to the bloodstream. As previously discussed, the kidneys also secrete renin, which eventually results in the production of angiotensin II and the retention of water. Water is drawn out of the salivary glands in the mouth in an attempt to further dilute the concentration of substances in the blood; this causes the mouth and throat to become even drier. Together, these mechanisms prevent a further loss of body fluid and help avoid dehydration.

Although the thirst mechanism can trigger an increase in fluid intake, this mechanism alone is not always sufficient: people tend to drink until they are no longer thirsty, but the amount of fluid consumed may not be enough to achieve fluid balance. This is particularly true when body water is rapidly lost, such as during intense exercise in the heat or high humidity. Because the thirst mechanism has some limitations, it is important that you drink regularly throughout the day and not wait to drink until you become thirsty, especially if you are active.

Foods provide water, too. Of course, you can clearly see that beverages are mostly water, but it isn't as easy to see the water content in most foods. For example, iceberg lettuce is almost 96% water, and even almonds contain a small amount of water (**Figure 9.7**).

Metabolic water is the water formed from the body's metabolic reactions. In the breakdown of fat, carbohydrate, and protein, adenosine triphosphate (ATP), carbon dioxide, and water are produced. The water that is formed during metabolic reactions contributes about 10% to 14% of the water the body needs each day.

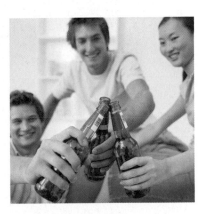

Drinking alcoholic beverages causes an increase in water loss because alcohol is a diuretic.

We Lose Fluids through Urine, Sweat, Evaporation, Exhalation, and Feces

Fluid loss that is noticeable, such as through urine output and sweating, is referred to as **sensible fluid loss.** Most of the water we consume is excreted through the kidneys in the form of urine. When we consume more water than we need, the kidneys process and excrete it in the form of dilute urine.

The second type of sensible fluid loss is via sweat. The sweat glands produce more sweat during exercise or when a person is in a hot environment. The evaporation of sweat from the skin releases heat, which cools the skin and reduces the body's core temperature.

metabolic water The water formed as a by-product of the body's metabolic reactions.

sensible fluid loss Body fluid loss that is noticeable, such as through urine output and sweating.

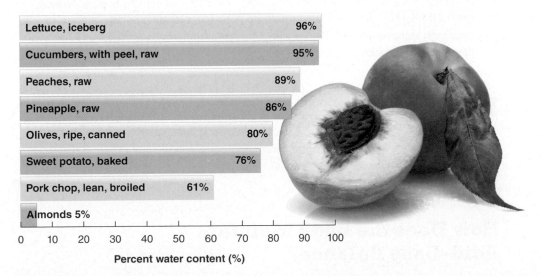

Food	Percent water content (%)
Lettuce, iceberg	96%
Cucumbers, with peel, raw	95%
Peaches, raw	89%
Pineapple, raw	86%
Olives, ripe, canned	80%
Sweet potato, baked	76%
Pork chop, lean, broiled	61%
Almonds	5%

Percent water content (%)

FIGURE 9.7 Water content of different foods. Much of your daily water intake comes from the foods you eat. (*Source*: Data from U.S. Department of Agriculture, Agricultural Research Service. 2009. USDA Nutrient Database for Standard Reference, Release 22. Nutrient Data Laboratory Home Page. www.ars .usda.gov/ba/bhnrc/ndl.)

Fluid is continuously evaporated from the skin even when a person is not consciously sweating, and fluid is continuously exhaled from the lungs. Fluid loss through these avenues is referred to as **insensible fluid loss,** as it is not perceived by the person. Under normal resting conditions, insensible fluid loss is less than 1 liter (L) each day; during heavy exercise or in hot weather, a person can lose up to 2 L of fluid per hour from insensible water loss.

Under normal conditions, only about 150 to 200 mL of fluid is lost each day in the feces. The gastrointestinal tract typically reabsorbs much of the large amounts of fluids that pass through it each day. However, when someone suffers from extreme diarrhea due to illness or from consuming excess laxatives, fluid loss in the feces can be as high as several liters per day.

In addition to these five common routes of fluid loss, certain situations can cause a significant loss of fluid from the body:

- Illnesses that involve fever, coughing, vomiting, diarrhea, and a runny nose significantly increase fluid loss. This is why doctors advise people to drink plenty of fluids when they are ill.
- Traumatic injury, internal hemorrhaging, blood donation, and surgery also increase loss of fluid because of the blood loss involved.
- Exercise increases fluid loss via sweat and respiration; although urine production typically decreases during exercise, fluid losses increase through the skin and lungs.
- Environmental conditions that increase fluid loss include high altitudes, cold and hot temperatures, and low humidity, such as in a desert or on an airplane. We breathe faster at higher altitudes due to the lower oxygen pressure; this results in greater fluid loss via the lungs. We sweat more in the heat, thus losing more water. Cold temperatures can trigger hormonal changes that result in an increased fluid loss.
- Pregnancy increases fluid loss for the mother, because fluids are continually diverted to the fetus and amniotic fluid.
- Breastfeeding requires a significant increase in fluid intake to make up for the loss of fluid as breast milk.
- Consumption of diuretics can result in dangerously excessive fluid loss. Diuretics include certain prescription medications and alcohol. Many over-the-counter weight-loss remedies are really just diuretics. In the past, it was believed that the caffeine in beverages such as coffee, tea, and cola could cause serious dehydration, but recent research suggests that caffeinated drinks do not have a significant impact on the hydration status of adults.[2] The caffeine content of numerous beverages and foods is listed in Appendix E.

RECAP

A healthy fluid level is maintained in the body by balancing intake with excretion. Primary sources of fluids include water and other beverages, foods, and the production of metabolic water in the body. Fluid losses occur through urination, sweating, the feces, evaporation from the skin, and exhalation from the lungs.   ■

 LO 5 Explain how the body maintains acid–base balance.

insensible fluid loss The unperceived loss of body fluid, such as through evaporation from the skin and exhalation from the lungs during breathing.

How Does the Body Maintain Acid–Base Balance?

Recall (from Chapter 3) that an acid is a compound that releases hydrogen ions in solution, whereas a base is a substance that takes up hydrogen ions. The body's cellular processes, including energy metabolism, result in the constant production of both acids and bases.

These substances are neutralized through the addition of buffers or through actions of the lungs or the kidneys. These homeostatic mechanisms enable the body to maintain control over the pH—or acid–base balance—of the blood, which normally is slightly alkaline, ranging from about 7.35 to 7.45. (For a review of the pH scale, see **You Do the Math**, Chapter 3, page 83.)

If the blood pH moves beyond this narrow range, life-threatening complications develop. The body goes into a state called *acidosis* when the blood pH drops below 7.35. *Alkalosis* results if the blood pH rises above 7.45. Both acidosis and alkalosis can be caused by disorders affecting metabolism, respiration, or kidney function. For example, uncontrolled diabetes can result in a buildup of ketones, which are weak acids, and prompt acidosis, whereas the loss of gastric acid following repeated episodes of vomiting can cause alkalosis. Acidosis and alkalosis can cause coma and death by denaturing vital body proteins, such as enzymes and hemoglobin.

Three major systems account for the body's ability to regulate acid–base balance: blood buffers, the lungs, and the kidneys.

- *Blood buffers*. The blood transports many natural buffers. Proteins are excellent buffers, having the ability to take up excess hydrogen ions during acidosis and to release hydrogen ions when the blood becomes too basic. Another blood buffer is the bicarbonate-carbonic acid system. Carbon dioxide (CO_2), one of the end products of energy metabolism, dissolves in the bloodstream to form carbonic acid (H_2CO_3), which itself dissociates into hydrogen (H^+) and bicarbonate ions (HCO_3^-):

$$CO_2 + H_2O \longleftrightarrow H_2CO_3 \longleftrightarrow H^+ + HCO_3^-$$

  Notice that this reaction is reversible: the bicarbonate ions are able to take up excess hydrogen ions or release hydrogen ions as needed in order to maintain acid–base balance.

- *Respiratory compensation*. Although fast acting, blood buffers don't have enough buffering capacity to correct large or long-term acid–base imbalances. The second line of defense is the lungs. By increasing or decreasing the rate of respiration, the lungs regulate the amount of carbonic acid in the blood. High levels of carbonic acid (acidosis) trigger hyperventilation. Excess carbon dioxide is forced out, helping to increase blood pH. In a state of alkalosis, with high blood levels of bicarbonate, respiration slows, carbon dioxide is retained, and more carbonic acid is formed, decreasing blood pH.

- *Renal compensation*. Since there is a limit to how fast or slow a person can breathe, the ability of the lungs to regulate acid–base balance is also limited. The last line of defense is the kidneys. Healthy kidneys have the capacity to either secrete into blood or excrete into urine significant bicarbonate to correct acid–base imbalances. They can also use nonbicarbonate buffers, such as ammonia or hydrogen phosphate, to excrete excess hydrogen ions.

By working together, blood buffers, the lungs, and the kidneys are usually able to maintain blood pH in a homeostatic range. When these mechanisms fail, clinical intervention, such as the intravenous administration of bicarbonate to a patient with diabetic ketoacidosis, may be necessary to save the patient's life.

RECAP

Three primary mechanisms account for the body's ability to regulate acid–base balance: Blood buffers, such as blood proteins and the bicarbonate-carbonic acid system, can take up or release hydrogen ions under acidic or alkaline conditions. In the lungs, increased or decreased respiration can influence the blood level of carbonic acid. Finally, renal secretion or excretion of bicarbonate can influence the pH of blood. ■

LO 6 Identify the DRIs for water and compare the nutritional quality of several common beverages.

How Much Water Should We Drink, and What Are the Best Sources?

Water is essential for life. Although we can live for weeks without food, we can survive only a few days without water, depending on environmental temperature. We do not have the capacity to store water, so we must continuously replace the water lost each day.

Our Requirements for Water Are Individualized

The need for water varies greatly depending on age, body size, health status, physical activity level, and exposure to environmental conditions. It is important to pay attention to how much the need for water changes under various conditions, so that dehydration can be avoided.

Fluid requirements are very individualized. For example, a highly active male athlete training in a hot environment may require up to 10 L of fluid per day to maintain healthy fluid balance, whereas an inactive, petite woman who lives in a mild climate and works in a temperature-controlled office building may require only about 3 L of fluid per day. The DRI for adult men aged 19 to 50 years is 3.7 L of total water per day. This includes approximately 3.0 L (13 cups) as total water, other beverages, and food. The DRI for adult women aged 19 to 50 is 2.7 L of total water per day. This includes about 2.2 L (9 cups) as total water, other beverages, and food.[3]

Figure 9.8 shows the amount and sources of water intake and output for a woman expending 2,500 kcal per day. Based on current recommendations, this woman needs about 3,000 mL of water per day:

- Water from metabolism provides 300 mL of water.
- The food she eats provides her with an additional 500 mL of water each day.
- The beverages she drinks provide the remainder of water needed, which is equal to 2,200 mL.

An 8-oz glass of water is equal to 240 mL. In this example, the woman would need to drink nine glasses of fluid to meet her needs. You may have read or heard that drinking eight glasses of fluid each day is recommended for most people. Drinking this amount will provide most people with enough fluid to maintain proper fluid balance. Remember, however, that this recommendation of eight glasses of fluid each day is a general guideline.

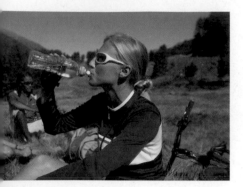

Vigorous exercise causes significant water loss, which must be replenished to optimize performance and health.

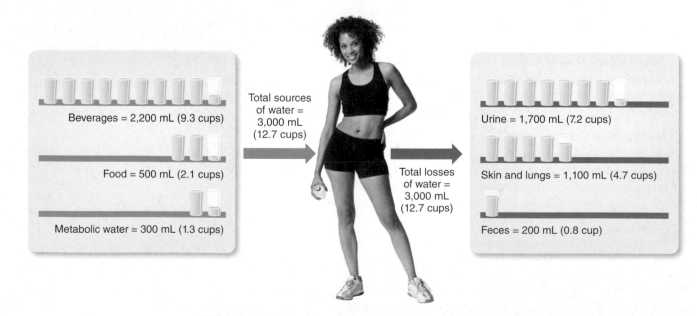

Beverages = 2,200 mL (9.3 cups)

Food = 500 mL (2.1 cups)

Metabolic water = 300 mL (1.3 cups)

Total sources of water = 3,000 mL (12.7 cups)

Total losses of water = 3,000 mL (12.7 cups)

Urine = 1,700 mL (7.2 cups)

Skin and lungs = 1,100 mL (4.7 cups)

Feces = 200 mL (0.8 cup)

FIGURE 9.8 Amounts and categories of water sources and losses for a woman expending 2,500 kcal per day.

For some people, that amount of fluid may be too high, or it may fluctuate with certain environmental conditions or changes in physical activities.

In contrast, athletes and others who are highly active, especially those working in very hot environments, may require more fluid than the current recommendations. The amount of sweat lost during strenuous activity is very individualized and depends on body size, activity intensity, level of fitness, environmental temperature, and humidity. We do know that some people can lose as much as 10% of body weight or mass during a marathon held in extreme heat[4] and that professional and collegiate football players can lose up to 2 L of sweat per hour.[5] Thus, these individuals need to drink more to replace the fluid they lose. Sodium is the major electrolyte lost in sweat; we also lose some potassium and small amounts of iron and calcium in sweat.

Because of fluid and electrolyte losses during exercise, some athletes drink sports beverages instead of plain water to help them maintain fluid balance. Recently, however, sports beverages have also become popular with recreationally active people and non-athletes, including an increasing number of children and adolescents.[6] For these groups, there is really no health benefit to consuming these beverages instead of plain water.

Public Tap Water Is Safe to Drink

So many types of drinking water are available in the United States, how can we distinguish among them? Tap water is available from private wells and municipal water systems in homes and public places. Carbonated water contains carbon dioxide gas that either occurs naturally or is added to the water. Mineral water contains 250 to 500 parts per million (ppm) of minerals. Many people prefer the unique taste of mineral water; however, a number of brands contain high amounts of sodium and so should be avoided by people who are trying to reduce their sodium intake.

Two types of water not used for drinking are distilled water and purified water. Distilled water is processed in such a way that all dissolved minerals are removed. It is sometimes used in steam irons and automobile cooling systems to prevent mineral buildup, but it has a flat taste. Purified water has been treated so that all dissolved minerals and contaminants are removed. It is used in research and medical procedures.

One of the major changes in the beverage industry during the past two decades has been the growth in sales of bottled water, now estimated at $13 billion per year. Americans now consume about 34 gallons of bottled water per person, per year.[7] This meteoric rise in bottled water production and consumption is most likely due to the convenience of drinking bottled water, to the health messages related to drinking more water, to the recognition that water is more beneficial than other packaged beverages, and to the public's fears related to the safety of tap water. While environmental concerns related to disposal of water bottles continue to grow, the bottled water industry has responded with several environmental initiatives, such as smaller bottle caps, thinner bottles, and greater use of recyclable containers. Is bottled water safer or more healthful than tap water? Refer to the *Highlight* box on page 356 to find out.

All Beverages Are Not Created Equal

Many commercial beverages contain several important nutrients in addition to their water content, whereas others provide water and refined sugar but very little else. Let's review the health benefits of and potential concerns about some of the most popular beverages on the market.

Milk and Milk Substitutes

Low-fat and skim milk are healthful beverage choices for many people, because they provide protein, calcium, phosphorus, vitamin D, and usually vitamin A. Many brands of fluid milk are now "specialized" and provide additional calcium, vitamin E, essential fatty acids, and/or plant sterols (to lower serum cholesterol). Kefir, a blended yogurt drink, is

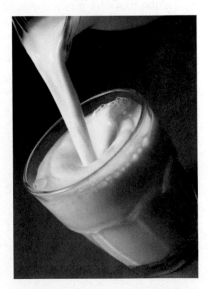

Low-fat and skim milk are healthful beverage choices for many people.

HIGHLIGHT

Which Is Better, Bottled Water or Tap?

Americans consume 34 gallons of bottled water per person every year.[1] Although some people choose bottled water for its convenience, and some say they prefer the taste, many people believe that bottled water is safer and more healthful than tap water. Is this true?

The water we drink generally comes from either surface water (from lakes, rivers, and reservoirs) or groundwater (from underground rock formations called *acquifers*). Surface water can be contaminated by animal and industrial wastes, pesticides, and runoff from highways. Groundwater can be tainted by garbage dumps, landfills, and oil or gas pipelines as well as natural contaminants such as arsenic and high levels of iron.

Thanks to the widespread use of water treatment plants, the United States has one of the safest water systems in the world. Chlorine and ozone, the most common purifying agents, are effective in killing many contaminants. Water treatment plants routinely check our water supplies for hazardous chemicals, minerals, and other contaminants. In addition, many water treatment plants fluoridate the water to prevent dental decay and optimize oral health.

The Environmental Protection Agency (EPA) sets and monitors the standards for municipal water systems. The EPA does not monitor water from private wells, but it publishes recommendations for well owners to help them maintain a safe water supply.

In contrast, the Food and Drug Administration (FDA) regulates bottled water. Its quality standards are no higher than those for public water. Most bottling plants use an

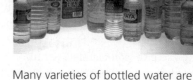

Many varieties of bottled water are available to consumers.

ozone treatment to disinfect water and many people feel this produces water that tastes better than chlorine-treated water.

There is no evidence that bottled water is safer to drink, even by most consumers with compromised immunity. On the other hand, some people do not have access to safe tap water where they live. Mining by-products, lead, and other contaminants are major long-term concerns in some parts of the United States, while natural disasters may temporarily interrupt the supply of safe tap water. For these people, bottled water may be the safer choice.

Is bottled water more healthful? While some brands may contain more nutrient minerals than tap water, bottled water has no other nutritional advantages over tap water. In addition, most bottled waters fail to provide optimal levels of fluoride, increasing the risk for dental decay in children.

After reading this discussion, if you still choose to drink bottled water, look for brands with the International Bottled Water Association (IBWA) trademark. For more information on drinking water safety, go to the EPA website at www.epa.gov; for information on bottled water, go to www.bottledwater.org.

References

1. International Bottled Water Association. 2014. Bottled Water Sales and Consumption Projected to Increase in 2014, Expected to be the Number One Packaged Drink by 2016. Available at: www.bottledwater.org/bottled-water-sales-and-consumption-projected-increase-2014-expected-be-number-one-packaged-drink. (accessed April 2015).

also a good source of most of these nutrients, and provides beneficial probiotic bacteria. Many brands of soy milk are fortified with calcium and vitamins A and D and provide about 6 grams of protein per cup. In contrast, most commercial almond, cashew, and rice milks are low in protein, with only 1 gram or less per cup.

When purchasing flavored milk, kefir, or milk substitutes, check the Nutrition Facts panel for the sugar content. Some brands of chocolate milk, for example, can contain 6 or more teaspoons of refined sugar in a single cup.

Hot Beverages Containing Caffeine

Coffee made without cream or nondairy creamer can be a healthful beverage choice if consumed in moderation. As mentioned earlier, recent research suggests that its caffeine content does not significantly decrease the body's hydration status, and the calcium in coffee drinks made with milk, such as café con leche and café latte, can be significant. Coffee (regular or decaffeinated) is known to provide several types of phytochemicals (beneficial plant chemicals) that may actually lower the risk for certain chronic diseases, such as type 2 diabetes.[8] There is also growing evidence that people who drink moderate amounts of coffee have a lower risk for stroke, and some evidence of a lower risk for age-related dementia, although not all research supports these hypotheses.[9,10] While some people are sensitive to the caffeine in coffee, moderate consumption is safe and potentially healthful.

Tea is second only to water as the most commonly consumed beverage in the world. With the exception of red tea and herbal teas, which do not contain caffeine, all forms of tea come from the same plant, *Camellia sinesis*. Black tea is the most highly processed (the tea leaves are fully fermented), whereas oolong tea leaves are only partially fermented, and green and white tea leaves have been dried but not fermented. Both green and white teas have higher levels of phytochemicals than black and oolong teas. These phytochemicals are thought to contribute to the health-promoting qualities of tea, including decreased risk for hypertension,[11] heart disease and stroke,[9] diabetes, and certain cancers; decreased levels of LDL-cholesterol; and increased levels of HDL-cholesterol. All teas derived from *Camellia sinesis* provide caffeine, but the amount in brewed tea is usually half the amount in most brewed coffee. If consumed without added sugar, tea is an excellent source of fluid that may have unexpected long-term health benefits.

Chocolate and cocoa-based beverages provide small amounts of a compound called theobromine, which has effects similar to but milder than those of caffeine and is present in amounts lower than those found in coffee, tea, or colas. Chocolate, especially dark chocolate, is rich in phytochemicals known as flavanols, which may lower risk for heart failure.[12] Hot chocolate made with dark cocoa powder and skim or low-fat milk is a nutritious and satisfying drink.

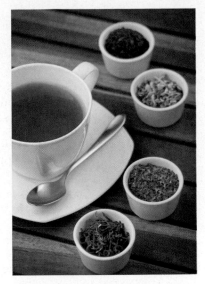

After water, tea is the most commonly consumed beverage in the world.

Energy Drinks

Energy drinks are another popular beverage option, with over $13.5 billion in sales in 2015. These products advertise their ability to provide a boost, jump start, buzz, punch, or rocket-powered blast! As many as half of all adolescents and young adults consume these products, although nutrition experts and consumer groups have raised significant concerns.[13] Many of these beverages contain more than three times the amount of caffeine in a comparable serving of cola, and a few contain up to 10 times the caffeine in cola. In addition, many energy drinks contain guarana seed extract: guarana seeds contain more caffeine than coffee beans, so their "extract" is simply a potent source of additional caffeine. Some also contain *taurine,* an amino acid associated with muscle contraction, or bitter orange, a compound known to increase blood pressure and heart rate.[13] Moreover, unlike hot coffee and tea, which are sipped slowly, energy drinks can be consumed quickly, releasing a large amount of caffeine into the bloodstream in a short period of time.

There is little research on the effects of these ingredients, either alone or in combination with one another, particularly in children and adolescents. We do know that these substances can significantly increase blood pressure and heart rate. Moreover, mood swings, behavioral disorders, insomnia, dizziness, tremors, seizures, caffeine dependency, dehydration, and other problems have been linked to consumption of energy drinks. Between 2007 and 2011, the number of emergency department visits related to energy drinks doubled and now exceed 20,000 per year.[14] Patients are more likely to be between the ages of 18 and 39 years than any other age group. Although the FDA limits the amount of caffeine in soft drinks, it has no legal authority to regulate the ingredients, including caffeine, in energy drinks, since they are classified as dietary supplements, not food.

Energy drinks are also a source of significant added sugar. For example, a 16-ounce bottle of Rockstar Original contains 62 grams—more than 15 teaspoons—of sugar and 248 empty Calories. In short, as a source of fluid, energy drinks have a high potential for undesirable side effects and should be avoided by children and adolescents and used sparingly by adults.

Beverages with Added Sugars

MyPlate advises us to "Drink water instead of sugary drinks," and there's a simple reason: Most soft drinks, juice drinks, flavored waters, energy drinks, and bottled teas and coffees are

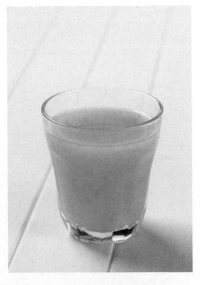

Many fruit juices are made from juice concentrate that is little more than pure sugar and, thus, are Calorie dense.

loaded with added sugars. Although many beverage manufacturers are switching from high-fructose corn syrup to "pure cane sugar" to sweeten their products, all forms of added sugars provide the same number of Calories per gram, no matter their molecular structure. Similarly, some beverage producers have begun to use "fruit juice concentrate" as a source of added sugar. Although it sounds like a healthy option, the concentrate is little more than pure sugar, with none of the fiber or other nutrients that make fruit a nutritious food. Honey is another popular source of added sugar, but it is also Calorie dense and low in nutrient value.

Fruit juices themselves are also high in empty Calories. For example, you might think of cranberry juice cocktail as a healthful beverage, but did you know that one 8-oz serving contains more than 7 teaspoons of added sugar, providing 112 Calories? Even 100% fruit juice with no added sugar can be high in Calories. For instance, an 8-ounce serving of a popular brand of premium orange juice provides the same number of Calories as cranberry juice cocktail.

Specialty Waters

So-called designer waters are made with added nutrients and/or herbs that supposedly enhance memory, delay aging, boost energy levels, or strengthen the immune response. Many of these products are labeled with disclaimers such as "This statement has not been evaluated by the FDA. This product is not intended to diagnose, treat, cure, or prevent any disease." This disclaimer is required by the FDA whenever a food manufacturer makes a structure–function claim (see Chapter 2). In other words, manufacturers must acknowledge that the statements made on the labels of these waters are not based on research!

In fact, the amounts of vitamins or other substances added to these waters are usually so low, compared to what can be obtained from foods, that they are unlikely to make an impact on the consumer's health or well-being. In addition, specialty waters made with added sugars can increase the consumer's energy intake by more than 300 Calories.

Another specialty water being marketed through online sites and "health" stores is alkaline water. Promoted as a way to counteract the build-up of free radicals in the body, alkaline water supposedly slows aging, improves digestion, fights cancer, and minimizes bone loss. Alkaline water has a slightly higher pH than most forms of tap or bottled water. However, as soon as alkaline water is swallowed and moves into the stomach, the highly acidic gastric juice immediately reduces the water's pH; moreover, as discussed earlier, blood buffers, the lungs, and the kidneys respond to fluctuations in the body's pH, maintaining a healthy balance even when we drink black coffee or other acidic beverages. In short, no scientific evidence supports the health claims made for alkaline water.

Sports Beverages and Coconut Water

We noted earlier that, because of the potential for fluid and electrolyte imbalances during rigorous exercise, many endurance athletes drink sports beverages, which provide water, electrolytes, and a source of carbohydrate, before, during, and after workouts. Others are turning to coconut water, marketed as a good source of electrolytes and "natural sugars." Coconut water, while growing in popularity, is still viewed primarily as a specialty product and is significantly more expensive than traditional sports beverages. As a general rule, only people who exercise or do manual labor vigorously for 60 minutes or more benefit from consuming either sports beverages or coconut water.

As you can see, American consumers have a wide range of beverage choices available to them. Poor choices can increase total caloric intake and lower daily nutrient intake. Although the caloric contribution of beverages to our total energy intake nearly doubled over the past 40 years, there is some evidence that caloric intake from beverages is now decreasing.[15] Plain drinking water is available free of charge, contributes no Calories, contains no additives, is highly effective in quenching thirst and maintaining hydration status, and poses no health threat. For most of us, most of the time, water really is the perfect beverage choice.

Theo

Nutri-Case

"Our basketball coach keeps reminding us how important it is to drink at least 8 cups of fluid a day, even on days when we don't have practice or a game. At first that seemed like an awful lot, but after keeping track of what I drank yesterday, I figure I'm good. I had a 16-ounce energy drink on my way to classes, a 12-ounce coffee mocha on my morning break, a 16-ounce Coca-Cola with lunch, and a 12-ounce bottle of Gatorade when I finished working out at the gym. With dinner in the cafeteria, I had an 8-ounce carton of chocolate milk. Then while I was studying in the dorm, I got a 12-ounce Mountain Dew from the vending machine. I'm not sure what all that adds up to, but I know it's more than 8 cups. It's not as hard as I thought to get enough fluid!"

How many ounces are in 8 cups of fluid? How many ounces of fluid did Theo drink? Did he meet, or exceed, the recommended fluid intake? What do you think of the nutritional quality of his fluid choices?

Answers are located in the MasteringNutrition Study Area.

RECAP

Fluid requirements are highly individualized and depend on body size, age, physical activity, health status, and environmental factors. All beverages provide water, and some, such as milk and calcium-fortified drinks, provide other important nutrients as well. Some beverages contain excessive amounts of caffeine, added sugars, or other potentially harmful ingredients and should be consumed only in moderation if at all. Pure water remains an ideal beverage choice.

How Do Four Major Minerals Contribute to Fluid Balance?

The major minerals sodium, potassium, chloride, and phosphorus make significant contributions to the body's fluid balance. The recommended intake for these nutrients is identified in **Table 9.1**.

LO 7 Identify the functions, DRIs, and common dietary sources of sodium, potassium, chloride, and phosphorus.

LO 8 Distinguish between *hypernatremia* and *hyponatremia* and identify factors that can cause these conditions.

Sodium Is the Body's Major Extracellular Cation

Over the past 20 years, researchers have linked high sodium intake to an increased risk for hypertension (HTN) in some individuals. Because of this possible link to HTN, many

TABLE 9.1 Overview of Nutrients Involved in Hydration and Neuromuscular Function

To see the full profile of micronutrients, turn to Chapter 7.5, In Depth, Vitamins and Minerals: Micronutrients with Macro Powers, *pages 292–303*.

Nutrient	Recommended Intake
Sodium	1.5 g/day*
Potassium	4.7 g/day*
Chloride	2.3 g/day*
Phosphorus	700 mg/day[7]

*Adequate Intake (AI).
[7]RDA.

Nutrition
MILESTONE

Sodium does not occur by itself in nature. Instead, it forms compounds such as table salt, baking soda, and lye. So how and when did it come to be recognized as an independent mineral? In the early 1800s, the English chemist Sir Humphry Davy began experimenting with a new device—a forerunner of our modern battery—that could generate an electrical current. He used the device to run an electrical current through a variety of chemical compounds, thereby forcing a chemical reaction that wouldn't otherwise have occurred. He discovered that the current caused the compounds to break down into their component minerals.

In **1807**, Davy used his technique to separate the components of a powdery salt commonly called potash. In doing so, he isolated potassium. Shortly thereafter, he used the same technique on lye and isolated sodium, which until that time had not been considered distinct from potassium. The following year, he succeeded in isolating calcium and magnesium. For these reasons, Davy is considered a pioneer of electrochemistry.

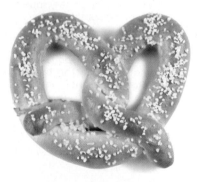

Many popular snack foods, such as pretzels, are high in sodium.

people have come to believe that sodium is harmful to the body. That oversimplification, however, is just not true: sodium is essential for survival. Moreover, as discussed in this chapter's **Nutrition Myth or Fact?** this hypothesis linking high sodium intake and HTN is widely debated.

Functions of Sodium

Sodium has a variety of functions. As discussed earlier in this chapter, as the major cation in the extracellular fluid, it allows cells to maintain proper fluid balance. Renal sodium excretion and reabsorption contribute to blood pressure regulation. Sodium also assists with the transmission of nerve signals and aids in muscle contraction and relaxation. Finally, sodium assists in the absorption of glucose from the small intestine. Glucose is absorbed via active transport that involves sodium-dependent glucose transporters.

How Much Sodium Should We Consume?

Virtually all of the dietary sodium consumed is absorbed by the body. Most is absorbed from the small intestine, although some can be absorbed in the large intestine. As discussed earlier in this chapter, the kidneys reabsorb sodium when it needs to be retained by the body and excrete excess sodium in the urine. Although many people are concerned about consuming too much sodium, it should not be completely eliminated from the diet, nor should it be excessively limited.

Recommended Dietary Intake for Sodium The AI for sodium is 1.5 g/day (1,500 mg/day) for adult men and women aged 19 to 50 years, which is equivalent to just over half a teaspoon of salt.[4] The AI drops to 1.3 g/day for those 51 to 70 years of age and 1.2 g/d for persons over the age of 70 years. Most people in the United States greatly exceed this guideline: the usual U.S. intake is nearly 3.5 g of sodium per day, with many adults consuming up to 6 g per day. Most health organizations recommend a daily sodium intake of no more than 2.3 or 2.4 g per day. The current Dietary Guidelines recommend limiting sodium intake to less than 2.3 g per day.[16]

Food Sources of Sodium Sodium is found naturally in many common foods, and many processed foods and restaurant meals contain large amounts of added sodium. Thus, it is easy to consume excess amounts in our daily diets. Try to guess which of the following foods contains the most sodium: 1 cup of tomato juice, 1 oz of potato chips, or 4 saltine crackers. Now look at **Table 9.2** to find the answer. This table shows foods that are high in sodium and gives lower-sodium alternatives. Are you surprised to find out that, of all these food items, the tomato juice has the most sodium? When eating processed foods, such as lunch meats, canned soups and beans, vegetable juices, and prepackaged rice and pasta dishes, look for labels with the words "low-sodium" or "no added salt," as these foods are lower in sodium than the original versions.

What Happens If We Consume Too Much Sodium?

Some people who consume high-sodium diets are at increased risk for HTN, especially if their potassium intake is low.[17] This finding has prompted many, but not all, health

TABLE 9.2 High-Sodium Foods and Lower-Sodium Alternatives

High-Sodium Food	Sodium (mg)	Lower-Sodium Food	Sodium (mg)
Dill pickle (1 large, 4 in.)	1,731	Low-sodium dill pickle (1 large, 4 in.)	25
Ham, cured, roasted (3 oz)	1,177	Pork, loin roast (3 oz)	54
Chipped beef (3 oz)	913	Beef chuck roast, cooked (3 oz)	53
Tomato juice, regular (1 cup)	654	Tomato juice, lower sodium (1 cup)	24
Tomato sauce, canned (½ cup)	741	Fresh tomato (1 medium)	11
Canned cream corn (1 cup)	730	Cooked corn, fresh (1 cup)	28
Tomato soup, canned (1 cup)	695	Lower-sodium tomato soup, canned (1 cup)	480
Potato chips, salted (1 oz)	168	Baked potato, unsalted (1 medium)	14
Saltine crackers (4 each)	156	Saltine crackers, unsalted (4 each)	100

Source: Data from U.S. Department of Agriculture. 2005. U.S.D.A. National Nutrient Database for Standard Reference, Release 18. Nutrient Data Laboratory Home Page. www.ars.usda.gov/ba/bhnrc/ndl.

organizations to recommend a population-wide reduction in sodium intakes.[16] The questions of whether high-sodium diets actually cause or contribute to HTN and whether low-sodium diets reduce the risk of HTN remain the subject of much controversy; many researchers believe a high sodium-to-potassium ratio is the primary dietary pattern leading to increased risk while others believe a low sodium intake actually increases overall mortality.[16,17]

Also controversial is the effect of high sodium intake on bone loss: while some studies have linked high sodium intakes to increased urinary excretion of calcium and lower bone density, recent research suggests that a high sodium intake does not negatively impact bone health in people with adequate calcium intake.[18]

Hypernatremia refers to an abnormally high blood sodium concentration. It is usually caused by a rapid intake of high amounts of sodium, such as when a shipwrecked sailor drinks seawater. Eating a high-sodium diet does not usually cause hypernatremia in a healthy person, as the kidneys are able to excrete excess sodium in the urine. But people with congestive heart failure or kidney disease are not able to excrete sodium effectively, making them more prone to the condition. Hypernatremia is dangerous, because it causes an abnormally high blood volume, leading to edema (swelling) of tissues and raising blood pressure to unhealthy levels.

What Happens If We Don't Consume Enough Sodium?

Because dietary sodium intake is so high in the United States, deficiencies are extremely rare, except in individuals who sweat heavily or consume little or no sodium in the diet. Nevertheless, certain conditions can cause dangerously low blood sodium levels. **Hyponatremia,** abnormally low blood sodium concentration, can occur during periods of intense activity, such as a marathon run or all-day hike, when people drink large volumes of water and fail to replace sodium. Hazing rituals in which people are forced to drink excessive amounts of plain water can also dilute blood sodium to the point of hyponatremia. Severe diarrhea, vomiting, or excessive, prolonged sweating can also cause hyponatremia.

Symptoms of hyponatremia include headaches, dizziness, fatigue, nausea, vomiting, and muscle cramps. If hyponatremia is left untreated, it can lead to seizures, coma, and death. Treatment for hyponatremia includes the ingestion of liquids and foods high in sodium and may even require the intravenous administration of electrolyte rich solutions if the person has lost consciousness or is not able to consume beverages and foods by mouth.

hypernatremia A condition in which blood sodium levels are dangerously high.

hyponatremia A condition in which blood sodium levels are dangerously low.

RECAP

Sodium is the primary cation in the extracellular fluid. It works to maintain fluid balance and blood pressure, and transmission of nerve signals, aids muscle contraction, and assists in the absorption of glucose from the small intestine. The AI for sodium is 1.5 g per day. Deficiencies are rare, because the typical American diet is high in sodium. Excessive sodium intake, particularly when potassium intake is low, has been related to an increased risk for hypertension and loss of bone density, but these associations are the subject of controversy. Hypernatremia is a dangerous condition characterized by a high blood sodium level. ■

Potassium Is the Body's Major Intracellular Cation

As we discussed previously, potassium is the major cation in the intracellular fluid. It is a major constituent of all living cells and is found in both plants and animals. About 85% of dietary potassium is absorbed, and, as with sodium, the kidneys regulate reabsorption and urinary excretion of potassium.

Functions of Potassium

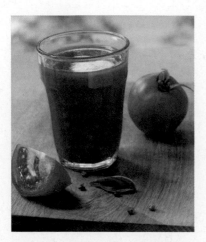

Fresh tomatoes have only 4 mg of sodium per ½ cup serving whereas the same amount of tomato juice has 327 mg of sodium; both are excellent sources of potassium.

Potassium and sodium work together to maintain proper fluid balance, to regulate the transmission of nerve impulses, and to assist in muscle contraction. Potassium also assists in maintaining blood pressure. In contrast with a high-sodium diet, eating a diet high in potassium actually helps maintain a lower blood pressure.

How Much Potassium Should We Consume?

We can reduce our risk for high blood pressure by consuming adequate potassium in our diets. The AI for potassium for adult men and women aged 19 to 50 years is 4.7 g/day (4,700 mg/day).[3] Unlike sodium, which is abundant in the typical American diet, potassium is abundant in foods that many Americans fail to consume in adequate amounts, particularly fresh fruits and vegetables. **Figure 9.9** identifies foods that are high in potassium. Processing foods generally increases their amount of sodium and decreases their amount of potassium. Thus, you can optimize your potassium intake and reduce your sodium intake by avoiding processed foods and eating more fresh fruits,

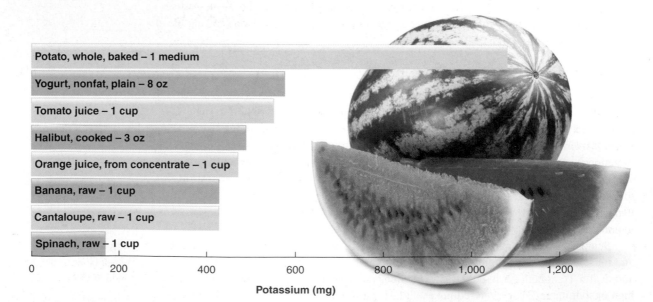

Potato, whole, baked – 1 medium

Yogurt, nonfat, plain – 8 oz

Tomato juice – 1 cup

Halibut, cooked – 3 oz

Orange juice, from concentrate – 1 cup

Banana, raw – 1 cup

Cantaloupe, raw – 1 cup

Spinach, raw – 1 cup

0   200   400   600   800   1,000   1,200

Potassium (mg)

FIGURE 9.9 Common food sources of potassium. The AI for potassium is 4.7 g/day. (*Source:* Data from U.S. Department of Agriculture, Agricultural Research Service. 2009. USDA Nutrient Database for Standard Reference, Release 22. Nutrient Data Laboratory Home Page. www.ars.usda.gov/ba/bhnrc/ndl.)

vegetables, legumes, and whole grains. Following these tips can also help you increase your consumption of potassium:

- For breakfast, look for cereals containing bran and/or wheat germ, or sprinkle fruit and yogurt with wheat germ.
- Toss a banana, some dried apricots, or a bag of sunflower seeds into your backpack for a mid-morning snack.
- Instead of soft drinks, choose low-fat milk, kefir, soy milk, or low-sodium vegetable juice, or blend low-fat vanilla yogurt with ice cubes and a banana.
- Serve avocado or bean dip with veggie slices.
- Make a tropical salad with avocado, papaya, and grapefruit.
- Make sweet potato fries (toss potato slices in olive oil and bake at 400° for 15–20 minutes), or bake a wedge of acorn squash.

Salmon and other fish, lean cuts of beef, and tomato juice are other foods that can boost your potassium intake. As discussed ahead, the Dietary Approaches to Stop Hypertension (DASH) diet is designed to provide an optimal intake of potassium.

What Happens If We Consume Too Much Potassium?

People with healthy kidneys are able to excrete excess potassium effectively. However, people with kidney disease are not able to regulate their blood potassium levels. **Hyperkalemia,** or high blood potassium concentration, occurs when potassium is not efficiently excreted from the body. Because of potassium's role in cardiac muscle contraction, severe hyperkalemia can alter the normal rhythm of the heart, resulting in heart attack and death. People with kidney disease must monitor their potassium intake very carefully and should avoid consuming salt substitutes, as these products are high in potassium.

What Happens If We Don't Consume Enough Potassium?

Because potassium is common in many foods, a dietary potassium deficiency is rare. However, potassium deficiency is not uncommon among people who have serious medical disorders. Kidney disease, diabetic ketoacidosis, and other illnesses can lead to potassium deficiency.

In addition, people with high blood pressure who are prescribed certain diuretic medications to treat their disease are at risk for potassium deficiency. As we noted earlier, diuretics promote the excretion of fluid as urine through the kidneys. Some diuretics also increase the body's urinary excretion of potassium. People who are taking diuretic medications should have their blood potassium monitored regularly and should eat foods that are high in potassium to prevent **hypokalemia,** or low blood potassium concentration. This is not a universal recommendation, however, because some diuretics are specially formulated to spare or retain potassium; therefore, people taking diuretics should consult their physician regarding dietary potassium intake.

Extreme dehydration, vomiting, and diarrhea can also cause hypokalemia, as can long-term consumption of natural licorice, which contains glycyrrhizic acid (GZA), a substance that increases urinary excretion of potassium. Because the majority of foods that contain licorice flavoring in the United States do not contain GZA, licorice-induced hypokalemia is rarely seen here. People who abuse alcohol or laxatives can suffer from hypokalemia. Symptoms include confusion, loss of appetite, and muscle weakness. Severe cases of hypokalemia result in fatal changes in heart rate; many deaths attributed to extreme dehydration or an eating disorder are caused by abnormal heart rhythms due to hypokalemia.

RECAP

Potassium is the major cation inside of the cell. It regulates fluid balance, blood pressure, and the transmission of nerve impulses, and assists in muscle contraction. The AI for potassium is 4.7 g per day. Potassium is found in abundance in fresh foods, particularly fruits and vegetables, but is typically low in processed foods. Both hyperkalemia and hypokalemia can result in heart failure and death. ■

hyperkalemia A condition in which blood potassium levels are dangerously high.

hypokalemia A condition in which blood potassium levels are dangerously low.

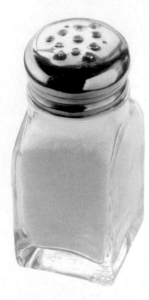

Almost all dietary chloride is consumed through table salt.

Chloride Is the Body's Major Extracellular Anion

Chloride is an anion obtained almost exclusively from sodium chloride, or table salt. It should not be confused with *chlorine*, which is a poisonous gas used to kill germs in our water supply. As with sodium, the majority of dietary chloride is absorbed in the small intestine. The kidneys regulate urinary excretion of chloride.

Coupled with sodium in the extracellular fluid, chloride assists with the maintenance of fluid balance. Chloride is also a component of hydrochloric acid (HCl) in the stomach. Chloride also works with the white blood cells during an immune response to help kill bacteria, and it assists in the transmission of nerve impulses.

The AI for chloride for adult men and women aged 19 to 50 years is 2.3 g/day (2,300 mg/day).[3] As chloride is coupled with sodium to form table salt, our primary dietary source of chloride is salt in our foods. Chloride is also found in some fruits and vegetables. Keep in mind that salt is composed of about 60% chloride; thus, you can calculate the content of chloride in processed foods by multiplying its salt content by 0.60 (60%). For instance, a food that contains 500 mg of salt would contain 300 mg of chloride (500 mg $\times$ 0.60 = 300 mg).

Because we consume virtually all of our dietary chloride in the form of sodium chloride, there is no known toxicity symptom for chloride alone, although consuming excess amounts of sodium chloride over a prolonged period contributes to HTN in salt-sensitive individuals. Chloride deficiency is rare, even in people who consume a low-sodium diet. It can occur, however, during conditions of severe dehydration and frequent vomiting. This is sometimes seen in people with eating disorders who regularly vomit to rid their bodies of unwanted energy.

Phosphorus Is the Body's Major Intracellular Anion

Phosphorus is the body's major intracellular anion, and is most commonly found combined with oxygen in the form of hydrogen phosphate, HPO_4^{2-}. Phosphorus is an essential constituent of all cells and is found in both plants and animals. Adults absorb about 55% to 70% of dietary phosphorus, primarily in the small intestine. The active form of vitamin D (1,25-dihydroxyvitamin D, or calcitriol) facilitates the absorption of phosphorus, whereas consumption of aluminum-containing antacids and high doses of calcium carbonate reduce its absorption. The kidneys regulate reabsorption and urinary excretion of phosphorus.

Phosphorus works with potassium inside the cell to maintain proper fluid balance. It also plays a critical role in bone formation, as it is a part of the mineral complex of bone. In fact, about 85% of the body's phosphorus is stored in the bones.

As a primary component of ATP, phosphorus plays a key role in creating energy for the body through the reactions in glycolysis and oxidative phosphorylation. It also helps regulate many biochemical reactions by activating and deactivating enzymes during phosphorylation. Phosphorus is a part of both DNA and RNA, and it is a component of cell membranes (as phospholipids) and of lipoproteins.

The RDA for phosphorus is 700 mg per day.[19] The average U.S. adult consumes about twice this amount each day; thus, phosphorus deficiencies are rare. Phosphorus is widespread in many foods; high protein foods such as milk, meats, and eggs are good sources of phosphorus (**Figure 9.10**).

It is important to note that phosphorus from animal sources is absorbed more readily than phosphorus from plant sources. Much of the phosphorus in plant foods such as beans, whole-grain cereals, and nuts is found in the form of **phytic acid,** a plant storage form of phosphorus. Our bodies do not produce enzymes that can break down phytic acid, but we are still able to absorb up to 50% of the phosphorus found in plant foods because the bacteria in the large intestine can break down phytic acid. Soft drinks are another common source of phosphorus in the American diet.

People suffering from kidney disease and people taking too many vitamin D supplements or too many phosphorus-containing antacids can suffer from high blood phosphorus levels. Severely high levels of blood phosphorus cause muscle spasms and convulsions.

phytic acid The form of phosphorus stored in plants.

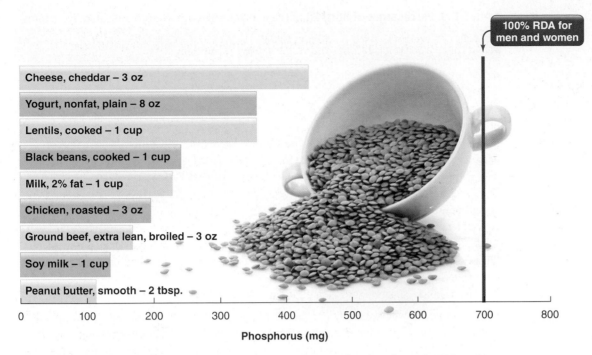

100% RDA for
men and women

Cheese, cheddar – 3 oz

Yogurt, nonfat, plain – 8 oz

Lentils, cooked – 1 cup

Black beans, cooked – 1 cup

Milk, 2% fat – 1 cup

Chicken, roasted – 3 oz

Ground beef, extra lean, broiled – 3 oz

Soy milk – 1 cup

Peanut butter, smooth – 2 tbsp.

| 0 | 100 | 200 | 300 | 400 | 500 | 600 | 700 | 800 |

Phosphorus (mg)

FIGURE 9.10 Common food sources of phosphorus. The RDA for phosphorus is 700 mg/day. (*Source:* Data from U.S. Department of Agriculture, Agricultural Research Service. 2009. USDA Nutrient Database for Standard Reference, Release 22. Nutrient Data Laboratory Home Page. www.ars.usda.gov/ba/bhnrc/ndl.)

As previously noted, deficiencies of phosphorus are rare. People who may suffer from low blood phosphorus levels include premature infants, elderly people with poor diets, and people who abuse alcohol. People with vitamin D deficiency or hyperparathyroidism (oversecretion of parathyroid hormone), and those who overuse antacids that bind with phosphorus may also have low blood phosphorus levels.

RECAP

Chloride is the major anion outside the cell, and phosphorus is the major anion inside the cell. Both are important for fluid balance. Chloride is also a component of HCl, and phosphorus is a component of bone. The AI for chloride is 2.3 g per day. Our main dietary source of chloride is sodium chloride. There are no known toxicity symptoms. The RDA for phosphorus is 700 mg per day, and it is commonly found in high-protein foods. High blood phosphorus levels can cause muscle spasms and convulsions. Deficiencies of either chloride or phosphorus are rare. ■

What Disorders Are Related to Fluid and Electrolyte Imbalances?

A number of serious, and potentially fatal, disorders can result from an imbalance of fluid and electrolytes in the body, while other disorders contribute to fluid and electrolyte imbalance. We review some of these here.

Dehydration Develops When Fluid Loss Exceeds Fluid Intake

Dehydration is a serious health problem that results when fluid losses exceed fluid intake. It can occur as a result of heavy exercise or exposure to high environmental temperatures, when the body loses significant amounts of water through increased sweating

LO 9 Describe several disorders related to fluid and electrolyte imbalance and identify their signs and symptoms.

LO 10 Define *hypertension* and list three lifestyle changes that can reduce it.

dehydration The depletion of body fluid, which results when fluid excretion exceeds fluid intake.

Adequate hydration

Minor dehydration

Severe dehydration

FIGURE 9.11 Urine color chart. Color variations indicate levels of hydration.

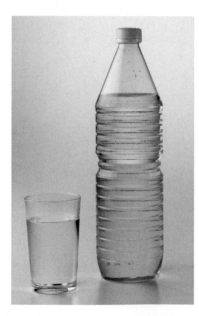

Dehydration occurs when fluid losses exceed fluid intake.

heat stroke A potentially fatal heat illness characterized by hot, dry skin; rapid heart rate; vomiting; diarrhea; elevated body temperature; hallucinations; and coma.

TABLE 9.3 Percentages of Body Fluid Loss Correlated with Weight Loss and Symptoms

% Body Fluid Loss	Weight Lost If You Weigh 160 lb	Weight Lost If You Weigh 130 lb	Symptoms
1–2	1.6 lb–3.2 lb	1.3 lb–2.6 lb	Strong thirst, loss of appetite, feeling uncomfortable
3–5	4.8 lb–8.0 lb	3.9 lb–6.5 lb	Dry mouth, reduced urine output, greater difficulty working and concentrating, flushed skin, tingling extremities, impatience, sleepiness, nausea, emotional instability
6–8	9.6 lb–12.8 lb	7.8 lb–10.4 lb	Increased body temperature that doesn't decrease, increased heart rate and breathing rate, dizziness, difficulty breathing, slurred speech, mental confusion, muscle weakness, blue lips
9–11	14.4 lb–17.6 lb	11.7 lb–14.3 lb	Muscle spasms, delirium, swollen tongue, poor balance and circulation, kidney failure, decreased blood volume and blood pressure

and breathing. However, elderly people and infants can get dehydrated even when inactive, as their risk for dehydration is much higher than that of healthy young and middle-aged adults. The elderly are at increased risk because they have a lower total amount of body fluid and their thirst mechanism is less effective than that of a younger person; they are therefore less likely to meet their fluid needs. Infants, on the other hand, excrete urine at a higher rate, cannot tell us when they are thirsty, and have a greater ratio of body surface area to body core, causing their bodies to respond more dramatically to heat and cold and to lose more body fluid than older children.

Dehydration is classified in terms of the percentage of weight loss that is exclusively due to the loss of fluid. As indicated in **Table 9.3,** relatively small losses in body fluid result in symptoms such as thirst, discomfort, and loss of appetite. More severe fluid losses result in symptoms that include sleepiness, nausea, flushed skin, and problems with mental concentration. Severe losses of body fluid can result in delirium, coma, cardiac arrest, and death.

We discussed earlier the importance of fluid replacement when you are exercising. How can you tell whether you are drinking enough fluid before, during, and after your exercise sessions? First, you can measure your body weight before and after each session. If you weighed in at 160 lb before basketball practice, and immediately afterward you weigh 158 lb, then you have lost 2 lb of body weight. This is equal to 1.3% of your body weight prior to practice. As you can see in Table 9.3, you are most likely feeling strong thirst, diminished appetite, and even general discomfort. Your goal is to consume enough water and other fluids to fully rehydrate prior to your next exercise session. This would require drinking about 1.5 times as much fluid as was lost (1 pound of weight loss equals 2 cups of fluid).[20]

A simpler method of monitoring your fluid levels is to observe the color of your urine (**Figure 9.11**). If you are properly hydrated, your urine should be clear to pale yellow in color, similar to diluted lemonade. Urine that is medium to dark yellow in color, similar to apple juice, indicates an inadequate fluid intake. Very dark or brown-colored urine, such as the color of a cola beverage, is a sign of severe dehydration and indicates potential muscle breakdown and kidney damage. People should strive to maintain a urine color that is clear or pale yellow.

Heat Stroke Is a Medical Emergency

Heat stroke is a potentially fatal heat illness characterized by failure of the body's heat-regulating mechanisms. Symptoms include rapid pulse; hot, dry skin; high temperature; vomiting; diarrhea; hallucinations; and loss of consciousness (coma).

Recall that evaporative cooling is less efficient in a humid environment, because sweat is less able to evaporate. Therefore, athletes who work out in hot, humid weather are particularly vulnerable to heat stroke. Over the past decade, 31 football players have died of heat-related complications, most of them high school players.[21] These deaths are more common in overweight or obese athletes for two reasons. Significant muscle mass produces a lot of body heat, while excess body fat adds an extra layer of insulation that makes it more difficult to dissipate that heat. Tight-fitting uniforms and helmets also trap warm air and blunt the body's ability to cool itself.

Heat-related deaths also occur among other collegiate and professional athletes, such as endurance runners. These deaths have prompted national attention and resulted in strict guidelines encouraging regular fluid breaks and cancellation of events or changing the time of the event to avoid high heat and humidity. In addition, people who are active in a hot environment should stop exercising if they feel dizzy, light-headed, disoriented, or nauseated. When these symptoms are accompanied by hot, dry skin, the person needs immediate cooling, preferably by immersion in an ice bath, and emergency medical care. Heat illnesses can be avoided by following established guidelines for fluid intake before, during, and after exercise.

Water Intoxication Can Be Fatal

Overhydration, or *water intoxication,* is rare. It generally occurs only in people with health problems that cause the kidneys to retain too much water, causing overhydration and hyponatremia, which were discussed earlier. However, individuals have died of overhydration while following a fad diet or participating in a hazing ritual or competition involving excessive water intake. In 2012, for example, a 12-year-old girl died after participating in a card game with friends in which the loser of each hand had to drink a glass of water. Thus, the overconsumption of water can be deadly and should never be thought of as a prank or a joke.

A Majority of Americans Have Hypertension or Prehypertension

One of the major chronic diseases in the United States, **hypertension (HTN)** is estimated to affect nearly 70 million U.S. adults, or about one-third of the population. Another 1 in 3 have *prehypertension,* a condition in which blood pressure is above normal but not yet high enough to be diagnosed as HTN.[22] The prevalence of HTN is even higher (43–46%) among African American adults.[22] Although HTN itself is often without symptoms, it increases a person's risk for many other serious conditions, including heart disease, stroke, and kidney disease; it can also reduce brain function, impair physical mobility, and cause death.

Diagnosis

There are no obvious symptoms of HTN. For this reason, it is important that people get their blood pressure checked on a regular basis. Blood pressure is measured in two phases: systolic and diastolic. *Systolic blood pressure* represents the pressure exerted in the arteries at the moment that the heart contracts, sending blood into the blood vessels. *Diastolic blood pressure* represents the pressure in the arteries between contractions, when the heart is relaxed. You can also think of diastolic blood pressure as the resistance in the arteries that the heart must pump against every time it beats. Blood pressure is measured in millimeters of mercury (mm Hg). When your blood pressure is measured, the systolic pressure is given first, followed by the diastolic pressure. For example, your reading might be given as "115 (systolic) over 75 (diastolic)." Here are the clinical classifications of blood pressure measurements:

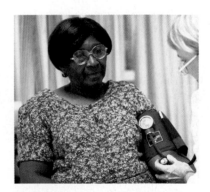

Hypertension is a major chronic disease in the United States, affecting more than 50% of adults over 65 years of age.

- Optimal blood pressure is a systolic blood pressure *less than* 120 mm Hg and a diastolic blood pressure *less than* 80 mm Hg.
- Pre-hypertension is defined as a systolic blood pressure between 120 and 139 mm Hg or a diastolic blood pressure between 80 and 89 mm Hg.
- Hypertension is a systolic blood pressure greater than or equal to 140 mm Hg or a diastolic blood pressure greater than or equal to 90 mm Hg.

Causes and Risk Factors

For about 90% to 95% of people who have HTN, the cause is unknown.[23] This type is referred to as *primary,* or *essential, hypertension.* For the other 5% to 10% of people with HTN, the causes include kidney disease, sleep apnea (a sleep disorder that affects

overhydration The dilution of body fluid. It results when water intake or retention is excessive.

hypertension A chronic condition characterized by above-average blood pressure readings—specifically, systolic blood pressure over 140 mm Hg or diastolic blood pressure over 90 mm Hg.

breathing), and chronic alcohol abuse. It is estimated that about two-thirds of all adults with HTN have a condition known as **salt sensitivity.** These people respond to a high salt intake by experiencing an increase in blood pressure; they also experience a decrease in blood pressure when salt intake is low. People who do not experience changes in blood pressure with changes in salt intake are referred to as **salt resistant.**

Risk factors associated with HTN include overweight and obesity, as increased blood volume leads to increased pressure on blood vessel walls. A sedentary lifestyle also increases the risk. Tobacco use is a primary risk factor, because it immediately raises blood pressure, and chronic use damages the lining of the blood vessels, increasing the likelihood of plaque deposition. Excessive alcohol intake and a diet high in sodium and low in potassium are also risk factors.

Prevention

Although we do not know what causes most cases of HTN, certain lifestyle changes can help reduce it:[23, 24]

- Lose excess weight. Losing just 10 pounds can lower blood pressure although, in general, the more you lose, the lower your blood pressure.
- Exercise regularly. The amount and intensity of exercise needed to improve blood pressure are easily achievable for most people. Regular physical activity, such as brisk walking, lasting at least 30 minutes per day most days of the week, can help lower blood pressure.
- Limit your alcohol intake. Because alcohol consumption can worsen HTN, it is suggested that people with this disease abstain from drinking alcohol or limit their intake to no more than one (women) or two (men) drinks per day.
- Reduce your sodium intake, especially if you are salt sensitive. Some people who are not salt sensitive also benefit from eating lower-sodium diets.
- Eat more whole grains, fruits, vegetables, and low-fat dairy foods.
- Avoid all tobacco products. If you currently use tobacco, quit.

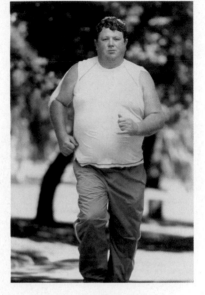

Losing weight and increasing physical activity can help fight hypertension.

To download a comprehensive guide to the DASH diet, go to www.nhlbi.nih.gov.

The Role of the DASH Diet Plan

The **DASH diet** was developed according to research sponsored by the National Institutes of Health. DASH stands for Dietary Approaches to Stop Hypertension. The diet emphasizes high fiber, low fat foods that are rich in potassium, calcium, and magnesium, including 10 servings of fruits and vegetables each day along with whole-grain foods and low-fat or nonfat milk and dairy products. The sodium content of the DASH diet is about 3 g (or 3,000 mg) of sodium, which is slightly less than the average sodium intake in the United States. **Figure 9.12** (page 369) shows the DASH diet plan for an energy intake of 2,000 kcal per day.

Numerous studies have demonstrated the effectiveness of the DASH diet in lowering both systolic and diastolic blood pressure. The greatest reductions occur in those with higher baseline blood pressure and BMI values, in males, and in persons combining a lower sodium intake with the DASH diet.[25,26] In addition, the DASH diet, compared to the typical American diet, reduces cardiovascular risk factors such as total and LDL cholesterol levels and inflammation.[25] Finally, a dietary pattern that mimics the DASH diet has been shown to be particularly beneficial in reducing mortality among African Americans, a population group at very high risk for HTN and its complications.[27]

The Role of Medications

For some individuals, lifestyle changes are not completely effective in normalizing blood pressure. When this is the case, medications are typically prescribed. Individuals taking medications to control blood pressure also are advised to continue to practice the healthful lifestyle changes identified earlier.

Hypertension is called "the silent killer" because people commonly fail to take their prescribed medication because they do not feel sick. Some of these people eventually suffer a fatal heart attack or stroke.

salt sensitivity A condition in which certain people respond to a high salt intake by experiencing an increase in blood pressure; these people also experience a decrease in blood pressure when salt intake is low.

salt resistant A condition in which certain people do not experience changes in blood pressure with changes in salt intake.

DASH diet The Dietary Approaches to Stop Hypertension diet plan emphasizing fruits and vegetables, whole grains, low/no-fat milk and dairy, and lean meats.

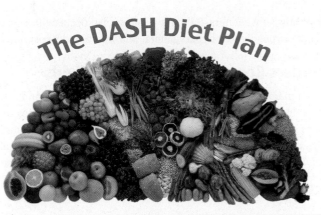

The DASH Diet Plan

FIGURE 9.12 The DASH diet plan. The plan is based on a 2,000-kcal-per-day diet. The number of servings in a food group may differ from the number listed here, depending on your own energy needs. (*Source:* "Healthier Eating with DASH," National Institutes of Health from National Heart, Lung and Blood Institute website.)

Food Group	Daily Servings	Serving Size
Grains and grain products	7–8	1 slice bread 1 cup ready-to-eat cereal* ½ cup cooked rice, pasta, or cereal
Vegetables	4–5	1 cup raw leafy vegetables ½ cup cooked vegetable 6 fl. oz vegetable juice
Fruits	4–5	1 medium fruit ¼ cup dried fruit ½ cup fresh, frozen, or canned fruit 6 fl. oz fruit juice
Low-fat or fat-free dairy foods	2–3	8 fl. oz milk 1 cup yogurt 1½ oz cheese
Lean meats, poultry, and fish	2 or less	3 oz cooked lean meats, skinless poultry, or fish
Nuts, seeds, and dry beans	4–5 per week	⅓ cup or 1½ oz nuts 1 tbsp. or ½ oz seeds ½ cup cooked dry beans
Fats and oils†	2–3	1 tsp. soft margarine 1 tbsp. low-fat mayonnaise 2 tbsp. light salad dressing 1 tsp. vegetable oil
Sweets	5 per week	1 tbsp. sugar 1 tbsp. jelly or jam ½ oz jelly beans 8 fl. oz lemonade

*Serving sizes vary between ½ and 1¼ cups. Check the product's nutrition label.

†Fat content changes serving counts for fats and oils: for example, 1 tablespoon of regular salad dressing equals 1 serving; 1 tablespoon of a low-fat dressing equals ½ serving; 1 tablespoon of a fat-free dressing equals 0 servings.

Electrolyte Imbalances Can Cause Seizures

Because electrolytes are necessary for the initiation and transmission of nerve impulses, electrolyte imbalances commonly affect the nervous system. In fact, the first sign of an electrolyte imbalance may be a **seizure,** a sudden and usually transient episode of abnormal electrical activity in the brain. Because nerves synapse with muscles, seizures typically trigger uncontrollable muscle spasms that may be localized to one area of the body, such as the face, or can violently wrack a person's entire body. The person may lose consciousness, and confusion and memory loss is common following the seizure.

Muscle cramps are involuntary, spasmodic, and painful muscle contractions that last for many seconds or even minutes. They do not affect the brain. Muscle cramps are common with imbalances of calcium and magnesium, as well as with hypernatremia that occurs

seizures A sudden episode of abnormal electrical activity in the brain that can result from electrolyte imbalances or a chronic disease, such as epilepsy.

muscle cramps Involuntary, spasmodic, and painful muscle contractions that last for many seconds or even minutes; electrolyte imbalances are often the cause of muscle cramps.

with dehydration. Muscle weakness and paralysis can also occur with severe electrolyte imbalances, such as hypokalemia, hyperkalemia, and low blood phosphorus levels.

Kidney Disorders Commonly Affect Body Fluids

The kidneys play a major role in the regulation of fluid, electrolyte, and acid–base balance, so it is not surprising that diseases of the kidneys result in abnormalities throughout the body. Many forms of kidney disease lead to edema and abnormal retention of body fluid, since the kidneys are no longer able to effectively excrete excess fluid. Similarly, blood levels of many electrolytes, such as sodium, potassium, and phosphorus, increase to dangerously high concentrations. High levels of potassium can lead to abnormal heart rhythms and heart failure, while increased levels of phosphorus can drive down serum calcium levels.

Congestive Heart Failure May Be Managed with Fluid Restriction

Congestive heart failure (CHF) is a condition in which the heart can no longer pump an adequate supply of blood to the rest of the body and, as venous return to the heart slows, fluid accumulates in body tissues. It can develop following an infection involving the heart or from coronary artery disease, heart valve disease, or other disorders. Fluid can accumulate in the legs and feet, as well as the abdominal area, and in the lungs, causing shortness of breath and inability to maintain activity levels. Management of congestive heart failure often includes restriction of sodium and fluids to reduce blood volume and strain on the heart. To calculate appropriate fluid restriction for a client with CHF, see the *You Do the Math* box (below).

Intake of Sugary Drinks Can Promote Obesity

Among many Americans, inappropriate beverage choices contribute significantly to overweight and obesity. Until about 50 years ago, beverage choices were fairly limited and serving sizes were small—the original bottles of Coca-Cola held just 6 to 7 ounces! The introduction of a very cheap sweetener, high-fructose corn syrup, and dramatic changes in the sizing, marketing, and sales of beverages, has led to a surge in the popularity of super-size sodas and other sugary drinks. Today, a convenience-store soda may hold 64 ounces, with 59 teaspoons of sugar and 800 Calories!

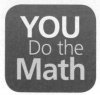

Calculating Fluid Restriction

Fluid restriction is often required in the management of congestive heart failure (CHF). A typical fluid "prescription" is 30 mL/kg body weight/day. Suppose that one of your older relatives suffers from CHF and asks you to help figure out a day's worth of beverages. (In this example, we will ignore the water content of foods, although many dietitians include foods when calculating the fluid intake of seriously ill patients.) Your relative weighs 168 lb and enjoys drinking milk, orange juice, and plain water.

In order to calculate how many fluid ounces are permitted each day, you will first need to convert body weight from pounds to kilograms:

$$168 \text{ lb} \div 2.2 \text{ lb/kg} = 76.4 \text{ kg}$$

Next, multiply the fluid allowance of 30 mL/kg by body weight:

$$30 \text{ mL/kg} \times 76.4 \text{ kg} = 2,292 \text{ mL}$$

Finally, convert mL to fluid ounces. There are roughly 30 mL/fl. oz:

$$2,292 \text{ mL} \div 30 \text{ mL/fl. oz} = \text{around } 76 \text{ fl. oz}$$

Your relative could drink 12 fl. oz of milk, 8 fl. oz of orange juice, and 56 fl. oz of water or other beverages.

Here is a similar problem for you to solve: a young woman is restricted to 25 mL/kg body weight/day. She weighs 122 lb. How much total fluid (in fluid ounces) is she allowed to drink each day?

Answers are located online in the MasteringNutrition Study Area.

Although sales of sugary drinks have dropped considerably over the past few years and Americans are now getting fewer Calories from them,[6,15] beverages continue to account for approximately 20% of our daily energy intake. The major culprits are sweetened soft drinks and fruit juices. As we discussed earlier, sweetened bottled waters, bottled teas, energy drinks, and specialty coffee drinks have also contributed to the problem: a "frappucino" at one prominent national coffee chain provides 520 Calories, which is more than one-fourth of an average adult's total daily Calorie needs.

Beverages with a high Calorie content do little to curb appetite, so most people do not compensate for the extra Calories they drink by eating less. In addition, sugary drinks displace more nutritious beverages, such as milk, which provides protein, calcium, vitamin D, and other nutrients important for bone health.

In the past, very few people realized how many Calories were in the sugary drinks they consumed, and how such beverages were contributing to the growing problem of obesity. Recently, however, public health agencies have been raising awareness of the empty Calorie content of sugary drinks, and some are advocating that a first step in any weight-loss program should be to entirely eliminate these products from the diet. Members of the American Beverage Association launched a "Clear on Calories" campaign, which prominently displays Calorie information on the front of the product. All beverages packaged in containers 20 fl. oz or smaller now display the total Calories per package, not just per serving. Thus, when consumers buy a 20-oz bottle of sweetened tea, they know they'll be consuming, for example, 250 Calories if they drink the whole bottle.

RECAP

Dehydration, heat stroke, and even death can occur when water loss exceeds water intake. Hypertension is a major chronic illness in the United States; it can often be controlled by losing weight if overweight, increasing physical activity, avoiding smoking, decreasing alcohol intake, and making specific dietary changes, such as those in the DASH diet. Electrolyte imbalances can lead to seizures and muscle cramps. Fluid and electrolyte imbalances can result from diseases such as certain forms of kidney and heart failure. Excessive intake of sugary beverages can contribute significantly to obesity.

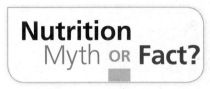

Low Sodium Diets: Fit for All or Just a Few?

For decades, U.S. and international public health organizations have almost unanimously recommended a "low" sodium diet to prevent and treat hypertension (HTN) and reduce the risk for heart disease.[1] Many still do. Yet recently, some organizations have modified their sodium intake recommendations in response to recent research suggesting that a low sodium intake may not benefit the population as a whole, and may even increase health risks. So who should reduce their sodium intake? Should you? Keeping in mind that nutrition research is always providing new information, let's explore our current understanding of this issue.

How Have Sodium Intake Recommendations Evolved Over Time?

Prior to 2005, the *Dietary Guidelines for Americans* (DGA) used only descriptive phrases, not specific numerical targets, for their sodium intake recommendations:

1980 and 1985: "Avoid too much sodium."
1990: "Use salt and sodium only in moderation."
1995: "Choose a diet moderate in salt and sodium."
2000: "Choose and prepare foods with less salt."[2]

But in 2005, the recommendations changed, specifying precise intake levels. Both the 2005 and 2010 DGA recommended a sodium intake of less than 2,300 mg per day, with a further reduction to 1,500 mg per day for those Americans 51 years of age and older and those who are African American or have hypertension, diabetes, or chronic kidney disease.[1]

Why the change? As with all national dietary recommendations, the 2005 and 2010 guidelines were set after a thorough and careful review of human research available at the time, including epidemiologic or observational studies, double-blind clinical trials, and community based

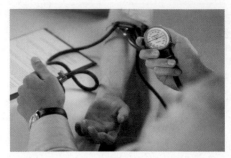

intervention studies. As discussed (in Chapter 1), all of these types of research studies have different advantages and disadvantages. Moreover, many of the research studies reviewed had specific flaws. For example, some researchers "measured" dietary sodium intake (notoriously inaccurate!) or used a one-time morning urine sample instead of the gold-standard measure of 24-hour urinary sodium excretion. Other studies included both sodium restriction and weight loss to assess the impact of lifestyle change on risk of heart disease, which then made it difficult to determine the effect of sodium restriction alone. Some studies focused on men only, or just older adults, or one specific ethnic group. After reviewing hundreds of different studies and summarizing the strengths and limitations of their results, the DGA panel rated the evidence and formed a consensus agreement about what their recommendations should be.

Not all public health organizations agreed with the 2005 and 2010 DGA numerical targets. In 2009, the American Heart Association (AHA) stated that the DGA recommendation of 2,300 mg of sodium per day was "too high" and proposed "no more than 1,500 mg of sodium per day" for everyone.[3] In 2012, the World Health Organization (WHO) recommended a target intake of 2,000 mg per day—300 mg per day lower than the DGA guideline—for all adults not under medical care.[4]

Why these disagreements? The AHA and the WHO each had their own experts review the research and they simply came up with different conclusions. And, as new research became available each year, the controversy over sodium guidelines continued.

What Changes in Sodium Intake Did the 2015 DGA Advisory Committee Recommend?

In 2015, the Dietary Guidelines Advisory Committee published guidelines that differed from the 2005 and 2010 recommendations in four key ways.[5]

■ Instead of addressing the U.S. population as a whole, the Advisory Committee aimed their advice at "adults who would benefit from a reduction in blood pressure."

■ The final 2015 *Dietary Guidelines* recommend limiting sodium intake to no more than 2,300 mg per day. And instead of identifying specific populations who should reduce sodium to 1,500 mg per day, the Advisory Committee simply acknowledged that reducing sodium intake to 1,500 mg per day would lower blood pressure even more.

■ Recognizing that Americans consume, on average, nearly 3,500 mg of sodium per day (well above the AI of 1,200–1,500 mg per day, depending upon age), the Advisory Committee argued that even if the 2,300 or 1,500 mg goals could not be met, a reduction of 1,000 mg of sodium per day, regardless of intake, would effectively lower blood pressure.

■ The Advisory Committee acknowledged the importance of one's total dietary patterns, in addition to single nutrients such as sodium, by confirming that the DASH diet combined with a lower sodium intake would also help reduce blood pressure.

The members of the 2015 Dietary Guidelines Advisory Committee made these changes in light of new information from recent research studies that they could evaluate and "grade" in terms of the strength of the evidence. For example, the Committee felt there was "strong" evidence to support the statement that "adults who would benefit from blood pressure lowering should lower sodium intake" but found only "limited" evidence that "higher dietary sodium intake is associated with a greater risk for fatal and nonfatal stroke and CVD (cardiovascular disease)." In part, the Committee 's report reflected the findings of a 2013 Institute of Medicine (IOM) report on sodium and cardiovascular disease. The IOM report confirmed that the risk of CVD increased as sodium intake increased; however, it did not find significant benefits of limiting sodium intake to 1,500 mg per day for either the population as a whole or the high risk groups described above.[6] In addition, it identified certain health risks associated with a sodium intake of 1,500 mg per day among people with diabetes, kidney disease, or cardiovascular disease, including increased risk of "all cause mortality." In short, in the years following the 2010 DGAs, enough new research had been published to support a change in recommendations.

How Do Other Organizations' Sodium Recommendations Differ?

Many public health organizations' sodium recommendations related to the prevention and treatment of hypertension conflict at least in part with the 2015 DGA Advisory Committee:

■ The American Heart Association continues to recommend that ALL Americans consume less than 1,500 mg of sodium per day to lower the incidence of high blood pressure and heart disease.[7]

■ The American Society of Hypertension and the International Society of Hypertension also continue to recognize high dietary salt as a major factor in the causation of hypertension, particularly among persons of African ancestry. While not establishing a specific numerical goal, their guidelines state that, "reduction of salt intake is recommended because it can reduce blood pressure and decrease the need for medications in patients who are 'salt sensitive,' which may be a fairly common finding in black communities."[8]

- The World Health Organization (WHO) continues to recommend the consumption of no more than 2,000 mg of sodium per day.[4]

  Here are a few factors that contribute to the differences in recommendations:

- As previously discussed, the research studies used in developing the recommendations vary widely in their design, the populations measured, and the measures taken. With thousands of research articles reporting on dietary sodium and health, it is not surprising that there are different interpretations.

- Different organizations have different goals. The American Heart Association is most concerned with preventing CVD among Americans, while the World Health Organization's goal is to relieve the global burden of disease.

- Some recommendations account for the highly beneficial effect of dietary potassium when establishing sodium guidelines, while others do not. It is well known that higher intakes of dietary potassium lower risk of HTN, especially among those with high sodium intakes.

- Each advisory panel is made up of a different group of scientists, each of whom has a unique bias. Although well trained in the scientific method, some researchers simply interpret the data in ways that differ from those of their peers.

Should You Reduce Your Sodium Intake?

Given the level of uncertainty regarding the most healthful sodium intake, what steps can you take to apply the different opinions to your own situation?

- First, recognize that lifestyle interventions, including food choices, are low risk, low cost approaches to preventing chronic diseases and, for people already affected, can be effective treatments. Thus, most Americans would do well to reduce their current intake of sodium by at least 1,000 mg per day.

- Second, since most of us have no idea how much sodium we actually eat, the most practical approach is to look at dietary patterns. Following the DASH or Mediterranean diet can greatly reduce sodium intake with no known health risks. These diets will also increase potassium intake, a proven lifestyle change to lower risk of HTN.

- Third, limit the use of highly processed foods such as packaged or frozen dinners and choose low/no salt canned products. Emphasize fresh foods as much as possible.

- Fourth, remember that the benefits of lowering sodium intake will be even stronger when combined with other lifestyle interventions such as increased physical activity, smoking cessation, weight management, and moderation of alcohol intake.[8]

- Finally, focus on gradual change. A modest increase in fruit and vegetable intake and regular physical activity along with fewer restaurant meals can make a significant and lasting impact.

In addition to the steps just described, people with diagnosed medical conditions and/or a strong family history of specific diseases should always consult with their health care team, including a Registered Dietitian Nutritionist (RDN), to determine the best dietary pattern for their unique needs.

Critical-Thinking Questions

- After reading about the sodium controversy, do you plan to cut back on your sodium intake? If so, what are three dietary changes you could make?

- Now that you know the health benefits of the DASH diet, would you be willing to try and increase your fruit and vegetable intake to 10 servings a day? Why or why not?

- Would you rather have one set of dietary guidelines, even if they aren't perfect, or be able to evaluate the different opinions of various health organizations and come to your own conclusions?

References

1. U.S. Department of Agriculture and U.S. Department of Health and Human Services. *Dietary Guidelines for Americans, 2010*. 7th Edn. Washington, DC.: U.S. Government Printing Office, December 2010.
2. Center for Nutrition and Health Policy. 2000. *Dietary Guidelines for Americans,* 1980-2000. Available at http://www.health.gov/dietaryguidelines/1980_2000_chart.pdf. (accessed May 2015).
3. Gardner, T. J. 2009. Letter to C. Davis, U.S. Department of Agriculture and K. McMurry, Department of Health and Human Services. Available at http://www.heart.org/idc/groups/heart-public/@wcm/@adv/documents/downloadable/ucm_312853.pdf (Accessed May 2015).
4. World Health Organization. *Guideline: Sodium intake for adults and children*. Geneva, World Health Organization (WHO), 2012. Available at http://www.who.int/nutrition/publications/guidelines/sodium_intake_printversion.pdf.
5. Institute of Medicine. 2015. Dietary Guidelines Advisory Committee *Scientific Report of the 2015 Dietary Guidelines Advisory Committee*. Washington DC: National Academies Press; 2015. Available at http://www.health.gov/dietaryguidelines/2015-scientific-report/02-executive-summary.asp (Accessed April 2015).
6. Institute of Medicine. 2013. *Sodium Intake in Populations: Assessment of Evidence*. Washington, DC.: National Academies Press.
7. American Heart Association. 2013. New IOM report an incomplete review of sodium's impact, says American Heart Association. Available from http://newsroom.heart.org/news/new-iom-report-an-incomplete-review-of-sodiums-impact-says-american-heart-association. (accessed April 2015).
8. Weber, M. A., E. L. Schiffrin, W. B. White, S. Mann, L. H. Lindholm, J. G. Kenerson,…, and S. B. Harrap. 2014. Clinical practice guidelines for the management of hypertension in the community. *J. Clin. Hypertension*. 16:12–26.

STUDY PLAN MasteringNutrition™

Customize your study plan—and master your nutrition!—in the Study Area of MasteringNutrition.

TEST YOURSELF | ANSWERS

1. **T** Between approximately 50% and 70% of our body weight consists of fluid.

2. **F** Sodium is a nutrient necessary for health, but we should not consume more than recommended amounts.

3. **F** Children rarely exercise to the point of needing the added sugar and electrolytes found in sports beverages. Pure water is almost always the best choice.

4. **F** There is no evidence that bottled water consistently offers any additional health or nutrition benefits compared to tap water.

5. **F** We do not know the precise cause of high blood pressure in most people. A high-sodium diet, however, can contribute to high blood pressure in a subset of people who are sensitive to sodium.

summary

Scan to hear an MP3 Chapter Review in **MasteringNutrition**.

LO 1 ■ Approximately 50% to 70% of a healthy adult's body weight is fluid. Two-thirds of this fluid is intracellular fluid, meaning that it is enclosed within the membrane of body cells. One-third is extracellular fluid. This includes interstitial—or tissue—fluid as well as intravascular fluid found within the blood and lymphatic vessels.

■ Electrolytes are electrically charged atoms—cations and anions—found in body fluid that assist in maintaining fluid balance and the normal functioning of cells and the nervous system. Six major minerals form the body's most important electrolytes. These are sodium, potassium, chloride, and phosphorus, which are critical to fluid balance, and calcium and magnesium, which are important in muscle contraction and bone health.

LO 2 ■ Water acts as a solvent and a transport fluid. It also acts to maintain blood volume, blood pressure, and body temperature, and provides protection and lubrication for organs and tissues.

■ The health of body cells and tissues depends on maintaining a balance between water and electrolytes on both sides of the cell membrane. Electrolytes help maintain this balance by exerting osmotic pressure, the extent of which cells can regulate by using transport proteins to pump electrolytes across their membrane. The movement of sodium and potassium ions across the cell membrane is essential in the transmission of nerve impulses, and the release of calcium ions from their intracellular storage site is essential for muscle contraction.

LO 3 ■ The kidneys play a key role in regulating blood volume and blood pressure by shifting their excretion and retention of water and electrolytes.

LO 4 ■ The two primary sources of fluid intake are beverages and foods we consume and the metabolic water produced by chemical reactions during metabolism.

■ The primary avenues of fluid excretion are sensible water loss (urine and sweat), insensible water loss (via evaporation from the skin and exhalation from the lungs), and feces.

- Conditions that significantly increase fluid loss from our bodies include fever, vomiting, diarrhea, hemorrhage, blood donation, heavy exercise, and exposure to heat, cold, and altitude. During pregnancy and breastfeeding, the mother loses fluids and requires increased intake. Diuretics, including certain prescription and over-the-counter drugs, some dietary supplements, and alcohol, can cause excessive fluid losses.

LO 5
- The body relies on blood buffers, the respiratory system, and the kidneys to maintain normal acid–base balance. Blood buffers, such as blood proteins and the bicarbonate-carbonic acid system, can take up hydrogen ions, increasing blood pH, or release hydrogen ions, reducing pH. In the lungs, increased or decreased respiration can influence the blood level of carbonic acid. Finally, renal secretion or excretion of bicarbonate can influence the pH of blood.

LO 6
- Fluid intake needs are highly variable and depend on body size, age, physical activity, health status, and environmental conditions. The DRI for adult men is 3.7 L of total water per day, an amount that includes about 3.0 L (or 13 cups) in beverages and food. The DRI for adult women is 2.7 L of total water, which is about 2.2 L (9 cups) in beverages and food.
- Some beverages, such as milk and milk alternatives, provide important nutrients. Hot coffee and tea, especially when made with milk, can be nutritious, and their phytochemicals may have health benefits. Moreover, moderate caffeine intake has not been shown to significantly decrease fluid status. Many other beverages, from soft drinks to specialty waters, provide little more than empty Calories. Sports drinks are most appropriate for athletes. Energy drinks have been associated with seizures, cardiac arrest, and death, as well as other health problems. They are inappropriate for children and adolescents, and should be consumed only in limited amounts, if at all, by adults.

LO 7
- Sodium is the primary cation in the extracellular fluid. It assists in maintaining fluid balance, blood pressure, transmission of nerve impulses, and muscle contraction. It also assists the absorption of glucose from the small intestine.
- The AI for sodium is 1.5 g per day. Consuming excess sodium can contribute to hypertension in some people.
- Potassium is the primary cation in the intracellular fluid. It thereby works with sodium in maintaining fluid balance, healthy blood pressure, and the transmission of nerve impulses, and aids in muscle contraction.
- The AI for potassium is 4.7 g per day, more than triple the AI for sodium. Potassium is found in

a variety of fresh foods, especially fruits and vegetables, and is low in most processed foods.
- Hyperkalemia is high blood potassium, and typically occurs as a result of kidney disease. Hypokalemia is low blood potassium and can occur as a result of kidney disease, diabetic acidosis, and the use of some diuretic medications.
- Chloride is the primary anion in the extracellular fluid. It assists in maintaining fluid balance, normal nerve-impulse transmission, and the chemical digestion of food via the action of HCl in the stomach. It also has antibacterial functions.
- Phosphorus is the primary anion in the intracellular fluid. It assists in maintaining fluid balance and transferring energy via ATP. It is also a component of bone, phospholipids, genetic material, and lipoproteins. Vitamin D boosts phosphorus absorption, whereas consumption of aluminum-containing antacids and high doses of calcium carbonate reduce its absorption.

LO 8
- A high blood sodium level is called hypernatremia. Eating a high-sodium diet does not usually cause hypernatremia in a healthy person, as the kidneys are able to excrete excess sodium in the urine. But people with congestive heart failure or kidney disease are not able to excrete sodium effectively, making them more prone to the condition. Sodium deficiencies are rare, but hyponatremia can occur when excessive fluid intake is not accompanied by adequate sodium intake, such as during intense exercise of long duration, such as a marathon run. It can also occur when excessive intake of plain water dilutes blood sodium to dangerous levels.

LO 9
- Dehydration occurs when fluid losses exceed fluid intake. Individuals at risk include the elderly, infants, people exercising heavily for prolonged periods in the heat, and individuals suffering from prolonged vomiting and diarrhea.
- Heat stroke occurs when the body's core temperature rises above 100°F. Heat stroke can lead to death if left untreated.
- Overhydration, or water intoxication, is caused by consuming too much water. Hyponatremia can also result, as water intoxication dilutes blood sodium.
- Certain forms of kidney disease and heart failure contribute to fluid and electrolyte imbalance and require specific dietary controls.
- An excessive intake of sugary drinks can, over time, result in overweight and obesity, not only because sugary drinks are high in empty Calories, but also because consumers fail to compensate for the Calories by eating less. In addition, sugary drinks tend to displace more nutritious beverages such as milk.

LO 10 ■ Hypertension, or high blood pressure, increases the risk for heart disease, stroke, and kidney disease. Consuming excess sodium is associated with hypertension in some, but not all, people.

■ Avoiding all tobacco use, consuming alcohol in moderation if at all, maintaining a healthful body weight, and engaging in regular physical activity are all important in reducing the risk for hypertension. In addition, following the DASH diet, a lower-sodium diet rich in fruits and vegetables, has been shown to reduce blood pressure.

review questions

LO 1 1. Plasma is one example of
a. extracellular fluid.
b. intracellular fluid.
c. tissue fluid.
d. metabolic water.

LO 2 2. The cell membrane
a. is freely permeable to water.
b. is freely permeable to electrolytes.
c. is freely permeable to both water and electrolytes.
d. is freely permeable to neither water nor electrolytes.

LO 3 3. Makoto went hiking with friends, but forgot to bring along a bottle of water. At the end of a two-hour hike, he is mildly dehydrated. His kidneys
a. release antidiuretic hormone (ADH).
b. secrete renin.
c. secrete aldosterone.
d. decrease water reabsorption.

LO 4 4. The body loses fluid through
a. urine and feces.
b. sweat.
c. evaporation and exhalation.
d. all of the above.

LO 5 5. In a state of acidosis
a. the blood pH is elevated above 7.45.
b. blood proteins release hydrogen ions.
c. an individual is likely to hyperventilate.
d. all of the above are true.

LO 6 6. Which of the following beverages contains added sugars?
a. red wine
b. fresh-squeezed orange juice
c. chocolate milk
d. lime-flavored sparkling water

LO 7 7. Which of the following is a characteristic of potassium?
a. It is a critical component of the mineral complex of bone.
b. It can be found in fresh fruits and vegetables.
c. It is the major cation in the extracellular fluid.
d. It is the major anion in the extracellular fluid.

LO 8 8. Hyponatremia
a. is characterized by excessive blood sodium.
b. is common in people who take prescription diuretics.
c. is a significant risk in an individual with congestive heart failure.
d. is a significant risk in an individual experiencing severe and persistent vomiting.

LO 9 9. Dehydration
a. is characterized by colorless urine.
b. may prompt an increased appetite.
c. is a greater risk for older adults than for younger adults.
d. is due to failure of the body's heat-regulating mechanisms.

LO 10 10. Which of the following statements about hypertension is true?
a. More than 70% of African American adults have hypertension.
b. For people who are overweight and hypertensive, losing 10 pounds can reduce blood pressure.
c. A blood pressure reading of 120 over 80 is normal.
d. All of the above statements are true.

true or false?

LO 1 11. **True or false?** Interstitial fluid is extracellular fluid.

LO 4 12. **True or false?** A decreased concentration of electrolytes in our blood stimulates the thirst mechanism.

LO 6 13. **True or false?** The DRI for water is about 9 cups per day (in beverages and food) for adult women and about 13 cups for adult men.

LO 7 14. **True or false?** A major mineral essential to the chemical digestion of food is chloride.

LO 9 15. **True or false?** Drinking lots of plain water throughout a marathon will prevent fluid and electrolyte imbalances.

short answer

LO 2   **16.** List at least four functions of water critical to body functioning.

LO 4   **17.** Your cousin, who is breastfeeding her 3-month-old daughter, confesses to you that she has resorted to taking over-the-counter weight-loss pills to help her lose the weight she gained during pregnancy. What concerns might this raise?

LO 7   **18.** For lunch today, your choices are (a) chicken soup, a ham sandwich, and a can of tomato juice or (b) potato salad, a tuna-fish sandwich, and a bottle of mineral water. You have hockey practice in mid-afternoon. Which lunch should you choose, and why?

LO 8   **19.** Explain why severe diarrhea in a young child can lead to death from heart failure.

LO 9   **20.** While visiting your grandmother over the holidays, you notice that she avoids drinking any beverage with her evening meal or in the hours prior to bedtime. You ask her about it, and she explains that she avoids fluids so that she won't have to get up and go to the bathroom during the night. "Though I still don't get a good night's sleep," she sighs. "Many nights I wake up with cramps in my legs and have to get up and walk around, anyway!" Could there be a link here? If so, explain.

math review

LO 9   **21.** Your roommate comes home after basketball practice and tells you he has lost 3 lb. Knowing that 1 pound of body weight loss represents the loss of 2 cups of fluid, how much fluid should he consume over the next few hours in order to fully rehydrate? (Recall that the goal of rehydration is to consume 1.5 times *more* fluid than is lost).

Answers to Review Questions and Math Review can be found online in the MasteringNutrition Study Area.

web links

water.epa.gov
U.S. Environmental Protection Agency (EPA)
Go to the EPA's water site for more information about drinking-water quality, standards, and safety.

www.bottledwater.org
International Bottled Water Association
Find current information about bottled water from this trade association that represents the bottled water industry.

www.nlm.nih.gov/medlineplus
Medline Plus Health Information
Search for "dehydration" and "heat stroke" to obtain additional resources and the latest news about the dangers of these heat-related illnesses.

www.nhlbi.nih.gov
National Heart, Lung, and Blood Institute
Go to this site to learn more about heart disease, including how to prevent high blood pressure.

www.americanheart.org
American Heart Association
The American Heart Association provides plenty of tips on how to lower your blood pressure.

www.nih.gov
National Institutes of Health (NIH)
Search this site to learn more about the DASH Diet (Dietary Approaches to Stop Hypertension).

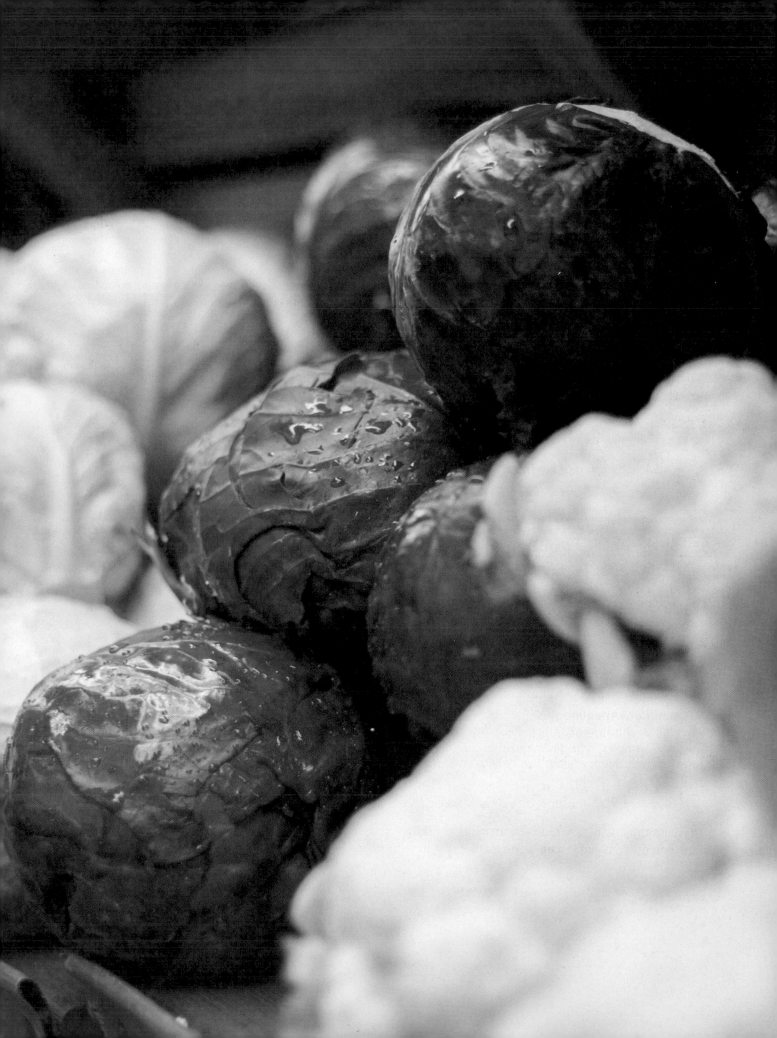

10 Nutrients Involved in Antioxidant Function and Vision

Learning Outcomes

After studying this chapter, you should be able to:

1 Explain how free radicals form, why they are a health concern, and how antioxidants oppose them, *pp. 380–383.*

2 Identify the most potent form of vitamin E in foods, and describe how it functions as an antioxidant, *pp. 383–384.*

3 Discuss at least three critical functions of vitamin C and identify good food sources, *pp. 387–390.*

4 Discuss the roles of five trace minerals in opposing oxidation, *pp. 391–394.*

5 Classify beta-carotene and describe its key functions in the body, *pp. 394–395.*

6 Explain how vitamin A works to ensure healthy vision, *pp. 398–400.*

7 Identify the functional and health problems associated with vitamin A toxicity and deficiency, *pp. 402–404.*

8 Describe the three stages of cancer development, *pp. 404–406.*

9 Identify a variety of factors, including consumption of antioxidant nutrients and phytochemicals, that influence cancer risk, *pp. 406–407.*

10 Discuss the role of free radical damage in cardiovascular disease and the potential benefit of consuming a diet rich in antioxidant nutrients, *pp. 408–409.*

M
ika, a first-year student at a university hundreds of miles from home, just opened another care package from her mom. As usual, it contained an assortment of healthful snacks, herbal teas, and several types of supplements: echinacea extract to ward off colds, powdered papaya for good digestion, and antioxidant vitamins. "Wow, Mika!" her roommate laughed. "Can you let your mom know I'm available for adoption?"

"I guess she just wants me to stay healthy," Mika sighed. She wondered what her mother would think if she ever found out how much junk food Mika had been eating since she'd started college, that she'd been binge drinking every weekend, or that she'd been smoking since high school. "Still," Mika reminded herself, "at least I take the vitamins she sends."

What do you think of Mika's current lifestyle? Why do you think Mika's mom included a bottle of antioxidant vitamins in her care package, and do you think they'll reduce— or increase—her health risks? If your health-food store were promoting an antioxidant supplement, would you buy it?

It isn't easy to sort fact from fiction when it comes to antioxidants—especially when they're in the form of supplements. Internet ads and articles in fitness and health magazines tout their benefits, yet some researchers claim that they don't protect us from diseases and in some cases may even be harmful. In this chapter, you'll learn what antioxidants are and how they work in the body. We'll also discuss the multiple roles of vitamin A in promoting healthy vision, cell differentiation, and other key functions.

LO 1 Explain how free radicals form, why they are a health concern, and how antioxidants oppose them.

What Are Antioxidants and How Does the Body Use Them?

Antioxidants are compounds that protect cells from the damage caused by oxidation. *Anti* means "against," and antioxidants work *against*, or *prevent*, oxidation. Before we can go further in our discussion of antioxidants, we need to review what oxidation is and how it damages cells.

Oxidation Is a Chemical Reaction in Which Atoms Lose Electrons

As you can see in **Figure 10.1a,** during metabolic reactions, atoms may lose electrons. This loss of electrons is called **oxidation,** because it is fueled by oxygen. Atoms are also capable of gaining electrons, through a complementary process called *reduction* (**Figure 10.1b**). Because oxidation–reduction reactions typically result in an even exchange of electrons, scientists call them *exchange reactions*.

Stable atoms have an even number of electrons orbiting in pairs at successive distances (called *shells* or *rings*) from the nucleus. When a stable atom loses an electron during oxidation, it is left with an odd number of electrons in its outermost shell. In other words, it now has an *unpaired electron*. In most exchange reactions, atoms with unpaired electrons immediately pair up, making newly stabilized molecules, but in some cases, atoms with unpaired electrons in

antioxidant A compound that has the ability to prevent or repair the damage caused by oxidation.

oxidation A chemical reaction in which molecules of a substance are broken down into their component atoms. During oxidation, the atoms involved lose electrons.

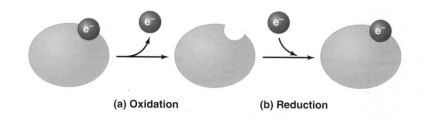

(a) Oxidation   **(b) Reduction**

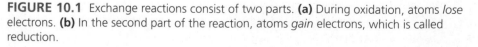

FIGURE 10.1 Exchange reactions consist of two parts. **(a)** During oxidation, atoms *lose* electrons. **(b)** In the second part of the reaction, atoms *gain* electrons, which is called reduction.

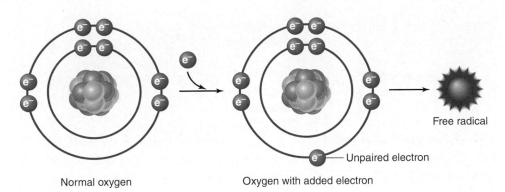

Normal oxygen   Oxygen with added electron

Unpaired electron

Free radical

FIGURE 10.2 Normally, an oxygen atom contains eight electrons. Occasionally, oxygen will accept an unpaired electron during the oxidation process. This acceptance of a single electron causes oxygen to become an unstable atom called a free radical.

their outermost shell remain unpaired. Atoms with an unpaired electron—and the molecules in which they occur—are highly unstable and are called **free radicals.**

Free radicals can also form as a result of energy metabolism. As cells use oxygen and hydrogen to generate energy (ATP), single electrons are sometimes released. Occasionally, oxygen accepts one of these single electrons (**Figure 10.2**). When it does so, the newly unstable oxygen atom becomes a free radical because of the added unpaired electron. This type of free-radical production is common during energy metabolism.

Free radicals are also formed from other metabolic processes, such as when our immune system produces inflammation to fight allergens or infections. Other factors that cause free-radical formation include exposure to air pollution, ultraviolet (UV) rays from the sun, other types of radiation, tobacco smoke, industrial chemicals, and asbestos. Continual exposure to these factors leads to uncontrollable free-radical formation, cell damage, and disease, as discussed next.

Free Radicals Can Destabilize Other Molecules and Damage Cells

Why are we concerned with the formation of free radicals? Simply put, it is because of their destabilizing power. If you were to think of paired electrons as a married couple, a free radical would be an extremely seductive outsider. Its unpaired electron exerts a powerful attraction toward all stable molecules around it. In an attempt to stabilize itself, a free radical will "steal" an electron from stable compounds, in turn generating more unstable free radicals. This is a dangerous chain reaction, because the free radicals generated can damage or destroy cells.

One of the most significant sites of free-radical damage is the cell membrane. As shown in **Figure 10.3a** (page 382), free radicals that form within the phospholipid bilayer of cell membranes steal electrons from the stable lipid heads. When the lipid heads, which are hydrophobic, are destroyed, they no longer repel water. With the cell membrane's integrity lost, its ability to regulate the movement of fluids and nutrients into and out of the cell is also lost. This loss of cell integrity causes damage to the cell and to all systems affected by the cell.

Other sites of free-radical damage include low-density lipoproteins (LDLs), cell proteins, and DNA. Damage to LDLs and cell proteins disrupts the transport of substances into and out of cells and alters cell function, whereas defective DNA results in faulty protein synthesis. These changes can also cause harmful changes (mutations) in cells or prompt cells to die prematurely. Free radicals also promote blood-vessel inflammation, which you learned (in Chapter 5) is an early step in the process of atherosclerosis, a risk factor for cardiovascular disease. In addition, they promote the formation of blood clots. When this occurs within arteries serving the heart or brain, the individual can experience a heart attack or stroke. Other diseases linked with free-radical production include cancer, type 2 diabetes, arthritis, cataracts, and Alzheimer's and Parkinson's diseases.

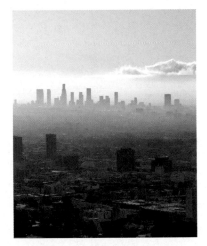

Exposure to pollution from car exhaust and industrial waste increases our production of free radicals.

free radical A highly unstable atom with an unpaired electron in its outermost shell, or the molecule in which such an atom occurs.

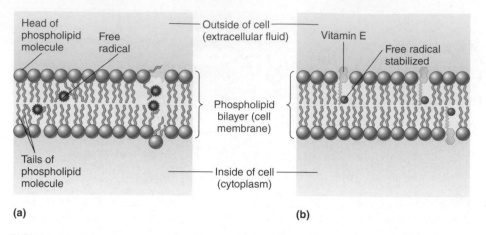

FIGURE 10.3 **(a)** The formation of free radicals in the lipid portion of our cell membranes can cause a dangerous chain reaction that damages the integrity of the membrane and can cause cell death. **(b)** Vitamin E is stored in the lipid portion of our cell membranes. By donating an electron to free radicals, it protects the lipid molecules in our cell membranes from being oxidized and stops the chain reaction of oxidative damage.

Antioxidants Work by Stabilizing Free Radicals or Opposing Oxidation

How does the body fight free radicals and repair the damage they cause? These actions are performed by antioxidant vitamins, minerals, and phytochemicals and other compounds. These antioxidants perform their role in three ways:

1. Antioxidant vitamins work independently by donating their electrons or hydrogen atoms to free radicals to stabilize them and reduce the damage caused by oxidation (see Figure 10.3b).
2. Antioxidant minerals, including selenium, copper, iron, zinc, and manganese, act as cofactors within complex *antioxidant enzyme systems* that convert free radicals to less damaging substances that are excreted by the body. They also work to break down fatty acids that have become oxidized, thereby destroying the free radicals associated with them. Antioxidant enzyme systems also make more vitamin antioxidants available to fight other free radicals. The following are examples of antioxidant enzyme systems:
   - Superoxide dismutase converts superoxide free radicals to less damaging substances, such as hydrogen peroxide, which can then be degraded by other enzyme systems.
   - Catalase promotes the elimination of hydrogen peroxide from the body by converting it to water and oxygen.
   - Glutathione peroxidase also promotes the elimination of hydrogen peroxide from the body by reducing it to water and stops the production of free radicals in lipids.
3. *Phytochemicals* (beneficial plant chemicals), such as *beta-carotene* and other compounds, help stabilize free radicals and prevent damage to cells and tissues.

In summary, free-radical formation is generally kept safely under control by certain vitamins, minerals working within antioxidant systems, and phytochemicals. Next, we take a look at the specific vitamins and minerals involved, including vitamins E, C, and A; the minerals selenium, copper, iron, zinc, and manganese; and beta-carotene (a phytochemical that is a precursor to vitamin A) (**Table 10.1**). For a detailed discussion of phytochemicals, see In Depth 10.5 immediately following this chapter.

TABLE 10.1 Nutrients Involved in Antioxidant Function and Vision

To see the full profile of all micronutrients, turn to Chapter 7.5, In Depth: Vitamins and Minerals: Micronutrients with Macro Powers, pages 292–303.

Nutrient	Recommended Intake
Vitamin E (fat soluble)	RDA: Women and men = 15 mg alpha-tocopherol
Vitamin C (water soluble)	RDA: Women = 75 mg Men = 90 mg Smokers = 35 mg more per day than RDA
Beta-carotene (fat-soluble provitamin for vitamin A)	None at this time
Vitamin A (fat soluble)	RDA: Women: 700 µg Men: 900 µg
Selenium (trace mineral)	RDA: Women and men = 55 µg

RECAP

Free radicals are formed when a stable atom loses or gains an electron and this electron remains unpaired. They can be produced as a normal by-product of oxidation reactions, when our immune system fights allergens or infections, and when we are exposed to radiation or toxic substances. Free radicals can damage our cell membranes, low-density lipoproteins (LDLs), cell proteins, and DNA and are associated with many chronic diseases, including heart disease, various cancers, and type 2 diabetes. Antioxidant vitamins donate electrons or hydrogen atoms to free radicals to stabilize them. Antioxidant minerals function as part of antioxidant enzyme systems that convert free radicals to less damaging substances. Some phytochemicals also have antioxidant properties. ◼

What Makes Vitamin E a Key Antioxidant?

LO 2 Identify the most potent form of vitamin E in foods, and describe how it functions as an antioxidant.

Vitamin E is one of the fat-soluble vitamins. It is absorbed with dietary fat and incorporated into the chylomicrons. As the chylomicrons are broken down, most of the vitamin E remains in their remnants and is transported to the liver. There, vitamin E is incorporated into very-low-density lipoproteins (VLDLs) and released into the blood. As previously described (in Chapter 5), VLDLs are transport vehicles that ferry triglycerides from their source to the body's cells. After VLDLs release their triglyceride load, they become LDLs. Vitamin E is a part of both VLDLs and LDLs and is transported to the tissues and cells by both of these lipoproteins.

Vitamin E and the other fat-soluble vitamins are stored in the body. The liver serves as a storage site for vitamins A and D, and about 90% of the vitamin E in the body is stored in our adipose tissue. The remaining vitamin E is found in cell membranes.

There Are Several Forms of Vitamin E

Vitamin E is actually two separate families of compounds, **tocotrienols** and **tocopherols.** None of the four tocotrienol compounds—alpha, beta, gamma, and delta—appears to play an active role in the body. The tocopherol compounds are the biologically active forms. Four tocopherol compounds have been discovered; as with tocotrienol, these have been designated alpha, beta, gamma, and delta. Of them, the most active, or potent, vitamin E compound found in food and supplements is *alpha-tocopherol* (**Figure 10.4**, page 384). The RDA for vitamin E is expressed as alpha-tocopherol in milligrams per day (α-tocopherol, mg per day).

tocotrienols A family of vitamin E that does not play an important biological role in our bodies.

tocopherols A family of vitamin E that is the active form in our bodies.

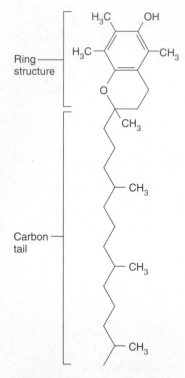

FIGURE 10.4 Chemical structure of α-tocopherol. Note that α-tocopherol is composed of a ring structure and a long carbon tail. Variations in the spatial orientation of the carbon atoms in this tail and in the composition of the tail itself are what result in forming the different tocopherol and tocotrienol compounds.

Food labels and vitamin and mineral supplements may express vitamin E in units of alpha-tocopherol equivalents (α-TE), in milligrams, and as International Units (IU). Supplements may contain either the natural form of vitamin E (called d-alpha-tocopherol) or the synthetic form (dl-alpha-tocopherol). The following can be used for conversion purposes:

- In food, 1 α-TE is equal to 1 mg of active vitamin E.
- In supplements containing the natural form of vitamin E, 1 IU is equal to 0.67 mg α-TE.
- In supplements containing the synthetic form of vitamin E, 1 IU is equal to 0.45 mg α-TE.

Vitamin E Donates an Electron to Free Radicals

The primary function of vitamin E is as an antioxidant: it donates an electron to free radicals, stabilizing them and preventing them from destabilizing other molecules. Once vitamin E is oxidized, it is either excreted from the body or recycled back into active vitamin E through the help of other antioxidant nutrients, such as vitamin C.

Because vitamin E is prevalent in adipose tissue and cell membranes, its action specifically protects polyunsaturated fatty acids (PUFAs) and other fatty components of our cells and cell membranes from being oxidized (see Figure 10.3b). Vitamin E also protects LDLs from being oxidized, thereby lowering the risk for cardiovascular disease. (The relationship between antioxidants and cardiovascular disease is reviewed later in this chapter.) In addition to protecting PUFAs and LDLs, vitamin E protects the membranes of red blood cells from oxidation and plays a critical role in protecting the cells of our lungs, which are constantly exposed to oxygen and the potentially damaging effects of oxidation. Vitamin E's role in protecting PUFAs and other fatty components also explains why it is added to many oil-based foods and skincare products—by preventing oxidation in these products, it reduces rancidity and spoilage.

Vitamin E serves many other roles essential to human health. It has anticoagulant properties, and thus opposes excessive clot formation of blood that is promoted by free radicals. It is critical for normal fetal and early childhood development of nerves and muscles, as well as for maintenance of their functions. It protects white blood cells and other components of the immune system, thereby helping the body defend against acute infection and disease. It also improves the absorption of vitamin A if the dietary intake of vitamin A is low.

How Much Vitamin E Should We Consume?

Considering the importance of vitamin E to our health, you might think that you need to consume a huge amount daily. In fact, the Recommended Dietary Allowance (RDA) is modest, and the food sources are plentiful.

Recommended Dietary Allowance for Vitamin E

The RDA for vitamin E for men and women is 15 mg alpha-tocopherol per day. This is the amount determined to be sufficient to prevent **erythrocyte hemolysis,** or the rupturing (*lysis*) of red blood cells (*erythrocytes*). The Tolerable Upper Intake Level (UL) is 1,000 mg alpha-tocopherol per day. Remember that one of the primary roles of vitamin E is to protect PUFAs from oxidation. Thus, our need for vitamin E increases as we eat more oils and other foods that contain PUFAs. Fortunately, these foods also contain vitamin E, so we typically consume enough vitamin E within them to protect their PUFAs from oxidation.

Good Food Sources of Vitamin E

Vitamin E is widespread in foods from plant sources (**Figure 10.5**). Much of the vitamin E that we consume comes from products such as spreads, salad dressings, and mayonnaise made from vegetable oils, including safflower oil, sunflower oil, canola oil, and soybean oil. Nuts, seeds, soybeans, and some vegetables—including spinach, broccoli, and avocados—also contribute vitamin E to our diets. Although no single fruit or vegetable contains very

erythrocyte hemolysis The rupturing or breakdown of red blood cells, or erythrocytes.

high amounts of vitamin E, eating the recommended amounts of fruits and vegetables each day will help ensure adequate intake of this nutrient. Cereals are often fortified with vitamin E, and other grain products contribute modest amounts to our diets. Animal and dairy products are poor sources. Here are some tips for eating more vitamin E:

- Eat cereals high in vitamin E for breakfast or as a snack.
- Add sunflower seeds to salads and trail mixes, or just have them as a snack.
- Add sliced almonds to salads, granola, and trail mixes to boost vitamin E intake.
- Pack a peanut butter sandwich for lunch.
- Eat veggies throughout the day—for snacks, for sides, and in main dishes.
- When dressing a salad, use vitamin E—rich oils, such as sunflower, safflower, or canola.
- Enjoy some fresh, homemade guacamole: mash a ripe avocado with a squeeze of lime juice and a sprinkle of garlic salt.

Vitamin E is destroyed by exposure to oxygen, metals, ultraviolet light, and heat. Although raw (uncooked) vegetable oils contain vitamin E, heating these oils destroys vitamin E. Thus, foods that are deep-fried and processed contain little vitamin E; this includes most fast foods.

What Happens If We Consume Too Much Vitamin E?

Until recently, standard supplemental doses (1 to 18 times the RDA) of vitamin E were not associated with any adverse health effects. However, a 2005 study found that, among adults 55 years of age or older with vascular disease or diabetes, a daily intake of 268 mg

Nutrition
MILESTONE

In **1922**, Herbert M. Evans from UC Berkeley and Katharine Scott Bishop from Johns Hopkins University School of Medicine published a landmark paper in the journal *Science* identifying the existence of "an unrecognized dietary factor essential for reproduction." Similar studies were being conducted by Henry Mattill and colleagues at the University of Iowa, who in 1923 discovered that wheat germ is a rich source of this dietary factor. In 1924, research scientist Bennet Sure named this factor vitamin E, as vitamins A, B, C, and D had already been identified.

For the next decade, the research teams of both Evans and Mattill worked independently to identify the antioxidant properties of vitamin E. In 1936, Evans' team isolated vitamin E from wheat germ oil and chemically characterized it, naming it *tocopherol* from the Greek words *phero* ("to bring") and *tocos* ("childbirth"). In 1937, collaboration between Mattill's and Evans' research groups confirmed that alpha-, beta-, and gamma-tocopherols are effective antioxidants. The antioxidant function of vitamin E is still recognized as one of its primary roles in human physiology and health.

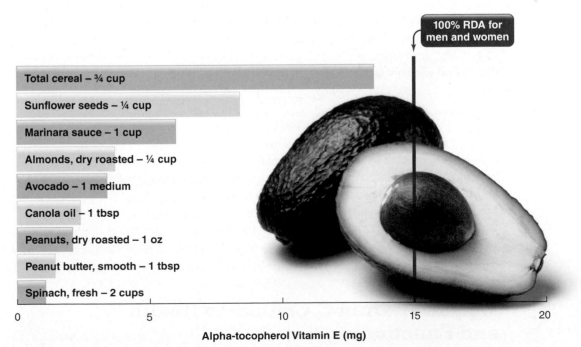

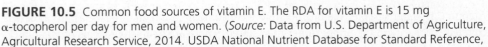

FIGURE 10.5 Common food sources of vitamin E. The RDA for vitamin E is 15 mg α-tocopherol per day for men and women. (*Source:* Data from U.S. Department of Agriculture, Agricultural Research Service, 2014. USDA National Nutrient Database for Standard Reference, Release 27. www.ars.usda.gov/ba/bhnrc/ndl.)

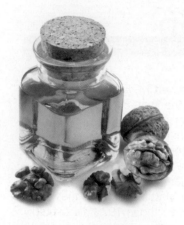

Vegetable oils, nuts, seeds, and avocados are good sources of vitamin E.

of vitamin E per day (about 18 times the RDA) for approximately 7 years resulted in a significant increase in heart failure.[1] A recent systematic review has also shown a significant increase in premature mortality in adults taking vitamin E supplements in doses ranging from 10 IU to 5,000 IU per day,[2] and the Selenium and Vitamin E Cancer Prevention Trial (SELECT) found that taking 400 IU per day of vitamin E supplements increased the risk for prostate cancer by 17% in healthy U.S. men from the general population.[3]

Some individuals report side effects such as nausea, intestinal distress, and diarrhea with vitamin E supplementation. In addition, certain medications interact negatively with vitamin E. The most important of these are the *anticoagulants*, substances that stop blood from clotting excessively. Aspirin is an anticoagulant, as is the prescription drug Coumadin. Vitamin E supplements can augment the action of these substances, uncontrollable bleeding. In addition, evidence suggests that in some people, long-term use of standard vitamin E supplements may cause hemorrhaging in the brain, leading to a hemorrhagic stroke.[4]

What Happens If We Don't Consume Enough Vitamin E?

True vitamin E deficiencies are uncommon in humans. This is primarily because vitamin E is fat soluble, so we typically store adequate amounts in our fatty tissues, even when our current intakes are low. Vitamin E deficiencies are usually a result of diseases that cause malabsorption of fat, such as those that affect the small intestine, liver, gallbladder, and pancreas. As noted earlier (in Chapter 3), the liver makes bile, which is stored in the gallbladder until released into the small intestine, where it emulsifies fats. The pancreas makes fat-digesting enzymes. Thus, when the liver, gallbladder, or pancreas is not functioning properly, fat and the fat-soluble vitamins, including vitamin E, cannot be absorbed, leading to their deficiency.

Research suggests that the diets of most Americans do not provide the RDA for vitamin E.[5] However, these intake estimates may be low, as the amounts and types of fat added during cooking are often not known and thus are not included in survey estimates.

Despite the rarity of true vitamin E deficiencies, they do occur. One vitamin E deficiency symptom is erythrocyte hemolysis. This rupturing of red blood cells leads to *anemia*, a condition in which the red blood cells cannot carry and transport enough oxygen to the tissues, leading to fatigue, weakness, and a diminished ability to perform physical and mental work. (Anemia is discussed in more detail in Chapter 12.) Vitamin E deficiency can also cause loss of muscle coordination and reflexes, leading to impairments in vision, speech, and movement, and can reduce immune function, especially when body stores of the mineral selenium are low.

RECAP

Vitamin E is a fat-soluble vitamin stored primarily in adipose tissue. Of its several forms, alpha-tocopherol is the most potent. Vitamin E protects cell membranes from oxidation, enhances immune function, and improves the absorption of vitamin A if dietary intake is low. The RDA for vitamin E is 15 mg alpha-tocopherol per day for men and women. Vitamin E is found primarily in vegetable oils and nuts. Toxicity is uncommon, but taking very high doses can cause excessive bleeding, and supplementation has been linked to premature mortality in some studies. A genuine deficiency is rare, but symptoms include anemia and impaired vision, speech, and movement. ∎

 LO 3 Discuss at least three critical functions of vitamin C and identify good food sources.

Why Is Vitamin C Critical to Health and Functioning?

Vitamin C is water soluble. We must therefore consume it on a regular basis, as any excess is excreted (primarily in the urine) rather than stored. There are two active forms of vitamin C: ascorbic acid and dehydroascorbic acid (**Figure 10.6**). Interestingly, most animals can make

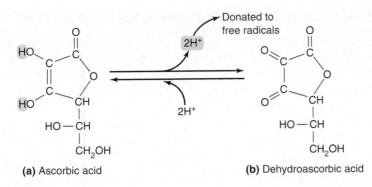

FIGURE 10.6 Chemical structures of ascorbic acid and dehydroascorbic acid. **(a)** By donating two of its hydrogens to free radicals, ascorbic acid protects against oxidative damage and becomes **(b)** dehydroascorbic acid. In turn, dehydroascorbic acid can accept two hydrogens to become ascorbic acid.

their own vitamin C from glucose. Humans and guinea pigs cannot synthesize their own vitamin C and must consume it in the diet.

At low concentrations, vitamin C is absorbed in the intestines via active transport; at high concentrations, it is absorbed via simple diffusion. Between consumptions of 30 to 80 mg/day, about 70% to 90% of dietary vitamin C is absorbed, but absorption falls to less than 50% when more than 1 g per day is consumed.[4] The kidneys regulate excretion of vitamin C, with increased excretion occurring during periods of high dietary intake and decreased excretion when dietary intakes are low.

Vitamin C Helps Synthesize Tissues and Functional Compounds

Vitamin C is probably best known for its role in preventing scurvy, a disease that ravaged sailors on long sea voyages centuries ago. In fact, the derivation of the term *ascorbic acid* means a ("without") *scorbic* ("having scurvy"). Scurvy was characterized by bleeding tissues, especially of the gums, and is thought to have caused more than half of the deaths that occurred at sea. During these long voyages, the crew ate all of the fruits and vegetables early in the trip, then had only grain and animal products available until they reached land to resupply. In 1740 in England, Dr. James Lind discovered that consumption of citrus fruits prevents scurvy. This is due to their high vitamin C content. Fifty years after the discovery of the link between citrus fruits and prevention of scurvy, the British navy finally required all ships to provide daily lemon juice rations for each sailor to prevent the onset of scurvy. A century later, sailors were given lime juice rations, earning them the nickname "limeys." It wasn't until 1930 that vitamin C was discovered and identified as a nutrient.

One reason that vitamin C prevents scurvy is that it assists in the synthesis of **collagen.** Collagen, a protein, is a critical component of all connective tissues in the body, including bone, teeth, skin, tendons, and blood vessels. Collagen assists in preventing bruises, and it ensures proper wound healing, as it is a part of scar tissue and a component of the tissue that mends broken bones. Without adequate vitamin C, the body cannot form collagen, and tissue hemorrhage, or bleeding, occurs. Vitamin C may also be involved in the synthesis of other components of connective tissues, such as elastin and bone matrix.

In addition to connective tissues, vitamin C assists in the synthesis of DNA, bile, neurotransmitters such as serotonin, and carnitine, which transports long-chain fatty acids from the cytosol into the mitochondria for energy production. Vitamin C also helps ensure appropriate levels of thyroxine, a hormone produced by the thyroid gland, to support basal metabolic rate and maintain body temperature. Other hormones that are synthesized with assistance from vitamin C include epinephrine, norepinephrine, and steroid hormones.

collagen A protein found in all connective tissues in the body.

Vitamin C Acts as an Antioxidant and Boosts Absorption of Iron

Vitamin C also acts as an antioxidant. Because it is water soluble, it is an important antioxidant in the extracellular fluid. Like vitamin E, it donates electrons to free radicals, thus preventing the damage of cells and tissues (see Figure 10.6a). It also protects LDL-cholesterol from oxidation, which may reduce the risk for cardiovascular disease. Vitamin C acts as an important antioxidant in the lungs, helping protect us from the damage caused by ozone and cigarette smoke. It also enhances immune function by protecting the white blood cells from the oxidative damage that occurs in response to fighting illness and infection. But contrary to popular belief, it is not a miracle cure (see the *Highlight* box). In the stomach, vitamin C reduces the formation of *nitrosamines*, cancer-causing agents found in foods such as cured and processed meats. We discuss the role of vitamin C and other antioxidants in preventing some forms of cancer later in this chapter.

Vitamin C also regenerates vitamin E after it has been oxidized. This occurs when ascorbic acid donates electrons to vitamin E radicals, becoming dehydroascorbic acid (**Figure 10.7**). The regenerated vitamin E can then continue to protect cell membranes and other tissues. In turn, dehydroascorbic acid is regenerated as an antioxidant by gaining an electron from the reduced form of **glutathione (GSH),** which is a tripeptide composed of glycine, cysteine, and glutamic acid. Glutathione is then restored to its antioxidant form by the enzyme *glutathione reductase*, in a reaction (not shown in Figure 10.7) that is dependent on the mineral selenium, which is discussed later in this chapter.

Vitamin C also enhances the absorption of iron. It is recommended that people with low iron stores consume vitamin C–rich foods along with iron sources to improve absorption.

glutathione (GSH) A tripeptide composed of glycine, cysteine, and glutamic acid that assists in regenerating vitamin C into its antioxidant form.

Can Vitamin C Prevent the Common Cold?

What do you do when you feel a cold coming on? If you are like many people, you drink a lot of orange juice or take vitamin C supplements to ward it off. Do these tactics really help prevent a cold?

It is well known that vitamin C is important for a healthy immune system. A deficiency of vitamin C can seriously weaken the immune cells' ability to detect and destroy invading microbes, increasing susceptibility to many diseases and illnesses—including the common cold. Many people have taken vitamin C supplements to prevent the common cold, basing their behavior on its actions of enhancing our immune function. Nevertheless, scientific studies do not support this action. A recent review of many of the studies of vitamin C and the common cold found that people taking vitamin C regularly in an attempt to ward off the common cold experienced as many colds as people who took a placebo. However, the *duration* of their colds was modestly reduced—by 8% in adults and 14% in children.[1] Timing appears to be important, though: taking vitamin C after the onset of cold symptoms did not reduce either the duration or severity of the cold. Interestingly, taking vitamin C supplements regularly did reduce the number of colds experienced in marathon runners, skiers, and soldiers participating in exercises done under extreme environmental conditions.

The amount of vitamin C taken in these studies was at least 200 mg per day, with many using doses as high as 4,000 mg per day (more than 40 times the RDA), with no harmful effects noted in those studies that reported adverse events.

In summary, it appears that, for most people, taking vitamin C supplements regularly will not prevent colds but may reduce their duration. Consuming a healthful diet that includes excellent sources of vitamin C will also help you maintain a strong immune system. Taking vitamin C after the onset of cold symptoms does not appear to help, so next time you feel a cold coming on, you may want to think twice before taking extra vitamin C.

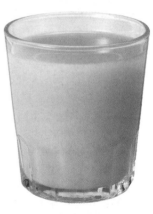

References

1. Hemilä, H., and E. Chalker. 2013. Vitamin C for preventing and treating the common cold. *Cochrane Database Syst. Rev.* Issue 1. Art. No. CD000980. DOI: 10.1002/14651858.CD000980.pub4.

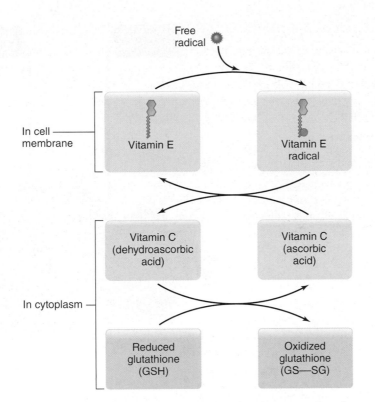

In cell membrane

Free radical

Vitamin E

Vitamin E radical

In cytoplasm

Vitamin C (dehydroascorbic acid)

Vitamin C (ascorbic acid)

Reduced glutathione (GSH)

Oxidized glutathione (GS—SG)

FIGURE 10.7 Regeneration of vitamin E by vitamin C. Vitamin E neutralizes free radicals in the cell membrane, and vitamin C (in the form of ascorbic acid) regenerates vitamin E from the resulting vitamin E radical. Vitamin C (in the form of dehydroascorbic acid) is regenerated to ascorbic acid by the reduced form of glutathione (GSH).

For people with high iron stores, this practice can be dangerous and lead to iron toxicity (see Chapter 12, page 473).

How Much Vitamin C Should We Consume?

Although popular opinion suggests that our needs for vitamin C are high, we really only require amounts that are easily obtained when we eat the recommended amounts of fruits and vegetables daily.

Recommended Dietary Allowance for Vitamin C

The RDA for vitamin C is 90 mg per day for men and 75 mg per day for women. The Tolerable Upper Intake Level (UL) is 2,000 mg per day for adults. Smoking increases a person's need for vitamin C; thus, the RDA for smokers is 35 mg more per day than for nonsmokers. This equals 125 mg per day for men and 110 mg per day for women. Other high-stress situations that may increase the need for vitamin C include healing from a traumatic injury, surgery, or burns and the use of oral contraceptives among women; there is no consensus as to how much extra vitamin C is needed in these circumstances.

Good Food Sources of Vitamin C

Fruits and vegetables are the best sources of vitamin C. Because heat and oxygen destroy vitamin C, fresh sources of these foods have the highest content. Cooking foods, especially boiling them, leaches their vitamin C, which is then lost when we strain them. The forms of cooking that are least likely to compromise the vitamin C content of foods are steaming, microwaving, and stir-frying.

As indicated in **Figure 10.8**, (page 390) many fruits and vegetables are high in vitamin C. Citrus fruits (such as oranges, lemons, and limes), potatoes, strawberries, tomatoes, kiwifruit,

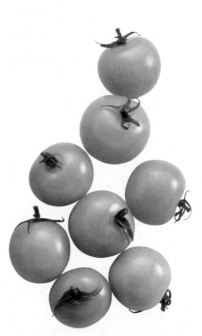

Many fruits, such as these yellow tomatoes, are high in vitamin C.

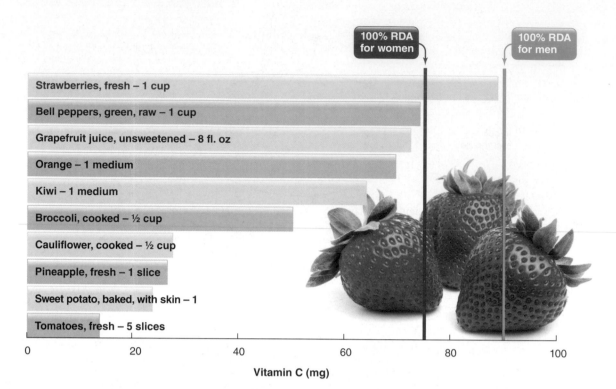

FIGURE 10.8 Common food sources of vitamin C. The RDA for vitamin C is 90 mg per day for men and 75 mg per day for women. (*Source:* Data from U.S. Department of Agriculture, Agricultural Research Service, 2014. USDA National Nutrient Database for Standard Reference, Release 27. http://www.ars.usda.gov/ba/bhnrc/ndl.)

broccoli, spinach and other leafy greens, cabbage, green and red peppers, and cauliflower are excellent sources of vitamin C. Fortified beverages and cereals are also good sources. Dairy foods, meats, and nonfortified cereals and grains provide little or no vitamin C.

Here are some tips for selecting foods high in vitamin C:

- Mix strawberries, kiwifruit, melon, and oranges for a tasty fruit salad loaded with vitamin C.
- Include tomatoes on salads, wraps, and sandwiches for more vitamin C.
- Make your own fresh-squeezed orange or grapefruit juice.
- Add your favorite vitamin C–rich fruits, such as strawberries, to smoothies.
- Buy ready-to-eat vegetables, such as baby carrots and cherry tomatoes, and toss some in a zip-lock bag to take to school or work.
- Put a few slices of romaine lettuce on your sandwich.
- Throw a small container of orange slices, fresh pineapple chunks, or berries into your backpack for an afternoon snack.
- Store some 100% juice boxes in your freezer to pack with your lunch. They'll thaw slowly, keeping the rest of your lunch cool, and many brands contain a full day's supply of vitamin C in just 6 oz.
- Enjoy raw bell peppers with low-fat dip for a crunchy snack.

By eating the recommended amounts of fruits and vegetables daily, we can easily meet the body's requirement for vitamin C. A serving of vegetables is ½ cup of cooked or 1 cup of raw vegetables or 6 oz of vegetable juice, and a serving of fruit is one medium fruit, 1 cup of chopped or canned fruit, or 6 oz of 100% fruit juice.

What Happens If We Consume Too Much Vitamin C?

Because vitamin C is water soluble, we usually excrete any excess. Consuming excess amounts in food sources does not lead to toxicity, and only supplements can lead to toxic doses. Taking megadoses of vitamin C is not fatal; however, the side effects of doses exceeding 2,000 mg per day for a prolonged period include nausea, diarrhea, nosebleeds, and abdominal cramps.

There are rare instances in which consuming even moderately excessive doses of vitamin C can be harmful. As mentioned earlier, vitamin C enhances the absorption of iron. This action is beneficial to people who need to increase iron absorption. It can be harmful, however, to people with a disease called *hemochromatosis,* which causes an excess accumulation of iron in the body. Such iron toxicity can damage tissues and lead to a heart attack. In people who have preexisting kidney disease, taking excess vitamin C can lead to the formation of kidney stones. This does not appear to occur in healthy individuals.

Critics of vitamin C supplementation claim that taking the supplemental form of the vitamin is "unbalanced" nutrition and leads vitamin C to act as a prooxidant. A **prooxidant,** as you might guess, is a substance that promotes oxidation. It does this by pushing the balance of exchange reactions toward oxidation, which promotes the production of free radicals. Although the results of a few studies suggested that vitamin C acts as a prooxidant, these studies were found to be flawed or irrelevant for humans. At the present time, there appears to be no strong scientific evidence that vitamin C, either from food or dietary supplements, acts as a prooxidant in humans.

What Happens If We Don't Consume Enough Vitamin C?

Vitamin C deficiencies are rare in developed countries but can occur in developing countries. Scurvy is the most common vitamin C–deficiency disease. The symptoms of scurvy appear after about 1 month of a vitamin C–deficient diet and include bleeding gums, loose teeth, weakness, wounds that fail to heal, swollen ankles and wrists, bone pain and fractures, diarrhea, weakness, and depression. Anemia can also result from vitamin C deficiency. People most at risk are those who eat few fruits and vegetables, including impoverished or homebound individuals, and people who abuse alcohol and drugs.

RECAP

Vitamin C prevents scurvy and assists in the synthesis of collagen, hormones, neurotransmitters, and DNA. It also acts as an antioxidant, scavenging free radicals and regenerating vitamin E after it has been oxidized. Vitamin C also enhances iron absorption. The RDA for vitamin C is 90 mg per day for men and 75 mg per day for women. Many fruits and vegetables are high in vitamin C. Toxicity is uncommon with dietary intake but may occur with supplements; symptoms include nausea, diarrhea, and nosebleeds. Deficiency can lead to scurvy and anemia. ■

What Minerals Act in Antioxidant Enzyme Systems?

LO 4 Discuss the roles of five trace minerals in opposing oxidation.

Several trace minerals play key roles in antioxidant enzyme systems, including selenium, copper, iron, zinc, and manganese. Keep in mind that, although we need only minute amounts of trace minerals, they are just as important to our health as the vitamins and the major minerals.

Selenium Is a Critical Component of the Glutathione Peroxidase Enzyme System

Selenium is a trace mineral, and it is found in varying amounts in soil and thus in the food grown there. Selenium is efficiently absorbed, with about 50% to 90% of dietary selenium absorbed from the small intestine.[4]

prooxidant A nutrient that promotes oxidation and oxidative damage of cells and tissues.

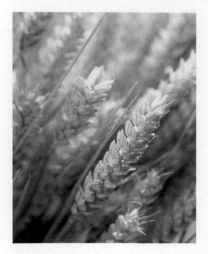

Wheat is a rich source of selenium.

Functions of Selenium

It is only recently that we have learned about the critical role of selenium as a nutrient in human health. In 1979, Chinese scientists reported an association between a heart disorder called **Keshan disease** and selenium deficiency. This disease occurs in children in the Keshan province of China, where the soil is depleted of selenium. The scientists found that Keshan disease can be prevented with selenium supplementation.

The selenium in our bodies is contained in amino acids. Two amino acid derivatives contain the majority of selenium in our bodies: **selenomethionine** is the storage form for selenium, and **selenocysteine** is the active form of selenium. Selenocysteine is a critical component of the glutathione peroxidase enzyme system, mentioned earlier. As shown in **Figure 10.9**, glutathione peroxidase breaks down the peroxides (such as hydrogen peroxide) that are formed by the body, so that they cannot form free radicals; this decrease in the number of free radicals spares vitamin E. Thus, selenium helps spare vitamin E and prevents oxidative damage to cell membranes.

Like vitamin C, selenium is needed for the production of *thyroxine*, or thyroid hormone. By this action, selenium is involved in the maintenance of basal metabolism and body temperature. Selenium appears to play a role in immune function, and poor selenium status is associated with higher rates of some forms of cancer.

How Much Selenium Should We Consume?

The content of selenium in foods is highly variable. As it is a trace mineral, we need only minute amounts to maintain health. The RDA for selenium is 55 μg per day for both men and women. The UL is 400 μg per day.

Selenium is present in both plant and animal food sources but in variable amounts. Because it is stored in the tissues of animals, selenium is found in reliably consistent amounts in animal foods. Organ meats, such as liver and kidney, as well as pork and seafood, are particularly good sources (**Figure 10.10**).

In contrast, the amount of selenium in plants is dependent on the selenium content of the soil in which the plant is grown. Many companies marketing selenium supplements warn that the agricultural soils in the United States are depleted of selenium and inform us

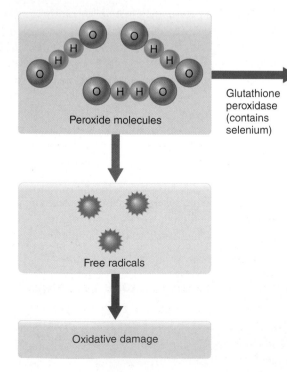

FIGURE 10.9 Selenium is part of glutathione peroxidase, which neutralizes peroxide molecules that are formed by the body, so that they cannot form free radicals; this decrease in the number of free radicals spares vitamin E and prevents oxidative damage.

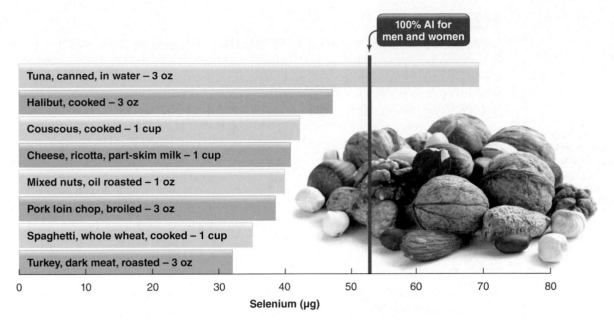

100% AI for men and women

Tuna, canned, in water – 3 oz

Halibut, cooked – 3 oz

Couscous, cooked – 1 cup

Cheese, ricotta, part-skim milk – 1 cup

Mixed nuts, oil roasted – 1 oz

Pork loin chop, broiled – 3 oz

Spaghetti, whole wheat, cooked – 1 cup

Turkey, dark meat, roasted – 3 oz

0   10   20   30   40   50   60   70   80

Selenium (µg)

FIGURE 10.10 Common food sources of selenium. The RDA for selenium is 55 µg per day. (*Source:* Data from U.S. Department of Agriculture, Agricultural Research Service, 2014. USDA National Nutrient Database for Standard Reference, Release 27. www.ars.usda.gov/ba/bhnrc/ndl.)

that we need to take selenium supplements. In reality, the selenium content of soil varies greatly across North America, and because we obtain our food from a variety of geographic locations, few people in the United States suffer from selenium deficiency. This is especially true for people who eat even small quantities of meat or seafood.

Selenium toxicity does not result from eating foods high in selenium. However, supplementation can cause toxicity. Toxicity symptoms include brittle hair and nails that can eventually break and fall off. Other symptoms include skin rashes, nausea, vomiting, weakness, and cirrhosis of the liver.

As discussed previously, selenium deficiency is associated with a form of heart disease called Keshan disease. Selenium deficiency does not cause the disease, but selenium is necessary to help the immune system effectively fight the viral infection that causes the disease.[4] Selenium supplements significantly reduce the incidence of Keshan disease, but they cannot reduce the damage to the heart muscle once it occurs.

Another deficiency disorder is *Kashin-Beck disease,* a disease of the cartilage that results in deforming arthritis (**Figure 10.11**). Kashin-Beck disease is found in selenium-depleted areas in China and Tibet. Other deficiency symptoms include impaired immune responses, infertility, depression, impaired cognitive function, and muscle pain and wasting. Deficiencies of both selenium and iodine in pregnant women can cause a form of *cretinism* in the infant. (The condition of cretinism is discussed in Chapter 8.)

Copper, Iron, Zinc, and Manganese Assist in Antioxidant Function

As discussed earlier, there are numerous antioxidant enzyme systems in our bodies. Copper, zinc, and manganese are a part of the superoxide dismutase antioxidant enzyme system. Iron is part of the structure of catalase. In addition to their role in protecting against oxidative damage, these trace minerals play major roles in the optimal functioning of many other enzymes in the body. Manganese, for example, is an important cofactor in protein, fat, and carbohydrate metabolism. Copper, iron, and zinc help us maintain the health of our blood (these nutrients are discussed in detail in Chapter 12).

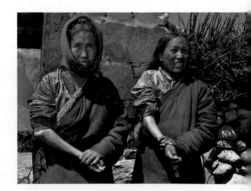

FIGURE 10.11 Selenium deficiency can lead to a type of deforming arthritis called Kashin-Beck disease.

RECAP

Selenium is a trace mineral that is part of the glutathione peroxidase enzyme system. It indirectly spares vitamin E from oxidative damage, and it assists with immune function and the production of thyroid hormone. Organ meats, pork, and seafood are good sources. The selenium content of plants is dependent on the amount of selenium in the soil in which they are grown. Toxicity symptoms include brittle hair and nails, nausea, vomiting, and liver cirrhosis. Deficiency can result in Keshan disease, Kashin-Beck disease, impaired immune function, infertility, and muscle wasting. Copper, zinc, and manganese are cofactors for the superoxide dismutase antioxidant enzyme system. Iron is a cofactor for the catalase antioxidant enzyme. These minerals play other critical roles in the body, including in blood health and energy metabolism.

> Watch a video on enzymes and cofactors and their role in neutralizing peroxides at www.bozemanscience.com. Type in the search bar "048 enzymes" and click on the link.

LO 5 Classify beta-carotene and describe its key functions in the body.

What Is Beta-Carotene, and What Are Its Roles in the Body?

Beta-carotene is not considered an essential nutrient; rather, it is a phytochemical classified as a **carotenoid,** a group of plant pigments that are the basis for the red, orange, and deep-yellow colors of many fruits and vegetables. (Even dark-green, leafy vegetables contain plenty of carotenoids, but the green pigment, chlorophyll, masks their color.) Although there are more than 600 carotenoids in nature, only about 50 are found in the typical human diet. We are just beginning to learn how carotenoids function in our bodies and how they may affect our health.

Beta-Carotene Is a Provitamin

Although not a nutrient, beta-carotene is considered a **provitamin**; that is, an inactive form of vitamin that the body cannot use until it is converted to its active form. Our bodies convert beta-carotene to an active form of vitamin A, *retinol;* thus, beta-carotene is a precursor of retinol.

The most common carotenoids found in human blood are alpha-carotene, beta-carotene, beta-cryptoxanthin, lutein, lycopene, and zeaxanthin. Of these, the body can convert only alpha-carotene, beta-carotene, and beta-cryptoxanthin to retinol. These are referred to as *provitamin A carotenoids.*

One molecule of beta-carotene can be split to form two molecules of active vitamin A (**Figure 10.12**); nevertheless, 12 g of beta-carotene are considered equivalent to just 1 g of vitamin A. Several factors account for this. Sometimes a beta-carotene

carotenoid A fat-soluble plant pigment that the body stores in the liver and adipose tissues. The body is able to convert certain carotenoids to vitamin A.

provitamin An inactive form of a vitamin that the body can convert to an active form. An example is beta-carotene.

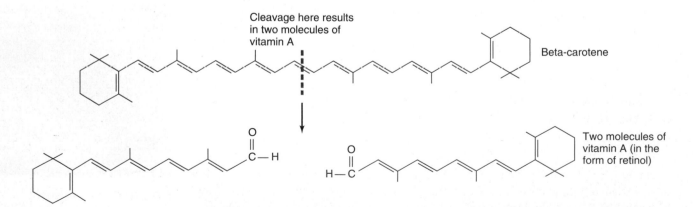

Cleavage here results in two molecules of vitamin A

Beta-carotene

Two molecules of vitamin A (in the form of retinol)

FIGURE 10.12 Chemical structure of beta-carotene. Cleavage of beta-carotene can result in the formation of two molecules of vitamin A.

molecule is cleaved in such a way that only one molecule of vitamin A is produced. In addition, not all of the dietary beta-carotene that is consumed is converted to vitamin A, and the absorption of beta-carotene from the intestines is not as efficient as our absorption of vitamin A.

Nutritionists express the units of beta-carotene in a food as Retinol Activity Equivalents, or RAEs. This measurement indicates how much active vitamin A is available to the body after it has converted the beta-carotene in the food.

Beta-Carotene Has Antioxidant Properties

Beta-carotene and some other carotenoids are recognized to have antioxidant properties. Like vitamin E, they are fat soluble and fight the harmful effects of oxidation in the lipid portions of the cell membranes and in LDLs; however, compared to vitamin E, beta-carotene is a relatively weak antioxidant. In fact, other carotenoids, such as lycopene and lutein, may be stronger antioxidants.

Through their antioxidant action, carotenoids play other important roles in the body as well, such as:

- enhancing the immune system
- protecting skin from the damage caused by the sun's ultraviolet rays
- protecting our eyes from damage, preventing or delaying age-related vision impairment

A diet rich in carotenoids is associated with a decreased risk for certain types of cancer. We will discuss the roles of carotenoids and other antioxidants in cancer later in this chapter.

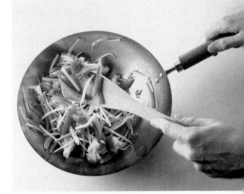

Fresh vegetables are good sources of vitamin C and beta-carotene.

How Much Beta-Carotene Should We Consume?

Nutritional scientists do not consider beta-carotene and other carotenoids to be essential nutrients, as they play no known essential roles in our bodies and are not associated with any deficiency symptoms. Thus, no RDA for these compounds has been established. Eating the recommended five servings of fruits and vegetables each provides approximately 6 to 8 mg of beta-carotene.[6]

Good Food Sources of Beta-Carotene

Fruits and vegetables that are red, orange, yellow, and deep green are generally high in beta-carotene and other carotenoids, such as lutein and lycopene. Eating the recommended amounts of fruits and vegetables each day ensures an adequate intake of carotenoids. Because of its color, beta-carotene is used as a natural coloring agent for many foods, including margarine, yellow cheddar cheese, cereal, cake mixes, gelatins, and soft drinks. However, these foods are not significant sources of beta-carotene. **Figure 10.13** (page 396) identifies common foods that are high in beta-carotene. The following are some ways to boost your intake of dietary beta-carotene:

- Start your day with an orange, a grapefruit, a pear, a banana, an apple, or a slice of cantaloupe. All are good sources of beta-carotene.
- Pack a zip-lock bag of carrot slices or dried apricots in your lunch.
- Instead of french fries, think orange! Slice raw sweet potatoes, toss the slices in olive or canola oil, and bake.
- Add veggies to homemade pizza.
- Add shredded carrots to cake and muffin batters.
- Taking dessert to a potluck? Make a pumpkin pie! It's easy if you use canned pumpkin and follow the recipe on the can.
- Go green, too! The next time you have a salad, go for the dark-green, leafy vegetables instead of iceberg lettuce.
- Add raw spinach or other green, leafy vegetables to wraps and sandwiches.

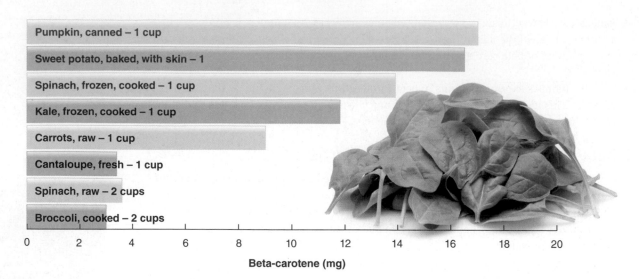

FIGURE 10.13 Common food sources of beta-carotene. There is no RDA for beta-carotene. (*Source:* Data from U.S. Department of Agriculture, Agricultural Research Service, 2014. USDA National Nutrient Database for Standard Reference, Release 27. www.ars.usda.gov /ba/bhnrc/ndl.)

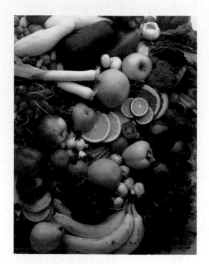

Foods that are high in carotenoids are easy to recognize by their bright colors.

We generally absorb only between 20% and 40% of the carotenoids present in the foods we eat. In contrast to vitamins E and C, carotenoids are better absorbed from cooked foods. Carotenoids are bound in the cells of plants, and the process of lightly cooking these plants breaks chemical bonds and can rupture cell walls, which humans don't digest. These actions result in more of the carotenoids being released from the plant. For instance, one cup of raw carrots provides approximately 10 mg of beta-carotene, whereas the same amount of cooked frozen carrots provides approximately 12 mg.[7]

What Happens If We Consume Too Much Beta-Carotene?

Consuming large amounts of beta-carotene or other carotenoids in foods does not appear to cause toxic symptoms. However, your skin can turn yellow or orange if you consume large amounts of foods that are high in beta-carotene. This condition is referred to as *carotenosis* or *carotenodermia,* and it appears to be both reversible and harmless.

Supplements containing beta-carotene are very popular, and several studies have investigated claims that beta-carotene supplementation can reduce the risk for chronic diseases, particularly cancer. However, evidence from large, randomized, controlled trials, such as the Alpha-Tocopherol Beta-Carotene (ATBC) Cancer Prevention Study and the Beta-Carotene and Retinol Efficacy Trial (CARET), has found that, contrary to expectations, taking beta-carotene supplements, typically in doses of 15 to 30 mg daily, *increased* the rates of premature death from lung cancer, heart disease, and stroke.[8,9] A recent systematic review of the available published studies reports that beta-carotene supplementation has no effect on the incidence of all cancers combined, pancreatic cancer, colorectal cancer, prostate cancer, breast cancer, and skin cancer. However, the incidence of lung and stomach cancers was significantly increased in those taking high doses, as well as in smokers and asbestos workers.[10]

What Happens If We Don't Consume Enough Beta-Carotene?

There are no known deficiency symptoms for beta-carotene or other carotenoids apart from beta-carotene's function as a precursor for vitamin A.

RECAP

Beta-carotene is a carotenoid and a provitamin of vitamin A. It protects the lipid portions of cell membranes and LDL-cholesterol from oxidative damage. It also enhances immune function and protects vision. There is no RDA for beta-carotene. Orange, red, and deep-green fruits and vegetables are good sources of beta-carotene. There are no known toxicity or deficiency symptoms of beta-carotene when consumed from food, but yellowing of the skin can occur if too much beta-carotene is consumed. Taking beta-carotene supplements has been associated with increased rates of premature death from lung cancer, heart disease, and stroke.

■

How Does Vitamin A Support Health and Functioning?

LO 6 Explain how vitamin A works to ensure healthy vision.

LO 7 Identify the functional and health problems associated with vitamin A toxicity and deficiency.

As early as AD 30, the Roman writer Aulus Cornelius Celsus described in his medical encyclopedia, *De Medicina*, a condition called *night blindness* and recommended as a cure the consumption of liver. We now know that night blindness is due to a deficiency of vitamin A, a fat-soluble vitamin stored primarily in the liver of animals.

There Are Three Active Forms of Vitamin A

There are three active forms of vitamin A in the body: **retinol** is the alcohol form, **retinal** is the aldehyde form, and **retinoic acid** is the acid form. These three forms are collectively referred to as the *retinoids* (**Figure 10.14**). Of the three, retinol has the starring role in maintaining the body's physiologic functions.

Remember from the previous section that beta-carotene is a precursor to vitamin A. When we eat foods that contain beta-carotene, it is converted to retinol in the wall of the small intestine. Preformed vitamin A is present in foods in the form of retinol and as *retinyl ester-compounds*, in which retinol is attached to a fatty acid. These retinyl ester-compounds are hydrolyzed in the small intestine, leaving retinol in its free form. Free retinol is then absorbed into the wall of the small intestine, where a fatty acid is attached to form new retinyl ester-compounds. These compounds are then packaged into chylomicrons and enter into the lymphatic system. The chylomicrons transport vitamin A to the cells as needed or into the liver for storage. About 90% of the vitamin A we absorb is stored in the liver; the remainder is stored in adipose tissue, the kidneys, and the lungs.

Because fat-soluble vitamins cannot dissolve in the blood, they require proteins that can bind with and transport them from their storage sites through the bloodstream to target

retinol An active, alcohol form of vitamin A that plays an important role in healthy vision and immune function.

retinal An active, aldehyde form of vitamin A that plays an important role in healthy vision and immune function.

retinoic acid An active, acid form of vitamin A that plays an important role in cell growth and immune function.

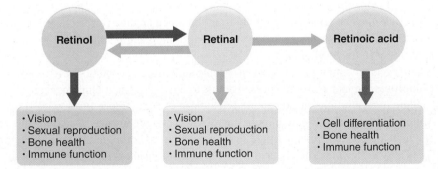

FIGURE 10.14 The three active forms of vitamin A in our bodies are retinol, retinal, and retinoic acid. Retinol and retinal can be converted interchangeably; retinoic acid is formed from retinal, and this process is irreversible. Each form of vitamin A contributes to many of our bodily processes.

tissues and cells. *Retinol-binding protein* is one such carrier protein for vitamin A. Retinol-binding protein carries retinol from the liver to the cells that require it.

The unit of expression for vitamin A is Retinol Activity Equivalents (RAE). You may still see the expression Retinol Equivalents (RE) or International Units (IU) for vitamin A on food labels or dietary supplements. The conversions to RAE from various dietary forms of retinol are as follows:

- 1 RAE = 1 microgram (µg) retinol
- 1 RAE = 12 µg beta-carotene
- 1 RAE = 24 µg alpha-carotene or beta-cryptoxanthin
- 1 RAE = 1 RE
- 1 RAE = 3.3 IU

Conversion rates from IU to µg RAE are as follows:

- 1 IU retinol from food or supplements = 0.3 µg RAE
- 1 IU beta-carotene from supplements = 0.15 µg RAE
- 1 IU beta-carotene from food = 0.05 µg RAE
- 1 IU alpha-carotene or beta-cryptoxanthin = 0.025 µg RAE

Vitamin A Is Essential to Sight

The known functions of vitamin A are numerous, and researchers speculate that many are still to be discovered. Let's begin with its critical role in the maintenance of healthy vision. Vitamin A affects our sight in two ways: it enables us to react to changes in the brightness of light, and it enables us to distinguish between different wavelengths of light—in other words, to see different colors. Let's take a closer look at this process.

Light enters the eyes through the cornea, travels through the lens, and then hits the **retina,** which is a delicate membrane lining the back of the inner eyeball (**Focus Figure 10.15**). You might already have guessed how *retinal* got its name: it is found in—and is integral to—the retina. In the retina, retinal combines with a protein called **opsin** to form **rhodopsin,** a light-sensitive pigment. Rhodopsin is found in the **rod cells,** which are cells that react to dim light and interpret black-and-white images.

When light hits the retina, the rod cells go through a **bleaching process.** In this reaction, rhodopsin is split into retinal and opsin, and the rod cells lose their color. The retinal component also changes spatial orientation from a *cis* configuration, which is bent, into a *trans* configuration, which is straight. The opsin component also changes shape. These changes in retinal and opsin during the bleaching process generate a nerve impulse that travels to the brain, resulting in the perception of a black-and-white image. Most of the retinal is converted back to its original *cis* form and binds with opsin to regenerate rhodopsin, allowing the visual cycle to begin again. However, some of the retinal is lost with each cycle and must be replaced by retinol from the bloodstream. This visual cycle goes on continually, allowing our eyes to adjust moment to moment to subtle changes in our surroundings or in the level of light.

When levels of vitamin A are deficient, people suffer from a condition referred to as **night blindness,** an inability of the eyes to adjust to dim light. Night blindness can also result in the failure to regain sight quickly after a bright flash of light (**Figure 10.16**, page 400).

At the same time that we are interpreting black-and-white images, the **cone cells** of the retina, which are only effective in bright light, use retinal to interpret different wavelengths of light as different colors. The pigment involved in color vision is **iodopsin.** Iodopsin experiences similar changes during the color vision cycle as rhodopsin does during the black-and-white vision cycle. As with the rod cells, the cone cells can also be affected by a deficiency of vitamin A, resulting in color blindness.

In summary, the abilities to adjust to dim light, recover from a bright flash of light, and see in color are all critically dependent on adequate levels of retinal in the eyes.

retina The delicate, light-sensitive membrane lining the inner eyeball and connected to the optic nerve. It contains retinal.

opsin A protein that combines with retinal in the retina to form rhodopsin.

rhodopsin A light-sensitive pigment found in the rod cells that is formed by retinal and opsin.

rod cells Light-sensitive cells found in the retina that contain rhodopsin and react to dim light and interpret black-and-white images.

bleaching process A reaction in which the rod cells in the retina lose their color when rhodopsin is split into retinal and opsin.

night blindness A vitamin A–deficiency disorder that results in loss of the ability to see in dim light.

cone cells Light-sensitive cells found in the retina that contain the pigment iodopsin and react to bright light and interpret color images.

iodopsin A color-sensitive pigment found in the cone cells of the retina.

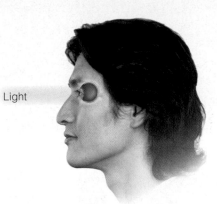

Light

Vitamin A is a component of two light-sensitive proteins, rhodopsin and iodopsin, that are essential for vision. Here we examine rhodopsin's role in vision. Although the breakdown of iodopsin is similar, rhodopsin is more sensitive to light than iodopsin and is more likely to become bleached.

EYE STRUCTURE

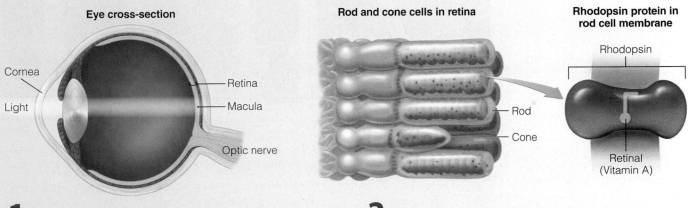

Eye cross-section

Cornea

Light

Retina

Macula

Optic nerve

Rod and cone cells in retina

Rod

Cone

Rhodopsin protein in rod cell membrane

Rhodopsin

Retinal (Vitamin A)

1 After light enters your eye through the cornea, it travels to the back of your eye to the macula, which is located in the retina. The macula allows you to see fine details and things that are straight in front of you.

2 Inside the retina are two types of light-absorbing cells, rods and cones. Rods contain the protein rhodopsin, while cones contain the protein iodopsin.

EFFECT OF LIGHT ON RHODOPSIN

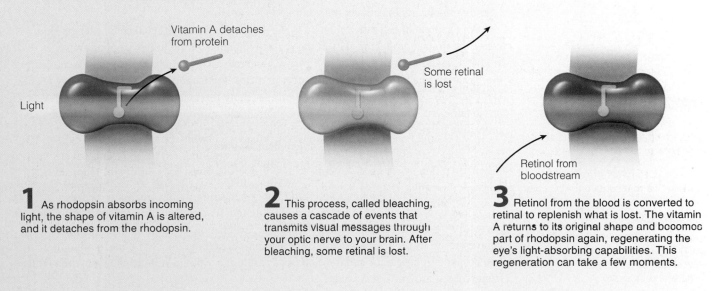

Vitamin A detaches from protein

Light

Some retinal is lost

Retinol from bloodstream

1 As rhodopsin absorbs incoming light, the shape of vitamin A is altered, and it detaches from the rhodopsin.

2 This process, called bleaching, causes a cascade of events that transmits visual messages through your optic nerve to your brain. After bleaching, some retinal is lost.

3 Retinol from the blood is converted to retinal to replenish what is lost. The vitamin A returns to its original shape and becomes part of rhodopsin again, regenerating the eye's light-absorbing capabilities. This regeneration can take a few moments.

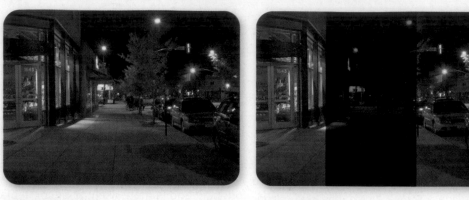

(a) Normal night vision   Poor night vision

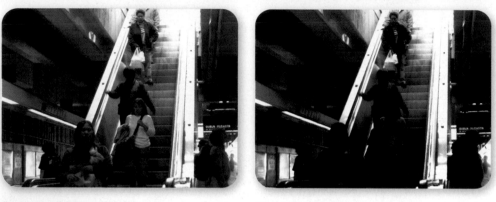

(b) Normal light adjustment   Slow light adjustment

FIGURE 10.16 A deficiency of vitamin A can result in night blindness. This condition results in **(a)** diminished side vision and overall poor night vision and **(b)** difficulty in adjusting from bright light to dim light.

Vitamin A Contributes to Cell Differentiation and Many Other Body Functions

Another important role of vitamin A is its contribution to **cell differentiation,** the process by which stem cells mature into highly specialized cells that perform unique functions. The retinoic acid form of vitamin A interacts with the receptor sites on a cell's DNA. This interaction influences gene expression and the determination of the type of cells that the stem cells eventually become. Obviously, this process is critical to the development of healthy organs and effectively functioning body systems.

An example of cell differentiation is the development of epithelial cells, such as skin cells, and mucus-producing cells of the protective linings of the lungs, vagina, intestines, stomach, bladder, urinary tract, and eyes. The mucus that epithelial cells produce lubricates the tissue and helps propel microbes, dust particles, foods, and fluids out of the body tissues (for example, when we cough up secretions or empty the bladder). When vitamin A levels are insufficient, the epithelial cells fail to differentiate appropriately, and we lose these protective barriers against infectious microbes and irritants.

Vitamin A is also critical to the differentiation of specialized immune cells called *T-lymphocytes,* or *T cells.* T cells assist in fighting infections. You can therefore see why vitamin A deficiency can lead to a breakdown of immune responses and to infections and other disorders of the lungs and respiratory tract, urinary tract, vagina, and eyes.

Vitamin A is involved in reproduction. Although its exact role is unclear, it appears necessary for sperm production in men and for fertilization to occur in women. It also contributes to healthy bone growth by assisting in breaking down old bone, so that new, longer, and stronger bone can develop. As a result of a vitamin A deficiency, children suffer from stunted growth and wasting.

cell differentiation The process by which immature, undifferentiated stem cells develop into highly specialized functional cells of discrete organs and tissues.

Past limited research indicated that vitamin A may act as an antioxidant by scavenging free radicals and protecting LDLs from oxidation. However, in the absence of recent research confirming this view, we can only say that it is unclear if vitamin A makes some minimal contribution to antioxidant function.

Search the Internet and you'll find plenty of sites claiming a direct link between vitamin A deficiency and acne and insisting that vitamin A supplements can successfully treat it. Should you believe the hype?

Early research into this topic reported an association between low blood levels of vitamin A and the presence of acne: the more severe the acne, the lower the levels of vitamin A.[11] Although these findings may seem suggestive, this study was conducted with a very small number of participants who were not randomly selected. Also, plasma levels of vitamin A were assessed to indicate vitamin A status; however, the Institute of Medicine states that plasma levels of vitamin A are not necessarily an indicator of vitamin A status.[12] To date, these results have not been replicated by other researchers, and there appears to be no evidence that vitamin A deficiency causes acne.

Interestingly, two effective treatments for acne are synthetic derivatives of vitamin A. Retin-A, or tretinoin, is a treatment applied to the skin. Accutane, or isotretinoin, is taken orally. These medications are available only by prescription and, because they increase a person's sensitivity to the sun and can cause severe birth defects, their use must be monitored by a licensed physician. Contrary to what you might read on the Internet, vitamin A itself has no effect on acne; thus, vitamin A supplements are not recommended in its treatment.

How Much Vitamin A Should We Consume?

Vitamin A toxicity can occur readily, because it is a fat-soluble vitamin, so it is important to consume only the amount recommended for your gender and age range.

Recommended Dietary Intake for Vitamin A

The RDA for vitamin A is 900 µg per day for men and 700 µg per day for women. The UL is 3,000 µg per day of preformed vitamin A in women (including those pregnant and lactating) and men.

How can you determine the µg RAE when expressed as IU units that come from various food and supplement sources? Refer to the *You Do the Math* box to learn how to apply these conversions.

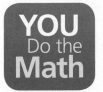

Vitamin A Unit Conversions from Food and Supplement Sources

Shaleen is a 24-year-old female who is neither pregnant nor lactating, and she wants to better understand how the various forms of vitamin A she may consume from food and supplements contribute to her RDA. The information she has available is in IU units, and she wants to calculate how these sources contribute to her RDA of 700 µg RAE. (To do the math, Shaleen refers to the conversion rates listed on page D-1.)

On the same page, she saw that the conversion rates from IU to µg RAE are as follows:

- 1 IU retinol from food or supplements – 0.3 µg RAE
- 1 IU beta-carotene from supplements = 0.15 µg RAE
- 1 IU beta-carotene from food = 0.05 µg RAE
- 1 IU alpha-carotene or beta-cryptoxanthin = 0.025 µg RAE

a. If Shaleen were to consume all of her vitamin A as retinol from food or supplements, how many IU units would she need to consume to meet her RDA?

As Shaleen's RDA is 700 µg RAE, and 1 IU retinol from food or supplements is equal to 0.3 µg RAE, this is equal to 700 µg RAE ÷ 0.3 µg RAE per 1 IU = 2,333 IU of retinol.

b. If Shaleen consumed a vegetarian diet and consumed all of her vitamin A as beta-carotene from food, how many IU units would she need to consume to meet her RDA?

1 IU retinol from beta-carotene from food is equal to 0.05 µg RAE. Thus, 700 µg RAE ÷ 0.05 µg RAE per 1 IU = 14,000 IU of retinol.

c. In reality, Shaleen consumes a mixed diet in which she gets her vitamin A from a variety of food sources. She uses MyDietAnalysis to analyze her diet and finds she is currently consuming 600 µg RAE, which is 85.7% of the RDA, where (600 µg RAE ÷ 700 µg RAE) × 100 = 85.7%. She is considering taking a beta-carotene supplement to reach her RDA. She finds a supplement advertised on the Internet that contains 10,000 IU of beta-carotene and is enriched with carrots, parsley, and watercress. She knows that 1 IU of beta-carotene from supplements is equal to 0.15 µg RAE. Thus, the total amount of µg RAE she would get by taking this supplement is

10,000 IU × 0.15 µg RAE = 1,500 µg RAE, which is well above the 100 µg RAE she needs to meet the RDA!

Shaleen would be much wiser to consume this 100 µg RAE from fruits and vegetables high in beta-carotene.

As 1 µg RAE = 12 µg beta-carotene from food, she determines that she needs to consume 1,200 µg of beta-carotene from food (12 µg beta-carotene × 100 µg RAE needed to meet the RDA). She refers to the U.S. Department of Agriculture Nutrient Database Standard Reference 27 on the Internet at http://ndb.nal.usda.gov/, looks at the report of food sources specifically for beta-carotene, and discovers she can simply and more safely consume 1 cup of cooked broccoli (1,450 µg beta-carotene) or one raw carrot (5,965 µg beta-carotene) to easily and inexpensively meet her RDA for vitamin A.

Now use your own diet assessment to determine *your* intake of vitamin A. What percentage of the RDA for vitamin A do you currently consume? If you were to consume the same beta-carotene supplement that Shaleen considered, how many could you take before exceeding the UL for vitamin A based on your current dietary intake of vitamin A?

Answers will vary depending on individual body criteria and intake levels.

Good Food Sources of Vitamin A

Vitamin A is present in both animal and plant sources. To calculate the total RAE in a person's diet, you must take into consideration both the amount of retinol and the amount of provitamin A carotenoids that are present in the foods eaten. Remember that 12 µg of beta-carotene yields 1 µg of RAE, and 24 µg of alpha-carotene or beta-cryptoxanthin yields 1 µg of RAE. Thus, if a person consumes 400 µg retinol, 1,200 µg beta-carotene, and 3,000 µg alpha-carotene, the total RAE is equal to 400 µg + (1,200 µg ÷ 12) + (3,000 µg ÷ 24), or 625 µg RAE.

The most common sources of dietary preformed vitamin A are animal foods such as beef liver, chicken liver, eggs, and whole-fat dairy products. Vitamin A is also found in fortified reduced-fat milks, margarine, and some breakfast cereals (**Figure 10.17**). The other sources of the vitamin A we consume are foods high in beta-carotene and other carotenoids that can be converted to vitamin A. As discussed earlier in this chapter, dark-green, orange, and deep-yellow fruits and vegetables are good sources of beta-carotene and thus of vitamin A. Carrots, spinach, mango, cantaloupe, and tomato juice are excellent sources of vitamin A because they contain beta-carotene.

What Happens If We Consume Too Much Vitamin A?

Vitamin A is highly toxic, and toxicity symptoms develop after consuming only three to four times the RDA. Toxicity rarely results from food sources, but vitamin A supplementation is known to have caused severe illness and even death. In pregnant women, it can cause serious birth defects and spontaneous abortion. Other toxicity symptoms include fatigue, loss of appetite, blurred vision, hair loss, skin disorders, bone and joint pain, abdominal pain, nausea, diarrhea, and damage to the liver and nervous system. If caught in time, many of these symptoms are reversible once vitamin A supplementation is stopped. However, permanent damage can occur to the liver, eyes, and other organs. Because liver contains such a high amount of vitamin A, children and pregnant women should not consume liver on a daily or weekly basis.

What Happens If We Don't Consume Enough Vitamin A?

As discussed earlier, night blindness and color blindness can result from vitamin A deficiency. How severe a problem is night blindness? Although much less common among

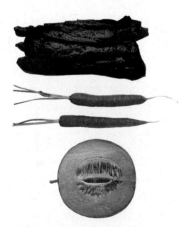

Liver, carrots, and cantaloupe all contain carotenoids that can be converted to vitamin A.

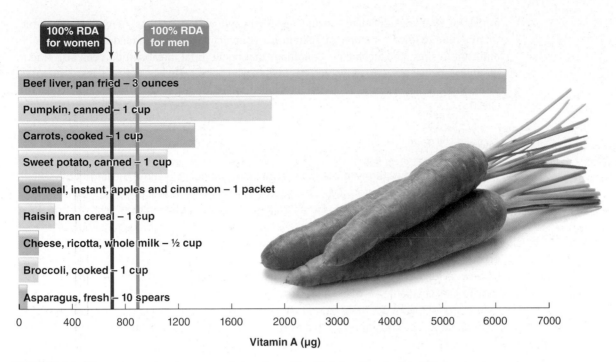

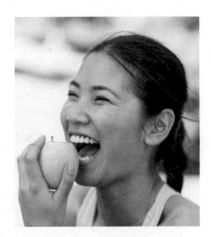

100% RDA for women

100% RDA for men

Beef liver, pan fried – 3 ounces

Pumpkin, canned – 1 cup

Carrots, cooked – 1 cup

Sweet potato, canned – 1 cup

Oatmeal, instant, apples and cinnamon – 1 packet

Raisin bran cereal – 1 cup

Cheese, ricotta, whole milk – ½ cup

Broccoli, cooked – 1 cup

Asparagus, fresh – 10 spears

0   400   800   1200   1600   2000   3000   4000   5000   6000   7000

Vitamin A (μg)

FIGURE 10.17 Common food sources of vitamin A. The RDA for vitamin A is 900 μg per day for men and 700 μg per day for women. (*Source:* Data from U.S. Department of Agriculture, Agricultural Research Service, 2014. USDA National Nutrient Database for Standard Reference, Release 27. www.ars.usda.gov/ba/bhnrc/ndl.)

people of developed nations, vitamin A deficiency is a severe public health concern in developing countries. According to the World Health Organization, approximately 250 million preschool children suffer from vitamin A deficiency.[13] Of the children affected, 250,000 to 500,000 become permanently blinded every year. At least half of these children are likely to die within 1 year of losing their sight, typically from infectious diseases such as measles and diarrhea, which are easily prevented and treated in more affluent countries. Vitamin A deficiency is also a tragedy for pregnant women in many developing countries. They often suffer from night blindness, are more likely to transmit HIV to their child if HIV-positive, and run a greater risk for maternal mortality.

If vitamin A deficiency progresses, it can result in irreversible blindness due to hardening of the cornea (the transparent membrane covering the front of the eye), a condition called **xerophthalmia.** The prefix of this word, *xero-*, comes from a Greek word meaning "dry." Lack of vitamin A causes the epithelial cells of the cornea to lose their ability to produce mucus, causing the eye to become very dry. This leaves the cornea susceptible to damage, infection, and hardening. Once the cornea hardens in this way, the resulting blindness is irreversible. This is why it is critical to catch vitamin A deficiency in its early stages and treat it with either the regular consumption of fruits and vegetables that contain beta-carotene or with vitamin A supplementation.

Vitamin A deficiency can also lead to follicular **hyperkeratosis,** a condition characterized by the excess accumulation of the protein keratin in the hair follicles. Keratin is usually found only on the outermost surface of skin, hair, nails, and tooth enamel. With hyperkeratosis, keratin clogs hair follicles, makes skin rough and bumpy; prevents proper sweating through the sweat glands; and causes skin to become very dry and thick. Hyperkeratosis can also affect the epithelial cells of various tissues, including the mouth, urinary tract, vagina, and eyes, reducing the production of mucus by these tissues and leading to an increased risk for infection. Hyperkeratosis can be reversed with vitamin A supplementation.

Other deficiency symptoms include impaired immunity, increased risk for illness and infections, reproductive system disorders, and failure of normal growth. Individuals who are

Eating plenty of fruits and vegetables can help prevent vitamin A deficiency.

xerophthalmia An irreversible blindness due to hardening of the cornea and drying of the mucous membranes of the eye.

hyperkeratosis A condition resulting in the excess accumulation of the protein keratin in the follicles of the skin; this condition can also impair the ability of epithelial tissues to produce mucus.

at risk for vitamin A deficiency include elderly people with poor diets, newborns, premature infants (due to low liver stores of vitamin A), young children with inadequate vegetable and fruit intakes, and alcoholics. Conditions that result in fat malabsorption can also lead to vitamin A deficiency. These include cystic fibrosis, Crohn's disease, celiac disease, diseases of the liver, pancreas, or gallbladder, and consumption of large amounts of the fat substitute Olestra.

RECAP

There are three active forms of vitamin A in the body: retinol, which has the largest physiologic role; retinol; and retinoic acid. They are collectively referred to as the retinoids. Vitamin A is critical for maintaining our vision. It is also necessary for cell differentiation, reproduction, and growth. The role of vitamin A as an antioxidant is still under investigation. The RDA for vitamin A is 900 µg per day for men and 700 µg per day for women. Animal liver, dairy products, and eggs are good animal sources of vitamin A; fruits and vegetables are high in beta-carotene, which is used to synthesize vitamin A. Supplementation can be dangerous, as toxicity is reached at levels of only three to four times the RDA. Toxicity symptoms include birth defects, spontaneous abortion, blurred vision, and liver damage. Deficiency symptoms include night blindness, color blindness, impaired immune function, and growth failure. ■

LO 8 Describe the three stages of cancer development.

LO 9 Identify a variety of factors, including consumption of antioxidant nutrients and phytochemicals, that influence cancer risk.

LO 10 Discuss the role of free radical damage in cardiovascular disease and the potential benefit of consuming a diet rich in antioxidant nutrients.

Watch a 6-minute video from the MD Anderson Cancer Center providing a basic overview of cancer. Go to www.mdanderson.org. Enter "'What Is Cancer' video" into the search box, then click on the link.

cancer A group of diseases characterized by cells that reproduce spontaneously and independently and may invade other tissues and organs.

tumor Any newly formed mass of immature, undifferentiated cells with no physiologic function.

What Disorders Are Related to Free-Radical Damage?

You've probably encountered a plethora of health claims related to the functions of antioxidants—for instance, that they slow the effects of aging or prevent heart disease and cancer. In opposition to these claims, there is some evidence that taking antioxidant supplements may be harmful (refer to the previous discussion on beta-carotene, pages 394–396).

In this section, we will review what is currently known about the role of antioxidant nutrients in cancer and heart disease.

Cancer Is a Group of Diseases Characterized by Cells Growing Out of Control

Before we explore how antioxidants affect the risk for cancer, let's take a closer look at precisely what cancer is and how it spreads. **Cancer** is actually a group of diseases that are all characterized by cells that grow "out of control." By this we mean that cancer cells reproduce spontaneously and independently, and they are not inhibited by the boundaries of tissues and organs. Thus, they can aggressively invade tissues and organs far away from those in which they originally formed.

Most forms of cancer result in one or more **tumors,** which are newly formed masses of undifferentiated cells that are immature and have no physiologic function. Although the word *tumor* sounds frightening, it is important to note that not every tumor is *malignant*, or cancerous. Many are *benign* (not harmful to us) and are made up of cells that will not spread widely.

Cancer Develops in Three Stages

Figure 10.18 shows how changes to normal cells prompt a series of other changes that can progress into cancer. There are three primary stages of cancer development: initiation, promotion, and progression. These stages occur as follows:

1. *Initiation:* The initiation of cancer occurs when a cell's DNA is *mutated* (changed). This mutation may be random, inherited, or due to environmental factors, such as exposure to the chemicals in tobacco smoke, UV radiation, or certain viruses. Such factors

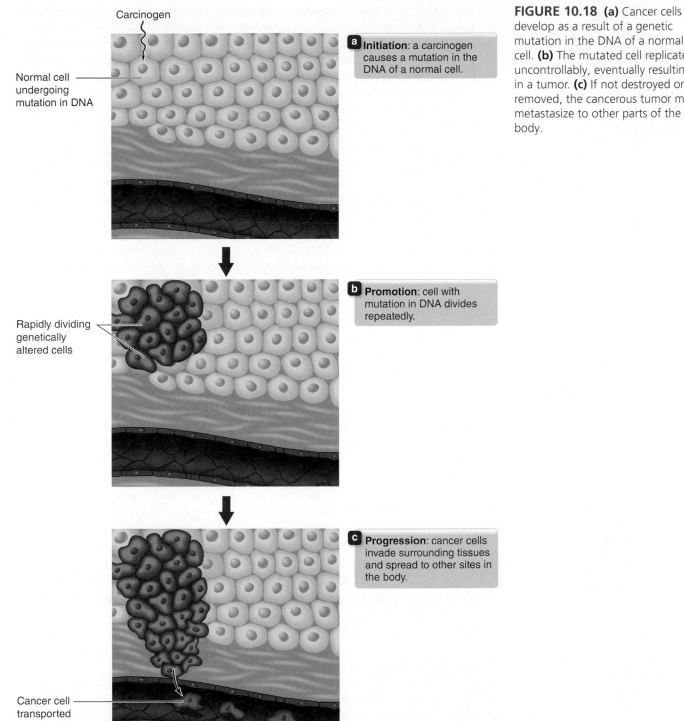

Carcinogen

Normal cell undergoing mutation in DNA

a **Initiation:** a carcinogen causes a mutation in the DNA of a normal cell.

Rapidly dividing genetically altered cells

b **Promotion:** cell with mutation in DNA divides repeatedly.

c **Progression:** cancer cells invade surrounding tissues and spread to other sites in the body.

Cancer cell transported in blood vessel

FIGURE 10.18 (a) Cancer cells develop as a result of a genetic mutation in the DNA of a normal cell. **(b)** The mutated cell replicates uncontrollably, eventually resulting in a tumor. **(c)** If not destroyed or removed, the cancerous tumor may metastasize to other parts of the body.

are called *carcinogens,* substances that can generate cancer. Cells with mutated DNA may engage in self-repair or self-destruction, or they may be destroyed by the body's immune system; if they escape destruction, they can develop characteristics that enable their promotion.

2. *Promotion:* During this stage, the genetically altered cell is stimulated to divide. A single mutated cell divides in two, and these double to four, and so on. The mutated DNA is locked into each new cell's genetic instructions. Because the enzymes that normally work to repair damaged cells cannot detect alterations in the DNA, the cells can continue to divide uninhibited. Typically, it takes many years for a mutated cell to

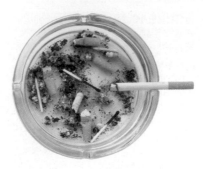

Using tobacco is a risk factor for cancer.

double repeatedly into a tumor mass large enough to be detectable (about the size of a grape), and promotion is the longest stage in cancer development.

3. *Progression:* During this stage, the cancerous cells grow out of control. They grow their own blood vessels, which supply them with blood and nutrients, and invade adjacent tissues. In this early stage of progression, the immune system can sometimes detect these cancerous cells and destroy them. However, if the cells continue to grow, they develop into malignant tumors, disrupting body functioning at their primary site and invading the circulatory and lymphatic systems to *metastasize* (spread) to distant sites in the body.

Although cancer is often fatal, a majority of people who develop cancer survive. In 2015, the American Cancer Society reported that the 5-year survival rate for all cancers was 68%.[14] Of course, cancers can be more or less aggressive, some are more readily detectable than others, and some tissues and organs are more vulnerable to cancer. All these factors influence the overall mortality rate associated with different cancers. The type of cancer with the highest mortality rate is lung cancer, with an estimated 158,000 deaths in 2015. Even when it has not invaded regional tissues, the survival rate is just 54%, and with metastasis, this drops to just 4%. Cancer of the colon and/or rectum ranks second (an estimated 49,700 deaths in 2015), and pancreatic cancer ranks third (40,560 deaths).[14]

A Variety of Factors Influence Cancer Risk

Researchers estimate that about half of all men and one-third of all women will develop cancer during their lifetime.[14] But what factors cause cancer? Are you and your loved ones at risk, and is there anything you can do to lower your risk? The answers to these questions depends on several factors, including your family history of cancer, your exposure to environmental agents, various lifestyle choices, and possibly even "bad luck."

Random Mutations A 2015 study published in the journal *Science* reported the results of a mathematical analysis comparing the incidence of various cancers with an estimate of the number of stem cell divisions in corresponding tissues over a lifetime. The results of this analysis suggest that about two-thirds of all cancers are a result of random mutations that arise during replication of DNA in noncancerous stem cells.[15] Based on these findings, the authors of the study concluded that the majority of cancers are due to "bad luck," and are not due to heredity, environment, or lifestyle choices.

These findings created a media storm, and various health organizations questioned them. For instance, the International Agency for Research on Cancer (IARC), which is the World Health Organization's specialized cancer agency, strongly disagreed and stated, "Concluding that 'bad luck' is the major cause of cancer would be misleading and may detract from efforts to identify the causes of the disease and effectively prevent it."[16] They further state that nearly half of all cancers worldwide can be prevented.

*Nutri-*Case

Gustavo

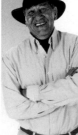

"Last night, there was an actress on TV talking about having colon cancer and saying everybody over age 50 should get tested. It brought back all the memories of my father's cancer, how thin and weak he got before he went to the doctor, so that by the time they found the cancer it had already spread too far. But I don't think I'm at risk. I only eat red meat two or three times a week, and I eat a piece of fruit or a vegetable at every meal. I don't smoke, and I get plenty of exercise, sunshine, and fresh air working in the vineyard."

What lifestyle factors reduce Gustavo's risk for cancer? What factors increase his risk? Think especially about possible occupational risk factors. Would you recommend he increase his consumption of fruits and vegetables? Why or why not? If Gustavo were your father, would you encourage him to have the screening test for colon cancer that the actress on television recommended?

Heredity   There is strong evidence that heredity can play a role in the development of cancer, because inherited "cancer genes," such as the *BRC* genes for breast cancer, increase the risk that an individual with those genes will develop cancer. However, only about 5% of all cancers are strongly hereditary.[14] In addition, it is important to bear in mind that a family history of cancer does not guarantee you will get cancer, too. It just means that you are at an increased risk and should take all preventive actions available to you. While some risk factors are out of your control, others are modifiable, which means that you can take positive steps to reduce your risk.

Tobacco Use   The American Cancer Society has identified six modifiable risk factors that have been shown to have the greatest impact on an individual's cancer risk.[17] Foremost among these is tobacco use. More than forty compounds in tobacco and tobacco smoke are known carcinogens, and smoking is the single major cause of cancer deaths, accounting for 30% of all cancer deaths and 80% of lung cancer deaths. Moreover, it increases the risk for acute myeloid leukemia and cancers of the nasopharynx, nasal cavity, paranasal sinus, lip, oral cavity, pharynx, larynx, lung, esophagus, pancreas, uterine cervix, ovaries, kidney, bladder, stomach, and colorectum (**Figure 10.19**).[17] Smoking can also cause heart disease and stroke, and is the primary cause of chronic obstructive pulmonary disease (COPD). Overall, tobacco use accounts for about one in five deaths each year. The positive news is that tobacco use is a modifiable risk factor. If you smoke or chew tobacco, you can reduce your risk for cancer considerably by quitting.

Weight, Diet, and Physical Activity   Researchers estimate that one-third of cancer deaths are related to overweight or obesity, poor nutrition, and physical inactivity and thus could be prevented.[17] Nutritional factors that are protective against cancer include the consumption of foods rich in antioxidant micronutrients and phytochemicals, and fiber. Diets high in saturated fats and low in fruits and vegetables increase the risk for cancers of the esophagus, colon, breast, and prostate. Consumption of alcohol and compounds found in cured and charbroiled meats can also increase the risk for cancer.

A sedentary lifestyle increases the risk for colon cancer and possibly other forms of cancer. There is convincing evidence that regular physical activity decreases the risk for colon cancer, as well as probable evidence of a protective effect for endometrial cancer and postmenopausal breast cancer. There is limited evidence that suggests physical activity may also be protective against cancers of the lung, pancreas, and breast (premenopausal). At this time, we do not know how exercise reduces the overall risk for cancer or for certain types of cancers. However, these findings have prompted the American Cancer Society and the National Cancer Institute to promote increased physical activity as a way to reduce our risk for cancer.

Infectious Agents   Infectious agents account for 15% to 20% of cancers worldwide, with this figure lower in the United States but higher in developing countries. For example, infection with the sexually transmitted high-risk human papillomaviruses (high-risk HPVs) causes virtually all cervical cancers and most anal cancers (**Figure 10.20**), and infection with the bacterium *Helicobacter pylori* is linked not only to ulcers but also to stomach cancer. As microbial research advances, it is thought that more cancers will be linked to infectious agents.

Ultraviolet Radiation   Skin cancer is the most common form of cancer in the United States and accounts for over half of all cancers diagnosed each year. Most skin cancer cases are linked to exposure to ultraviolet (UV) rays from the sun and indoor tanning beds. UV rays damage the DNA of immature skin cells, which then reproduce uncontrollably. Research has shown that a person's risk for skin cancer doubles if he or she has had five or more sunburns; however, your risk for skin cancer still increases with UV exposure even if you do not get sunburned. Exposure to tanning beds before age 35 increases by 75% your risk of developing the most invasive form of skin cancer.[18]

Skin cancer includes the nonmelanoma cancers (basal cell and squamous cell cancers), which are not typically invasive, and malignant melanoma, which is one of the most deadly of all types of cancer (**Figure 10.21**, page 408). Limiting exposure to sunlight to no more than 20 minutes between 10 AM and 4 PM can help reduce your risk for skin cancer while allowing your body to synthesize adequate vitamin D. After that, wear sunscreen with at least a 15 SPF (sun protection factor) rating and protective clothing.

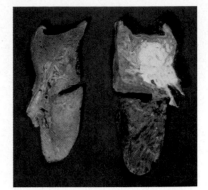

FIGURE 10.19 Cigarette smoking significantly increases our risk for lung and other types of cancer. The risk for lung cancer is twenty-three times higher in men who smoke and twelve times higher in women who smoke. **(a)** A normal, healthy lung; **(b)** the lung of a smoker. Notice the deposits of tar, as well as the areas of tumor growth.

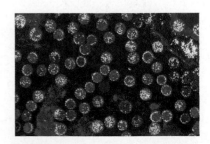

FIGURE 10.20 High-risk human papillomaviruses (high-risk HPVs) are a group of viruses that can cause cancer.

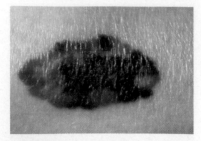

FIGURE 10.21 A lesion associated with malignant melanoma is characterized by asymmetry; uneven or blurred borders; mixed shades of tan, brown, black, and sometimes red or blue; and a diameter larger than a pencil eraser (6 mm).

Antioxidants Play a Role in Preventing Cancer

There is a large and growing body of evidence that antioxidants consumed in food play an important role in cancer prevention, but how? The following are some proposed mechanisms:

- Enhancing the immune system, which assists in the destruction and removal of precancerous cells from the body
- Preventing oxidative damage to the cells' DNA by scavenging free radicals and stopping the formation and subsequent chain reaction of oxidized molecules
- Inhibiting the growth of cancer cells and tumors
- Inhibiting the capacity of cancer cells to avoid aging and apoptosis (programmed cell death)

Eating whole foods—especially fruits, vegetables, and whole grains—that are high in antioxidant phytochemicals is linked with probable evidence of decreased risk for various cancers. (See the In Depth following this chapter for a detailed look at phytochemicals.) For example, several recent studies have suggested that consuming fruits, vegetables, spices, and teas high in a phytochemical called apigenin, a type of flavonoid, might alter gene regulation in cancer cells in a way that impairs their ability to avoid aging and apoptosis.[19,20] Another group of flavonoids, anthocyanins, are plant pigments thought to have antioxidant and anti-inflammatory properties. Produce with intense colors, such as blue corn and blackberries, has higher levels of anthocyanin pigments. Finally, glucosinolates, a group of phytochemicals found in cruciferous vegetables like Brussels sprouts and broccoli, as well as in bitter greens such as arugula, inhibit cell division and stimulate apoptosis in tumor cells.[21]

In addition, populations eating diets low in antioxidant micronutrients have a higher risk for cancer. These studies show varying levels of association between these factors, but they do not prove cause and effect. Nutrition experts agree that there are important interactions between antioxidant nutrients and phytochemicals, fiber, and other substances in foods, all of which may work together to reduce the risk for many types of cancers. Studies are now being conducted to determine whether eating foods high in antioxidants directly causes lower rates of cancer.

As noted previously, growing evidence over the past 20 years indicates that antioxidant supplementation does not reduce cancer risk; in fact, it may increase risks for various cancers and other chronic diseases.[22] Why have antioxidant supplements failed to bring the health benefits one might expect? It has been speculated that antioxidants taken in supplement form may act as prooxidants in some situations, whereas antioxidants consumed in foods may be more balanced.

Thus, it appears that the best way to try to reduce our risk for cancer is to eat a diet with ample fruits and vegetables, maintain a healthy body weight, stay regularly physically active, quit smoking if applicable, and avoid exposure to infectious agents and UV radiation. Refer to the *Nutrition Myth or Fact?* at the end of the chapter to gain a better understanding of situations that may warrant vitamin and mineral supplementation.

Free Radical Damage Plays a Role in Cardiovascular Disease

The details of *cardiovascular disease* (*CVD*) and its relationship to cholesterol and lipoproteins were presented earlier in this text (see Chapter 5). A brief review of CVD is presented here, focusing on the question of how antioxidants may reduce the risk for CVD.

Cardiovascular disease is the leading cause of death for adults in the United States. CVD encompasses all diseases of the heart and blood vessels, including coronary heart disease, hypertension (high blood pressure), cerebrovascular disease, and many more. The two primary manifestations of CVD are heart attack and stroke. About 610,000 people die each year from CVD, and it is estimated that CVD costs the United States about $109 billion each year in healthcare costs and lost work revenue.[23,24]

Remember that the major risks for CVD are smoking, hypertension, high blood levels of LDL-cholesterol, obesity, and a sedentary lifestyle. Other risk factors include a low level of HDL-cholesterol, diabetes, family history (CVD in males younger than

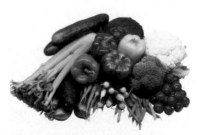

These vegetables provide antioxidant nutrients, fiber, and phytochemicals, all of which reduce the risk for some cancers.

55 years of age and females younger than 65 years of age), being a male older than 45 years of age, and being a postmenopausal woman. Although we cannot alter our gender, family history, or age, we can change our nutrition and physical activity habits to reduce our risk for CVD.

Research has recently identified a risk factor for CVD that may be even more important than elevated cholesterol levels: a condition called *low-grade inflammation*.[25] This condition weakens the atherosclerotic plaque in the blood vessels, making it more fragile. As the plaque becomes more fragile, it is more likely to burst, breaking away from the arterial lining and traveling freely in the bloodstream. It may then lodge in the blood vessels of the heart or brain, closing them off and leading to a heart attack or stroke, respectively.

In laboratory blood tests, the marker that indicates the degree of inflammation is C-reactive protein (CRP). Having higher levels of CRP increases the risk for a heart attack even if people do not have elevated cholesterol levels. For people with high levels of CRP and cholesterol, the risk for a heart attack is almost nine times higher than that for someone with normal levels of both. These findings have prompted the medical community to develop standards for measuring CRP along with cholesterol as a test for CVD risk. We noted earlier in this chapter that, among other reasons, free radicals are harmful because they promote blood-vessel inflammation. Thus, it is possible that an elevated level of CRP may reflect oxidative stress, and that a diet rich in antioxidants might help.

We also said earlier that free radicals promote the formation of blood clots—including within the coronary and cerebrovascular arteries serving the heart and brain. Clot formation in these sites can trigger a heart attack or stroke. You might know that physicians sometimes prescribe low-dose aspirin—an anticoagulant—for patients at high risk for CVD. An adequate intake of antioxidant-rich foods may have a similar effect.

Epidemiological studies find consistent associations between consumption of foods high in antioxidants and a decreased risk for CVD. What mechanisms might explain this reduced risk? Laboratory studies suggest that some antioxidants, specifically vitamin E and the phytochemical lycopene, work in a variety of ways that reduce damage to blood vessels. This, in turn, reduces an individual's risk for a heart attack or stroke. One way antioxidants protect blood vessels is by scavenging free radicals. As discussed earlier in this chapter, this protects cell membranes, including those of endothelial (blood vessel lining) cells. In addition, studies suggest that an antioxidant-rich diet is associated with lower levels of inflammation.[26,27] Finally, we just noted that certain antioxidants, like vitamin E, have anticoagulant properties. They might therefore protect blood vessels by reducing the formation of blood clots.

It is important to note that other compounds (besides antioxidants) found in fruits, vegetables, and whole grains can reduce our risk for CVD. For instance, soluble fiber has been shown to reduce elevated LDL-cholesterol and total cholesterol. The most successful effects have been found in people eating oatmeal and oat-bran cereals. Dietary fiber in general has been shown to reduce blood pressure, lower total cholesterol levels, and improve blood glucose and insulin levels. Folate is found in fortified cereals, bananas, legumes, orange juice, and green, leafy vegetables. Folate is known to reduce homocysteine levels in the blood, and a high concentration of homocysteine in the blood is a known risk factor for CVD. Thus, it appears that there are a plethora of nutrients and other components in fruits, vegetables, and whole-grain foods that may be protective against CVD.

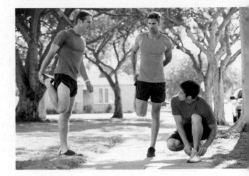

Staying physically active may help reduce our risk for some cancers.

Hear the real stories of people living with smoking-related diseases and disability by going to the Centers for Disease Control and Prevention "Tips from Former Smokers at http://www .cdc.gov/tobacco/campaign/tips/

RECAP

Cancer is a group of diseases in which genetically mutated cells grow out of control. Its three stages include initiation, promotion, and progression. Tobacco use, obesity, dietary factors, low physical activity levels, infectious agents, and UV radiation are related to a higher risk for some cancers. Eating foods high in antioxidants is associated with lower rates of cancer and cardiovascular disease (CVD), but studies of antioxidant supplements, cancer, and CVD indicate that taking these supplements is not helpful and may even increase your health risks. ■

Nutrition Myth OR Fact?

Dietary Supplements: Necessity or Waste?

In April of 2015, 14 U.S. Attorneys General signed a letter to the congressional subcommittee responsible for consumer product safety requesting that Congress launch an investigation of the dietary supplements industry. The action came after DNA testing of certain supplements brands found that they did not contain the ingredients promised on the labels; some were contaminated with high levels of heavy metals like lead and mercury; and some contained allergens such as wheat and grass not identified on the label. In response, the Natural Products Association trade group called the action "harassment."

The use of dietary supplements in the United States has skyrocketed in recent years. The National Institutes of Health cites annual sales of supplements in the United States at $32.5 billion.[1] Currently, about half of American adults report using one or more dietary supplements.[2] However, many say they don't report the use of these products to their physicians because they feel their physicians have little knowledge of supplements and may discourage their use.

Is it smart to use supplements? Dangerous? Who, if anyone, *should* be taking them? To answer these questions, you need to make sure you know what a dietary supplement is.

What Are Dietary Supplements?

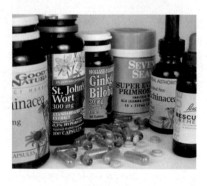

According to the U.S. Food and Drug Administration (FDA), a dietary supplement is "a product intended for ingestion that contains a 'dietary ingredient' intended to add further nutritional value to (supplement) the diet."[3] Supplements may contain vitamins, minerals, herbs or other botanicals, amino acids, enzymes, tissues from animal organs or glands, or a concentrate, a metabolite, a constituent, or an extract. Supplements come in many forms, including pills, capsules, liquids, and powders.

How Are Dietary Supplements Regulated?

As presented in the Dietary Supplement Health and Education Act (DSHEA) of 1994, dietary supplements are categorized within the general group of foods, not drugs. This means that the regulation of supplements is much less rigorous than the regulation of drugs. As an informed consumer, you should know the following:

- Dietary supplements do not need approval from the FDA before they are marketed.
- The company that manufactures a supplement is responsible for determining that the supplement is safe;

the FDA does not test any supplement for safety prior to marketing.

- Supplement companies do not have to provide the FDA with any evidence that their supplements are safe unless the company is marketing a new dietary ingredient that was not sold in the United States prior to 1994.
- There are at present no federal guidelines on practices to ensure the purity, quality, safety, and composition of dietary supplements.
- There are no rules to limit the serving size or amount of a nutrient in any dietary supplement.
- Once a supplement is marketed, the FDA must prove it unsafe before the product will be removed from the market.

Despite these limitations in supplement regulation, supplement manufacturers are required to follow dietary supplement labeling guidelines. There are specific requirements for the information that must be included on supplement labels. Federal advertising regulations also require that any claims on the label must be truthful and not misleading and that advertisers must be able to substantiate all label claims. In addition, labels bearing a claim must also include the disclaimer "This statement has not been evaluated by the FDA. This product is not intended to diagnose, cure, or prevent any disease." Any products not meeting these guidelines can be removed from the market.

How Can You Avoid Fraudulent or Dangerous Supplements?

Although many of the supplement products sold today are safe, some are not. A 2014 study, for example, found that, over a 10-year period, eight U.S. medical centers reported over 100 cases of drug-induced liver injury caused by dietary supplements. Many of these cases resulted in the need for a liver transplant, and 13% of the cases resulted in death.[4] In addition, as the 2015 study of supplement DNA revealed, some companies are less than forthright about the true content of their supplements. How can you avoid purchasing dangerous or fraudulent supplements? The FDA suggests that consumers do the following when evaluating dietary supplements:[5]

1. Check with your healthcare provider or a registered dietician nutritionist about any nutrients you may need in addition to your regular diet.
2. Ask your healthcare provider for help distinguishing between reliable and questionable information.
3. Look for the Pharmacopeia (USP) Verified Mark on the label. This mark indicates that the manufacturer followed the standards that the USP has established for features such as purity, strength, quality, packaging, labeling, and acceptable length of storage.
4. Consider buying recognized brands of supplements. Although not guaranteed, products made by nationally

recognized companies more likely have well-established manufacturing standards.

5. Do not assume that the word *natural* on the label means that the product is safe. Arsenic, lead, and mercury are all natural substances that can kill you if consumed in large enough quantities.

6. Be skeptical of anecdotal information or personal testimonials.

7. Ask yourself if the claims for the supplement sound too good to be true. Warning signs include exaggerated, unrealistic, or extreme claims; for example, promising that the supplement will enable you to lose a large amount of weight in a short amount of time, or that it can cure a chronic disease.

8. Do not hesitate to question a company about how it makes its products. Reputable companies have nothing to hide and are more than happy to inform their customers about the safety and quality of their products.

What About Botanicals?

A common saying in India cautions that "A house without ginger is a sick house." Indeed, ginger, echinacea, lavender, and many other *botanicals* have been used by different cultures throughout the world for centuries to promote health and treat discomfort and disease. The National Institutes of Health Office of Dietary Supplements defines a *botanical* as a plant or plant part valued for its medicinal or therapeutic properties, flavor, and/or scent.[6] They are commonly referred to as "herbs." Currently, 20% of adults in the United States use a dietary supplement with at least one herbal ingredient, either in combination with another dietary supplement, such as a vitamin/mineral supplement with echinacea, or alone.[2]

There are hundreds of different herbs on the market. If you're considering purchasing an herbal remedy, the National Center for Complimentary and Integrative Health (NCCIH) evaluates dozens of the most common in their "Herbs at a Glance" fact sheets, available online (see **Web Links** at the end of this chapter). In addition to the tips listed previously, which apply to all types of dietary supplements, the following precautions are specific to the use of herbs.

Consult a healthcare provider before using any herbal supplement. Herbs can act the same way as drugs; therefore, they can cause medical problems if not used correctly or if taken in large amounts. It's especially important to check with your healthcare provider if you are taking any prescription medications. Some herbal supplements are known to interact with medications in ways that cause health problems.

Avoid using herbs if you are pregnant or nursing unless your physician has approved their use. Some can promote miscarriage or birth defects or can enter breast milk. This caution also applies to treating children with herbal supplements.

Finally, be aware that the active ingredients in many herbs and herbal supplements are not known. There may be dozens, even hundreds, of unknown compounds in an herbal supplement. Also, published analyses of herbal supplements have found differences between what's listed on the label and what's in the bottle. This means you may be taking less— or more—of the supplement than what the label indicates or ingesting substances not mentioned on the label. Some herbal supplements have been found to be contaminated with metals, unlabeled prescription drugs, microorganisms, and other substances.[7] Be aware that the words *standardized, certified,* or *verified* on a label are no guarantee of product quality; in the United States, these terms have no legal definition for supplements.

Should You Take a Dietary Supplement?

Contrary to what some people believe, not all people need to supplement their diets all of the time. In fact, foods contain a diverse combination of compounds that are critical to our health, and vitamin and mineral supplements do not contain the same amount or variety of substances found in foods. Thus, dietary supplements are not substitutes for whole foods. In fact, in 2013, an editorial appeared in the *Annals of Internal Medicine* that advised most Americans to stop wasting their money on multivitamin-mineral supplements.[8] This editorial highlighted three articles published in that issue of the journal that independently illustrated no clear evidence of a beneficial effect of dietary supplementation on all-cause mortality, CVD, cancer,[9] cognitive decline,[10] or recurrence of cardiovascular events in adults who had experienced a previous myocardial infarction (or heart attack).[11] Thus, the U.S. Preventive Services Taskforce has concluded that current evidence is insufficient to support the use of multivitamins, or single- or paired-nutrient supplements, and they recommend against using beta-carotene or vitamin E supplements, in the prevention of CVD or cancer.[9]

However, our nutritional needs change throughout our life spans, so you may benefit from taking a supplement at certain times for certain reasons. For instance, if you adopt a vegan diet in your college years, your healthcare provider might prescribe a supplement providing riboflavin, vitamin B_{12}, vitamin D, calcium, iron, and zinc. Animal products are high in these nutrients, so if you eliminate these foods, you might not get enough of these nutrients in the other foods you are eating. Or if you're a member of your college soccer team, your team's sport dietitian might advise taking a supplement formulated to provide micronutrients that support intense physical activity.

Dietary supplements include hundreds of thousands of products sold for many purposes, and it is impossible to discuss here all of the various situations in which their use may be advisable. So let's focus on identifying the groups of people who may or may not benefit from taking vitamin and mineral supplements.

Table 10.2 (page 412) lists groups of people who may benefit from supplementation. But even if you fall within one of these groups, it's still important to analyze your total diet to determine whether you need to take the vitamin or mineral supplement indicated. It is also a good idea to check with your healthcare provider or a registered dietitian (RD) before taking any supplements, as supplements can interfere with some prescription and over-the-counter medications.

Of course, many people who do not need to take supplements do so anyway. The following are instances in which taking vitamin and mineral supplements is unnecessary, or even harmful:

1. Providing fluoride supplements to children who already drink fluoridated water

2. Taking supplements in the belief that they will cure a disease, such as cancer, diabetes, or heart disease

TABLE 10.2 Individuals Who May Benefit from Dietary Supplementation

Type of Individual	Specific Supplements That May Help
Newborns	Routinely given a single dose of vitamin K at birth
Infants	Depends on age and nutrition; may need iron, vitamin D, or other nutrients
Children not drinking fluoridated water	Fluoride supplements
Children on strict vegetarian diets	Vitamin B_{12}, iron, zinc, vitamin D (if not exposed to sunlight)
Children with poor eating habits or overweight children on an energy-restricted diet	Multivitamin-multimineral supplement that does not exceed the RDA for the nutrients it contains
Pregnant teenagers	Iron and folic acid; other nutrients may be necessary if diet is very poor
Women who may become pregnant	Multivitamin or multivitamin-multimineral supplement that contains 0.4 mg of folic acid
Pregnant or lactating women	Multivitamin-multimineral supplement that contains iron, folic acid, zinc, copper, calcium, vitamin B_6, vitamin C, vitamin D
People on prolonged weight-reduction diets	Multivitamin-multimineral supplement
People recovering from serious illness or surgery	Multivitamin-multimineral supplement
People with HIV/AIDS or other wasting diseases; people addicted to drugs or alcohol	Multivitamin-multimineral supplement or single-nutrient supplements
People who do not consume adequate calcium	Calcium supplements: for example, teens need to consume 1,300 mg of dietary calcium per day; thus, supplements may be necessary
People whose exposure to sunlight is inadequate to allow synthesis of adequate vitamin D	Vitamin D
People eating a vegan diet	Vitamin B_{12}, riboflavin, calcium, vitamin D, iron, zinc
People who have had portions of the intestinal tract removed; people who have a malabsorptive disease	Depends on the exact condition; may include various fat-soluble and/or water-soluble vitamins and other nutrients
People with lactose intolerance	Calcium supplements
Elderly people	Multivitamin-multimineral supplement, vitamin B_{12}

3. Taking supplements with certain medications. For instance, people who take the blood-thinning drug Coumadin should not take vitamin E or K supplements, as this can cause excessive bleeding. People who take aspirin daily should check with their physicians before taking vitamin E or K supplements, as aspirin also thins the blood.

4. Taking nonprescribed supplements if you have liver or kidney disease. Physicians may prescribe vitamin and mineral supplements for their patients, because many nutrients are lost during treatment for these diseases. However, these individuals cannot properly metabolize certain supplements and should not take any that are not prescribed by their physicians because of a high risk for toxicity.

5. Taking beta-carotene supplements, particularly if you are a smoker. As already mentioned, there is evidence that beta-carotene supplementation increases the risk for lung and other cancers and increases the risk for premature mortality. Moreover, a recent systematic review and meta-analysis examining randomized, controlled trials on antioxidant supplements found that taking beta-carotene, vitamin E, and vitamin A increases the risk for premature mortality from all causes.[12] The review examined

randomized controlled trials where these nutrients were taken separately, or in combination with each other, with other vitamins, or with trace elements with no known antioxidant function.

6. Taking vitamins and minerals in an attempt to improve physical appearance or athletic performance. There is no evidence that vitamin and mineral supplements enhance appearance or athletic performance in healthy adults who consume a varied diet with adequate energy.

7. Taking supplements to increase energy level. Vitamin and mineral supplements do not provide energy, because they do not contain fat, carbohydrate, or protein (sources of Calories). Although many vitamins and minerals are necessary for us to produce energy, taking dietary supplements in place of eating food will not provide us with the energy necessary to live a healthy and productive life.

8. Taking single-nutrient supplements, unless a qualified healthcare practitioner prescribes a single-nutrient supplement for a diagnosed medical condition (iron supplements for someone with anemia). These products contain very high amounts of the given nutrient, and taking them can quickly lead to toxicity.

The Academy of Nutrition and Dietetics advises that the ideal nutritional strategy for optimizing health is to eat a healthful diet that contains a variety of whole foods.[13] If you do use a supplement, select one that contains no more than 100% of the recommended levels for the nutrients it contains. Avoid taking single-nutrient supplements unless advised to do so by your healthcare practitioner. Finally, avoid taking supplements that contain substances known to cause illness or injuries. Some of these substances are listed in **Table 10.3**.

TABLE 10.3 Supplement Ingredients Associated with Illnesses and Injuries

Ingredient	Potential Risks
Herbal Ingredients	
Gingko	Headache, nausea, gastrointestinal upset, diarrhea, dizziness, allergic skin reactions, increased bleeding risk
Kava (also known as kava kava)	Severe liver toxicity
Ephedra (also known as ma huang, Chinese ephedra, and epitonin)	High blood pressure, irregular heartbeat, nerve damage, insomnia, tremors, headaches, seizures, heart attack, stroke, possible death
Lobelia	Breathing problems, nausea, vomiting, diarrhea, cough, dizziness, tremors, excessive sweating, convulsions, rapid heartbeat, low blood pressure, coma, possible death
Willow bark	Reye's syndrome (a potentially fatal disease that may occur when children take aspirin), allergic reaction in adults
Yohimbe	High blood pressure, increased heart rate, headache, anxiety, dizziness, vomiting, tremors, and sleeplessness
Vitamins and Essential Minerals	
Vitamin A (when taking 25,000 IU or more per day)	Birth defects, bone abnormalities, severe liver disease
Vitamin B$_6$ (when taking more than 100 mg per day)	Loss of balance, injuries to nerves that alter touch sensation
Niacin (when taking slow-release doses of 500 mg or more per day or when taking immediate-release doses of 750 mg or more per day)	Stomach pain; nausea; vomiting; bloating; cramping; diarrhea; liver disease; damage to the muscles, eyes, and heart
Selenium (when taking 800 to 1,000 µg per day)	Tissue damage
Other Ingredients	
Germanium (a nonessential mineral)	Kidney damage
L-tryptophan (an amino acid)	Eosinophilia-myalgia syndrome (a potentially fatal blood disorder that causes high fever)

Sources: Data from NIH National Center for Complementary and Integrative Health. 2015. Herbs at a Glance. https://nccih.nih.gov/health/herbsataglance .htmand; WebMD. 2015. Vitamins & Supplements. http://www.webmd.com /vitamins-supplements/.

Critical Thinking Questions

■ Do you think that the FDA should more closely regulate supplement manufacturers? If so, how?

■ Have you decided whether taking a supplement is right for you? Why or why not?

References

1. National Institutes of Health (NIH). Office of Dietary Supplements. 2013. *Multivitamin/mineral Supplements.* http://ods.od.nih.gov/factsheets/MVMS-HealthProfessional/.
2. Bailey, R. L., J. J Gahche, C. V. Lentino, J. T. Dwyer, J. S. Engel, P. R. Thomas,…, and M. F. Picciano. 2011. Dietary supplement use in the United States, 2003–2006. *J. Nutr.* 141(2):261–266.
3. U.S. Food and Drug Administration (FDA). 2015. What is a dietary supplement? http://www.fda.gov/AboutFDA /Transparency/Basics/ucm195635.htm
4. Navarro, V. J., H. Barnhart, H. L. Bonkovsky, T. Davern, R. J. Fontana, L. Grant,…, and R. Vuppalanchi. 2014. Liver injury from herbals and dietary supplements in the U.S. Drug-Induced Liver Injury Network. *Hepatol.* 60(4):1399–1408.
5. U.S. Food and Drug Administration (FDA). 2013. 6 Tip-offs to Rip-offs: Don't Fall for Health Fraud Scams. http://www.fda .gov/ForConsumers/ConsumerUpdates/ucm341344.htm.
6. National Institutes of Health. Office of Dietary Supplements. 2011. Botanical Dietary Supplements. http://ods.od.nih.gov /factsheets/BotanicalBackground-HealthProfessional/.
7. Newmaster, S. G., M. Grguric, D. Shanmughanandhan, S. Ramalingam, and S. Ragupahty. 2013. DNA barcoding detects contamination and substitution in North American herbal products. *BMC Med.* 11:222, http://www. biomedcentral.com/1741-7015/11/222.
8. Guallar, E., S. Stranges, C. Mulrow, L. J. Appel, and E. R. Miller III. 2013. Enough is enough: stop wasting money on vitamin and mineral supplements. *Ann. Intern. Med.* 159(12):850–851.
9. Fortmann S. P., B. U. Burda, C. A. Senger, J. S. Lin, and E. P. Whitlock. 2013. Vitamin and mineral supplements in the primary prevention of cardiovascular disease and cancer: an updated systematic evidence review for the U.S. Preventive Services Task Force. *Ann. Intern. Med.* 159:824–834.
10. Grodstein F., J. O'Brien, J. H. Kang, R. Dushkes, N. R. Cook, O. Okereke O,…, and H. D. Sesso. 2013. Long-term multivitamin supplementation and cognitive function in men. A randomized trial. *Ann. Intern. Med.* 159:806–814.
11. Lin J. S., E. O'Connor, R. C. Rossom, L. A. Perdue, E. Eckstrom. 2013. Screening for cognitive impairment in older adults: a systematic review for the U.S. Preventive Services Task Force. *Ann. Intern. Med.* 159:601–612.
12. Bjelakovic, G., D. Nikolova, L. L. Gluud, R. G. Simonetti, and C. Gluud. 2012. Antioxidant supplements for prevention of mortality in healthy participants and patients with various diseases. *Cochrane Database Syst. Rev.* Issue 3. Art. No.: CD007176. DOI: 10.1002/14651858. CD007176.pub2.
13. Freeland Graves, J. H., S. Nitzke, Academy of Nutrition and Dietetics. 2013. Position of the Academy of Nutrition and Dietetics: Total diet approach to healthy eating.

STUDY PLAN   MasteringNutrition™

Customize your study plan—and master your nutrition!—
in the Study Area of MasteringNutrition.

summary

 Scan to hear an MP3 Chapter Review in **MasteringNutrition**.

LO 1 ■ Antioxidants are compounds that protect our cells from oxidative damage.

■ Free radicals are produced under many situations, including when a stable atom loses an electron during oxidation reactions, when oxygen gains a free electron released during the generation of ATP, when the immune system fights infection, and when we are exposed to environmental toxins, such as pollution, radiation, and tobacco smoke.

■ Free radicals are dangerous because they can damage the lipid portion of our cell membranes, destroying their integrity. Free radicals also damage LDLs, cell proteins, and DNA.

■ Antioxidant vitamins donate their electrons or hydrogen atoms to free radicals to neutralize them. Antioxidant minerals are cofactors in antioxidant enzyme systems, which convert free radicals to less damaging substances that our bodies excrete. Some phytochemicals have antioxidant properties.

LO 2 ■ Vitamin E is an antioxidant fat-soluble vitamin. Of its several forms, the most active vitamin E compound found in food and supplements is *alpha-tocopherol.*

■ Vitamin E protects the fatty components of cell membranes from oxidation. It also protects LDLs, vitamin A, and our lungs from oxidative damage. Other functions of vitamin E are the development of nerves and muscles, enhancement of the immune function, and improvement of the absorption of vitamin A if intake of vitamin A is low.

■ Good food sources of vitamin E include plant oils, nuts, seeds, soybeans, and some vegetables. Vitamin E supplementation has been linked to premature mortality. Vitamin E deficiency is uncommon except in people with malabsorption disorders.

LO 3 ■ Vitamin C is a water-soluble vitamin essential for the synthesis of collagen and the prevention of scurvy. It is also required for the synthesis of carnitine, various hormones, neurotransmitters, and DNA. Vitamin C is oxidized by free radicals and prevents the damage of cells and tissues. Vitamin C also regenerates vitamin E after it has been oxidized. Other functions of vitamin C include enhancing immune function and increasing the absorption of iron.

■ Fruits and vegetables are excellent sources of vitamin C, as are 100% fruit juices. Toxicity is rare except in people taking high-dose supplements. Deficiency leads to scurvy and can contribute to anemia.

LO 4 ■ Five trace minerals have antioxidant functions. These include selenium, copper, iron, zinc, and manganese.

■ Selenium is a trace mineral that is part of the structure of glutathione peroxidases, a family of antioxidant enzymes. Other functions of selenium include assisting in the production of thyroid hormone and enhancing immune function. Selenium is found in variable amounts in many plant and animal foods; organ meats, pork, and seafood are reliable sources.

■ Copper, iron, zinc, and manganese are trace minerals that act as cofactors for antioxidant enzyme systems. Copper, zinc, and manganese are part of the superoxide dismutase complex, whereas iron is part of catalase. These minerals also play important roles in energy metabolism, and iron, zinc, and copper are critical in blood formation.

LO 5 ■ The phytochemical beta-carotene is one of about 600 carotenoids identified to date. Beta-carotene is a provitamin, or precursor, to vitamin A, meaning it is an inactive form of vitamin A that is converted to vitamin A in the body.

■ Beta-carotene protects the lipid portions of cell membranes and LDL-cholesterol from oxidative damage. Other functions of beta-carotene include enhancing our immune system, protecting our skin from sun damage, and protecting our eyes from oxidative damage. Eating foods high in carotenoids may help reduce our risk for some forms of cancer.

■ Yellowing of the skin can occur if too much beta-carotene is consumed; however, this is harmless and reversible. Taking beta-carotene supplements can increase the risk for premature death from lung cancer, heart disease, and stroke.

LO 6 ■ Vitamin A is a fat-soluble vitamin. The three active forms of vitamin A are retinol, retinal, and retinoic acid. They are collectively referred to as the retinoids. Of the three, retinol has the main role in physiologic functioning. Beta-carotene is converted to vitamin A in the small intestine.

■ Vitamin A is essential for healthy vision. Found in the retina, it combines with a protein called opsin to form rhodopsin, a light-sensitive pigment. When vitamin A detaches from rhodopsin, a cascade of changes occur that result in the transmission of visual messages to the brain. Vitamin A thereby enables the eyes to adjust to changes in the brightness of light and to recover from a bright flash of light. Through a related process, vitamin A also helps maintain color vision.

■ Vitamin A was once considered an antioxidant, but this role is not supported by recent research evidence. Other functions of vitamin A include assistance in cell differentiation, maintenance of healthy immune function, sexual reproduction, and proper bone growth.

LO 7 ■ Vitamin A toxicity can develop after consuming only three to four times the RDA. It can damage the liver and nervous system, and even be fatal. In pregnant women, vitamin A toxicity can cause birth defects and spontaneous abortion.

■ Deficiency of vitamin A can result in night blindness, color blindness, and xerophthalmia, a hardening of the cornea that causes irreversible blindness. Deficiency also leads to hyperkeratosis, impaired immunity, reproductive system disorders, and failure of normal growth.

■ Antioxidants play a role in cancer and CVD prevention. Eating foods high in antioxidants results in lower rates of some cancers and risk for CVD, but taking antioxidant supplements can cause cancer and increase the risk for premature mortality.

LO 8 ■ Cancer is a group of diseases that are all characterized by cells that grow "out of control." It is initiated when a cell's DNA is mutated; during promotion, the genetically altered cell is stimulated to divide and, after many years, it may form a detectable tumor; during progression, the tumor develops its own blood supply, invades nearby tissues, and may release malignant cells that travel through blood or lymph to distant body sites.

LO 9 ■ Random mutations and heredity play roles in the development of cancer. Modifiable risk factors include tobacco use, body weight, diet, physical activity, infection, and exposure to ultraviolet radiation also influence cancer risk.

■ There is evidence that consuming a diet rich in fruits, vegetables, and whole grains, all of which provide antioxidants, plays an important role in cancer prevention. In contrast, taking antioxidant supplements does not influence cancer risk, and taking high doses of antioxidant supplements has been shown to increase risk.

LO 10   ■ Free radicals play a role in increasing our risks for CVD by injuring the membranes of endothelial cells; promoting low-grade inflammation, which damages blood vessel walls; and increasing the formation of blood clots. Consuming antioxidant-rich foods is associated with a decreased risk for CVD. It is hypothesized that the antioxidant vitamins and minerals and phytochemicals in these foods act to scavenge free radicals, and reduce inflammation, blood vessel damage, and excessive blood clot formation.

review questions

LO 1   **1.** Oxidation is best described as a process in which
  a. a carcinogen causes a mutation in a stem cell's DNA.
  b. an atom loses an electron.
  c. two atoms exchange electrons.
  d. a complex compound is broken apart with the addition of water.

LO 2   **2.** Which of the following is a characteristic of vitamin E?
  a. It enhances the absorption of iron.
  b. It can be manufactured from beta-carotene.
  c. It is a critical component of the glutathione peroxidase system.
  d. It protects the lipid molecules in cell membranes from oxidation.

LO 3   **3.** Which of the following is a critical function of vitamin C?
  a. It is required for the formation of collagen.
  b. It regenerates glutathione to its antioxidant form.
  c. It reduces the incidence, duration, and severity of the common cold.
  d. It promotes the conversion of beta-carotene to vitamin A.

LO 4   **4.** Which of the following trace minerals is part of the structure of catalase?
  a. iodine
  b. iron
  c. copper
  d. manganese

LO 5   **5.** Beta-carotene is
  a. a weak antioxidant phytochemical.
  b. a carotenoid.
  c. a provitamin for vitamin A.
  d. all of the above.

LO 6   **6.** Vitamin A
  a. participates in the conversion of iodopsin to rhodopsin, a key step in both black-and-white and color vision.
  b. opposes oxidation of the pigment in rod cells during the bleaching process.
  c. is a key component of the pigment in rod cells that enables us to perceive black-and-white images.
  d. is a key player in the process by which humans see in the dark.

LO 7   **7.** Deficiency of vitamin A is associated with
  a. scurvy and anemia
  b. erythrocyte hemolysis and impaired movement
  c. xerophthalmia and hyperkeratosis
  d. carotenosis and carotenodermia

LO 8   **8.** Within a year or two of its initiation, cancer develops to the point at which it is able to
  a. invade surrounding tissues.
  b. establish its own blood supply.
  c. release malignant cells into the blood or lymph.
  d. none of the above is true.

LO 9   **9.** The modifiable factor that most significantly increases the risk for cancer is
  a. random mutation.
  b. heredity.
  c. tobacco use.
  d. poor nutrition.

LO 10   **10.** A diet rich in antioxidant nutrients may help reduce the risk for CVD by
  a. causing body cells with mutated DNA to self-repair or self-destruct.
  b. protecting endothelial cell membranes and reducing inflammation and coagulation.
  c. promoting the synthesis of homocysteine and CRP.
  d. all of the above.

true or false?

LO 1   **11. True or false?** Free-radical formation can occur as a result of normal cellular metabolism.

LO 2   **12. True or false?** Vitamin C helps regenerate vitamin A.

LO 3   **13. True or false?** As part of glutathione peroxidase, selenium neutralizes peroxide molecules and spares vitamin E.

LO 4   **14. True or false?** Pregnant women are advised to consume plentiful quantities of beef liver.

LO 5   **15. True or false?** Cervical cancer is caused by a sexually transmitted virus.

short answer

LO 1 16. Explain how free radicals damage cell membranes and lead to cell death.

LO 2 17. Explain how vitamin E reduces our risk for cardiovascular disease.

LO 4 18. Discuss the contribution of trace minerals, such as selenium, to the prevention of oxidation.

LO 5 19. Nico's father is 66 years old, smokes, is overweight, sedentary, and has a family history

of cancer. He mentions to Nico that, given his cancer risks, he is planning to start taking an antioxidant supplement on sale at his local drug store. One capsule of the supplement contains 200 mg of vitamin C, 30 mg of beta-carotene and 100 µg of selenium. What advice should Nico give his father?

LO 8 20. Describe the process by which cancer occurs, beginning with initiation and ending with metastasis of the cancer to widespread body tissues.

math review

LO 2 21. Joey is home, visiting his parents for the weekend, and he finds a bottle of vitamin E supplements in the medicine cabinet. He asks his parents about them, and his mother says that she is worried about having a weak immune system and read on the Internet that vitamin E can boost immunity. As Joey's mother eats plenty of plant foods and oils that are good sources of vitamin E, he is worried she may be consuming too much by adding these supplements to her diet. Each supplement capsule contains 400 IU of dl-alpha-tocopherol,

and she takes one capsule each day. Answer the following questions:

a. How much vitamin E in mg is Joey's mother consuming each day from these supplements?

b. What percentage of the RDA for vitamin E do these supplements provide?

c. Based on what you've learned in this chapter about vitamin E, should Joey's mother be worried about vitamin E toxicity? Would your answer be different if you learned that she is taking aspirin each day, as prescribed by her doctor?

Answers to Review Questions and Math Review can be found online in the MasteringNutrition Study Area.

web links

www.who.int/en
World Health Organization (WHO)
Click on "Health Topics" and select "nutrition disorders" and then "Nutrition: micronutrients" to find out more about vitamin A deficiency around the world.

www.heart.org/HEARTORG
American Heart Association
Discover the best way to lower your risk for cardiovascular disease.

www.cancer.org
American Cancer Society (ACS)
Get ACS recommendations for nutrition and physical activity for cancer prevention.

www.cancer.gov
National Cancer Institute
Learn more about the nutritional factors that can influence your risk for cancer.

www.fda.gov
U.S. Food and Drug Administration
Select "Food" on the pull-down menu and then click on "Dietary Supplements" under the heading "Navigate

the Food Section" for more information on how to make informed decisions and evaluate information related to dietary supplements.

fnic.nal.usda.gov
Food and Nutrition Information Center, U.S. Department of Agriculture National Agricultural Library
Click on the "Dietary Supplements" link in the "Browse By Subject" box to obtain information on vitamin and mineral supplements, including consumer reports and industry regulations.

ods.od.nih.gov
Office of Dietary Supplements
Go to this site to obtain current research results and reliable information about dietary supplements.

nccih.nih.gov
National Centre for Complementary and Integrative Health
Go to this site to learn more about botanicals, herbs, and other forms of dietary supplements.

Phytochemicals: Another Advantage of Plants

After studying this In Depth, you should be able to:

1 Define phytochemicals and identify a few of the most common phytochemical groups, pp. 419–420.

2 Identify at least three health-promoting functions associated with phytochemicals, pp. 419–421.

3 State three reasons that there is no RDA for phytochemicals, pp. 421–422.

4 Explain why phytochemical supplements should be avoided, pp. 422–423.

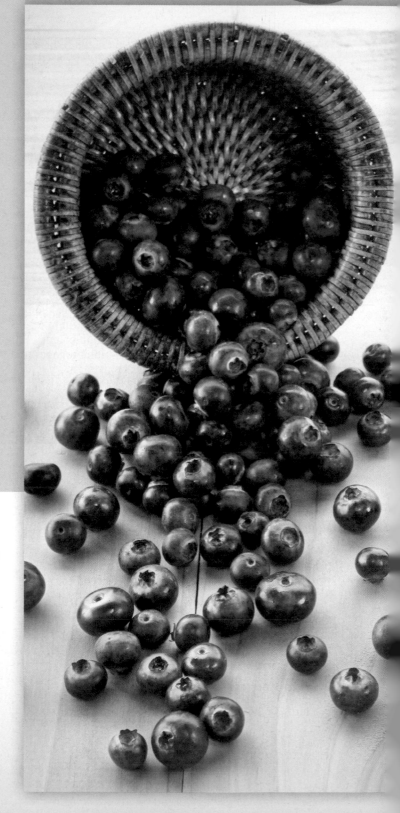

Imagine a patient visiting his physician for his annual exam. He is 20 pounds overweight and has a family history of heart disease. The physician measures his blood pressure and finds it modestly elevated. She diagnoses prehypertension. At the close of the visit, she hands the patient a prescription: *one apple; two servings of dark-green, leafy vegetables; ½ cup of oatmeal; and 2 cups of soy milk daily.* The patient accepts the prescription gratefully, assuring his physician as he says goodbye, "I'll stop at the market on my way home!"

Sound unreal? As researchers uncover more evidence of a link between plant foods and health, it's possible that scenarios like this might become familiar. Here, we explore *In Depth* some of the reasons that certain chemicals occurring naturally in plants are thought to promote human health. Who knows? When you finish reading, you might find yourself writing up your own health-promoting grocery list!

What Are Phytochemicals?

LO 1 Define phytochemicals and identify a few of the most common phytochemical groups

Plant foods are loaded with nutrients, including carbohydrates, vitamins, minerals, and water; moreover, they're a great source of dietary fiber. You've also learned (in Chapter 3) that many plant foods classify as "prebiotics," meaning that they help promote the growth and health of your GI flora. But another advantage of plants is their phytochemicals. *Phyto* means "plant," so **phytochemicals** are literally plant chemicals. While plants are growing, these naturally occurring compounds are believed to protect them from pests, the UV radiation they capture, and the oxygen they produce. What makes them important to nutrition scientists is that phytochemicals are believed to have health-promoting properties for humans who consume them.

Thousands of different phytochemicals have been identified, and researchers believe there may be thousands more.[1] They are present in whole grains, fruits, legumes and other vegetables, mushrooms, nuts, seeds, coffee, tea, wine, beer, herbs, spices, and many other plant-based foods. Any one food can contain hundreds. **Figure 1** (page 420) identifies a few of the most common phytochemical groups.

How Might Phytochemicals Help Prevent or Treat Disease?

LO 2 Identify at least three health-promoting functions associated with phytochemicals

Eating a plant-based diet rich in a variety of phytochemicals is thought to reduce the risk for many diseases. The evidence supporting this claim stems mainly from large epidemiological studies in which people report their usual food intake to researchers, who then look for relationships between specific dietary patterns and common diseases. Recall (from Chapter 1) that epidemiological studies can reveal only *associations* between diet and health; they cannot prove that a food component, food, or dietary pattern directly *causes* a health outcome. Nevertheless, these large studies often find that the reduced disease risk from high intakes of plant foods cannot be attributed solely to differences in intake of macro- and micronutrients. This suggests that other compounds in plant foods may be playing a role.

Moreover, thousands of laboratory studies also suggest that plants have non-nutrient health-promoting compounds. For example, laboratory experiments have shown that, at least in the test tube, many phytochemicals have antioxidant

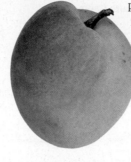

Apricots contain carotenoids, a type of phytochemical.

properties; that is, they have the capacity to neutralize the free radicals that damage our cells. However, human biology can't be reduced to a few simple chemical reactions. Phytochemicals are modified during digestion and after absorption. As a result, body cells are exposed to metabolites that are structurally different from the phytochemicals extracted from foods and studied in labs. Moreover, phytochemicals are thought to work in synergy with one another and with other compounds in foods, in medications, and in the human body.[2] Thus, the test tube can only hint at what is happening inside the body.

Fortunately, researchers have also employed cellular and animal studies, which have provided further evidence that phytochemicals have antioxidant properties, as well as a broad range of other health-promoting functions. Among the multitude of beneficial actions associated with phytochemicals, they are thought to:

- Reduce inflammation, which is linked to the development of cardiovascular disease, cancer, and Alzheimer's disease and is symptomatic of allergies and arthritis.[1-5]
- Impede the initiation and progression of cancer by enhancing the activity of enzymes that detoxify carcinogens, slowing tumor cell growth, inhibiting signaling pathways among cancer cells, and instructing cancer cells to self-destruct.[1,5-8]
- Combat infections by enhancing our immune function, reducing bacterial resistance to antibiotics, and acting as antibacterial and antiviral agents.[9-10]
- Protect against cardiovascular disease by protecting cardiac muscle cells, modulating blood lipids, and reducing blood pressure, platelet aggregation, blood clotting, and blockage of blood vessels.[11-13]
- Inhibit lipid synthesis and increase fatty acid oxidation, thereby potentially acting as an "antiobesity" agent.[14,15]

In addition, research over the past decade has increasingly focused on the beneficial role of phytochemicals in increasing the effectiveness of medications used to treat disease. When administered in concentrated doses along with traditional medications, certain phytochemicals work synergistically to enhance or prolong the effectiveness of those medications. Most such research is still in the stage of clinical trials, but this synergistic effect has been shown in the treatment of bacterial infections that have developed resistance to traditional antibiotics, as well as with chemotherapy drugs in the treatment of cancer.[16,17]

phytochemicals Compounds found in plants and believed to have health-promoting effects in humans.

Phytochemical	Health Claims	Food Source
Carotenoids: alpha-carotene, beta-carotene, lutein, lycopene, zeaxanthin, etc.	Diets with foods rich in these phytochemicals may reduce the risk for cardiovascular disease, certain cancers (e.g., prostate), and age-related eye diseases (cataracts, macular degeneration).	Red, orange, and deep-green vegetables and fruits, such as carrots, cantaloupe, sweet potatoes, apricots, kale, spinach, pumpkin, and tomatoes 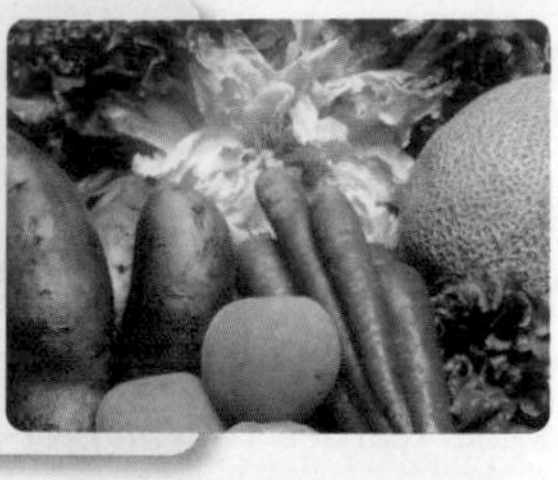
Flavonoids:[1] flavones, flavonols (e.g., quercetin), catechins (e.g., epigallocatechin gallate or EGCG), anthocyanidins, isoflavonoids, etc.	Diets with foods rich in these phytochemicals are associated with lower risk for cardiovascular disease and cancer, possibly because of reduced inflammation, blood clotting, and blood pressure and increased detoxification of carcinogens or reduction in replication of cancerous cells.	Berries, black and green tea, chocolate, purple grapes and juice, citrus fruits, olives, soybeans and soy products (soy milk, tofu, soy flour, textured vegetable protein), flaxseed, whole wheat, nuts 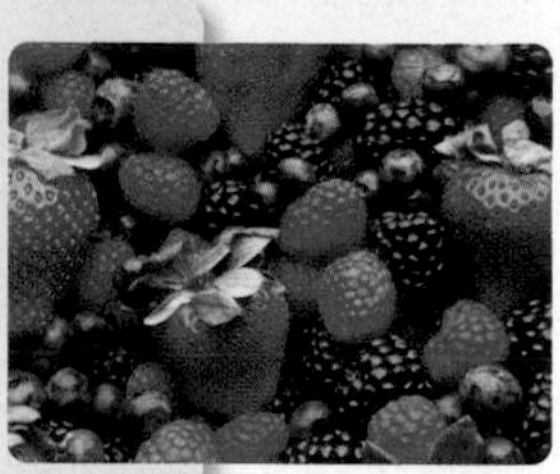
Phenolic acids:[1] ellagic acid, ferulic acid, caffeic acid, curcumin, etc.	Similar benefits as flavonoids.	Coffee beans, fruits (apples, pears, berries, grapes, oranges, prunes, strawberries), potatoes, mustard, oats, soy 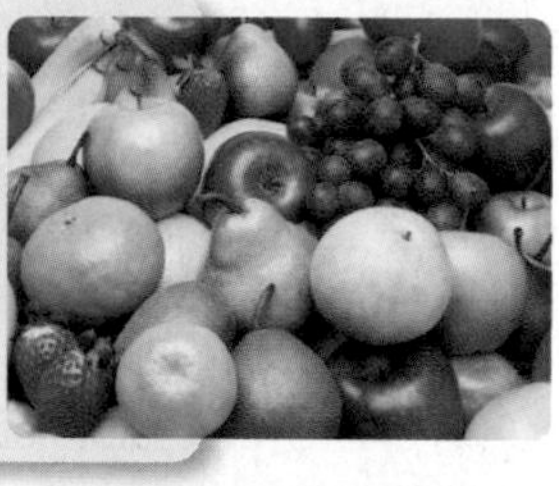
Phytoestrogens:[2] genistein, diadzein, lignans	Foods rich in these phytochemicals may provide benefits to bones and reduce the risk for cardiovascular disease and cancers of reproductive tissues (e.g., breast, prostate).	Soybeans and soy products (soy milk, tofu, soy flour, textured vegetable protein), flaxseed, whole grains 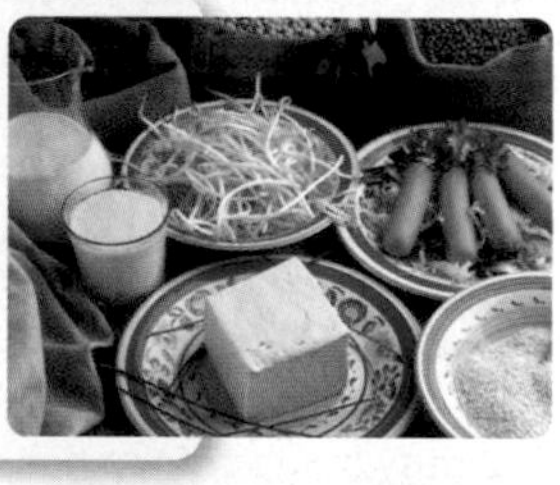
Organosulfur compounds: allylic sulfur compounds, indoles, isothiocyanates, etc.	Foods rich in these phytochemicals may protect against a wide variety of cancers.	Garlic, leeks, onions, chives, cruciferous vegetables (broccoli, cabbage, cauliflower), horseradish, mustard greens 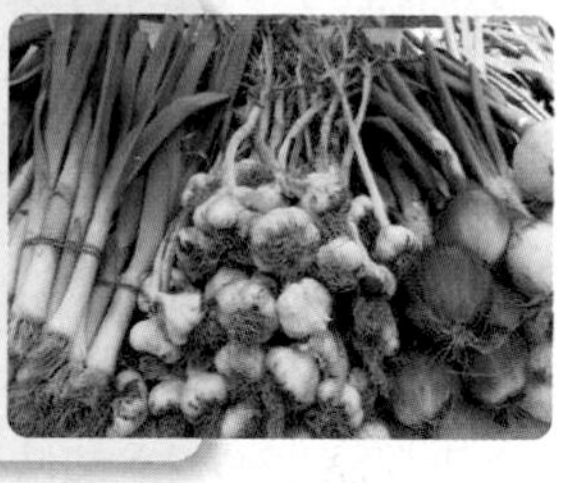

[1] Flavonoids, phenolic acids, and stilbenes are three groups of phytochemicals called phenolics. The phytochemical Resveratrol is a stilbene. Flavonoids and phenolic acids are the most abundant phenolics in our diet.

[2] Phytoestrogens include phytochemicals that have mild or anti-estrogenic action in our body. They are grouped together based on this similarity in biological function, but they also can be classified into other phytochemical groups, such as isoflavonoids.

FIGURE 1 Health claims and food sources of phytochemicals.

Will a PB&J Keep the Doctor Away?

Whole-grain bread, natural peanut butter, and grape jelly: how could a food that tastes so good be good for the body, too? We've known for decades about the fiber-rich carbohydrates, plant proteins, healthful unsaturated fats, and micronutrients a peanut butter and jelly (PB&J) sandwich provides. But recently, research has revealed that the comforting PB&J is a good source of phytochemicals, too, especially those in the phenolics group, which includes flavonoids, phenolic acids, and a small group called stilbenes.

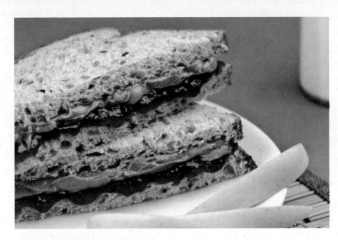

Peanut butter, peanuts, and other nuts, as well as grapes and whole-wheat bread, are all rich in flavonoids. In clinical studies, participants who added nuts to their diet experienced an improved lipid profile and blood vessel function, as well as reduced inflammation, all factors associated with reduced risk for cardiovascular disease. They also experienced no weight gain![1] Other studies have shown that regular consumption of nuts, including peanuts, significantly reduces risk for cardiovascular disease and premature mortality from a range of causes.[2,3]

Phenolic acids are also present in your sandwich, in the grapes, peanuts, and whole-wheat bread. They're free-radical scavengers active against mechanisms involved in the development of cardiovascular disease, cancer, inflammatory bowel disorders, and other chronic diseases.[4]

Among the stilbenes, the most famous is probably resveratrol, which is found in wine as well as in the peanuts and grapes (including—in minute amounts—grape jelly) in your sandwich. A chemical with antimicrobial and anti-inflammatory properties, resveratrol is thought to have protective effects against cancer, heart disease, obesity, infections, and degenerative neurologic diseases.[5,6]

Despite the host of phytochemicals in a PB&J, no one knows what an effective "dose" of any one of them might be, or whether the amounts in a PB&J would qualify as protective, even if you ate one every day. What we do know is that a PB&J makes a highly nutritious meal or snack, doesn't need refrigeration, is inexpensive, and tastes great.

References

1. Vinson, J. A., and Y. Cal. 2012. Nuts, especially walnuts, have both antioxidant quantity and efficacy and exhibit significant potential health benefits. *Food Func.* 3(2): 134–140.
2. Bao, Y., J. Han, F. B. Hu, E. L. Giovannucci, M. J. Stampfer, W. C. Willett, and C. S. Fuchs. 2013. Association of nut consumption with total and cause-specific mortality. *N. Engl. J. Med.* 369: 2001–2011.
3. Lu, H. N., W. J. Blot, Y-B. Xiang, H. Cai, M. K. Hargreaves, H. Li,…, and X-O. Shu. 2015. Prospective evaluation of the association of nut/peanut consumption with total and cause-specific mortality. *JAMA Intern. Med.* Epub ahead of print, DOI:10.1001/jamainternmed.2014.8347.
4. Saxena, M., J. Saxena, and A. Pradhan. 2012. Flavonoids and phenolic acids as antioxidants in plants and human health. *Int. J. Pharm. Sci. Rev. Res.* 16(2): 130–134. Available at http://globalresearchonline.net/journalcontents/v16-2/28.pdf.
5. Whitlock, N. C., and S. J. Baek. 2012. The anti-cancer effects of resveratrol: modulation of transcription factors. *Nutr. Cancer.* 64(4): 493–502.
6. Svajger, U., and M. Geras. 2012. Anti-inflammatory effects of resveratrol and its potential use in therapy of immune-mediated diseases. *Int. Rev. Immunol.* 31(3): 202–222.

When the results of such studies are published, we read about them in the popular press: one day we're advised to eat blueberries, another day cinnamon, purple potatoes, or—as we explored in the *Highlight* box on the previous page—peanut butter and jelly sandwiches! But is it wise to focus on a single food? How much of any one phytochemical do we really need? Let's take a look.

What's the Best "Dose" of Phytochemicals?

LO 3 State three reasons that there is no RDA for phytochemicals

LO 4 Explain why phytochemical supplements should be avoided

Given the many benefits of phytochemicals in helping prevent and treat disease, why is there no RDA? First, phytochemicals are not considered nutrients—that is, substances necessary for sustaining life. Whereas a total lack of vitamin C or iron is incompatible with life, a total lack of lutein or allylic sulfur compounds is not known to be fatal. Even for carotenoids, probably the most studied class, the Institute of Medicine has affirmed that there is not enough evidence to identify with confidence a possible impact of these compounds on chronic disease and thus establish a daily recommended intake.[18]

Second, as noted earlier, phytochemicals interact with each other and with other substances in foods and in the body

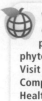

Want to learn more about carotenoids, phytoestrogens, pomegranates, soy, or other phytochemical groups or foods? Visit the National Center for Complementary and Integrative Health's *Health Topics* index at https://nccih.nih.gov and click away!

to produce a synergistic effect that is greater than the sum of the effects of individual phytochemicals. Teasing out the different contributions and determining precise therapeutic ratios would thus be essentially impossible.

Third, phytochemicals can act in different ways under different circumstances in the body. For example, certain phytoestrogens and phenolic acids—when consumed in foods—appear to reduce the risk for breast cancer in healthy women; however, the same compounds, even at low concentrations, may actually stimulate breast cancer cells already present.[19]

For all of these reasons, no RDA for phytochemicals can safely be established for any life stage group. The same is true for establishing a Tolerable Upper Intake Level (UL). This

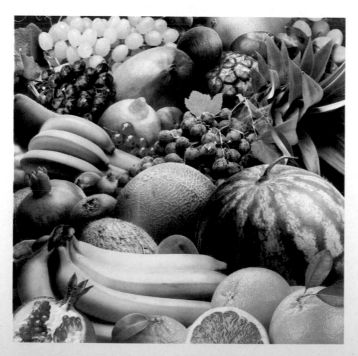

Avoid phytochemical supplements in favor of whole foods.

Nutri-Case

Hannah

"On my way home from campus today, I was really hungry, and when I passed by a convenience store about halfway home, I just had to go in. I looked around for something healthy, like a banana or an apple or something, but they didn't have anything fresh. So I bought some pretzels. I know pretzels aren't exactly a health food, but at least they're low-fat."

Hannah and her mother, Judy, live in an urban neighborhood that has 11 different fast-food outlets and four convenience stores but lacks a standard grocery store. There is no local farmers' market or community garden. To purchase fresh produce, they have to travel to one of the more affluent neighborhoods several miles away. Given the importance of phytochemicals to a healthful diet, suggest at least two strategies Hannah and Judy could undertake to increase their access to affordable fresh produce.

lack of guidance on safe phytochemical intake is particularly concerning because, although phytochemicals appear to be beneficial in the low doses commonly provided by foods, they may be ineffective or even harmful when consumed as supplements.[2,12,20] This may be due to their mode of action: Scientists believe that, in plants, many phytochemicals act as toxins; for example, as intrinsic pesticides, helping the plant ward off harmful insects and microbes. Thus, instead of *protecting* our cells, phytochemicals we consume might benefit our health by *stressing* our cells, causing them to rev up their internal defense systems. Cells are very well equipped to deal with minor stresses, but not with excessive stress, which may explain why clinical trials with phytochemical supplements do not show the same benefits as a plant-based diet.[20,21]

So are phytochemical supplements harmful? A basic principle of toxicology is that any compound can be toxic if the dose is high enough. Dietary supplements are no exception. For example, a classic study found that supplementing with 20 to 30 mg/day of beta-carotene for 4 to 6 years *increased* lung cancer risk by 16% to 28% in smokers.[22,23] Based on these and other results, experts recommend against beta-carotene supplementation and, in fact, against phytochemical supplementation in general.[20,24] In short, whereas there is ample evidence to support the health benefits of a plant-based diet, no recommendations for amounts of any precise foods or phytochemicals can be given, and phytochemical supplements should be avoided.

To increase your phytochemical intake, build a rainbow of colors on your plate; for instance, black beans, onions, peppers, and tomatoes over brown rice, a green salad sprinkled with nuts or seeds—and why not fruit salad for dessert! Eat this way at most meals, most days of the week, to ensure you're getting nutrients, fiber, prebiotics, and phytochemicals—in short, all the advantages of plants.

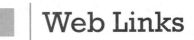

Web Links

www.aicr.org
American Institute for Cancer Research (AICR)
Search for "phytochemicals" to learn about the AICR's position and recommendations on phytochemicals, and their role in cancer prevention.

www.lpi.oregonstate.edu
Linus Pauling Institute
This extensive website covers not only phytochemicals but also nutrients and other cutting-edge health and nutrition topics.

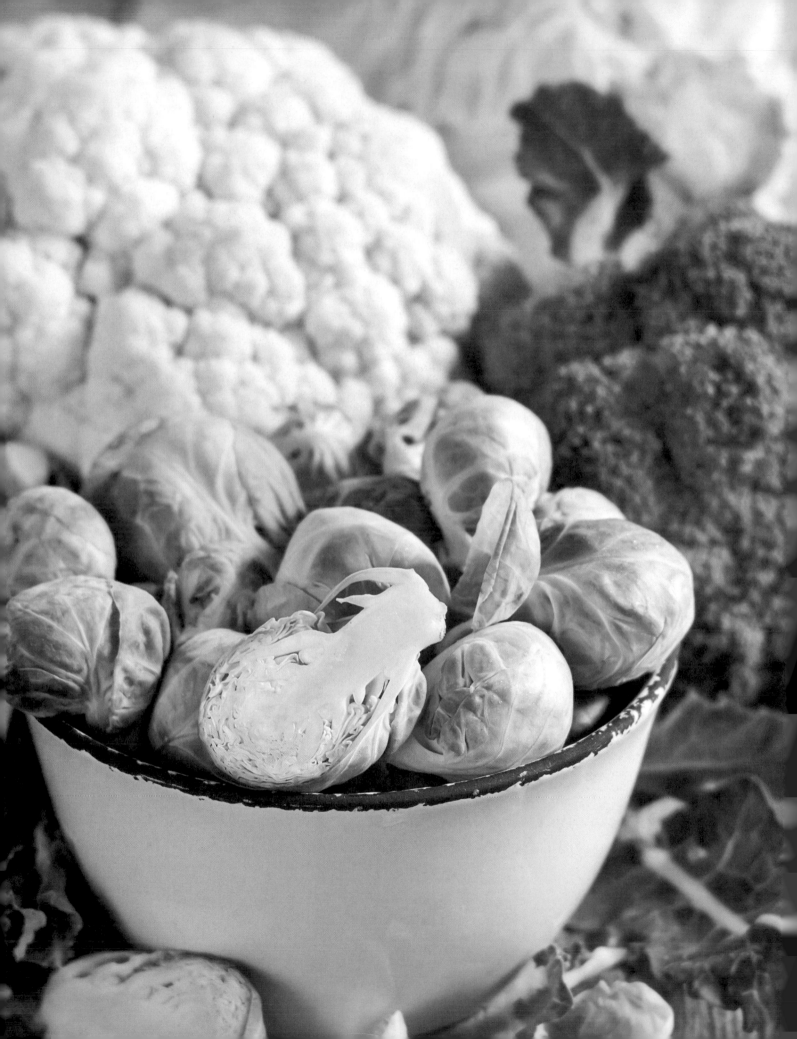

11 Nutrients Involved in Bone Health

Learning Outcomes

After studying this chapter, you should be able to:

1. Identify the functions of bone in the human body and distinguish between cortical and trabecular bone, *pp. 426–427.*
2. Describe the processes of bone growth, modeling, and remodeling, *pp. 427–429.*
3. Identify the most accurate tool for assessing bone density and the significance of the T-score, *pp. 429–430.*
4. Explain the critical role of calcium in maintaining bone health and other body functions, *pp. 430–431.*
5. Discuss foods that are good sources of calcium and factors that affect its absorption, *pp. 432–435.*
6. Discuss the contributions of vitamin D to bone health, and the process by which the body synthesizes vitamin D from exposure to sunlight, *pp. 437–438.*
7. Identify the contributions of vitamin K, phosphorus, and magnesium to bone health, as well as good food sources, *pp. 442–447.*
8. Describe the main functions of fluoride in the development and maintenance of teeth and bones, and the results of consuming too much and too little fluoride, *pp. 447–449.*
9. Define *osteoporosis*, and identify the factors that influence the risk for developing the disease, *pp. 449–453.*
10. Describe osteoporosis treatment, *pp. 453–454.*

TEST YOURSELF

True or False?

1. As long as we stay active, we can continue to increase bone density throughout our lives. **T** *or* **F**
2. Very few foods—except milk, yogurt, and cheese—provide calcium. **T** *or* **F**
3. We are capable of making vitamin D within our body and do not necessarily have to consume it in our diet. **T** *or* **F**
4. Osteoporosis is a disease that affects only elderly women. **T** *or* **F**
5. Being overweight or obese may increase a person's risk for osteoporosis. **T** *or* **F**

Test Yourself answers are located in the Study Plan.

MasteringNutrition™

Go online for chapter quizzes, pre-tests, interactive activities, and more!

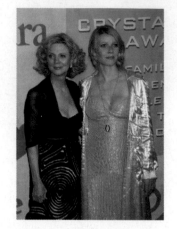

Mother–daughter actresses Blythe Danner and Gwyneth Paltrow share not only a career, but a medical diagnosis: low bone density. Maintaining a slender and youthful appearance is important to both women; so did a strict diet, intense physical activity, and sun avoidance contribute to their condition? Or given their shared family history, are genes to blame? Danner has osteoporosis, a disease characterized by abnormally fragile, "porous" bones. Paltrow has a more modest thinning of the bones called osteopenia. As you might suspect, the less dense the bone, the more likely it is to break, and indeed, both women have suffered fractures.

Do only slender females develop bone disease? What roles do age, genetics, and other factors play? We begin this chapter with a quick look at the components and activities of bone tissue. Then we'll discuss the nutrients, dietary choices, and other factors critical to maintaining bone health.

LO 1 Identify the functions of bone in the human body, and distinguish between cortical and trabecular bone.

LO 2 Describe the processes of bone growth, modeling, and remodeling.

How Does the Body Maintain Bone Health?

Contrary to what most people think, the skeleton is not an inactive collection of bones that simply holds the body together. Bones are living organs that contain several tissues, including two types of bone tissue, cartilage, and connective tissue. Nerves and blood vessels run within channels in bone tissue, supporting its activities. Bones have many important functions in the body, some of which might surprise you (**Table 11.1**). For instance, did you know that most blood cells are formed deep within the bones?

Given the importance of bones, it is critical that we maintain their health. Bone health is achieved through complex interactions among nutrients, hormones, and environmental factors. To better understand these interactions, we first need to learn about how bone structure and the constant activity of bone tissue influence bone health throughout our lifetime.

The Composition of Bone Provides Strength and Flexibility

We tend to think of bones as totally rigid, but if they were, how could we twist and jump our way through a basketball game or even carry an armload of books up a flight of stairs? Bones need to be both strong and flexible, so that they can resist the compression, stretching, and twisting that occur throughout our daily activities. Fortunately, the composition of bone is ideally suited for its complex job: about 65% of bone tissue is made up of an assortment of minerals (mostly calcium and phosphorus) that provide hardness, but the remaining 35% is a mixture of organic substances that provide strength, durability, and flexibility. The most important of these is the fibrous protein collagen. You might be surprised to learn that collagen fibers are actually stronger than steel fibers of similar size! Within bones, the minerals form tiny crystals (called *hydroxyapatite*) that cluster around the collagen fibers. This design enables bones to bear weight while responding to our demands for movement.

TABLE 11.1 Functions of Bone in the Human Body

Functions Related to Structure and Support	Functions Related to Metabolic Processes
• Bones provide physical support for organs and body segments. • Bones protect vital organs; for example, the rib cage protects the lungs, the skull protects the brain, and the vertebrae of the spine protect the spinal cord. • Bones work with muscles and tendons to allow movement—muscles attach to bones via tendons, and their contraction produces movement at the body's joints.	• Bone tissue acts as a storage reservoir for many minerals, including calcium, phosphorus, and fluoride. The body draws on such deposits when these minerals are needed for various body processes; however, this can reduce bone mass. • Most blood cells are produced in the red bone marrow.

If you examine a bone very closely, you will notice two distinct types of tissue (**Figure 11.1**): cortical bone and trabecular bone. **Cortical bone,** which is also called **compact bone,** is very dense. It constitutes approximately 80% of the skeleton. The outer surface of all bones is cortical; plus, many small bones of the body, such as the bones of the wrists, hands, and feet, are made entirely of cortical bone. Although cortical bone looks solid to the naked eye, it actually contains many microscopic openings, which serve as passageways for blood vessels and nerves.

In contrast, **trabecular bone** makes up only 20% of the skeleton. It is found within the ends of the long bones (such as the bones of the arms and legs), vertebral bones, the sternum (breastbone), the ribs, most bones of the skull, and the pelvis. Trabecular bone is sometimes referred to as **spongy bone,** because to the naked eye it looks like a sponge, with cavities and no clear organization. The microscope reveals that trabecular bone is, in fact, aligned in a precise network of columns that protect the bone from stress. You can think of trabecular bone as the scaffolding of the inside of the bone that supports the outer cortical bone.

Cortical and trabecular bone also differ in their rate of turnover—that is, in how quickly the bone tissue is broken down and replenished. Trabecular bone has a faster turnover rate than cortical bone. This makes trabecular bone more sensitive to changes in hormones and nutritional deficiencies. It also accounts for the much higher rate of age-related fractures in the spine and pelvis (including the hip)—both of which contain a significant amount of trabecular bone. Let's investigate how bone turnover influences bone health.

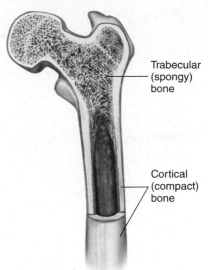

FIGURE 11.1 The structure of bone. Notice the difference in density between the trabecular (spongy) bone and the cortical (compact) bone.

Trabecular (spongy) bone

Cortical (compact) bone

The Constant Activity of Bone Tissue Promotes Bone Health

Bones develop through a series of three processes: bone growth, bone modeling, and bone remodeling (**Figure 11.2**). Bone growth and modeling begin during the early months of fetal life, when the skeleton is forming, and continue until early adulthood. Bone remodeling predominates during adulthood; this process helps us maintain a healthy skeleton as we age.

Bone Growth

Through the process of *bone growth*, the size of bones increases. The first period of rapid bone growth is from birth to age 2, but growth continues in spurts throughout childhood and into adolescence. Although most girls reach their adult height by age 18, some continue to increase in height past age 19, although the rate of growth slows considerably. Most boys continue to grow up to the age of 21, although their rate of growth also slows over time. In the later decades of life, some loss in height usually occurs because of decreased bone density in the spine.[1]

Bone Modeling

Bone modeling is the process by which the shape of bones is determined, from the round "pebble" bones that make up the wrists to the uniquely shaped bones of the face to the long bones of the arms and legs. Even after bones stop growing in length, they can still increase

cortical bone (compact bone) A dense bone tissue that makes up the outer surface of all bones, as well as the entirety of most small bones of the body.

trabecular bone (spongy bone) A porous bone tissue that makes up only 20% of the skeleton and is found within the ends of the long bones, inside the spinal vertebrae, inside the flat bones (sternum, ribs, and most bones of the skull), and inside the bones of the pelvis.

Bone growth	Bone modeling	Bone remodeling
· Determines bone size · Begins in the womb · Continues until early adulthood	· Determines bone shape · Begins in the womb · Continues until early adulthood	· Maintains integrity of bone · Replaces old bone with new bone to maintain mineral balance · Involves bone resorption and formation · Occurs predominantly during adulthood

FIGURE 11.2 Bone develops through three processes: bone growth, bone modeling, and bone remodeling.

in thickness if we stress them by engaging in repetitive exercise, such as weight training, or by being overweight or obese.

Although the size and shape of bones do not change significantly after puberty, our **bone density,** or the compactness of our bones, continues to develop into early adulthood. *Peak bone density* is the point at which our bones are strongest because they are at their highest density. The following factors are associated with a lower peak bone density:[1]

- Late pubertal age in boys and late onset of menstruation in girls
- Inadequate calcium intake
- Low body weight
- Physical inactivity during adolescence

About 90% of a woman's bone density has been built by 17 years of age, whereas the majority of a man's bone density has been built by his twenties. However, male or female, before we reach the age of 30 years, our bodies have reached peak bone mass, and we can no longer significantly add to our bone density. In our thirties, our bone density remains relatively stable, but by age 40, it has begun its irreversible decline.

Bone Remodeling

Although our bones cannot increase in density after our twenties, bone tissue still remains very active throughout adulthood, balancing the breakdown of older bone tissue and the formation of new bone tissue. This bone recycling process is called **remodeling.** Remodeling is also used to repair fractures and to strengthen bone regions that are exposed to higher physical stress. The process of remodeling involves two steps: resorption and formation.

Bone is broken down through the process of **resorption** (**Figure 11.3a**). During resorption, cells called **osteoclasts** erode the bone surface by secreting enzymes and acids that dig grooves into the bone matrix. One of the primary reasons the body regularly breaks down bone is to release calcium into the bloodstream. As discussed in more detail later in this chapter, calcium is critical for many physiologic processes, and bone is an important calcium reservoir. The body also breaks down bone that is fractured and needs to be repaired. Resorption at the injury site smoothes the rough edges created by the break. Bone may also be broken down in areas away from the fracture site to obtain the minerals that are needed to repair the damage. Regardless of the reason, once bone is broken down, the resulting products are transported into the bloodstream and used for various body functions.

New bone is formed through the action of cells called **osteoblasts,** or "bone builders" (see Figure 11.3b). These cells work to synthesize new bone matrix by laying down the

bone density The degree of compactness of bone tissue, reflecting the strength of the bones. *Peak bone density* is the point at which a bone is strongest.

remodeling The two-step process by which bone tissue is recycled; includes the breakdown of existing bone and the formation of new bone.

resorption The process by which the surface of bone is broken down by cells called osteoclasts.

osteoclasts Cells that erode the surface of bones by secreting enzymes and acids that dig grooves into the bone matrix.

osteoblasts Cells that prompt the formation of new bone matrix by laying down the collagen-containing component of bone, which is then mineralized.

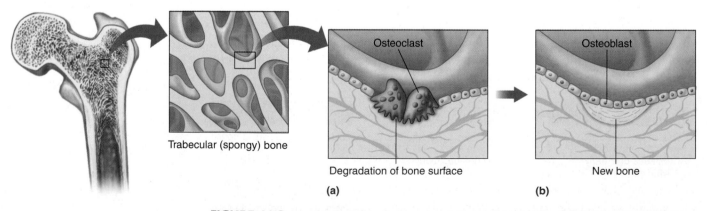

Trabecular (spongy) bone

Osteoclast

Degradation of bone surface

(a)

Osteoblast

New bone

(b)

FIGURE 11.3 Bone remodeling involves resorption and formation. **(a)** Osteoclasts erode the bone surface by degrading its components, including calcium, other minerals, and collagen; these components are then transported to the bloodstream. **(b)** Osteoblasts work to build new bone by filling the pit formed by the resorption process with new bone.

collagen-containing organic component of bone. Within this substance, the hydroxyapatite crystallizes and packs together to create new bone where it is needed.

In young, healthy adults, the processes of bone resorption and formation are equal, so that just as much bone is broken down as is built, maintaining bone mass. Around 40 years of age, bone resorption begins to occur more rapidly than bone formation, and this imbalance results in an overall loss in bone density. Because this affects the vertebral bones, people tend to lose height as they age. As discussed shortly, achieving a high peak bone mass through proper nutrition and exercise when we are young provides us with a stronger skeleton before the loss of bone begins. It can therefore reduce our risk for *osteoporosis*, a disorder characterized by low-density bones that fracture easily. Osteoporosis is discussed later in this chapter.

To learn more about bone biology, watch any of the several videos at www .bonebiology.amgen.com.

RECAP

Bones are organs that contain metabolically active tissues composed primarily of minerals and collagen. Of the two types of bone, cortical bone is more dense and trabecular bone is more porous. Trabecular bone is also more sensitive to hormonal and nutritional factors and turns over more rapidly than cortical bone. The three types of bone activity are growth, modeling, and remodeling. During remodeling, osteoclasts break down old bone in a process called resorption, and osteoblasts synthesize new organic matrix upon which hydroxyapatite crystallizes. Bones reach their peak bone mass by the late teenage years into the twenties; bone mass begins to decline around age 40.

How Do We Assess Bone Health?

LO 3 Identify the most accurate tool for assessing bone density and the significance of the T-score.

Over the past 40 years, technological advancements have led to the development of a number of affordable methods for measuring bone health. **Dual-energy x-ray absorptiometry (DXA** or **DEXA)** is considered the most accurate assessment tool for measuring bone density. This method can measure the density of the bone mass over the entire body. Software is also available that provides an estimation of percentage of body fat.

The DXA procedure is simple, painless, and noninvasive and is considered to be of minimal risk. It takes just 15 to 30 minutes to complete. The person participating in the test remains fully clothed but must remove all jewelry or other metal objects. The participant lies quietly on a table, and bone density is assessed through the use of a very low level of x-ray (**Figure 11.4,** page 430).

DXA is a very important tool to determine a person's risk for osteoporosis. It generates a bone density score, which is compared to the average peak bone density of a healthy 30-year-old. Doctors use this comparison, which is known as a **T-score,** to assess the risk for fracture and to determine whether the person has osteoporosis. T-scores are interpreted as follows:

 Take a closer look at a DXA scan at www.webmd.com. Type "dr siris inside a bone density test" into the search bar to get started.

- A T score between +1 and −1 means that the individual's bone density is normal.
- A T-score between −1 and −2.5 indicates low bone mass and an increased risk for fractures.
- A T-score more negative than −2.5 indicates that the person has osteoporosis.

DXA tests are generally recommended for postmenopausal women, because they are at highest risk for osteoporosis and fracture. Men and younger women may also be recommended for a DXA test if they have significant risk factors for osteoporosis.

Other technologies have been developed to measure bone density. The quantitative ultrasound technique uses sound waves to measure the density of bone in the heel, shin, and kneecap. Peripheral dual-energy x-ray absorptiometry, or pDXA, is a form of DXA that measures bone density in the peripheral regions of our bodies, including the wrist, heel, or finger. Single-energy x-ray absorptiometry is a method that measures bone density at the

dual-energy x-ray absorptiometry (DXA, DEXA) Currently the most accurate tool for measuring bone density.

T-score A numerical score comparing an individual's bone density to the average peak bone density of a 30-year-old healthy adult, to determine the risk for osteoporosis.

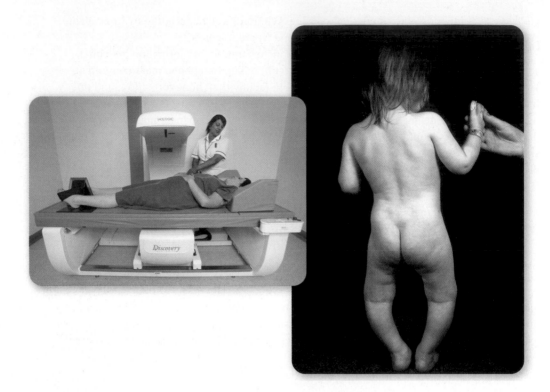

FIGURE 11.4 Dual-energy x-ray absorptiometry is a safe and simple procedure that assesses bone density.

wrist or heel. These technologies are frequently used at health fairs, because the machines are portable and provide scores faster than the traditional DXA.

RECAP

Dual-energy x-ray absorptiometry (DXA or DEXA) is the gold-standard measurement of bone mass. It is a simple, painless, and minimal-risk procedure. The results of a DXA include a T-score, which is a comparison of the person's bone density to that of a 30-year-old healthy adult. A T-score lower than −1 indicates poor bone density. Quantitative ultrasound, peripheral dual-energy x-ray absorptiometry, and single-energy x-ray absorptiometry are additional methods that can be used to measure bone density. ∎

 LO 4 Explain the critical role of calcium in maintaining bone health and other body functions.

 LO 5 Discuss foods that are good sources of calcium and factors that affect its absorption.

Why Is Calcium Critical to Healthy Bone?

Dietary calcium is absorbed in the intestines via active transport and passive diffusion across the intestinal mucosal membrane. The majority of the calcium consumed is absorbed from the duodenum, as this area of the small intestine is slightly more acidic than the more distal regions, and calcium absorption is enhanced in an acidic environment. Active transport of calcium is dependent on the active form of vitamin D, or 1,25-dihydroxyvitamin D; most of the absorption of calcium at low to moderate intake levels is accounted for by this vitamin D–enhanced active transport. Passive diffusion of calcium across the intestinal–mucosal membrane is a function of the calcium concentration gradient in the intestines, and this mechanism becomes a more important means of calcium absorption at high-calcium intakes.[2]

Recall (from Chapter 1) that the major minerals are those required in our diets in amounts greater than 100 mg per day. Calcium is by far the most abundant major mineral in the body, comprising about 2% of our entire body weight! Not surprisingly, it plays many critical roles in maintaining overall function and health.

Calcium Plays Many Roles Critical to Body Functioning

One of the primary functions of calcium is to provide structure to the bones and teeth. About 99% of the calcium in the body is stored in the hydroxyapatite crystals built up on the collagen foundation of bone. As noted earlier, the combination of crystals and collagen provides both the characteristic hardness of bone and the flexibility needed to support various activities.

The remaining 1% of calcium in the body is found in the blood and soft tissues. Calcium is alkaline, or basic, and plays a critical role in assisting with acid–base balance. We cannot survive for long if our blood calcium level rises above or falls below a very narrow range; therefore, the body maintains the appropriate blood calcium level at all costs.

Focus Figure 11.5 (page 432) illustrates how various organ systems and hormones work together to maintain blood calcium levels. When blood calcium levels fall, the parathyroid glands are stimulated to produce **parathyroid hormone (PTH).** Also known as parathormone, PTH stimulates the activation of vitamin D. PTH increases absorption of calcium in the kidneys, while PTH and vitamin D stimulate osteoclasts to break down bone, releasing more calcium into the bloodstream. In addition, vitamin D increases the absorption of calcium from the intestines. Through these mechanisms, blood calcium levels increase.

When blood calcium levels are too high, the secretion of PTH is inhibited, which then reduces the synthesis of vitamin D. This inhibits the actions of vitamin D, leading to decreased reabsorption of calcium by the kidneys, decreased calcium absorption from the intestines, and inhibition of the osteoclasts, which decreases the breakdown of bone.

As just noted, the body must maintain blood calcium levels within a very narrow range. Thus, when an individual does not consume or absorb enough calcium from the diet, osteoclasts erode bone, so that calcium can be released into the blood. To maintain healthy bone density, we need to consume and absorb enough calcium to balance the calcium taken from our bones.

Calcium is also critical for the normal transmission of nerve impulses. Calcium flows into nerve cells (neurons) and stimulates the release of molecules called neurotransmitters, which transfer the nerve impulses from one nerve cell to another. Without adequate calcium, the nerves' ability to transmit messages is inhibited. Not surprisingly, when blood calcium levels fall dangerously low, a person can experience convulsions.

A fourth role of calcium is to assist in muscle contraction, which is initiated when intracellular stores of calcium ions are released from the sarcoplasmic reticulum, the intracellular storage site for calcium. Conversely, muscles relax when calcium is pumped back into the sarcoplasmic reticulum. If calcium levels are inadequate, normal muscle contraction and relaxation are inhibited, and the person may suffer from twitching and spasms. This is referred to as **calcium tetany.** High levels of blood calcium can cause **calcium rigor,** an inability of muscles to relax, which leads to a hardening or stiffening of the muscles. These problems affect the function not only of skeletal muscles but also of heart muscle and can cause heart failure.

Other functions of calcium include the maintenance of healthy blood pressure, the initiation of blood clotting, and the regulation of various hormones and enzymes.

How Much Calcium Should We Consume?

Calcium requirements, and thus recommended intakes, vary according to age and gender. Many people of all ages fail to consume enough calcium to maintain bone health.

Recommended Dietary Intake for Calcium

The RDA for adult men aged 19 to 70 years and women aged 19 to 50 years is 1,000 mg of calcium per day. For men older than 70 years of age and women older than 50 years of age, the RDA increases to 1,200 mg of calcium per day. At 1,300 mg per day, the RDA for boys and girls aged 9 to 18 years is even higher, reflecting their developing bone mass. The Upper Limit (UL) for calcium is 2,500 mg for all age groups (**Table 11.2**, page 433).

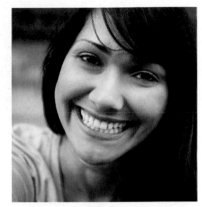

A major role of calcium is to form and maintain bones and teeth.

parathyroid hormone (PTH) A hormone secreted by the parathyroid gland when blood calcium levels fall. It is also known as parathormone, and it increases blood calcium levels by stimulating the activation of vitamin D, increasing reabsorption of calcium from the kidneys, and stimulating osteoclasts to break down bone, which releases more calcium into the bloodstream.

calcium tetany A condition in which muscles experience twitching and spasms due to inadequate blood calcium levels.

calcium rigor A failure of muscles to relax, which leads to a hardening or stiffening of the muscles; caused by high levels of blood calcium.

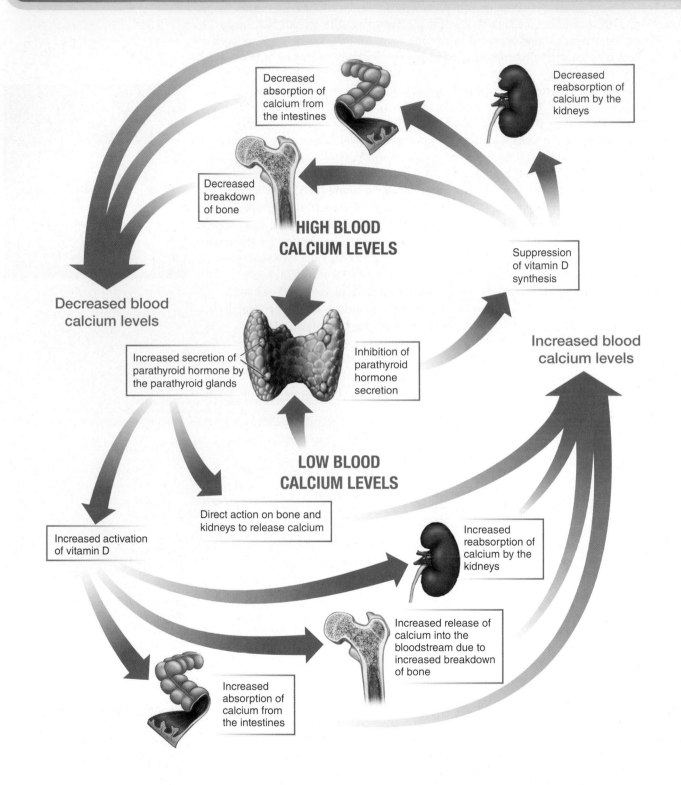

Decreased absorption of calcium from the intestines

Decreased reabsorption of calcium by the kidneys

Decreased breakdown of bone

HIGH BLOOD CALCIUM LEVELS

Suppression of vitamin D synthesis

Decreased blood calcium levels

Increased secretion of parathyroid hormone by the parathyroid glands

Inhibition of parathyroid hormone secretion

Increased blood calcium levels

LOW BLOOD CALCIUM LEVELS

Increased activation of vitamin D

Direct action on bone and kidneys to release calcium

Increased reabsorption of calcium by the kidneys

Increased release of calcium into the bloodstream due to increased breakdown of bone

Increased absorption of calcium from the intestines

TABLE 11.2 Overview of Nutrients Essential to Bone Health

To see the full profile of micronutrients, turn to Chapter 7.5, In Depth: Vitamins and Minerals: Micronutrients with Macro Powers, pages 292–303.

Nutrient	Recommended Intake
Calcium (major mineral)	RDA: Adults aged 19 to 50 years = 1,000 mg/day Men aged 51–70 = 1,000 mg/day; men aged .70 = 1,200 mg/day Women aged >50 = 1,200 mg/day UL = 2,500 mg/day
Vitamin D (fat-soluble vitamin)	RDA:* Adults aged 19 to 50 years = 600 IU/day Adults aged 50 to 70 years = 600 IU/day Adults aged >70 years = 800 IU/day
Vitamin K (fat-soluble vitamin)	AI: Women = 90 µg/day Men = 120 µg/day
Phosphorus (major mineral)	RDA: Adults = 700 mg/day
Magnesium (major mineral)	RDA: Women aged 19 to 30 years = 310 mg/day Women aged >30 years = 320 mg/day Men aged 19 to 30 years = 400 mg/day Men aged >30 years = 420 mg/day
Fluoride (trace mineral)	RDA: Women = 3 mg/day Men = 4 mg/day UL = 2.2 mg/day for children aged 4 to 8; children >8 = 10 mg/day

*Based on the assumption that a person does not get adequate sun exposure.

A nutrient's **bioavailability** is the degree to which the body can absorb and use any given nutrient. The bioavailability of calcium depends in part on a person's age and need for calcium. For example, infants, children, and adolescents can absorb more than 60% of the calcium they consume, as calcium needs are very high during these stages of life. In addition, pregnant and lactating women can absorb about 50% of dietary calcium. In contrast, healthy, young adults absorb only about 30% of the calcium consumed in the diet. When calcium needs are high, the body can generally increase its absorption from the small intestine. Although older adults have a high need for calcium, their ability to absorb calcium from the small intestine diminishes with age and can be as low as 25%. These variations in bioavailability and absorption capacity were taken into account when calcium recommendations were determined.

The bioavailability of calcium also depends on how much calcium is consumed throughout the day or at any one time. When diets are generally high in calcium, absorption of calcium is reduced. In addition, the body cannot absorb more than 500 mg of calcium at any one time, and as the amount of calcium in a single meal or supplement goes up, the fraction that is absorbed goes down. This explains why it is critical to consume calcium-rich foods throughout the day, rather than relying on a single, high-dose supplement. Conversely, when dietary intake of calcium is low, the absorption of calcium is increased.

Dietary factors can also affect the absorption of calcium. Binding factors, such as phytates and oxalates, occur naturally in some calcium-rich seeds, nuts, grains, and vegetables, such as spinach and Swiss chard. Such factors bind to the calcium in these foods and prevent its absorption from the small intestine. Additionally, consuming calcium with iron, zinc, magnesium, or phosphorus can interfere with the absorption and utilization of all these minerals. Despite these potential interactions, the Institute of Medicine has concluded that there is not sufficient evidence to suggest that these interactions cause deficiencies of calcium or other minerals in healthy individuals.[2]

Finally, because vitamin D is necessary for the absorption of calcium, a lack of vitamin D severely limits the bioavailability of calcium. We'll discuss this and other contributions of vitamin D to bone health shortly.

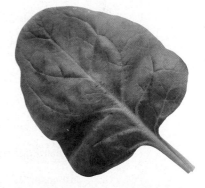

Although spinach contains high levels of calcium, binding factors in the plant prevent much of its absorption in the body.

bioavailability The degree to which the body can absorb and use any given nutrient.

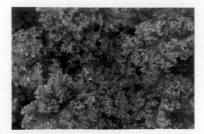

Kale is a good source of calcium.

Foods Rich in Calcium

Dairy products are among the most common sources of calcium in the U.S. diet. Skim milk, low-fat cheeses, and nonfat yogurt are nutritious sources of calcium (**Figure 11.6**). Ice cream, regular cheese, and whole milk also contain a relatively high amount of calcium, but these foods should be eaten in moderation because of their high saturated fat and energy content.

Other good sources of calcium are green, leafy vegetables, such as kale, collard greens, turnip greens, broccoli, cauliflower, green cabbage, brussels sprouts, and Chinese cabbage (bok choy). The bioavailability of the calcium in these vegetables is relatively high compared to spinach, as these vegetables contain low levels of oxalates. Many packaged foods are now available fortified with calcium. For example, you can buy calcium-fortified orange juice, soy milk, rice milk, and tofu processed with calcium. Some dairies have even boosted the amount of calcium in their brand of milk!

Figure 11.7 illustrates serving sizes of various calcium-rich foods that contain the equivalent amount of calcium as one glass (8 fl. oz) of skim milk. As you can see from this figure, a wide variety of foods can be consumed each day to contribute to adequate calcium intakes. When you are selecting foods that are good sources of calcium, it is important to remember that we do not absorb 100% of the calcium contained in our foods. For example, although a serving of milk contains approximately 300 mg of calcium, we do not actually absorb this entire amount. To learn more about how calcium absorption rates vary for select foods, see the ***Nutrition Label Activity*** (page 436).

In general, meats and fish are not good sources of calcium. An exception is canned fish with bones (for example, sardines or salmon), providing you eat the bones. Fruits (except dried figs) and nonfortified grain products are also poor sources of calcium.

As you can see, many foods are good sources of calcium. Nevertheless, many Americans do not have adequate intakes because they consume very few dairy-based foods and calcium-rich vegetables. Recent results from the NHANES survey found that calcium

To find out if you're getting enough calcium in your diet, take the calcium quiz at www .healthyeating.org. **Click on the Healthy Eating tab, then scroll down to the "Calcium Quiz."**

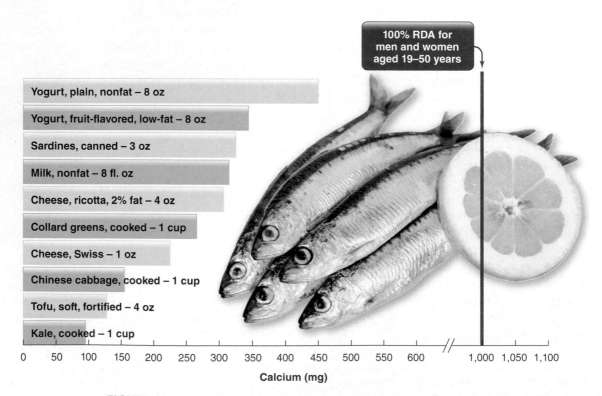

FIGURE 11.6 Common food sources of calcium. The RDA for calcium is 1,000 mg of calcium per day for men and women aged 19 to 50. (*Source:* Data from U.S. Department of Agriculture, Agricultural Research Service, 2014, USDA Nutrient Database for Standard Reference, Release 27. Nutrient Data Laboratory Home Page, www.ars.usda.gov/ba/bhnrc/ndl.)

intakes were lower than recommended for both men and women across the age ranges from 19 years to older than 80 years.[3] From the youngest to oldest age group, calcium intakes decreased by almost 23% in men and 14% in women.

A variety of quick, simple tools are available on the Internet to assist individuals in determining their daily calcium intake. Most of these tools are designed to provide an estimated calcium intake score based on the types and amounts of calcium-rich foods a person consumes. Refer to the **Nutrition Online** link (page 434, margin) to access one of these tools. In addition, follow these tips to help you add more calcium to your bone bank:

- At the grocery store, stock up on calcium-fortified juices and milk alternatives. Look for single-serving, portable "juice boxes" containing milk or calcium-fortified beverages.
- Purchase breakfast cereals and breads that are fortified with calcium.
- For quick snacks, purchase single-serving cups of yogurt, individually wrapped "cheese sticks," or calcium-fortified protein bars.
- Keep on hand shredded Parmesan or any other hard cheese, and sprinkle it on hot soups, chili, salads, pasta, and other dishes.
- In any recipe, replace sour cream or mayonnaise with nonfat plain yogurt.
- Add nonfat dry milk powder to hot cereals, soups, chili, recipes for baked goods, coffee, and hot cocoa. One-third of a cup of nonfat dry milk powder provides the same amount of calcium as a whole cup of nonfat milk.
- For a "guilt-free" dessert, try half a cup of plain nonfat Greek yogurt with a drizzle of maple syrup.
- Make a yogurt smoothie by blending nonfat plain or flavored yogurt with fresh or frozen fruit.
- At your favorite café, instead of black coffee, order a skim milk latte. Instead of black tea, order a cup of chai—spiced Indian tea brewed with milk.
- At home, brew a cup of strong coffee; then add half a cup of warm skim milk for a café au lait.
- When eating out, order skim milk instead of a soft drink with your meal.

If you do not consume enough dietary calcium, you might benefit from taking calcium supplements. Refer to the **Nutrition Myth or Fact?** at the end of this chapter (pages 455–457) to learn more about both calcium and vitamin D supplements, and how to determine if taking a calcium supplement is right for you.

What Happens If We Consume Too Much Calcium?

In general, consuming too much calcium in the diet does not lead to significant toxicity symptoms in healthy individuals. Much of the excess calcium is excreted in feces. However, excessive intake of calcium from supplements can lead to health problems. As mentioned earlier, one concern with consuming too much calcium is that it can lead to various mineral imbalances, because calcium interferes with the absorption of other minerals, including iron, zinc, and magnesium. This interference may only be of major concern in individuals vulnerable to mineral imbalance, such as the elderly and people who consume very low amounts of minerals in their diets. Another potential problem is kidney stone formation: calcium from foods does not increase the risk for kidney stones, but some studies suggest that taking calcium supplements can.[4]

Various diseases and metabolic disorders can alter the body's ability to regulate blood calcium. **Hypercalcemia** is a condition in which blood calcium levels reach abnormally high concentrations. Hypercalcemia can be caused by cancer and by the overproduction of PTH. Recall that PTH stimulates the osteoclasts to break down bone and release more calcium into the bloodstream. Symptoms of hypercalcemia include fatigue, loss of appetite, constipation, and mental confusion, and it can lead to coma and possibly death. Hypercalcemia can also result in an accumulation of calcium deposits in the soft tissues, such as the liver and kidneys, causing failure of these organs.

9 cups
lima beans
1,946 kcal

5.2 oz plain,
nonfat yogurt
83 kcal

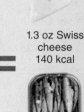

1.3 oz Swiss
cheese
140 kcal

8 fl. oz
nonfat milk
299 mg Ca
83 kcal

=

2.8 oz canned
sardines
165 kcal

7 oz tofu, soft,
with calcium
163 kcal

1 1/8 cup cooked
collard greens
(from frozen)
70 kcal

FIGURE 11.7 Serving sizes and energy content of various foods that contain the same amount of calcium as an 8-fl. oz glass of skim milk.

hypercalcemia A condition characterized by an abnormally high concentration of calcium in the blood.

Nutrition Label Activity

How Much Calcium Am I Really Consuming?

As you have learned in this chapter, we do not absorb 100% of the calcium contained in our foods. This is particularly true for individuals who eat a diet dominated by foods that are high in fiber, oxalates, and phytates, such as whole grains and certain vegetables. So if you want to design an eating plan that contains adequate calcium, it's important to understand how the rate of calcium absorption differs for the foods you include.

Estimates of the rate of calcium absorption have been established for a variety of common foods that are considered good sources of calcium. The following table shows some of these foods, their calcium content per serving, the calcium absorption rate, and the estimated amount of calcium absorbed from each food.

As you can see from this table, many dairy products have a similar calcium absorption rate, just over 30%. Interestingly, many green, leafy vegetables have a higher absorption rate of around 60%; however, because a typical serving of these foods contains less calcium than dairy foods, you would have to eat more vegetables to get the same calcium as you would from a standard serving of dairy foods. Note the relatively low calcium absorption rate for spinach, even though it contains a relatively high amount of calcium. This is due to the high levels of oxalates in spinach, which bind with calcium and reduce its bioavailability.

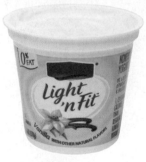

Remember that the RDA for calcium takes these differences in absorption rate into account. Thus, the 300 mg of calcium in a glass of milk counts as 300 mg toward your daily calcium goal. In general, you can trust that dairy products are good, absorbable sources of calcium, as are most dark-green, leafy vegetables. Other

Food	Serving Size	Calcium per Serving (mg)*	Absorption Rate (%)[7]	Estimated Amount of Calcium Absorbed (mg)
Yogurt, plain skim milk	8 fl. oz	452	32	145
Milk, skim	1 cup	299	32	96
Milk, 2%	1 cup	293	32	94
Kale, frozen, cooked	1 cup	179	59	106
Turnip greens, boiled	1 cup	197	52	103
Broccoli, frozen, chopped, cooked	1 cup	61	61	37
Cauliflower, boiled	1 cup	20	69	14
Spinach, frozen, cooked	1 cup	291	5	14

*Data from U.S. Department of Agriculture, Agricultural Research Service. 2014. USDA National Nutrient Database for Standard Reference, Release 27. www.ars.usda.gov/ba/bhnrc/ndl.

[7]Data from Weaver, C. M., W. R. Proulx, and R. Heaney. 1999. Choices for achieving adequate dietary calcium with a vegetarian diet. *Am. J. Clin. Nutr.* 70(suppl.):543S–548S; and Weaver, C. M., and K. L. Plawecki. 1994. Dietary calcium: adequacy of a vegetarian diet. *Am. J. Clin. Nutr.* 59(suppl.):1238S–1241S.

dietary sources of calcium with good absorption rates include calcium-fortified juices and milk alternatives, tofu processed with calcium, and fortified breakfast cereals. Armed with this knowledge, you will be better able to select food sources that can optimize your calcium intake and support bone health.

What Happens If We Don't Consume Enough Calcium?

There are no short-term symptoms associated with consuming too little calcium. Even when a person does not consume enough dietary calcium, the body continues to tightly regulate blood calcium levels by taking the calcium from bone. A long-term repercussion of inadequate calcium intake is osteoporosis. But because other nutrients and non-nutrient factors may be involved, we'll discuss this disease later in the chapter.

Hypocalcemia is the condition of having an abnormally low level of calcium in the blood. Hypocalcemia does not result from consuming too little dietary calcium, but is caused by various diseases, including kidney disease, vitamin D deficiency, and diseases that inhibit the production of PTH. Symptoms of hypocalcemia include muscle spasms and convulsions.

hypocalcemia A condition characterized by an abnormally low concentration of calcium in the blood.

RECAP

Calcium is the most abundant mineral in the body and a significant component of bones. It also helps the body maintain acid–base balance, and is necessary for normal nerve and muscle function. Blood calcium is maintained within a very narrow range, and bone calcium is used to maintain normal blood calcium if dietary intake is inadequate. The RDA for calcium is 1,000 mg per day for adults aged 19 to 50; the RDA increases to 1,200 mg per day for men older than 70 years of age and women older than 50 years of age, and goes up to 1,300 mg per day for adolescents. Bioavailability of calcium is affected by the individual's need, the amount of calcium consumed, dietary factors such as phytates and oxalates that may reduce absorption, and level of vitamin D. Dairy products, canned fish with bones, and some green, leafy vegetables are good sources of calcium. The most common long-term effect of inadequate calcium consumption is osteoporosis.

How Does Vitamin D Contribute to Bone Health?

LO 6 Discuss the contributions of vitamin D to bone health and the process by which the body synthesizes vitamin D from exposure to sunlight.

Vitamin D is like other fat-soluble vitamins in that excess amounts are stored in the liver and adipose tissue. But vitamin D is different from other nutrients in two ways. First, vitamin D does not always need to come from the diet. This is because the body can synthesize vitamin D using energy from exposure to sunlight. However, when we do not get enough sunlight, we must consume vitamin D in our diets. Second, in addition to being a nutrient, vitamin D is considered a *hormone*, because it is made in one part of the body yet regulates various activities in other parts of the body.

Figure 11.8 illustrates how the body makes vitamin D by converting a cholesterol compound in our skin to the active form of vitamin D that we need to function properly.

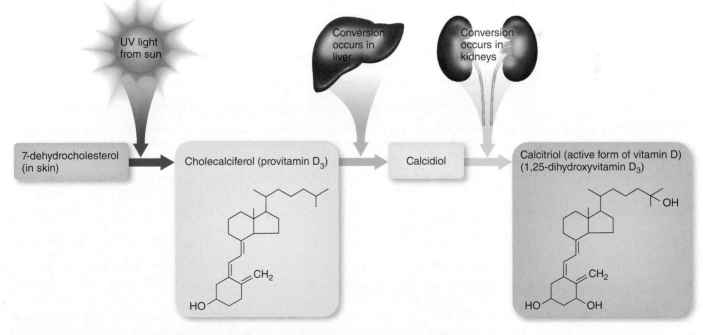

FIGURE 11.8 The process of converting sunlight into vitamin D in our skin. When the ultraviolet rays of the sun hit the skin, they react with 7-dehydrocholesterol. This compound is converted to cholecalciferol, an inactive form of vitamin D that is also called provitamin D_3. Cholecalciferol is then converted to calcidiol in the liver. Calcidiol travels to the kidneys, where it is converted into calcitriol, which is considered the primary active form of vitamin D in our bodies.

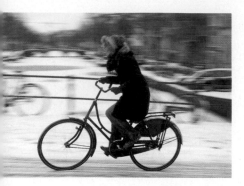

Vitamin D synthesis from the sun is not possible during most of the winter months for people living in high latitudes. Therefore, many people around the world need to consume vitamin D in their diets, particularly during the winter.

When the ultraviolet rays of the sun hit the skin, they react with 7-dehydrocholesterol. This cholesterol compound is converted into a precursor of vitamin D, **cholecalciferol,** which is also called provitamin D$_3$. This inactive form is then converted to calcidiol in the liver, where it is stored. When needed, calcidiol travels to the kidneys, where it is converted into **calcitriol,** which is considered the primary active form of vitamin D in the body. Calcitriol then circulates to various parts of the body, performing its many functions. Excess calcitriol can also be stored in adipose tissue for later use.

Vitamin D Has Many Regulatory Functions

As you've learned, vitamin D and PTH work together continuously to regulate blood calcium levels, which in turn maintains bone health. They do this by regulating the absorption of calcium and phosphorus from the small intestine, causing more to be absorbed when the need for them is higher and less when the need is lower. They also decrease or increase blood calcium levels by signaling the kidneys to excrete more or less calcium in the urine. Finally, vitamin D works with PTH to stimulate osteoclasts to break down bone when calcium is needed elsewhere in the body.

Vitamin D is also necessary for the normal calcification of bone. This means it assists the process by which minerals such as calcium and phosphorus are crystallized.

Vitamin D may also play a role in decreasing the formation of some cancerous tumors, as it can prevent certain types of malignant cells from growing out of control. Also, like vitamin A, vitamin D appears to play a role in cell differentiation in various tissues.

How Much Vitamin D Should We Consume?

If your exposure to the sun is adequate, then you do not need to consume any vitamin D in your diet. But how do you know whether you are getting enough sun?

Recommended Dietary Intake for Vitamin D

The RDA is based on the assumption that an individual does not get adequate sun exposure. Of the many factors that affect the ability to synthesize vitamin D from sunlight, latitude and time of year are most significant (**Table 11.3**). People living in very sunny climates relatively close to the equator, such as the southern United States and Mexico, may synthesize

cholecalciferol Vitamin D$_3$, a form of vitamin D found in animal foods and the form we synthesize from the sun.

calcitriol The primary active form of vitamin D in the body.

TABLE 11.3 Factors Affecting Sunlight-Mediated Synthesis of Vitamin D in the Skin

Factors That Enhance Synthesis of Vitamin D	Factors That Inhibit Synthesis of Vitamin D
Season—summer months, particularly June and July, during which most vitamin D is produced	Season—winter months (October through February), resulting in little or no vitamin D production
Latitude—locations closer to the equator, which get more sunlight throughout the year	Latitude—regions north of 37°N and south of 37°S, which get inadequate sunlight during the winter
Time of day—generally, between 10:00 AM and 3:00 PM (depending on latitude and time of year)	Time of day—early morning, late afternoon, and evening hours Age—older, due to reduced skin thickness with age
Age—younger	Use of sunscreen with SPF 8 or greater
Limited or no use of sunscreen	Cloudy weather
Sunny weather	Protective clothing
Exposed skin	Darker skin pigmentation
Lighter skin pigmentation	Glass and plastics—windows or other barriers made of glass or plastic (such as Plexiglas), which block the sun's rays Obesity—possible negative effect on metabolism and storage of vitamin D

enough vitamin D from the sun to meet their needs throughout the year—as long as they spend time outdoors. However, vitamin D synthesis from the sun is not possible during most of the winter months for people living in places located at a latitude of more than 37°N or more than 37°S. At these latitudes in winter, the sun never rises high enough in the sky to provide the amount of direct sunlight needed. The 37°N latitude runs like a belt across the United States from northern Virginia in the East to northern California in the West (**Figure 11.9**). In addition, entire countries, such as Canada and the United Kingdom, are affected, as are countries and regions in the far southern hemisphere. Thus, many people around the world need to consume vitamin D in their diets, particularly during the winter months.

Other factors influencing vitamin D synthesis include the time of day, skin color, age, and body weight status:

■ More vitamin D can be synthesized during the time of day when the sun's rays are strongest, generally between 10 AM and 3 PM. Vitamin D synthesis is severely limited or may be nonexistent on overcast days.

■ Darker skin contains more melanin pigment, which reduces the penetration of sunlight. Thus, people with dark skin have a more difficult time synthesizing vitamin D from the sun than do light-skinned people.

■ People 65 years of age or older experience a fourfold decrease in their capacity to synthesize vitamin D from the sun; they are also more likely to spend more time indoors and may have inadequate dietary intakes.[5]

■ Obesity has recently been found to cause lower levels of circulating vitamin D.[6] Although the exact mechanism for this finding is not clear, this study implicates variation in the genes associated with the synthesis and breakdown of vitamin D. Other possible contributors include a lower bioavailability of cholecalciferol from adipose tissue, decreased exposure to sunlight due to limited mobility or time spent outdoors with skin exposed, and alterations in vitamin D metabolism in the liver.

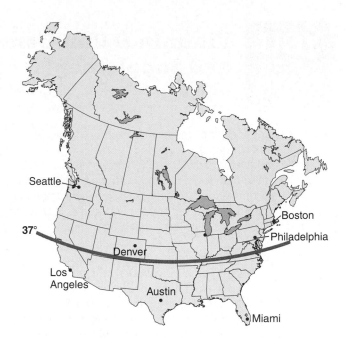

FIGURE 11.9 This map illustrates the geographic location of 37° latitude in the United States. In southern cities below 37° latitude, such as Los Angeles, Austin, and Miami, the sunlight is strong enough to allow for vitamin D synthesis throughout the year. In northern cities above 37° latitude, such as Seattle, Chicago, and Boston, the sunlight is too weak from about mid-October to mid-March to allow for adequate vitamin D synthesis.

Wearing protective clothing and sunscreen (with an SPF greater than 8) limits sun exposure, so it is suggested that we expose our hands, face, and arms to the sun two or three times per week for a period of time that is one-third to one-half of the amount it would take to get sunburned. This means that, if you normally sunburn in 1 hour, you should expose yourself to the sun for 20 to 30 minutes two or three times per week to synthesize adequate amounts of vitamin D. Again, this guideline does not apply to people living in more northern climates during the winter months; they can get enough vitamin D only by consuming it in their diets.

Because not everyone is able to get adequate sun exposure throughout the year, an RDA has been established for vitamin D. For men and women aged 19 to 70 years, the RDA is 600 IU, and for adults older than 70 years, it is 800 IU. The UL for vitamin D is 4,000 IU for everyone 9 years of age and older. Recent evidence suggests that the current RDA for vitamin D is not sufficient to maintain optimal bone health and reduce the risks for diseases such as cancer; the controversy surrounding the current recommendations for vitamin D intake are discussed in more detail in the ***Nutrition Myth or Fact?*** on page 455.

When reading labels, you will see the amount of vitamin D expressed on food and supplement labels in units of either µg or IU. For conversion purposes, 1 µg of vitamin D is equal to 40 IU of vitamin D. Refer to the ***You Do the Math*** (page 440) to learn how to convert vitamin D units from food and supplement sources.

YOU Do the Math

Vitamin D Unit Conversions from Foods and Supplements

Labels on foods and supplements may express vitamin D content in units of either IU or µg. Judy's physician is concerned about her vitamin D intake, because Judy is obese, rarely drinks milk, and doesn't spend much time outdoors in the sun. He recommends that she increase her consumption of foods that are good sources of vitamin D. Judy's RDA for vitamin D is 600 IU per day. Recall that 1 µg of vitamin D is equal to 40 IU.

Judy enjoys tuna sandwiches, and her doctor has explained that tuna is high in vitamin D. At the grocery store, she finds that 3 oz of canned tuna (packed in oil) contains 5.7 µg of vitamin D. Judy decides that she'll add a 1-oz slice of American cheese (fortified with vitamin D) to her sandwich. The cheese contains 2.1 µg of vitamin D.

a. How much vitamin D in IU units do these two foods contain?

Tuna: 5.7 µg × 40 IU = 228 IU of vitamin D
American cheese: 2 µg × 40 IU = 84 IU of vitamin D

Thus, these two foods contain a total of 312 IU of vitamin D.

b. Assuming Judy does not get adequate sun exposure and these two foods are the only sources of vitamin D she consumes today, how much of the RDA for vitamin D are these sources contributing to her diet?

Again, Judy's RDA for vitamin D is 600 IU per day:
(312 IU ÷ 600 IU) × 100 = 52% of the RDA is supplied by these foods.

c. If Judy decides to take a vitamin D supplement in addition to consuming these foods to meet her RDA, what amount of vitamin D (in µg) would be sufficient?

The amount of vitamin D not supplied by foods is
600 IU − 312 IU = 288 IU
288 IU ÷ 40 µg in 1 IU = 7.2 µg vitamin D in supplement form

Now use your own diet assessment to determine *your* intake of vitamin D. What percentage of the RDA for vitamin D do you currently consume? Do you get adequate sunlight to ensure you meet your needs for vitamin D? If not, what foods (and in what amounts) can you consume to meet your RDA for vitamin D?

Answers will vary depending on body type and individual nutrient needs.

Vitamin D: Fish, Fortified Foods, Supplements, or Sunlight

There are many forms of vitamin D, but only two can be converted into calcitriol. Vitamin D_2, also called **ergocalciferol,** is found exclusively in plant foods, such as green beans and mushrooms. Vitamin D_3, or cholecalciferol, is found in animal foods. As noted earlier, cholecalciferol also is the form of vitamin D we synthesize from the sun.

Most foods naturally contain very little vitamin D. The few exceptions are cod liver oil and fatty fish (such as salmon, mackerel, and sardines), foods that few Americans consume in adequate amounts. Egg yolks, beef liver, and cheese also provide small amounts of vitamin D, but we would have to eat very large amounts to consume enough vitamin D.

Thus, the primary source of vitamin D in the diet is from fortified foods, such as milk (**Figure 11.10**). In the United States, milk is fortified with 100 IU of vitamin D per cup.[5] Additional foods fortified with vitamin D include some milk alternatives, breakfast cereals, margarines, juices, and yogurts. Because plants contain very little vitamin D, vegetarians who consume no fortified dairy products need to obtain their vitamin D from sun exposure, fortified foods and beverages, or supplements.

What Happens If We Consume Too Much Vitamin D?

A person cannot get too much vitamin D from sun exposure, as the skin has the ability to limit its production. As noted, foods contain little natural vitamin D. Thus, the only way a person can consume too much vitamin D is through supplementation.

Consuming too much vitamin D causes hypercalcemia, or high blood calcium concentrations. As discussed in the section on calcium, symptoms of hypercalcemia include weakness, loss of appetite, constipation, mental confusion, vomiting, excessive urine output,

Fatty fish contain vitamin D.

ergocalciferol Vitamin D_2, a form of vitamin D found exclusively in plant foods.

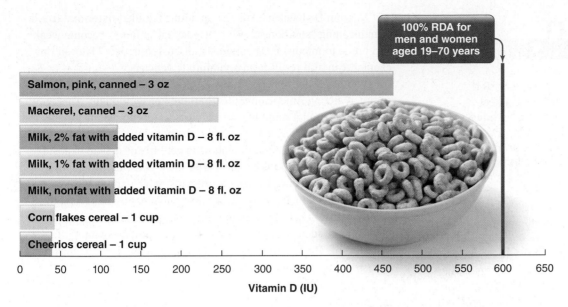

FIGURE 11.10 Common food sources of vitamin D. For men and women aged 19 to 70 years, the RDA for vitamin D is 600 IU per day. The RDA increases to 800 IU per day for adults over the age of 70 years. (*Source*: Data from U.S. Department of Agriculture, Agricultural Research Service, 2014, USDA Nutrient Database for Standard Reference, Release 27. Nutrient Data Laboratory Home Page, www.ars.usda.gov/ba/bhnrc/ndl.)

and extreme thirst. Hypercalcemia also leads to the formation of calcium deposits in soft tissues, such as the kidney, liver, and heart. In addition, toxic levels of vitamin D lead to increased bone loss, because calcium is then pulled from the bones and excreted more readily from the kidneys.

What Happens If We Don't Consume Enough Vitamin D?

The primary deficiency associated with inadequate vitamin D is loss of bone mass. In fact, when vitamin D levels are inadequate, the intestines can absorb only 10% to 15% of the calcium consumed. Vitamin D deficiencies occur most often in individuals who have diseases that cause intestinal malabsorption of fat and thus the fat-soluble vitamins. People with liver disease, kidney disease, Crohn's disease, celiac disease, cystic fibrosis, or Whipple's disease may suffer from vitamin D deficiency and require supplements.

Vitamin D–deficiency disease in children, called **rickets,** results in inadequate mineralization (or *demineralization*) of the skeleton. The classic sign of rickets is deformity of the skeleton, such as bowed legs and knocked knees (**Figure 11.11**). However, severe cases can be fatal. Rickets is not common in the United States because of fortification of milk products with vitamin D, but children with illnesses that cause fat malabsorption, or who drink no milk and get limited sun exposure, are at increased risk. There is no national surveillance program for rickets, and thus it is not clear what the prevalence of rickets is in the United States. However, a recent study conducted in Minnesota found an increase in cases of rickets in children 3 years of age and younger from zero in 1970 to 24 per 100,000 in 2000. Increased risk in these children was associated with having darker skin and breastfeeding.[7] Breast milk contains very little vitamin D, and none of the breast-fed children were reported to have received vitamin D supplementation before being diagnosed. Other contributing factors included poor feeding, limited sun exposure, limited milk intake, a predominantly vegetarian diet, and being born premature. Thus, rickets appears to occur more commonly in children with darker skin (their need for adequate sun exposure is higher than that of light-skinned children) and in breast-fed children who do not receive adequate vitamin D supplementation. Rickets is still a significant nutritional problem for children living outside the United States.

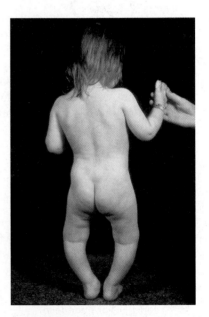

FIGURE 11.11 A vitamin D–deficiency causes a bone-deforming disease in children called rickets.

rickets A vitamin D–deficiency disease in children. Symptoms include deformities of the skeleton, such as bowed legs and knocked knees.

Nutrition
MILESTONE

The disease rickets has been reported throughout history, with the earliest descriptions in 1645 and 1650 credited to two English physicians, Daniel Whistler and Francis Glisson. In 1890, the British scientist T. A. Palm found a relationship between geographic distribution of rickets and sunlight, and he concluded that rickets is caused by inadequate exposure to sun. However, no major advances in the study and treatment of rickets were made until the early 20th century, when scientists began to explore how dietary factors might be used to treat rickets. Elmer McCollum, a nutritional biochemist at Johns Hopkins University, and his colleagues ran a series of experiments in rats in which cod liver oil was found to be an effective treatment for rickets.

In **1922**, McCollum and colleagues identified the effective *antirachitic* agent (an agent that cures rickets) in cod liver oil, which was named vitamin D, as it was the fourth vitamin to be discovered. By the 1930s, the use of cod liver oil to treat rickets was common throughout the United States, and the fortification of milk with vitamin D led to the almost complete eradication of rickets by the mid-1940s.

Vitamin D–deficiency disease in adults is called **osteomalacia,** a term meaning "soft bones." With osteomalacia, bones become weak and prone to fractures. Osteoporosis, discussed in detail later in this chapter, can also result from a vitamin D deficiency.

Vitamin D deficiencies have recently been found to be more common among American adults than previously thought. This may be partly due to jobs and lifestyle choices that keep people indoors for most of the day. Not surprisingly, the population at greatest risk is older, institutionalized individuals who get little or no sun exposure.

Various medications can also alter the metabolism and activity of vitamin D. For instance, glucocorticoids, which are medications used to reduce inflammation, can cause bone loss by inhibiting the ability to absorb calcium through the actions of vitamin D. Antiseizure medications, such as phenobarbital and Dilantin, alter vitamin D metabolism. Thus, people who are taking such medications may need to increase their vitamin D intake.

RECAP

Vitamin D is a fat-soluble vitamin and a hormone. It can be made in the skin using energy from sunlight; however, synthesis is impaired in older adults, people with darker skin, and at certain times of day and seasons of the year at northern latitudes. Vitamin D works with PTH to regulate blood calcium levels by influencing intestinal absorption and renal excretion, and with PTH to influence osteoclast activity. It also assists in the crystallization of minerals, in cell differentiation, and in other body functions. The RDA for vitamin D is 600 IU per day for adult men and women aged 19 to 70 years; the RDA increases to 800 IU per day for adults over the age of 70 years. Foods contain little vitamin D, with fortified milk being the primary source. Vitamin D toxicity causes hypercalcemia. Vitamin D deficiency can result in osteoporosis; rickets is vitamin D deficiency in children, whereas osteomalacia is vitamin D deficiency in adults.

LO 7 Identify the contributions of vitamin K, phosphorus, and magnesium to bone health, as well as good food sources.

LO 8 Describe the main functions of fluoride in the development and maintenance of teeth and bones, and the results of consuming too much and too little fluoride.

osteomalacia A vitamin D–deficiency disease in adults, in which bones become weak and prone to fractures.

phylloquinone The form of vitamin K found in plants.

menaquinone The form of vitamin K produced by bacteria in the large intestine.

osteocalcin A vitamin K–dependent protein that is secreted by osteoblasts and is associated with bone turnover.

What Other Nutrients Help Maintain Bone Health?

Although calcium and vitamin D are the most recognized nutrients associated with bone health, vitamin K, phosphorus, magnesium, and fluoride are also essential for strong bones. The roles of other vitamins, minerals, and phytochemicals are currently being researched.

Vitamin K Serves as a Coenzyme Contributing to Bone Health

Vitamin K, a fat-soluble vitamin stored primarily in the liver, is actually a family of compounds known as quinones. **Phylloquinone,** which is the primary dietary form of vitamin K, is also the form found in plants; **menaquinone** is the animal form of vitamin K produced by bacteria in the large intestine (**Figure 11.12**).

The absorption of phylloquinone occurs in the jejunum and ileum of the small intestine, and its absorption is dependent on the normal flow of bile and pancreatic juice. Dietary fat enhances its absorption. The absorption of phylloquinone has been reported to be as low as 10% from boiled spinach eaten with butter to as high as 80% when given in its free form.[8] It is transported through the lymph as a component of chylomicrons, and it circulates to the liver, where most of the vitamin K in the body is stored. Small amounts of vitamin K are also stored in adipose tissue and bone.[8] The absorption of menaquinone is not well understood, and its contribution to the maintenance of vitamin K status has been difficult to assess.[8]

Functions of Vitamin K

The primary function of vitamin K is to serve as a coenzyme during the production of specific proteins that play important roles in the coagulation of blood and in bone metabolism. (Refer to Chapter 12 for an in-depth description of the role of vitamin K in maintaining blood health.) Here, we limit our discussion to vitamin K's role in the production of two bone proteins, referred to as "Gla" proteins: **Osteocalcin** is a Gla protein that is secreted by osteoblasts and is associated with bone remodeling. **Matrix Gla protein** is located in the protein matrix of bone and is found in cartilage, blood-vessel walls, and other soft tissues. The specific role of vitamin K in maintaining bone health is unclear, with studies reporting conflicting results. A recent meta-analysis of randomized, controlled trials examining the effect of vitamin K on bone mineral density indicates that vitamin K has an overall modest effect, with gender, ethnicity, and type of vitamin K exerting variable effects on bone density.[9] Matrix Gla protein also appears to play a role in preventing the calcification of arteries, which may reduce the risk for cardiovascular disease.[10]

How Much Vitamin K Should We Consume?

We can obtain vitamin K from our diets, and we absorb the vitamin K produced by bacteria in the large intestine. These two sources of vitamin K usually provide adequate amounts of this nutrient to maintain health, and there is no RDA or UL for vitamin K. AI recommendations for adult men and adult women are 120 μg per day and 90 μg per day, respectively.

Only a few foods contribute substantially to our dietary intake of vitamin K. Green, leafy vegetables, including kale, spinach, collard greens, turnip greens, and lettuce, are good sources, as are broccoli, brussels sprouts, and cabbage. **Figure 11.13** identifies the micrograms per serving for these foods.

What Happens If We Consume Too Much Vitamin K?

Based on our current knowledge, for healthy individuals there appear to be no side effects associated with consuming large amounts of vitamin K. This seems to be true for both supplements and food sources. In the past, a synthetic form of vitamin K was used for therapeutic purposes and was shown to cause liver damage; thus, this form is no longer used.

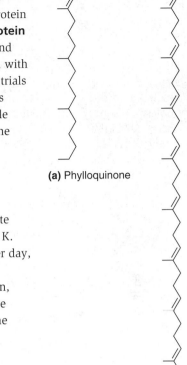

(a) Phylloquinone

(b) Menaquinone

FIGURE 11.12 The chemical structure of **(a)** phylloquinone, the plant form of vitamin K, and **(b)** menaquinone, the animal form of vitamin K.

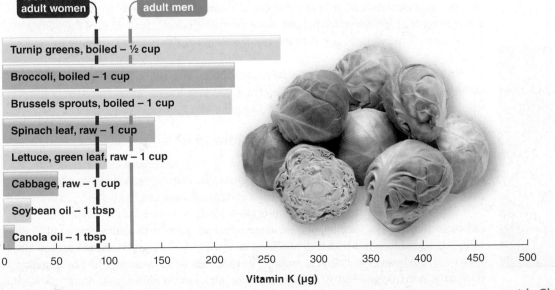

FIGURE 11.13 Common food sources of vitamin K. The AIs for adult men and adult women are 120 μg per day and 90 μg per day, respectively. (*Source:* Data from U.S. Department of Agriculture, Agricultural Research Service, 2014, USDA Nutrient Database for Standard Reference, Release 27. Nutrient Data Laboratory Home Page, www.ars.usda.gov/ba/bhnrc/ndl.)

matrix Gla protein A vitamin K–dependent protein located in the protein matrix of bone and in cartilage, blood-vessel walls, and other soft tissues.

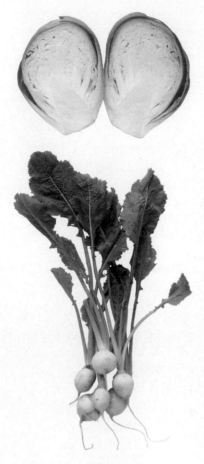

Green, leafy vegetables, including brussels sprouts and turnip greens, are good sources of vitamin K.

What Happens If We Don't Consume Enough Vitamin K?

Vitamin K deficiency is associated with a reduced ability to form blood clots, leading to excessive bleeding; however, primary vitamin K deficiency is rare in humans. People with diseases that cause malabsorption of fat, such as celiac disease, Crohn's disease, and cystic fibrosis, can suffer secondarily from a deficiency of vitamin K. Long-term use of antibiotics, which typically reduce bacterial populations in the colon, combined with limited dietary intake of vitamin K–rich food sources, can also lead to vitamin K deficiency. Newborns are typically given an injection of vitamin K at birth, as they lack the intestinal bacteria necessary to produce this nutrient.

The impact of vitamin K deficiency on bone health is controversial. As recently described, the effect of vitamin K on bone mineral density appears to be modest, and studies report inconsistent results.[9] Thus, there is not enough scientific evidence to support the contention that vitamin K deficiency directly causes osteoporosis. In fact, there is no significant impact on overall bone density in people who take anticoagulant medications that result in a relative state of vitamin K deficiency.

RECAP

Vitamin K is a fat-soluble vitamin and coenzyme that is important for blood clotting and bone metabolism. We obtain vitamin K largely from beneficial bacteria in the large intestine. The AIs for adult men and adult women are 120 μg per day and 90 μg per day, respectively. Green, leafy vegetables and vegetable oils contain vitamin K. There are no known toxicity symptoms for vitamin K in healthy individuals. Vitamin K deficiency is rare and may lead to excessive bleeding.

Phosphorus Is Part of the Mineral Complex of Bone

Phosphorus is the major negatively charged intracellular electrolyte (see Chapter 9). In the body, phosphorus is most commonly found combined with oxygen in the form of phosphate (PO_4^{3-}). Phosphorus is an essential constituent of all cells and is found in both plants and animals.

Functions of Phosphorus

Phosphorus plays a critical role in bone formation, as it is a part of the mineral complex of bone. As discussed earlier in this chapter, calcium and phosphorus crystallize to form hydroxyapatite crystals, which provide the hardness of bone. About 85% of the body's phosphorus is stored in bones, with the rest stored in soft tissues, such as muscles and organs.

In addition to its role in fluid balance, phosphorus also helps activate and deactivate enzymes, and it is a component of lipoproteins, cell membranes, DNA and RNA, and several energy molecules, including adenosine triphosphate (ATP).

How Much Phosphorus Should We Consume?

The RDA for phosphorus is 700 mg for adults. In general, phosphorus is widespread in many foods and is found in high amounts in foods that contain protein. Milk, meats, poultry, eggs, and legumes, including peanuts, are good sources.

Phosphorus is also found in many processed foods as a food additive, where it enhances smoothness, binding, and moisture retention. Moreover, in the form of phosphoric acid, it is added to soft drinks to give them a sharper, or more tart, flavor and to slow the growth of molds and bacteria. Our society has increased its consumption of phosphorus during the past 30 years due to consuming more processed foods and soft drinks. This could have detrimental effects on our health, as a recent study found that a high phosphorus intake is associated with increased risk of premature mortality in healthy adults.[11]

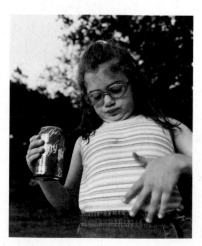

Phosphorus, in the form of phosphoric acid, is a major component of soft drinks.

In the past, some studies associated consumption of soft drinks with reduced bone mass or an increased risk for fractures in both youth and adults. The mechanisms speculated to explain this link were that the phosphoric acid and/or caffeine content of soft drinks causes an increased loss of calcium—supposedly because calcium is drawn from bone into the blood to neutralize the excess phosphoric acid, and caffeine increases the excretion of calcium in the urine. It was also hypothesized that drinking soft drinks led to a milk displacement effect; in other words, soft drinks take the place of milk in our diets. However, more recent evidence suggests that the most likely explanation for the link between soft drink consumption and poor bone health is that a high intake of soft drinks may be a marker of overall poor dietary quality. Researchers in Australia have found that a dietary pattern that included high consumption of refined cereals, soft drinks, fried potatoes, processed meats, fast foods, beer, and low consumption of vegetables, whole grains, tea, coffee, fruit, and breakfast cereals was associated with poorer bone health in women.[12] In contrast, a dietary pattern high in legumes, seafood, seeds, nuts, wine, rice, vegetables, and low in processed meats was associated with better bone health.

What Happens If We Consume Too Much Phosphorus?

People with kidney disease and those who take too many vitamin D supplements or too many phosphorus-containing antacids can suffer from high blood phosphorus levels; severely high levels of blood phosphorus can cause muscle spasms and convulsions.

What Happens If We Don't Consume Enough Phosphorus?

Phosphorus deficiencies are rare but can occur in people who abuse alcohol, in premature infants, and in elderly people with poor diets. People with vitamin D deficiency, those who have hyperparathyroidism (oversecretion of parathyroid hormone), and those who overuse antacids that bind with phosphorus may also have low blood phosphorus levels.

RECAP

Phosphorus is the major negatively charged electrolyte inside the cell. It helps maintain fluid balance and bone health. It also assists in regulating chemical reactions, and it is a primary component of ATP, DNA, and RNA. Phosphorus is commonly found in high-protein foods. Excess phosphorus can lead to muscle spasms and convulsions, whereas phosphorus deficiencies are rare.

Magnesium Builds Bone and Helps Regulate Calcium Balance

Magnesium is a major mineral. Approximately 50% of dietary magnesium is absorbed via both passive and active transport mechanisms; maximal absorption of magnesium occurs in the distal jejunum and ileum of the small intestine. The absorption of magnesium decreases with higher dietary intakes. The kidneys are responsible for the regulation of blood magnesium levels. Two forms of vitamin D, 25-hydroxyvitamin D and 1,25-dihydroxyvitamin D, can enhance the intestinal absorption of magnesium to a limited extent. Excessive alcohol intake can cause magnesium depletion, and some diuretic medications can lead to increased excretion of magnesium in the urine. Dietary fiber and phytates decrease intestinal absorption of magnesium.

Total body magnesium content is approximately 25 g. About 50% to 60% of the magnesium in the body is found in bones, with the rest located in soft tissues.

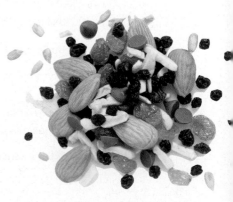

Trail mix with chocolate chips, nuts, and seeds is a common food source of magnesium.

Functions of Magnesium

Magnesium is one of the minerals that make up the structure of bone. It is also important in the regulation of bone and mineral status. Specifically, magnesium influences the formation of hydroxyapatite crystals through its regulation of calcium balance and its interactions with vitamin D and parathyroid hormone.

Magnesium is a critical cofactor for more than 300 enzyme systems. It is necessary for the production of ATP, and it plays an important role in DNA and protein synthesis and repair. Magnesium supplementation has been shown to improve insulin sensitivity, and there is epidemiological evidence that a high magnesium intake is associated with a modest decrease in the risk for colorectal cancer.[13,14] Magnesium supports normal vitamin D metabolism and action and is necessary for normal muscle contraction and blood clotting.

How Much Magnesium Should We Consume?

As magnesium is found in a wide variety of foods, people who are adequately nourished generally consume adequate magnesium in their diets. The RDA for magnesium changes across age groups and genders. For adult men 19 to 30 years of age, the RDA for magnesium is 400 mg per day; the RDA increases to 420 mg per day for men 31 years of age and older. For adult women 19 to 30 years of age, the RDA for magnesium is 310 mg per day; this value increases to 320 mg per day for women 31 years of age and older. There is no UL for magnesium consumed in food and water; the UL for magnesium from pharmacologic sources is 350 mg per day.

Magnesium is found in green, leafy vegetables, such as spinach; whole grains; seeds; and nuts. Other good food sources include seafood, beans, and some dairy products. Refined and processed foods are low in magnesium. **Figure 11.14** shows many foods that are good sources of magnesium.

The magnesium content of drinking water varies considerably. The "harder" the water, the higher its content of magnesium. This large variability in the magnesium content of water makes it impossible to estimate how much our drinking water contributes to the magnesium content of our diets.

The ability of the small intestine to absorb magnesium is reduced when one consumes a diet that is extremely high in fiber and phytates, because these substances bind with magnesium. Even though seeds and nuts are relatively high in fiber, they are excellent

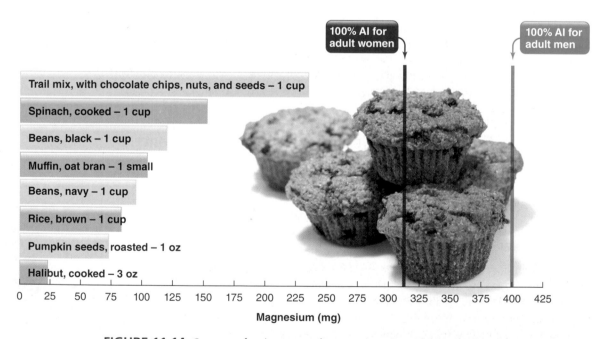

FIGURE 11.14 Common food sources of magnesium. For adult men 19 to 30 years of age, the RDA for magnesium is 400 mg per day; the RDA increases to 420 mg per day for men 31 years of age and older. For adult women 19 to 30 years of age, the RDA for magnesium is 310 mg per day; this value increases to 320 mg per day for women 31 years of age and older. (*Source:* Data from U.S. Department of Agriculture, Agricultural Research Service, 2014, USDA Nutrient Database for Standard Reference, Release 27. Nutrient Data Laboratory Home Page, www.ars.usda.gov/ba/bhnrc/ndl.)

sources of absorbable magnesium. Overall, our absorption of magnesium should be sufficient if we consume the recommended amount of fiber (20 to 35 g per day). In contrast, higher dietary protein intakes enhance the absorption and retention of magnesium.

What Happens If We Consume Too Much Magnesium?

There are no known toxicity symptoms related to consuming excess magnesium in the diet. The toxicity symptoms that result from pharmacologic use of magnesium include diarrhea, nausea, and abdominal cramps. In extreme cases, large doses can result in acid–base imbalances, massive dehydration, cardiac arrest, and death. High blood magnesium, or **hypermagnesemia,** occurs in individuals with impaired kidney function who consume large amounts of nondietary magnesium, such as antacids. Side effects include impairment of nerve, muscle, and heart function.

What Happens If We Don't Consume Enough Magnesium?

Hypomagnesemia, or low blood magnesium, results from magnesium deficiency. This condition may develop secondarily to kidney disease, chronic diarrhea, or chronic alcohol abuse. Elderly people seem to be at particularly high risk for low dietary intakes of magnesium and other micronutrients, because they have a reduced appetite and blunted senses of taste and smell. In addition, the elderly face challenges related to shopping and preparing micronutrient-dense meals, and their ability to absorb magnesium is reduced.

Low blood calcium levels are a side effect of hypomagnesemia. Other symptoms of magnesium deficiency include muscle cramps, spasms or seizures, nausea, weakness, irritability, and confusion. Considering magnesium's role in bone formation, it is not surprising that long-term magnesium deficiency is associated with osteoporosis. Magnesium deficiency is also associated with many other chronic diseases, including heart disease, high blood pressure, and type 2 diabetes.

RECAP

Magnesium is a major mineral found in fresh foods, including spinach, nuts, seeds, whole grains, and some fish. Magnesium is important for bone health, energy production, and muscle function. The RDA for magnesium is a function of age and gender. Hypermagnesemia can result in diarrhea, muscle cramps, and cardiac arrest. Hypomagnesemia causes hypocalcemia, muscle cramps, spasms, and weakness. Magnesium deficiencies are also associated with osteoporosis, heart disease, high blood pressure, and type 2 diabetes.

Fluoride Helps Develop and Maintain Teeth and Bones

Fluoride, a trace mineral, is the ionic form of the element fluorine. About 99% of the fluoride in the body is stored in teeth and bones.

Functions of Fluoride

Fluoride assists in the development and maintenance of teeth and bones. During the development of both baby and permanent teeth, fluoride combines with calcium and phosphorus to form **fluorohydroxyapatite,** which is more resistant to destruction by acids and bacteria than hydroxyapatite. Even after all of our permanent teeth are in, treating them with fluoride, whether at the dentist's office or by using fluoridated toothpaste, gives them more protection against dental caries (cavities) than teeth that have not been treated. That's because fluoride enhances tooth mineralization, decreases and reverses tooth demineralization, and inhibits the metabolism of acid-producing bacteria that cause tooth decay.

Fluoride also stimulates new bone growth, and it is currently being researched as a potential treatment for osteoporosis both alone and in combination with other medications.

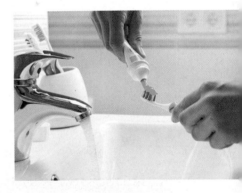

Fluoride is readily available in many communities in the United States through fluoridated water and dental products.

hypermagnesemia A condition marked by an abnormally high concentration of magnesium in the blood.

hypomagnesemia A condition characterized by an abnormally low concentration of magnesium in the blood.

fluorohydroxyapatite A mineral compound in human teeth that contains fluoride, calcium, and phosphorus and is more resistant to destruction by acids and bacteria than hydroxyapatite.

While early results are promising, more research needs to be conducted to determine if fluoride is an effective treatment for osteoporosis.[15]

How Much Fluoride Should We Consume?

Our need for fluoride is relatively small. There is no RDA for fluoride. The AI for children aged 4 to 8 years is 1 mg per day; this value increases to 2 mg per day for boys and girls aged 9 to 13 years. The AI for boys and girls aged 14 to 18 years is 3 mg per day. The AI for adults is 4 mg per day for men and 3 mg per day for women. The UL for fluoride is 2.2 mg per day for children aged 4 to 8 years; the UL for everyone older than 8 years of age is 10 mg per day.

Fluoride is readily available in many communities in the United States through fluoridated water and dental products. In the mouth, fluoride is absorbed directly into the teeth and gums, and it can be absorbed from the gastrointestinal tract once it has been ingested. In the early 1990s, there was considerable concern that our intake of fluoride was too high due to the consumption of fluoridated water and fluoride-containing toothpastes and mouthwashes; it was speculated that this high intake of fluoride could have been contributing to an increased risk for cancer, bone fractures, kidney and other organ damage, infertility, and Alzheimer's disease. After reviewing the potential health hazards of fluoride, the U.S. Department of Health and Human Services and the National Cancer Institute found that there is no reliable scientific evidence available to indicate that fluoride increases our risks for these illnesses.[16,17]

There are concerns that individuals who consume bottled water exclusively may be getting too little fluoride and increasing their risk for dental caries, as most bottled waters do not contain fluoride. However, these individuals may still consume fluoride through other beverages that contain fluoridated water and through fluoridated dental products. Toothpastes and mouthwashes that contain fluoride are widely marketed and used by most consumers in the United States, and these products can contribute as much, if not more, fluoride to our diets than fluoridated water. Fluoride supplements are available only by prescription, and these are generally given only to children who do not have access to fluoridated water. Incidentally, tea is a good source of fluoride: one 8-oz cup provides about 20% to 25% of the AI.

What Happens If We Consume Too Much Fluoride?

Consuming too much fluoride increases the protein content of tooth enamel, resulting in a condition called **fluorosis.** Because increased protein makes the enamel more porous, the teeth become stained and pitted (**Figure 11.15**). Teeth seem to be at highest risk for fluorosis during the first 8 years of life, when the permanent teeth are developing. To reduce their risk, children should not swallow oral care products that are meant for topical use only, and children under the age of 6 years should be supervised while using fluoride-containing products. Mild fluorosis generally causes white patches on the teeth, but it has no effect on tooth function. Although moderate and severe fluorosis causes greater discoloration of the teeth, there appears to be no adverse effect on tooth function.

Excess consumption of fluoride can also cause fluorosis of the skeleton. Mild skeletal fluorosis results in an increased bone mass and stiffness and pain in the joints. Moderate and severe skeletal fluorosis can be crippling, but it is extremely rare in the United States.

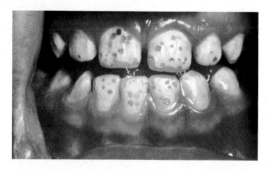

FIGURE 11.15 Consuming too much fluoride causes fluorosis, leading to staining and pitting of the teeth.

What Happens If We Don't Consume Enough Fluoride?

The primary result of fluoride deficiency is dental caries. Adequate fluoride intake appears necessary at an early age and throughout adult life to reduce the risk for tooth decay. Inadequate fluoride intake may also be associated with lower bone density, but there is not enough research available to support the widespread use of fluoride to prevent osteoporosis. Studies are currently being done to determine the role fluoride might play in reducing the risk for osteoporosis and fractures.

fluorosis A condition characterized by staining and pitting of the teeth; caused by an abnormally high intake of fluoride.

RECAP

Fluoride is a trace mineral whose primary function is to support the health of teeth and bones. The AI for fluoride is 4 mg and 3 mg per day for adult men and women, respectively. Primary sources of fluoride are fluoridated dental products and fluoridated water. Fluoride toxicity causes fluorosis of the teeth and skeleton, and fluoride deficiency causes an increase in tooth decay. ■

What Is Osteoporosis, and What Factors Influence the Risk?

 LO 9 Define osteoporosis and identify the factors that influence the risk for developing the disease.

LO 10 Describe osteoporosis treatment.

Of the many disorders associated with poor bone health, the most prevalent in the United States is **osteoporosis,** a disease characterized by low bone mass. The bone tissue of a person with osteoporosis deteriorates over time, becoming thinner and more porous than that of a person with healthy bone. These structural changes weaken the bone, leading to a significantly reduced ability of the bone to bear weight (**Figure 11.16**). This greatly increases the person's risk for a fracture. In the United States, more than 2 million fractures each year are attributed to osteoporosis.[18]

Because the hip and the vertebrae of the spinal column are common sites of osteoporosis, it is not surprising that osteoporosis is the single most important cause of fractures of the hip and spine in older adults (**Figure 11.17**). These fractures are extremely painful and can be debilitating, with many individuals requiring nursing home care. In addition, they increase a person's risk for infection and other related illnesses, which can lead to premature death. In fact, about 24% of adults 50 years and older who suffer a hip fracture die within 1 year after the fracture occurs, and because men are typically older at the time of fracture, death rates are higher for men than for women.[19]

Osteoporosis of the spine also causes a generalized loss of height and can be disfiguring and painful: gradual compression fractures in the vertebrae of the upper back lead to a shortening and hunching of the spine called *kyphosis,* commonly referred to as *dowager's hump* (**Figure 11.18**, page 450). The changes that kyphosis causes in the structure of the rib cage can impair breathing; moreover, back pain from collapsed or fractured vertebrae can be severe. However, especially in the early stages, osteoporosis can be a silent disease: the person may have no awareness of the condition until a fracture occurs.

Osteoporosis is a common disease: worldwide, one in three women and one in five men over the age of 50 are affected. In the United States, more than 10 million people have been diagnosed, and half of all women and one in four men over the age of 50 will suffer an osteoporosis-related fracture in their lifetime.[19,20]

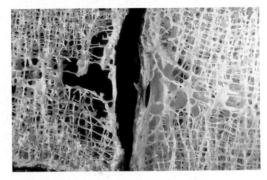

FIGURE 11.16 The vertebrae of a person with osteoporosis (left) are thinner and more collapsed than the vertebrae of a healthy person (right), in which the bone is more dense and uniform.

osteoporosis A disease characterized by low bone mass and deterioration of bone tissue, leading to increased bone fragility and fracture risk.

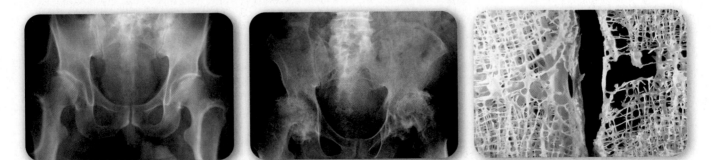

(a) Healthy hip bone **(b) Osteoporotic hip bone** **(c) Fractured hip bone**

FIGURE 11.17 These x-rays reveal the progression of osteoporosis in hip bones. **(a)** Healthy bone. **(b)** A hip bone weakened by osteoporosis.

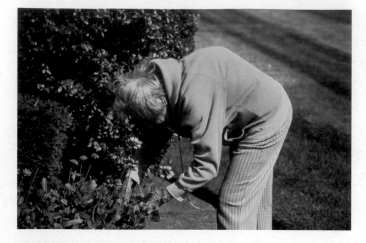

FIGURE 11.18 Gradual compression of the vertebrae in the upper back causes a shortening and rounding of the spine called *kyphosis*.

A Variety of Factors Influence Osteoporosis Risk

The risk for osteoporosis is influenced by age, gender, genetics, and certain lifestyle factors (**Table 11.4**). Let's review these factors and identify lifestyle changes that reduce the risk for osteoporosis.

Aging

Because bone density declines with age, low bone mass and osteoporosis are significant health concerns for older adults. The prevalence of osteoporosis and low bone mass is predicted to increase in the United States during the next 20 years, primarily because of increased longevity; as the U.S. population ages, more people will live long enough to suffer from osteoporosis.

Hormonal changes that occur with aging have a significant impact on bone loss. Average bone loss approximates 0.3% to 0.5% per year after 30 years of age; however, during menopause in women, levels of the hormone estrogen decrease dramatically and cause bone loss to increase to about 3% per year during the first 5 years of menopause. Both estrogen and testosterone play important roles in promoting the deposition of new bone and limiting the activity of osteoclasts. Thus, men can also suffer from osteoporosis, caused by age-related decreases in testosterone. In addition, reduced levels of physical activity in older people and a decreased ability to metabolize vitamin D with age exacerbate the hormone-related bone loss.

Gender

Approximately 80% of Americans with osteoporosis are women. There are three primary reasons for this:

- Women have a lower absolute bone density than men. From birth through puberty, bone mass is the same in girls as in boys. But during puberty, bone mass increases more in boys, probably because of their prolonged period of accelerated growth.

TABLE 11.4 Risk Factors for Osteoporosis

Modifiable Risk Factors	Nonmodifiable Risk Factors
Smoking	Older age (elderly)
Low body weight	Caucasian or Asian race
Low calcium intake	History of fractures as an adult
Low sun exposure	Family history of osteoporosis
Alcohol abuse	Gender (female)
History of amenorrhea (failure to menstruate) in women with inadequate nutrition	History of amenorrhea (failure to menstruate) in women, with no recognizable cause
Estrogen deficiency (females)	
Testosterone deficiency (males)	
Repeated falls	
Sedentary lifestyle	

Source: Information adapted from the National Osteoporosis Society. 2014. Factors that increase your risk of osteoporosis and fractures. https://www.nos.org.uk/healthy-bones-and-risks/are-you-at-risk; accessed April 14, 2015.

This means that, when bone loss begins around age 40, women have less bone stored in their skeleton; thus, the loss of bone that occurs with aging causes osteoporosis sooner and to a greater extent in women.

■ The hormonal changes that occur in men as they age do not have as dramatic an effect on bone density as those in women.

■ On average, women live longer than men, and because risk increases with age, more elderly women suffer from this disease.

A secondary factor that is gender-specific is the social pressure on girls to be thin. Extreme dieting is particularly harmful in adolescence, when bone mass is building and adequate consumption of calcium and other nutrients is critical. In many girls, weight loss causes both a loss of estrogen and reduced weight-bearing stress on the bones. In contrast, men experience pressure to "bulk up," typically by lifting weights. This puts healthful stress on the bones, resulting in increased density.

For a helpful video overview of osteoporosis, go to www .methodisthealthsystem.org. **Type "osteoporosis animation" in the search bar, then click on "Osteoporosis."**

Genetics

Some individuals have a family history of osteoporosis, which increases their risk for this disease. Particularly at risk are Caucasian women of low body weight who have a first-degree relative (mother or sister) with osteoporosis. Asian women are at higher risk than other non-Caucasian groups. Family studies have supported a strong genetic component in bone mineral density, and recently, a review study identified an assortment of genes that appear to influence postmenopausal estrogen levels and bone resorption rates, thereby affecting osteoporosis risk.[21]

Although we cannot change our genes, we can modify the lifestyle factors that affect our risk for osteoporosis. These include substance use, diet, and physical activity.

Tobacco, Alcohol, and Caffeine

Cigarette smoking is known to decrease bone density because of its effects on hormones that influence bone formation and resorption. For this reason, cigarette smoking increases the risk for osteoporosis and resulting fractures.

Chronic alcohol abuse is detrimental to bone health and is associated with high rates of fractures. In contrast, a recent review has reported that bone density may be higher in people who are *light* or *moderate* drinkers, but the findings differ depending upon a person's age, gender, and the form of alcohol consumed.[22] Although light-to-moderate alcohol intake may be protective for bone, the dangers of alcohol abuse for overall health warrant caution in considering any dietary recommendations. As is consistent with the alcohol intake recommendations related to heart disease, people should not start drinking if they are nondrinkers, and people who do drink should do so in moderation. That means no more than two drinks per day for men and one drink per day for women.

Some researchers consider excess caffeine consumption to be detrimental to bone health. Caffeine is known to increase calcium loss in the urine, at least over a brief period of time. Younger people are able to compensate for this calcium loss by increasing absorption of calcium from the intestine. However, older people are not always capable of compensating to the same degree. Although the findings have been inconsistent, a recent review states that the risk of hip fracture modestly increases with the consumption of caffeine equivalent to the amount found in greater than or equal to 2.5 cups of coffee or 6 cups of tea.[23] However, the negative effects of this level of caffeine intake can be offset by increasing calcium intake by 40 mg for every 1 cup of coffee or 0.5 cup of tea.[23] Thus, it appears important to bone health that we moderate our caffeine intake and consume an adequate amount of calcium.

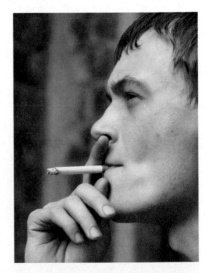

Smoking increases the risk for osteoporosis and resulting fractures.

Nutritional Factors

In addition to their role in reducing the risk for heart disease and cancer, diets high in fruits and vegetables are also associated with improved bone health.[24,25] This is most likely due to the fact that fruits and vegetables are good sources of the nutrients that play a role in bone

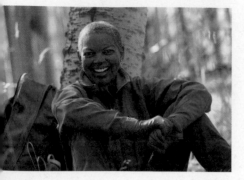

A healthy diet and regular physical activity can reduce your risk for osteoporosis.

and collagen health, including magnesium, vitamin C, and vitamin K. The effects of protein, calcium, vitamin D, and sodium on bone health have been the subject of extensive research.

Protein   The effect of high dietary protein intake on bone health is controversial. High protein intakes have been shown to have both a negative and a positive impact on bone health. Although it is well established that high protein intakes increase calcium loss, protein is a critical component of bone tissue and is necessary for bone health. As with caffeine, the key to this mystery appears to be adequate calcium intake. Early research on this topic illustrated that older adults taking calcium and vitamin D supplements and eating higher-protein diets were able to significantly increase bone mass over a 3-year period, whereas those eating more protein and not taking supplements lost bone mass over the same time period.[26] More recent research indicates that adequate intakes of both protein and calcium are necessary to maximize bone mass and prevent fractures in adolescents and older adults.[27] Thus, there appears to be an interaction between dietary calcium and protein, in that adequate amounts of each nutrient are needed together to support bone health.

Calcium and Vitamin D   Of the many nutrients that help maintain bone health, calcium and vitamin D have received the most attention for their role in the prevention of osteoporosis. It is clear that consuming adequate amounts of both nutrients in our diets is critical to optimize our bone health because people who do not consume enough of these two nutrients over a prolonged period of time have a lower bone density and thus a higher risk for bone fractures. Whether taking calcium and vitamin D supplements is effective in preventing osteoporosis is somewhat controversial. Refer to the **Nutrition Myth or Fact?** at the end of this chapter to learn more about this controversy.

Because bones reach peak density when people are young, it is very important that children and adolescents consume a high-quality diet that contains the proper balance of calcium, vitamin D, protein, and other nutrients to allow for optimal bone growth. Young adults also require a proper balance of these nutrients to maintain bone mass. In older adults, diets rich in calcium and vitamin D can help minimize bone loss.

Sodium   Higher intakes of sodium are known to increase the kidneys' excretion of calcium in the urine. Although some studies have found that diets moderate to high in salt increase excretion of urinary calcium and have a negative impact on bone calcium balance, there is no direct evidence that a high-sodium diet causes osteoporosis.[28] At this time, the Institute of Medicine states that there is insufficient evidence to warrant different calcium recommendations based on dietary salt intake.[2]

Regular Physical Activity

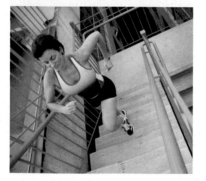

Regular weight-bearing exercises, such as jogging, can help increase and maintain bone mass.

Regular exercise is highly protective against bone loss and osteoporosis. Athletes are consistently shown to have more dense bones than nonathletes, and regular participation in weight-bearing exercises (such as walking, jogging, tennis, and strength training) can help increase and maintain bone mass. When we exercise, our muscles contract and pull on our bones; this stresses bone tissue in a healthful way that stimulates increases in bone density. In addition, carrying weight during activities such as walking and jogging stresses the bones of the legs, hips, and lower back, resulting in a healthier bone mass in these areas. It appears that people of all ages can improve and maintain bone health by consistent physical activity. For instance, a recent systematic review examining the role of exercise in preventing and treating osteoporosis in postmenopausal women found that overall, exercise resulted in small positive effect on bone density that could be clinically important. When examining the types of exercise that are most beneficial, this review found that doing combined types of exercise programs, such as resistance training combined with walking or jogging, improved bone density specifically at the neck of the femur, the spine, and the trochanter area of the femur. The risk of fractures was also lower in people doing combination exercises as compared to postmenopausal women who were not exercising.[29]

Can exercise ever be detrimental to bone health? Yes, exercise can be harmful when the body is not receiving the nutrients it needs to rebuild the hydroxyapatite and collagen broken down in response to physical activity. Thus, active people who are chronically malnourished, including people who are impoverished and those who suffer from eating disorders, are at increased fracture risk. Research has confirmed this association among nutrition, physical activity, and bone loss in the *female athlete triad,* a potentially serious condition characterized by the coexistence of three (a *triad* of) clinical conditions in some physically active females: low energy availability (with or without eating disorders), menstrual dysfunction, and low bone density. In the female athlete triad, inadequate food intake and regular strenuous exercise together result in a state of severe energy drain that causes a multitude of hormonal changes, including a reduction in estrogen production. Estrogen is important to maintaining healthy bone in women, so the loss of estrogen leads to low bone density and even osteoporosis in young women. (The female athlete triad is discussed *In Depth* on pages 548–549.)

Certain Treatments Can Slow Bone Loss

Although there is no cure for osteoporosis, a variety of treatments can slow and even reverse bone loss. First, individuals with osteoporosis are encouraged to consume adequate calcium and vitamin D and to exercise regularly in consultation with their healthcare provider. Studies have shown that the most effective exercise programs include a combination of weight-bearing exercises, such as jogging, stair climbing, and resistance training.[29,30]

In addition, several medications are available:

Want to calculate your risk for osteoporosis? Take the International Osteoporosis Foundation's One-Minute Osteoporosis risk quiz at www .osteofound.org/.

- *Bisphosphonates,* such as alendronate (brand name Fosamax), which decrease bone loss and can increase bone density and reduce the risk of spinal and nonspinal fractures in postmenopausal women with osteoporosis who have already had a fracture. However they do not appear to reduce risk for a postmenopausal woman's first osteoporotic fracture, suggesting these medications may not be effective for primary prevention of fractures in postmenopausal women.[31]
- *Selective estrogen receptor modulators,* such as raloxifene (brand name Evista), which have an estrogen-like effect on bone tissue, slowing the rate of bone loss and prompting some increase in bone mass.

*Nutri-*Case

Gustavo

"When my wife, Antonia, fell and broke her hip, I was shocked. You see, the same thing happened to her mother, but she was an old lady by then! Antonia's only 68, and she still seems young and beautiful—at least to me! As soon as she's better, her doctor wants to do some kind of scan to see how thick her bones are. But I don't think she has that disease everyone talks about. She's always watched her weight and keeps active with our kids and grandchildren. It's true she likes her coffee and diet colas, and doesn't drink milk, but that's not enough to make a person's bones fall apart, is it?"

Review Table 11.4, page 450. Which risk factors apply to Antonia? Which risk factors do not? Given what Gustavo has said about his wife's nutrition and lifestyle, should he encourage her to have a DXA test? Why or why not?

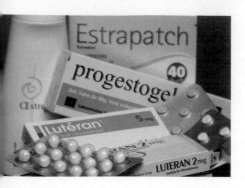

Hormone replacement medications come in a variety of forms.

- *Calcitonin* (brand name Calcimar or Miacalcin), a pharmacologic preparation of a hormone secreted by the thyroid hormone, which when given in pharmacologic doses can reduce the rate of bone loss.
- *Hormone replacement therapy (HRT)*, which combines estrogen with a hormone called progestin and can reduce bone loss, increase bone density, and reduce the risk of hip and spinal fractures.

All of these drugs can prompt side effects. For example, bisphosphonates are associated with several gastrointestinal side effects, including abdominal pain, constipation, diarrhea, heartburn, irritation of the esophagus, and difficulty swallowing. In addition there is evidence that long-term use of bisphosphonates may increase the risk for "atypical" fractures. Two recent studies found that these fractures are still quite rare and that the relative benefits of taking the medication outweigh the potential risks.[32,33] However, results from a systematic review published in 2015 found an increased risk for atypical fractures associated with bisphosphonates, and the authors conclude that the growing evidence about the risks of bisphosphonates warrants a comprehensive evaluation of patients before prescribing bisphosphonates, and that future studies need to examine the benefit of these medications over their potential harms.[34]

HRT also has side effects, including breast tenderness, changes in mood, vaginal bleeding, and an increased risk for gallbladder disease. The health benefits and risks of HRT are controversial based on current evidence. Until recently, it was believed that HRT protected women against heart disease. However, a landmark study published in 2002 found that one type of HRT actually increases a woman's risk for heart disease, stroke, and breast cancer.[35] The U.S. Preventive Services Task Force states that HRT does not affect one's risk for heart disease but increases the risk for stroke, blood clots in the legs, gallbladder disease, and urinary incontinence.[36] The type of HRT and the age and menopausal status of the woman appear to be important factors in affecting a person's risk of side effects; women over the age of 50 who are postmenopausal or who have had a hysterectomy (surgery to remove a woman's uterus) are advised against taking HRT to prevent chronic diseases.[36] As a result, hundreds of thousands of women in the United States have stopped taking HRT as a means to prevent or treat osteoporosis. However, despite the associated risks, it is recognized that HRT is still an effective treatment and prevention option for osteoporosis. It also reduces the risk for colorectal cancer. Thus, women should work with their physicians to weigh these benefits against the increased risks for breast cancer and heart disease when considering HRT as a treatment option for osteoporosis.

RECAP

Osteoporosis is a major disease of concern for elderly men and women in the United States. Osteoporosis increases the risk for fractures and premature death from subsequent illness. Factors that increase the risk for osteoporosis include advanced age, being female, being of the Caucasian or Asian race, a family history, low levels of estrogen, cigarette smoking, alcohol abuse, a sedentary lifestyle, and a diet low in calcium and vitamin D. Medications available for the prevention and treatment of osteoporosis include bisphosphonates, selective estrogen receptor modulators, calcitonin, and hormone replacement therapy; however, all can prompt side effects. Adequate intake of calcium and vitamin D is important, as is regular, weight-bearing exercise as prescribed by the patient's physician.

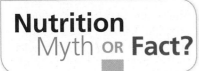

Preserving Bone Mass: Are Supplements the Solution?

Despite the fact that some risk factors for osteoporosis cannot be changed, consuming adequate calcium and vitamin D throughout the lifespan is an essential first step in preventing osteoporosis.

Consuming adequate calcium and vitamin D throughout the life span is an essential first step. Now that so many products are fortified with these nutrients, from cereals and energy bars to orange juice and milk alternatives, it is not difficult for most people, even vegans, to get sufficient calcium and vitamin D from the diet. Still, small or inactive people who eat less to maintain a healthful weight may not be able to consume enough food to provide adequate amounts, and elderly people may need more than they can obtain in their normal diet. In these circumstances, supplements may be warranted.

Which Calcium Supplements Are Best?

Numerous calcium supplements are available to consumers, but which are best? Most supplements come in the form of calcium carbonate, calcium citrate, calcium lactate, or calcium phosphate. Our body is able to absorb about 30% of the calcium from these various forms. Calcium citrate malate, which is the form of calcium used in fortified juices, is slightly more absorbable, at 35%. Many antacids are also good sources of calcium, and it appears that they are safe to take, as long as you consume only enough to get the recommended level of calcium.

What is the most cost-effective form of calcium? In general, supplements that contain calcium carbonate tend to have more calcium per pill than other types. Thus, you are getting more calcium for your money when you buy this type. However, be sure to read the label of any calcium supplement you are considering taking to determine just how much calcium it contains. Some very expensive calcium supplements do not contain a lot of calcium per pill, and you could be wasting your money.

The lead content of calcium supplements is an important public health concern. Those made from "natural" sources, such as oyster shell, bone meal, and dolomite, are known to be higher in lead, and some of these products can contain dangerously high levels. The Food and Drug Administration (FDA) has set an Upper Limit of 7.5 µg of lead per 1,000 mg calcium, but currently calcium supplements are not tested for lead content, and it is the manufacturer's responsibility to ensure that its supplements meet FDA standards. To avoid taking supplements that contain too much lead, look for supplements claiming to be lead-free, and make sure the word *purified* is on the label, in addition to the U.S. Pharmacopeia (USP) symbol.

Are Calcium Supplements Safe?

A concern that has emerged in recent years is the evidence suggesting that taking calcium supplements might increase the

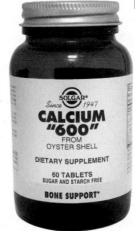

risk for a myocardial infarction (MI; a heart attack). Analyses based on the prospective observational data from the Women's Health Initiative study, in which almost 37,000 postmenopausal women were prescribed a calcium-vitamin D supplement or placebo over an average of 7 years, showed that the supplementation significantly increased total and hip bone density. However, there was no change in risk for fractures, and evidence suggested that taking these supplements could increase the risk for MI.[1] A subsequent study that re-analyzed the data from the randomized controlled trial phase of this large study found that among those women who were not already taking calcium or vitamin D supplements before the trial began, the supplement reduced the risk of hip fractures, and did not increase the risk of myocardial infarction.[2] Even more recently, researchers have proposed a mechanism by which an increased load of supplemental calcium in the bloodstream might promote the formation of calcium deposits in the coronary arteries and thereby increase MI risk.[3] Thus, this topic is contentious, and it may be that there is an interaction between history and level of calcium supplementation use and its impact on health.

If you decide to use a calcium supplement, how should you take it? Remember that the body cannot absorb more than 500 mg of calcium at one time. Thus, taking a supplement that contains 1,000 mg of calcium is no more effective than taking one that contains 500 mg. If at all possible, try to consume calcium supplements in small doses throughout the day. In addition, calcium is absorbed better with meals, because the calcium stays in the intestinal tract longer during a meal and more calcium can be absorbed.

Why Do Many People Need Supplemental Vitamin D?

No doubt about it: unless you live at a latitude within 37° of the equator and spend time outdoors without sunscreen, it's tough to get enough vitamin D. That's because, as you learned in this chapter, there are very few natural food sources of vitamin D, and even fortified food sources are limited to milk and a handful of other products. It is clear that meeting the Institute of Medicine's current RDA for vitamin D is posing a challenge to many Americans. Interestingly, some researchers are calling for an even higher intake recommendation. What is the evidence behind this call, and are supplements the only way to meet current recommendations?

The call for higher vitamin D intake recommendations arises from a growing concern about widespread vitamin D deficiency and its associated diseases, including rickets in children and osteomalacia and osteoporosis in adults. Data from the National Health and Examination Survey (NHANES) indicate that, from 2001 to 2006, about 25% of the U.S. population were at risk for vitamin D inadequacy, with 8% at risk for vitamin D deficiency.[4] In addition, since the Institute of Medicine set its vitamin D recommendations in 1997, new information has been published about vitamin D metabolism and its potential role in reducing the risks for diseases such as type 1 diabetes, some cancers, multiple sclerosis, and metabolic syndrome.[5,6] These discussions have resulted in a full review of the current research on vitamin D.

What is contributing to the dramatic increase in vitamin D insufficiency among Americans, and what can we do about it? Researchers have proposed the following three causative factors:[6]

■ A downward trend in the consumption of vitamin D–fortified milk products

■ A significant increase in sun avoidance and the use of sun protection products, such as sunscreen

■ An increased rate of obesity because obesity appears to alter the metabolism and storage of vitamin D such that vitamin D deficiency is more likely to occur

To address the first factor, people can increase their intake of vitamin D–fortified milk products; however, it is difficult to meet even the current RDA from consumption of milk alone. For instance, children and teens would have to drink a full quart each day to meet the recommendation! As a result, the use of vitamin D supplements is gaining wide support. Recently published clinical practice guidelines state that children and adolescents aged 1 to 18 years who are vitamin D deficient should be treated with 2,000 IU of vitamin D per day for at least 6 weeks, followed by a maintenance supplement of 600 to 1,000 IU per day.[6] Additionally, it is recommended that all adults who are vitamin D deficient should be treated with 6,000 IU of vitamin D per day for 8 weeks, followed by a maintenance supplement of 1,500 to 2,000 IU per day.[6]

The Office of Dietary Supplements at the National Institutes of Health states that vitamin D_2 and D_3 appear to be equally effective in raising and maintaining blood levels of vitamin D.[7] Make sure the word *purified* is on the label, in addition to the U.S. Pharmacopeia (USP) symbol. Because vitamin D is a fat-soluble vitamin, it is important to stay below the UL of 4,000 IU (for adults) per day. Supplementation with vitamin D is efficient, inexpensive, and effective. Used correctly, it is also very safe. Although vitamin D toxicity is rare, supplementation should be monitored to ensure both a safe and an adequate intake.

What about the second factor—lack of sufficient exposure to sunlight? Responsible, safe exposure to sunlight offers many advantages: it will never lead to vitamin D toxicity, it is easy and virtually cost-free, and sun exposure may offer benefits beyond that of improved vitamin D status. That's why many healthcare professionals advocate moderate sun exposure. They suggest that public health authorities soften the "sun avoidance" campaigns of recent years (see **Figure 11.19**); they would like to see "well-balanced" recommendations that promote brief (15 minutes or so) periods of sun exposure without sunscreen or sun-blocking clothing two or three times a week, with avoidance of mid-day sun during summer months.[8]

To address the third factor in vitamin D deficiency—obesity—the only solution is to maintain a healthful weight. That means losing weight if you are overweight or obese. By doing so, you'll reduce your risk not only for vitamin D deficiency but also for cardiovascular disease, type 2 diabetes, and many forms of cancer.

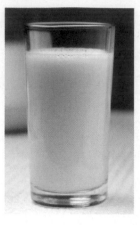

What's the Bottom Line?

By consuming foods high in calcium throughout the day, you can avoid the need for calcium supplements. However, even by getting regular, safe sun exposure, people living north or south of the 37° latitude line are unable to produce enough vitamin D during the winter months, and few of us can consume the recommended amounts each day. If you cannot consume enough calcium and vitamin D in your diet, and do not get adequate sun exposure, many inexpensive, safe, and effective supplements are available. The best supplement for you is the one that you can tolerate and is affordable, lead-free, and readily available when you need it. In addition, although vitamin D deficiency is becoming a public health issue in the United States, maintaining a healthy body weight can help to promote a healthy vitamin D status.

Critical Thinking Questions

■ Do you think you would benefit from calcium and vitamin D supplementation? Why or why not?

■ Would you prefer to try to increase your circulating levels of vitamin D through natural foods, fortified foods, supplements, or increased sun exposure? State your reasoning.

References

1. Bolland, M. J., A. Grey, A. Avenell, G. D. Gamble, and I. R. Reid. 2011. Calcium supplements with or without vitamin D and risk of cardiovascular events: reanalysis of the Women's Health Initiative limited dataset and meta-analysis. *BMJ* 342:d2040, doi:10.1136/bmj.d2040.
2. Prentice, R. L., M. B. Pettinger, R. D. Jackson, J. Wastawski-Wende, A. Z. LaCoix, G. L. Anderson,…, and J. E. Rossouw. 2013. Health risks and benefits from calcium and vitamin D supplementation: Women's Health Initiative clinical trial and cohort study. *Osteoporos. Int.* 24(12):567–580.
3. Paziana, K., and S. Pazaianas. 2015. Calcium supplements controversy in osteoporosis: a physiological mechanism supporting cardiovascular adverse effects. *Endocrine.* 48(3):776–778.
4. Looker, A. C., C. L. Johnson, D. A. Lacher, C. M. Pfeiffer, R. L. Schleicher, and C. T. Sempos. 2011. Vitamin D status: United States 2001–2016. NCHS data brief, no. 59. Hyattsville, MD: National Center for Health Statistics.
5. Adams, J. S., and M. Hewison. 2010. Update on vitamin D. *J. Clin. Endocrinol. Metab.* 95:471–478.
6. Holick, M. F., N. C. Binkley, H. A. Bischoff-Ferrari, C. M. Gordon, D. A. Hanley,…, and C. M. Weaver. 2011. Evaluation, treatment, and prevention of vitamin D deficiency: an Endocrine Society Clinical Practice Guideline. *J. Clin. Endocrinol. Metab.* 96:1911–1930.
7. National Institutes of Health. Office of Dietary Supplements. 2014. Vitamin D. Fact sheet for health professionals. http://ods.od.nih.gov/factsheets/VitaminD-HealthProfessional
8. International Osteoporosis Foundation. 2014. Are skin cancer prevention campaigns scaring people away from healthy sun exposure? News Stories, December 16, 2014. http://www.iofbonehealth.org/news/are-skin-cancer-prevention-campaigns-scaring-people-away-healthy-sun-exposure

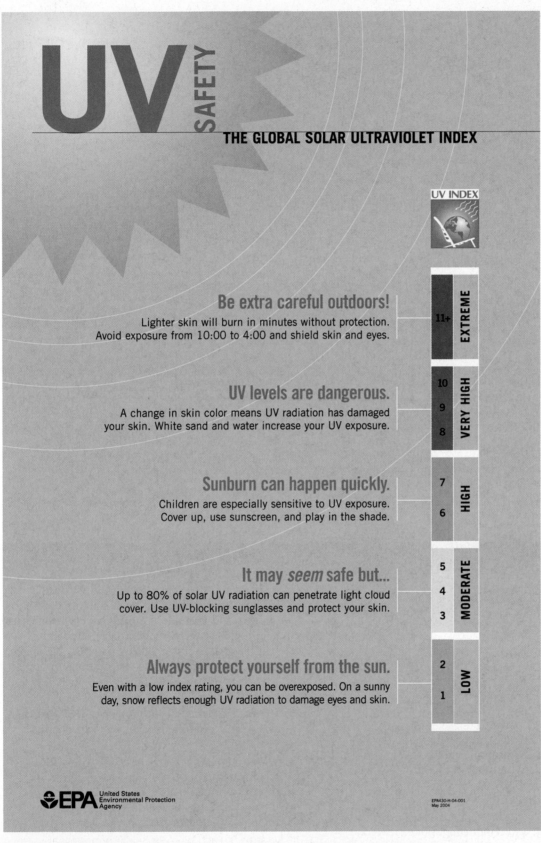

FIGURE 11.19 The Environmental Protection Agency is one of many public health agencies that warn Americans about the danger of exposure to even low levels of sun. (*Source:* UV Safety: The Global Solar Ultraviolet Index from the Environmental Protection Agency, May 2004.)

STUDY PLAN   MasteringNutrition™

Customize your study plan—and master your nutrition!—in the Study Area of MasteringNutrition.

summary

Scan to hear an MP3 Chapter Review in MasteringNutrition.

LO 1 ▪ Bones support the body's tissues and organs, work with muscles and tendons to provide movement, and protect vital organs such as the brain and lungs.

▪ Cortical bone is the dense outer layer of tissue of most bones and entirely makes up many small bones of the body. Trabecular bone is a more porous tissue within bones that provides scaffolding and flexibility.

LO 2 ▪ Bone develops through three processes: growth, modeling, and remodeling. Bone size is determined during growth, bone shape is determined during modeling and remodeling, and bone remodeling also affects the density of bone.

▪ Bone remodeling includes resorption, during which osteoclasts break down existing bone surface, and formation, during which osteoblasts synthesize new organic matrix upon which hydroxyapatite crystals pack together. As we age, bone resorption begins to exceed bone formation, leading to a gradual loss in bone density.

LO 3 ▪ Dual-energy x-ray absorptiometry (DEXA or DXA) is the most accurate tool for measuring bone density.

▪ The results of a DXA include a T-score, which is a comparison of the person's bone density to that of a 30-year-old healthy adult. A T-score lower than –1 indicates poor bone density, and lower than –2.5 indicates osteoporosis.

LO 4 ▪ Calcium is a major mineral that is an integral component of the hydroxyapatite crystals that, together with collagen, make up bones and teeth. Calcium also helps maintain acid–base balance, and levels are maintained in the blood at all times. Calcium is also necessary for normal nerve impulse transmission, muscle contraction, healthy blood pressure, and blood clotting.

LO 5
- The RDA for calcium is 1,000 mg per day for adult men and women aged 19 to 70 years, and 1,200 mg per day for adult men and women older than 70 years of age. The RDA is highest for adolescents, who require 1,300 mg per day.
- Calcium absorption is affected by an individual's needs, amount consumed, presence of binding factors, and availability of vitamin D. Good food sources include dairy products, many green leafy vegetables, and calcium-fortified juices and milk alternatives.
- Consuming excess calcium leads to mineral imbalance, and consuming inadequate calcium causes osteoporosis.

LO 6
- Vitamin D is a fat-soluble vitamin that can be produced from a cholesterol compound in skin using energy from sunlight. Vitamin D works with PTH to regulate blood calcium levels by regulating absorption of calcium and phosphorus from the intestine, and signaling the kidneys to excrete more or less calcium in urine. Vitamin D and PTH also stimulate osteoclasts to break down bone when calcium is needed elsewhere in the body. Vitamin D is also needed for crystallization of calcium and phosphorus.
- When the ultraviolet rays of the sun hit the skin, they react with 7-dehydrocholesterol. This is converted to cholecalciferol, which is then converted to calcidiol in the liver. Calcidiol travels to the kidneys, where it is converted into calcitriol, the primary active form of vitamin D in the body.
- Skin synthesis of vitamin D requires adequate exposure to sunlight, and is not possible in northern regions during winter months. Food sources of vitamin D include certain fish and fortified foods and beverages, including milk and milk alternatives. Supplements may be necessary to meet vitamin D needs.
- The RDA for vitamin D is 600 IU per day for adult men and women aged 19 to 70 years; the RDA increases to 800 IU per day for adults over the age of 70 years.
- Hypercalcemia results from consuming too much vitamin D, causing weakness, loss of appetite, diarrhea, vomiting, and formation of calcium deposits in soft tissues. Vitamin D deficiency leads to loss of bone mass, causing rickets in children or osteomalacia and osteoporosis in adults.

LO 7
- Vitamin K is a fat-soluble vitamin that is obtained in the diet and is produced in the large intestine by beneficial bacteria. Vitamin K serves as a coenzyme for blood clotting and bone metabolism. Green, leafy vegetables are good food sources.
- Phosphorus is a major mineral that is an important part of the structure of bone; phosphorus is also a component of ATP, DNA, RNA, cell membranes, and lipoproteins. It is widespread in foods and is abundant in meats, poultry, dairy, eggs, and legumes, including peanuts.
- Magnesium is a major mineral. It is part of the structure of bone, it influences the formation of hydroxyapatite crystals and bone health through its regulation of calcium balance and the actions of vitamin D and parathyroid hormone, and it is a cofactor for more than 300 enzyme systems. Magnesium is found in green, leafy vegetables; nuts, seeds, and legumes; whole grains; seafoods; and some dairy products.

LO 8
- Fluoride is a trace mineral that combines with calcium and phosphorus to form fluorohydroxyapatite in teeth, which increases their resistance to dental caries. It also stimulates new bone growth.
- Excessive intake of fluoride, whether from fluoridated water, dental products, or supplements, can cause fluorosis, a staining and pitting of teeth. Fluoride deficiency increases the risk for tooth decay and may promote osteoporosis.

LO 9
- Osteoporosis is a bone disease characterized by low bone mass and deterioration of bone tissue, leading to increased bone fragility and fracture risk. It affects more than 10 million Americans. About 80% of people with this disease are women; however, men over the age of 50 are also at risk.
- Osteoporosis increases the risk for bone fractures and premature disability and death due to subsequent illness.
- Factors that increase the risk for osteoporosis include increased age, being female, having a family history of osteoporosis, being of the Caucasian or Asian race, cigarette smoking, alcohol abuse, low calcium and vitamin D intakes, and a sedentary lifestyle.

LO 10
- Prescription medications available for osteoporosis treatment include bisphosphonates, selective estrogen receptor modulators, calcitonin, and hormone replacement therapy; however, all can prompt side effects. Adequate consumption of calcium and vitamin D is important, as is weight-bearing exercise as prescribed.

To further your understanding, go online and apply what you've learned to real-life case studies that will help you master the content!

review questions

LO 1   1. Which of the following statements about trabecular bone is true?

a. It accounts for about 80% of the skeleton.
b. It forms the core of all bones of the skeleton.
c. It is also called compact bone.
d. It provides the scaffolding for cortical bone.

LO 2   2. The shape of our facial bones is determined during the process of

a. bone growth
b. bone modeling
c. bone resorption
d. bone remodeling

LO 3   3. On a DXA test, a T-score of +1.0 indicates that the patient has

a. osteoporosis.
b. low bone density, but does not yet have osteoporosis.
c. normal bone density.
d. abnormally high bone density.

LO 4   4. Calcium is necessary for

a. demineralization of bone.
b. regulation of vitamin D levels.
c. opposition to blood clotting.
d. the body's regulation of acid–base balance.

LO 5   5. Which of the following foods provides the highest amount of bioavailable calcium?

a. a cup of cooked kale
b. a cup of cooked cauliflower
c. a cup of cooked spinach
d. a cup of red leaf lettuce

LO 6   6. Which of the following individuals is most likely to require vitamin D supplements?

a. a dark-skinned child living in Hawaii
b. a fair-skinned construction worker living in Florida
c. a dark-skinned retiree living in Illinois
d. a fair-skinned college student living in Oklahoma

LO 7   7. Which of the following nutrients is a major component of bone?

a. phosphorus
b. magnesium
c. both a and b
d. neither a nor b

LO 8   8. Fluoride

a. stimulates new bone growth.
b. is an important treatment for osteoporosis.
c. is an important treatment for fluorosis.
d. toxicity can impair the function of teeth.

LO 9   9. Which of the following behaviors is associated with an increased risk for osteoporosis?

a. smoking
b. high-impact exercise
c. occasional consumption of alcohol
d. all of the above

LO 10   10. Which of the following statements about osteoporosis treatment is true?

a. The most effective exercise programs for the treatment of osteoporosis involve stretching and balance exercises along with aerobic exercises such as swimming that do not stress bones.
b. Hormone replacement therapy is effective in preventing and treating osteoporosis.
c. Bisphosphonates and selective estrogen receptor modulators both work by increasing bone resorption.
d. Aspirin and other anti-inflammatory drugs are primary drug therapies for osteoporosis.

true or false?

LO 2   11. **True or false?** The process by which bone is formed through the action of osteoblasts and resorbed through the action of osteoclasts is called remodeling.

LO 5   12. **True or false?** The amount of calcium we absorb depends on our needs, our calcium intake, the types of calcium-rich foods we eat, and the body's supply of vitamin D.

LO 6   13. **True or false?** Given adequate exposure, sunlight is an excellent direct source of vitamin D.

LO 7   14. **True or false?** Green, leafy vegetables are our only significant sources of vitamin K.

LO 9   15. **True or false?** Although osteoporosis can lead to painful and debilitating fractures, it is not associated with an increased risk for premature death.

short answer

LO 2 16. Most people reach their peak height by the end of adolescence, maintain that height for several decades, and then start to lose height in their later years. Describe the two processes behind this phenomenon.

LO 5 17. The morning after reading this chapter, you are eating your usual breakfast cereal when you notice that the Nutrition Facts panel on the box states that one serving contains 100% of your DRI for calcium. In addition, you're eating the cereal with about ½ cup of skim milk. Does this meal ensure that your calcium needs for the day are met? Why or why not?

LO 6 18. Bert has light skin and lives in Buffalo, New York. How much time does Bert

need to spend out of doors with exposed skin on winter days to avoid the need for consuming vitamin D in the diet or from supplements?

19. Explain why people with diseases that cause a malabsorption of fat may suffer from deficiency of vitamin D.

LO 8 20. Mr. and Mrs. Erikson have asked their pediatrician to prescribe fluoride supplements for their 3-year-old son, Hans. The family lives in a community with fluoridated water, which they drink, and Hans brushes his teeth with fluoride toothpaste. Do you think the pediatrician would prescribe fluoride supplements? Why or why not?

math review

21. Refer to the table in the *Nutrition Label Activity* (page 436) on calcium absorption rates for various food sources. How much broccoli would you need to consume to absorb the same amount of calcium as in 1 cup of skim milk?

Answers to Review Questions and Math Review can be found online in the MasteringNutrition Study Area.

web links

www.nlm.nih.gov/medlineplus
Medline Plus Health Information
Search for "rickets" or "osteomalacia" to learn more about these vitamin D–deficiency diseases.

www.ada.org
American Dental Association
Look under "Advocacy," the "ADA Positions, Policies and Statements," and click on "Fluoride and Sealants" to learn more about the fluoridation of community water supplies and the use of fluoride-containing products.

nof.org
National Osteoporosis Foundation
Learn more about the causes, prevention, detection, and treatment of osteoporosis.

www.osteofound.org
International Osteoporosis Foundation
Find out more about this foundation and its mission to increase awareness and understanding of osteoporosis worldwide.

www.niams.nih.gov/Health_Info/Bone/
National Institutes of Health Osteoporosis and Related Bone Diseases—National Resource Center
Access this site for additional resources and information on metabolic bone diseases, including osteoporosis.

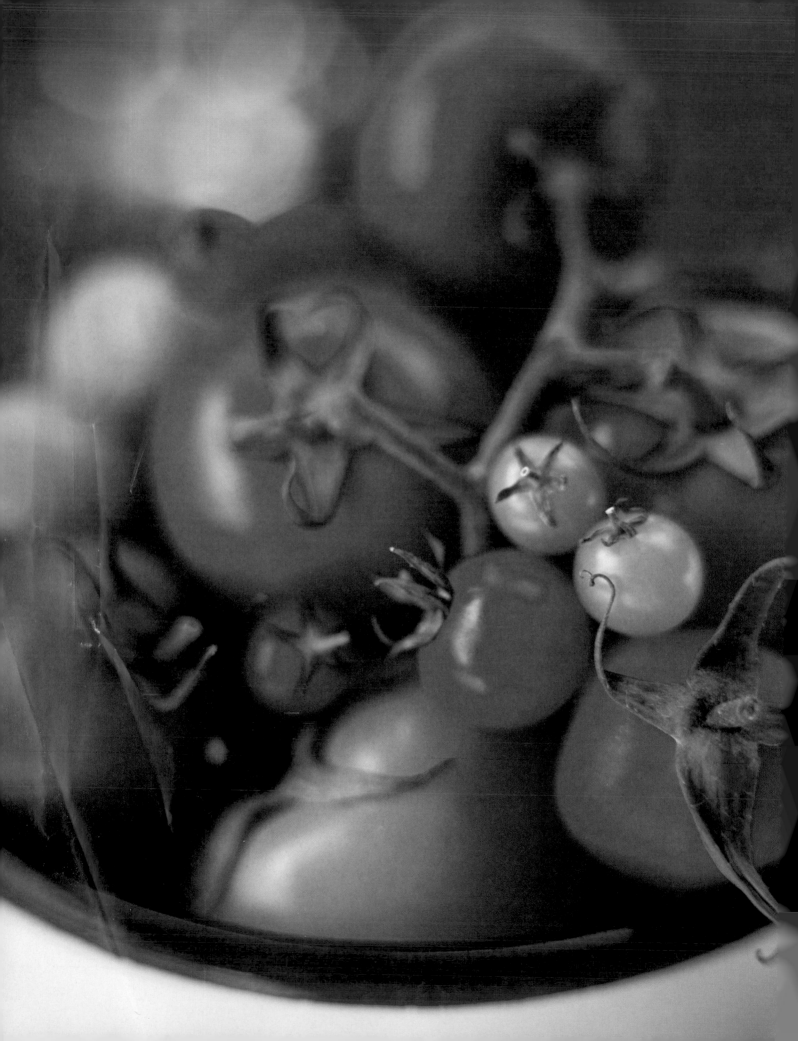

12 Nutrients Involved in Blood Health and Immunity

Learning Outcomes

After studying this chapter, you should be able to:

1. Identify the functions and components of blood and the micronutrients most critical to blood health, *pp. 464–465.*

2. Discuss the role that iron plays in maintaining blood health overall, and specifically in oxygen transport, *pp. 466–7.*

3. Explain how the body absorbs, transports, and stores iron, *pp. 467–70.*

4. Discuss the progression of iron deficiency from depletion to microcytic anemia, *pp. 474–75.*

5. Discuss the functions, RDA, and food sources of zinc, *pp. 476–480.*

6. Discuss the functions, RDA, and food sources of copper, *pp. 480–482.*

7. Discuss the functions and sources of vitamin K, *pp. 482–484.*

8. Discuss the contributions of vitamin B_6, folate, and vitamin B_{12} to blood health, *pp. 481–485.*

9. Compare and contrast nonspecific and specific immunity, *pp. 486–487.*

10. Describe the role of protein–energy malnutrition, obesity, essential fatty acids, and key micronutrients in immune function, *pp. 488–490.*

According to the World Health Organization, over 30% of the world's population is anemic.[1] As a result, millions of children experience poor physical and cognitive development and an increased risk for infection and early death. Pregnant women are also at increased risk: in developing nations, half of all pregnant women are anemic, and anemia contributes to 20% of maternal deaths. Even in the United States, anemia is a major cause of behavioral and cognitive delays in children.

What is anemia, and what is the role of nutrition in causing or preventing it? Which micronutrients make the greatest contribution to the formation and maintenance of the red blood cells of our cardiovascular system, as well as the white blood cells of our immune system? How do they function? We explore these questions here.

LO 1 Identify the functions and components of blood and the micronutrients most critical to blood health.

What Are the Functions and Components of Blood?

Blood transports to body cells virtually all the components necessary for life. No matter how much carbohydrate, fat, and protein we eat, we could not survive without healthy blood to transport these nutrients, and the oxygen to metabolize them, to our cells. In addition to transporting nutrients and oxygen, blood removes the waste products generated from metabolism, so that they can be properly excreted. Blood is also essential for body defenses; as we discuss later in this chapter, the white blood cells of our immune system defend against invasion by microorganisms such as bacteria and viruses, and can recognize and destroy cells with DNA mutations before they progress to cancer (see Chapter 10). Finally, you learned in Chapter 9 that circulating blood is an important mechanism for heat transfer from the body core to the cooler skin. In short, our health and our ability to perform daily activities are compromised if the quantity and quality of our blood is diminished.

Blood is actually a tissue, the only fluid tissue in the body. It has four components (**Figure 12.1**):

erythrocytes Red blood cells; they transport oxygen in the blood.

leukocytes White blood cells; they are important to immune functions.

- **Erythrocytes,** or red blood cells, are the cells that transport oxygen. They far outnumber white blood cells, and live much longer, typically about four months. Mature red blood cells lack both a nucleus and ribosomes, and so cannot synthesize proteins. They also lack mitochondria, and depend on the anaerobic breakdown of glucose for energy.
- **Leukocytes,** or white blood cells, are the key to our immune function, protecting us from infections and cancer. They also assist in tissue repair. They live, on average, from about one to three weeks, and therefore must be replaced at a faster rate than

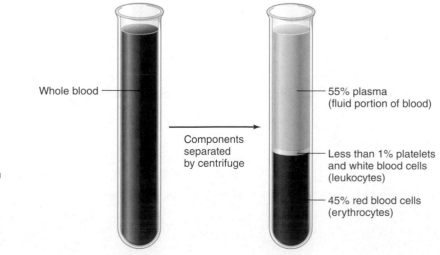

FIGURE 12.1 Blood has four components, which are visible when the blood is drawn into a test tube and spun in a centrifuge. The bottom layer is the erythrocytes, or red blood cells. The milky layer above the erythrocytes contains the leukocytes and platelets. The yellow fluid on top is the plasma.

Whole blood

Components separated by centrifuge

55% plasma (fluid portion of blood)

Less than 1% platelets and white blood cells (leukocytes)

45% red blood cells (erythrocytes)

erythrocytes. Unlike erythrocytes, which remain in the blood vessels, leukocytes can slip between adjacent cells in the blood vessel wall and move into tissues where they perform their functions.

- **Platelets** are cell fragments—essentially bundles of cytoplasm that survive only about one week. When a blood vessel breaks, they adhere to collagen present in the adjacent tissue, forming a blood clot that slows and helps stop bleeding.
- **Plasma** is the fluid portion of the blood. Made up mostly of water, plasma maintains adequate blood volume, so that blood can flow easily through the heart and blood vessels. It also contains important plasma proteins, the most abundant of which is albumin, which helps retain fluid in the bloodstream, preventing edema. Plasma also contains clotting proteins, hormones, glucose and other nutrients, gases, and dissolved wastes.

The cellular elements of blood—erythrocytes, leukocytes, and platelets—are formed in the bone marrow and all arise from the same bone marrow stem cells. Their production, and that of plasma, depends on a healthful diet. Specifically, adequate fluid intake is essential to maintain blood volume (see Chapter 8). Because blood is a tissue, adequate protein intake is also important (see Chapter 6). In this chapter, we discuss the micronutrients essential for blood health (**Table 12.1**). These include the trace minerals iron, zinc, and copper, which are essential for oxygen transport in blood. They also include fat-soluble vitamin K, which is necessary for the clotting function of blood, and the water-soluble vitamin B_6, folate, and vitamin B_{12}, which are critical to the formation of red blood cells. These nutrients are discussed in detail in the following section.

Watch a video of red blood cell production from the National Library of Medicine at www.nlm.nih.gov.

RECAP

Blood functions in delivery of nutrients and oxygen to cells, and elimination of metabolic wastes. It is also essential to body defenses and maintenance of a healthful body temperature. The four components of blood are erythrocytes, leukocytes, platelets, and plasma. Healthy blood requires adequate intake of fluids, protein, and several micronutrients, including the trace minerals iron, zinc, and copper and vitamins K, B_6, folate, and B_{12}. ◼

TABLE 12.1 Overview of Nutrients Essential to Blood Health

To see the full profile of nutrients essential to blood health, turn to Chapter 7.5, In Depth: Vitamins and Minerals. Micronutrients with Macro Powers, pages 292–303.

Nutrient	Recommended Intake (RDA or AI and UL)
Iron	RDA: Women aged 19 to 50 years = 18 mg/day Men aged 19 to 50 years = 8 mg/day UL = 45 mg/day
Zinc	RDA: Women aged 19 to 50 years = 8 mg/day Men aged 19 to 50 years = 11 mg/day UL = 40 mg/day
Copper	RDA for all people 19–50 years = 90 µg/day UL = 10,000 µg/day
Vitamin K	AI: Women 19–50 years = 90 µg/day Men 19–50 years = 120 µg/day UL = none determined
Vitamin B_6 (pyridoxine)	RDA for all people 19–50 years = 1.3 mg/day RDA for people 51 and older: women = 1.5 mg/day; men = 1.7 mg/day
Folate (folic acid)	RDA for all people 19–50 years = 400 µg/day UL = 1,000 µg/day
Vitamin B_{12} (cobalamin)	RDA for all people 19–50 years = 2.4 µg/day UL = not determined (ND)

platelets Cell fragments that aggregate to form blood clots that help slow or stop bleeding.

plasma The fluid (noncellular) portion of the blood.

LO 2 Discuss the role that iron plays in maintaining blood health overall, and specifically in oxygen transport.

LO 3 Explain how the body absorbs, transports, and stores iron.

LO 4 Discuss the progression of iron deficiency from depletion to microcytic anemia.

Why Is Iron Essential to Blood Health?

Iron (Fe) is a trace mineral found in very small amounts in the body. Despite our relatively small need for iron, the World Health Organization lists iron deficiency as the most common nutrient deficiency in the world, including in industrialized countries.[1,2] Iron is a unique mineral with a positive charge that can easily give up and/or gain an electron, thereby changing its state from ferrous iron (Fe^{2+}) to ferric iron (Fe^{3+}) and back again. Although other forms of iron exist, ferrous and ferric iron are the two most common forms in our diet. Iron also binds easily to negatively charged elements, such as oxygen, nitrogen, and sulfur, a capacity that is important for the various functions iron plays in the body. We will discuss more about the various oxidative states of iron shortly.

Iron Transports Oxygen

Iron is a component of numerous proteins in the body, including enzymes and other proteins involved in energy production and both hemoglobin and myoglobin, the proteins involved in the transport and metabolism of oxygen. **Hemoglobin** is the oxygen-carrying protein found in the erythrocytes. It transports oxygen to tissues and accounts for almost two-thirds of all of the body's iron. Every day, within the bone marrow, the body produces approximately 200 billion erythrocytes, which require more than 24 mg of iron.[3] Thus, it is easy to see that hemoglobin synthesis for the formation of red blood cells is a primary factor in iron homeostasis. In fact, healthy individuals use about 80% of their absorbed iron for hemoglobin synthesis.[4] **Myoglobin,** another oxygen-carrying protein that is similar to hemoglobin, transports and stores oxygen within the muscles, accounting for approximately 10% of total iron in the body.

We cannot survive for more than a few minutes without oxygen; thus, hemoglobin's ability to transport oxygen throughout the body is critical to life. To carry oxygen, hemoglobin depends on the iron in its **heme** groups. As shown in **Figure 12.2**, the

hemoglobin The oxygen-carrying protein found in red blood cells; almost two-thirds of all of the iron in the body is found in hemoglobin.

myoglobin An iron-containing protein found in muscle cells.

heme The iron-containing molecule found in hemoglobin and myoglobin.

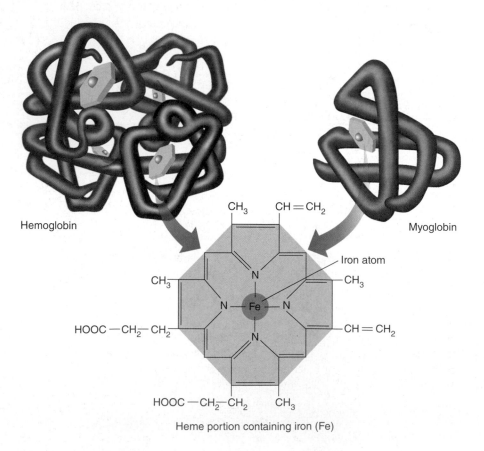

FIGURE 12.2 Iron is contained in the heme portion of hemoglobin and myoglobin. Notice the central iron atom (circled in red), which is surrounded by a porphyrin ring.

Heme portion containing iron (Fe)

hemoglobin molecule consists of four polypeptide chains studded with four iron-containing heme groups. Iron is able to bind with and release oxygen easily. It does this by transferring electrons to and from the other atoms as it moves between various oxidation states. In the bloodstream, iron acts as a shuttle, picking up oxygen from the environment, binding it during its transport in the bloodstream, and then dropping it off again in our tissues.

As noted, iron is also important in energy metabolism. It is a component of the cytochromes, electron carriers within the metabolic pathways, which result in the production of energy from carbohydrates, fats, and protein. Cytochromes contain heme and thus require iron. If iron is not available to form them, the production of energy is limited, especially during times of high energy demand, such as during physical activity. Iron is also involved in some of the key enzymes in the tricarboxylic acid (TCA) cycle and for enzymes required in amino acid and lipid metabolism.

As discussed in Chapter 10, iron is a part of the antioxidant enzyme system that assists in fighting free radicals. Interestingly, excess iron can also act as a prooxidant and promote the production of free radicals. Finally, iron is necessary for the enzymes involved in DNA synthesis and plays an important role in cognitive development and immune health (discussed later in this chapter).[5,6]

The Body Tightly Regulates Iron Homeostasis

The body contains relatively little iron; men have less than 4 g of iron in their body, and women have just over 2 g Iron is necessary for life, yet too much is toxic; therefore, the body maintains iron homeostasis primarily through regulating iron absorption, transport, storage, and excretion. **Figure 12.3** (page 468) provides an overview of iron absorption and transport.

Absorption of Iron

The body's ability to absorb dietary iron is influenced by a number of factors. The most important are the individual's iron status; the level of dietary iron consumption; the type of iron present in the foods consumed; the amount of stomach acid present to digest the foods; and the presence of the dietary factors that can either enhance or inhibit the absorption of iron.

Although the iron absorbed from the typical western diet is considered to be 14% to 18%,[6,7] the actual amount absorbed can vary widely depending on one's iron status (0.7–23%).[4] Thus, for an individual with poor iron status iron absorption can be as high as 23%. If iron status is good, iron absorption decreases to about 10% to 12%,[4,6] whereas if iron status is high, absorption can drop to as low as 2% to 4%.[4] Thus, people with poor iron status, such as those with iron deficiency, pregnant women, and people who have recently experienced blood loss (including menstruation) generally have the highest iron absorption rates. The typical Western diet of 2,000 kcal/day would contain about 10 to 14 mg of iron. In an individual with good iron status, only about 1.0 to 1.6 mg of this would be absorbed. However, an individual with poor iron status might absorb nearly twice this amount. By altering absorption rate, the body can improve iron status without dramatic increases in dietary iron intake.

Similarly, the total amount of iron consumed in the diet influences an individual's iron absorption rate. People who consume low levels of dietary iron absorb more iron from their foods than do those with higher dietary iron intakes. If the gut mucosal cells have a high iron pool, less iron is absorbed from the next meal.

The type of iron in foods is another major factor influencing iron absorption. There are two types:

- **Heme iron** is a part of hemoglobin and myoglobin and is found only in animal-based foods, such as meat, fish, and poultry.
- **Nonheme iron** is the form of iron that is not a part of hemoglobin or myoglobin. It is found in both plant-based and animal-based foods.

heme iron Iron that is a part of hemoglobin and myoglobin; it is found only in animal-based foods, such as meat, fish, and poultry.

nonheme iron The form of iron that is not a part of hemoglobin or myoglobin; it is found in animal-based and plant-based foods.

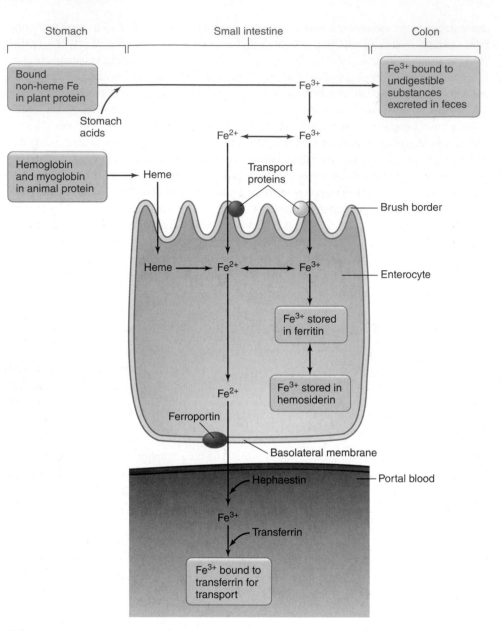

FIGURE 12.3 Overview of iron absorption and transport. (*Source:* "Advanced Nutrition and Human Metabolism (with InfoTrac®) 4e," by Gropper; Smith; Groff, 2005. Copyright © 2005 by Brooks/Cole, a part of Cengage Learning, Inc. Reproduced by permission. www.cengage .com/permissions.)

The major of iron (90–95%) in all diets is in the form of nonheme iron.[8] In individuals with high iron status (serum ferritin ≥100 µg/L), whole mixed diets containing high-bioavailable iron (heme + nonheme iron) have absorption rates of 2% to 4%, while low-bioavailable diets (primarily nonheme iron) have absorption rates closer to 1%.[4] Overall, dietary nonheme iron is less absorbable than heme iron. When foods containing heme iron are added to the diet with nonheme iron, total iron absorption will increase.[4] Once heme, which contains the ferrous form (Fe^{2+}), is released from either hemoglobin or myoglobin in the small intestine, it is rapidly bound to a specific receptor on the intestinal lumen and is taken into the enterocyte by endocytosis. Within the enterocyte, the heme group is broken down, and the iron that is released becomes part of a common iron pool within the cell. Because the iron in animal-based foods is about 50% to 60% heme iron (meat, fish, and poultry) and the rest nonheme iron, animal-based foods are good sources of absorbable iron.[6,7] Meat, fish, and poultry also contain a special **meat factor,** which enhances the absorption of nonheme iron in the diet.[9]

In contrast, all of the iron found in plant-based foods is nonheme iron. Its absorption is influenced by the amount of heme iron in the diet and by the individual's level of stomach acid. During digestion, nonheme iron–containing foods enter the stomach, where gastric juices containing pepsin and hydrochloric acid reduce the ferric iron (Fe^{3+}) to ferrous iron (Fe^{2+}), which is more soluble in the alkaline environment (higher pH) of the small intestine. Thus, adequate amounts of stomach acid are necessary for nonheme iron absorption. People with low levels of stomach acid, including many older adults and individuals who use medications that reduce stomach acid, may experience reduced iron absorption.

Once iron enters the duodenum, it is taken up by the enterocytes, with ferrous iron more rapidly absorbed than ferric iron. In addition, the solubility of nonheme iron in the small intestine is greatly modified by the presence of enhancing or inhibitory factors within the meal. Vitamin C enhances nonheme absorption from the gut by reducing dietary ferric to ferrous iron, which then forms a soluble iron–ascorbic acid complex in the stomach.[5] Conversely, iron absorption is impaired by oxalic acid, phytates, polyphenols, vegetable proteins, fiber, and calcium. Typically, these substances bind to the ferric iron and form complexes that cannot be digested. Phytates are found in legumes, rice, and whole grains; and polyphenols are found in oregano, red wine, tea, and coffee. Soybean protein, fiber, and minerals such as calcium inhibit iron absorption. Oxalic acid is found in spinach, some whole grains, chard, and rhubarb. Because of the influence of these dietary factors on iron absorption, it is estimated that the bioavailability of iron from a vegan diet is approximately 1% to 10%,[7] compared with the 14% to 18% absorption of the typical Western diet.[7] Of course, the iron absorption rates from these diets will change depending on the iron status of the individual.

To optimize absorption of the nonheme iron in plant foods, consume these foods either with foods rich in heme iron or in combination with foods high in vitamin C. For instance, eating meat with vegetables enhances the absorption of the nonheme iron found in the vegetables. Drinking a glass of orange juice with breakfast cereal will increase the absorption of the nonheme iron in the cereal. Avoid taking zinc or calcium supplements or drinking milk when eating iron-rich foods, as iron absorption will be impaired.

Finally, cooking foods in cast-iron pans will significantly increase the iron content of any meal. That's because the iron in the pan is released and combines with food during the cooking process.

Iron Transport

Regardless of the form, iron taken into the enterocytes becomes part of the total iron pool. From this pool the iron can be stored within the enterocytes, or it can be transported across the membrane of the enterocytes by **ferroportin** into the interstitial fluid, from which it can enter the circulation.[6,10] Ferroportin is an iron transporter that helps regulate intestinal iron absorption and release.[10] Iron crossing into the interstitial fluid is in the ferrous form (Fe^{2+}) but is quickly converted to ferric iron (Fe^{3+}) by either **hephaestin** in the intestinal basal cell membrane (see Figure 12.3) or **ceruloplasmin** in the blood. Both are copper-containing plasma proteins capable of oxidizing iron. The Fe^{3+} is rapidly bound to **transferrin,** the primary iron-transport protein in the blood, which transports the Fe^{3+} to the cells of the body. Transferrin receptors on the cells increase and decrease in number, depending on the cells need for iron. In this way, cells can regulate the amount of iron they take in from the blood.

Iron Storage

The body is capable of storing small amounts of iron in two storage forms: **ferritin** and **hemosiderin.** These storage forms of iron provide us with iron when our diet is inadequate

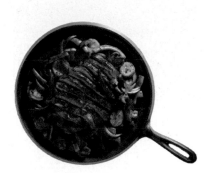

Cooking foods in cast-iron pans significantly increases their iron content.

meat factor A special factor found in meat, fish, and poultry that enhances the absorption of nonheme iron.

ferroportin An iron transporter that helps regulate intestinal iron absorption and the release of iron from the enterocyte into the general circulation.

hephaestin A copper-containing protein that oxidizes Fe^{2+} to Fe^{3+} once iron is transported across the basolateral membrane by ferroportin.

ceruloplasmin A copper-containing protein that transports copper in the body. It also plays a role in oxidizing ferrous to ferric iron (Fe^{2+} to Fe^{3+}).

transferrin The primary iron transport protein in the blood; transports iron to body cells.

ferritin A storage form of iron found primarily in the intestinal mucosa, spleen, bone marrow, and liver.

hemosiderin A storage form of iron found primarily in the intestinal mucosa, spleen, bone marrow, and liver.

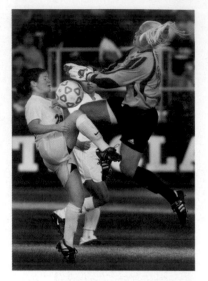

Athletes may have an increased need for iron.

or when our needs are high. Both ferritin and hemosiderin can be mobilized if the body needs iron.

Figure 12.3 shows iron storage in the enterocytes as ferritin or hemosiderin. Other common areas of iron storage are the liver, bone marrow, and spleen. Ferritin is the normal storage form, whereas hemosiderin storage occurs predominately in conditions of iron overload. However, if an iron overload occurs, and the excess iron is stored as hemosiderin in the heart and liver, organ damage can occur.

The amount of iron stored can vary dramatically between men and women, with women at greater risk of having low iron stores (from 300 to 1,000 mg). Average iron stores for men are estimated to be 500 to 1,500 mg. Women of childbearing age have one of the highest rates of iron deficiency, which is attributed to increased iron losses in menstrual blood, poor intakes of iron, and the additional iron requirements that accompany pregnancy. The iron "cost" of pregnancy is high; thus, a woman of childbearing age should have good iron stores prior to pregnancy and consume iron-rich foods during pregnancy. Iron supplements are routinely prescribed during the last two trimesters to ensure that there is adequate iron for the woman and her developing fetus. The iron needs of pregnancy are covered in more detail later in this text (see Chapter 17).

Regulation of Total Body Iron

The body regulates iron balance and homeostasis through three mechanisms:

- *Iron absorption.* As discussed earlier, the change in the iron absorption rate is based on the amount of iron consumed, the amount needed by the body, and the dietary factors that affect absorption.
- *Iron losses.* One of the major routes of iron loss is through the turnover of the gut enterocytes. Every 3 to 6 days, the gut cells are shed and lost into the lumen of the intestine. In this way, the iron stored as ferritin within the enterocytes is returned to the lumen, from which it is lost in the feces. The regulation of iron absorption in this way dramatically reduces the possibility of too much iron entering the system, regardless of the iron source. Iron can also be lost in blood (menses, blood donations, injury), sweat, and semen and passively from cells that are shed from the skin and urinary tract. The dietary recommendations for iron are based on an overall estimated daily iron turnover of 1.5 mg/d for menstruating women and 1.0 mg/d for sedentary men and postmenopausal women.[5] The typical menstruating female loses approximately 14 mg of iron per menstrual cycle; thus, the additional 0.5 mg/d would provide an extra 15 mg of iron per month to cover menstrual losses.[5] Women who experience heavy menstrual bleeding would have even greater iron losses, which would need to be covered by either dietary or supplemental iron. Active individuals can also have increased iron losses due to iron lost in urine, sweat, and increased red cell turnover.[5]
- *Storage and recycling of iron.* Stored iron gives the body access to iron to maintain health when intakes of dietary iron are low or losses are great. Conversely, once iron balance has been restored, the body will gradually increase the amount of iron stored, so that reserves are again available in times of need. The body is also efficient at recycling iron already within the system. The majority of the body's iron is bound to hemoglobin within the red blood cells, which have a life of 120 days. In order to prevent the body from losing this valuable source of iron, as old red cells are broken down, the iron is recycled and returned to the body's iron pool. The iron supplied through recycling is approximately 20 times greater than the amount of iron absorbed from the diet.[2] Thus, the body's ability to recycle iron is extremely important in maintaining iron homeostasis.

RECAP

Iron is a trace mineral that, as part of the hemoglobin and myoglobin proteins, plays a major role in the transport of oxygen in the body. Iron is also a cofactor in many metabolic pathways involved in energy production. The body tightly regulates iron homeostasis. Absorption of iron from a mixed diet averages about 14% to 18%. However, absorption varies according to the individual's iron status, level of dietary iron consumption, type of iron present in foods consumed, amount of stomach acid, and presence of dietary factors that enhance or inhibit iron absorption. Animal-based foods contain 50% to 60% of their iron as heme iron, which is more readily absorbed than the nonheme iron found in both animal and plant-based foods. Iron can be stored within the enterocytes, or transported across the membrane of the enterocytes and into the circulation by ferroportin. The body is capable of storing small amounts of iron as ferritin and hemosiderin.

How Much Iron Should We Consume?

In determining the RDA for iron, researchers take into account the bioavailability of iron from food and absorption rates.

Recommended Dietary Intakes for Iron

The RDA for iron for men aged 19 years and older is 8 mg/day. The RDA for iron for women aged 19 to 50 years is 18 mg/day and decreases to 8 mg/day for women 51 years of age and older. The higher iron requirement for younger women is due to the excess iron and blood lost during menstruation. Pregnancy is a time of very high iron needs, and the RDA for pregnant women is 27 mg/day. The UL for iron for adults aged 19 and older is 45 mg/day.[5] Although it is difficult to get too much iron from whole foods, it is easy to get high doses of iron from supplements and/or the use of highly fortified processed foods, such as breakfast cereals, meal-replacement drinks, energy bars, and protein powders. See the ***You Do the Math*** box (on page 472) to learn how to calculate your iron intake. Special circumstances that significantly affect iron status and may increase requirements are identified in **Table 12.2.**

Food Sources of Iron

Foods rich in heme iron include meats, poultry, fish, and shellfish (**Figure 12.4**, page 472). Clams, oysters, and beef liver are particularly good sources, providing 5 to 11 mg of iron per

TABLE 12.2 Special Circumstances Affecting Iron Status

Circumstances That Improve Iron Status	Circumstances That Diminish Iron Status
Use of oral contraceptives—reduces menstrual blood loss in women.	**Use of hormone replacement therapy**—can cause uterine bleeding.
Breastfeeding—delays resumption of menstruation in new mothers and thereby reduces blood loss. It is therefore an important health measure, especially in developing nations.	**Eating a vegetarian diet**—reduces or eliminates sources of heme iron.
Consumption of iron-containing foods and supplements	**Intestinal parasite infection**—causes intestinal bleeding. Iron-deficiency anemia is common in people with intestinal parasite infection. **Blood donation**—reduces iron stores; people who donate frequently, particularly premenopausal women, may require iron supplementation. **Intense endurance exercise training**—appears to increase the risk for poor iron status because of many factors, including inflammation, suboptimal iron intake, and increased iron loss due to rupture of red blood cells and increased fecal losses.

Source: Data from Institute of Medicine, Food and Nutrition Board. 2002. *Dietary Reference Intakes for Vitamin A, Vitamin K, Arsenic, Boron, Chromium, Copper, Iodine, Iron, Manganese, Molybdenum, Nickel, Silicon, Vanadium, and Zinc.* Washington, DC: National Academies Press. © 2002 by the National Academy of Sciences.

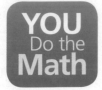

Calculating Daily Iron Intake

Determining whether you're getting the iron your body needs each day can be tricky, because the amount you consume may not be the amount that is absorbed. Food combinations, fortified foods, and supplements all make a difference. Determine the amount of iron available for absorption for Hannah, who is menstruating normally:

Foods with heme iron (15% available):

- Turkey, light meat (3 oz): 1.1 mg
- Tuna, light canned (3 oz): 1.3 mg

Foods with nonheme iron (5% available):

- Oatmeal, 1 instant packet: 11 mg
- Spinach, 1 cup raw: 6.4 mg
- Bread, whole-wheat, 2 slices: 1.4 mg

In addition, Hannah is taking a daily multivitamin/mineral supplement with 18 mg of Fe (5% available). This is the amount of iron in a typical 1-day multivitamin/mineral supplement designed for menstruating women.

What is the total available iron for absorption (mg/d)? Does it cover the amount of iron lost each day? If Hannah were not taking a daily supplement, would she still be getting adequate iron?

Answers are located online in the MasteringNutrition Study Area.

---

serving. Many breakfast cereals and breads are enriched or fortified with iron; although this nonheme iron is less absorbable, it is still significant because these foods are a major part of the Western diet. Legumes, such as lentils and beans, are also good sources of iron, as are some green, leafy vegetables such as spinach. The absorption of their nonheme iron can be enhanced by eating them with animal foods or vitamin C–rich foods. People who avoid animal products, especially pregnant and lactating women following a vegan diet, need to plan their diet carefully to ensure adequate iron intake, because heme iron sources are eliminated.

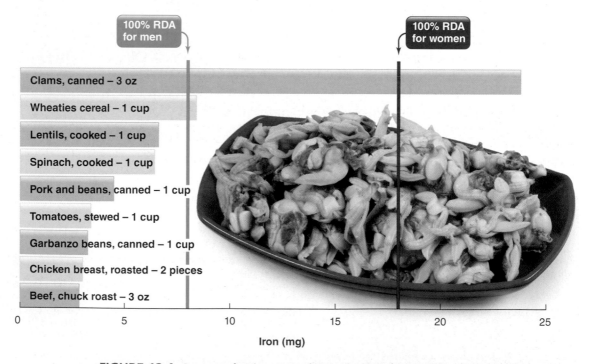

FIGURE 12.4 Common food sources of iron. The RDA for iron is 8 mg/day for men and 18 mg/day for women aged 19 to 50 years. (*Source:* Data from U.S. Department of Agriculture, Agricultural Research Service, 2009, USDA Nutrient Database for Standard Reference, Release 22. Nutrient Data Laboratory Home Page, www.ars.usda.gov/ba/bhnrc/ndl.)

Increasing Your Iron Intake

Simple changes in your daily diet can help you increase your daily intake of iron and avoid deficiency. Here are a few:

- Shop for iron-fortified breads and breakfast cereals. Check the Nutrition Facts panel!
- Consume a food or beverage that is high in vitamin C along with plant or animal sources of iron. For instance, drink a glass of orange juice with your morning toast to increase the absorption of the nonheme iron in the bread. Or add chopped tomatoes to beans or lentils or orange slices to your spinach salad. Or sprinkle lemon juice on fish.
- Add small amounts of meat, poultry, or fish to baked beans, vegetable soups, stir-fried vegetables, or salads to enhance the absorption of the nonheme iron in the plant-based foods.
- Cook foods in cast-iron pans to significantly increase the iron content of foods: the iron in the pan will be absorbed into the food during the cooking process.
- Avoid drinking red wine, coffee, or tea when eating iron-rich foods, as chemicals called polyphenols in these beverages will reduce iron absorption.
- Avoid drinking cow's milk or soymilk with iron-rich foods, as both calcium and soybean protein inhibit iron absorption.
- Avoid taking calcium supplements or zinc supplements with iron-rich foods, as these minerals decrease iron absorption.

What Happens If We Consume Too Much Iron?

Accidental iron overdose is the most common cause of poisoning deaths in children younger than 6 years of age in the United States.[11] It is important for parents to take the same precautions with dietary supplements as they would with other drugs, keeping them in a locked cabinet or well out of reach of children. Symptoms of iron toxicity include nausea, vomiting, diarrhea, dizziness, confusion, and rapid heartbeat. If iron toxicity is not treated quickly, significant damage to the heart, central nervous system, liver, and kidneys can result in death.

Many adults who take iron supplements, even at prescribed doses, commonly experience constipation and gastrointestinal distress.[5] High doses of iron supplements can also cause nausea, vomiting, and diarrhea. Taking iron supplements with food can reduce these adverse effects in most, but not all, people.

As mentioned (in Chapter 10), some individuals suffer from a hereditary disorder called *hemochromatosis*. This disorder is the most common cause of severe iron overload[12] and affects approximately 5 in 1,000 individuals of Northern European orgin.[10] Hemochromatosis is characterized by excessive absorption of dietary iron and altered iron storage. In this disease, the transport of iron from the enterocytes into the circulation is not regulated appropriately, and iron transport continues even when it is not needed.[13] Because the body has no homeostatic mechanism for eliminating high amounts of iron from the system, iron accumulates in body tissues over many years, causing organ damage and other disease.[10] High levels of serum iron can also increase the risk for oxidative damage by stimulating the activity of free radicals, which are also associated with chronic diseases. Free radicals can damage coronary arteries and contribute to cardiovascular disease, and a build-up of iron in the liver can contribute to liver cancer.[10] Treatment includes reducing dietary intake of iron, avoiding high intakes of vitamin C, use of chelation drugs that bind iron and eliminate it in the urine, and blood removal, a process similar to the donation of blood except that the blood is not reused.

What Happens If We Don't Consume Enough Iron?

Iron deficiency can have a number of health consequences. People at particularly high risk include infants and young children, menstruating girls and women, and pregnant women. Refer to the nearby *Highlight: Iron Deficiency around the World* to learn more about the global impact of iron deficiency.

HIGHLIGHT

Iron Deficiency around the World

Iron deficiency is the most common nutritional deficiency in the world. According to the World Health Organization, approximately 2 billion people, or 30% of the world's population, are anemic, many due to iron deficiency.[1] Because of its high prevalence worldwide, iron deficiency is considered an epidemic.

Those who are particularly susceptible to iron deficiency include people living in developing countries, pregnant women, and young children. Among children, the health consequences of iron—deficiency anemia are particularly devastating. They include

- Premature birth
- Low birth weight
- Increased risk for infections
- Increased risk for premature death
- Impaired cognitive and physical development
- Behavioral problems and poor school performance

But the harmful consequences of iron deficiency are not limited to individuals. Because it results in increased healthcare needs, premature death, resultant family breakdown, and lost work productivity, it also damages communities and entire nations.

Research is currently examining the role of iron supplementation in improving cognitive function.

A meta-analysis of the current research literature suggests that iron supplementation in children suffering from iron-deficiency anemia can improve their intelligence quotient; however, the effect of supplementation on attention and concentration is not clear.[2]

The World Health Organization has developed a comprehensive plan to address all aspects of iron deficiency and anemia.[1,3] This plan, which is being implemented in several developing countries, not only is restoring personal health but also is estimated to be capable of raising national productivity levels by 20%.

References

1. World Health Organization. 2012. Nutrition. Micronutrient Deficiencies: Iron Deficiency Anemia. www.who.int/nutrition/topics/ida/en/index.html.
2. Falkingham, M., A. Abdelhamid, P. Curtis, A. Fairweather-Tait, L. Dye, and L. Hooper. 2010. The effects of oral iron supplementation on cognition in older children and adults: a systemic review and meta-analysis. *J Nut.* 9:4.
3. Baltussen, R., C. Knai, and M. Sharan. 2004. Iron fortification and iron supplementation are cost-effective interventions to reduce iron deficiency in four subregions of the world. *J. Nut.* 134:2678–2684.

Many Factors Contribute to Iron Deficiency For some individuals, iron deficiency is simply due to poor dietary intakes of iron. Other factors can include high iron losses in blood and sweat, a diet high in fiber or phytates that bind iron, low stomach acid, and poor iron absorption due to poor gut health or the consumption of dietary supplements containing high levels of minerals, such as calcium, that compete with iron absorption binding sites. Significant blood losses through blood donations, surgery, or heavy menstrual periods can contribute to poor iron status. Thus, the causes of iron deficiency and/or depletion can be numerous and may involve a number of issues that need to be addressed before iron status can be improved.

Iron Deficiency Progresses through Three Stages As shown in **Figure 12.5**, **stage I** of iron deficiency is called **iron depletion**.[6,14] It is caused by a decrease in iron *stores*, resulting in reduced levels of circulating ferritin in the blood. As discussed earlier, ferritin is one form of stored iron. Small amounts of ferritin circulate in the blood, and these concentrations are highly correlated with iron stores.

During iron depletion, there are generally no physical symptoms because hemoglobin levels are not yet affected. However, when iron stores are low, the amount of iron available to mitochondrial proteins and enzymes appears to be depleted. This reduces the individual's ability to produce energy during periods of high demand. For example, research has shown that, when sedentary women with poor ferritin levels participated in an exercise-training program, they did not experience the same improvements in fitness as women who had adequate ferritin levels.[15] This same effect has been observed in female athletes; those with low ferritin levels had lower aerobic capacity, which improved with iron supplementation.[16,17]

iron depletion (stage I) The first phase of iron deficiency, characterized by a decrease in stored iron, which results in a decrease in blood ferritin levels.

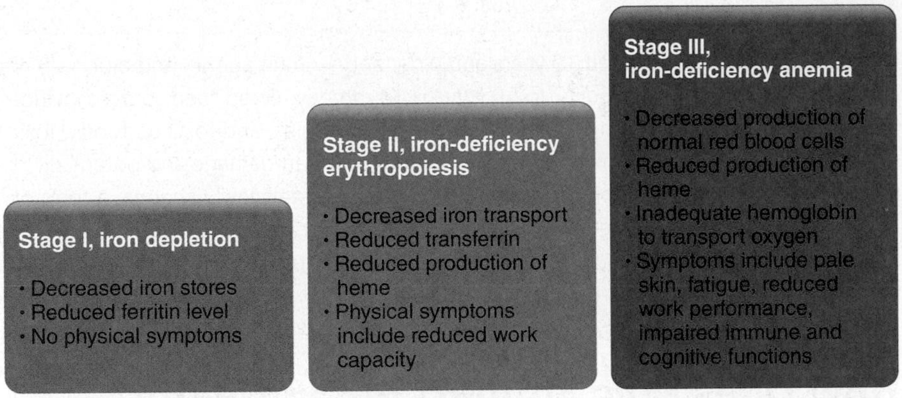

Stage I, iron depletion

- Decreased iron stores
- Reduced ferritin level
- No physical symptoms

Stage II, iron-deficiency erythropoiesis

- Decreased iron transport
- Reduced transferrin
- Reduced production of heme
- Physical symptoms include reduced work capacity

Stage III, iron-deficiency anemia

- Decreased production of normal red blood cells
- Reduced production of heme
- Inadequate hemoglobin to transport oxygen
- Symptoms include pale skin, fatigue, reduced work performance, impaired immune and cognitive functions

FIGURE 12.5 Iron deficiency passes through three stages. The first stage is identified by decreased iron stores and reduced ferritin levels. The second stage is identified by decreased iron transport and a reduction in transferrin. The final stage is iron-deficiency anemia, which is identified by decreased production of normal, healthy red blood cells and inadequate hemoglobin levels.

The second stage of iron deficiency causes a decrease in the *transport* of iron and is called **iron-deficiency erythropoiesis (stage II)**. This stage is manifested by a reduction in the saturation of transferrin with iron. Transferrin, the transport protein for iron, has the ability to bind two iron molecules and transport them to the cells of the body. During this stage, the iron binding sites on transferrin are left empty, because there is no iron available for binding. This results in transferrin having an increased ability to bind iron, which is called *total iron binding capacity (TIBC)*. In addition, transferrin receptors on the cells increase to promote uptake of iron by the cell. Overall, then, individuals with iron-deficiency erythropoiesis have low serum ferritin and iron concentrations, a low level of iron saturation, and a high TIBC and transferrin receptors. The production of heme and the ability to make new red blood cells (red blood cell production is called *erythropoiesis*) starts to decline during this stage, leading to symptoms of reduced work capacity, because fewer red blood cells are being made.

During the third, and final, stage of iron deficiency, **iron-deficiency anemia (stage III)** results. In iron-deficiency anemia, the production of normal, healthy red blood cells has decreased, the cell size decreases by as much as a third, and hemoglobin levels are inadequate. Not only are too few red blood cells made, but those that are produced cannot bind and transport oxygen adequately. Individuals with stage III iron-deficiency anemia will still have abnormal values for all the assessment parameters measured in stages I and II.

Iron-Deficiency Anemia Is a Microcytic Anemia The term *anemia* literally means "without blood"; it is used to refer to any condition in which hemoglobin levels are low, regardless of the cause.

Microcytic anemias are a group of anemias characterized by red blood cells that are smaller than normal (*micro-* means "small," and *–cyte* means "cell"). As just noted, red blood cells that are synthesized in an iron-deficient environment will be as much as a third smaller than normal and will not contain enough hemoglobin to transport adequate oxygen or to allow the proper transfer of electrons to produce energy. Microcytic anemia is sometimes referred to as *microcytic hypochromic anemia*, because reduced levels of hemoglobin deprive the cells of their bright red color (*hypo-* means "low," and *–chromic* refers to "color").

In iron-deficiency anemia, as normal red blood cell death occurs over time, more and more healthy red blood cells are replaced by microcytic cells. At the same time, fewer red blood cells are made. These changes prompt classic symptoms of oxygen and energy deprivation, including general fatigue, pale skin, depressed immune function, and impaired cognitive and nerve function, work performance, and memory. Pregnant women with severe anemia are at higher risk for low-birth-weight infants, premature delivery, and increased infant and maternal mortality.

Watch an interview from the National Heart, Lung, and Blood Institute with a woman recovering from severe iron-deficiency anemia at **www.nhlbi.nih.gov**.

iron-deficiency erythropoiesis (stage II) The second stage of iron deficiency, characterized by a decrease in the transport of iron in the blood and an increase in total iron binding capacity.

iron-deficiency anemia (stage III) A form of anemia that results from severe iron deficiency.

microcytic anemia A form of anemia manifested as the production of smaller than normal red blood cells containing insufficient hemoglobin, which reduces the red blood cell's ability to transport oxygen; it can result from iron deficiency or vitamin B_6 deficiency.

RECAP

The RDA for iron for men aged 19 years and older and women age 51 and older is 8 mg/day. The RDA for women aged 19 to 50 years is 18 mg/day. Good food sources include meat, poultry, seafood, legumes and certain other vegetables, and fortified foods. Toxicity symptoms for iron range from nausea and vomiting to organ damage and potentially death. If left untreated, iron depletion can eventually lead to iron-deficiency anemia, a form of microcytic anemia in which red blood cells are smaller than normal and will not contain enough hemoglobin to transport adequate oxygen or to allow the proper transfer of electrons to produce energy.

LO 5 Discuss the functions, RDA, and food sources of zinc.

How Does Zinc Support Blood Health?

Zinc (Zn^{2+}) is a positively charged trace mineral that, like iron, is found in very small amounts in the body (1.5–2.5 g). Most of the zinc found in the body is concentrated in the muscles and bone. However, in contrast with iron and other minerals, zinc has no dedicated storage sites within the body. Instead a small, exchangeable pool of zinc is found in the bone, liver, and blood. Loss of zinc from this pool, if not replaced, leads to zinc deficiency.

Zinc Has Enzymatic, Structural, and Regulatory Functions

Zinc has multiple functions within nearly every body system.[18] As a component of various enzymes, zinc helps maintain the structural integrity of proteins and assists in the regulation of gene expression.[5,18] Without zinc, the body cannot grow, develop, or function properly. It is easiest to review the many roles of zinc in the body by dividing them into three categories: enzymatic, structural, and regulatory.

Enzymatic Functions

It is estimated that more than 300 different enzymes within the body require zinc for their functioning.[18] If zinc is not present, these enzymes cannot function properly and lose their activity. For example, we require zinc to metabolize alcohol (alcohol dehydrogenase), digest our food (carboxypeptidase C, aminopeptidase, phospholipase C), help form bone (collagenase), provide the body with energy through glycolysis, and synthesize the heme

Liz *Nutri*-Case

"It was really hard spending last summer with my parents, because we kept arguing over food! Even though I'd told them that I'm a vegetarian, they kept serving meals with meat! Then they'd get mad when I'd fix myself a hummus sandwich! When it was my turn to cook, I made lentils with brown rice, whole-wheat pasta primavera, vegetarian curries, and lots of other yummy meals, but my father still complained. He kept insisting, 'You have to eat meat or you won't get enough iron!' I told him that plant foods have lots of iron, but he wouldn't listen. Was I ever glad to get back onto campus this fall!"

Recall that Liz is a ballet dancer who trains daily. If she eats a vegetarian diet, including meals such as the ones she describes here, will she be at risk for iron deficiency? Why or why not? Are there any other micronutrients that might be low in Liz's diet because she avoids meat? If so, what are they? Overall, will Liz get enough energy to support her high level of physical activity on a vegetarian diet? How would she know if she were low on energy?

structure in hemoglobin. Thus, zinc, like iron, is required to make the oxygen-carrying component of hemoglobin. In this way, zinc contributes to the maintenance of blood health.

Structural Functions

Zinc helps maintain the structural integrity and shape of proteins. If proteins lose their shape, they lose their function, much like a plastic spoon that has melted into a ball. Zinc helps stabilize the structure of certain DNA-binding proteins, called *zinc fingers*, which help regulate gene expression by facilitating the folding of proteins into biologically active molecules used in gene regulation.[6] Zinc fingers also help stabilize vitamin A receptors in the retina of the eye, thereby facilitating night vision. Another function associated with zinc fingers is the sequencing of hormone receptors for vitamin D and thyroid hormone.[6,19]

Zinc's role in stabilizing protein structures includes maintaining the integrity of some enzymes. For example, zinc helps maintain the integrity of copper–zinc superoxide dismutase, which is important in helping prevent oxidative damage caused by free radicals. Zinc also helps maintain the integrity of enzymes involved in the development and activation of certain immune cells (discussed shortly). In fact, zinc has received so much attention for its contribution to immune system health that zinc lozenges have been formulated to fight the common cold. The *Nutrition Myth or Fact?* essay at the end of this chapter explores the question of whether these lozenges are effective.

Regulatory Functions

As a regulator of gene expression, zinc helps turn genes "on" and "off," thus regulating the body functions these genes control. For example, if zinc is not available to activate certain genes related to cellular growth during fetal development and early childhood, growth is stunted. Zinc also plays a role in cell signaling. For example, zinc helps maintain blood glucose levels by interacting with insulin and influencing the way fat cells take up glucose. Zinc also helps regulate the activity of a number of other hormones, such as human growth hormone, sex hormones, and corticosteroids.[6]

A number of biological actions require zinc in all three of the functions just covered. The major example of this is in reproduction. Zinc is critical for cell replication and normal growth. In fact, zinc deficiency was discovered in the early 1960s when researchers were trying to determine the cause of severe growth retardation, anemia, and poorly developed genitalia in some Middle Eastern males. These symptoms of zinc deficiency illustrate its critical role in normal growth and sexual maturation.

Several Factors Influence Zinc Absorption and Transport

Overall, the body absorbs from 20% to 30% of dietary zinc.[20] As with iron, absorption rates can vary widely (from 10 to 80%), depending on zinc status.[6] People with poor zinc status absorb more zinc than individuals with optimal zinc status, and zinc absorption increases during times of growth, sexual development, and pregnancy.

As shown in **Figure 12.6** (page 478), zinc is absorbed from the lumen of the intestine into the enterocytes through both active transport by carriers and simple diffusion, with the efficiency of absorption decreasing as the amount of zinc in the diet increases. Once inside the enterocytes, zinc can be released into the interstitial fluid (as discussed shortly) or bound to a protein called **metallothionein,** which prevents zinc from moving out of the enterocyte into the system.

Nutrition MILESTONE

In **1958**, Drs. James Halsted and Ananda Prasad, American physicians working in Iran, consulted together on the case of a 21-year-old Iranian man who looked like a 10-year-old boy. In addition to his abnormally small size, he had underdeveloped genitalia; rough, dry skin; and cognitive deficits. Blood tests revealed that he was iron deficient. At first the physicians considered the possibility that the patient had a pituitary disorder, but when 10 more such cases were brought to their attention within a short period of time, they discarded the hypothesis in favor of a dietary explanation. They noted that the bread the patients ate was unleavened, that their diet included almost no animal protein, and that they practiced geophagia—they ate clay. These factors were known to contribute to iron deficiency.

Although the effects of zinc deficiency in humans were unknown, they considered that the same factors might also have decreased the availability of zinc. Further experiments supported the hypothesis. The physicians found that patients administered supplemental zinc developed normal genitalia and secondary sexual characteristics within 6 months and an increase in height of 5 to 6 inches within 1 year. This research showed for the first time that zinc is essential to human health.

metallothionein A zinc-containing protein within the enterocyte; it assists in the regulation of zinc homeostasis.

FIGURE 12.6 Overview of zinc absorption and transport. (*Source: "Advanced Nutrition and Human Metabolism (with InfoTrac®) 4e,"* by Gropper; Smith; Groff, 2005. Copyright © 2005 by Brooks/Cole, a part of Cengage Learning, Inc. Reproduced by permission. www.cengage.com/permissions.)

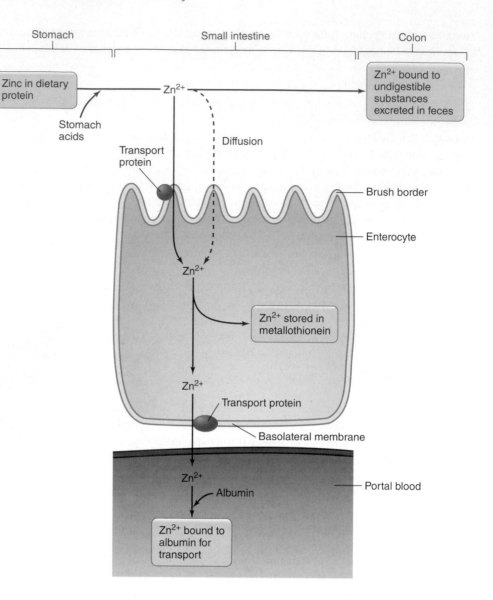

In this way, the body can regulate the amount of absorbed zinc that actually enters the total zinc pool of the body. When the enterocytes are sloughed off into the intestine, the zinc bound to metallothionein is lost in the feces. In this way, the body can maintain total zinc homeostasis.

Several dietary factors influence zinc absorption. High nonheme iron intakes can inhibit zinc absorption, which is a primary concern with iron supplementation, particularly during pregnancy and lactation. (Iron supplements typically contain nonheme iron.) High intakes of heme iron, however, appear to have no effect on zinc absorption. Although calcium is known to inhibit zinc absorption in animals, the effect in humans appears to depend on the form and amount of calcium given and the study population used.[6] The phytates and fiber found in whole grains and beans strongly inhibit zinc absorption. In contrast, dietary protein enhances zinc absorption, with animal-based proteins increasing the absorption of zinc to a much greater extent than plant-based proteins. It's not surprising, then, that the primary cause of the zinc deficiency in the Middle Eastern men mentioned earlier was their low consumption of meat and high consumption of beans and unleavened breads (also called *flat breads*). In leavening bread, the baker adds yeast to the dough. This not only makes the bread rise but also helps reduce the phytate content of the bread.

Zinc crosses the basolateral enterocyte membrane via a process of active transport using both a zinc transporter and energy (ATP). Upon reaching the interstitial fluid, zinc is picked up by albumin, a transport protein in the plasma, and carried via the portal vein to the liver. Once in the liver, some of the zinc is repackaged and released back into the blood, bound to either albumin (about 60%) or other transport proteins (about 40%).[6] The bound zinc can then be delivered to the cells, where it is taken up by energy-dependent carriers.

How Much Zinc Should We Consume?

As with iron, our need for zinc is relatively small, but our dietary intakes and level of absorption are variable. Absorption factors were considered when the RDA for zinc was set.[5] The RDA values for zinc for adult men and women aged 19 and older are 11 mg/day and 8 mg/day, respectively. The UL for zinc for adults aged 19 and older is 40 mg/day.

Good food sources of zinc include red meats, some seafood, whole grains, and enriched grains and cereals. The dark meat of poultry has a higher content of zinc than white meat. As zinc is significantly more absorbable from animal-based foods, zinc deficiency is a concern for people eating a vegetarian or vegan diet. **Figure 12.7** shows various foods that are relatively high in zinc.

Eating high amounts of dietary zinc does not appear to lead to toxicity; however, toxicity can occur from consuming high amounts of supplemental zinc. Toxicity symptoms include intestinal pain and cramps, nausea, vomiting, loss of appetite, diarrhea, and headaches. Excessive zinc supplementation has also been shown to depress immune function and decrease high-density lipoprotein concentrations. High intakes of zinc (five to six times the RDA) can also reduce copper and iron status, as zinc absorption interferes with the absorption of these minerals.

Zinc deficiency is uncommon in the United States, occurring more often in countries in which people consume predominantly grain-based foods. When zinc deficiency does occur, it is primarily associated with growth retardation in children, in which the lack of zinc disrupts functions associated with cell division.[6] Other symptoms of zinc deficiency include diarrhea, delayed sexual maturation and impotence, eye and skin lesions, hair loss, and impaired appetite. As zinc is critical to a healthy immune system, zinc deficiency results in increased incidence of infections and illnesses.

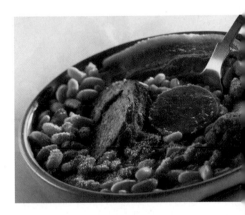

Zinc can be found in pork and beans.

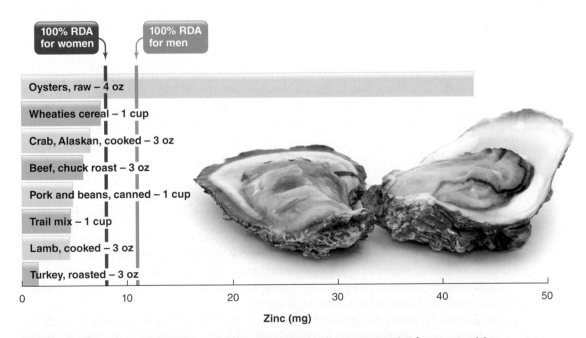

FIGURE 12.7 Common food sources of zinc. The RDA for zinc is 11 mg/day for men and 8 mg/day for women. (*Source:* Data from U.S. Department of Agriculture, Agricultural Research Service, 2009, USDA Nutrient Database for Standard Reference, Release 22. Nutrient Data Laboratory Home Page, www.ars.usda.gov/ba/bhnrc/ndl.)

Because we do not have good assessment parameters for zinc, we have no way of recognizing poor zinc status until deficiency symptoms occur. In developed countries, those at greatest risk for zinc deficiencies are individuals with malabsorption syndromes and adults and children who eliminate high-zinc foods from their diet while consuming diets high in fiber. A recent systematic review examined the effect of zinc supplementation on the prevention of mortality, morbidity and growth failure of children in middle- and low-income countries. They found that zinc supplementation significantly reduced death due to diarrhea, respiratory infection and malaria and modestly improved height.[21]

RECAP

Zinc is a trace mineral that is a part of almost 300 enzymes that affect virtually every body system. Zinc also helps maintain the structural integrity and shape of proteins, and regulates gene expression and cell signaling. Overall, zinc plays roles in hemoglobin synthesis, physical growth and sexual maturation, immune function, and antioxidant defenses. For adult men and women, the RDA for zinc is 11 and 8 mg/day. Good food sources of zinc include red meats, some seafood, whole grains, and enriched grains and cereals. ▪

LO 6 Discuss the functions, RDA, and food sources of copper.

What Is the Role of Copper in Blood Health?

Copper is a trace mineral required for a number of oxidation reactions, including those involved in iron transport. Fortunately, copper is widely distributed in foods and deficiency is rare.

Copper Functions in Blood Health and Energy Metabolism

In the body, copper is primarily found as a component of ceruloplasmin, a protein that is critical for its transport. Indeed, an individual's copper status is typically assessed by measuring plasma levels of ceruloplasmin. As we mentioned in the discussion of iron, ceruloplasmin is important for the oxidation of ferrous to ferric iron ($Fe^{2+} \rightarrow Fe^{3+}$), which is necessary before iron can bind to transferrin and be transported in the plasma.[5] Because of ceruloplasmin's role in iron metabolism, it is also called ferroxidase I. When ceruloplasmin is inadequate, the transport of iron for heme formation is impaired and anemia can result. Because iron cannot be transported properly, iron accumulates in the tissues, causing symptoms similar to those of the genetic disorder hemochromatosis (page 473).

Copper also functions as a cofactor in the metabolic pathways that produce energy, in the production of the connective tissues collagen and elastin, and as part of the superoxide dismutase enzyme system that fights the damage caused by free radicals. Copper is also necessary for the regulation of certain neurotransmitters, especially serotonin, important to nervous system function.

Several Factors Influence Copper Absorption and Transport

The major site of copper absorption is in the small intestine, with small amounts also absorbed in the stomach. As with zinc and iron, the amount of copper absorbed is related to the amount of copper in the diet, with absorption decreasing on high-copper diets and increasing on low-copper diets. Thus, regulation of copper absorption is one of the primary ways the body maintains good copper balance.

Copper is transported into the enterocytes through the use of carrier proteins. Once in the enterocytes copper is bound to amino acids or proteins, where it can be used within the enterocyte, stored, or actively transported out of the enterocyte.[6] Copper is then transported in the portal blood to the liver bound to albumin (as with zinc). In the liver, about 60% to 70% of the copper is incorporated into ceruloplasmin, where it is then released into the plasma for general circulation and distribution to other tissues.[6] Copper is lost in the feces when enterocytes are sloughed off into the lumen. When the copper in bile is not reabsorbed, it, too, is lost in the feces.

How Much Copper Should We Consume?

As with iron and zinc, our need for copper is small, but our dietary intakes are variable and, as we have seen, absorption is influenced by a number of factors. People who eat a varied diet can easily meet their requirements for copper. High zinc intakes can reduce copper absorption and, subsequently, copper status. In fact, zinc supplementation is used as a treatment for a rare genetic disorder called Wilson's disease, in which copper toxicity occurs. High iron intakes can also interfere with copper absorption. The RDA for copper for men and women aged 19 years and older is 900 µg/day. The UL for adults aged 19 years and older is 10 mg/day.[5]

Good food sources of copper include organ meats, seafood, nuts, and seeds. Whole-grain foods are also relatively good sources. **Figure 12.8** reviews some foods relatively high in copper.

The long-term effects of copper toxicity are not well studied in humans. However, accidental copper toxicity has occurred by drinking beverages that have come into contact with copper.[6] Toxicity symptoms include abdominal pain and cramps, nausea, diarrhea, and vomiting. Liver damage occurs in the extreme cases of copper toxicity seen with Wilson's disease and other health conditions associated with excessive copper levels. In Wilson's disease, the copper accumulates in the liver because the liver cells cannot incorporate the copper into ceruloplasmin or eliminate it in the bile.[6]

Copper deficiency is rare but can occur in premature infants fed milk-based formulas and in adults fed prolonged formulated diets that are deficient in copper. Deficiency symptoms include anemia, reduced levels of white blood cells, and osteoporosis in infants and growing children, in whom the lack of copper contributes to bone demineralization.

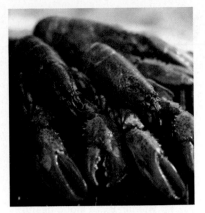

Lobster is a food that contains copper.

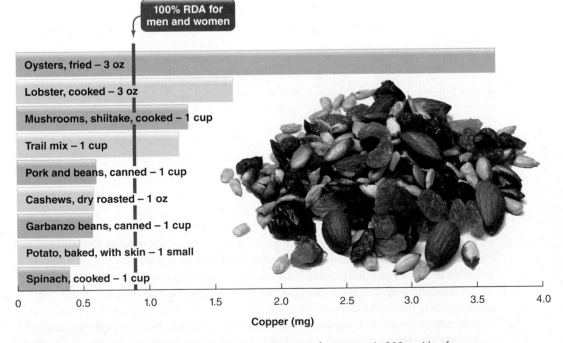

FIGURE 12.8 Common food sources of copper. The RDA for copper is 900 µg/day for men and women. (*Source:* Data from U.S. Department of Agriculture, Agricultural Research Service. 2005. USDA -Nutrient Database for Standard Reference, Release 21. www.ars.usda .gov/Services/docs.htm?docid=8964.)

Watch a video from the National Library of Medicine to learn more about blood clotting at http://www.nlm.nih.gov.

LO 7 Discuss the functions and sources of vitamin K.

LO 8 Discuss the contributions of vitamin B_6, folate, and vitamin B_{12} to blood health.

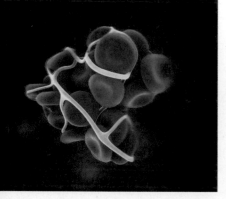

Blood clotting. Without enough vitamin K, the blood will not clot properly.

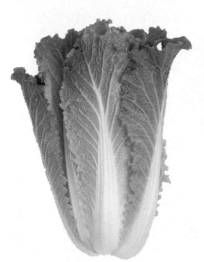

Green, leafy vegetables are a good source of vitamin K.

RECAP

Copper is a component of ceruloplasmin, a protein that is critical for the proper transport of iron. This trace mineral is also a cofactor in energy metabolism, in the production of the connective tissues collagen and elastin, and in the superoxide dismutase antioxidant enzyme system. For adults, the RDA for copper is 900 µg/day. Good food sources of copper include organ meats, seafood, nuts, and seeds. ∎

What Vitamins Help Maintain Blood Health?

The vitamins recognized as playing a critical role in maintaining blood health include vitamin K, vitamin B_6, folate, and vitamin B_{12} (see Table 12.1, page 465). Each of these vitamins has multiple functions, some of which were discussed in previous chapters. Here, we focus on their role in blood health.

Vitamin K Assists in the Synthesis of Clotting Factors

Vitamin K is a fat-soluble vitamin important for both bone and blood health. Although a number of compounds exhibit vitamin K activity, the primary forms are phylloquinones and menaquinones. Phylloquinones are the form of vitamin K found in green plants and the primary form of vitamin K in our diet, whereas menaquinones are primarily consumed in foods that contain fat (plant oils, eggs, fish, and butter) and are synthesized in the body from phylloquinones or in the intestine from bacteria. Dietary menaquinones account for about 25% of dietary vitamin K[22] and are the primary form of vitamin K in the body.[23] The role of vitamin K in the synthesis of proteins involved in maintaining bone density was discussed in Chapter 11. In this section, we focus on its role in blood health.

Vitamin K derives its name from the Danish word *koagulation*, which means "coagulation."[6] Vitamin K acts as a coenzyme that assists in the synthesis of a number of proteins involved in the coagulation of blood, including *prothrombin* and the *procoagulants, factors VII, IX,* and *X.* Without adequate vitamin K, the blood does not clot properly: clotting time can be delayed or clotting may even fail to occur. The failure of the blood to clot can lead to increased bleeding from even minor wounds, as well as internal hemorrhaging.

Because vitamin K is a fat-soluble vitamin, it is absorbed into the enterocyte, incorporated into chylomicrons, and then released into the lymphatic system with other dietary fats and fat-soluble vitamins. Any factors, either dietary or intestinal, that disrupt fat absorption will also disrupt vitamin K absorption. Vitamin K is found in all the circulating lipoproteins; therefore, vitamin K status is typically assessed by measuring plasma phylloquinones.[24] Research on the role of menaquinones in human health is more limited, thus, the RDA for vitamin K was based on plasma levels of phylloquinones.[22]

Although both forms of vitamin K are found in the liver, the phylloquinones are rapidly turned over and lost in the urine and bile. The liver does not store large amounts of vitamin K as it does other fat-soluble vitamins. The majority of vitamin K is stored in cell membranes of tissues such as the lungs, kidney, and bone marrow.[6]

The AI for vitamin K for men and women 19 years of age and older is 120 µg/day and 90 µg/day, respectively. There is no UL established for vitamin K at this time.[5]

Although our needs for vitamin K are relatively small, intakes of this nutrient in the United States are highly variable because vitamin K is found in relatively few foods.[5] In general, green, leafy vegetables are the major sources of vitamin K in our diet. Good sources include collard greens, kale, spinach, broccoli, brussels sprouts, and cabbage. Soybean and canola oils are also good sources.

Healthful bacteria residing in the large intestine produce vitamin K, providing us with an important nondietary source; thus, the amount of vitamin K needed from the diet will depend on intestinal health. Factors that reduce the ability of the gastrointestinal bacteria to produce vitamin K—such as excessive use of broad-spectrum antibiotics—also reduce our total vitamin K status.[6]

There are no known side effects associated with consuming large amounts of vitamin K from supplements or from food.[5] In the past, a synthetic form of vitamin K was used for therapeutic purposes and was shown to cause liver damage; this form is no longer used.

Vitamin K deficiency inhibits the blood's ability to clot, resulting in excessive bleeding and even severe hemorrhaging in some cases. Fortunately, vitamin K deficiency is rare in humans. People with diseases that cause malabsorption of fat, such as celiac disease, Crohn's disease, and cystic fibrosis, can suffer secondarily from a deficiency of vitamin K. Newborns are typically given an injection of vitamin K at birth, as they lack the intestinal bacteria necessary to produce this nutrient.

RECAP

Vitamin K is a fat-soluble vitamin and coenzyme that is important for blood clotting and bone metabolism. The AI for vitamin K for men and women 19 years of age and older is 120 µg/day and 90 µg/day, respectively. Green, leafy vegetables are the major source of vitamin K in our diet. Bacteria manufacture vitamin K in the large intestine. Deficiency inhibits the blood's ability to clot. ◼

Vitamin B$_6$ Is Essential for the Synthesis of Heme

Vitamin B$_6$ is essential for the synthesis of heme, the importance of which you learned about in the discussion of iron earlier in this chapter. It is required for the formation of the porphyrin ring that surrounds iron (see the lower portion of Figure 12.2) and therefore is an integral part of the heme complex. Without vitamin B$_6$, heme synthesis is impaired, just as it is with iron deficiency. For this reason, although we associate microcytic hypochromic anemia with iron deficiency, a deficiency in vitamin B$_6$ can also cause it. However, iron deficiency is the more common cause.

The RDA for vitamin B$_6$ for adult men and women aged 19 to 50 is 1.3 mg/day. In older adults, the RDA increases to 1.5 mg for women and 1.7 mg/day for men. The UL for vitamin B$_6$ is 100 mg/day.

Vitamin B$_6$ is abundant in meats, poultry, fish, and soy-based meat substitutes. Ready-to-eat cereals and starchy vegetables are also good sources. As discussed (in Chapter 8), high-dose supplements of vitamin B$_6$ can be toxic to nerves; however, toxicity is not seen with the consumption of B$_6$ in foods. In addition to inhibiting red blood cell production, vitamin B$_6$ deficiency impairs protein metabolism and the synthesis of neurotransmitters.

Folate Is Essential for the Production of Red Blood Cells

Folate is one of the B-vitamins (discussed in Chapter 8). The generic term *folate* is used for all the various forms of food folate that demonstrate biological activity. Folic acid (pteroylglutamate; see Figure 8.12, page 317) is the form of folate found in most supplements and used in the enrichment and fortification of foods.

Folate is important for synthesis of DNA and amino acids, and folate deficiency impairs the normal production of red blood cells. Much of the folate circulating in the blood is attached to transport proteins, especially albumin, for transport to cells of the body. The red blood cells also contain folate attached to hemoglobin. Because this folate is not transferred out of the red blood cells to other tissues, it may be a good measure of folate status over the past 4 months—the life of red blood cells.[6] If red blood cell folate levels begin to drop, this indicates that when the red blood cells were being formed, folate was inadequate in the body.

The RDA for folate for adult men and women aged 19 years and older is 400 µg/day. The RDA for pregnant women is 600 µg/day.[25] These levels reflect the importance of folate in the earliest weeks of pregnancy, when folate deficiency is linked to an increased risk for

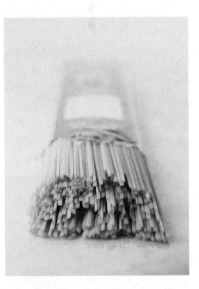

Ready-to-eat grain products, such as pasta, are often fortified with folic acid.

birth defects, including neural tube defects. (The role of folate during pregnancy is discussed in detail in Chapter 17.) UL for folate is 1,000 µg/day.

Folate is so important for good health and the prevention of birth defects that in 1998 the U.S. Department of Agriculture (USDA) mandated the fortification with folic acid of enriched breads, flours, corn meals, rice, pastas, and other grain products. Because folic acid is highly available for absorption, the goal of this fortification was to increase folate intake in all Americans and thus decrease the risk for the birth defects and chronic diseases associated with low folate intakes (see **Figure 12.9**).

Because of fortification, ready-to-eat cereals, bread, and other grain products are among the primary sources of folate in the United States; however, you need to read the label of processed grain products to make sure they contain folate. Other good food sources include liver, spinach, lentils, oatmeal, asparagus, and romaine lettuce.

Folate deficiency progresses in stages similar to those seen with iron:[26]

- *Stage I, or negative folate balance:* As the body has less and less folate available to it, the serum levels of folate begin to decline.
- *Stage II, or folate depletion:* If folate is not increased in the diet or through supplementation, then folate depletion occurs, characterized by both low serum and red blood cell folate, with slightly elevated serum homocysteine concentrations.
- *Stage III, or folate-deficiency erythropoiesis:* The folate levels in the body are low enough that the ability to synthesize new red blood cells (erythropoiesis) is inhibited.
- *Stage IV, or folate-deficiency anemia:* The number of red blood cells has declined because folate is not available for DNA synthesis, and macrocytic anemia develops.

Macrocytic anemias are characterized by the production of larger-than-normal red blood cells (macrocytes) containing insufficient hemoglobin to transport adequate oxygen. Symptoms of macrocytic anemias are similar to those of microcytic anemias and include weakness, fatigue, difficulty concentrating, irritability, headache, shortness of breath, and reduced work tolerance. Because vitamin B_{12} deficiency also causes macrocytic anemia, it is important for healthcare providers to determine if a patient's symptoms are due to a folate or a vitamin B_{12} deficiency.

Vitamin B_{12} Is Necessary for the Proper Formation of Red Blood Cells

Vitamin B_{12} is part of coenzymes that assist with DNA synthesis, which is necessary for the proper formation of red blood cells.[25] It also assists in the regeneration of folic acid during red blood cell formation. As discussed (in Chapter 8), alterations in total body vitamin B_{12} status mimic those seen with iron and folate, with states of deficiency developing as the amount of vitamin B_{12} decreases in the body.[25,26] As vitamin B_{12} status decreases, the body's ability to synthesize new red blood cells decreases:

- *Stage I, or negative vitamin B_{12} balance:* a decline in the blood level of cobalamin attached to its transport protein. This occurs as vitamin B_{12} absorption declines, decreasing the amount of total vitamin B_{12} available to the body.
- *Stage II, or vitamin B_{12} depletion.* If vitamin B_{12} absorption is not increased or B_{12} supplementation provided, then blood levels of cobalamin attached to its transport protein continue to decline, resulting in a decreased saturation of the transport protein with cobalamin.
- *Stage III, or vitamin B_{12}–deficiency erythropoiesis.* The body's level of vitamin B_{12} is so low that the ability to synthesize new red blood cells is inhibited.
- *Stage IV, called vitamin B_{12}–deficiency anemia.* The number of red blood cells has declined because vitamin B_{12} is not available for DNA synthesis, and macrocytic anemia develops.

The RDA for vitamin B_{12} for adult men and women aged 19 and older is 2.4 µg/day. Vitamin B_{12} is found primarily in dairy products, eggs, meats, poultry, fish, and shellfish.

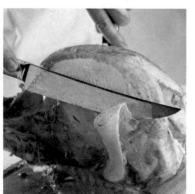

Turkey contains vitamin B_{12}.

macrocytic anemia A form of anemia manifested as the production of larger than normal red blood cells containing insufficient hemoglobin; also called megaloblastic anemia. Macrocytic anemia can be caused by folate deficiency or vitamin B_{12} deficiency.

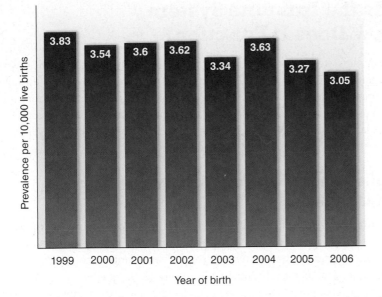

FIGURE 12.9 Prevalence of spina bifida in the years following mandatory folate fortification. (*Source:* Centers for Disease Control and Prevention, Spina bifida, data and statistics, 2011.)

Individuals consuming a vegan diet need to eat foods that are fortified with vitamin B_{12} or take vitamin B_{12} supplements or injections.

Pernicious anemia is classified as a type of macrocytic anemia and is associated with vitamin B_{12} deficiency. Pernicious anemia occurs at the end stage of an autoimmune disorder that causes the loss of various cells in the stomach, including the parietal cells that produce intrinsic factor. As you learned (in Chapter 8), intrinsic factor binds to vitamin B_{12} in the small intestine and aids its absorption into the enterocyte. Without intrinsic factor, vitamin B_{12} cannot be absorbed from the gut. It is estimated that approximately 1% to 3% of adults over age 60 have pernicious anemia due to lack of intrinsic factor.[27,28]

Macrocytic anemia can also occur in people who consume little or no vitamin B_{12} in their diet, such as people following a vegan diet. It is also commonly seen in people with malabsorption disorders, such as people with tapeworm infestation of the gut, as the worms take up the vitamin B_{12} before it can be absorbed by the intestines.

In addition to the symptoms associated with all anemias—such as pale skin, reduced energy and exercise tolerance, fatigue, and shortness of breath—lack of B_{12} also causes the destruction of the myelin sheath covering nerve cells, which facilitates nerve impulse transmission. As we saw in the scenario of Mr. Katz (in Chapter 8), after the onset of neurological deficits, even prompt intramuscular injections of vitamin B_{12} cannot entirely reverse the decline.

As mentioned earlier, a deficiency of either folate or vitamin B_{12} causes similar symptoms, and high doses of folate supplements can mask the physical symptoms of vitamin B_{12} deficiency, so that this deficiency progresses unchecked and causes neurologic damage.[25] Thus, before treatment for macrocytic anemia can occur, the cause must be identified.

RECAP

Three B vitamins, vitamin B_6, folate, and vitamin B_{12}, are essential to blood health. All are involved in the synthesis of new red blood cells. Deficiency of vitamin B_6 can result in a form of microcytic anemia, whereas deficiency of folate or B_{12} can result in macrocytic anemia. Meat, poultry, and fish are excellent sources of vitamins B_6 and B_{12}, whereas green vegetables and fortified grain products are our primary sources of folate.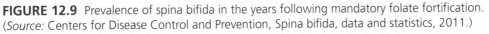

pernicious anemia A form of macrocytic anemia that is the primary cause of a vitamin B_{12} deficiency; occurs at the end stage of an autoimmune disorder that causes the loss of various cells in the stomach.

LO 9 Compare and contrast nonspecific and specific immunity.

What Is the Immune System, and How Does It Function?

A healthy immune system protects the body from infectious diseases, helps heal wounds, and guards against the development of cancers. Made up of cells and tissues throughout the body, the immune system acts as an integrated network to carry out surveillance against invaders such as bacteria and viruses, as well as enemies within, such as infected body cells and cancer cells, and destroy them before they can cause significant disease. There are two basic types of immune function: nonspecific or specific immunity.

Nonspecific Immune Function Protects against All Potential Invaders

Nonspecific immune function is the body's first line of defense against microbes, airborne particles, venom, and ingested toxins. Nonspecific immunity is active even if you are encountering the invader for the first time. Because even infants have all of the cells and tissues required for it to operate effectively, it is also called *innate immunity*.

Nonspecific defenses include intact skin and healthy mucous membranes, which block invaders from entering the blood, lungs, and other deeper tissues. Coughing, sneezing, vomiting, and diarrhea all expel harmful agents before they can multiply. Foodborne microbes can also be destroyed by stomach acid. Even tears contain enzymes that attack potentially harmful microbes and wash them out of the eyes.

In addition, a variety of immune cells, including macrophages, neutrophils, and natural killer (NK) cells, work together to directly kill a wide variety of harmful microbes, or to kill infected body cells or cells with damaged DNA that otherwise could multiply to form a tumor.

Finally, our nonspecific defenses include the release of inflammatory chemicals that cause discomfort, loss of appetite, fatigue, and fever: most disease-causing microbes thrive at normal body temperature, whereas a high temperature inhibits their growth. Fever also facilitates the actions of cells and chemicals involved in repair.

Together, our nonspecific defenses can inhibit the penetration and reproduction of invaders until the slower-acting, but more effective, specific immune system is activated.

Specific Immune Function Protects against Identified Antigens

Specific immune function is directed against recognized **antigens**—that is, large proteins on microbes or other foes that the immune system has encountered before and recognizes as foreign, or *non-self*. But how does this recognition occur?

The first time the immune system encounters a substance with an antigen that is detected as non-self, it produces a primary immune response. This response takes several days to peak, but eventually, in most cases, it destroys the invader. A key process within that primary immune response is the production of **memory cells** dedicated to the task of seeking out and destroying any substance bearing that particular antigen. Memory cells remain in circulation (in some cases, for life), so that any subsequent encounter with the same antigen causes a faster and stronger response. Often, the response is so fast that the person does not even feel sick.

Cells of Specific Immunity

In specific immune responses, two primary types of immune cells are activated:

- **B cells** are a type of white blood cell. During a primary immune response, B cells differentiate into two types: the memory cells just described and **plasma cells.** The job of plasma cells is to produce thousands of *antibodies,* proteins that attach to recognized antigens on invaders and flag them for destruction. In fact, the term *antigen* reflects this antibody-generating response.

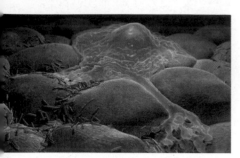

A macrophage is a type of nonspecific immune cell. The one shown here is about to engulf an invading microbe.

nonspecific immune function Generalized body defenses including tissues, mechanisms, and cells that protect against the entry or reproduction of non-self agents, such as microbes, toxins, and body cells with mutated DNA; also called *innate immunity*.

specific immune function The strongest defense against pathogens. It requires adaptation of white blood cells that recognize antigens and that multiply to protect against the pathogens carrying those antigens; also called *adaptive immunity* or *acquired immunity*.

antigens Parts of a molecule, usually large proteins, from microbes, toxins, or other substances that are recognized by immune cells and activate an immune response.

memory cells White blood cells that recognize a particular antigen and circulate in the body, ready to respond if the antigen is encountered again. The purpose of vaccination is to create memory cells.

B cells White blood cells that can become either antibody-producing plasma cells or memory cells.

plasma cells White blood cells that have differentiated from activated B cells and produce millions of antibodies to an antigen during an infection.

- **T cells** are also white blood cells. They differentiate into several types, the most important of which are cytotoxic T cells and helper T cells. As their name suggests, **cytotoxic T cells** are toxic to body cells harboring microbes or any other non-self substances. For instance, by killing body cells that have been infected by a flu virus, they keep the virus from multiplying and spreading. **Helper T cells** don't kill directly. Rather, they manufacture chemicals that call in macrophages to consume microbes, prompt B cells to speed up their production of antibodies, and activate cytotoxic T cells to kill cells displaying non-self markers.

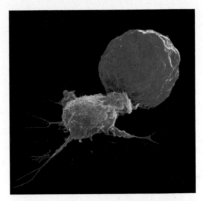

Natural killer (NK) cells are part of our nonspecific defenses. Here, an NK cell attacks one cancer cells.

Acquisition of Specific Immunity

There are four primary ways in which humans acquire immunity to specific invaders:

- One natural way is to have a disease once. For example, if you had mumps as a child, you will never get it again, because memory cells against mumps are continuously circulating throughout your body.
- **Vaccinations** (also called *immunizations*) are another way to develop immunity. When you are vaccinated, a small amount of weakened, killed, or inactivated microbe or toxin is injected into your body. Your plasma cells produce antibodies against this antigen, and memory cells begin to circulate. If you encounter the microbe or toxin later, your immune response will protect you from getting sick.
- When a woman is pregnant, antibodies from her blood pass into the bloodstream of her fetus. These maternal antibodies protect a newborn during the first few months of life while the specific immune system is maturing. In addition, breast milk contains antibodies that protect the infant for as long as he or she nurses.
- The injection of **antiserum** can provide immediate protection from a specific foe—for instance, to snake venom in the bloodstream of a victim of a snakebite. Antiserum is a pharmacologic preparation containing antibodies to specific antigens, such as those in snake venom. Injection of this antibody-rich serum provides immediate protection. Without it, the snake venom would be fatal before the victim's immune system could produce antibodies.

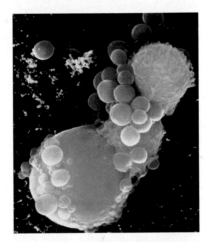

Two cytotoxic T cells (orange) killing another cell (mauve).

Immune System Disorders

A malfunctioning immune system can damage body tissues or prevent the resolution of infection. For example, during allergic reactions, the immune system "interprets" harmless proteins that enter the body from the environment or food as dangerous and produces a hypersensitivity immune response. This can provoke a variety of symptoms, from a rash to wheezing to intestinal inflammation. Autoimmune responses occur when the body's own proteins are mistaken for pathogens. This occurs, for example, in type 1 diabetes and results in destruction of the insulin-producing cells of the pancreas.

In some people, the immune system is compromised and cannot effectively quell infections. Chronic infection is commonly seen in malnourished individuals, as well as in people with immunodeficiency diseases. Cancer patients and transplant recipients also are more susceptible to infection when they are taking immunosuppressive drugs.

T cells White blood cells that are of several varieties, including cytotoxic T cells and helper T cells.

cytotoxic T cells Activated T cells that kill infected body cells.

helper T cells Activated T cells that secrete chemicals needed to recruit, promote, or activate other immune cells.

vaccination The method of administering a small amount of antigen to elicit an immune response for the purpose of developing memory cells that will protect against the disease at a later time.

antiserum Human or animal serum that contains antibodies to a particular antigen because of previous exposure to the disease or to a vaccine containing antigens from that infectious agent.

RECAP

The main function of the immune system is to protect the body against foreign agents. Nonspecific defenses include skin, mucous membranes, enzymes, inflammatory chemicals, and certain defensive cells. Specific immunity is provided by B cells and T cells. B cells include plasma cells, which produce antibodies, and memory cells, which persist in the body, seeking the antigens to which they are sensitized. Cytotoxic T cells directly kill body cells displaying non-self markers, such as cells infected with a virus, whereas helper T cells help macrophages, B cells, and cytotoxic T cells perform their roles. Specific immunity can be acquired by experiencing a disease, by vaccination, from maternal antibodies, and from antiserum. Immune disorders include hypersensitivity reactions, autoimmune diseases, and compromised immunity.

LO 10 Describe the role of protein–energy malnutrition, obesity, essential fatty acids, and key micronutrients in immune function.

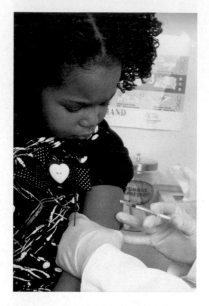

Vaccinations provide active immunity.

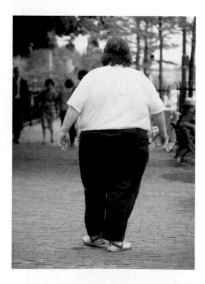

Obesity has been linked to disorders involving chronic inflammation, such as asthma, hypertension, heart disease, and type 2 diabetes.

immunocompetence The body's ability to adequately produce an effective immune response to an antigen.

How Does Nutrition Affect the Immune System?

A nourishing diet provides all the nutrients the immune system needs to carry out its defense of the body. Single-nutrient deficiencies or subclinical deficiencies can cause subtle, but important, abnormalities in immune function, even in apparently healthy people. This type of malnutrition is common in hospitalized individuals and the elderly.[29] Research has demonstrated that viruses multiplying in malnourished hosts actually become more infective and destructive than viruses multiplying in well-nourished hosts.[30]

Protein–Energy Malnutrition Impairs Immune Function

Malnutrition and infection participate in a vicious cycle: malnutrition increases the risk for infection; infection depresses appetite and often causes vomiting and diarrhea; decreased appetite, vomiting, and diarrhea cause malnutrition, which increases vulnerability to infection. Infection diverts needed nutrients toward mounting an immune response to the infection, further decreasing nutrition status in already compromised individuals.[31] Specifically, protein–energy malnutrition (see Chapter 6) is known to severely diminish the ability of the immune system to respond to antigens. Malnourished children show reduced production of antibodies and diminished capacity of their immune cells to kill bacteria.[32] In addition, a healthy immune response requires energy and amino acids, two things that are in short supply in a malnourished individual. By inhibiting the immune response to infection, malnutrition is estimated to kill 3.1 million children worldwide per year.[33]

The synergistic effect of protein–energy malnutrition and infection in diminishing both the capacity of the immune response and nutritional status is now widely recognized. Because even moderate nutrient deficiencies impair immune function, it has been suggested that decreased **immunocompetence** is a sensitive indicator of reduced nutritional status.

Obesity Increases the Incidence and Severity of Infections

Obesity has become a public health issue much more recently than the problem of protein–energy malnutrition. Therefore, fewer studies have been done on the effects of obesity on immune function. However, obesity has been associated with increased susceptibility to and poorer outcomes from infection.[34] In the 2009–2010 influenza pandemic in the United Kingdom, obesity was identified as one of the major comorbidities associated with death.[35]

The mechanisms underlying lower immune function in obese individuals are unclear. Research suggests a reduced ability of B and T cells to multiply in response to stimulation, and a decrease in the activity of NK cells.[34] Overall, obesity is associated with a persistent low-grade inflammatory response, resulting in elevated levels of macrophages, inflammatory chemicals, and immune proteins.[34,36] This inflammatory state is currently thought to increase the likelihood that obese individuals will develop chronic diseases associated with inflammation such as asthma, hypertension, cardiovascular disease, and type 2 diabetes.[34] Weight loss is associated with a decrease in inflammatory markers in the blood.[34]

Essential Fatty Acids Make Signaling Molecules for the Immune System

As previously noted (in Chapter 5), the essential fatty acids are precursors for important signaling molecules called eicosanoids. The immune system requires certain eicosanoids to respond appropriately to threatening agents. Experimental dietary deficiency of essential fatty acids in animals impairs aspects of the immune response. In humans, research shows that supplementation of the diet with EPA and DHA reduces inflammation and may be useful in treating some chronic inflammatory conditions such as rheumatoid arthritis, inflammatory bowel disease, and cardiovascular disease.[31,34]

Certain Vitamins and Minerals Are Critical to a Strong Immune Response

Although all essential nutrients are likely needed in some measure for effective immune function, certain micronutrient deficiencies and toxicities have been recognized as particularly important:

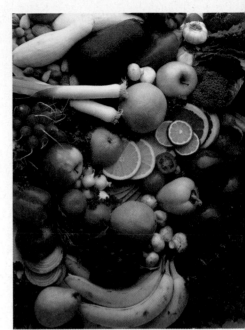

- *Vitamin A.* As early as the 1920s, vitamin A was called "the anti-infective vitamin" because it is needed to maintain the mucosal surfaces of the respiratory, gastrointestinal, and genitourinary tracts and for differentiation of immune system cells. Clinical trials have clearly shown that vitamin A supplementation in populations with low vitamin A status reduces the incidence and fatality of respiratory infections and infections of measles, malaria, and diarrheal diseases.[31] Correspondingly, infections can increase the risk of vitamin A deficiency. Diarrhea, respiratory infections, measles, chickenpox and human immunodeficiency virus (HIV) are all associated with an increased risk of developing vitamin A deficiency.[31]

- *Vitamins C and E.* The immune activities of defensive cells such as macrophages require oxygen and generate a highly reactive molecule, called a *reactive oxygen species*, that can damage the cell membrane if there is insufficient antioxidant protection. Both vitamin C and vitamin E provide this protection.

Vitamins E and C, found in fruits and vegetables, can contribute to immune system health.

- *Zinc.* As discussed earlier, the importance of zinc to immune function was suggested by the observation that Middle Easteners whose growth was stunted by zinc deficiency also died of infections by their early twenties. Zinc is also important for antioxidant defenses, gene expression, and enzyme activation for B and T cell proliferation.[31] Even marginal zinc deficiency impairs immune response. In fact, low plasma levels of zinc are used to predict development of respiratory infection and diarrhea in malnourished populations, among whom diarrhea is considered a symptom of zinc deficiency.[31] However, excessive zinc supplementation depresses immunity, possibly by causing copper deficiency.

- *Selenium.* In trace amounts, selenium is necessary for the synthesis of 25 selenoproteins within the body many of which are important enzymes.[37] Selenium has two roles in immune function. It is a required coenzyme for glutathione peroxidase and thioredoxin reductase, two important antioxidant enzymes in immune cells. It also promotes proper B and T cell proliferation and antibody production. Selenium deficiency in an infected host also permits viruses to multiply over a longer time period and to mutate into more pathogenic strains.[38]

- *Iron and Copper.* Both iron and copper are part of two important antioxidant enzymes, superoxide catalase and dismutase.[38] Thus, deficiencies of these nutrients have numerous effects on the body's immune response, especially the functions of B and T cells. Macrophages take up and store iron during an infection and seem unaffected by deficiency. This storage is thought to be beneficial because it keeps iron away from invading microbes, which require iron to multiply. This may explain why some studies show that iron supplementation given to children during infection is detrimental, and why iron toxicity increases the rate of infections.[31,38] In addition, excessive iron is a potent pro-oxidant that can damage immune-cell membranes.

We've said that infections such as diarrhea can sometimes prompt deficiencies of specific micronutrients such as vitamin A. Moreover, infection can alter nutritional status overall in the following ways:[31]

- *Reduced food intake.* Illness or infections frequently reduce appetite and overall energy intake by as little 5% to total cessation of food intake. Of course, not eating during a time when nutrient demands are high can lead to decreases in nutritional status. If this condition persists, nutrient deficiencies can occur.

■ *Increased nutrient loss, or malabsorption.* If an infection causes diarrhea or vomiting, nutrients, especially fluids and electrolytes, will be lost. Inflammation of the gut can also decrease nutrient absorption.

■ *Increased resting metabolic rate.* When infection is accompanied by fever, metabolic rate increases. For every 1°C increase in temperature, metabolic rate increases by 13%, a significant increase in energy needs. Even if illness is accompanied by reduced activity, increased energy expenditure at a time when food intake is low or diarrhea or vomiting are present can dramatically increase the loss of weight and lean tissue.

■ *Redistribution of energy and nutrients.* At the onset of infection, energy and nutrients are redirected to enhance the immune response. The energy and nutrients are then unavailable for other tissues to utilize for important biological functions. If it persists, this situation can result in decreased metabolic functioning and loss of lean tissue. Especially in individuals who are already malnourished when the infection occurs, this redistribution of important resources can slow recovery and compromise health.

RECAP

A nourishing diet is important in optimizing immune response. Protein–energy malnutrition increases the frequency and severity of infection. Obesity compromises immune response, exacerbating infection and inflammation. Essential fatty acids, vitamins A, C, and E and the minerals zinc, copper, iron, and selenium are all necessary for appropriate immune function. Correspondingly, infection can reduce appetite and food intake, promote loss or malabsorption of nutrients, increase energy expenditure by increasing resting metabolic rate, and redistribute energy and nutrients to favor immune responses at the expense of other body functions. ■

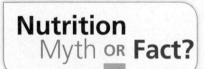

Nutrition Myth OR **Fact?**

Do Zinc Lozenges Help Fight the Common Cold?

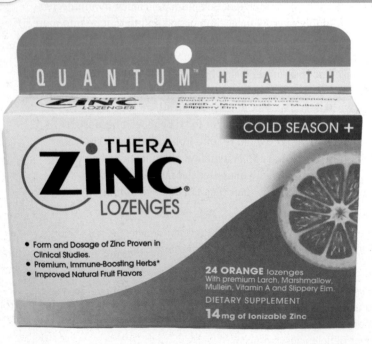

The common cold has plagued human beings since the beginning of time. Millions of colds occur each year in the United States.[1] Adults average 2 to 3 colds per year, whereas children under 2 have about six infections per year.[2] Although colds are typically benign, they cause discomfort and stress and result in approximately 22 million school days and 22 million work days lost each year.[3] Colds are also the most common reason people visit a medical professional, accounting for over 100 million primary care visits per year.[4] Finding a cure for the common cold has been at the forefront of modern medicine for many years.

It is estimated that more than 200 different viruses can cause a cold. The most frequent causes of adult colds are a group of viruses called rhinoviruses, which account for approximately half of all colds.[4] Even within the rhinovirus category, there are over a 100 different distinct viruses; thus, finding treatments or potential cures for a cold is extremely challenging.

The role of zinc in the overall health of our

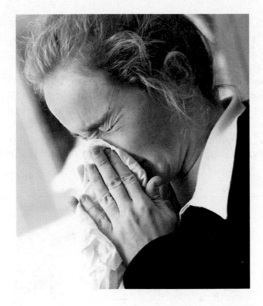

immune system is well known, but zinc has also been shown to inhibit the replication of rhinoviruses and other viruses that cause the common cold. These specific findings have suggested that taking zinc supplements may reduce the length and severity of colds.[4,5] Consequently, zinc lozenges have been formulated as a means of providing potential relief from cold symptoms. These lozenges are readily found in a variety of formulations and dosages in most drugstores.

Does taking zinc in lozenge form actually reduce the length and severity of a cold? During the past 25 years, numerous research studies have been conducted to try to answer this question. Unfortunately, the results have been mixed.[5] Three recent reviews examined between 13 and 17 randomized controlled trials (RCT) with over 966 to 2,121 participants.[4-6] The first study found a reduction in the severity and duration of the common cold with zinc lozenges or syrups (30–160 mg/day) if administered within 24 to 48 hours of the onset of the cold. Overall, the duration of the cold was reduced by about 1 day. Assessment of the severity of cold symptoms is more difficult, because there is no objective measure, but they did find that severity scores were very modestly reduced with supplementation. However, study participants reported significant negative effects from zinc supplementation as well, including a bad taste and nausea.[6] The second review divided the studies by zinc dose. It found that, if 75 mg/day or less of zinc was given, no effect occurred; however, in three studies in which 75 mg/day of zinc acetate was given, there was a 42% reduction in cold duration. There were five studies that gave over 75 mg/day of zinc salts other than zinc acetate. In these studies there was a 20% reduction in cold duration.[4] The third study reviewed all RCTs that administered zinc with placebo or no treatment in adults and children. Compared to a placebo, adults taking zinc supplements reported a shorter duration of their cold by 2.6 days, but there was no effect in children.

Unfortunately, we will probably never know the true effect of zinc lozenges on colds for the following reasons:

- *It is difficult to truly "blind" participants to the treatment.* Because zinc lozenges have a unique taste, it may be difficult to truly "blind" the research participants as to whether they are getting zinc lozenges or a placebo. Knowledge of which lozenge they are taking would bias study participants.

- *Self-reported symptoms are subject to inaccuracy.* Many studies had the research participants self-report changes in symptoms, which may be inaccurate and influenced by mood and other emotional factors.

- *Subject compliance may be suspect.* Typically, participants are required to take the lozenges on a set schedule for 6 to 10 days. Unless they monitor all participants, researchers are forced to rely on the participants' self-reports of their compliance with the study protocol. Differences in compliance could lead to differences in outcomes.

- *A wide variety of viruses cause the common cold.* More than 200 viruses can cause a cold. It is highly unlikely that zinc can combat all of them. It is possible that people who do not respond favorably to zinc lozenges are suffering from a cold virus that does not respond to zinc.

- *Zinc formulations and dosages differ.* The type of zinc formulation and the dosages of zinc consumed by study participants differ across studies, which may determine how quickly the zinc ions are delivered to the tissues in the mouth. These differences most likely have contributed to various responses across studies. As mentioned, it is estimated that, for zinc to be effective, at least 75 to 80 mg of zinc should be consumed each day and that people should begin using the lozenges within 24 to 48 hours of the onset of cold symptoms. Also, the sweeteners and flavorings found in many zinc lozenges, such as citric acid, sorbitol, and mannitol, may bind the zinc and inhibit its ability to be absorbed into the body, limiting its effectiveness.

Because there is suggestive, but not conclusive, evidence supporting modest effectiveness of zinc lozenges in combating colds, the debate over whether people should take them will most likely continue.

Critical Thinking Questions

- Have you ever tried zinc lozenges for a cold? If so, did you find them effective? Were you bothered by any unpleasant side effects, such as a persistent bad taste, alteration in your sense of smell, or nausea?

- Even if you have only about a 50/50 chance of reducing the length of your cold by 20% to 40% by taking zinc lozenges, do you think they're worth a try?

A word of caution: if you decide to use zinc lozenges, more is not necessarily better. Excessive or prolonged zinc supplementation can cause other mineral imbalances. Check the label of the product you are using, and do not exceed its recommended dosage or duration of use.

References

1. Center for Disease Control and prevention (CDC). 2015. Common Colds: Protect Yourself and Others. http://www.cdc.gov/features/rhinoviruses/ Accessed February 2015.

2. Allan, G. M., and B. Arroll. 2014. Prevention and treatment of the common cold: making sense of the evidence. *CMAJ* 186(3):190–199. DOI: http://dx.doi.org/10.1503/cmaj.121442

3. National Institute of Allergy and Infectious Diseases. National Institutes of Health. 2011. The Common Cold. www.niaid.nih.gov/topics/commonCold/Pages/overview.aspx. Accessed March 2012.

4. Singh, M., and R. R. Das. 2012. Zinc for the common cold. *Cochrane Database Syst. Rev.*. Issue 2. Art. No. Cd001364. DOI: 10.1002/14651858.

5. Science, M., J. Johnstone, D. E. Roth, G. Guyatt, and M. Loeb. 2012. Zinc for the treatment of the common cold: a systematic review and meta-analysis of randomized controlled trials. *CMAJ* 184(10):E551–561. DOI: http://dx.doi.org/10.1503/cmaj.111990

6. Hemila, H. 2011. Zinc lozenges may shorten the duration of colds: a systematic review. *Open Respir. Med. J.* 5:51–58.

STUDY **PLAN** MasteringNutrition™

Customize your study plan—and master your nutrition!—in the Study Area of MasteringNutrition.

TEST YOURSELF | *ANSWERS*

1 **T** Iron deficiency is particularly common in infants, children, and women of childbearing age.

2 **F** In addition to folate, vitamin B$_6$ and vitamin B$_{12}$ promote blood health.

3 **T** People who consume a vegan diet need to pay particularly close attention to consuming enough vitamin B$_{12}$, iron, and zinc. In some cases, these individuals may need to take supplements to consume adequate amounts of these nutrients.

4 **F** The term *anemia* means "without blood" and can refer to any condition in which hemoglobin levels are low. Iron-deficiency anemia is just one type.

5 **T** Fever increases body temperature, making the internal environment inhospitable to microbes and increasing the rate of protective immune reactions. Vomiting and diarrhea expel microbes and toxins from the gastrointestinal tract before they can cause widespread tissue damage.

summary

Scan to hear an MP3 Chapter Review in **MasteringNutrition**.

LO 1 ▪ Blood is critical for transporting oxygen and nutrients to cells and for removing waste products from cells so that these products can be properly excreted. It is also important in maintenance of a healthful body temperature.

▪ Blood is the only fluid tissue in the body. It has four components: erythrocytes, or red blood cells, which transport nutrients and oxygen; leukocytes, or white blood cells, which are the cells responsible for immune defenses; platelets, cell fragments important in blood clotting; and plasma, or the fluid portion of blood. Blood cells and platelets arise from stem cells in the bone marrow.

- Healthy blood requires adequate intake of fluids, protein, and several micronutrients, most importantly the trace minerals iron, zinc, and copper and vitamins K, B_6, folate, and B_{12}.

LO 2
- Iron is a trace mineral. Almost two-thirds of the iron in the body is found in hemoglobin, the oxygen-carrying protein in blood. One of the primary functions of iron is to assist with the transportation of oxygen in blood. Iron in hemoglobin picks up oxygen in the lungs and deposits it in body tissues.

LO 3
- The body tightly regulates iron absorption, transport, and storage. Absorption of iron from a mixed diet averages about 14% to 18%. However, absorption rates are influenced by multiple factors, including the individual's iron status, and the level and type of dietary iron consumed. Heme iron, available only from animal-based foods, is more absorbable than nonheme iron, which can be found in both animal and plant foods, as well as supplements. Consuming foods with a source of vitamin C can enhance iron absorption, whereas intake of calcium, fiber, and certain binding factors can reduce absorption.
- Iron can be stored within the enterocytes, or it can be transported across the membrane of the enterocytes by ferroportin. The body is capable of storing small amounts of iron as ferritin and hemosiderin.

LO 4
- Iron deficiency progresses from depletion of iron stores, a state that may only decrease ability to perform vigorous physical activity, to reduced iron transport and erythropoiesis, to iron-deficiency anemia, a form of microcytic anemia. In iron-deficiency anemia, the production of normal, healthy red blood cells with adequate hemoglobin levels decreases. The individual experiences fatigue, pale skin, depressed immune function, and impaired cognitive and nerve function, work performance, and memory. Deficiency of vitamin B_6 can also cause microcytic anemia.

LO 5
- Zinc is a trace mineral that acts as a cofactor in the production of hemoglobin; in the superoxide dismutase antioxidant enzyme system; in the metabolism of carbohydrates, fats, and proteins; and in activating vitamin A in the retina. Zinc is also critical for cell reproduction and growth and for proper development and functioning of the immune system.
- For adult men and women, the RDA for zinc is 11 and 8 mg/day. Good food sources of zinc include red meats, some seafood, whole grains, and enriched grains and cereals.

LO 6
- Copper is a trace mineral that functions as a cofactor in the metabolic pathways that produce energy, in the production of collagen and elastin, and as part of the superoxide dismutase antioxidant enzyme system. Copper is also a component of ceruloplasmin, a protein needed for the proper transport of iron.
- For adults, the RDA for copper is 900 µg/day. Good food sources of copper include organ meats, seafood, nuts, and seeds.

LO 7
- Vitamin K is a fat-soluble vitamin that acts as a coenzyme important for the synthesis of several clotting factors, proteins necessary for the coagulation of blood. Vitamin K is also a coenzyme in the synthesis of proteins that assist in maintaining bone density.
- Sources of vitamin K include green, leafy vegetables, soybean and canola oils, and production by the healthful bacteria residing in the large intestine.

LO 8
- Three B-vitamins involved in the synthesis of red blood cells are vitamin B_6, folate, and vitamin B_{12}. Vitamin B_6 is necessary for the synthesis of heme in hemoglobin. Folate is important for synthesis of DNA and amino acids, and folate deficiency impairs the normal production of red blood cells. Vitamin B_{12} is part of coenzymes that assist with DNA synthesis, which is necessary for the proper formation of red blood cells. It also assists in the regeneration of folate.
- Macrocytic anemia results from folate or vitamin B_{12} deficiency and causes the formation of excessively large red blood cells that have reduced hemoglobin. Symptoms are similar to those of microcytic anemia. One form of macrocytic anemia, called pernicious anemia, is caused by a deficit of intrinsic factor, which in turn results in vitamin B_{12} deficiency.

LO 9
- A healthy immune system is a network of cells and tissues that protects us from harmful invaders such as bacteria and their toxins, as well as from proliferation of cells with mutated DNA.
- Nonspecific defenses include the skin and mucosal membranes; protective molecules, such as mucus, stomach acid, and enzymes; and immune cells, such as macrophages, neutrophils, and NK cells.
- Specific immune function is directed against specific antigens. An initial encounter with a foreign agent triggers the development of immune cells that recognize that agent. On subsequent encounters with the same agent, these cells mount a faster, stronger immune response.

- The two primary types of cells involved in specific immunity are B cells and T cells. B cells include plasma cells, which produce antibodies that mark antigens for destruction, and memory cells that, after becoming sensitized to a specific antigen, circulate in the body, seeking that antigen. Cytotoxic T cells destroy body cells displaying non-self markers, and helper T cells assist macrophages, B cells, and cytotoxic T cells to respond.

- Human beings can acquire immunity by experiencing an infection, being vaccinated, receiving maternal antibodies, or receiving an injection of antiserum.

- Malfunctions of the immune system include allergies, autoimmune diseases, chronic inflammation, and immunodeficiencies.

LO 10
- Protein–energy malnutrition is linked to a greatly increased risk for infection and diminished capacity to respond to infection. Obesity can impair immune responses, and is associated with persistent, low-grade inflammation that is thought to play a role in many chronic diseases.

- Essential fatty acids are important for regulating immune function.

- Critical to immune function are vitamins A, C, and E and the minerals zinc, copper, iron, and selenium. For some nutrients, both deficiency and toxicity can impair immune response.

To further your understanding, go online and apply what you've learned to real-life case studies that will help you master the content!

review questions

LO 1 **1.** Erythrocytes
a. are essential for the transport of glucose, albumin, and many other solutes throughout the body.
b. lack a nucleus and mitochondria, and are filled with hemoglobin, which is essential for oxygen transport.
c. are involved in both non-specific and specific immunity.
d. are produced in the liver, whereas leukocytes and platelets are produced in the bone marrow.

LO 2 **2.** Which of the following statements about iron is true?
a. Every molecule of hemoglobin contains one atom of iron.
b. Iron is a component of hemoglobin, the oxygen-transport protein within red blood cells.
c. Iron in myoglobin accounts for about one-third of total iron in the body.
d. All of these statements are true.

LO 3 **3.** Jenna is an ovo-lacto vegetarian concerned about her iron intake. From which of the following breakfasts is she likely to absorb the greatest percentage of iron?
a. a bowl of iron-fortified cereal with cow's milk, and a cup of coffee
b. a bowl of iron-fortified cereal with soy milk, and a cup of tea
c. an iron-fortified breakfast bar with a glass of orange juice
d. a cheese croissant and a diet coke

LO 4 **4.** A classic sign of stage I iron-deficiency is
a. reduced levels of circulating ferritin.
b. a significantly elevated total iron binding capacity.
c. smaller than normal red blood cells that are pale in color.
d. exhaustion, impaired cognitive functions, and increased risk for infection.

LO 5 **5.** Zinc plays an important role in
a. heme synthesis.
b. maintaining the structural integrity of iron.
c. preventing copper deficiency.
d. reducing the risk for pernicious anemia.

LO 6 **6.** Good food sources of copper include
a. green, leafy vegetables and fortified grain products.
b. green, leafy vegetables and dairy products.
c. red, orange, and yellow fruits and vegetables.
d. organ meats, seafood, nuts, and seeds.

LO 7 **7.** The physiologic function most closely associated with vitamin K is
a. synthesis of heme.
b. blood clotting.
c. formation of the embryonic neural tube.
d. maintenance of the myelin sheath.

LO 8 **8.** Vitamin B_6, folate, and vitamin B_{12} are all required for
a. the formation of the porphyrin rings in heme.
b. the function of platelets.
c. erythropoiesis.
d. hemochromatosis.

LO 9 **9.** Which of the following cells produce antibodies involved in specific immune responses?
a. plasma cells
b. NK cells
c. macrophages
d. neutrophils

LO 10 **10.** A sensitive indicator of reduced nutritional status is
a. nausea and vomiting.
b. fatigue and weakness.
c. inflammation.
d. decreased immunocompetence.

true or false?

LO 1 **11. True or false?** Blood has four components: erythrocytes, leukocytes, platelets, and plasma.

LO 4 **12. True or false?** Iron deficiency causes pernicious anemia.

LO 6 **13. True or false?** Wilson's disease occurs when copper deficiency allows the accumulation of iron in the body.

LO 8 **14. True or false?** Macrocytic anemias can result from deficiency of either folate or vitamin B_{12}.

LO 10 **15. True or false?** Studies suggest that excessive vitamin A, iron, or selenium can impair immune function.

short answer

LO 3 **16.** Jessica is 11 years old and has just begun menstruating. She and her family members are vegans (that is, they consume only plant-based foods). Explain why Jessica's parents should be careful that their daughter consumes not only adequate iron and zinc but also adequate vitamin C.

LO 7 **17.** Explain why newborns are routinely given an injection of vitamin K shortly after birth.

LO 8 **18.** Janine is 23 years old and engaged to be married. She is 40 lb overweight, she has

hypertension, and her mother suffered a mild stroke recently, at age 45. For all these reasons, Janine is highly motivated to lose weight and has put herself on a strict, low-carbohydrate diet recommended by a friend. She now scrupulously avoids breads, cereals, pastries, pasta, rice, and "starchy" fruits and vegetables. Identify two reasons Janine should begin taking a folate supplement.

LO 10 **19.** What health risk do people who are emaciated and people who are obese have in common? Why?

math review

LO 5 **20.** About 2 g of zinc are stored in the body of an average adult. An adult male consumes 20 mg of zinc each day. He thereby builds his total body store of zinc every 100 days. Is this statement true or false, and why?

Answers to Review Questions and Math Review can be found online in the MasteringNutrition Study Area.

web links

www.ars.usda.gov/ba/bhnrc/ndl
Nutrient Data Laboratory Home Page
Click on "Reports for Single Nutrients" to find reports listing food sources for selected nutrients.

www.webmd.com
Web ME
Visit this site and search on anemia to learn about anemia and its various treatments.

http://www.unicef.org/nutrition/index. html http://www.unicef.org/search/search .php?q=Micronutrients&type=Main
UNICEF—Nutrition
This site provides information about micronutrient deficiencies in developing countries and the efforts to combat them.

www.nlm.nih.gov/medlineplus/
Medline Plus, U.S. National Library of Medicine, National Institutes of Health

Search this site for "neural tube defects" and find a wealth of information on the development and prevention of these conditions.

www.kidshealth.org/parent
Kidshealth.org
Search for "immune system" to find a good overview of the immune system.

www.fda.gov
U.S. Food and Drug Administration (FDA)
Click on "Food" and then "Dietary Supplements" for a wealth of information about various dietary supplements and the FDA's regulation of them.

www.dietary-supplements.info.nih.gov
Office of Dietary Supplements (ODS)
Go to this site to obtain current research results and reliable information about dietary supplements.

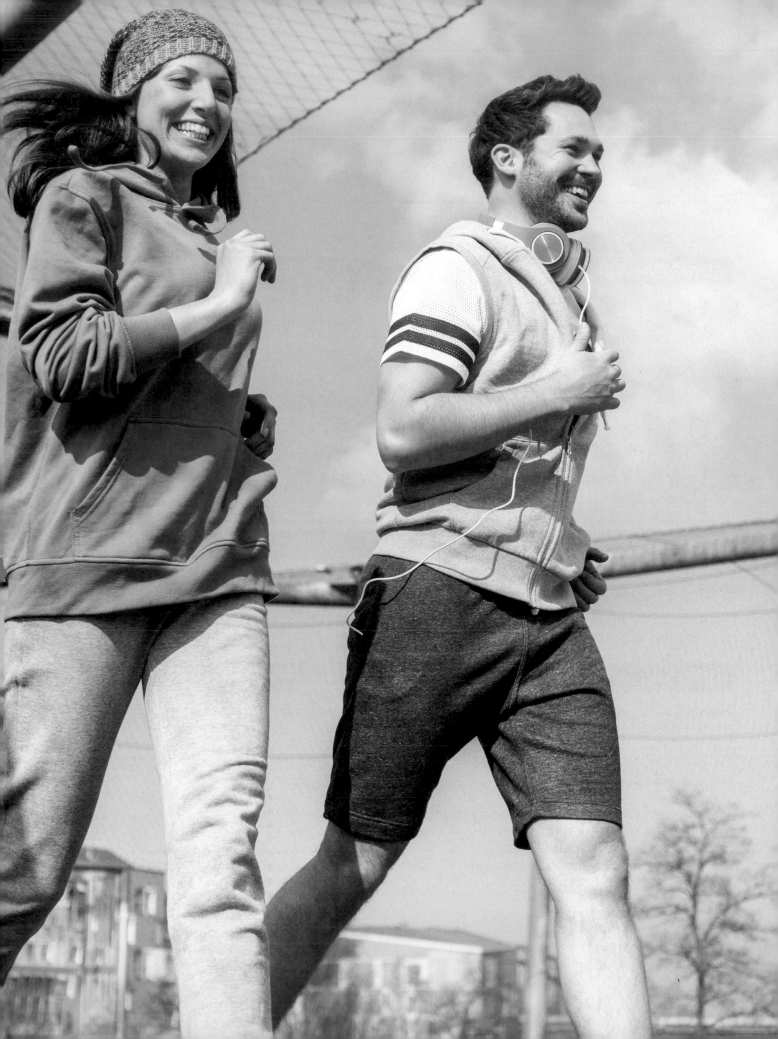

13 Achieving and Maintaining a Healthful Body Weight

Learning Outcomes

After studying this chapter, you should be able to:

1 Explain what is meant by a healthful weight, *p. 498.*

2 Define the terms *underweight, normal weight, overweight, obesity,* and *morbid obesity* and describe three methods you can use to evaluate your body weight, *pp. 499–503.*

3 Explain the concept of energy balance, *pp. 504–509.*

4 Discuss techniques used to measure energy expenditure, and three ways that the body expends energy, *pp. 504–511.*

5 List and describe several biological influences on body weight, *pp. 511–515.*

6 Discuss cultural, economic, and social influences on body weight, *pp. 515–518.*

7 Discuss several health risks of obesity and explain why it is considered a multifactorial disease, *pp. 518–521.*

8 Describe four treatment options for obesity, *pp. 521–525.*

9 Develop a diet, exercise, and behavioral plan for healthful weight loss, *pp. 525–532.*

10 Identify four key strategies for gaining weight safely and effectively, *pp. 532–533.*

I n 2012, British pop singer Adele became only the second woman in history to win six Grammy Awards in one night. At age 27, she has won critical acclaim from musicians of various genres and the adoration of millions of fans worldwide. Still, some critics—perhaps most famously the fashion designer Karl Lagerfeld—focus not on her powerful, soulful voice but on her weight. Is Adele overweight? A size "14 to 16," she exudes supreme confidence in her large, curvy body and insists she's not interested in losing weight just because someone else thinks she should. Rather than worry about something as "petty" as what one looks like, Adele suggests, "The first thing to do is be happy with yourself and appreciate your body."[1]

Are you happy with your weight, shape, body composition, and fitness level? If not, what needs to change—your diet, your level of physical activity, or maybe just your attitude? How much of your body size and shape is due to genetics? What influence does society have on your weight? And if you decide that you do need to lose weight, what's the best way to do it? In this chapter, we will explore these questions and provide some answers.

> **Watch an interview in which Adele talks about her body image and weight at** http://www.cbsnews.com. **In the Search bar, type "the year of Adele."**

LO 1 Explain what is meant by a healthful weight.

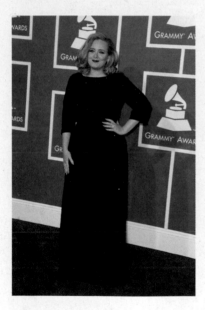

One's perception of a healthful body weight varies from person to person. British singer Adele is comfortable with her body weight.

What Is a Healthful Body Weight?

Throughout history, our standards of physical attraction, especially regarding body shape and weight, have changed. In the 1600s, the full-figured females and muscular males of Flemish Baroque painter Peter Paul Rubens were considered ideal. Fast forward to the 1960s, when skinny stars such as Twiggy and Mick Jagger were the rage. These ideals shifted again in the 1980s, when physically fit bodies were in style for both women and men, and again in the 1990s, when the emaciated look of "heroin chic" was touted as beautiful for women, whereas the ideal man had broad shoulders and "six-pack abs." There are also cultural differences in body shape and weight standards; in many cultures, being larger is associated with possessing greater wealth, health, fertility, and sexual desirability. These examples illustrate that opinions regarding what may be an ideal body shape and weight are influenced by social and cultural norms, fashion, and personal preferences, but they are not necessarily consistent with a body weight that is healthful.

As you begin to think about achieving and maintaining a healthful weight, it's important to make sure you understand what a healthful body weight actually is. We can define a healthful weight as all of the following:

- A weight that is appropriate for your age and physical development
- A weight that you can achieve and sustain without severely curtailing your food intake or constantly dieting
- A weight that is compatible with normal blood pressure, lipid levels, and glucose tolerance
- A weight that is based on your genetic background and family history of body shape and weight
- A weight that is supported by good eating habits and regular physical activity
- A weight that is acceptable to you

As you can see, a healthful weight is one at which you don't have to be extremely thin or overly muscular. In addition, there is no *one* body type that can be defined as healthful. Thus, achieving a healthful body weight should not be dictated by the latest fad or current societal expectations of what is acceptable.

RECAP

Standards of ideal body weight have changed over the course of human history, and vary from one culture to another. A healthful body weight is appropriate for your age, physical development, genetics, and family history; achievable without constant dieting; compatible with normal blood pressure, lipids, and glucose; supported by good eating and regular physical activity habits; and acceptable to you. ∎

How Can You Evaluate Your Body Weight?

Define the terms *under-weight, normal weight, overweight, obesity,* and *morbid obesity* and describe three methods you can use to evaluate your body weight.

Various methods are available to help you determine whether you are currently maintaining a healthful body weight. Let's review a few of these methods.

Determine Your Body Mass Index (BMI)

Body mass index (BMI, or *Quetelet's index*) is a commonly used index representing the ratio of a person's body weight to the square of his or her height. A person's BMI can be calculated using the following equation:

$$\text{BMI (kg/m}^2) = \text{weight (kg)/height (m)}^2$$

For those less familiar with the metric system, there is an equation to calculate BMI using weight in pounds and height in inches:

$$\text{BMI (kg/m}^2) = [\text{weight (lb)/height (inches)}^2] \times 703$$

A less exact but practical method is to use the graph in **Figure 13.1,** which shows approximate BMIs for a person's height and weight and whether a given BMI is in a healthful range.

Why Is BMI Important?

BMI provides an important clue to a person's overall health because it is associated with one of five weight categories, each of which involves a certain level of health risk:

- **Underweight** is defined as having a BMI less than 18.5 kg/m². This weight is below an acceptably defined standard for a given height. A person who is underweight has too little body fat to maintain health and therefore has an increased risk for many health problems.

body mass index (BMI) A measurement representing the ratio of a person's body weight to his or her height (kg/m²).

underweight Having too little body fat to maintain health, causing a person to have a weight that is below an acceptable defined standard for a given height; a BMI less than 18.5 kg/m².

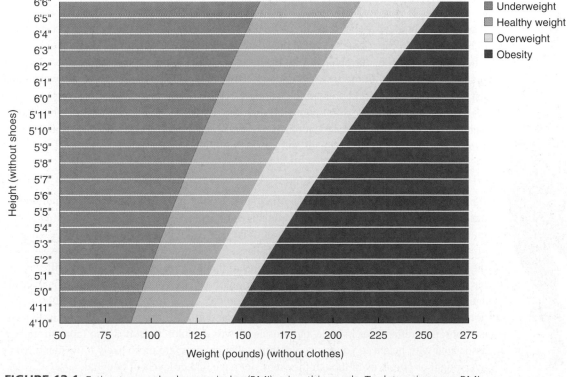

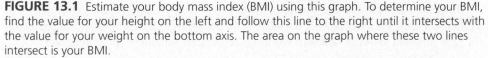

FIGURE 13.1 Estimate your body mass index (BMI) using this graph. To determine your BMI, find the value for your height on the left and follow this line to the right until it intersects with the value for your weight on the bottom axis. The area on the graph where these two lines intersect is your BMI.

- **Normal weight** ranges from 18.5 to 24.9 kg/m². This weight is associated with the lowest disease risk.
- **Overweight** is a BMI between 25 and 29.9 kg/m². It is defined as having a moderate amount of excess body fat, resulting in a person having a weight that is greater than some accepted standard for a given height but is not considered obese.
- **Obesity** is a BMI value between 30 and 39.9 kg/m². Clinicians define obesity as having an excess of body fat that adversely affects health, resulting in a person having a weight that is substantially greater than some accepted standard for a given height. Research studies show that a person's risk for type 2 diabetes, cardiovascular disease, and many other diseases increases significantly when BMI is above a value of 30.
- **Morbid obesity** is defined as a BMI greater than or equal to 40 kg/m²; in this case, the person's body weight exceeds 100% of normal, putting him or her at very high risk for serious health consequences.

normal weight Having an adequate but not excessive level of body fat for health.

overweight Having a moderate amount of excess body fat, resulting in a person having a weight that is greater than some accepted standard for a given height but is not considered obese; a BMI of 25 to 29.9 kg/m².

obesity Having an excess of body fat that adversely affects health, resulting in a person having a weight that is substantially greater than some accepted standard for a given height; a BMI of 30 to 39.9 kg/m².

morbid obesity A condition in which a person's body weight exceeds 100% of normal, putting him or her at very high risk for serious health consequences; a BMI = 40 kg/m².

In addition to the effect of body weight on disease risk, researchers study the relationship between body weight and risk for premature death. Until recently, data from national surveys have indicated that having a BMI value within the healthful range means that your risk of dying prematurely is within the expected average. Thus, if your BMI value fell outside this range, either higher or lower, your risk of dying prematurely was considered greater than the average risk. However, recent evidence suggests that having a BMI in the overweight category may actually be protective against premature death. A 2013 analysis of 97 previously published studies found that people who are overweight (BMI of 25 to 29.99 kg/m²) but not obese have a 6% *lower* risk of dying prematurely than those with a normal BMI.[2]

The publication of these findings created a firestorm of controversy among health professionals and prompted numerous scientists to question the study.[3] Most notably, Dr. Walter Willett of the Harvard School of Public Health called the findings "rubbish" and warned that they would confuse health care providers and discourage overweight and obese people from losing weight. In contrast, an editorial published in the journal *Nature* questioned the motives and views of these critics, emphasizing that the topic is highly complex, and concluding that "a bit of extra weight" does appear to be protective for people who are middle-aged or older or who are already sick.[4] This controversy has drawn international attention to *how* research findings are reported in the media, leading to questions such as: Is it acceptable to reject major research findings when they don't agree? Do we risk misleading the public when we oversimplify our public health messages and fail to report the complexities of an issue such as obesity? Until future research findings clarify the relationship between body weight and risk for chronic disease and premature death, this topic will continue to be controversial.

Theo always worries about being too thin, and he wonders if he is underweight. Theo calculates his BMI (see the calculations in the **You Do the Math** box, page 501) and is surprised to find that it is 22 kg/m² and falls within the normal range.

Limitations of BMI

While calculating your BMI can be very helpful in estimating your health risk, this method has a number of limitations that should be taken into consideration. BMI cannot tell us how much of a person's body mass is composed of fat, nor can it give us an indication of where on the body excess fat is stored. As we'll discuss shortly, upper-body fat stores increase the risk for chronic disease more than fat stores in the lower body. A person's age affects his or her BMI; BMI does not give a fair indication of overweight or obesity in people over the age of 65 years, as the BMI standards are based on data from younger people, and BMI does not accurately reflect the differential rates of bone and muscle loss in older people. BMI also cannot reflect differences in bone and muscle growth in children. BMI is also more strongly associated with height in young people; thus, taller children are more likely to be identified as overweight or obese, even though they may not have higher levels of body fat.

BMI also does not take into account physical and metabolic differences between people of different ethnic backgrounds. At the same BMI, people from different ethnic backgrounds will have different levels of body fat. For instance, African American and Polynesian

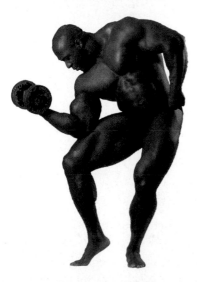

BMI is not an accurate indicator of overweight for certain populations, including heavily muscled people.

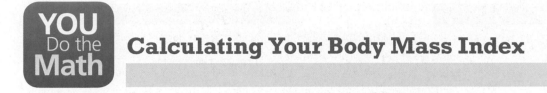

Calculating Your Body Mass Index

Calculate your personal BMI value based on your height and weight. Let's use Theo's values as an example:

$$BMI = weight\ (kg)/height\ (m)^2$$

1. Theo's weight is 200 lb. To convert his weight to kilograms, divide his weight in pounds by 2.2 lb per kg:

200 lb/2.2 lb per kg = 90.91 kg

2. Theo's height is 6 feet 8 inches, or 80 inches. To convert his height to meters, multiply his height in inches by 0.0254 meters/inch:

80 in. × 0.0254 m/in. = 2.03 m

3. Find the square of his height in meters:

2.03 m × 2.03 m = 4.13 m²

4. Then, divide his weight in kilograms by his height in square meters to get his BMI value:

90.91 kg/4.13 m² = 22.01 kg/m²

Is Theo underweight according to this BMI value? No. As you can see in Figure 13.1, this value shows that he is maintaining a normal, healthful weight!

---

people have less body fat than white people at the same BMI value, while Indonesian, Thai, and Ethiopian people have more body fat than white people at the same BMI value. There is also evidence that, even at the same BMI level, Asian, Hispanic, and African American women have a higher risk for diabetes than white women.[5,6] A landmark study examining this topic found that when Asian and Hispanic women gained weight, their risk of developing diabetes over a 20-year period was approximately twice as high as it was for white and African American women who gained the same amount of weight.[6]

Finally, BMI is limited when used with people who have a disproportionately higher muscle mass for a given height, such as certain types of athletes, and with pregnant and lactating women. For example, one of Theo's friends, Randy, is a 23-year-old weight lifter who is 5'7" and weighs 210 pounds. According to our BMI calculations, Randy's BMI is 32.9, placing him in the obese category. Is Randy really obese? In cases such as his, an assessment of body composition is necessary.

Measure Your Body Composition

There are many methods available to assess your **body composition,** or the amount of **body fat mass** (*adipose tissue*) and **lean body mass** (*lean tissue*) you have. **Figure 13.2** (page 502) lists and describes some of the more common methods. It is important to remember that measuring body composition provides only an *estimate* of your body fat and lean body mass; it cannot determine your exact level of these tissues. Because the range of error of these methods can be from 3% to more than 20%, body composition results should not be used as the only indicator of health status.

Let's return to Randy, whose BMI of 32.9 kg/m² places him in the obese category. Is he obese? Randy trains with weights 4 days per week, rides the exercise bike for about 30 minutes per session three times per week, and does not take drugs, smoke cigarettes, or drink alcohol. Through his local gym, Randy contacted a trained technician who assesses body composition. The results of his skinfold measurements show that his body fat is 9%. This value is within the healthful range for men. Randy is an example of a person whose BMI appears very high but who is not actually obese.

Assess Your Fat Distribution Patterns

To evaluate the health of your current body weight, it is also helpful to consider the way fat is distributed throughout your body. This is because your fat distribution pattern is known to affect

You can also calculate your BMI more precisely on the Internet using the BMI calculator from the U.S. Centers for Disease Control. Just enter "CDC BMI calculator" into your Internet browser and click on Adult BMI Calculator. Enter your data and the program will calculate your BMI.

body composition The ratio of a person's body fat to lean body mass.

body fat mass The amount of body fat, or adipose tissue, a person has.

lean body mass The amount of fat-free tissue, or bone, muscle, and internal organs, a person has.

Method		Limitations

Underwater weighing:
Considered the most accurate method. Estimates body fat within a 2–3% margin of error. This means that if your underwater weighing test shows you have 20% body fat, this value could be no lower than 17% and no higher than 23%. Used primarily for research purposes.

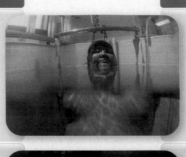

- Subject must be comfortable in water.
- Requires trained technician and specialized equipment.
- May not work well with extremely obese people.
- Must abstain from food for at least 8 hours and from exercise for at least 12 hours prior to testing.

Skinfolds:
Involves "pinching" a person's fold of skin (with its underlying layer of fat) at various locations of the body. The fold is measured using a specially designed caliper. When performed by a skilled technician, it can estimate body fat with an error of 3–4%. This means that if your skinfold test shows you have 20% body fat, your actual value could be as low as 16% or as high as 24%.

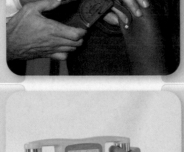

- Less accurate unless technician is well trained.
- Proper prediction equation must be used to improve accuracy.
- Person being measured may not want to be touched or to expose their skin.
- Cannot be used to measure obese people, as their skinfolds are too large for the caliper.

Bioelectrical impedance analysis (BIA):
Involves sending a very low level of electrical current through a person's body. As water is a good conductor of electricity and lean body mass is made up of mostly water, the rate at which the electricity is conducted gives an indication of a person's lean body mass and body fat. This method can be done while lying down, with electrodes attached to the feet, hands, and the BIA machine. Hand-held and standing models (which look like bathroom scales) are now available. Under the best of circumstances, BIA can estimate body fat with an error of 3–4%.

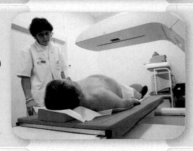

- Less accurate.
- Body fluid levels must be normal.
- Proper prediction equation must be used to improve accuracy.
- Should not eat for 4 hours and should not exercise for 12 hours prior to the test.
- No alcohol should be consumed within 48 hours of the test.
- Females should not be measured if they are retaining water due to menstrual cycle changes.

Dual-energy x-ray absorptiometry (DXA):
The technology is based on using very-low-level x-rays to differentiate among bone tissue, soft (or lean) tissue, and fat (or adipose) tissue. It involves lying for about 30 minutes on a specialized bed fully clothed, with all metal objects removed. The margin of error for predicting body fat ranges from 2% to 4%.

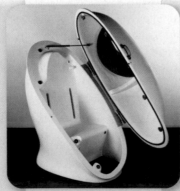

- Expensive; requires trained technician with specialized equipment.
- Cannot be used to measure extremely tall, short, or obese people, as they do not fit properly within the scanning area.

Bod Pod:
A machine that uses air displacement to measure body composition. This machine is a large, egg-shaped chamber made from fiberglass. The person being measured sits inside, wearing a swimsuit. The door is closed and the machine measures how much air is displaced. This value is used to calculate body composition. It appears promising as an easier and equally accurate alternative to underwater weighing in many populations, but it may overestimate body fat in some African American men.

- Expensive.
- Less accurate in some populations.

FIGURE 13.2 Overview of various body composition assessment methods.

your risk for various diseases. **Figure 13.3** shows two types of fat patterning. *Apple-shaped fat patterning,* or upper-body obesity, is known to significantly increase a person's risk for many chronic diseases, such as type 2 diabetes and cardiovascular disease. It is thought that the apple-shaped patterning causes problems with the metabolism of fat and carbohydrate, leading to unhealthful changes in blood cholesterol, insulin, glucose, and blood pressure. In contrast, *pear-shaped fat patterning,* or lower-body obesity, does not seem to significantly increase your risk for chronic diseases. Women tend to store fat in their lower body, and men in their abdominal region.

You can use the following three-step method to determine your type of fat patterning:

1. Ask a friend to measure the circumference of your natural waist, that is, the narrowest part of your torso as observed from the front (**Figure 13.4a**).
2. Then, have that friend measure your hip circumference at the maximal width of the buttocks as observed from the side (Figure 13.4b).
3. Then, divide the waist value by the hip value. This measurement is called your *waist-to-hip ratio.* For example, if your natural waist is 30 inches and your hips are 40 inches, then your waist-to-hip ratio is 30 divided by 40, which equals 0.75.

Once you figure out your ratio, how do you interpret it? An increased risk for chronic disease is associated with the following waist-to-hip ratios:

- In men, a ratio higher than 0.90
- In women, a ratio higher than 0.80

These ratios suggest an apple-shaped fat distribution pattern. In addition, waist circumference alone can indicate your risk for chronic disease. For males, your risk of chronic disease is increased if your waist circumference is above 40 inches (102 cm). For females, your risk is increased at measurements above 35 inches (88 cm).

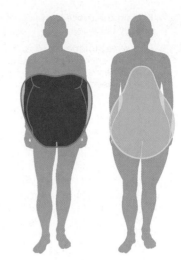

(a) Apple-shaped fat patterning   **(b) Pear-shaped fat patterning**

FIGURE 13.3 Fat distribution patterns. **(a)** An apple-shaped fat distribution pattern increases an individual's risk for many chronic diseases. **(b)** A pear-shaped fat distribution pattern does not seem to be associated with an increased risk for chronic disease.

RECAP

Body mass index, body composition, and the waist-to-hip ratio and waist circumference are tools that can help you evaluate the health of your current body weight. **Body mass index** (BMI) represents the ratio of a person's body weight to the square of his or her height. A BMI in the normal weight category ranges from 18.5 to 24.9 kg/m². This weight is associated with the lowest disease risk. Body composition measurements help you estimate your fat-to-lean tissue mass. A waist-to-hip ratio higher than 0.90 for males and 0.80 for females is associated with an apple-shaped fat distribution pattern, which increases your risk for several chronic diseases. None of these methods is completely accurate, but most may be used appropriately as general health indicators. ■

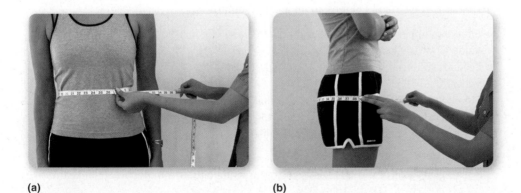

(a)   **(b)**

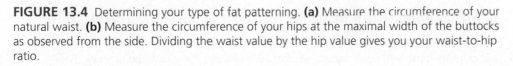

FIGURE 13.4 Determining your type of fat patterning. **(a)** Measure the circumference of your natural waist. **(b)** Measure the circumference of your hips at the maximal width of the buttocks as observed from the side. Dividing the waist value by the hip value gives you your waist-to-hip ratio.

LO 3 Explain the concept of energy balance.

LO 4 Discuss techniques used to measure energy expenditure, and three ways that the body expends energy.

How Does Energy Balance Influence Body Weight?

Have you ever wondered why some people are thin and others are overweight, even though they seem to eat about the same diet? If so, you're not alone. For hundreds of years, researchers have puzzled over what makes us gain and lose weight. In this section, we explore some information and current theories that may shed light on this complex question.

Fluctuations in body weight are a result of changes in **energy intake** (the food and beverages consumed) and **energy expenditure** (the amount of energy expended at rest and during physical activity). This relationship between what we eat and what we do is defined by the energy balance equation:

Energy balance occurs when *energy intake = energy expenditure*

Although the concept of energy balance appears simple, it is a dynamic process.[7] This means that, over time, factors that impact the energy intake side of the equation (including total energy consumed and the macronutrient composition of this energy) need to balance with the factors that impact the energy expenditure side of the equation. **Focus Figure 13.5** is a simplistic representation of how our weight changes when either side of this equation is altered. From this figure, you can see that, in order to lose body weight, we must expend more energy than we consume. In contrast, to gain weight, we must consume more energy than we expend. Unless we purposefully change one side of the equation, weight change is typically gradual and occurs over an extended period of time. Finding the proper balance between energy intake and expenditure allows someone to maintain a healthful body weight.

Energy Intake Is the Food We Eat Each Day

Energy intake is equal to the amount of energy in the foods and beverages we consume each day. Daily energy intake is expressed as *kilocalories per day* (*kcal/day*, or *kcal/d*). Energy intake can be estimated manually by using food composition tables or computerized dietary analysis programs. Remember (from Chapter 1) that the energy value of carbohydrate and protein is 4 kcal/g and the energy value of fat is 9 kcal/g. The energy value of alcohol is 7 kcal/g. By multiplying the energy value (in kcal/g) by the amount of the nutrient (in g), you can calculate how much energy is in a particular food. For instance, 1 cup of quick oatmeal has an energy value of 142 kcal, because it contains 6 g of protein, 25 g of carbohydrate, and 2 g of fat.

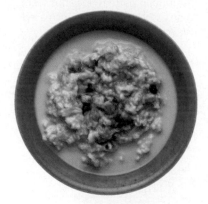

The energy provided by a bowl of oatmeal is derived from its protein, carbohydrate, and fat content.

Over a period of time, when someone's total daily energy intake exceeds the amount of energy that person expends, then weight gain results. Without exercise, this gain will likely be mostly fat. How many Calories are in a pound of fat?

To determine how much energy you consumed in one meal or on one day, log on to **ChooseMyPlate at** www .choosemyplate.gov. **Click on the tab for SuperTracker & Other Tools, then get started!**

- First, it is important to remember that there are 454 g in 1 pound and that the energy value of fat is 9 kcal/g.
- Second, you need to know that adipose tissue contains 87% fat (the remainder is water).
- Finally, to calculate the amount of kcal that will result in a gain of 1 pound (454 g), you need to multiply the amount of weight, 454 g, by the proportion of fat in adipose tissue (87%, or 0.87) and then multiply this value by the energy value of fat (9 kcal/g):

$$454 \text{ g} \times 0.87 = 395 \text{ g of fat}$$
$$395 \text{ g} \times 9 \text{ kcal/g} = 3,555 \text{ kcal (which, for simplicity, is rounded to 3,500 kcal)}$$

energy intake The amount of energy a person consumes; in other words, the number of kcal consumed from food and beverages.

energy expenditure The energy the body expends to maintain its basic functions and to perform all levels of movement and activity.

Energy Expenditure Includes More Than Just Physical Activity

Energy expenditure (also known as energy output) is the energy the body expends to maintain its basic functions and to perform all levels of movement and activity. Total 24-hour energy expenditure is calculated by estimating the energy used during rest and

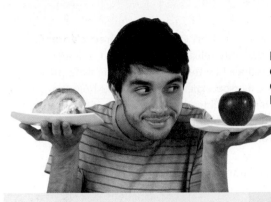

Energy balance is the relationship between the food we eat and the energy we expend each day. Finding the proper balance between energy intake and energy expenditure allows us to maintain a healthy body weight.

ENERGY INTAKE < ENERGY EXPENDITURE = WEIGHT LOSS

ENERGY DEFICIT

When you consume fewer Calories than you expend, your body will draw upon your stored energy to meet its needs. You will lose weight. When you are in a state of energy deficit the body can become more metabolically efficient, which can slow weight loss based on predicted changes.

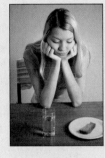

Calories in   Calories out

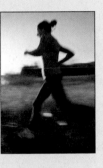

ENERGY INTAKE = ENERGY EXPENDITURE = WEIGHT MAINTENANCE

ENERGY BALANCE

When the Calories you consume meet your needs, you are in energy balance. Your weight will be stable.

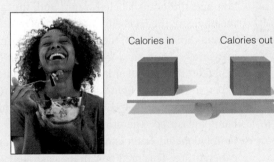

Calories in   Calories out

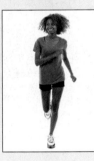

ENERGY INTAKE > ENERGY EXPENDITURE = WEIGHT GAIN

ENERGY EXCESS

When you take in more Calories than you need, the surplus Calories will be stored as fat. You will gain weight. However, when some people consume excess energy their body may attempt to increase energy expenditure through heat to slow weight gain. These people have a hard time gaining weight.

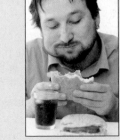

Calories in   Calories out

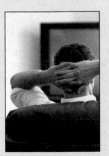

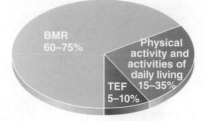

Components of energy expenditure

FIGURE 13.6 The components of energy expenditure are basal metabolic rate (BMR), the thermic effect of food (TEF), and the energy cost of physical activity and activities of daily living. BMR accounts for 60% to 75% of our total energy output, whereas TEF and physical activity together account for 25% to 40%.

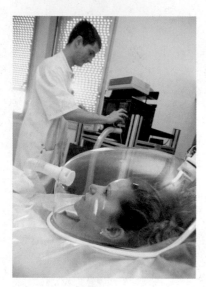

Indirect calorimetry can be used to measure the components of energy expenditure.

direct calorimetry A method used to determine energy expenditure by measuring the amount of heat released by the body.

indirect calorimetry A method used to estimate energy expenditure by measuring oxygen consumption and carbon dioxide production.

doubly labeled water A form of indirect calorimetry that measures total daily energy expenditure through the rate of carbon dioxide production. It requires the consumption of water that is labeled with nonradioactive isotopes of hydrogen (deuterium, or ^2H) and oxygen (^{18}O).

as a result of physical activity. There are three components of energy expenditure: basal metabolic rate (BMR), thermic effect of food (TEF), and energy cost of physical activity and activities of daily living (**FIGURE 13.6**). We discuss these components in detail shortly.

Measuring Energy Expenditure

Energy expenditure can be measured using direct or indirect calorimetry. **Direct calorimetry** is a method that measures the amount of heat the body releases. This method is done using an air-tight chamber in which the heat produced by the body warms the water that surrounds the chamber. The amount of energy a person expends is calculated from the changes in water temperature. The minimum period of time that a person must stay in a direct calorimetry chamber is 24 hours; because of the burden to the individual, the high cost, and the complexity of this method, it is rarely used to measure energy expenditure in humans.

Indirect calorimetry estimates energy expenditure by measuring oxygen consumption and carbon dioxide production. Because there is a predictable relationship between the amount of heat produced (energy expended) by the body and the amount of oxygen consumed and carbon dioxide produced, this method can be used to indirectly determine energy expenditure. This method involves the use of a whole-body chamber, mask, hood, or mouthpiece to collect expired air over a specified period of time. The expired air is analyzed for oxygen and carbon dioxide content. This method is much less expensive and more accessible than direct calorimetry, so it is most commonly used to measure energy expenditure under both resting and physically active conditions.

Both direct and indirect calorimetry require a person to be confined to a laboratory setting or special metabolic chamber, which limits the ability to determine a person's energy expenditure in a free-living environment. This limitation is overcome in a technique using **doubly labeled water,** that is, water labeled with isotopes of hydrogen (deuterium, or ^2H) and oxygen (^{18}O). In this method, the research subject consumes controlled amounts of doubly labeled water. Both the labeled hydrogen and oxygen are used during metabolism; the ^2H is eliminated in water, and the ^{18}O is eliminated in both water and carbon dioxide. Thus, the difference between the elimination rates of these labeled isotopes measures carbon dioxide production, which in turn can be used to estimate energy expenditure. The advantages of this method are that it can be used to measure energy expenditure in free-living situations, over longer periods of time (3 days to 3 weeks), requires only periodic collection of urine, and requires little inconvenience to the person being measured. The primary disadvantages of the method are that it is expensive, the doubly labeled water is difficult to acquire, and it only measures total 24-hour energy expenditure. This method cannot separately measure the three components of energy expenditure discussed next: BMR, TEF, and the energy cost of physical activity and activities of daily living.

Basal Metabolic Rate

Basal metabolic rate, or **BMR,** is the energy expended just to maintain the body's *basal,* or *resting,* functions. These functions include respiration, circulation, body temperature, synthesis of new cells and tissues, secretion of hormones, and nervous system activity. The majority of our energy output each day (about 60% to 75%) is a result of our BMR. This means that 60% to 75% of our energy output goes to fuel the basic activities of staying alive, aside from any physical activity.

BMR varies widely among people. The primary determinant of our BMR is the amount of lean body mass we have. People with a higher lean body mass have a higher BMR, as lean body mass is more metabolically active than body fat. Thus, it takes more energy to support this active tissue. One common assumption is that obese people have a depressed BMR. This is usually not the case. Most studies of obese people show that the amount of energy they expend for every kilogram of lean body mass is similar to that of a non-obese person. Moreover, people who weigh more also have more lean body mass and consequently have a *higher* BMR. See **Figure 13.7** for an example of how lean body mass can vary for people with different body weights and body fat levels.

BMR decreases with age, approximately 3% to 5% per decade after age 30. This age-related decrease results partly from hormonal changes, but much of this change is due to the loss of lean body mass resulting from physical inactivity. Thus, a large proportion of this decrease may be prevented with regular physical activity. Of the many other factors that can affect a person's BMR, some of the most common are listed in **Table 13.1** (page 508).

How can you estimate the amount of energy you expend for your BMR? One of the simplest methods is to multiply your body weight in kilograms by 1.0 kcal per kilogram of body weight per hour for men or by 0.9 kcal per kilogram of body weight per hour for women. A little later in this chapter, you will have an opportunity to calculate your BMR and determine your total daily energy needs.

The Thermic Effect of Food

The **thermic effect of food (TEF)** is the energy we expend to digest, absorb, transport, metabolize, and store the nutrients we need. The TEF is equal to about 5% to 10% of the energy content of a meal, a relatively small amount. Thus, if a meal contains 500 kcal, the thermic effect of that meal is about 25 to 50 kcal, depending upon how processed the foods contained in the meal happen to be. These values apply to eating what is referred to as a mixed diet, or a diet containing carbohydrate, fat, and protein. Individually, the processing of each nutrient takes a different amount of energy. Whereas fat requires very little energy to digest, transport, and store in our cells, protein and carbohydrate require relatively more energy to process. Finally, the more processed a food is prior to consumption, the less energy it takes to digest this food. For example, it requires more energy to digest an orange than it does to digest orange juice.

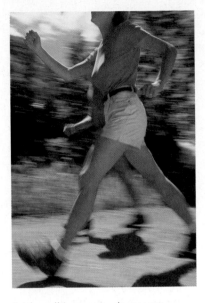

Brisk walking expends energy.

basal metabolic rate (BMR) The energy the body expends to maintain its fundamental physiologic functions.

thermic effect of food (TEF) The energy expended as a result of processing food consumed.

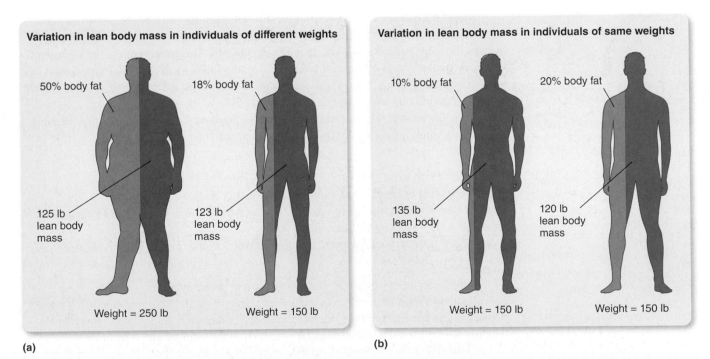

(a)
Variation in lean body mass in individuals of different weights

50% body fat
18% body fat

125 lb lean body mass
123 lb lean body mass

Weight = 250 lb
Weight = 150 lb

(b)
Variation in lean body mass in individuals of same weights

10% body fat
20% body fat

135 lb lean body mass
120 lb lean body mass

Weight = 150 lb
Weight = 150 lb

FIGURE 13.7 Lean body mass varies in people with different body weights and body fat levels. **(a)** The person on the left has a higher body weight, body fat, and lean body mass than the person on the right. **(b)** The two people are the same weight but the person on the right has more body fat and less lean body mass than the person on the left.

TABLE 13.1 Factors Affecting Basal Metabolic Rate (BMR)

Factors That Increase BMR	Factors That Decrease BMR
Higher lean body mass	Lower lean body mass
Greater height (more surface area)	Lower height
Younger age	Older age
Elevated levels of thyroid hormone	Depressed levels of thyroid hormone
Stress, fever, illness	Starvation, fasting or very-low-Calorie diets
Male gender	Female gender due to decreased lean tissue
Pregnancy and lactation	
Certain drugs, such as stimulants, caffeine, and tobacco	

The Energy Cost of Physical Activity

The **energy cost of physical activity** represents about 15% to 35% of our total energy output each day. This is the energy we expend in any movement or work above basal levels. *Non-exercise activity thermogenesis (NEAT)* is a term used to refer to the energy we expend to do all activities above BMR and TMF, but excluding volitional sporting activities. This also includes *spontaneous physical activity,* which includes subconscious activities such as fidgeting and shifting in one's seat. The energy cost of physical activity also includes the energy we expend participating in higher-intensity activities such as running, skiing, and bicycling. One of the most obvious ways to increase how much energy we expend as a result of physical activity is to do more activities for a longer period of time. For example, the energy cost of physical activity in a highly trained athlete may represent 50% of their total energy expenditure, compared to lower values for those who are not as active.

Table 13.2 lists the energy costs for certain activities. As you can see, activities such as running, swimming, and cross-country skiing, which involve moving our larger muscle groups (or more parts of the body) require more energy. The amount of energy we expend during activities is also affected by our body size, the intensity of the activity, and how long we perform the activity. This is why the values in Table 13.2 are expressed as kcal of energy per kilogram of body weight per minute.

Using the energy value for running at 6 miles per hour (a 10-minute-per-mile running pace) for 30 minutes, let's calculate how much energy Theo would expend doing this activity:

- Theo's body weight (in kg) = 200 lb/2.2 lb/kg = 90.91 kg
- Energy cost of running at 6 mph = 0.163 kcal/kg body weight/min
- At Theo's weight, the energy cost of running per minute = 0.163 kcal/kg body weight/min × 90.91 kg = 14.82 kcal/min
- If Theo runs at this pace for 30 minutes, his total energy output = 14.82 kcal/min × 30 min = 445 kcal

Given everything we've discussed so far, you're probably asking yourself, "How many kcal do I need each day to maintain my current weight?" This question is not easy to answer, as our energy needs fluctuate from day-to-day according to our activity level, environmental conditions, and other factors, such as the amount and type of food we eat and our intake of caffeine, which temporarily increases our BMR. However, you can get a general estimate of how much energy your body needs to maintain your present weight. The **You Do the Math** box (on page 510) describes how you can estimate your total daily energy needs.

energy cost of physical activity The energy that is expended on body movement and muscular work above basal levels.

TABLE 13.2   **Energy Costs of Various Physical Activities**

Activity	Intensity	Energy Cost (kcal/kg body weight/min)
Sitting, studying (including reading or writing)	Light	0.022
Cooking or food preparation (sitting or standing)	Light	0.033
Walking (e.g., to neighbor's house)	Light	0.042
Stretching—Hatha yoga	Moderate	0.042
Cleaning (dusting, straightening up, vacuuming, changing linen, carrying out trash)	Moderate	0.058
Weight lifting (free weights, Nautilus, or universal type)	Light or moderate	0.050
Bicycling, 10 mph	Leisure (work or pleasure)	0.067
Walking, 4 mph (brisk pace)	Moderate	0.083
Aerobics	Low impact	0.083
Weight lifting (free weights, Nautilus, or universal type)	Vigorous	0.100
Bicycling, 12 to 13.9 mph	Moderate	0.133
Running, 5 mph (12 minutes per mile)	Moderate	0.138
Running, 6 mph (10 minutes per mile)	Moderate	0.163
Running, 8.6 mph (7 minutes per mile)	Vigorous	0.205

Source: Data from The Compendium of Physical Activities Tracking Guide. Healthy Lifestyles Research Center, College of Nursing & Health Innovation, Arizona State University.

Research Suggests Limitations of the Energy Balance Equation

As researchers have learned more about the factors that regulate body weight, the accuracy and usefulness of the classic energy balance equation illustrated in Focus Figure 13.5 has been called into question. Many researchers point out that the equation in its current form is static and can only be applied when one is weight stable—meaning it does not account for many factors that can alter energy intake and expenditure when one side of the equation is changed, nor does it help explain why people gain and lose weight differently.

For example, if an individual were to consume an additional 100 kcal each day above the energy needed to maintain weight (the energy content of 8 fl oz of a cola beverage) for 10 years, he or she would consume an extra intake of 365,000 kcal! Based on the static energy balance equation, and assuming that no other changes occur in energy expenditure, this individual should gain 104 pounds. However, the static energy balance calculation does not take into account the increase in energy expenditure that would occur, including increased BMR and increased cost of moving a larger body, as weight increased. Thus, after a short period of positive energy balance, body weight would increase, resulting in an increase in energy expenditure that would eventually balance the increased energy intake. The individual would then achieve energy balance and become weight stable at a higher body weight. Thus, the extra 100 kcal/d would actually result in a more realistic weight gain of a few pounds. To maintain this larger body size the individual would need to continue to eat these additional kcals. Of course, the amount of weight an individual gains when overeating will depend on the number of extra kcals consumed, the macronutrient composition of these kcals (i.e., the amount of fat, carbohydrate, protein, or alcohol), and overall energy expenditure.

The inadequacy of the classic energy balance equation to explain individual differences in weight loss or weight gain has prompted experts to propose a dynamic equation of energy balance that takes into account the rates of energy intake and expenditure and their effect

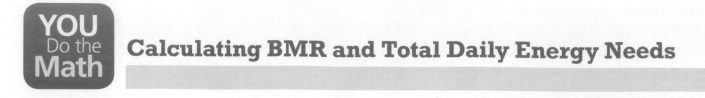

Calculating BMR and Total Daily Energy Needs

One potential way to estimate how much energy you need each day is to record your total food and beverage intake for a defined period of time, such as 3 or 7 days. You can then use a food composition table or computer dietary assessment program to estimate the amount of energy you eat each day. Assuming that your body weight is stable over this period of time, your average daily energy intake should represent how much energy you need to maintain your present weight.

Unfortunately, many studies of energy intake in humans have shown that dietary records estimating energy needs are not very accurate. Most studies show that humans underestimate the amount of energy they eat by 10% to 30%. Overweight people tend to underestimate by an even higher margin, at the same time overestimating the amount of activity they do. This means that someone who really eats about 2,000 kcal/day may record eating only 1,400 to 1,800 kcal/day. So one reason many people are confused about their ability to lose weight is that they are eating more than they realize.

A simpler and more accurate way to estimate your total daily energy needs is to calculate your BMR, then add the amount of energy you expend as a result of your activity level. Refer to the following example to learn how to do this. As the energy cost for the thermic effect of food is very small, you don't need to include it in your calculations.

1. *Calculate your BMR.* If you are a man, you will need to multiply your body weight in kilograms by 1 kcal per kilogram of body weight per hour. Assuming you weigh 175 pounds, your body weight in kilograms would be 175 lb/2.2 lb/kg $\times$ 79.5 kg. Next, multiply your weight in kilograms by 1 kcal per kilogram body weight per hour:

   1 kcal/kg body weight/hour $\times$ 79.5 kg = 79.5 kcal/hour

   Calculate your BMR for the total day (or 24 hours):

   79.5 kcal/hour $\times$ 24 hours/day = 1,909 kcal/day

   If you are a woman, multiply your body weight in kg by 0.9 kcal/kg body weight/hour.

2. *Estimate your activity level by selecting the description that most closely fits your general lifestyle.* The energy cost of activities is expressed as a percentage of your BMR. Refer to the values in the following table when estimating your own energy output.

3. *Multiply your BMR by the decimal equivalent of the lower and higher percentage values for your activity level.* Let's use the man referred to in step 1. He is a college student who lives on campus. He walks to classes located throughout campus, carries his book bag, and spends

most of his time reading and writing. He does not exercise on a regular basis. His lifestyle would be defined as lightly active, meaning he expends 50% to 70% of his BMR each day in activities. You want to calculate how much energy he expends at both ends of this activity level. How many kcal does this equal?

   1,909 kcal/day $\times$ 0.50 (50%) = 955 kcal/day
   1,909 kcal/day $\times$ 0.70 (70%) = 1,336 kcal/day

   These calculations show that this man expends about 955 to 1,336 kcal/day doing daily activities.

4. *Calculate total daily energy output by adding together BMR and the energy needed to perform daily activities.* In this man's case, his total daily energy output is

   1,909 kcal/day + 955 kcal/day – 2,864 kcal/day

   or

   1,909 kcal/day + 1,336 kcal/day – 3,245 kcal/day

   Assuming this man is maintaining his present weight, he requires between 2,864 and 3,245 kcal/day to stay in energy balance!

	Men	Women
Sedentary/Inactive	25–40%	25–35%
Involves mostly sitting, driving, or very low levels of activity		
Lightly Active	50–70%	40–60%
Involves a lot of sitting; may also involve some walking, moving around, and light lifting		
Moderately Active	65–80%	50–70%
Involves work plus intentional exercise, such as an hour of walking or walking 4 to 5 days per week; may have a job requiring some physical labor		
Heavily Active	90–120%	80–100%
Involves a great deal of physical labor, such as roofing, carpentry work, and/or regular heavy lifting and digging		
Exceptionally Active	130–145%	110–130%
Involves a lot of physical activities for work and intentional exercise; also applies to athletes who train for many hours each day, such as triathletes and marathon runners or other competitive athletes performing heavy, regular training		

on rate of change of energy stores (including fat and lean tissues) in the body, not simply on body weight overall.[7]

Predict a realistic time course for kcal intake, exercise, and weight loss or weight gain using the human metabolism simulator at http://bwsimulator .niddk.nih.gov.

RECAP

The energy balance equation states that energy balance occurs when energy intake equals energy expenditure. Over time, consuming more energy than you expend causes weight gain, while consuming less energy than you expend causes weight loss. Although energy expenditure can be measured using direct calorimetry, which measures the amount of heat the body releases, this method is costly and complex and is rarely used. Indirect calorimetry estimates energy expenditure by measuring oxygen consumption and carbon dioxide production, and can be done in a laboratory setting. Doubly labeled water can be used to measure energy expenditure in free-living situations over longer periods of time. The three components of energy expenditure are basal metabolic rate, which is the energy expended to maintain basic physiologic functions; the thermic effect of food, which is the energy expended to process food; and the energy cost of physical activity, which is the energy expended in movement above basal levels. Research has called into question the accuracy and usefulness of the classic energy balance equation because it fails to account for many factors that can alter energy intake and expenditure or to explain why people gain and lose weight differently. ∎

What Factors Influence Body Weight?

A variety of types of research studies over many decades suggest that the greatest influence on body weight is our genetic inheritance. However, many nongenetic factors also contribute.

LO 5 List and describe several biological influences on body weight.

LO 6 Discuss cultural, economic, and social influences on body weight.

Genes May Influence Body Weight in Different Ways

Our genetic background influences our height, weight, body shape, and metabolic rate. Research indicates that the body weights of adults who were adopted as children are similar to the weights of their biological parents, not their adoptive parents.[8] How much of our BMI can be accounted for by genetic influences remains controversial, however, with proposed values ranging from 50% to 90%.[9] This means that 10% to 50% of our BMI is accounted for by nongenetic, environmental factors and lifestyle choices, such as exposure to cheap, high-energy food and low levels of physical activity.

The message that our genes strongly influence our BMI could prove to be detrimental to our efforts to convince people that they can reduce their weight by changing their lifestyle. Bloss and colleagues found that individuals who were genetically tested and found to have higher genetic risk for obesity were more likely to report a higher fat intake and lower levels of physical activity 6 months after they received these results.[10]

Exactly how do genetic factors influence body weight? We discuss here some theories attempting to explain this link.

The FTO Gene

The existing evidence on genetics and obesity indicate that there is no one single "obesity gene." Instead, more than 120 genes currently are thought to be associated with an increased risk for obesity.[11] Nevertheless, one gene that has received a great deal of attention is the fat mass and obesity (FTO)–associated gene. This gene is relatively common: Approximately 44% to 65% of people are estimated to have at least one copy. The gene appears to stimulate excessive food intake and may diminish feelings of satiety; thus, it's not surprising that people who carry the gene weigh more, on average, than people who do not. A recent study indicates that physical activity can attenuate the influence of the FTO gene on obesity risk in adults and children by 27%. These results highlight the importance of regular physical activity in reducing risk for obesity in people who are genetically predisposed.[12]

The Thrifty Gene Theory

The **thrifty gene theory** suggests that some people possess a gene (or genes) that causes them to be energetically thrifty. This means that at rest and even during active times these individuals expend less energy than people who do not possess this gene. The proposed purpose of this gene is to protect a person from starving to death during times of extreme food shortages. This theory has been applied to some Native American tribes, as these societies were exposed to centuries of feast and famine. Those with a thrifty metabolism survived when little food was available, and this trait was passed on to future generations. Although an actual thrifty gene (or genes) has not yet been identified, researchers continue to study this explanation as a potential cause of obesity.

If this theory is true, think about how people who possess this thrifty gene might respond to today's environment. Low levels of physical activity, inexpensive food sources that are high in fat and energy, and excessively large serving sizes are the norm in our society. People with a thrifty metabolism would experience a great amount of weight gain, and their body would be more resistant to weight loss.

The Set-Point Theory

The **set-point theory** suggests that our body is designed to maintain our weight within a narrow range, or at a "set point." In many cases, the body appears to respond in such a way as to maintain a person's current weight. When we dramatically reduce energy intake (such as with fasting or strict diets), the body responds with physiologic changes that cause BMR to drop. This results in a significant slowing of our energy output. In addition, being physically active while fasting or starving is difficult, because a person just doesn't have the energy for it. These two mechanisms of energy conservation may contribute to some of the rebound weight gain many dieters experience after they quit dieting.

Conversely, overeating in some people may cause an increase in BMR, thought to be due to an increased TEF and increase in spontaneous physical activity. This in turn increases energy output and prevents weight gain. These changes may help to explain the limitations of the classic energy balance equation, mentioned earlier, in predicting how much weight people will gain from eating excess food.

In addition, we don't eat exactly the same amount of food each day; some days we overeat, and other days we eat less. When you think about how much our daily energy intake fluctuates (about 20% above and below our average monthly intake), our ability to maintain a certain weight over long periods of time suggests that there is some evidence to support the set-point theory.

Can we change our weight set point? It appears that, when we maintain changes in our diet and activity level over a long period of time, weight change does occur. This is obvious in the case of obesity, since many people who were normal weight as young adults become obese during middle adulthood. Also, many people do successfully lose weight and maintain that weight loss over long periods of time. Thus, the set-point theory cannot entirely account for the body's resistance to weight loss. On the other hand, although some children who are obese grow up to have a normal body weight, obese children and adolescents are more likely to remain obese as adults.[13]

A classic study on weight gain in twins demonstrated how genetics may affect our tendency to maintain a set point.[14] Twelve pairs of male identical twins volunteered to stay in a dormitory, where they were supervised 24 hours a day for 120 consecutive days. Researchers measured how much energy each man needed to maintain his body weight at the beginning of the study. For 100 days, the subjects were fed 1,000 kcal more per day than they needed to maintain body weight. Daily physical activity was limited, but each person

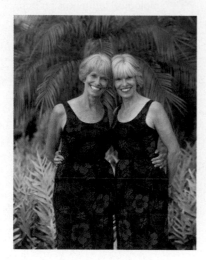

Identical twins tend to maintain a similar weight throughout life.

thrifty gene theory A theory suggesting that some people possess a gene (or genes) that causes them to be energetically thrifty, resulting in their expending less energy at rest and during physical activity.

set-point theory A theory suggesting that the body raises or lowers energy expenditure in response to increased and decreased food intake and physical activity. This action maintains an individual's body weight within a narrow range.

was allowed to walk outdoors for 30 minutes each day, read, watch television and videos, and play cards and video games. The research staff stayed with these men to ensure that they did not stray from the study protocol.

Although all these men were overfed enough energy to gain about 26 pounds, the average weight gain they experienced was only 18 pounds. They gained mostly fat but also about 6 pounds of lean body mass. Interestingly, while each twin gained an amount similar to that of his brother, there was a very wide range of weight gained overall: the lowest weight gain was 9.5 pounds, while the highest was more than 29 pounds! Keep in mind that the food these men ate and the activities they performed were tightly controlled.

This study shows that, when people overeat by the same amount of food, they can gain very different amounts of weight. Researchers theorize that those who are more resistant to weight gain when they overeat have the ability to increase BMR, store more excess energy as lean body mass instead of fat, and increase spontaneous physical activity. Thus, genetic differences may explain why some people are better able to maintain a certain weight set point.

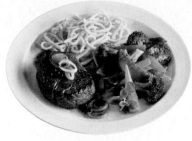

A balanced diet contains protein, carbohydrate, and fat.

Metabolic Factors Influence Weight Loss and Gain

Six metabolic factors are thought to be predictive of a person's risk for weight gain and resistance to weight loss.[7] These factors are:

- *Relatively low metabolic rate.* As discussed previously, obese individuals weigh more and have a higher amount of lean tissue than people of normal weight and, thus, will have a higher absolute BMR. However at any given size, people vary in their relative BMR—it can be high, normal, or low. People who have a relatively low BMR are more at risk for weight gain and are resistant to weight loss.
- *Low level of spontaneous physical activity.* People who exhibit less spontaneous physical activity are at increased risk for weight gain.
- *Low sympathetic nervous system activity.* The sympathetic nervous system plays an important role in regulating all components of energy expenditure, and people with lower rates of sympathetic nervous system activity are more prone to obesity and more resistant to weight loss.
- *Low fat oxidation.* Some people oxidize relatively more carbohydrate for energy, which means that less fat will be oxidized. Thus, relatively more fat will be stored in adipose tissue, so these people are more prone to weight gain. People who oxidize relatively more fat for energy are more resistant to weight gain and are more successful at maintaining weight loss.
- An *abnormally low level of thyroid hormone,* or an elevated level of the hormone cortisol, both of which play roles in metabolism, can lead to weight gain and obesity. A physician can check a patient's blood for levels of these hormones.
- *Certain prescription medications,* including steroids used for asthma and other disorders, seizure medications, and some antidepressants, can slow basal metabolic rate or stimulate appetite, leading to weight gain.[15]

Physiologic Factors Influence Body Weight

Numerous physiologic factors affect body weight, including hypothalamic regulation of hunger and satiety, specific hormones, and other factors. Together, these contribute to the complexities of weight regulation.

Hypothalamic Cells

As previously reviewed (in Chapter 3), cells in the hypothalamic *feeding center* respond to conditions of low blood glucose, causing hunger and driving a person to eat. Once one has eaten and the body has responded accordingly, cells in the hypothalamic *satiety center* are triggered, and the desire to eat is reduced. Some people may have an insufficient satiety mechanism, which prevents them from feeling full after a meal, allowing them to overeat. It is important to recognize that people with a sufficient satiety mechanism can and do override these signals and overeat even when they are not hungry.

Energy-Regulating Hormones

Leptin is a protein produced by adipose cells. It functions as a hormone. First discovered in mice, leptin acts to reduce food intake and to cause a decrease in body weight and body fat. Obese people tend to have very high amounts of leptin in their body but are insensitive to its effects. Researchers are currently studying the role of leptin in starvation and overeating, as well as the role it might play in cardiovascular and kidney complications that result from obesity and related diseases.

In addition to leptin, numerous proteins affect the regulation of appetite and storage of body fat. Primary among these is **ghrelin,** a protein synthesized in the stomach. It acts as a hormone and plays an important role in appetite regulation through its actions in the hypothalamus. Ghrelin stimulates appetite and increases the amount of food one eats. Ghrelin levels increase before a meal and fall within about 1 hour after a meal. This action indicates that ghrelin may be a primary contributor to both hunger and satiety. Ghrelin levels appear to increase after weight loss, and researchers speculate that this factor could help explain why people who have lost weight have difficulty keeping it off.[16] We noted earlier that obese people seem to lose their sensitivity to leptin, but this is not true for ghrelin: obese people are just as sensitive to the effects of ghrelin as non-obese people.[17] For this reason, potential mechanisms that can block the actions of ghrelin are currently a prime target of research into the treatment of obesity.

Peptide YY, or PYY, is a protein produced in the gastrointestinal tract. It is released after a meal, in amounts proportional to the energy content of the meal. In contrast with ghrelin, PYY decreases appetite and inhibits food intake in animals and humans. Interestingly, obese individuals have lower levels of PYY when they are fasting and show less of an increase in PYY after a meal, compared with non-obese individuals, which suggests that PYY may be important in the manifestation and maintenance of obesity.[18]

Uncoupling proteins have recently become the focus of research into body weight. These proteins are found in the inner membrane of the mitochondria, which you may recall (from Chapter 7) are organelles present within cells that generate ATP, including skeletal muscle cells and adipose cells. Some research suggests that uncoupling proteins uncouple certain steps in ATP production; when this occurs, the process produces heat instead of ATP. This production of heat increases energy expenditure and results in less storage of excess energy. Thus, a person with more uncoupling proteins or a higher activity of these proteins would be more resistant to weight gain and obesity.

Three forms of uncoupling proteins have been identified: UCP1 is found exclusively in **brown adipose tissue,** a type of adipose tissue that has more mitochondria than white adipose tissue. It is found in significant amounts in animals and newborn humans. It was traditionally thought that adult humans have very little brown adipose tissue. However, recent evidence suggests that humans may have substantially more brown adipose tissue than previously assumed,[19] and obesity is associated with a reduction in the amount and activity of brown adipose tissue.[19] These findings suggest a possible role of brown adipose tissue in obesity. Two other uncoupling proteins, UCP2 and UCP3, are known to be important to energy expenditure and resistance to weight gain. These proteins are found in various tissues, including white adipose tissue and skeletal muscle. The roles of brown adipose tissue and uncoupling proteins in human obesity are currently being researched.

leptin A hormone, produced by body fat, that acts to reduce food intake and to decrease body weight and body fat.

ghrelin A protein synthesized in the stomach that acts as a hormone and plays an important role in appetite regulation by stimulating appetite.

peptide YY (PYY) A protein produced in the gastrointestinal tract that is released after a meal in amounts proportional to the energy content of the meal; it decreases appetite and inhibits food intake.

brown adipose tissue A type of adipose tissue that has more mitochondria than white adipose tissue and can increase energy expenditure by uncoupling oxidation from ATP production. It is found in significant amounts in animals and newborn humans.

Other Physiologic Factors

The following other physiologic factors are known to increase satiety (or decrease food intake):

- The hormones serotonin and cholecystokinin (CCK); serotonin is made from the amino acid tryptophan, and CCK is produced by the intestinal cells and stimulates the gallbladder to secrete bile
- An increase in blood glucose levels, such as that normally seen after the consumption of a meal
- Stomach expansion
- Nutrient absorption from the small intestine

The following other physiologic factors can decrease satiety (or increase food intake):

- Beta-endorphins, which are hormones that enhance a sense of pleasure while eating, increasing food intake
- Neuropeptide Y, an amino-acid-containing compound produced in the hypothalamus; neuropeptide Y stimulates appetite
- Decreased blood glucose levels, such as the decrease that occurs after an overnight fast

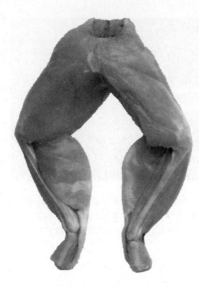

Food preferences often depend on culture. Some cultures enjoy foods such as frogs' legs, whereas others do not.

Cultural and Economic Factors Affect Food Choices and Body Weight

Both cultural and economic factors can contribute to obesity. As previously discussed (in detail in Chapter 3), cultural factors (including religious beliefs and learned food preferences) affect our food choices and eating patterns. In addition, the customs of many cultures put food at the center of celebrations of festivals and holidays, and overeating is tacitly encouraged. In addition, as both parents now work outside the home in most American families, more people are embracing the "fast-food culture," eating highly processed and highly Caloric fast foods from restaurants and grocery stores rather than lower-kcal, home-cooked meals.

Coinciding with these cultural influences on food intake are cultural factors that promote inactivity. These include the shift from manual labor to more sedentary jobs and increased access to laborsaving devices in all areas of our lives. Even seemingly minor changes—such as texting someone in your dorm instead of walking down the hall to chat or walking through an automated door instead of pushing a door open—add up to a lower expenditure of energy by the end of the day. Research with sedentary ethnic minority women in the United States indicates that other common barriers to increasing physical activity include lack of time due to placing family responsibilities first, lack of confidence to be physically active, no physically active role models to emulate, acceptance of larger body size, exercise being considered culturally unacceptable, and fear for personal safety.[20,21] In short, cultural factors influence both food consumption and levels of physical activity and can contribute to weight gain.

Economic status is known to be related to health status, particularly in developed countries, such as the United States: people of lower economic status have higher rates of obesity and related chronic diseases than people of higher incomes.[22] Income influences access to healthcare, food choices, eating behaviors, activity levels, and certain health-related aspects of our environment. For example, it has been proposed that pollution from vehicular exhaust may increase a person's risk for obesity. A 2014 study published in the journal *Environmental Health* found that higher levels of traffic pollution were associated with a higher BMI in children 5 to 11 years of age.[23] The authors speculate that various factors could contribute to this association, including:

- Reduced levels of physical activity and active travel due to pollution and perceived safety risks;

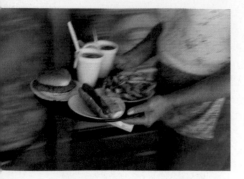

Easy-access and fast foods may be inexpensive and filling, but they are often also high in fat and sugar.

- Increased stress levels due to higher noise and vibration levels and feeling less safe, which disrupt sleep and increase energy intake; and
- Potential direct effects of pollution itself on hormone regulation and insulin resistance, which could affect appetite and basal metabolic rate.

Closely related to economic status is educational attainment: affluent families tend to live in neighborhoods with better schools, and their children are more likely to pursue higher education. Some studies suggest an association between level of educational attainment and BMI: a recent study of first-generation U.S. Latinos, for example, found that children had a 55% lower risk of abdominal obesity if their parents had more than 6 years of education and they had more than 12 years.[24] And a study of Caucasian women in the United States found that relative increases in obesity since the early 1980s have been disproportionately larger for women who did not complete high school compared to college-educated women.[25] Refer to the Chapter 16 for a more thorough discussion of the links between poverty and obesity.

Social Factors Influence Behavior and Body Weight

Previously (in Chapter 3), we explored the concept that *appetite* can be experienced in the absence of hunger and therefore may be considered a psychological drive to eat, being stimulated by learned preferences for food and particular situations that promote eating. People may also follow social cues related to the timing and size of meals. Mood can also affect appetite, as some people will eat more or less if they feel depressed or happy. As you can imagine, appetite leads many people to overeat.

Social Factors and Overeating

Social factors—such as pressure from family and friends to eat the way they do—can encourage people to overeat. For example, the pressure to overeat on holidays is high, as family members or friends offer extra servings of favorite holiday foods and follow a very large meal with a rich dessert.

Americans also have numerous opportunities to overeat because of easy access throughout the day to foods high in fat and energy. Vending machines selling junk foods are everywhere: at some schools, in office buildings, and even at fitness centers. Shopping malls are filled with fast-food restaurants, where inexpensive, large serving sizes are the norm. Food manufacturers are producing products in ever-larger serving sizes: Hardee's ½ lb Thickburger® El Diablo packs 1,380 kcal—which is approximately 65% of the Calorie intake recommended for an average adult for an entire day! Even some foods traditionally considered healthful, such as some brands of peanut butter, yogurt, chicken soup, and flavored milks, are filled with added sugars and other ingredients that are high in energy. This easy access to large servings of high-energy meals and snacks leads many people to overeat.

Social Factors and Inactivity

Social factors can also cause people to be less physically active. For instance, we don't even have to spend time or energy preparing food anymore, as everything is either ready-to-serve or requires just a few minutes to cook in a microwave oven. Other social factors restricting physical activity include living in an unsafe community; watching a lot of television; coping with family, community, and work responsibilities that do not involve physical activity; and living in an area with harsh weather conditions. Many overweight people identify such factors as major barriers to maintaining a healthful body weight, and research seems to confirm their influence.

Certainly, social factors are contributing to decreased physical activity among children. There was a time when children played outdoors regularly and physical education was offered daily in school. Today, many children cannot play outdoors due to safety concerns and lack of recreational facilities, and few schools have the resources to regularly offer physical education to children.

Another social factor promoting inactivity in both children and adults is the increasing dominance of technology in our choices of entertainment. Instead of participating in sports or gathering for a dance at the community hall, we go to the movies or stay at home, watching television, surfing the Internet, and playing with video games, smart phones, and other hand-held devices. By reducing energy expenditure, these behaviors contribute to weight gain. For instance, a study of 11- to 13-year-old schoolchildren found that the children who watched more than 2 hours of television per night were more likely to be overweight or obese than the children who watched less than 2 hours of television per night. Similarly, television watching in adults has been shown to be associated with weight gain over a 4-year period.[26]

Social Pressures and Underweight

On the other hand, social pressures to maintain a lean body are great enough to encourage many people to undereat or to avoid foods that are perceived as "bad," especially fats. Our society ridicules and often ostracizes overweight people, many of whom face discrimination in housing, employment, and other areas of their lives. A recent study found that children who are obese are 60% more likely to experience bullying than children of normal weight.[27] Moreover, media images of waiflike fashion models and men in tight jeans with muscular chests and abdomens encourage many people—especially adolescents and young adults—to skip meals, resort to crash diets, and exercise obsessively. Even some people of normal body weight push themselves to achieve an unrealistic and unattainable weight goal, in the process threatening their health and even their lives (see Chapter 13.5, "In Depth: Disordered Eating," immediately following this chapter, for information on the consequences of disordered eating).

It should be clear that how a person gains, loses, and maintains body weight is a complex matter. Most people who are overweight have tried several diet programs but have been unsuccessful in maintaining their weight loss. A significant number of these people have consequently given up all weight-loss attempts. Some even suffer from severe depression related to their body weight. Should we condemn these people as failures and continue to pressure them to lose weight? Should people who are overweight but otherwise healthy (for example, low blood pressure, cholesterol, triglycerides, and glucose levels) be advised to lose weight? As we continue to search for ways to help people achieve and

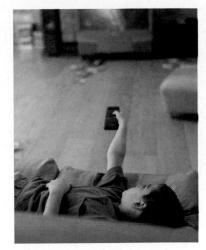

Behaviors learned as a child can affect adult weight and physical activity patterns.

*Nutri-*Case

Hannah

"I wonder what it would be like to be able to look in the mirror and not feel fat. Like my friend Kristi—she's been skinny since we were kids. I'm just the opposite: I've felt bad about my weight ever since I can remember. One of my worst memories is from the YMCA swim camp the summer I was 10 years old. Of course, we had to wear a swimsuit, and the other kids picked on me so bad I'll never forget it. One of the boys called me 'fatso,' and the girls were even meaner, especially when I was changing in the locker room. That was the last year I was in the swim camp, and I've never owned a swimsuit since."

Think back to your own childhood. Were you ever teased for some aspect of yourself that you felt unable to change? How might organizations that work with children, such as schools, YMCAs, scout troops, and church-based groups, increase their leaders' awareness of social stigmatization of overweight children and reduce incidents of teasing, bullying, and other insensitivity?

maintain a healthful body weight, our society must take measures to reduce the social pressures facing people who are overweight or obese.

RECAP

Many factors affect our ability to gain and lose weight. Our genetic background influences our height, weight, body shape, and metabolic rate. The FTO gene variant appears to prompt overeating and weight gain. The thrifty gene theory suggests that some people possess a thrifty gene, or set of genes, that causes them to expend less energy at rest and during physical activity than people who do not have this gene (or genes). The set-point theory suggests that our body is designed to maintain weight within a narrow range, also called a set point. Metabolic factors, such as low relative resting metabolic rate, low spontaneous physical activity, low sympathetic nervous system activity, and low fat oxidation, increase the risk for weight gain. Physiologic factors, such as various energy-regulating hormones, impact body weight by their effects on hunger, satiety, appetite, and energy expenditure. Cultural and economic factors can significantly influence the amounts and types of food we eat. Poverty limits access to healthcare, can encourage purchase of less healthful foods, and can force families to reside in less healthful neighborhoods and reduce access to education. Social factors influencing weight include pressure to eat the way family members eat, the ready availability of large portions of high-energy foods, our reduced levels of physical activity, and the dominance of technology in our leisure time. Social pressures on those who are overweight can drive people to use harmful methods to achieve an unrealistic body weight. ■

LO 7 Discuss several health risks of obesity and explain why it is considered a multifactorial disease.

What Makes Obesity Harmful, and Why Does It Occur?

Recall that obesity is defined as having an excess body fat that adversely affects health, resulting in a person having a weight for a given height that is substantially greater than some accepted standard. People with a BMI between 30 and 39.9 kg/m^2 are considered obese. Morbid obesity occurs when a person's body weight exceeds 100% of normal; people who are morbidly obese have a BMI greater than or equal to 40 kg/m^2.

Obesity Is Linked to Chronic Diseases and Premature Death

Obesity rates have increased more than 50% during the past 20 years, and it is now estimated that about 34.9% of adults 20 years and older are obese.[28] This alarming rise in obesity is a major health concern because it is linked to many chronic diseases and complications:

- Hypertension
- Dyslipidemia, including elevated total cholesterol, triglycerides, and LDL-cholesterol and decreased HDL-cholesterol
- Type 2 diabetes
- Heart disease
- Stroke
- Gallbladder disease
- Osteoarthritis
- Sleep apnea
- Certain cancers, such as colon, breast, endometrial, and gallbladder cancer
- Menstrual irregularities and infertility
- Gestational diabetes, premature fetal deaths, neural tube defects, and complications during labor and delivery
- Depression
- Alzheimer's disease, dementia, and cognitive decline

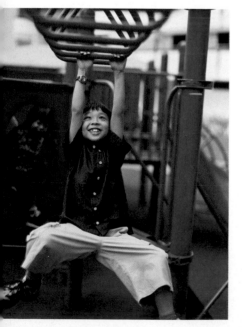

Adequate physical activity is instrumental in preventing childhood obesity.

Abdominal obesity, specifically a large amount of visceral fat that is stored deep within the abdomen (**Figure 13.8**), is one of five risk factors collectively referred to as **metabolic syndrome.** A diagnosis of metabolic syndrome—which is typically made if a person has three or more of the factors—increases one's risk for heart disease, type 2 diabetes, and stroke. These risk factors include the following:

■ Abdominal obesity (defined as a waist circumference greater than or equal to 40 inches for men and 35 inches for women)

■ Higher-than-normal triglyceride levels (greater than or equal to 150 mg/dL)

■ Lower-than-normal HDL-cholesterol levels (less than 40 mg/dL in men and 50 mg/dL in women)

■ Higher-than-normal blood pressure (greater than or equal to 130/85 mm Hg)

■ Fasting blood glucose levels greater than or equal to 100 mg/dL, including people with diabetes[29]

Metabolic syndrome is one of a number of components of global cardiometabolic risk, which includes the factors of metabolic syndrome and the additional factors of elevated LDL-cholesterol (≥130 mg/dL), smoking, inflammation, and insulin resistance.[30,31]

People with metabolic syndrome are twice as likely to develop heart disease and five times as likely to develop type 2 diabetes as people without metabolic syndrome. About 23% of adults in the United States have metabolic syndrome, and rising rates of elevated blood glucose and abdominal obesity are major contributors to the syndrome.[32]

Obesity is also associated with an increased risk for premature death: mortality rates for people with a BMI of 30 kg/m² or higher are 50% to 100% above the rates for those with a BMI between 20 and 25 kg/m². As discussed (in Chapter 1), several of the leading causes of death in the United States are associated with obesity.

As discussed earlier in this chapter, overweight (a BMI between 25 and 29.9 kg/m²) may actually be protective against dying prematurely.[2] However, some evidence suggests that being overweight can increase our risk for hypertension and osteoarthritis. Overweight people also have a higher risk of becoming obese than people of normal weight. Because of these concerns, health professionals recommend that people who are overweight adopt a lifestyle that incorporates healthful eating and regular physical activity to prevent additional weight gain, to reduce body weight to a normal level, and/or to support long-term health even if body weight is not significantly reduced.

Multiple Factors Contribute to Obesity

Obesity is a **multifactorial disease;** that is, all of the genetic, metabolic, physiologic, and environmental factors discussed in the previous section potentially contribute to the condition. In fact, a landmark report published in 2007 from the Government Office for Science in the United Kingdom revealed that the causes of obesity are embedded within highly complex biological and sociological systems. The authors of this report used a systems-mapping approach to identify over 100 variables that directly or indirectly influence energy balance (**Focus Figure 13.9**, page 520).[33] These variables

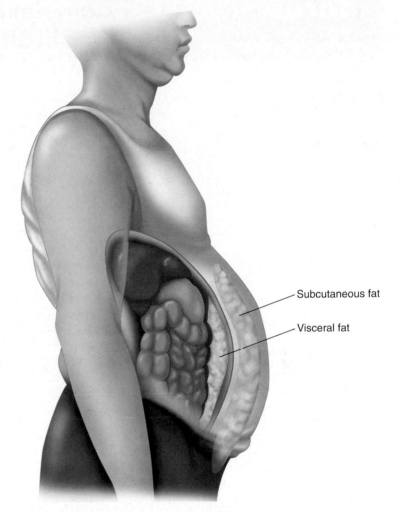

Subcutaneous fat

Visceral fat

FIGURE 13.8 Abdominal obesity, specifically a high amount of visceral fat stored deep within the abdomen, is one of the risk factors for metabolic syndrome.

metabolic syndrome A clustering of risk factors that increase one's risk for heart disease, type 2 diabetes, and stroke, including abdominal obesity, higher-than-normal triglyceride levels, lower-than-normal HDL-cholesterol levels, higher-than-normal blood pressure (greater than or equal to 130/85 mm Hg), and elevated fasting blood glucose levels.

multifactorial disease A disease that may be attributable to one or more of a variety of causes.

focus figure 13.9 | Complexities of the Contributors to Obesity

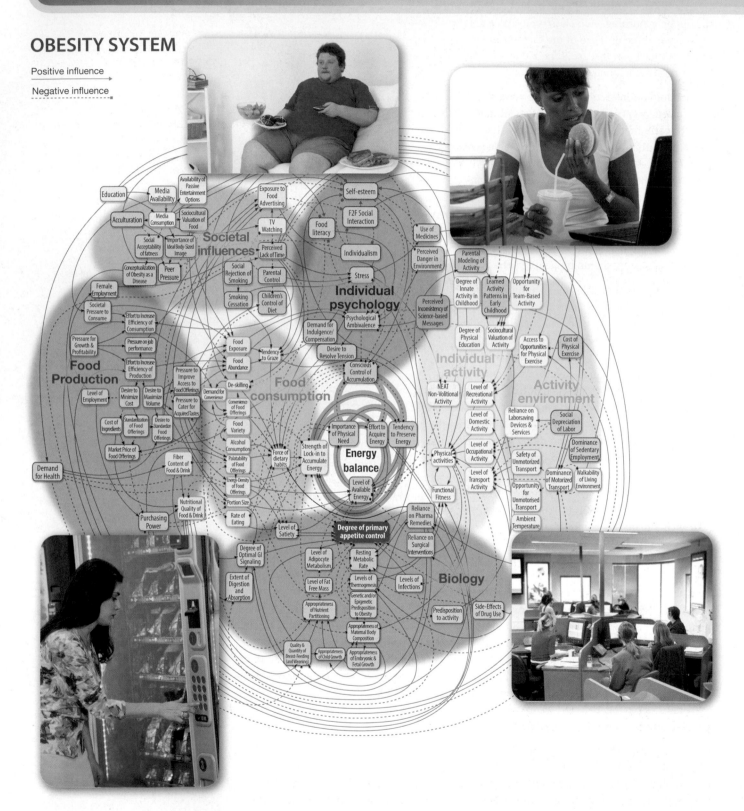

are grouped into seven predominant themes, some of which we explore in more detail ahead:

- Biology—including variables such as genetic predisposition to obesity, resting metabolic rate, and levels of certain hormones;
- Physical Activity Environment—includes variables that can promote or inhibit physical activity such as cost, perceived safety, and reliance on laborsaving devices;
- Individual Physical Activity—includes variables such as parental modeling of activity, level of fitness, and engagement in recreational or occupational physical activity;
- Individual Psychology—includes self-esteem, stress, level of food literacy, pressure to overindulge, and level of parental control over children's diet;
- Societal Influences—includes level of education, TV watching, and societal acceptance of obesity;
- Food Environment—includes variables related to food production such as industry pressure for growth and marketability, market price of food, and pressure to consume via advertisements; and
- Food Consumption—includes variables such as level of food abundance and variety, nutritional quality of food and beverages, and the energy density and portion sizes of foods.

RECAP

Obesity increases the risk for type 2 diabetes, cardiovascular disease, certain cancers, depression, dementia, and many other diseases. Abdominal obesity is one of the most significant factors in metabolic syndrome, which is in turn part of an individual's overall cardiometabolic risk. Obesity itself is a **multifactorial disease**; that is, over 100 variables directly or indirectly influence energy balance. These include biological variables and individual, environmental, and social influences on food consumption and physical activity. ■

Nutrition
MILESTONE

In **2007**, researchers from Harvard University and the University of California, San Diego, published evidence that obesity may be spread via social networks. Dr. Nicolas Christakis and Dr. James Fowler evaluated data involving over 12,000 people who participated in the Framingham Heart Study, a longitudinal cohort initiated in 1948. Data on BMI from 1971 to 2003 and statistical models were used to examine whether weight gain in participants was associated with weight gain in friends, siblings, spouses, or neighbors. The results showed that a person's chance of becoming obese was 57% higher if a friend became obese; 40% higher if a sibling became obese; and 37% higher if a spouse became obese. There was no evidence that neighbors had any effect on a person's obesity risk. Social distance was found to be much more important than geographic distance, suggesting that it was not exposure to the same environmental factors that caused people in close social networks to become obese. It may be that a person's perceptions of the acceptability of obesity changes when those close to him or her become obese. The researchers also theorized that, if social networks can increase obesity, they could be used as a means to spread positive health behaviors and reduce obesity.

How Is Obesity Treated?

Ironically, up to 40% of women and 25% of men are dieting at any given time. How can obesity rates be so high when there are so many people dieting? Although relatively few studies have tracked maintenance of weight loss, existing evidence suggests a wide range of success, with 20% to 59% of obese people from the general U.S. population maintaining long-term weight loss over 1 to 5 years.[34] These results suggest that about 41% to 80% of obese people who are dieting are somehow failing to lose weight or to keep it off. Although these statistics might suggest that obesity somehow resists intervention, that's not the case. Bearing in mind that 20% to 59% of people do succeed in long-term maintenance of weight loss, the question becomes "How do they do it?"

Obesity Does Respond to Diet and Exercise

The first line of defense in treating obesity in adults is a low-energy diet and regular physical activity. Overweight and obese individuals should work with their healthcare provider to design and maintain a healthy diet that has a deficit of 500 to 1,000 kcal/day. Physical activity should be increased gradually, so that the person can build a program in which

LO 8 Describe three treatment options for obesity.

 To view a detailed interactive graphic of the seven predominant themes highlighted in the Foresight Obesity map, go to http://www.shiftn.com.

To learn more about the complex factors contributing to the rise in obesity in the United States, watch a video from CDC-TV, the video channel of the U.S. Centers for Disease Control and Prevention, at http://www.cdc.gov/.

he or she is exercising at least 30 minutes per day, five times per week. The Institute of Medicine[35] concurs that 30 minutes a day, five times a week is the minimum amount of physical activity needed, but up to 60 minutes per day may be necessary for many people to lose weight and to sustain a body weight in the healthy range over the long term.

Counseling and support groups, such as Overeaters Anonymous (OA), can help people maintain these dietary and activity changes. Psychotherapy can be particularly helpful in challenging clients to examine the underlying thought patterns, situations, and stressors that may be undermining their efforts at weight loss.

Weight Loss Can Be Enhanced with Prescription Medications

The biggest complaint about the lifestyle recommendations for healthful weight loss is that these behaviors are difficult to maintain. Many people have tried to follow them for years but have not been successful. In response to this challenge, prescription drugs have been developed to assist people with weight loss. These drugs typically act as appetite suppressants and may also increase satiety.

Weight-loss medications should be used only with proper supervision from a physician, and while simultaneously following the diet and physical activity recommendations under which the drugs were tested. Physician involvement is so critical because many drugs developed for weight loss have serious side effects. Some have even proven deadly. These life-threatening drugs have been banned, yet they still serve as examples illustrating that the treatment of obesity through pharmacological means is neither simple nor risk-free.

Nine prescription weight-loss drugs are currently available.[36] The long-term safety of many of these drugs is still being explored:

- Diethylpropion (brand name Tenuate), phentermine (brand name Adipex-P or Suprenza), benzphetamine (brand name Didrex), and phendimetrazine (brand name Bontril) are drugs that decrease appetite and increase feelings of fullness. These are approved for only short-term use (typically less than 12 weeks) because of their potential to be abused. Side effects include increased blood pressure and heart rate, nervousness, insomnia, dry mouth, and constipation.
- Lorcaserin (brand name Belviq) also works by decreasing appetite and increasing feelings of fullness. Side effects include increased heart rate, headache, dizziness, and nausea.
- Naltrexone and bupropion extended-release (brand name Contrave) decreases appetite and increases feelings of fullness, with side effects including nausea, constipation, headache, vomiting and dizziness.
- Liraglutide (brand name Saxenda) slows gastric emptying and increases feelings of fullness. Side effects include nausea, vomiting, and inflammation of the pancreas (or pancreatitis).
- Orlistat (brand name Xenical) is a drug that acts to inhibit the absorption of dietary fat from the intestinal tract. Orlistat is also available in a reduced-strength form (brand name Alli) that is available without a prescription. Side effects include intestinal cramps, gas, diarrhea, and oily spotting. Although rare, liver injury can occur; thus, people taking orlistat should be aware of symptoms of liver injury, which include itching, loss of appetite, yellow eyes or skin, light-colored stools, or brown urine.
- Combination phentermine–topiramate (brand name Qsymia) decreases appetite and increases feelings of fullness. Side effects include increased heart rate, tingling of hands and feet, dry mouth, constipation, anxiety, and birth defects. Because of this increased risk for birth defects, women of childbearing years must avoid getting pregnant while taking this medication. Although it has been approved for long-term use, Qsymia contains phentermine and thus has the potential for abuse.

Although the use of prescribed weight-loss medications is associated with side effects and a certain level of risk, they are justified for people who are obese. That's because the health risks of obesity override the risks of the medications. They are also advised for people who have a BMI greater than or equal to 27 kg/m² who also have other significant health risk factors such as heart disease, hypertension, and type 2 diabetes.

Many Supplements Used for Weight Loss Contain Stimulants

The Office of Dietary Supplements (ODS) of the U.S. National Institutes of Health reports that the use of various supplements and alternative treatments for weight loss is common (20.6% among women and 9.7% among men). The ODS has reports that there is insufficient evidence of effectiveness for many of these products, including bitter orange, chromium, chitosan (derived from the exoskeleton of crustaceans), conjugated linoleic acid, guar gum, raspberry ketone, and yohimbe.[37] Yet these products continue their brisk sales to people desperate to lose weight.

Some products marketed for weight loss do indeed increase metabolic rate and decrease appetite; however, they prompt these effects because they contain *stimulants*, substances that speed up physiologic processes. Use of these products may be dangerous because abnormal increases in heart rate and blood pressure can occur. Stimulants commonly found in weight loss supplements include caffeine, phenylpropanolamine (PPA), and ephedra:

- **Caffeine**. In addition to being a stimulant, caffeine is addictive; nevertheless, it is legal and unregulated in most countries and is considered safe when consumed in moderate amounts (up to the equivalent of three to four cups of coffee). Adverse effects of high doses of caffeine include nervousness, irritability, anxiety, muscle twitching and tremors, headaches, elevated blood pressure, and irregular or rapid heartbeat. Long-term overuse of high doses of caffeine can lead to sleep and anxiety disorders that require clinical attention. Deaths due to caffeine toxicity have been associated primarily with caffeine tablets and energy drinks.
- **Phenylpropanolamine (PPA)**. In the year 2000, in response to several deaths, the FDA banned over-the-counter medications containing PPA, an ingredient that had been used in many cough and cold medications as well as in weight-loss formulas. However, PPA may still be present in dietary supplements marketed for weight loss because these are beyond FDA control.
- **Ephedra**. The use of ephedra has been associated with dangerous elevations in heart rate, blood pressure, and death. The FDA has banned the manufacture and sale of ephedra in the United States; however, some weight-loss supplements still contain *mahuang*, the so-called herbal ephedra. *Mahuang* is simply the Chinese name for ephedra. Some weight-loss supplements contain a combination of *mahuang*, caffeine, and aspirin.

As you can see, using weight-loss dietary supplements entails serious health risks.

Surgery Can Be Used to Treat Morbid Obesity

For people who are morbidly obese, surgery may be recommended. Generally, **bariatric surgery** (from the Greek word *baros* meaning "weight") is advised for people with a BMI greater than or equal to 40 kg/m² or for people with a BMI greater than or equal to 35 kg/m² who have other life-threatening conditions, such as diabetes, hypertension, or elevated cholesterol levels. The three most common types of weight-loss surgery are sleeve gastrectomy, gastric bypass, and gastric banding (**Figure 13.10**, page 524).

Bariatric surgery is considered a last resort for morbidly obese people who have not been able to lose weight with energy restriction, exercise, and medications. This is because the risks of surgery in people with morbid obesity are extremely high. They include an increased rate of infections, formation of blood clots, and adverse reactions to anesthesia.

However, bariatric surgery is not a simple procedure or a guaranteed cure for obesity. As a form of major surgery, risks associated with the various forms of bariatric surgery

bariatric surgery Surgical alteration of the gastrointestinal tract performed to promote weight loss.

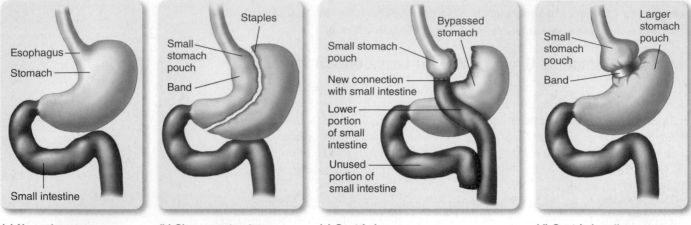

(a) Normal anatomy

(b) Sleeve gastrectomy

(c) Gastric bypass

(d) Gastric banding

FIGURE 13.10 Various forms of bariatric surgery alter the normal anatomy **(a)** of the gastrointestinal tract to result in weight loss. Sleeve gastrectomy **(b)**, gastric bypass **(c)**, and gastric banding **(d)**, are three surgical procedures used to reduce morbid obesity.

include excessive bleeding, infection, adverse reaction to anesthesia, blood clots, leaking from the gastrointestinal tract, and in relatively rare cases, death. After the surgery, many recipients face a lifetime of problems with chronic diarrhea, vomiting, intolerance to dairy products and other foods, dehydration, and nutritional deficiencies resulting from alterations in nutrient digestion and absorption that occur with bypass procedures. Additional longer-term complications include bowel obstruction, gallstones, hernias, hypoglycemia, ulcers, and perforation of the stomach. Thus, the potential benefits of the procedure must outweigh the risks. It is critical that each surgery candidate be carefully screened by a trained bariatric surgical team, which includes assessments of physical and psychological readiness for the surgery itself, and also for the lifestyle changes that need to be followed to ensure weight loss and maintenance of weight loss post-surgery. If the immediate threat of serious disease and death is more dangerous than the risks associated with surgery, then the procedure is justified.

About one-third to one-half of people who undergo bariatric surgery lose significant amounts of weight, and the limited research examining longer-term maintenance of weight loss indicate people are able to maintain weight loss for 3 to 5 years.[38] They also substantially reduce their risk for type 2 diabetes, and in many cases type 2 diabetes is fully resolved. Hypertension, elevated blood lipids, cardiovascular disease, and sleep apnea are also significantly reduced following the surgery.[38] The reasons that one-half to two-thirds do not experience long-term success include the following:

- Inability to eat less over time, even with a smaller stomach
- Loosening of staples and gastric bands and sleeves and enlargement of the stomach pouch
- Failure to survive the surgery or the postoperative recovery period

Liposuction is a cosmetic surgical procedure that removes fat cells from localized areas in the body. It is not recommended or typically used to treat obesity or morbid obesity. Instead, it is often used by normal or mildly overweight people to "spot reduce" fat from various areas of the body. This procedure is not without risks, however; blood clots, skin and nerve damage, adverse drug reactions, and perforation injuries can and do occur as a result of liposuction. It can also cause deformations in the area where the fat is removed. This procedure is not the solution to long-term weight loss, because the millions of fat cells that remain in the body after

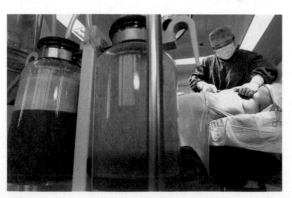

Liposuction removes fat cells from specific areas of the body.

liposuction enlarge if the person continues to overeat. In addition, although liposuction may reduce the fat content of a localized area, it does not reduce a person's risk for the diseases that are more common among overweight or obese people. Only traditional weight loss with diet and exercise can reduce body fat and the risks for chronic diseases.

RECAP

The first line of defense in treating obesity in adults is a low-energy diet and regular physical activity. Counseling and support groups can also help. Nine prescription weight-loss medications are currently available, but these should be used only with proper supervision from a physician because many have serious side effects, and some can even be deadly. Use of dietary supplements for weight loss is common; however, many are stimulants that cause abnormal increases in heart rate and blood pressure and can therefore be dangerous or even deadly. Bariatric surgery is typically reserved for people with a BMI greater than or equal to 40 kg/m² or for people with a BMI greater than or equal to 35 kg/m² who have other life-threatening conditions. The three most common types of weight-loss surgery are sleeve gastrectomy, gastric bypass, and gastric banding. Only about one-third to one-half of people who undergo bariatric surgery lose weight, maintain their weight loss, and reduce their chronic disease risks. Liposuction, localized removal of fat cells, is not recommended or typically used to treat obesity. ∎

How Can You Lose Weight Safely and Keep It Off?

LO 9 Develop a diet, exercise, and behavioral plan for healthful weight loss.

Achieving and maintaining a healthful body weight involve three primary strategies:

- Reasonable reductions in energy intake
- Incorporation of regular and appropriate physical activity
- Application of behavior modification techniques

In this section, we first discuss popular diet plans, which may or may not incorporate these strategies. We then explain how to design a personalized weight-loss plan that includes all three of them.

Avoid Fad Diets

If you'd like to lose weight and feel more comfortable following an established plan, many are available. How can you know whether or not it is based on sound dietary principles, and whether its promise of long-term weight loss will prove true for *you*? Look to the three strategies just identified: Does the plan promote gradual reductions in energy intake? Does it advocate increased physical activity? Does it include strategies for modifying your eating and activity-related behaviors? Reputable diet plans incorporate all of these strategies. Unfortunately, many dieters are drawn to fad diets, which do not.

Fad diets are simply what their name implies—fads that do not result in long-term, healthful weight changes. To be precise, fad diets are programs that enjoy short-term popularity and are sold based on a marketing gimmick that appeals to the public's desires and fears. Of the hundreds of such diets on the market today, most will "die" within a year, only to be born again as a "new and improved" fad diet. The goal of the person or company designing and marketing a fad diet is to make money.

How can you tell if the program you are interested in qualifies as a fad diet? Here are some pointers to help you:

- The promoters of the diet claim that the program is new, improved, or based on some new discovery; however, no scientific data are available to support these claims.

- The program is touted for its ability to promote rapid weight loss or body fat loss, usually more than 2 pounds per week, and may include the claim that weight loss can be achieved with little or no physical exercise.
- The diet includes special foods and supplements, many of which are expensive and/or difficult to find or can be purchased only from the diet promoter. Common recommendations for these diets include avoiding certain foods, eating only a special combination of certain foods, and including "magic" foods in the diet that "burn fat" and "speed up metabolism."
- The diet may include a rigid menu that must be followed daily or may limit participants to eating a few select foods each day. Variety and balance are discouraged, and restriction of certain foods (such as particular fruits, vegetables, or whole grains) is encouraged.
- Many programs promote supplemental foods and/or nutritional supplements that are described as critical to the success of the diet. They usually include claims that these supplements can cure or prevent a variety of health ailments or that the diet can stop the aging process.

In a world where many of us feel we have to meet a certain physical standard to be attractive and "good enough," fad diets flourish, with millions of people trying one each year.[39] Unfortunately, the only people who usually benefit from them are their marketers, who can become very wealthy promoting programs that are highly ineffectual.

Many Diets Focus on Macronutrient Composition

The three main types of weight-loss diets that have been most seriously and comprehensively researched all encourage increased consumption of certain macronutrients and restrict the consumption of others. Provided here is a brief review of these diets and their general effects on weight loss and health parameters.

Diets High in Carbohydrate and Moderate in Fat and Protein

Nutritionally balanced high-carbohydrate (that are less processed), moderate-fat and moderate-protein diets typically contain 55% to 60% of total energy intake as carbohydrate, 20% to 30% of total energy intake as fat, and 15% to 20% of energy intake as protein. These diets include Weight Watchers, Jenny Craig, and others that follow the general guidelines of the DASH diet and the USDA Food Guide. Typical energy deficits are between 500 and 1,000 kcal/day. A substantial amount of high-quality scientific evidence (from randomized controlled trials) indicates that these diets may be effective in decreasing body weight—at least initially. In addition, the people who lose weight on these diets may also decrease their LDL-cholesterol, reduce their blood triglyceride levels, and decrease their blood pressure. However, in 2006 a series of studies reporting results from a randomized controlled trial following almost 50,000 U.S. women for 7 years found that, contrary to established beliefs, this type of diet did not result in significant long-term weight loss or reduce the risks for breast and colorectal cancers or cardiovascular disease.[40–43] Is it possible that diets high in carbohydrate and moderate in fat and protein are not as effective as we'd come to believe? Refer to the *Nutrition Myth or Fact?* essay at the end of this chapter (pages 533–535) to learn more about this controversy.

Diets Low in Carbohydrate and High in Fat and Protein

Low-carbohydrate, high-fat and protein diets cycle in and out of popularity on a regular basis. By definition, these types of diets generally contain about 55% to 65% of total energy intake as fat and most of the remaining balance of daily energy intake as protein. Examples of these types of diets include Dr. Atkins' Diet Revolution, Sugar Busters, and the Paleo Diet. These diets minimize the role of restricting total energy intake on weight loss. They

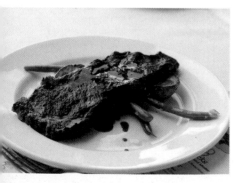

"Low-carb" diets may lead to weight loss, but they can be nutritionally inadequate in some cases.

instead advise participants to restrict carbohydrate intake, proposing that carbohydrates are addictive and that they cause significant overeating, insulin surges leading to excessive fat storage, and an overall metabolic imbalance that leads to obesity. The goal is to reduce carbohydrates enough to cause ketosis, which will decrease blood glucose and insulin levels and can reduce appetite.

Countless people claim to have lost substantial weight on these types of diets. The current limited evidence that has examined their effectiveness suggests that individuals following them, in both free-living and experimental conditions, do lose weight and improve their metabolic risk factors (such as blood lipid levels) for a period of at least 6 months.[44] However, the long-term health benefits of this type of a diet are unknown at this time, and more research must be conducted in this area.

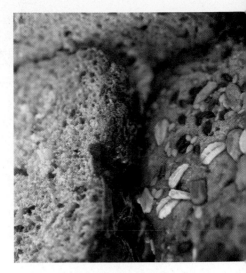

Low-fat and very-low-fat diets emphasize eating foods higher in complex carbohydrates and fiber.

Low-Fat and Very-Low-Fat Diets

Low-fat diets contain 11% to 19% of total energy as fat, whereas very-low-fat diets contain less than 10% of total energy as fat. Both of these types of diets are high in carbohydrate and moderate in protein, and tend to emphasize eating foods high in complex carbohydrates and fiber. Examples include Dr. Dean Ornish's Program for Reversing Heart Disease, which is vegetarian, and the New Pritikin Program, which allows 3.5 oz of lean meat per day. These programs were not originally designed for weight loss but, rather, were developed to decrease or reverse heart disease.

Consumers view these diets as too restrictive and difficult to follow; thus, there are limited data on their effects. However, high-quality evidence suggests that people following these diets do lose weight, and some data suggest that they also experience decreased blood pressure, LDL-cholesterol, blood triglyceride, glucose, and insulin levels. Few side effects have been reported; however, these diets are typically low in essential fatty acids, vitamins B_{12} and E, and zinc. Thus, supplementation is needed. These types of diets are not considered safe for people with diabetes who are insulin dependent (either type 1 or type 2) or for people with carbohydrate-malabsorption illnesses.

If You Design Your Own Diet Plan, Include the Three Strategies

As we noted earlier, a healthful and effective weight-loss plan involves implementing a modest reduction in energy intake, incorporating physical activity into each day, and practicing changes in behavior that can assist you in reducing your energy intake and increasing your energy expenditure. Following are some guidelines for designing your own personalized diet plan that incorporates these strategies.

Set Realistic Goals

The first key to safe and effective weight loss is setting realistic, achievable goals related to how much weight to lose and how quickly to lose it. Although making gradual changes in body weight is frustrating for most people, this slower change is much more effective in maintaining weight loss over the long term. Ask yourself the question "How long did it take me to gain this extra weight?" If you are like most people, your answer is that it took 1 or more years, not just a few months. A fair expectation for weight loss is similarly gradual: experts recommend a pace of about 0.5 to 2 pounds per week. A weight-loss plan should never provide less than 1,200 kcal/day unless you are under a physician's supervision. For most individuals, you do not want a diet that provides less than your energy needs to cover your BMR. Your weight-loss goals should also take into consideration any health-related concerns you have. After checking with your physician, you may decide initially to set a goal of simply maintaining your current weight and preventing additional weight gain. After your weight has remained stable for several weeks, you might then write down realistic goals for weight loss.

Goals that are more likely to be realistic and achievable share the following characteristics:

- *They are specific.* Telling yourself "I will eat less this week" is not helpful because the goal is not specific. An example of a specific goal is "I will eat only half of my restaurant entrée tonight and take the rest home and eat it tomorrow for lunch."
- *They are reasonable.* If you are not presently physically active, it would be unreasonable to set off a goal of exercising for 30 minutes every day. A more reasonable goal would be to exercise for 15 minutes per day, 3 days per week. Once you've achieved that goal, you can increase the frequency, intensity, and time of exercise according to the improvements in fitness that you have experienced.
- *They are measurable.* Effective goals are ones you can measure. An example is "I will lose at least 1 pound by May 1st."

Recording and monitoring your goals will help you better determine whether you are achieving them, or whether you need to revise them based on accomplishments or challenges that arise.

Eat Smaller Portions of Lower-Fat Foods

 Portion sizes have grown over the last few decades. To find out how much, take the Portion Distortion quiz from the National Institutes of Health at www.nhlbi.nih.gov/.

The portion sizes of foods offered and sold in restaurants and grocery stores have expanded considerably over the past 40 years. One of the most challenging issues related to food is understanding what a healthful portion size is and knowing how to reduce the portion sizes of the foods we eat.

Studies indicate that larger portions sizes of various foods and beverages are associated with eating more energy in both children and adults.[45,46] Thus, it has been suggested that effective weight-loss strategies include reducing both the portion size and the energy density of foods consumed, as well as replacing sugary drinks with low-Calorie or non-Calorie beverages.

What specific changes can you make to reduce your energy intake and stay healthy? Here are some suggestions:

- Follow the serving sizes recommended in the USDA Food Patterns (ChooseMyPlate .gov). Making this change involves understanding what constitutes a portion and measuring foods to determine whether they meet or exceed the recommended amounts.
- To help increase your understanding of the portion sizes of packaged foods, measure out the amount of food that is identified as 1 serving on the Nutrition Facts panel, and eat it from a plate or bowl instead of straight out of the box or bag.
- Try using smaller dishes, bowls, and glasses. This will make your portion appear larger, and you'll be eating or drinking less.
- When cooking at home, put a serving of the entrée on your plate; then freeze any leftovers in single-serving containers. This way, you won't be tempted to eat the whole batch before the food goes bad, and you'll have ready-made servings for future meals.
- To help fill you up, take second helpings of plain vegetables. That way, dessert may not seem so tempting!
- When buying snacks, go for single-serving, prepackaged items. If you buy larger bags or boxes, divide the snack into single-serving bags.
- Avoid or strictly limit your alcohol consumption. Remember, alcohol packs 7 kcal/gram, and it is preferentially used as an energy source, since we have no alcohol "storage" in the body. As a result, more of the fat in a meal that is consumed with alcohol can be stored as body fat. In addition, many mixed drinks have added sugars and cream, contributing even more Calories to the diet.

In addition to controlling portion sizes, try to increase the number of times each day that you choose foods that are relatively low in energy density. This includes salads (with low- or non-Calorie dressings), whole fruits and vegetables, whole grains, low-fat and nonfat dairy products, lean meats, and broth-based soups. Research indicates that eating a diet low in energy density results in greater weight loss than simply reducing portion sizes.[47] Because low energy-dense foods are relatively high in water and fiber than more energy-dense foods, they have a greater volume and occupy more space in the stomach, helping a person to feel full. In addition, low energy-dense foods are just as satiating as those higher in energy density, but they are lower in energy for every gram of food consumed. Thus, the energy content of an energy-dense eating plan is lower but equally as satisfying.

Meal Focus Figure 13.11 (page 530) illustrates two sets of meals, one higher in energy density and one lower in energy density. You can see from this figure that simple changes to a meal, such as choosing lower-fat dairy products and leaner meats, and reducing portion sizes, can reduce energy intake without sacrificing taste, pleasure, or nutritional quality!

Participate in Regular Physical Activity

The *Dietary Guidelines for Americans* emphasize the role of physical activity in maintaining a healthful weight. Why? Of course, we expend extra energy during physical activity, but there's more to it than that, because exercise alone (without a reduction of energy intake) does not result in dramatic weight loss. Instead, one of the most important reasons for being regularly active is that it helps us maintain or increase our lean body mass and our BMR. In contrast, energy restriction alone causes us to lose lean body mass. As you've learned, the more lean body mass we have, the more energy we expend over the long term.

Although very few weight-loss studies have documented long-term maintenance of weight loss, those that have find that only people who are regularly active are able to maintain most of their weight loss. The National Weight Control Registry is an ongoing project documenting the habits of people who have lost at least 30 pounds and kept their weight off for at least 1 year. Of the people studied thus far, the average weight loss was 66 pounds over 5.5 years.[48] Almost all of the people (98%) reported changing their dietary intake to lose weight, and 94% report increasing their physical activity, with walking being the most commonly reported form of activity. These successful "losers" reported doing an average of at least 1 hour of physical activity per day.

In addition to expending energy and maintaining lean body mass and BMR, regular physical activity improves our mood, results in a higher quality of sleep, increases self-esteem, and gives us a sense of accomplishment. All of these changes enhance our ability to engage in long-term healthful lifestyle behaviors.

What specific changes can you make to your level of physical activity? Although plenty of practical suggestions will be offered (in Chapter 14), here are some ideas that can help you start identifying—and overcoming—your barriers to an active life:

- "I don't have enough time!" An active lifestyle doesn't have to consume all your free time. Try to do a minimum of 30 minutes of moderate activity most—preferably all—days of the week. If you can, do 45 minutes. But remember, you don't have to get in all of your daily activity in one go! Be active for a few minutes at a time throughout your day. Walk from your dorm or apartment to classes, if possible. Instead of meeting friends for lunch, meet them for a lunchtime walk, jog, or workout. Break up study sessions with 3 minutes of jumping jacks. Skip the elevator and take the stairs. When you're talking on the phone, pace instead of sitting still.
- "I can't manage the details!" Bust this excuse by keeping clean clothes, shoes, water, and equipment for physical activity in a convenient place. If time management is an obstacle, enroll in a scheduled fitness class, yoga class, sports activity, walking group, or running club. Put it on your schedule of academic classes and make it part of your weekly routine.
- "I just don't like to work out!" You don't have to! Try dancing, roller blading, walking, hiking, swimming, tennis, or any other activity you enjoy.
- "I can't stay motivated!" Friends can help. Use the "buddy" system by exercising with a friend and calling each other when you need encouragement to stay motivated.

a day of meals

about 3,300 calories (kcal)

about 1,700 calories (kcal)

BREAKFAST

1½ cups Fruit Loops cereal
1 cup 2% milk
1 cup orange juice
2 slices white toast
1 tbsp. butter (on toast)

1½ cups Cheerios cereal
1 cup skim milk
½ fresh pink grapefruit

LUNCH

McDonald's Big Mac hamburger
French fries, extra large
3 tbsp. ketchup
Apple pie

Subway cold-cut trio 6" sandwich
Granola bar, hard, with chocolate chips, 1 bar (24 g)
1 fresh medium apple

DINNER

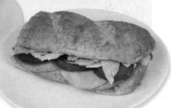

5 oz ground turkey, cooked
2 soft corn tortillas
1 oz low-fat cheddar cheese
4 tbsp. store-bought salsa
1 cup shredded lettuce
1 cup cooked mixed veggies

4.5 oz ground beef (80% lean, crumbled), cooked
2 medium taco shells
2 oz cheddar cheese
2 tbsp. sour cream
4 tbsp. store-bought salsa
1 cup shredded lettuce
½ cup refried beans
6 Oreos

nutrient analysis

3,319 kcal
44.1% of energy from carbohydrates
44.2% of energy from fat
15.6% of energy from saturated fat
12.5% of energy from protein
31.4 grams of dietary fiber
4,752 milligrams of sodium

nutrient analysis

1,753 kcal
44.6% of energy from carbohydrates
31.5% of energy from fat
10.6% of energy from saturated fat
21% of energy from protein
24.9 grams of dietary fiber
3,161 milligrams of sodium

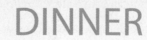

Saves 1,600 kcals!

Or keep a journal or log of your daily physical activity. Write your week's goal at the top of the page (such as "Walk to and from campus each day, and at least 10 minutes on campus at lunch"). Then track your progress. If you achieve your goal for the week, reward yourself with a film, a new song for your iPod, or some other non-food treat.

Incorporate Appropriate Behavior Modifications into Daily Life

Successful weight loss and long-term maintenance of a healthful weight require people to modify their behaviors. Some of the behavior modifications related to food and physical activity were discussed in the previous sections. Here are a few more tips on modifying behavior that will assist you in losing weight and maintaining a healthful weight:

- Shop for food only when you're not hungry.
- Avoid buying problem foods—that is, high-fat, high-sugar foods or foods that you may have difficulty eating in moderate amounts. Save high-kcal sweets, such as ice cream, doughnuts, and cakes, for occasional special treats.
- Avoid feelings of deprivation by eating small, regular meals throughout the day.
- Always use appropriate utensils.
- Stop at once if you begin to feel full. Leave food on your plate or store it for the next meal.
- Keep a log of what you eat, when, and why. Try to identify social or emotional cues that cause you to overeat, such as getting a poor grade on an exam or feeling lonely. Then strategize about non-food-related ways to cope, such as phoning a sympathetic friend.
- Whether at home or dining out, share food with others.
- Prepare healthful snacks to take along with you, so that you won't be tempted by foods from vending machines, food kiosks, and so forth.
- Don't punish yourself for deviating from your plan (and you will—everyone does). Ask others to avoid responding to any slips you make.

Interest has been growing about the effects of applying mindfulness to our eating practices. *Mindfulness* refers to the nonjudgmental awareness of the present moment. **Mindful eating** refers to a nonjudgmental awareness of the emotional and physical sensations one experiences while eating or in a food-related environment. Several recently published pilot studies conducted with small numbers of participants have indicated that mindful eating may help to promote healthy eating practices when eating out; enhance weight loss and psychological well-being in people with obesity; and improve dietary intake and blood glucose control in adults with type 2 diabetes.[49–51]

Interested in exploring mindful eating practices? Here are some tips to help get you started:

- Focus only on eating: Turn off the television, put away your cell phone, tune out distractions, and focus on your food and the process of eating.
- Savor each bite: Take your time, slow down, and chew slowly.
- Recruit all of your senses: Focus your attention on the smell, taste, texture, and even the temperature of your food. Pay attention to any sensations of satisfaction or fullness.
- Pause and rest between bites: Take a few breaths, sit back, and relax between each mouthful of food.
- Try 10 minutes of silence: If eating with others, try to avoid conversations in order to enhance your ability to be more aware of your food and the experience of eating.

Incorporating mindful eating into your life doesn't have to be a chore. Try practicing mindful eating during one meal each week. With practice, you may be inspired to do it more often!

mindful eating The nonjudgmental awareness of the emotional and physical sensations one experiences while eating or in a food-related environment.

RECAP

If you would like to lose weight and maintain that weight loss, a first step is to set a realistic, achievable goal. Experts recommend a pace of about 0.5 to 2 pounds of weight loss per week. You can achieve this by making gradual reductions in energy intake, such as by eating smaller portion sizes and choosing foods low in energy density and high in nutrient density. The precise macronutrient composition of the diet is thought to matter less than reduction in your energy intake. Avoid fad diets, programs that enjoy short-term popularity but do not incorporate sensible energy, activity, and behavioral strategies. A second step is to engage in regular physical activity, typically at least 30 minutes a day at least 5 days a week. This will not only burn energy but also help maintain or increase your lean body mass and BMR. Third and finally, apply appropriate behavior modification techniques, such as keeping a food log, avoiding shopping when you're hungry, and engaging in mindful eating. ■

 Identify four key strategies for gaining weight safely and effectively.

What If You Need to Gain Weight?

As defined earlier in this chapter, underweight occurs when a person has too little body fat to maintain health. People with a BMI of less than 18.5 kg/m² are typically considered underweight. Being underweight can be just as unhealthful as being obese, because it increases the risk for infections and illness and impairs the body's ability to recover. Some people are healthy but underweight because of their genetics and/or because they are very physically active and consume adequate energy to maintain their underweight status, but not enough to gain weight. In others, underweight is due to heavy smoking; an underlying disease, such as cancer or HIV infection; or an eating disorder, such as *anorexia nervosa* (see Chapter 13.5, "In Depth: Disordered Eating").

For Safe and Effective Weight Gain, Choose Nutrient-Dense Foods

With so much emphasis in the United States on obesity and weight loss, some find it surprising that many people are trying to gain weight. People looking to gain weight include those who are underweight to the extent that it is compromising their health and many athletes who are attempting to increase strength and power for competition.

To gain weight, people must eat more energy than they expend. While overeating large amounts of foods high in saturated fats (such as bacon, sausage, and cheese) can cause weight gain, doing this without exercising is not considered healthful because most of the weight gained is fat, and high-fat diets increase our risks for cardiovascular and other diseases. However, diets that are relatively higher in mono- and polyunsaturated fats, such as a Mediterranean-style diet, can be a healthful approach to weight gain. Recommendations for weight gain include:

- Eat a diet that includes about 500 to 1,000 kcal/day more than is needed to maintain present body weight. Although we don't know exactly how much extra energy is needed to gain 1 pound, estimates range from 3,000 to 3,500 kcal. Thus, eating 500 to 1,000 kcal/day in excess should result in a gain of 1 to 2 pounds of weight each week.
- Eat frequently, including meals and numerous snacks throughout the day. Many underweight people do not take the time to eat often enough.
- Avoid the use of tobacco products, as they depress appetite and increase metabolic rate, and both of these effects oppose weight gain. Tobacco use also causes lung, mouth, esophageal and other cancers and is a factor in cardiovascular disease.
- Exercise regularly and incorporate weight lifting or some other form of resistance training into your exercise routine. This form of exercise is most effective in increasing muscle mass. Performing aerobic exercise (such as walking, running, bicycling, or swimming) at least 30 minutes for 3 days per week will help maintain a healthy cardiovascular system.

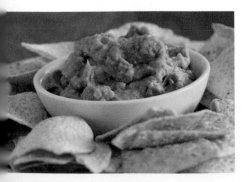

Eating frequent nutrient-dense snacks can help promote weight gain.

The key to gaining weight is to eat frequent meals throughout the day and to select healthful energy-dense foods. For instance, smoothies and milkshakes made with low-fat milk or yogurt are a great way to take in a lot of energy. Eating peanut butter with fruit or celery and including salad dressings on your salad are other ways to increase the energy density of foods. The biggest challenge to weight gain is setting aside time to eat; by packing a lot of foods to take with you throughout the day, you can enhance your opportunities to eat more.

Amino Acid and Protein Supplements Do Not Increase Muscle Mass

As with weight loss, there are many products marketed for weight gain. Many of these products are said to be *anabolic,* that is, to increase muscle mass. The most common of these include amino acid and protein supplements, often powders used to make protein "shakes." Do these substances really work?

As discussed earlier (in Chapter 6), current evidence illustrates that amino acid and protein supplements are not necessary to enhance muscle gain; adequate intake of energy, protein from high-quality food sources, and resistance training promote healthy increases in muscle mass. The health consequences of using them are unknown. Moreover, although they are legal to sell in the United States, all potentially anabolic substances are banned by the National Football League, the National Collegiate Athletic Association, and the International Olympic Committee. We also know that buying these substances can have a substantial slenderizing effect—on your wallet!

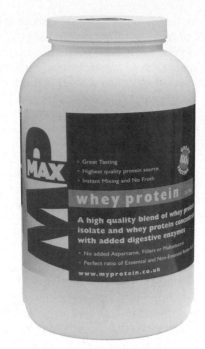

Protein powders or amino acid supplements will not enhance muscle growth or make you stronger.

RECAP

Weight gain can be achieved by increasing your kcal intake by about 500 to 1,000 kcal/day more than is needed to maintain present body weight. Focus on eating more nutrient-dense foods. Engage in regular resistance training to build and maintain muscle mass, and aerobic exercise to preserve your cardiovascular fitness. Avoid tobacco use, as it depresses appetite and increases metabolic rate, and is associated with an increased risk of cancer and many other diseases. Protein and amino acid supplements do not increase muscle mass, and their potential side effects are unknown. Anabolic substances are banned by major sports governing organizations. ■

Nutrition Myth OR Fact?

High-Carbohydrate, Moderate-Fat Diets—Have They Been Oversold?

For the past 30 years, dietary fat has been demonized as the cause of obesity, cardiovascular disease, type 2 diabetes, and many types of cancers. As a result, nutrition professionals have emphasized the health benefits of eating a moderate-fat, high-carbohydrate diet, and national dietary guidelines have promoted this message. However in 2006, published results from the Women's Health Initiative (WHI) Dietary Modification Trial shook the nutrition and health world and caused experts to seriously question the existing beliefs that moderate-fat diets are the key to reducing our risks for many chronic diseases.

The WHI Dietary Modification Trial involved 48,835 ethnically diverse postmenopausal women aged 50 to 79 years.[1] Women were randomized into either a control group that received a copy of the *Dietary Guidelines for Americans* and other health materials or an intervention group. Women

randomized to the intervention group received an intensive behavioral modification program involving eighteen group sessions in the first year of the study, followed by quarterly maintenance sessions. The intervention promoted dietary changes to achieve a goal of 20% of energy intake from fat (7% of energy intake from saturated fat), an increase in fruit and vegetable intake to at least five servings per day, and an increase in whole grains to at least 6 servings per day. However, the diet was not intended to reduce energy intake or induce weight loss. The average length of time to follow up participants was 8 years.

The results from this study, which is the most expensive study of diet conducted to date, surprised many experts. At the end of the follow-up period, there was no significant health benefit in the intervention group—there was no reduction in risk for cardiovascular disease, breast cancer, or colorectal cancer.[1-3] One benefit that was observed was that women in the intervention group lost weight during the first year (a loss of approximate 4.8 pounds), and they maintained a lower weight than women in the control group over 7.5 years.[4] Some women in the control group also lost weight, and the greatest amount of weight lost in both groups occurred in those who decreased their percentage of energy intake from fat.

What do these results mean? Should we no longer be concerned about the risks of dietary fat? Should we eat however we choose? The study had a number of limitations that need to be recognized, and an editorial published by the Harvard School of Public Health has helped put these findings into perspective.[5] Although participants in the intervention reduced their fat intake from 38% to 29% of total energy intake, they did not reach the target goal of consuming no more than 20% of energy intake from fat. Thus, it has been suggested that a lower-fat diet might be more effective in reducing the risk for chronic diseases. In addition, the participants were postmenopausal women, and it might be that intervening at this age is too late to prevent the development of cardiovascular disease and various cancers. Because dietary intake was self-reported, it might also be possible that the women over-reported the actual dietary changes they made, meaning that they did not improve their diet as reported and thus no health changes would result. Another issue is that it may take longer than 8 years to see the health benefits of this type of diet, and thus a much longer study would be needed to detect health benefits.

However there is now a growing body of evidence that the key to reducing chronic disease risks is focusing on changing the *type* of dietary fat consumed, not the total amount.[5] The challenge with reducing dietary fat is that many people choose to substitute low-fiber, highly refined carbohydrate foods in place of fat. This substitution leads to negative changes in blood lipids and blood glucose. In fact, the detrimental health effects resulting from the over-

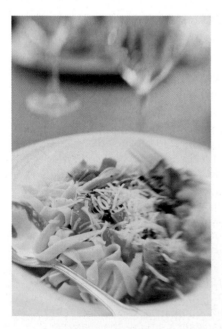

consumption of processed foods and grain-fed animals is a key factor driving the popularity of the Paleo (or Paleolithic) Diet. The Paleo Diet claims that the human body today is in the same evolutionary state as it was in prehistoric times, and thus we should eat the same diet that our prehistoric ancestors ate if we want to lose weight and optimize our health.[6] The Paleo Diet emphasizes the consumption of only those foods that can be hunted, fished, or gathered. This includes fresh lean meats and fish (ideally wild game and fish), eggs, fruits, some vegetables, nuts and seeds, and olive and coconut oils. All refined foods are prohibited, along with all grains, legumes, dairy, and processed vegetable oils such as canola. To date, no scientifically sound research studies have been conducted on the long-term effects of the Paleo Diet on weight loss or health. In theory, this diet could result in positive health changes due to consumption of plant foods, lean meats and fish, and reduced intake of sodium and added sugars. However, the Academy of Nutrition and Dietetics emphasizes that this diet exceeds the recommend dietary guidelines for saturated fat and protein intake and is deficient in carbohydrates; moreover, the exclusion of whole grains, legumes, and dairy could lead to deficiencies in micronutrients such as calcium and vitamin D, as well as dietary fiber.[7]

So what is the most healthful approach to losing weight and maintaining weight loss? Most reputable sources, including the *Dietary Guidelines for Americans*, recommend reducing intake of saturated and *trans* fats, and increasing intake of plant oils and food sources high in poly- and monounsaturated fats. Lowering total fat intake may not be critically important unless a person is trying to reduce total energy intake. Even under these circumstances, people should be encouraged to optimize their intake of healthy fats and avoid replacing fat with refined carbohydrates.

Another take-home message is that too many Calories from any source will lead to weight gain. In contrast, any diet that reduces energy intake below energy expenditure, and that people can maintain healthfully and comfortably over a long period of time, will lead to weight loss. Add regular aerobic activity and resistance training, and the weight loss and health benefits will be even greater.

Critical Thinking Questions

- Is a high-carb, moderate-fat diet compatible with your personal needs, preferences, health risks, and lifestyle?
- Do you think that higher-fat diets, such as the Paleo Diet, are better or worse alternatives to higher-carbohydrate, lower-fat diets? Why or why not?
- What diet do you think would be easiest for you to follow long-term; incorporate most of your food preferences; work best to help you either lose weight, gain weight, or maintain a healthful weight; and provide enough energy and nutrients to maintain your lifestyle, your lean-body mass, and your long-term health? Consider not only the several diets discussed in this chapter (Atkins, Ornish, etc.) but also the many diets discussed elsewhere in this text (Mediterranean, vegetarian, etc.).

References

1. Howard, B. V., L. Van Horn, J. Hsia, J. E. Manson, M. L. Stefanick, S. Wassertheil-Smoller,…, and J. M. Kotchen. 2006. Low-fat dietary pattern and risk of cardiovascular disease. The Women's Health Initiative Randomized Controlled Dietary Modification Trial. *JAMA* 295(6):655–666.

2. Prentice, R. L., B. Caan, R. T. Chlebowski, R. Patterson, L. H. Kuller, J. K. Ockene,…, and M. M. Henderson. 2006. Low-fat dietary pattern and risk of invasive breast cancer. The Women's Health Initiative Randomized Controlled Dietary Modification Trial. *JAMA* 295(6): 629–642.

3. Beresford, S. A. A., K. C. Johnson, C. Ritenbaugh, N. L. Lasser, L. G. Snetselaar, H. R. Black,…, and E. Whitlock. 2006. Low-fat dietary pattern and risk of colorectal cancer. The Women's Health Initiative Randomized Controlled-Dietary Modification Trial. *JAMA* 295(6): 643–654.

4. Howard, B. V., J. E. Manson, M. L. Stefanick, S. A. Beresford, G. Frank, B. Jones,…, and R. Prentice. 2006. Low-fat dietary pattern and weight change over 7 years.

The Women's Health Initiative Randomized Controlled Dietary Modification Trial. *JAMA* 295(6): 39–49.

5. Harvard School of Public Health. 2012. Low-Fat Diet Not a Cure-All. *The Nutrition Source.* www.hsph.harvard.edu /nutritionsource/nutrition-news/low-fat/. (Accessed May 2015.)

6. Cordain, L. 2001. *The Paleo Diet: Lose Weight and Get Healthy by Eating the Foods You Were Designed to Eat.* New York: Wiley.

7. Academy of Nutrition and Dietetics. 2015. Should We Eat Like Our Caveman Ancestors? http://www.eatright.org /resource/health/weight-loss/fad-diets/should-we-eat-like-our-caveman-ancestors. (Accessed May, 2015).

STUDY **PLAN**   MasteringNutrition™

Customize your study plan—and master your nutrition!—in the Study Area of MasteringNutrition.

TEST YOURSELF | ANSWERS

1 (T) Being underweight increases our risk for illness and premature death and in many cases can be just as unhealthful as being obese.

2 (F) Body composition assessments can help give us a general idea of body fat levels, but most methods are not extremely accurate.

3 (T) Health can be defined in many ways. An individual who is overweight but who exercises regularly and has no additional risk factors for chronic diseases is considered a healthy person.

4 (F) It is currently estimated that approximately 34.9% of all adults in the United States are considered obese.

5 (F) Obesity is a multifactorial disease with many contributing factors. Although eating too much food and not getting enough exercise can lead to being overweight or obese, the disease of obesity is complex and is not simply caused by overeating.

summary

Scan to hear an MP3 Chapter Review in **MasteringNutrition**.

LO 1 ■ Ideals for body weight and shape are influenced by culture, and have changed throughout history and in different regions. Definitions of a healthful body weight include one that is appropriate for someone's age, level of development, and heredity; promotes healthful blood pressure, lipids, and glucose; can be achieved and sustained without constant dieting; is supported by promotes good eating habits and regular physical activity; and is acceptable to you.

LO 2 ■ Body mass index (BMI) is an index of weight per height squared. It is useful to indicate health risks associated with different weight categories in groups of people.

- Underweight is defined as having too little body fat to maintain health, causing a person to have a weight for a given height that is below an acceptably defined standard. A BMI below 18.5 kg/m² is considered underweight.

- Overweight is defined as having a moderate amount of excess body fat, resulting in a person having a weight for a given height that is greater than some accepted standard but is not considered obese. A BMI of 25 to 29.9 kg/m² is considered overweight.

- Obesity is defined as having excess body fat that adversely affects health, resulting in a person having a weight for a given height that is substantially greater than some accepted standard. A BMI of 30 to 39.9 kg/m² is considered obese. Morbid obesity occurs when a person's body weight exceeds 100% of normal, which puts him or her at very high risk for serious health consequences. A BMI of 40 kg/m² or above is considered morbidly obese.

- Body composition assessments, such as underwater weighing or skinfold tests, estimate your ratio of fat-to-lean body tissue, but have a significant range of error.

- The waist-to-hip ratio and waist circumference are used to determine patterns of fat distribution. People with large waists (as compared to the hips) have an apple-shaped fat pattern. People with large hips (as compared to the waist) have a pear-shaped fat pattern. Having an apple-shaped pattern increases your risk for heart disease, type 2 diabetes, and other chronic diseases.

LO 3 - We lose or gain weight based on changes in our energy intake (the food and beverages we consume) and our energy expenditure (both at rest and when physically active). The energy balance equation states that energy balance occurs when energy intake = energy expenditure.

LO 4 - Energy expenditure can be measured using direct calorimetry, which measures the amount of heat the body releases; however, the technique is costly and complex and is rarely used. In contrast, indirect calorimetry, which measures oxygen consumption and carbon dioxide production, is used to estimate energy expenditure in laboratory settings. Doubly labeled water can be used to measure energy expenditure in free-living situations, over longer periods of time, and with less inconvenience to study participants.

- The three components of energy expenditure are basal metabolic rate (BMR), the thermic effect of food (TEF), and the energy cost of physical activity. Basal metabolic rate (BMR) is the energy needed to maintain the body's resting functions. BMR accounts for 60% to 75% of our total daily energy needs.

- The thermic effect of food is the energy we expend to digest food, and to absorb, transport, metabolize, and store nutrients. It accounts for 5% to 10% of the energy content of a meal and is higher for processing proteins and carbohydrates than for fats.

- The energy cost of physical activity represents energy that we expend for physical movement or work we do above basal levels, including non-exercise activity thermogenesis as well as volitional exercise. It typically accounts for 15% to 35% of our total daily energy output.

- Research has called into question the accuracy and usefulness of the classic energy balance equation because it fails to account for many factors that alter energy intake and expenditure and to explain why people gain and lose weight differently.

LO 5 - Our genetic heritage influences our body weight and shape. The FTO gene variant appears to prompt overeating and weight gain. The thrifty gene theory suggests that some people possess a thrifty gene, or set of genes, that causes them to expend less energy at rest and during physical activity than people who do not have this gene (or genes). The set-point theory suggests that our body is designed to maintain weight within a narrow range, also called a set point.

- Eating a diet proportionally higher in fat may increase the risk for obesity, as dietary fat is stored more easily as adipose tissue than is dietary carbohydrate or protein.

- Metabolic factors, such as low BMR, low spontaneous physical activity, low sympathetic nervous system activity, low fat oxidation, a low level of thyroid hormone, or use of certain prescription medications that slow metabolism can promote weight gain.

- Physiologic factors that influence body weight include various hormones and other functional compounds that influence hunger, satiety, and energy expenditure, and fat storage. These include leptin, ghrelin, peptide YY, uncoupling proteins, beta-endorphins, serotonin, and cholecystokinin.

LO 6 - Cultural factors such as learned food preferences and our current "fast-food culture" influence food intake, and the shift from manual to sedentary labor is one of many cultural factors promoting inactivity. Income strongly influences food intake patterns, activity patterns, and body weight. Social factors, such as easy access to large portions of inexpensive and high-fat foods and excessive use of electronic devices for entertainment, also contribute to obesity.

LO 7 ■ Obesity increases the risk for type 2 diabetes, cardiovascular disease, depression, certain cancers, and many other diseases. Abdominal obesity is one of the most significant factors in metabolic syndrome, which is in turn part of an individual's overall cardiometabolic risk. Obesity also increases the risk of premature death.

■ Obesity itself is a multifactorial disease; that is, over 100 variables directly or indirectly influence energy balance, including not only biological but individual, environmental, and social influences on food consumption and physical activity.

■ Overweight is not as detrimental to health as obesity, but it is associated with an increased risk for hypertension, osteoarthritis, and obesity.

LO 8 ■ The first line of defense in treating obesity in adults is a low-energy diet and regular physical activity. Counseling and support groups can also help.

■ Nine prescription weight-loss medications are currently available, but they are prescribed only for people who are obese or for people with a BMI greater than or equal to 27 kg/m² who also have other significant health risk factors. This is because many drugs developed for weight loss have serious side effects. Some have even proven deadly. Physician involvement and monitoring is critical.

■ The use of dietary supplements for weight loss is common, and yet there is insufficient evidence of effectiveness for many. Those containing stimulants do increase metabolic rate and decrease appetite, but their use is dangerous because they can prompt abnormal increases in heart rate and blood pressure, and some have caused death. The FDA has removed several stimulant weight-loss supplements from the market.

■ Bariatric surgery is typically reserved for people with a BMI greater than or equal to 40 kg/m² or for people with a BMI greater than or equal to 35 kg/m² who have other life-threatening conditions. The three most common types of weight-loss surgery are sleeve gastrectomy, gastric bypass, and gastric banding. Only about one-third to one-half of people who undergo bariatric surgery lose weight, maintain their weight loss, and reduce their chronic disease risks. Liposuction, localized removal of fat cells, is not recommended or typically used to treat obesity.

LO 9 ■ Fad diets are weight-loss programs that enjoy short-term popularity and are sold based on a marketing gimmick that appeals to the public's desires and fears. They typically promise rapid weight loss, often without increased physical activity or long-term behavioral modification, and they rarely result in long-term maintenance of weight loss.

■ Diet plans that restrict intake of certain macronutrients can help many people lose weight, but some have unhealthful side effects. Overall, the reduction in energy that these diets prescribe is probably more important than the macronutrient composition.

■ If you would like to lose weight and maintain that weight loss, a first step is to set a realistic, achievable goal. Experts recommend a pace of about 0.5 to 2 pounds of weight loss per week.

■ A sound weight-loss plan involves gradually reducing energy intake, incorporating physical activity into each day, and practicing changes in behavior that can assist in meeting realistic weight-change goals. You can reduce your energy intake by eating smaller portion sizes and choosing foods low in energy density and high in nutrient density. Avoid or strictly limit sugary drinks and alcohol. Engage in at least 30 minutes of physical activity a day, at least 5 days a week. This will not only burn energy but also help maintain or increase your lean body mass and BMR. Appropriate behavior modification techniques include keeping a food log, avoiding shopping when you're hungry, avoiding purchasing high-energy "problem" foods such as chips and sweets, and engaging in mindful eating.

LO 10 ■ Being underweight can be detrimental to one's health. Most of the products marketed for weight gain have been shown to be ineffective, and many are harmful.

■ Healthful weight gain involves consuming more energy than expended by selecting ample servings of nutrient-dense, high-energy foods. An increase of about 500 to 1,000 kcal/day is advised. Eat more frequently during each day, including small, nutritious snacks. Individuals attempting to gain weight should also engage in resistance training to build muscle and aerobic exercise to preserve cardiovascular fitness. Smoking and other forms of tobacco use should be strictly avoided, not only because they depress appetite and increase metabolic rate, but also because they increase the risk for cancer and other serious diseases.

To further your understanding, go online and apply what you've learned to real-life case studies that will help you master the content!

review questions

LO 1   1. A healthful weight is a weight that
a. is very close to that of other members of your immediate family.
b. you can maintain if you keep your kcal intake no higher than your BMR.
c. is acceptable to your peers.
d. none of the above.

LO 2   2. The ratio of a person's body weight to height is represented as his or her
a. body mass index.
b. fat distribution pattern.
c. basal metabolic rate.
d. fat-to-lean tissue ratio.

LO 3   3. All people gain weight when they
a. eat a high-fat diet ($>35\%$ fat).
b. take in more energy than they expend.
c. fail to exercise.
d. consume more energy, on average, than they did the previous year.

LO 4   4. Energy balance occurs when
a. energy expended via basal metabolism, the thermic effect of food, and physical activity equals energy intake.
b. energy expended via basal metabolism, temperature regulation, and exercise is greater than energy intake.
c. energy expended via the body mass index, basal metabolism, and physical activity equals energy intake.
d. energy expended via the body mass index, the thermic effect of food, and physical activity is greater than energy intake.

LO 5   5. Which of the following increases appetite?
a. leptin
b. ghrelin
c. PYY
d. uncoupling proteins

LO 6   6. Which of the following individuals is most likely to have a BMI over 30?
a. an investment banker who has time to exercise with his personal trainer twice weekly

b. a high school home economics teacher who loves to cook and rides her bicycle to work each day
c. a low-income single mother who provides child care to other families in her urban apartment block
d. a college student who smokes and gets no exercise other than walking to and from campus

LO 7   7. Obesity increases the risk for
a. certain types of cancer.
b. dementia.
c. premature death.
d. all of the above.

LO 8   8. Bariatric surgery
a. results in significant weight loss and long-term maintenance of weight loss in one-half to two-thirds of patients.
b. is considered too risky for people with morbid obesity (a BMI greater than or equal to 40 kg/m^2).
c. is justified if the immediate threat of serious obesity-related disease and death is more dangerous than the associated risks.
d. all of the above.

LO 9   9. A plan for healthful weight loss begins with
a. a realistic, achievable goal.
b. behavioral counseling or enrollment in a support group.
c. a low-fat diet.
d. a low-carb diet.

LO 10   10. Which of the following would be the most nutritious snack choice for someone who wishes to gain weight healthfully?
a. a slice of pepperoni pizza with extra cheese
b. four chocolate-chip cookies
c. a peanut-butter sandwich on whole-grain bread with an apple
d. a strawberry shake made with protein powder mixed into strawberry milk

true or false?

LO 1   11. **True or false?** Pear-shaped fat patterning is known to increase a person's risk for many chronic diseases, including diabetes and heart disease.

LO 3   12. **True or false?** One pound of fat is equal to about 3,500 kcal.

LO 4   13. **True or false?** About 60% to 75% of our energy output goes to fuel the basic activities of staying alive.

LO 8   14. **True or false?** Prescription weight-loss medications are typically advised for people who have a body mass index greater than or equal to 25.0 kg/m^2.

LO 10   15. **True or false?** Recommendations for weight gain include avoiding both aerobic and resistance exercise for the duration of the weight-gain program.

short answer

LO 1 16. Identify at least four characteristics of a healthful weight.

LO 4 17. Can you increase your basal metabolic rate? Is it wise to try? Defend your answer.

LO 6 18. Explain the relationship between abdominal obesity, metabolic syndrome, and cardiometabolic risk.

LO 7 19. Identify at least four societal factors that may have influenced the rise in obesity rates in the United States since 1963.

LO 9 20. Describe a sound weight-loss program, including recommendations for diet, physical activity, and behavioral modifications.

math review

LO 3 21. Your friend Misty joins you for lunch and confesses that she is discouraged about her weight. She says that she has been trying "really hard" for 3 months to lose weight but that, no matter what she does, she cannot drop below 148 lb. Based on her height of 5'8", calculate Misty's BMI. Is she overweight? What questions would you suggest she think about? How would you advise her? Misty's level of physical activity would classify her as moderately active. Approximately how many kcal does she need each day to maintain her current body weight?

Answers to Review Questions and Math Review are located in the MasteringNutrition Study Area.

web links

www.ftc.gov
Federal Trade Commission
Click on "Tips & Advice" and select "For Consumers" and then "Health and Fitness" to find how to avoid false weight-loss claims.

www.nutrition.gov/weight-management
Nutrition.gov
Visit this site to learn about successful strategies for achieving and maintaining a healthy weight.

www.eatright.org
Academy of Nutrition and Dietetics
Go to this site to learn more about fad diets and nutrition facts.

http://www.niddk.nih.gov/health-information /Pages/default.aspx
National Institute of Diabetes and Digestive and Kidney Diseases
Find out more about healthy weight loss and how it pertains to diabetes and digestive and kidney diseases.

www.sneb.org
Society for Nutrition Education and Behavior
Click on "Nutrition Resources" and then "Weight Realities Division Resource List" for additional resources related to positive attitudes about body image and healthful alternatives to dieting.

www.oa.org
Overeaters Anonymous
Visit this site to learn about ways to reduce compulsive overeating.

Disordered Eating

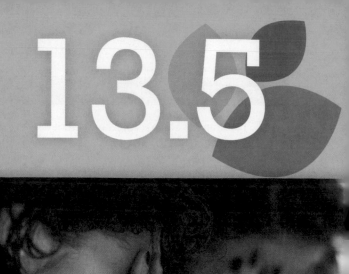

Learning Outcomes

After studying this In Depth, you should be able to:

1 Discuss the observation that eating behaviors occur on a continuum, p. 541.

2 Identify several factors that contribute to the development of eating disorders, pp. 541–543.

3 Identify the most common characteristics and health risks of anorexia nervosa, bulimia nervosa, and binge-eating disorder, pp. 543–547.

4 Describe night-eating syndrome and the female athlete triad, pp. 548–549.

5 Compare treatment options for disordered eating behaviors, pp. 549–550.

6 Role-play a discussion with a friend about his or her disordered eating behaviors, p. 550.

On November 17, 2010, French fashion model Isabelle Caro died at age 28. She had suffered from anorexia nervosa, a potentially deadly eating disorder, since age 13. In response to the deaths of several models over the past three decades, fashion shows and modeling agencies have begun to implement weight and health standards for models. For example, early in 2012, the Council of Fashion Designers of America (CFDA) released new guidelines for the hiring of runway models, including measures such as educating staff to recognize the warning signs of an eating disorder.

Of course, eating disorders aren't limited to fashion models. They can develop in anyone, male or female, including people like you. When does normal dieting cross the line into disordered eating? What early warning signs might tip you off that a friend was crossing that line? If you noticed the signs in a friend or family member, what—if anything—would you say? In the following pages, we explore *In Depth* some answers to these important questions.

Eating Behaviors Occur on a Continuum

LO 1 Discuss the observation that eating behaviors occur on a continuum.

Disordered eating is a general term used to describe a variety of atypical eating behaviors that people use to achieve or maintain a lower body weight. These behaviors may be as simple as going on and off diets or as extreme as refusing to eat any fat. Such behaviors don't usually continue for long enough to make the person seriously ill, nor do they significantly disrupt the person's normal routine.

In contrast, some people alter their eating behaviors so much and for so long that they become dangerously ill. These people have an **eating disorder,** a psychiatric condition that involves extreme body dissatisfaction and long-term eating patterns that negatively affect body functioning. Three clinically diagnosed eating disorders are anorexia nervosa, bulimia nervosa, and binge-eating disorder. Whereas anorexia nervosa is characterized by severe food restriction, bulimia nervosa and binge-eating disorder involve extreme overeating. These disorders will be discussed in more detail shortly.

Eating behaviors occur on a *continuum*, a spectrum that can't be divided neatly into parts. An example is a rainbow—where exactly does the red end and the orange begin? Thinking about eating behaviors as a continuum makes it easier to understand how a person can progress from relatively normal eating behaviors to a pattern that is disordered. For instance, let's say that for several years you've skipped breakfast in favor of a midmorning snack, but now you find yourself avoiding the cafeteria until early afternoon. Is this normal? To answer that question, you'd need to consider your feelings about food and your **body image**—the way you perceive your body.

Take a moment to study the Eating Issues and Body Image Continuum (**Figure 1**, page 542). Which of the five columns best describes your feelings about food and your body? If you find

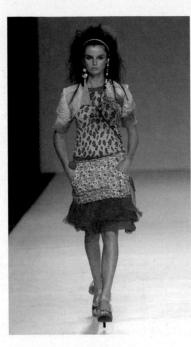

Brazilian model Ana Carolina Reston, who died in 2006 at the age of 21, was one of several models who have died as a result of eating disorders.

yourself identifying with the statements on the left side of the continuum, you probably have few issues with food or body image. Most likely you accept your body size and view food as a normal part of maintaining your health and fueling your daily physical activity. As you progress to the right side of the continuum, food and body image become bigger issues, with food restriction becoming the norm. If you identify with the statements on the far right, you are probably afraid of eating and dislike your body. If so, what can you do to begin to move toward the left side of the continuum? How can you begin to develop a more healthful approach to food selection and to view your body in a more positive light? Before you can begin to find solutions, you need to understand the many complex factors that contribute to eating disorders and disordered eating.

Many Factors Contribute to Disordered Eating Behaviors

LO 2 Identify several factors that contribute to the development of eating disorders.

The factors that contribute to the development of disordered eating in any particular individual are very complex.

Influence of Genetic Factors

Overall, the diagnosis of an eating disorder is several times more common in siblings and other blood relatives who also have the diagnosis than in the general population.[1,2] Data from twin studies estimate that genetic factors account for 50–83% of the variance in eating disorders.[1] These observations might imply the existence of an "eating disorder gene"; however, it is difficult to separate the contribution of genetic and environmental factors within families.

disordered eating A general term used to describe a variety of abnormal or atypical eating behaviors that are used to keep or maintain a lower body weight.

eating disorder A clinically diagnosed psychiatric disorder characterized by severe disturbances in body image and eating behaviors.

body image A person's perception of his or her body's appearance and functioning.

• I am not concerned about what others think regarding what and how much I eat. • When I am upset or depressed I eat whatever I am hungry for without any guilt or shame. • I feel no guilt or shame no matter how much I eat or what I eat. • Food is an important part of my life but only occupies a small part of my time. • I trust my body to tell me what and how much to eat.	• I pay attention to what I eat in order to maintain a healthy body. • I may weigh more than what I like, but I enjoy eating and balance my pleasure with eating with my concern for a healthy body. • I am moderate and flexible in goals for eating well. • I try to follow Dietary Guidelines for healthy eating.	• I think about food a lot. • I feel I don't eat well most of the time. • It's hard for me to enjoy eating with others. • I feel ashamed when I eat more than others or more than what I feel I should be eating. • I am afraid of getting fat. • I wish I could change how much I want to eat and what I am hungry for.	• I have tried diet pills, laxatives, vomiting, or extra time exercising in order to lose or maintain my weight. • I have fasted or avoided eating for long periods of time in order to lose or maintain my weight. • I feel strong when I can restrict how much I eat. • Eating more than I wanted to makes me feel out of control.	• I regularly stuff myself and then exercise, vomit, or use diet pills or laxatives to get rid of the food or Calories. • My friends/family tell me I am too thin. • I am terrified of eating fat. • When I let myself eat, I have a hard time controlling the amount of food I eat. • I am afraid to eat in front of others.
FOOD IS NOT AN ISSUE	**CONCERNED/WELL**	**FOOD PREOCCUPIED/ OBSESSED**	**DISRUPTIVE EATING PATTERNS**	**EATING DISORDERED**
BODY OWNERSHIP	**BODY ACCEPTANCE**	**BODY PREOCCUPIED/ OBSESSED**	**DISTORTED BODY IMAGE**	**BODY HATE/ DISASSOCIATION**
• Body image is not an issue for me. • My body is beautiful to me. • My feelings about my body are not influenced by society's concept of an ideal body shape. • I know that the significant others in my life will always find me attractive. • I trust my body to find the weight it needs to be at so I can move and feel confident about my physical body.	• I base my body image equally on social norms and my own self-concept. • I pay attention to my body and my appearance because it is important to me, but it only occupies a small part of my day. • I nourish my body so it has the strength and energy to achieve my physical goals. • I am able to assert myself and maintain a healthy body without losing my self-esteem.	• I spend a significant amount time viewing my body in the mirror. • I spend a significant amount of time comparing my body to others. • I have days when I feel fat. • I am preoccupied with my body. • I accept society's ideal body shape and size as the best body shape and size. • I believe that I'd be more attractive if I were thinner, more muscular, etc.	• I spend a significant amount of time exercising and dieting to change my body. • My body shape and size keep me from dating or finding someone who will treat me the way I want to be treated. • I have considered changing or have changed my body shape and size through surgical means so I can accept myself. • I wish I could change the way I look in the mirror.	• I often feel separated and distant from my body—as if it belongs to someone else. • I hate my body and I often isolate myself from others. • I don't see anything positive or even neutral about my body shape and size. • I don't believe others when they tell me I look OK. • I hate the way I look in the mirror.

FIGURE 1 The Eating Issues and Body Image Continuum. The progression from normal eating (far left) to disordered eating (far right) occurs on a continuum. (*Source:* Data from Smiley, L., L. King, and H. Avery. University of Arizona Campus Health Service. Original Continuum, C. Shlaalak. Preventive Medicine and Public Health. Copyright © 1997 Arizona Board of Regents.)

Influence of Family

Research suggests that family conditioning, structure, and patterns of interaction can influence the development and maintenance of an eating disorder. Based on observational studies, compared to families without a member with an eating disorder, there are three traits that run within families of people with eating disorders:[3]

■ *Anxiety.* Within families, anxiety can be contagious and can maintain or even exacerbate a pattern of disordered eating. For example, parents may display a high level of anxiety in response to a child's disordered eating behaviors. The child senses this anxiety and responds by intensifying the behavior.

■ *Compulsivity.* The families of individuals who develop eating disorders are typically characterized by inflexibility, rigidity, and the need for order. Thus, when the family experiences an unpredictable event, the individual may turn to compulsive behaviors—such as refusing food or obsessively exercising—to adapt.

■ *Abnormal eating behavior in one family member.* A pattern of disordered eating may already be present within the family, leading other family members to view this behavior as normal or acceptable.

Influence of Media

We now know media can play an important role in the formation of body image, especially in young females, and can create unrealistic expectations for body weight.[4,5] Every day, we are confronted with advertisements in which computer-enhanced images of lean, beautiful women and muscular men promote everything from beer to cars. Most adults understand that these images are unrealistic, but adolescents, who are still developing a sense of their identity and body image, lack the same ability to distance themselves from what they see.[4] Because body image influences eating behaviors, it is likely that this barrage of unrealistic media models may be contributing to the increase in eating disorders. However, scientific evidence demonstrating that the media are *causing* increased eating disorders is difficult to obtain.

Influence of Social and Cultural Values

Eating disorders are significantly more common in white females in Western societies than in other women worldwide.[2] This may be due in part to the white Western culture's association of slenderness with attractiveness, wealth, and high fashion. In contrast, until recently, the prevailing view in developing societies has been that excess body fat is desirable as a sign of health and material abundance.

The members of society with whom we most often interact—our family members, friends, classmates, and co-workers—also influence the way we see ourselves. Their comments related to our body weight or shape can be particularly hurtful—enough so to cause some people to start

down the path of disordered eating.[2] Peer relationships also appear to be highly influential in the development of anorexia. A 2011 study from the London School of Economics concluded that anorexia is primarily socially induced. The higher the BMI of one's peers, the lower the risk of developing anorexia.[6] In another study, when college women believed they were competing with a thin peer during a '"mock dating game" in which a male would choose which woman they wanted to "date," the women experienced decreased body satisfaction and confidence.[7] Data such as these support research suggesting a higher level of eating disorders among college women compared to high school girls.

Influence of Personality

Besides the focus on over-evaluation of eating, body shape, and weight, behaviors that are associated with eating disorders include perfectionism, low self-esteem, moodiness, and interpersonal difficulties.[1] Individuals with an eating disorder, especially those with anorexia nervosa, often have comorbidity with other psychological disorders such as obsessive-compulsive disorder.[8] Thus, anorexic patients frequently follow strict food and exercise routines, compulsively checking and counting.[8] They also express excessive anxiety over situations or events, and have a high need for control. This makes it difficult to complete tasks since nothing is ever quite good enough or done well enough.[9] Conversely, those with bulimia nervosa may respond more negatively or erratically to problems or issues. These negative moods may trigger overeating.[1,10]

Unfortunately, many studies observe these behaviors only in individuals who are very ill and in a state of starvation, which may affect personality. Thus, it is difficult to determine if personality is the cause or effect of the disorder.

> Think that families—or mothers—are to blame for eating disorders? Or that they develop only in teenage girls? Guess again. Visit the National Institute of Mental Health at www.nimh.nih.gov and type in the search bar "eating disorders myths" to find a series of short videos busting nine myths about disordered eating.

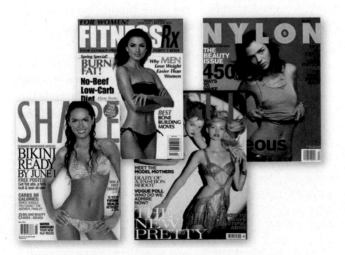

Photos of models and celebrities are routinely airbrushed or altered to "enhance" physical appearance. Unfortunately, many young people believe these portrayals are accurate and, hence, strive to meet unrealistic physical goals.

Eating Disorders Are Psychiatric Diagnoses

LO 3 Identify the most common characteristics and health risks of anorexia nervosa, bulimia nervosa, and binge-eating disorder.

Recall that eating disorders are psychiatric conditions. The clinical manual of the *American Psychiatric Association*, which is the world's largest psychiatric organization, recognizes three such eating disorders. These are anorexia nervosa, bulimia nervosa, and binge-eating disorder.[1]

Anorexia Nervosa

Anorexia nervosa is a potentially life-threatening eating disorder that is characterized by an extremely low body weight achieved through self-starvation, which eventually leads to a severe nutrient deficiency. According to the Office of Women's Health, 85% to 95% of people with anorexia nervosa are young girls or women.[11] Approximately 0.5% to 3.7% of American females develop anorexia, and 20% of these women will die prematurely from complications related to their disorder, including suicide and heart problems.[12] These statistics make anorexia nervosa the most common and most deadly psychiatric disorder diagnosed in women and one of the leading causes of death in females between the ages of 15 and 24 years.[12] As the statistics indicate, anorexia nervosa also occurs in males, but the prevalence is much lower than in females.[12,13]

Signs and Symptoms of Anorexia Nervosa

The classic sign of anorexia nervosa is an extremely restrictive eating pattern that leads to self-starvation. People with this disorder may fast completely, restrict energy intake to only a few kilocalories per day, or eliminate all but one or two food groups from their diet. They also have an intense fear of weight gain, and even small amounts (for example, 1–2 lb) trigger high stress and anxiety.

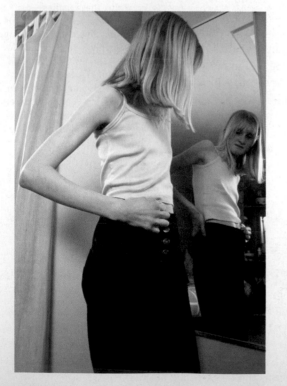

People with anorexia nervosa experience an extreme drive for thinness, resulting in potentially fatal weight loss.

In females, **amenorrhea** (the condition of having no menstrual periods for at least 3 continuous months) is a common feature of anorexia nervosa. It occurs when a young woman consumes insufficient energy to maintain normal body functions.

The American Psychiatric Association identifies the following conditions of anorexia nervosa:[14]

- Refusal to maintain body weight at or above a minimally normal weight for age and height
- Intense fear of gaining weight or becoming fat, even though considered underweight by all medical criteria
- Disturbance in the way in which one's body weight or shape is experienced, undue influence of body weight or shape on self-evaluation, or denial of the seriousness of the current low body weight

The signs of an eating disorder such as anorexia nervosa may be somewhat different in males. Females say they feel fat and wish to be thinner even though they typically are normal weight or even underweight before they develop the disorder.[15] In contrast, males are more focused on being lean and muscular.[15] Males with disordered eating are less concerned with actual body weight (scale weight) than females but are more concerned with body composition (percentage of muscle mass compared to fat mass). Their goals typically include avoiding teasing related to being obese, improving sports performance, avoiding weight-related medical complications, and improving homosexual relationships.[15]

The methods that men and women use to achieve weight loss also appear to differ. Males are more likely to use excessive exercise as a means of weight control, whereas females tend to use severe energy restriction, vomiting, and laxative abuse. These weight-control differences may stem from sociocultural biases; that is, dieting is considered to be more acceptable for women, whereas the overwhelming sociocultural belief is that "real men don't diet."[16] For more information on eating disorders in men, see the nearby *Highlight* box.

Health Risks of Anorexia Nervosa

Left untreated, anorexia nervosa eventually leads to a deficiency in energy and other nutrients that are required by the body to function normally. The body will then use stored fat and lean tissue (for example, organ and muscle tissue) as an energy source to maintain brain tissue and vital body functions. The body will also shut down or reduce nonvital body functions to conserve energy. Electrolyte imbalances can lead to heart failure and death. **Figure 2** (page 546) highlights many of the health problems that occur with anorexia nervosa. The best chance for recovery is when an individual receives intensive treatment early.

anorexia nervosa A serious, potentially life-threatening eating disorder that is characterized by self-starvation, which eventually leads to a deficiency in the energy and essential nutrients required by the body to function normally.

amenorrhea The absence of menstruation. In females who had previously been menstruating, it is defined as the absence of menstrual periods for 3 or more continuous months.

Muscle Dysmorphia: The Male Eating Disorder?

Is there a reverse form of anorexia nervosa unique to men? For decades, bodybuilders have recognized that some men view themselves as "puny" even when they are normal size or even very muscular; work out obsessively; and adhere to an extremely restrictive diet. Recognizing the syndrome they observed as a sort of "reverse anorexia" they coined the name "bigorexia."[1,2]

Recently, many psychiatric researchers and clinicians have confirmed that this disorder exists. They call it *muscle dysmorphia* (in medicine, a *dysmorphia* is an abnormality of structure). Some classify the disorder as a subtype of *body dysmorphic disorder*, a psychiatric illness in which the person is preoccupied with a physical flaw that is either extremely minor or doesn't actually exist. Others classify it as an eating disorder, pointing out that the patients' pathological pursuit of increased muscularity causes them to engage in highly disordered eating behaviors quite similar to those of patients with anorexia. They also note that the risk factors for muscle dysmorphia and anorexia nervosa and the approaches found to be successful in treating the two disorders are similar.[1,3]

No matter how the disorder is classified, the fundamental characteristic, as with anorexia nervosa, is a body image distortion. Men with muscle dysmorphia perceive themselves as small and frail even though they may actually be quite large and muscular. As a result, they are pathologically preoccupied with muscularity, spend long hours lifting weights, and follow a meticulous diet, often consisting of excessive high-protein foods and dietary supplements, such as protein powders and abuse anabolic steroids.[4] But no matter how "buff" they become, their reflection in the mirror does not match their idealized body size and shape. That said, studies suggest that as many as half of men with muscle dysmorphia do recognize at least to a "fair" extent that their perceptions about their physique are flawed.[3]

Men with muscle dysmorphia also share other characteristics with men and women with anorexia. For instance, they also report "feeling fat" and express significant discomfort with the idea of having to expose their body to others (for example, take off their clothes in the locker room). They also have increased rates of other psychiatric illnesses, including anxiety and depression.[5]

There are some outward indications that someone may be struggling with muscle dysmorphia. Not all of them

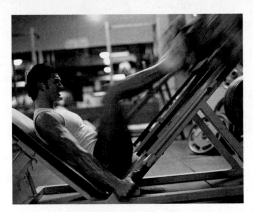

Men are more likely than women to exercise excessively in an effort to control their weight.

apply to all men with the disorder. If you notice any of these behaviors in a friend or relative, talk about it with him and let him know that help is available.

- Rigid and excessive schedule of weight training
- Strict adherence to a high-protein, muscle-enhancing diet
- Use of anabolic steroids, protein powders, or other muscle-enhancing drugs or supplements
- Poor attendance at work, school, or sports activities because of interference with a rigid weight-training schedule
- Avoidance of social engagements in which the person will not be able to follow his strict diet
- Avoidance of situations in which the person would have to expose his body to others
- Frequent and critical self-evaluation of body composition

Like anorexia nervosa, muscle dysmorphia can cause significant distress and despair, and can even be life-threatening. Men with the disorder are more likely to report substance abuse—including the use of anabolic steroids—and are more likely to have attempted suicide. In one study, half of the men diagnosed with muscle dysmorphia had attempted suicide. Therapy—especially participation in an all-male support group—can help.

References

1. Jones, W. R., and J. F. Morgan. 2010. Eating disorders in men: a review of the literature. *J. Public Ment. Health.* 9(2):23–31.
2. Kanayama, G., and H. G. Pope, Jr. 2011. Gods, men, and muscle dysmorphia. *Harv. Rev. Psychiat.*, 19(2):95–98.
3. Murray, S. B., E. Rieger, S. W. Touyz, and Y. de la Garza Garcia. 2010. Muscle dysmorphia and the DSM-V conundrum: where does it belong? *Int. J. Eat. Disord.* 43(6):483–491.
4. Choi, P. Y., H. G. Pope, Jr., and Olivardia, R. 2002. Muscle dysmorphia: a new syndrome in weightlifters. *Brit. J. Sports Med.*, 36(5):375–376.
5. Weltzin, T. E. 2012. A Silent Problem: Males with Eating Disorders in the Workplace. National Association of Anorexia Nervosa and Associated Disorders. www .anad.org/get-information/males-eating-disorders /medical-director-on-males-with-eds-in-the-workplace/. (Accessed March 2015.)

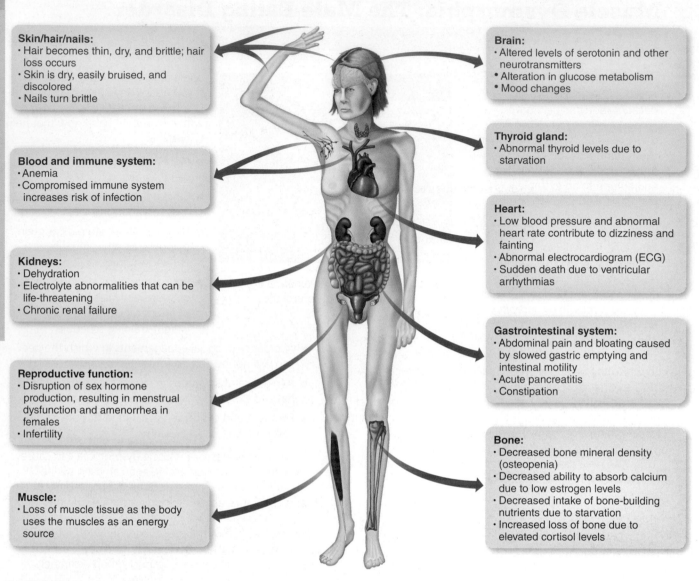

Skin/hair/nails:
- Hair becomes thin, dry, and brittle; hair loss occurs
- Skin is dry, easily bruised, and discolored
- Nails turn brittle

Blood and immune system:
- Anemia
- Compromised immune system increases risk of infection

Kidneys:
- Dehydration
- Electrolyte abnormalities that can be life-threatening
- Chronic renal failure

Reproductive function:
- Disruption of sex hormone production, resulting in menstrual dysfunction and amenorrhea in females
- Infertility

Muscle:
- Loss of muscle tissue as the body uses the muscles as an energy source

Brain:
- Altered levels of serotonin and other neurotransmitters
- Alteration in glucose metabolism
- Mood changes

Thyroid gland:
- Abnormal thyroid levels due to starvation

Heart:
- Low blood pressure and abnormal heart rate contribute to dizziness and fainting
- Abnormal electrocardiogram (ECG)
- Sudden death due to ventricular arrhythmias

Gastrointestinal system:
- Abdominal pain and bloating caused by slowed gastric emptying and intestinal motility
- Acute pancreatitis
- Constipation

Bone:
- Decreased bone mineral density (osteopenia)
- Decreased ability to absorb calcium due to low estrogen levels
- Decreased intake of bone-building nutrients due to starvation
- Increased loss of bone due to elevated cortisol levels

FIGURE 2 The impact of anorexia nervosa on the body.

Bulimia Nervosa

Bulimia nervosa is characterized by repeated episodes of binge eating and purging:

- **Binge eating** is usually defined as consumption of a quantity of food that is large for the person and for the amount of time in which it is eaten. For example, a person may eat a dozen brownies with 2 quarts of ice cream in a period of just 30 minutes. While binge eating, the person feels a loss of self-control, including an inability to end the binge once it has started.[17,18] At the same time, the person feels a sense of euphoria not unlike a drug-induced high.
- **Purging** is a compensatory behavior used to prevent weight gain. Methods of purging include vomiting, laxative or diuretic abuse, enemas, fasting, and excessive exercise. For example, after a binge, a runner may increase her daily mileage to equal the "calculated" energy content of the binge.

bulimia nervosa A serious eating disorder characterized by recurrent episodes of binge eating and recurrent inappropriate compensatory behaviors in order to prevent weight gain, such as self-induced vomiting, fasting, excessive exercise, or misuse of laxatives, diuretics, enemas, or other medications.

binge eating Consumption of a large amount of food in a short period of time, usually accompanied by a feeling of loss of self-control.

purging An attempt to rid the body of unwanted food by vomiting or other compensatory means, such as excessive exercise, fasting, or laxative abuse.

Signs and Symptoms of Bulimia Nervosa

The American Psychiatric Association has identified the following criteria for diagnosis of bulimia nervosa:[14]

- Recurrent episodes of binge eating (for example, eating a large amount of food in a short period, such as within 2 hours).
- Recurrent inappropriate compensatory behavior in order to prevent weight gain, such as self-induced vomiting; misuse of laxatives, diuretics, enemas, or other medications; fasting; or excessive exercise.
- Binge eating occurs on average at least twice a week for 3 months.
- Body shape and weight unduly influence self-evaluation.
- The disturbance does not occur exclusively during episodes of anorexia nervosa. Some individuals will have periods of binge eating and then periods of starvation, which makes classification of their disorder difficult.

Moreover, an individual with bulimia nervosa typically purges after most episodes but not necessarily on every occasion. Weight gain as a result of binge eating can therefore be significant.

How can you tell if someone has bulimia nervosa? In addition to the recurrent and frequent binge eating and purging episodes, the National Institutes of Health have identified the following symptoms of bulimia nervosa:[19]

- Chronically inflamed and sore throat
- Swollen glands in the neck and below the jaw
- Worn tooth enamel and increasingly sensitive and decaying teeth as a result of exposure to stomach acids
- Gastroesophageal reflux disorder
- Intestinal distress and irritation from laxative abuse
- Kidney problems from diuretic abuse
- Severe dehydration from purging of fluids

Health Risks of Bulimia Nervosa

The destructive behaviors of bulimia nervosa can lead to illness and even death. The most common health consequences associated with bulimia nervosa are:

- *Electrolyte imbalance:* typically caused by dehydration and the loss of potassium and sodium from the body with frequent vomiting. This can lead to irregular heartbeat and even heart failure and death.
- *Gastrointestinal problems:* inflammation, ulceration, and possible rupture of the esophagus and stomach from frequent bingeing and vomiting. Chronic irregular bowel

movements and constipation may result in people with bulimia who chronically abuse laxatives.

- *Dental problems:* tooth decay and staining from stomach acids released during frequent vomiting

As with anorexia nervosa, the chance of recovery from bulimia nervosa increases, and the negative effects on health decrease, if the disorder is detected at an early stage. Familiarity with the warning signs of bulimia nervosa can help you identify friends and family members who might be at risk.

Binge-Eating Disorder

When was the last time a friend or relative confessed to you about "going on an eating binge"? Most likely, he or she explained that the behavior followed some sort of stressful event, such as a problem at work, the breakup of a relationship, or a poor grade on an exam. Many people have one or two binge episodes every year or so, in response to stress. But in people with **binge-eating disorder,** the behavior occurs frequently. Because it is not usually followed by purging, the person tends to gain a lot of weight. This lack of compensation for the binge distinguishes binge-eating disorder from bulimia nervosa.

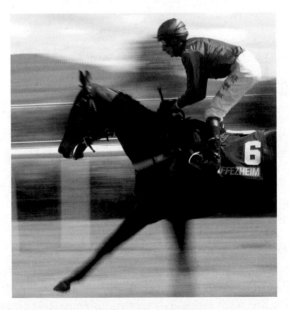

Men who participate in "thin-build" sports, such as jockeys, have a higher risk for bulimia nervosa than men who do not.

binge-eating disorder A disorder characterized by binge eating an average of twice a week or more, typically without compensatory purging.

The prevalence of binge-eating disorder is estimated to be 2% to 5% of the adult female population and 8% of the obese population.[12,20] In contrast to anorexia and bulimia, binge-eating disorder is also common in men. Our current food environment, which offers an abundance of good-tasting, cheap food any time of the day, makes it difficult for people with binge-eating disorder to avoid food triggers.

As you would expect, the increased energy intake associated with binge eating significantly increases a person's risk of being overweight or obese. In addition, the types of foods individuals typically consume during a binge episode are high in fat and sugar, which can increase blood lipids. Finally, the stress associated with binge eating can have psychological consequences, such as low self-esteem, avoidance of social contact, depression, and negative thoughts related to body size.

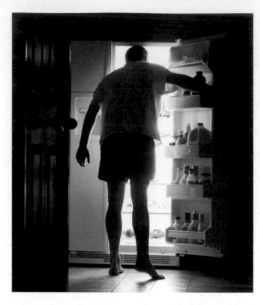

People with night-eating syndrome consume most of their daily energy between 8 PM and 6 AM.

nighttime and not being hungry at breakfast time. Thus, night-eating syndrome is diagnosed by one or both of the following criteria:[21]

- Eating at least 25% of daily food intake after the evening meal
- Experiencing at least two episodes per week of night eating; that is, getting up to eat after going to bed

Night eating is also characterized by a depressed mood and insomnia.[22] In short, this syndrome combines three unique disorders: an eating disorder, a sleep disorder, and a mood disorder.[21] Many night eaters are obese, and many experience anxiety or engage in substance abuse. Some engage in other disordered eating behaviors.

Night-eating syndrome is important clinically because of its association with obesity, which increases the risk for several chronic diseases, including heart disease, high blood pressure, stroke, type 2 diabetes, and arthritis. Obesity also increases the risk for sleep apnea, which can further disrupt the night eater's already abnormal sleeping pattern.

Disordered Eating Can Be Part of a Syndrome

LO 4 Describe night-eating syndrome and the female athlete triad.

A *syndrome* is a type of disorder characterized by the presence of two or more distinct health problems that tend to occur together. Two syndromes involving disordered eating behaviors are night-eating syndrome and the female athlete triad.

Night-Eating Syndrome

Night-eating syndrome was first described in a group of patients who were not hungry in the morning but spent the evening and night eating and reported insomnia. Like binge-eating disorder, it is associated with obesity because, although night eaters don't binge, they do consume significant energy in their frequent snacks, and they don't compensate for the excess energy intake.

The distinguishing characteristic of night-eating syndrome is the time during which most of the day's energy intake occurs. Night eaters have a daily pattern of significantly increasing their energy intake in the evening and/or at

The Female Athlete Triad

The **female athlete triad** is a serious syndrome that consists of three clinical conditions in some physically active females (**Figure 3**):[23]

- Low energy availability (such as inadequate energy intake to maintain menstrual function or to cover energy expended in exercise) with or without eating disorders
- Menstrual dysfunction, such as amenorrhea (the absence of menstruation for 3 months or more)
- Low bone density

Certain sports that strongly emphasize leanness or a thin body build may place a young girl or a woman at risk for the female athlete triad. These sports typically include figure skating, gymnastics, and diving; classical ballet dancers are also at increased risk for the disorder.

night-eating syndrome Disorder characterized by intake of the majority of the day's energy between 8:00 PM and 6:00 AM. Individuals with this disorder also experience mood and sleep disorders.

female athlete triad A syndrome that consists of three clinical conditions in some physically active females: low energy availability (with or without eating disorders), menstrual dysfunction, and low bone density.

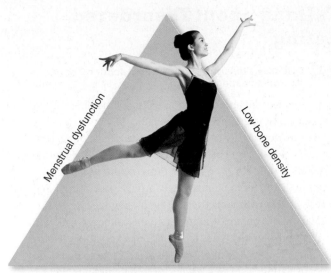

FIGURE 3 The female athlete triad is a syndrome composed of three coexisting disorders: low energy availability (with or without eating disorders), menstrual dysfunction (such as amenorrhea), and low bone density (such as osteoporosis). Energy availability is defined as dietary energy intake minus exercise energy expenditure.

Active women experience the general social and cultural demands placed on women to be thin, as well as pressure from their coach, teammates, judges, and/or spectators to meet weight standards or body-size expectations for their sport. Failure to meet these standards can result in severe consequences, such as being cut from the team, losing an athletic scholarship, or decreased participation with the team.

As the pressure to be thin mounts, active women may restrict their energy intake, typically by engaging in disordered eating behaviors. Energy restriction combined with high levels of physical activity can disrupt the menstrual cycle and result in amenorrhea. Menstrual dysfunction can also occur in active women who are not dieting and don't have an eating disorder. These women are just not eating enough to cover the energy costs of their exercise training and all the other energy demands of the body and daily living. Female athletes with menstrual dysfunction, regardless of the cause, typically have reduced levels of the reproductive hormones estrogen and progesterone. When estrogen levels in the body are low, it is difficult for bone to retain calcium, and gradual loss of bone mass occurs. Thus, many female athletes develop premature bone loss (osteoporosis) and are at increased risk for fractures.

Recognition of an athlete with one or more of the components of the female athlete triad can be difficult, especially if the athlete is reluctant to be honest when questioned about her eating behaviors and symptoms. For this reason, familiarity with the early warning signs is critical. These include excessive dieting and/or weight loss, excessive exercise, stress fractures, and comments suggesting that self-esteem appears to be dictated by body weight and shape. (See Chapter 11, page 453, for additional information on this topic.)

Treatment Requires a Multidisciplinary Approach

LO 5 Compare treatment options for disordered eating behaviors.

As with any health problem, prevention is the best treatment for disordered eating. People having trouble with eating and body image issues need help to deal with these issues before they develop into something more serious.

Inpatient Nutritional Therapies

Patients who are severely underweight, display signs of malnutrition, are medically unstable, or are suicidal may require immediate hospitalization. The goals of nutritional therapies are to restore the individual to a healthy body weight and normal eating patterns, teach the individual to identify hunger and satiety cues, and resolve the nutrition-related health issues.[24] For stable hospitalized patients, the expected weight gain per week ranges from 2 to 3 pounds. For outpatient settings, the expected weight gain is much lower

Nutri-Case

Liz

"I used to dance with a really cool modern company, where everybody looked sort of healthy and 'real.' No waifs! When they folded after Christmas, I was really bummed, but this spring, I'm planning to audition for the City Ballet. My best friend dances with them, and she told me that they won't even look at anybody over 100 pounds. So I've just put myself on a strict diet. Most days, I come in under 1,200 Calories, though some days I cheat and then I feel so out of control. Last week, my dance teacher stopped me after class and asked me whether or not I was menstruating. I thought that was a pretty weird question, so I just said sure, but then when I thought about it, I realized that I've been so focused and stressed out lately that I really don't know! The audition is only a week away, so I'm going on a juice fast this weekend. I've just got to make it into the City Ballet!"

What factors increase Liz's risk for the female athlete triad? What, if anything, do you think Liz's dance teacher should do? Is intervention even necessary, since the audition is only a week away?

(0.5 to 1 pound/week). However, determining the energy intake needed to achieve these levels of weight gain can be difficult because energy estimates used for healthy individuals of normal weight may not be appropriate for people who are underweight.

Patients frequently try a variety of methods to avoid consuming the food presented to them. They may discard the food, vomit, exercise excessively, or engage in a high level of nonexercise motor activity to eliminate the Calories they have just consumed. For this reason, patients are carefully watched by hospital staff or family members. In addition to increasing amounts of food, patients may be given vitamin and mineral supplements to ensure that adequate micronutrients are consumed.

Nutrition counseling is an important aspect of inpatient treatment, especially to deal with the body image issues that occur as weight is regained. Once the patient reaches an acceptable body weight, nutrition counseling will address issues such as the acceptability of certain foods; dealing with food situations, such as family gatherings and eating out; and learning to put together a healthful food plan for weight maintenance.

Outpatient Nutrition Counseling

Patients with anorexia nervosa who are underweight but medically stable may be able to enter an outpatient program designed to meet their specific needs. Outpatient programs are also an option for patients with other forms of disordered eating who are of normal weight or overweight. Some outpatient programs are extremely intensive, requiring patients to come in each day for treatment, whereas others are less rigorous, requiring only weekly visits for counseling.

Nutrition counseling generally focuses on identifying and dealing with events and feelings that trigger food restriction, or binge eating, or purging. Another goal is to establish structured eating behaviors that can enable the patient to maintain a healthful body weight. In addition, nutrition counseling will address factors specific to the individual, such as negative feelings about foods or fears associated with uncontrolled binge eating.

Talking about Disordered Eating

LO 6 Role-play a discussion with a friend about his or her disordered eating behaviors.

If you're concerned about a friend's or family member's eating behaviors, raising the subject can be difficult.

Before you do, learn as much as you can about eating disorders. Make sure you know the difference between the facts and myths. Locate a health professional specializing in eating disorders to whom you can refer your friend, and be ready to go with your friend if he or she does not want to go alone. If you are at a university or college, check with your campus health center to see if it has an eating disorder specialist or team or can recommend someone to you. The National Eating Disorders Association recommends the following steps to take during your discussion:[25]

- *Schedule a time to talk.* Set aside a time and place for a private discussion in which you can share your concerns openly and honestly in a caring and supportive way.
- *Communicate your concerns.* Share your memories of specific times when you felt concerned about your friend's eating or exercise behaviors. Explain that you think these things may indicate that there is a problem that needs professional attention.
- *Ask your friend to explore these concerns with a counselor, doctor, nutritionist, or other health professional* who is knowledgeable about eating issues. If you feel comfortable doing so, offer to help your friend make an appointment or accompany your friend on the first visit.
- *Avoid conflicts or a "battle of the wills."* If your friend refuses to acknowledge that there is any reason for you to be concerned, restate your feelings and the reasons for them and leave yourself available as a supportive listener.
- *Avoid placing shame, blame, or guilt* on your friend. Do not use accusatory "you" statements, such as "You just need to eat" or "You are acting irresponsibly." Instead, use "I" statements—for example, "I'm concerned about you because I never see you in the cafeteria anymore" or "It makes me afraid when I hear you vomit."
- *Avoid giving simple solutions* —for example, "If you would just stop, everything would be fine."
- *Express your continued support.* Remind your friend that you care and want your friend to be healthy and happy.

Web Links

www.massgeneral.org
Harris Center for Education and Advocacy in Eating
Disorders, Massachusetts General Hospital
*Enter "Harris Center" into the search box on the main page.
This site provides information about current eating disorder
research as well as sections on understanding eating disorders
and resources for those with eating disorders.*

www.nimh.nih.gov
National Institute of Mental Health (NIMH) Office of Communications and Public Liaison

*Search this site for "disordered eating" or "eating disorders" to
find numerous articles on the subject.*

www.anad.org
National Association of Anorexia Nervosa and Associated
Disorders
*Visit this site for information and resources about eating
disorders.*

www.nationaleatingdisorders.org
National Eating Disorders Association
*This site is dedicated to expanding public understanding of
eating disorders and promoting access to treatment for those
affected and support for their families.*

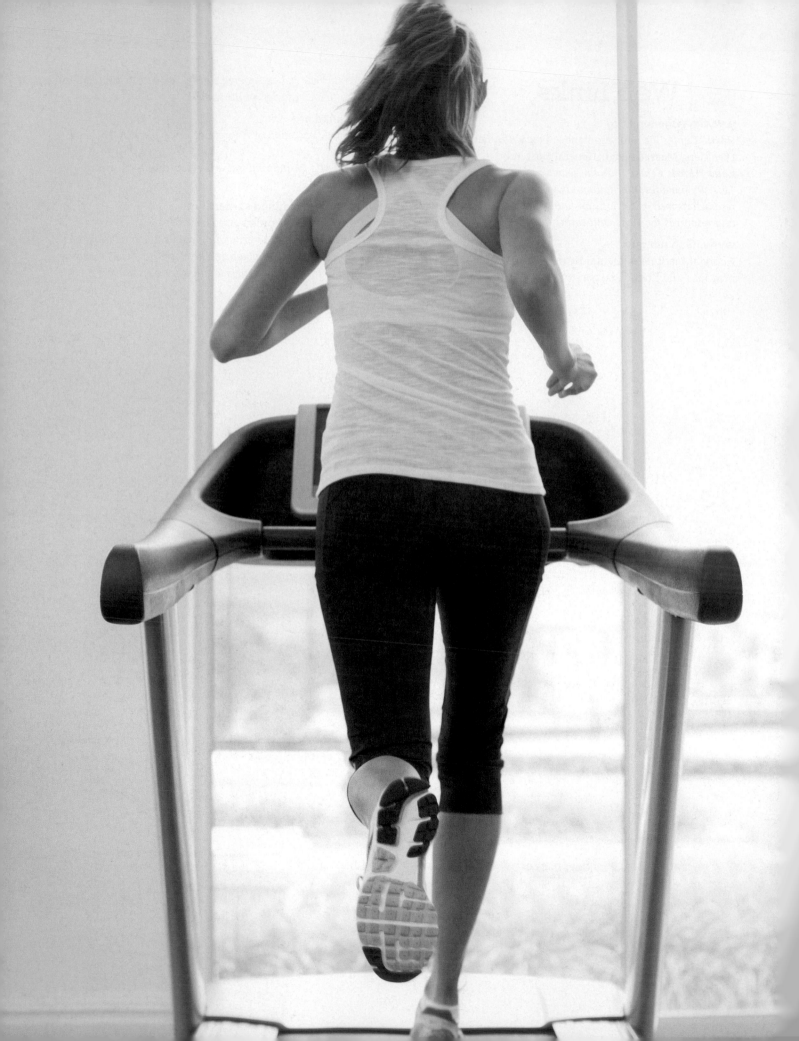

14 Nutrition and Physical Activity: Keys to Good Health

Learning Objectives

After studying this chapter, you should be able to:

1 Discuss the health benefits of being physically active on a regular basis, *pp. 554–556.*

2 Identify the four components of fitness and the forms of exercise necessary to achieve them, *pp. 554–555.*

3 Compare national recommendations for frequency, intensity, and duration of physical activity, *pp. 557–558.*

4 Identify six strategies for developing a sound fitness program, *pp. 558–564.*

5 Describe the FITT principle, and calculate your maximal and training heart rate range, *pp. 560–562.*

6 List and describe at least three metabolic processes cells use to fuel physical activity, *pp. 564–570.*

7 Explain how an increase in physical activity or athletic training can affect energy and macronutrient needs, *pp. 571–578.*

8 Define carbohydrate loading, and discuss situations in which this practice may enhance athletic performance, *pp. 576–577.*

9 Explain how an increase in physical activity or athletic training can affect fluid and micronutrient needs, *pp. 578–581.*

10 Compare heat syncope, heat cramps, heat exhaustion, and heat stroke, *pp. 578–579.*

TEST YOURSELF

True or False?

1 Only about half of all Americans perform adequate levels of physical activity. **T** *or* **F**

2 Physical activity of moderate intensity, such as walking, water aerobics, or gardening, does not yield significant health benefits. **T** *or* **F**

3 Carbohydrate loading before a 1,500-meter run can improve performance. **T** *or* **F**

4 Taking protein supplements is necessary if your goal is to build muscle. **T** *or* **F**

5 During exercise, our desire to drink is enough to prompt us to consume enough water or fluids. **T** *or* **F**

Test Yourself answers are located in the Study Plan.

MasteringNutrition™

Go online for chapter quizzes, pre-tests, interactive activities, and more!

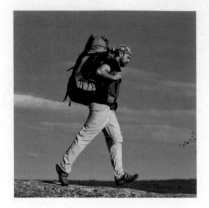

Hiking is a leisure-time physical activity that can contribute to your physical fitness.

 Discuss the health benefits of being physically active on a regular basis.

 Identify the four components of fitness and the forms of exercise necessary to achieve them.

physical activity Any movement produced by muscles that increases energy expenditure; includes occupational, household, leisure-time, and transportation activities.

leisure-time physical activity Any activity not related to a person's occupation; includes competitive sports, recreational activities, and planned exercise training.

exercise A subcategory of leisure-time physical activity; any activity that is purposeful, planned, and structured.

physical fitness The ability to carry out daily tasks with vigor and alertness, without undue fatigue, and with ample energy to enjoy leisure-time pursuits and meet unforeseen emergencies.

aerobic exercise Exercise that involves the repetitive movement of large muscle groups, increasing the body's use of oxygen and promoting cardiovascular health.

resistance training Exercise in which our muscles act against resistance.

stretching Exercise in which muscles are gently lengthened using slow, controlled movements.

I n the summer of 2013, Lillian Web of Florida and Harold Bach of North Dakota each won a gold medal for the 100-meter dash in track and field at the National Senior Games. Web did it in just over 38 seconds, and Bach's time was less than 22 seconds. If these performance times don't amaze you, perhaps they will when you consider these athletes' ages: Web was 99 years old, and Bach was 93!

There's no doubt about it: regular physical activity can dramatically improve a person's strength, stamina, health, and longevity. But what qualifies as "regular physical activity"? In other words, how much does a person need to do to reap the benefits? And if people do become more active, do their diets have to change too?

You may be asking yourself why a nutrition textbook includes a chapter on physical activity. One reason is that a healthful diet and regular physical activity are like two sides of the same coin, interacting in a variety of ways to improve strength and stamina and to increase resistance to many chronic diseases and acute illnesses. Physical activity also affects how we store and metabolize various nutrients, and our nutritional status impacts our ability to perform physical activity. In this chapter, we define physical activity, identify its many benefits, and discuss the nutrients needed to maintain an active life.

What Are the Benefits of Physical Activity?

The term **physical activity** describes any movement produced by muscles that increases energy expenditure. Different categories of physical activity include occupational, household, leisure-time, and transportation.[1] **Leisure-time physical activity** is any activity not related to a person's occupation, and includes competitive sports, planned exercise training, and recreational activities, such as hiking, walking, and bicycling. **Exercise** is therefore considered a subcategory of leisure-time physical activity and is activity that is purposeful, planned, and structured.[2]

Physical Activity Increases Our Fitness

A lot of people are looking for a "magic pill" that will help them maintain weight loss, reduce their risk for diseases, boost their mood, and improve their quality of sleep. Although they may not be aware of it, regular physical activity is this "magic pill." That's because it promotes **physical fitness**: the ability to carry out daily tasks with vigor and alertness, without undue fatigue, and with ample energy to enjoy leisure-time pursuits and meet unforeseen emergencies.[1]

The four components of physical fitness are cardiorespiratory fitness, which is the ability of the heart, lungs, and blood vessels to supply working muscles; musculoskeletal fitness, which is fitness of the muscles and bones; flexibility; and body composition (**Table 14.1**).[3] These are achieved through three types of exercise:

- **Aerobic exercise** involves the repetitive movement of large muscle groups, which increases the body's use of oxygen and promotes cardiorespiratory fitness. In your daily life, you get aerobic exercise when you walk to school, work, or a bus stop or take the stairs to a third-floor classroom.
- **Resistance training** is a form of exercise in which our muscles work against resistance, such as against handheld weights. It strongly promotes musculoskeletal fitness. Carrying grocery bags or books and moving heavy objects are everyday activities that make our muscles work against resistance.
- **Stretching** exercises are those that increase flexibility, as they involve lengthening muscles using slow, controlled movements. You can perform stretching exercises even while you're sitting in a classroom by flexing, extending, and rotating your neck, limbs, and extremities.

Both aerobic and resistance training promote a healthy body composition and body weight. Although stretching exercises are not associated with optimizing body composition and

TABLE 14.1 The Components of Fitness

Fitness Component	Examples of Activities One Can Do to Achieve Fitness in Each Component
Cardiorespiratory	Aerobic-type activities, such as walking, running, swimming, cross-country skiing
Musculoskeletal fitness	Resistance training, weight lifting, calisthenics, sit-ups, push-ups
Muscular strength	Weight lifting or related activities using heavier weights with few repetitions
Muscular endurance	Weight lifting or related activities using lighter weights with more repetitions
Flexibility	Stretching exercises, yoga
Body composition	Aerobic exercise, resistance training

body weight, they are critical to supporting one's ability to engage in all forms of exercise and activities of daily living.

Physical Activity Reduces Our Risk for Chronic Diseases

In addition to contributing to our fitness, physical activity can reduce our risk for certain diseases. Specifically, the health benefits of physical activity include (see **Figure 14.1**, page 556):

- *Reduces our risk for, and complications of, heart disease, stroke, and high blood pressure.* Regular physical activity increases high-density lipoprotein (HDL) cholesterol and lowers triglycerides in the blood, improves the strength of the heart, helps maintain healthy blood pressure, and limits the progression of atherosclerosis.

- *Reduces our risk for obesity.* Regular physical activity maintains lean body mass and promotes more healthful levels of body fat, may help in appetite control, and increases energy expenditure and the use of fat as an energy source.

- *Reduces our risk for type 2 diabetes.* Regular physical activity enhances the action of insulin, which improves the cells' uptake of glucose from the blood, and it can improve blood glucose control in people with diabetes, which in turn reduces the risk for, or delays the onset of, diabetes-related complications.

- *May reduce our risk for colon cancer.* Although the exact role that physical activity may play in reducing colon cancer risk is still unknown, we do know that regular physical activity enhances gastric motility, which reduces the transit time of potential cancer-causing agents through the gut.

- *Reduces our risk for osteoporosis.* Regular physical activity, especially weight-bearing exercise, increases bone density and enhances muscular strength and flexibility, thereby reducing the likelihood of falls and the incidence of fractures and other injuries when falls occur.

Regular physical activity is also known to improve our sleep patterns, reduce our risk for upper respiratory infections by improving immune function, and reduce anxiety and mental stress. It also can be effective in treating mild and moderate depression.

 Sitting too long, studying for tomorrow's exam? Stretching can help! Learn some simple stretches by watching the how-to video collection from the Mayo Clinic at **www.mayoclinic.com**. Enter "health," and then "office stretches" into the search bar.

Nutrition
MILESTONE

Although the benefits of exercise have been touted throughout history, it wasn't until **1953** that a significant link between physical health and exercise was confirmed. After returning from military service in World War II, Dr. Jeremiah "Jerry" Morris and other public health researchers in the United Kingdom became aware of the growing modern epidemic of coronary heart disease. Some evidence suggested that a person's occupation may play a key role in their risk of having a heart attack. Dr. Morris was able to prove his hypothesis in a landmark paper, published in *The Lancet*, which discussed his research on London transport employees.

This study showed that the heart attack rates of the bus drivers (who sat most of the day) were more than twice as high as those of conductors (who ran up and down the stairs of double-decker buses all day). He documented the waist circumferences of the bus employees via their pant waistband sizes, which indicated that the physically active conductors had a significantly lower risk for heart attack, no matter what the size of their waist! Dr. Morris is recognized as the father of physical activity epidemiology, and he continued to be an avid exerciser and active public health researcher until his death in 2009 at the age of 99.

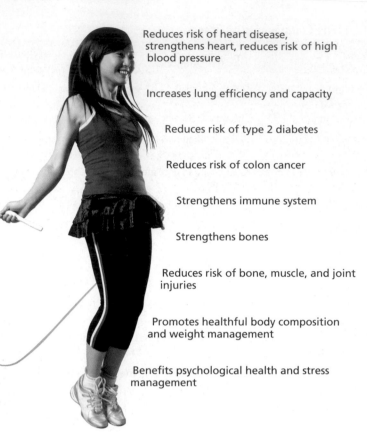

Reduces risk of heart disease, strengthens heart, reduces risk of high blood pressure

Increases lung efficiency and capacity

Reduces risk of type 2 diabetes

Reduces risk of colon cancer

Strengthens immune system

Strengthens bones

Reduces risk of bone, muscle, and joint injuries

Promotes healthful body composition and weight management

Benefits psychological health and stress management

FIGURE 14.1 Health benefits of regular physical activity.

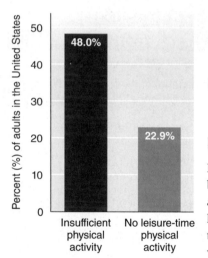

FIGURE 14.2 Rates of physical inactivity in the United States. Almost 50% of the U.S. population does not do enough physical activity to meet national health recommendations, and another 22.9% report doing no leisure-time physical activity. (*Sources*: Centers for Disease Control and Prevention. 2014. Facts about Physical Activity, http://www.cdc.gov/physicalactivity /data/facts.html and Centers for Disease Control and Prevention. Office of Surveillance, Epidemiology, and Laboratory Services. Behavioral Risk Factor Surveillance System. 2012. Prevalence and Trends Data. Exercise - 2012. http://apps.nccd.cdc .gov/brfss/list.asp?cat=EX&yr =2012&qkey=8041&state=All.)

Most Americans Are Inactive

For most of our history, humans were very physically active. This was not by choice but because their survival depended on it. Prior to the industrial age, humans expended a considerable amount of energy each day foraging and hunting for food, planting and harvesting food, preparing food once it was acquired, and securing shelter. In addition, their diet was composed primarily of small amounts of lean meats and naturally grown vegetables, fruits, and nuts. This lifestyle pattern contrasts considerably with today's, which is characterized by sedentary jobs, easy access to an overabundance of energy-dense foods, and few opportunities for or little interest in expending energy through occupational or recreational activities.

Given these changes, it isn't surprising that most people find the "magic pill" of physical activity hard to swallow. The Centers for Disease Control and Prevention reports that nearly half (or 48%) of adults in the United States do not do enough physical activity to meet national health recommendations, and another 22.9% admit to doing no leisure-time physical activity at all (**Figure 14.2**).[4,5] These statistics mirror the reported increases in obesity, heart disease, and type 2 diabetes in the United States.

This trend toward inadequate physical activity levels is also occurring in young people. Among high school students, only 17.7% of girls and 36.6% of boys are meeting the recommended 60 minutes per day on each of the 7 days before completing the survey.[6] Although physical education (PE) is part of the mandated curriculum in most states, only 24.0% of girls and 34.9% of boys participate in daily PE. Since our habits related to eating and physical activity are formed early in life, it is imperative that we provide opportunities for children and adolescents to engage in regular, enjoyable physical activity. An active lifestyle during childhood increases the likelihood of an active, healthier life as an adult.

RECAP

Physical activity increases our fitness and reduces our risk for chronic disease. It is defined as any movement produced by muscles that increases energy expenditure. Physical fitness is the ability to carry out daily tasks with vigor and alertness, without undue fatigue, and with ample energy to enjoy leisure-time pursuits and meet unforeseen emergencies. The four components of physical fitness are cardiorespiratory fitness, musculoskeletal fitness, flexibility, and body composition. These types of fitness can be achieved through aerobic exercise, resistance training, and stretching. Specific health benefits of physical activity include a reduced risk for obesity and other chronic diseases, as well as stress management, improved sleep, and many others. Nearly half of all people in the United States, including many children, are insufficiently active. ■

How Much Physical Activity Is Enough?

LO 3 Compare national recommendations for frequency, intensity, and duration of physical activity.

As you've just read, most Americans do not engage in enough regular physical activity to meet current national recommendations. But what are the current recommendations, and what must a person do to achieve them?

In 1996, a report of the Surgeon General recommended that Americans engage in at least 30 minutes of physical activity on most days of the week.[1] Then, in 2002, the Institute of Medicine (IOM), which is part of the National Academy of Sciences, released a recommendation that Americans be active 60 minutes per day to optimize health.[7] As this amount and frequency of physical activity was significantly higher than the Surgeon General's recommendation, it caused a great deal of confusion and controversy. What was the basis for this more challenging recommendation?

The IOM recommendation was derived from metabolic studies specifically examining the energy expenditure associated with maintaining a healthful body weight (defined as a BMI of 18.5 to 25 kg/m^2). After reviewing a large number of studies that assessed energy expenditure and BMI, the IOM concluded that participating in about 60 minutes of moderately intense physical activity per day will move people to an active lifestyle and will allow them to maintain a healthful body weight.

The IOM recommendation was not based on evidence supporting the wider range of health benefits that result when a person moves from doing no physical activity to at least some level of physical activity. The growing body of evidence regarding the health benefits of physical activity clearly indicates that doing at least some physical activity is better than doing none, and doing more physical activity is better than doing less.

In 2008, the United States Department of Health and Human Services (HHS) released the *Physical Activity Guidelines for Americans*.[8] These include guidelines for children and adolescents, adults, and older adults, with additional information for women who are pregnant; people with disabilities, type 2 diabetes, or osteoarthritis; and people who are cancer survivors. These guidelines build upon the Surgeon General's recommendation of 30 minutes per day on most, if not all, days of the week. Specifically, the 2008 HHS guidelines for adults state the following:

- Inactivity should be avoided. Participating in any amount of physical activity will provide some health benefits.
- To gain substantial health benefits, adults should do a minimum of 150 minutes per week of moderate-intensity activity, or 75 minutes per week of vigorous intensity activity, or an equivalent combination of these two intensities of activity. The activities should be aerobic in nature and performed in episodes of at least 10 minutes' duration, spread throughout the week.
- To gain additional and more extensive health benefits, adults should increase their aerobic activity level to 300 minutes per week of moderate-intensity activity, or

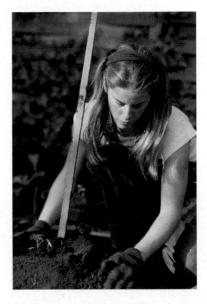

Moderate physical activity, such as gardening, helps maintain overall health.

150 minutes per week of vigorous-intensity activity, or an equivalent combination of these two intensities.

- Adults should also participate in muscle-strengthening activities that are moderate or vigorous in intensity and involve all major muscle groups on at least 2 days per week.

Notice that these guidelines promote a *minimum* of 150 minutes per week of moderate-intensity aerobic physical activity, with additional encouragement to increase both the intensity and the duration of activity throughout the week to gain even more health benefits. Two recent studies tracking hundreds of thousands of individuals over several years support these recommendations. They found that those who exercised moderately for at least 150 minutes a week had about a 30% to 47% lower risk of dying during the study period, and that those who exercised longer (up to 450 minutes a week) or more vigorously at least occasionally during the week experienced an even greater reduction in mortality risk.[9,10] This research supports the reliability of the 2008 HHS guidelines while helping to illustrate that the IOM and Surgeon General's recommendations are not really that different after all.

RECAP

A 1996 report of the Surgeon General recommended engaging in at least 30 minutes of moderate physical activity most days of the week, whereas a 2002 report from the IOM recommended 60 minutes. The *2008 Physical Activity Guidelines for Americans* suggest that adults do a minimum of 150 minutes of moderate-intensity aerobic activity per week or 75 minutes of vigorous-intensity aerobic activity per week, or an equivalent combination of the two. For greater benefits, adults should increase their level of activity. The guidelines also recommend that adults engage in moderate- or vigorous-intensity muscle strengthening exercises at least 2 days per week. The reliability of the 2008 guidelines has been supported by recent studies examining large populations. ■

LO 4 Identify six strategies for developing a sound fitness program.

LO 5 Describe the FITT principle, and calculate your maximal and training heart rate range.

How Can You Improve Your Fitness?

Several widely recognized qualities of a sound fitness program, as well as guidelines to help people design one that is right for them, are explored in this section. Keep in mind that people with heart disease, high blood pressure, diabetes, obesity, asthma, osteoporosis, or arthritis should get approval to exercise from their healthcare practitioner prior to starting a fitness program. In addition, a medical evaluation should be conducted before starting an exercise program for an apparently healthy but currently inactive man 40 years or older or woman 50 years or older.

Assess Your Current Level of Fitness

Before beginning any fitness program, it is important to know your initial level of fitness. This information can then be used to help you design a fitness program that meets your goals and is appropriate for you. How can you go about estimating your current fitness level? The President's Council on Fitness, Sports and Nutrition can help! Check out the **Web Links** at the end of the chapter to take The President's Challenge Adult Fitness test.

Identify Your Personal Fitness Goals

A fitness program that may be ideal for someone else may not be right for you. Before designing any program, it is important to define your personal fitness goals. Do you want to prevent osteoporosis, diabetes, or another chronic disease that runs in your family? Do you simply want to increase your energy and stamina? Or do you intend to compete in athletic events? Each of these scenarios requires a unique fitness program. This concept is referred to as the *specificity principle*: specific actions yield specific results.

Training is generally defined as activity leading to skilled behavior. Training is very specific to any activity or goal. For example, if you want to train for athletic competition, a traditional approach that includes planned, purposive exercise sessions under the guidance of a trainer or coach would be beneficial. If you wanted to achieve cardiorespiratory fitness, you might be advised to participate in an aerobics class at least three times per week or jog for at least 20 minutes three times per week.

In contrast, if your goal is to transition from doing no regular physical activity to doing enough physical activity to maintain your overall health, you could follow the minimum recommendations put forth in the *2008 Physical Activity Guidelines for Americans*.[8] To gain significant health benefits, including reducing your risk for chronic diseases, you can engage in at least 30 minutes per day of moderate-intensity aerobic physical activity (such as gardening, brisk walking, or basketball). The activity need not be completed in one session. You can divide the 30 minutes into two or more shorter sessions throughout the day (for example, brisk walking for 10 minutes three times per day). Again, performing physical activities at a higher intensity and for longer duration will confer even greater health benefits.

Make Your Program Varied, Consistent, and Fun!

A number of factors motivate us to be active. Some are *intrinsic* factors, which are those done for the satisfaction a person gains from engaging in the activity. Others are *extrinsic,* which are those done to obtain rewards or outcomes that are separate from the behavior itself.[11] Examples of intrinsic factors that motivate us to engage in physical activity include the desire to gain competence, the desire to be challenged by the activity and enhance our skills, and enjoyment. Some of the most common extrinsic factors are desires to improve appearance, to increase fitness, and to avoid feelings of guilt and shame. Recently, some employers have been offering financial incentives to log in time at the company's fitness center, another example of an extrinsic factor.

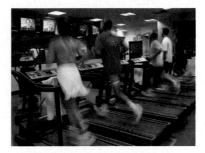

Watching television or listening to music can provide variety while running on a treadmill.

Whether we are more motivated by intrinsic or extrinsic factors is related to the type of activity in which we engage and whether we're a regular or infrequent exerciser. People who are regularly active tend to be more motivated by intrinsic factors, whereas extrinsic factors appear to be more important to people who are not regularly active or are engaging in activity for the first time. Being intrinsically motivated to be physically active has also been shown to positively influence eating behaviors and promote healthy weight control.[12]

Thus, an important motivator in maintaining regular physical activity is enjoyment—or fun! People who enjoy being active find it easy to maintain their physical fitness. What activities do you consider fun? If you enjoy the outdoors, hiking, camping, fishing, and rock climbing are potential activities for you. If you would rather exercise with friends between classes, walking, climbing stairs, jogging, roller-blading, or bicycle riding may be more appropriate. Or you may prefer to use the programs and equipment at your campus or community fitness center or purchase your own treadmill and free weights.

Variety is also important. Although some people enjoy doing similar activities day after day, many get bored with the same fitness routine. Incorporating a variety of activities into your fitness program will help maintain your interest and increase your enjoyment while promoting the various types of fitness identified in Table 14.1. Variety can be achieved in the following ways:

- Combining aerobic exercise, resistance training, and stretching
- Combining indoor and outdoor activities throughout the week
- Taking different routes when you walk or jog each day
- Watching a movie, reading a book, or listening to music while you ride a stationary bicycle or walk on a treadmill
- Participating in different activities each week, such as walking, dancing, bicycling, yoga, weight lifting, swimming, hiking, and gardening

This "smorgasbord" of activities can increase your fitness without leading to monotony and boredom.

Appropriately Overload Your Body

In order to improve your fitness, you need to increase the physical demands you make on your body. This is referred to as the **overload principle.** A word of caution is in order here: *the overload principle does not advocate subjecting the body to inappropriately high stress,* because this can lead to exhaustion and injuries. In contrast, an appropriate overload on various body systems will result in healthy improvements in fitness. For example, a gain in muscle strength and size that results from repeated work that overloads the muscle is referred to as **hypertrophy.** When muscles are not worked adequately, they **atrophy,** or decrease in size and strength.

To achieve an appropriate overload, four factors should be considered, collectively known as the **FITT principle:** *f*requency, *i*ntensity, *t*ime, and *t*ype of activity. The FITT principle can be used to design either a general physical fitness program or a performance-based exercise program. **Figure 14.3** shows how the FITT principle can be applied to a cardiorespiratory and muscular fitness program.

Let's consider each of the FITT principle's four factors in more detail.

Frequency

Frequency refers to the number of activity sessions per week. Depending on the goals for fitness, the frequency of activities will vary. The *Physical Activity Guidelines for Americans* recommend engaging in aerobic (cardiorespiratory) activities for at least 150 minutes a week. To achieve cardiorespiratory fitness, training should be at least 3 to 5 days per week. On the other hand, training 7 days a week does not cause significant gains in fitness but can

overload principle Placing an extra physical demand on your body in order to improve your fitness level.

hypertrophy The increase in strength and size that results from repeated work to a specific muscle or muscle group.

atrophy A decrease in the size and strength of muscles that occurs when they are not worked adequately.

FITT principle The principle used to achieve an appropriate overload for physical training; FITT stands for *f*requency, *i*ntensity, *t*ime, and *t*ype of activity.

frequency Refers to the number of activity sessions per week you perform.

	Frequency	Intensity	Time and Type
Cardiorespiratory fitness	At least 30 minutes most days of the week	50–70% maximal heart rate for moderate intensity; 70–85% maximal heart rate for vigorous intensity	At least 30 consecutive minutes Choose swimming, walking, running, cycling, dancing, or other aerobic activities
Muscular fitness	2–3 days per week	70–85% maximal weight you can lift	1–3 sets of 8–12 lifts for each set A minimum of 8–10 exercises involving the major muscle groups such as arms, shoulders, chest, abdomen, back, hips, and legs, is recommended.
Flexibility	2–4 days per week	Stretching through full range of motion	For stretching, perform 2–4 repetitions per stretch. Hold each stretch for 15–30 seconds. Or try yoga, tai chi, or other flexibility programs.

FIGURE 14.3 Using the FITT principle to achieve cardiorespiratory and musculoskeletal fitness and flexibility. The recommendations in this figure follow the 2008 Physical Activity Guidelines for Americans (still in effect today).

substantially increase the risks for injury. Training 3 to 6 days per week appears optimal to achieve and maintain cardiorespiratory fitness. In contrast, only 2 to 3 days of resistance training are needed to achieve muscular fitness.

Intensity

Intensity refers to the amount of effort expended, or to how difficult the activity is to perform. We can describe the intensity of activity as low, moderate, or vigorous:

- **Low-intensity activities** are those that cause very mild increases in breathing, sweating, and heart rate. Examples include walking at a leisurely pace, fishing, and light house-cleaning.
- **Moderate-intensity activities** cause moderate increases in breathing, sweating, and heart rate. For instance, you can carry on a conversation, but not continuously. Examples include brisk walking, water aerobics, doubles tennis, ballroom dancing, and bicycling slower than 10 miles per hour.
- **Vigorous-intensity activities** produce significant increases in breathing, sweating, and heart rate, so that talking is difficult when exercising. Examples include jogging, running, racewalking, singles tennis, aerobics, bicycling 10 miles per hour or faster, jumping rope, and hiking uphill with a heavy backpack.

Traditionally, heart rate has been used to indicate level of intensity during aerobic activities. You can calculate the range of exercise intensity that is appropriate for you by estimating your **maximal heart rate,** which is the rate at which your heart beats during maximal-intensity exercise. Maximal heart rate is estimated by subtracting your age from 220.

Figure 14.4 shows an example of a heart rate training chart, which you can use to estimate the intensity of your own workout. The Centers for Disease Control and Prevention makes the following recommendations:[13]

- To achieve moderate-intensity physical activity, your target heart rate should be 50–70% of your estimated maximal heart rate. Older adults and anyone who has been inactive for a long time may want to exercise at the lower end of the moderate-intensity range.

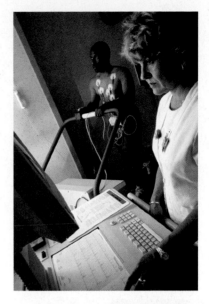

Testing in a fitness lab is the most accurate way to determine maximal heart rate.

 For a quick estimate of your training heart rate range, go to www.mayoclinic.com. **Enter "target heart rate" into the search box.**

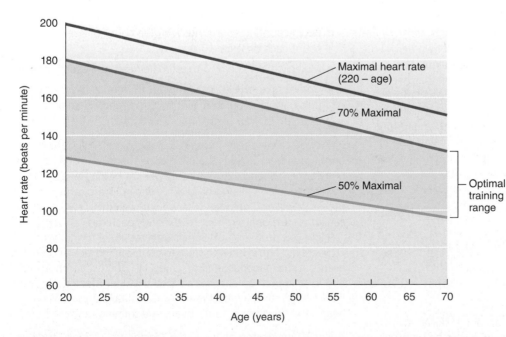

FIGURE 14.4 This heart rate training chart can be used to estimate aerobic exercise intensity. The top line indicates the predicted maximal heart rate value for a person's age (220 − age). The shaded area represents the heart rate values that fall between 50% and 70% of maximal heart rate, which is the range generally recommended to achieve aerobic fitness.

intensity The amount of effort expended during an activity, or how difficult the activity is to perform.

low-intensity activities Activities that cause very mild increases in breathing, sweating, and heart rate.

moderate-intensity activities Activities that cause moderate increases in breathing, sweating, and heart rate.

vigorous-intensity activities Activities that produce significant increases in breathing, sweating, and heart rate; talking is difficult when exercising at a vigorous intensity.

maximal heart rate The rate at which the heart beats during maximal-intensity exercise.

- To achieve vigorous-intensity physical activity, your target heart rate should be 70–85% of your estimated heart rate. Those who are physically fit or are striving for a more rapid improvement in fitness may want to exercise at the higher end of the vigorous-intensity range.
- Competitive athletes generally train at a higher intensity, around 80–95% of their maximal heart rate.

Although the calculation of *220 minus age* has been used extensively for years to predict maximal heart rate, it was never intended to accurately represent everyone's true maximal heart rate or to be used as the standard of aerobic training intensity. The most accurate way to determine your own maximal heart rate is to complete a maximal exercise test in a fitness laboratory; however, this test is not commonly conducted with the general public and can be very expensive. Although not completely accurate, the estimated maximal heart rate method can still be used to give you a general idea of your aerobic training range.

So what is your maximal heart rate and training range? To find out, try the easy calculation in the ***You Do the Math*** box.

YOU Do the Math — Calculating Your Maximal and Training Heart Rate Range

Judy was recently diagnosed with type 2 diabetes, and her healthcare provider has recommended she begin an exercise program. She is considered obese, according to her body mass index, and she has not been regularly active since she was a teenager. Judy's goals are to improve her cardiorespiratory fitness and achieve and maintain a more healthful weight. Fortunately, Valley Hospital, where she works as a nurse's aide, recently opened a small fitness center for its employees. Judy plans to begin by either walking on the treadmill or riding the stationary bicycle at the fitness center during her lunch break.

Judy needs to exercise at an intensity that will help her improve her cardiorespiratory fitness and lose weight. She is 38 years of age, is obese, has type 2 diabetes, and has been approved to do moderate-intensity activity by her healthcare provider. Even though she does a lot of walking and lifting in her work as a nurse's aide, her doctor has recommended that she set her exercise intensity range to begin at a heart rate at the low end of the currently recommended moderate intensity, or 50% to 70% of estimated maximal heart rate.

Let's calculate Judy's maximal heart rate values:

- Maximal heart rate: 220 − age = 220 − 38 = 182 beats per minute (bpm)
- Lower end of intensity range: 50% of 182 bpm = 0.50 × 182 bpm = 91 bpm
- Higher end of intensity range: 70% of 182 bpm = 0.70 × 182 bpm = 127 bpm

Because Judy is a trained nurse's aide, she is skilled at measuring a heart rate, or pulse. To measure your own pulse, take the following steps:

- Place your second (index) and third (middle) fingers on the inside of your wrist, just below the wrist crease and near the thumb. Press lightly to feel your pulse. Don't press too hard, or you will occlude the artery and be unable to feel its pulsation.
- If you can't feel your pulse at your wrist, try the carotid artery at the neck. This is located below your ear, on the side of your neck directly below your jaw. Press lightly against your neck under the jaw bone to find your pulse.
- Begin counting your pulse with the count of "zero"; then count each beat for 15 seconds.
- Multiply that value by 4 to estimate heart rate over 1 minute.
- Do not take your pulse with your thumb, as it has its own pulse, which would prevent you from getting an accurate estimate of your heart rate.

As you can see from these calculations, when Judy walks on the treadmill or rides the bicycle, her heart rate should be between 91 and 127 bpm; this will put her in her aerobic training zone and allow her to achieve cardiorespiratory fitness. It will also help her lose weight, assuming she consumes less energy than she expends each day.

Now you do the math. Sam is a recreational runner who is 70 years old and wishes to train to compete in track and field events at the National Senior Games. His doctor has approved him for competition and has advised that Sam train at 75% to 80% of his maximal heart rate. (A) Calculate Sam's maximal heart rate. (B) What is Sam's heart rate training range in bpm?

Answers are located online in the MasteringNutrition Study Area.

Time of Activity

Time of activity refers to how long each session lasts. To achieve general health, a person can do multiple, short bouts of activity that add up to 30 minutes each day. However, to achieve higher levels of fitness, it is important that the activities be done for at least 20 to 30 consecutive minutes.

For example, let's say you want to compete in triathlons. To be successful during the running segment of the triathlon, you will need to be able to run quickly for at least 5 miles. Thus, it is appropriate for you to train so that you can complete 5 miles during one session and still have enough energy to swim and bicycle during the race. You will need to train consistently at a distance of 5 miles; you will also benefit from running longer distances.

Type of Activity

Type of activity refers to the range of physical activities a person can engage in to promote health and physical fitness. Many examples are listed in Table 14.1 (page 555) and Figure 14.3 (page 560). The types of activity you choose to engage in will depend on your goals for health and physical fitness, your personal preferences, and the range of activities available to you.

Include a Warm-Up and a Cool-Down Period

To properly prepare for and recover from an exercise session, warm-up and cool-down activities should be performed. **Warm-up,** also called preliminary exercise, includes general activities, such as gentle aerobics, calisthenics, and then stretching followed by specific activities that prepare a person for the actual activity, such as jogging or swinging a golf club. The warm-up should be brief (5 to 10 minutes), gradual, and sufficient to increase muscle and body temperature. It should not cause fatigue or deplete energy stores.

Warming up prior to exercise is important, as it properly prepares your muscles for exertion by increasing blood flow and body temperature. It enhances the body's flexibility and may also help prepare you psychologically for the exercise session or athletic event.

Cool-down activities are done after the exercise session. The cool-down should be gradual and allow the body to recover slowly. The cool-down should include some of the same activities performed during the exercise session, but at a low intensity, and should allow ample time for stretching. Cooling down after exercise assists in the prevention of injury and may help reduce muscle soreness.

Keep It Simple, Take It Slow

There are 1,440 minutes in every day. Spend just 30 of those minutes in physical activity, and you'll be taking an important step toward improving your health. Here are some tips for how you incorporate more regular physical activity into your daily life and, as a result, improve your health:

- Walk as often and as far as possible: Park your car farther away from your dorm, a lecture hall, or shops. Walk to school or work. Go for a brisk walk between classes. Get on or off the bus one stop away from your destination. And don't be in such a rush to reach your destination—take the long way and burn a few more Calories.
- At every opportunity, take the stairs instead of the escalator or elevator.
- When working on the computer for long periods of time, take a 3- to 5-minute break every hour to stretch, walk to another room, or make a cup of tea.
- Exercise while watching television—for example by doing sit-ups, stretching, or using a treadmill or stationary bike.
- While talking on your cell phone, memorizing vocabulary terms, or practicing your choral part, don't stand still—pace!
- Turn on some music and dance!

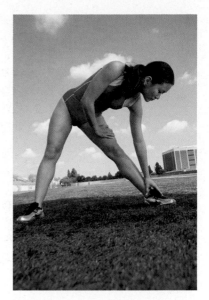

Stretching should be included in the warm-up and the cool-down for exercise.

 Want to learn more about the various tools used to measure physical activity levels? Go to the University of Pittsburgh Physical Activity Resource Center for Public Health at www.parcph .org to find out more.

time of activity How long each exercise session lasts.

type of activity The range of physical activities a person can engage in to promote health and physical fitness.

warm-up Also called preliminary exercise; includes activities that prepare you for an exercise bout, including stretching, calisthenics, and movements specific to the exercise bout.

cool-down Activities done after an exercise session is completed; should be gradual and allow your body to slowly recover from exercise.

- Get an exercise partner: join a friend for walks, hikes, cycling, skating, tennis, or a fitness class.
- Take up a group sport.
- Register for a class from the physical education department in an activity you've never tried before, maybe yoga or fencing.
- Register for a dance class, such as jazz, tap, or ballroom.
- Use the pool, track, rock-climbing wall, or other facilities at your campus fitness center, or join a health club, gym, or YMCA/YWCA in your community.
- Join an activity-based club, such as a skating, tennis, or hiking club.
- Play golf without using a golf cart—choose to walk and carry your clubs instead.
- Choose a physically active vacation that provides daily activities combined with exploring new surroundings.

If you have been inactive for a while, use a sensible approach by starting out slowly. The first month is an initiation phase, which is the time to start to incorporate relatively brief bouts of physical activity into your daily life and reduce the time you spend in sedentary activities. Gradually build up the time you spend doing the activity by adding a few minutes every few days until you reach 30 minutes a day.

The next 4 to 6 months is the improvement phase, in which you can increase the intensity and duration of the activities you engage in. As you become more fit, the 30-minute minimum becomes easier and you'll need to gradually increase either the length of time you spend in activity or the intensity of the activities you choose, or both, to continue to progress toward your fitness goals. Once you've reached your goals and a plateau in your fitness gains, you've entered into the maintenance phase. At this point you can either maintain your current activity levels, or you may choose to reevaluate your goals and alter your training accordingly.

RECAP

Before beginning any fitness program, assess your current level of fitness. Then set personal fitness goals using the specificity principle: specific actions yield specific results. Your program should be fun and include variety and consistency to help you maintain interest and achieve fitness in all components. It must also place an extra physical demand, or an appropriate overload, on your body. To achieve appropriate overload, follow the FITT principle: *Frequency* refers to the number of activity sessions per week. *Intensity* refers to how difficult the activity is to perform. *Time* refers to how long each activity session lasts. *Type* refers to the range of physical activities one can engage in. Warm-up exercises prepare the muscles for exertion by increasing blood flow and temperature. Cool-down activities help prevent injury and may help reduce muscle soreness. If you have been inactive for a while, start slowly and build gradually. ∎

 Map your walking, running, or cycling route and share it with friends—or check out dozens of fitness loops right in your neighborhood at www.livestrong.com. Enter "tools" into the search box, then scroll down to select the first choice under the Livestrong Search Results heading. Then select "Loops" to get underway.

LO 6 List and describe at least three metabolic processes cells use to fuel physical activity.

What Fuels Physical Activity?

In order to perform exercise, or muscular work, we must be able to generate energy. **Figure 14.5** provides an overview of all of the metabolic pathways that result in the generation of energy to support exercise. As this figure shows, the body can use carbohydrates, fats, and even relatively small amounts of proteins to fuel physical activity.

The common currency of energy for virtually all cells in the body is adenosine triphosphate, or ATP (see Chapter 7, Figure 7.2). Remember that, when one of the three phosphates in ATP is cleaved, energy is released. The products remaining after this reaction are adenosine diphosphate (ADP) and an independent inorganic phosphate group (Pi). In a mirror image of this reaction, the body regenerates ATP by adding a phosphate group back to ADP. In this way, energy is continually provided to the cells both at rest and during exercise.

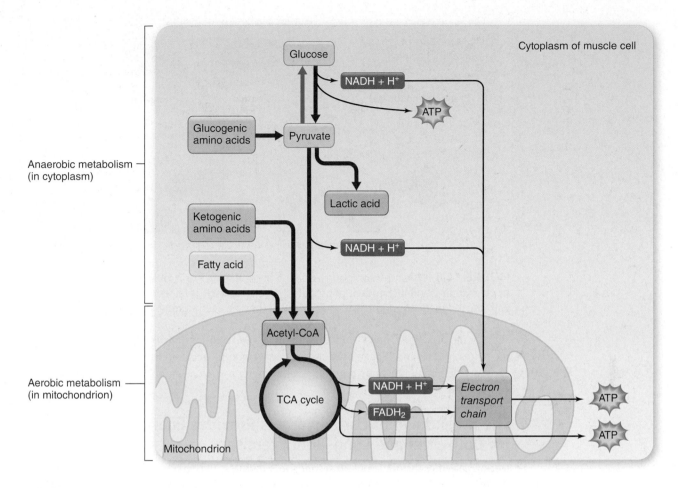

FIGURE 14.5 An overview of the metabolic pathways that result in ATP production during exercise. Carbohydrate, in the form of glucose, and proteins, in the form of amino acids, can be metabolized via anaerobic and aerobic pathways, whereas fatty acids are predominantly metabolized via aerobic pathways.

The amount of ATP stored in a muscle cell is very limited; it can keep the muscle active for only about 1 to 3 seconds. Thus, we need to generate ATP from other sources to fuel activities for longer periods of time. Fortunately, we are able to generate ATP from the breakdown of carbohydrate, fat, and protein, providing the cells with a variety of sources from which to receive energy. The primary energy systems that provide energy for physical activities are the adenosine triphosphate–creatine phosphate (ATP–CP) energy system and the anaerobic and aerobic breakdown of carbohydrates. Our bodies also generate energy from the breakdown of fats. As you will see, the type, intensity, and duration of the activities performed determine the amount of ATP needed and therefore the energy system that is used.

The ATP–CP Energy System Uses Creatine Phosphate to Regenerate ATP

As previously mentioned, muscle cells store only enough ATP to maintain activity for 1 to 3 seconds. When more energy is needed, a high-energy compound called **creatine phosphate (CP)** (also called phosphocreatine, or PCr) can be broken down to support the regeneration of ATP (**Figure 14.6**, page 566). Because this reaction can occur in the absence of oxygen, it is referred to as an anaerobic reaction (meaning "without oxygen").

Muscle tissue contains about four to six times as much CP as ATP, but there is still not enough CP available to fuel long-term activity. CP is used the most during very intense,

creatine phosphate (CP) A high-energy compound that can be broken down for energy and used to regenerate ATP.

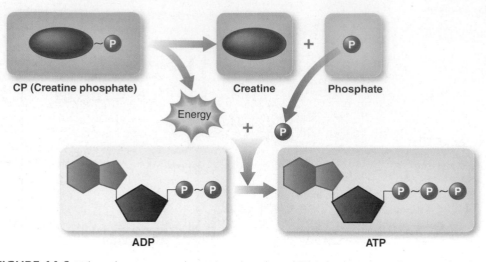

FIGURE 14.6 When the compound creatine phosphate (CP) is broken down into a molecule of creatine and an independent phosphate molecule, energy is released. This energy, along with the independent phosphate molecule, can then be used to regenerate ATP.

short bouts of activity, such as lifting, jumping, and sprinting (**Focus Figure 14.7**). Together, the stores of ATP and CP can only support a *maximal* physical effort for about 3 to 15 seconds. The body must rely on other energy sources, such as carbohydrate and fat, to support activities of longer duration.

The Breakdown of Carbohydrates Provides Energy for Both Brief and Long-Term Exercise

During activities lasting about 30 seconds to 3 minutes, the body needs an energy source that can be used quickly to produce ATP. The breakdown of carbohydrates, specifically glucose, provides this quick energy through glycolysis. The most common source of glucose during exercise comes from glycogen stored in the muscles and glucose found in the blood. For every glucose molecule that goes through glycolysis, two ATP molecules are produced (see Chapter 7, Figure 7.7). The primary end product of glycolysis is pyruvate, which is converted to lactic acid (lactate) when oxygen availability is limited in the cell.

For years it was assumed that lactic acid was a useless, even potentially toxic, by-product of high-intensity exercise. We now know that lactic acid is an important intermediate of glucose breakdown and that it plays a critical role in supplying fuel for working muscles, the heart, and resting tissues. But does lactic acid buildup cause muscle fatigue and soreness? See the ***Highlight*** (page 568) for the answer. Any excess lactic acid that is not used by the muscles is transported in the blood back to the liver, where it is converted back into glucose via the Cori cycle (**Figure 14.8**, page 568). The glucose produced in the liver via the Cori cycle can recirculate to the muscles and provide energy as needed.

The major advantage of glycolysis is that it is the fastest way to generate ATP for exercise, other than the ATP–CP system. However, this high rate of ATP production can be sustained only for a brief period of time, generally less than 3 minutes. To perform exercise that lasts longer than 3 minutes, the body relies on the aerobic energy system.

In the aerobic energy system, pyruvate goes through the additional metabolic pathways of the TCA cycle and the electron transport chain in the presence of oxygen (see Chapter 7, Figure 7.12). Although this process is slower than glycolysis occurring under anaerobic conditions, the breakdown of one glucose molecule going through aerobic metabolism yields 36 to 38 ATP molecules for energy, whereas the anaerobic process yields only two ATP molecules. Thus, this aerobic process supplies 18 times more energy! Another advantage of the aerobic process is that it does not result in the significant production of acids and other compounds that contribute to muscle fatigue, which means that a low-intensity activity can be performed for hours. Aerobic metabolism of glucose is the primary source of fuel for our muscles during activities lasting from 3 minutes to 4 hours.

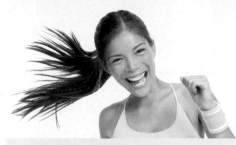

Depending on the duration and intensity of the activity, our bodies may use ATP-CP, carbohydrate, or fat in various combinations to fuel muscular work. Keep in mind that the amounts and sources shown below can vary based on the person's fitness level and health, how well fed the person is before the activity, and environmental temperatures and conditions.

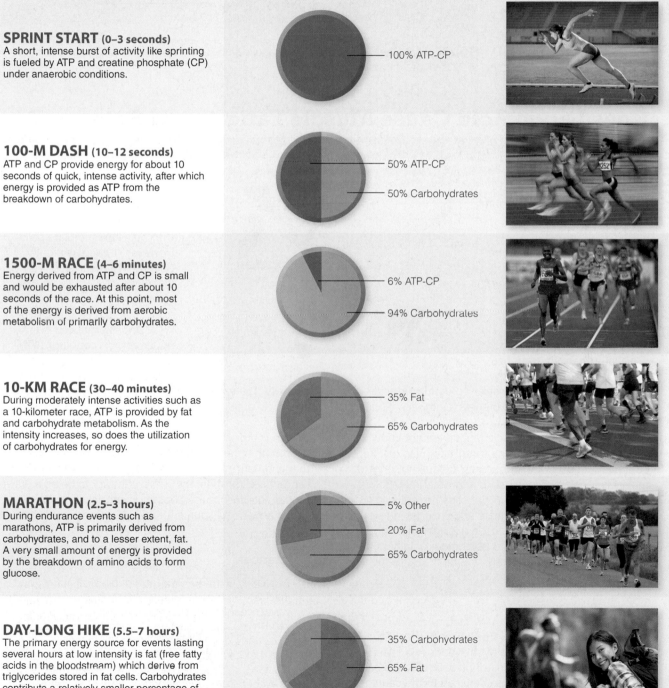

SPRINT START (0–3 seconds)
A short, intense burst of activity like sprinting is fueled by ATP and creatine phosphate (CP) under anaerobic conditions.

100% ATP-CP

100-M DASH (10–12 seconds)
ATP and CP provide energy for about 10 seconds of quick, intense activity, after which energy is provided as ATP from the breakdown of carbohydrates.

50% ATP-CP
50% Carbohydrates

1500-M RACE (4–6 minutes)
Energy derived from ATP and CP is small and would be exhausted after about 10 seconds of the race. At this point, most of the energy is derived from aerobic metabolism of primarily carbohydrates.

6% ATP-CP
94% Carbohydrates

10-KM RACE (30–40 minutes)
During moderately intense activities such as a 10-kilometer race, ATP is provided by fat and carbohydrate metabolism. As the intensity increases, so does the utilization of carbohydrates for energy.

35% Fat
65% Carbohydrates

MARATHON (2.5–3 hours)
During endurance events such as marathons, ATP is primarily derived from carbohydrates, and to a lesser extent, fat. A very small amount of energy is provided by the breakdown of amino acids to form glucose.

5% Other
20% Fat
65% Carbohydrates

DAY-LONG HIKE (5.5–7 hours)
The primary energy source for events lasting several hours at low intensity is fat (free fatty acids in the bloodstream) which derive from triglycerides stored in fat cells. Carbohydrates contribute a relatively smaller percentage of energy needs.

35% Carbohydrates
65% Fat

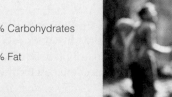

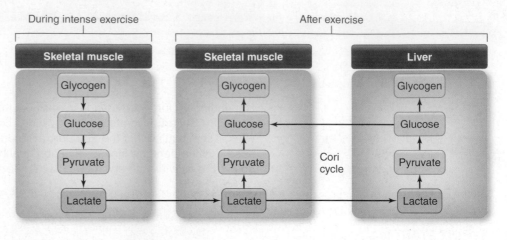

FIGURE 14.8 The Cori cycle is the metabolic pathway by which excess lactic acid can be converted into glucose in the liver.

Does Lactic Acid Cause Muscle Fatigue and Soreness?

Theo and his teammates won their basketball game last night, but just barely. With two of the players sick, Theo got more court time than usual, and when he got back to the dorm, he could hardly get his legs to carry him up the stairs. This morning, Theo's muscles ache all over, and he wonders if a buildup of lactic acid is to blame.

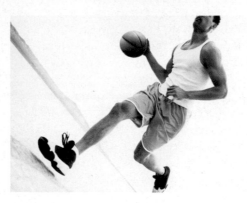

Lactic acid is a by-product of glycolysis. For many years, both scientists and athletes believed that lactic acid causes muscle fatigue and soreness. Does recent scientific evidence support this belief?

The exact causes of muscle fatigue are not known, and there appear to be many contributing factors. Recent evidence suggests that fatigue may be due not only to the accumulation of many acids and other metabolic by-products, such as inorganic phosphate, but also to the depletion of creatine phosphate and changes in calcium in muscle cells. Depletion of muscle glycogen, liver glycogen, and blood glucose, as well as psychological factors, can all contribute to fatigue.[1] Thus, it appears that lactic acid only contributes to fatigue and does not cause it independently.

So what factors cause muscle soreness? As with fatigue, there are probably many factors. It is hypothesized that soreness usually results from microscopic tears in the muscle fibers as a result of strenuous exercise. This damage triggers an inflammatory reaction, which causes an influx of fluid and various chemicals to the damaged tissue area. These substances work to remove damaged tissue and initiate tissue repair, but they may also stimulate pain. However, it appears highly unlikely that lactic acid is an independent cause of muscle soreness.

Recent studies indicate that lactic acid is produced even under aerobic conditions! This means it is produced at rest as well as during exercise at any intensity. The reasons for this constant production of lactic acid are still being studied. What we do know is that lactic acid is an important fuel for resting tissues, for working cardiac and skeletal muscles, and even for the brain both at rest and during exercise.[2,3] We also know that endurance training improves the muscle's ability to use lactic acid for energy. Thus, contrary to being a waste product of glucose metabolism, lactic acid is actually an important energy source for muscle cells during rest and exercise.

References

1. Bogdanis, G. C. 2012. Effects of physical activity and inactivity on muscle fatigue. *Front. Physiol.* 3:142. http://www.ncbi.nlm.nih.gov/pmc/articles/PMC3355468/
2. van Hall, G. 2010. Lactate kinetics in human tissues at rest and during exercise. *Acta Physiologica* 199(4):499–508.
3. Wyss, M. T., R. Jolivet, A. Buck, P. J. Magistretti, and B. Weber. 2011. *J. Neurosci.* 31(20):7477–7485.

The body can store only a limited amount of glycogen. An average, well-nourished man who weighs about 154 lb (70 kg) can store about 200 to 500 g of muscle glycogen, which is equal to 800 to 2,000 kcal of energy. Although trained athletes can store more muscle glycogen than the average person, even their bodies do not have enough stored glycogen to provide an unlimited energy supply for long-term activities. Thus, we also need a fuel source that is abundant and can be broken down under aerobic conditions, so that it can support activities of lower intensity and longer duration. This fuel source is fat.

Aerobic Breakdown of Fats Supports Exercise of Low Intensity and Long Duration

When we refer to fat as a fuel source, we mean stored triglycerides. Their fatty acid chains provide much of the energy needed to support long-term activity. The longer the fatty acid, the more ATP that can be generated from its breakdown. For instance, palmitic acid is a fatty acid with 16 carbons. If palmitic acid is broken down completely, it yields 129 ATP molecules! Obviously, far more energy is produced from this 1 fatty acid molecule than from the aerobic breakdown of a glucose molecule.

There are two major advantages of using fat as a fuel. First, fat is an abundant energy source, even in lean people. For example, a man who weighs 154 lb (70 kg) who has a body fat level of 10% has approximately 15 lb of body fat, which is equivalent to more than 50,000 kcal of energy! This is significantly more energy than can be provided by his stored muscle glycogen (800 to 2,000 kcal). Second, fat provides 9 kcal of energy per gram, more than twice as much energy per gram as carbohydrate. The primary disadvantage of using fat as a fuel is that the breakdown process is relatively slow; thus, fat is used predominantly as a fuel source during activities of lower intensity and longer duration. Fat is also our primary energy source during rest, sitting, and standing in place.

What specific activities are fueled by fat? Walking long distances uses fat stores, as does hiking, long-distance cycling, and other low- to moderate-intensity forms of exercise. Fat is also an important fuel source during endurance events such as marathons (26.2 miles) and ultra-marathon races (49.9 miles). Endurance exercise training improves our ability to use fat for energy, which may be one reason that people who exercise regularly tend to have lower body fat levels than people who do not exercise.

It is important to remember that we are almost always using some combination of carbohydrate and fat for energy. At rest, less carbohydrate is used, and the body relies mostly on fat. During maximal exercise (at 100% effort), the body uses mostly carbohydrate and very little fat. However, most activities done each day involve some use of both fuels (**Figure 14.9**).

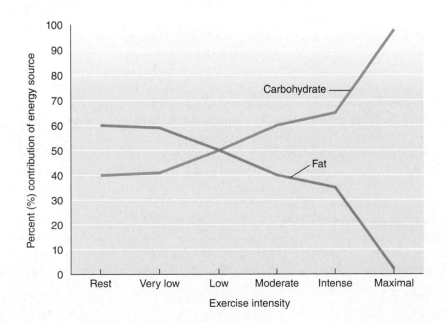

FIGURE 14.9 For most daily activities, including exercise, we use a mixture of carbohydrate and fat for energy. At lower exercise intensities, we rely more on fat as a fuel source. As exercise intensity increases, we rely more on carbohydrate for energy. (*Source*: Data adapted from Brooks, G. A., and J. Mercier. 1994. Balance of carbohydrate and lipid utilization during exercise: the "crossover" concept. *J. Appl. Physiol.* 76[6]:2253–2261.)

If you want to decrease body fat, is it better to do low-intensity exercise or moderate- and high-intensity exercises? The answer to this question depends on how long you are able to engage in an activity. Even though fat is the primary fuel source during low-intensity activities, such as sitting and standing, to decrease body fat you would obviously want to do activities of higher intensity to expend additional energy and decrease body fat stores. If you have a low fitness level and can walk for 20 minutes but can jog for only 2 minutes, then the overall amount of fat used and energy expended for walking is higher than for jogging; thus, walking would be the better choice to decrease body fat in this particular case. Recent evidence suggests that engaging in *high-intensity interval training* (*HIT*) is a time-efficient strategy to optimize aerobic fitness and the use of fat as a fuel to support exercise.[14] HIT involves engaging in brief, intermittent bouts of vigorous activity interspersed with bouts of rest or low-intensity exercise. Beneficial changes have been observed with only about 15 minutes of very intense exercise performed over 2 weeks; improvements in aerobic fitness have been observed in people with cardiovascular disease, congestive heart failure, metabolic syndrome, and obesity.[14]

When it comes to eating properly to support regular physical activity or exercise training, the nutrient to focus on is carbohydrate. This is because most people store more than enough fat to support exercise, whereas our storage of carbohydrate is limited. It is especially important that adequate stores of glycogen are maintained for moderate to intense exercise. Dietary recommendations for fat, carbohydrate, and protein are identified shortly.

Amino Acids Are Not Major Sources of Fuel During Exercise

Proteins—more specifically, amino acids—are not major energy sources during exercise. Although they can be used directly for energy if necessary, they are more often used to make glucose to maintain blood glucose levels during exercise. The carbon skeletons of amino acids can be converted into pyruvate or acetyl-CoA, or they can feed directly into the TCA cycle to provide energy during exercise if necessary. (See Chapter 7, Figure 7.19.) Amino acids also help build and repair tissues after exercise. Depending on the intensity and duration of the activity, amino acids may contribute about 3% to 6% of the energy needed.

Given this, why is it that so many active people are concerned about their protein intakes? As you've learned (in Chapter 6), appropriate physical training combined with an adequate intake of dietary protein is the optimal stimulus for muscles to grow and strengthen. The protein needs of athletes are higher than the needs of nonathletes, but most people eat more than enough protein to support even the highest requirements for competitive athletes! Thus, there is generally no need for recreationally active people or even competitive athletes to consume protein or amino acid supplements.

RECAP

The amount of ATP stored in a muscle cell is limited and can keep a muscle active for only about 1 to 3 seconds. For intense activities lasting about 3 to 15 seconds, creatine phosphate can be broken down to provide energy and support the regeneration of ATP. To support activities that last from 30 seconds to 2 minutes, energy is produced from glycolysis. Fatty acids can be broken down aerobically to support activities of low intensity and longer duration. The two major advantages of using fat as a fuel are that it is an abundant energy source and it provides more than twice the energy per gram as carbohydrate. Recent evidence suggests that high-intensity interval training (HIT) optimizes aerobic fitness and the use of fat as a fuel to support exercise. Amino acids may contribute from 3% to 6% of the energy needed during exercise, depending on the intensity and duration of the activity. Amino acids help build and repair tissues after exercise.

How Does Physical Activity Affect Energy and Macronutrient Needs?

 LO 7 Explain how an increase in physical activity or athletic training can affect energy and macronutrient needs.

LO 8 Define carbohydrate loading, and discuss situations in which this practice may enhance athletic performance.

Lots of people wonder "Do my nutrient needs change if I become more physically active?" The answer to this question depends on the type, intensity, and duration of the chosen activities. It is not necessarily true that our requirement for every nutrient is greater if we are physically active.

People who are performing moderate-intensity, daily activities for health can follow the general guidelines put forth in the USDA Food Patterns. For smaller or less active people, the lower end of the range of recommendations for each food group may be appropriate. For larger or more active people, the higher end of the range is suggested. Modifications may be necessary for people who exercise vigorously every day, and particularly for athletes training for competition. **Table 14.2** provides an overview of the nutrients that can be affected by regular, vigorous exercise training. Each of these nutrients is described in more detail in the following section.

Vigorous Exercise Increases Energy Needs

Athletes generally have higher energy needs than moderately active or sedentary people. The amount of extra energy needed to support regular training is determined by the type,

TABLE 14.2 Suggested Intakes of Nutrients to Support Vigorous Exercise

Nutrient	Functions	Suggested Intake
Energy	Supports exercise, activities of daily living, and basic body functions	Depends on body size and the type, intensity, and duration of activity. For many female athletes: 1,800 to 3,500 kcal/day For many male athletes: 2,500 to 7,500 kcal/day
Carbohydrate	Provides energy, maintains adequate muscle glycogen and blood glucose; high complex carbohydrate foods provide vitamins and minerals	45–65% of total energy intake Depending on sport and gender, should consume 6–10 g of carbohydrate per kg body weight per day
Fat	Provides energy, fat-soluble vitamins, and essential fatty acids; supports production of hormones and transport of nutrients	20–35% of total energy intake
Protein	Helps build and maintain muscle; provides building material for glucose; is an energy source during endurance exercise; aids recovery from exercise	10–35% of total energy intake Endurance athletes: 1.2–1.5 g per kg body weight Strength athletes: 1.3–1.8 g per kg body weight
Water	Maintains temperature regulation (adequate cooling); maintains blood volume and blood pressure; supports all cell functions	Consume fluid before, during, and after exercise Consume enough to maintain body weight Consume at least 8 cups (64 fl. oz) of water daily to maintain regular health and activity Athletes may need up to 10 liters (170 fl. oz) every day; more is required if exercising in a hot environment
B-vitamins	Critical for energy production from carbohydrate, fat, and protein	May need slightly more (1–2 times the RDA) for thiamin, riboflavin, and vitamin B_6
Calcium	Builds and maintains bone mass; assists with nervous system function, muscle contraction, hormone function, and transport of nutrients across cell membrane	Meet the current RDA: 14–18 yr: 1,300 mg/day 19–50 yr: 1,000 mg/day 51–70 yr: 1,000 mg/day (men); 1,200 mg/day (women) 71 yr and older: 1,200 mg/day
Iron	Primarily responsible for the transport of oxygen in blood to cells; assists with energy production	Consume at least the RDA: Males: 14–18 yr: 11 mg/day 19 and older: 8 mg/day Females: 14–18 yr: 15 mg/day 19–50 yr: 18 mg/day 51 and older: 8 mg/day

intensity, and duration of the activity. In addition, the energy needs of male athletes are higher than those of female athletes, because male athletes weigh more, have more muscle mass, and expend more energy during activity. This is relative, of course: a large woman who trains 3 to 5 hours each day will probably need more energy than a small man who trains 1 hour each day. The energy needs of athletes can range from only 1,500 to 1,800 kcal per day for a small female gymnast to more than 7,500 kcal per day for a male cyclist competing in the Tour de France cross-country cycling race.

Meal Focus Figure 14.10 shows an example of 1 day's meals and snacks, totaling about 1,800 kcal and 4,000 kcal, with the carbohydrate content of these foods meeting around 60% of total energy intake. As you can see, athletes who need more than 4,000 kcal per day need to consume very large quantities of food. However, the heavy demands of daily physical training, work, school, and family responsibilities often leave these athletes with little time to eat adequately. Thus, many athletes meet their energy demands by planning regular meals and snacks and **grazing** (eating small meals throughout the day) consistently. They may also take advantage of the energy-dense snack foods and meal replacements specifically designed for athletes participating in vigorous training. These steps help athletes maintain their blood glucose levels and energy stores.

If an athlete is losing body weight, his or her energy intake is inadequate. Conversely, weight gain may indicate that energy intake is too high. Weight maintenance is generally recommended to maximize performance. If weight loss is warranted, food intake should be lowered no more than 200 to 500 kcal per day, and athletes should try to lose weight prior to the competitive season, if at all possible. Weight gain may be necessary for some athletes and can usually be accomplished by consuming 500 to 700 kcal per day more than needed for weight maintenance. The extra energy should come from a healthy balance of carbohydrate (45% to 65% of total energy intake), fat (20% to 35% of total energy intake), and protein (10% to 35% of total energy intake).

Many athletes are concerned about their weight. Jockeys, boxers, wrestlers, judo athletes, and others are required to "make weight"—to meet a predefined weight category. Others, such as distance runners, gymnasts, figure skaters, and dancers, are required to maintain a very lean figure for performance and aesthetic reasons. These athletes tend to eat less energy than they need to support vigorous training, which puts them at risk for inadequate intakes of all nutrients. These athletes are also at a higher risk of suffering from health consequences resulting from poor energy and nutrient intake, including eating disorders, osteoporosis, menstrual disturbances (in women), dehydration, heat and physical injuries, and even death. It is also important to understand that athletes should not adopt low-carbohydrate diets in an attempt to lose weight. As we discuss next, carbohydrates are a critical energy source for maintaining exercise performance.

Carbohydrate Needs Increase for Many Active People

Carbohydrate (in the form of glucose) is one of the primary sources of energy for a body in training. Both endurance athletes and strength athletes require adequate carbohydrate to maintain their glycogen stores and provide quick energy.

DRIs for Carbohydrate for Athletes

Recall (from Chapter 4) that the AMDR for carbohydrate is 45% to 65% of total energy intake. Athletes should consume carbohydrate intakes within this recommended range. Although high-carbohydrate diets (greater than 60% of total energy intake) have been recommended in the past, this percentage value may not be appropriate for all athletes. In addition, it is recommended that athletes consume a daily carbohydrate intake of approximately 6 to 10 g of carbohydrate per kg body weight to optimize muscle glycogen stores. However, the need may be much greater in athletes who are training heavily daily, as they have less time to recover and require more carbohydrate to support both training and storage needs.

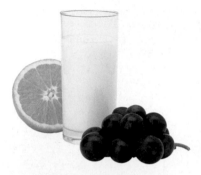

Small, healthful snacks can help you meet daily energy demands.

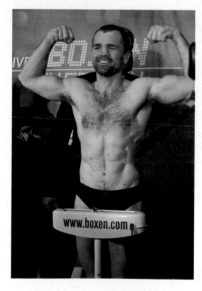

Some athletes diet to meet a predefined weight category.

grazing Consistently eating small meals throughout the day; done by many athletes to meet their high energy demands.

a day of meals

about 1,800 calories (kcal)

about 4,000 calories (kcal)

BREAKFAST

about 1,800:
1 cup Cheerios
4 oz skim milk
1 medium banana
6 fl. oz orange juice

about 4,000:
1-½ cups Cheerios
8 fl. oz skim milk
1 medium banana
2 slices whole-wheat toast
1 tbsp. butter
6 fl. oz orange juice

LUNCH

Turkey sandwich:
2 slices whole-wheat bread
3 oz turkey lunch meat
1 oz Swiss cheese slice
1 leaf iceberg lettuce
2 slices tomato
1 cup tomato soup
   (made with water)
1 large apple
8 oz nonfat fruit yogurt
¼ cup dried, sweetened
   cranberries

2 turkey sandwiches, each with:
2 slices whole-wheat bread
3 oz turkey lunch meat
1 oz Swiss cheese slice
1 leaf iceberg lettuce
2 slices tomato
2 cups tomato soup
   (made with water)
Two 8 oz containers of low-fat
   fruit yogurt
¼ cup trail mix
12 fl. oz Gatorade

DINNER

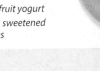

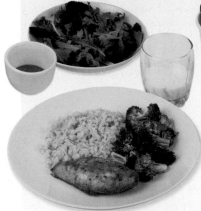

4 oz grilled skinless chicken breast
1-½ cups mixed salad greens
1 tbsp. French salad dressing
1 cup steamed broccoli
½ cup cooked brown rice
4 fl. oz skim milk
1 cup fresh blackberries

6 oz grilled skinless chicken breast
3 cups mixed salad greens
3 tbsp. French salad dressing
2 cups cooked spaghetti noodles
1 cup spaghetti sauce with meat
8 fl. oz skim milk
1 large apple
2 tbsp. peanut butter

nutrient analysis

1,797 kcal
60.8% of energy from carbohydrates
15.7% of energy from fat
4.7% of energy from saturated fat
23.5% of energy from protein
35 grams of dietary fiber
2,097 milligrams of sodium

More
energy
for activity!

nutrient analysis

3,984 kcal
59.4% of energy from carbohydrates
22.6% of energy from fat
7.0% of energy from saturated fat
18.0% of energy from protein
45.4 grams of dietary fiber
6019 milligrams of sodium

To illustrate the importance of carbohydrate intake for athletes, let's see what happens to Theo when he participates in a study designed to determine how carbohydrate intake affects glycogen stores during a period of heavy training. Theo was asked to go to the exercise laboratory at the university and ride a stationary bicycle for 2 hours a day for 3 consecutive days at 75% of his maximal heart rate. Before and after each ride, samples of muscle tissue were taken from his thighs to determine the amount of glycogen stored in the working muscles. Theo performed these rides under two different experimental conditions— once when he had eaten a high-carbohydrate diet (80% of total energy intake) and again when he had eaten a moderate- carbohydrate diet (40% of total energy intake). As you can see in **Figure 14.11**, Theo's muscle glycogen levels decreased dramatically after each training session. More important, his muscle glycogen levels did not recover to baseline levels over the 3 days when Theo ate the lower-carbohydrate diet. He was able to maintain his muscle glycogen levels only when he was eating the higher-carbohydrate diet. Theo also told the researchers that completing the 2-hour rides was much more difficult when he had eaten the moderate-carbohydrate diet as compared to when he was eating the diet that was higher in carbohydrate.

Timing of Carbohydrate Consumption

It is important for athletes not only to consume enough carbohydrate to maintain glycogen stores but also to time their intake optimally. The body stores glycogen very rapidly during the first 24 hours of recovery from exercise, with the highest storage rates occurring during the first few hours.[15] Higher carbohydrate intakes during the first 24 hours of recovery from exercise, particularly when consumed with a source high in protein (such as chocolate milk), are associated with higher amounts of glucose being stored as muscle glycogen and enhanced performance.[16]

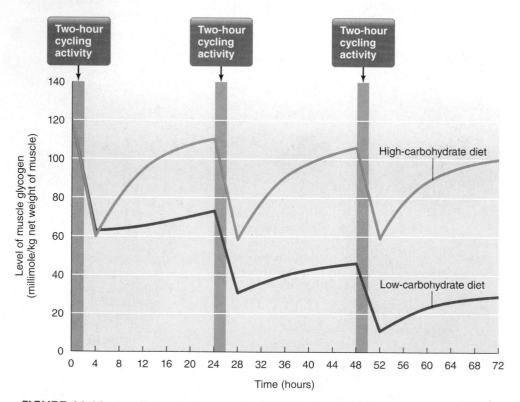

FIGURE 14.11 The effects of a low-carbohydrate diet on muscle glycogen stores. When a low-carbohydrate diet is consumed, glycogen stores cannot be restored during a period of regular, vigorous training. (*Source*: Data adapted from Costill, D. L., and J. M. Miller. 1980. Nutrition for endurance sport: CHO and fluid balance. *Int. J. Sports Med*. 1:2–14. Copyright © 1980 Georg Thieme Verlag. Used with permission.)

If an athlete has to perform or participate in training bouts that are scheduled less than 8 hours apart, then he or she should try to consume enough carbohydrate in the few hours after training to allow for ample glycogen storage. However, with a longer recovery time (generally 12 hours or more), the athlete can eat when he or she chooses, and glycogen levels should be restored as long as the total carbohydrate eaten is sufficient.

Interestingly, studies have shown that muscle glycogen can be restored to adequate levels in the muscle whether the food is eaten in small, multiple snacks or in larger meals,[15] although some studies show enhanced muscle glycogen storage during the first 4 to 6 hours of recovery when athletes are fed large amounts of carbohydrate every 15 to 30 minutes. There is also evidence that consuming high glycemic index foods during the immediate postrecovery period results in higher glycogen storage than is achieved as a result of eating low glycemic index foods. This may be due to a greater malabsorption of the carbohydrates in low glycemic index foods, as these foods contain more indigestible forms of carbohydrate.[14]

Fruit and vegetable juices can be a good source of carbohydrates.

Food Sources of Carbohydrates for Athletes

What are good carbohydrate sources to support vigorous training? In general, fiber-rich, less processed carbohydrate foods, such as whole grains and cereals, fruits, vegetables, and juices, are excellent sources that also supply fiber, vitamins, and minerals. Guidelines recommend that intake of simple sugars be less than 10% of total energy intake, but some athletes who need very large energy intakes to support training may need to consume more. In addition, as previously mentioned, glycogen storage can be enhanced by consuming foods with a high glycemic index immediately postrecovery. Thus, there are advantages to consuming a wide variety of carbohydrate sources.

As a result of time constraints, many athletes have difficulties consuming enough food to meet carbohydrate demands. Sports drinks and energy bars have been designed to help athletes increase their carbohydrate intake. **Table 14.3** identifies some energy bars and other simple, inexpensive snacks and meals that provide 50 to 100 g of carbohydrate.

TABLE 14.3 Carbohydrate and Total Energy in Various Foods

Food	Amount	Carbohydrate (g)	Energy from Carbohydrate (%)	Total Energy (kcal)
Sweetened applesauce	1 cup	50	97	207
Large apple with Saltine crackers	1 each 8 each	50	82	248
Whole-wheat bread with jelly and skim milk	1 oz slice 4 tsp 12 fl. oz	50	71	282
Spaghetti (cooked) with tomato sauce	1 cup ¼ cup	50	75	268
Brown rice (cooked) with mixed vegetables and apple juice	1 cup ½ cup 12 fl. oz	100	88	450
Grape-Nuts cereal with raisins and skim milk	½ cup 3/8 cup 8 fl. oz	100	84	473
Clif Bar (chocolate chip)	2.4 oz	43	75	230
Meta-Rx (fudge brownie)	100 g	41	41	400
Power Bar (chocolate)	1 bar	45	75	240
PR Bar Ironman	50 g	22	44	200

Source: Data adapted from Manore, M. M., N. L. Meyer, and J. L. Thompson. 2009. *Sport Nutrition for Health and Performance.* 2nd Edn. Champaign, IL: Human Kinetics.

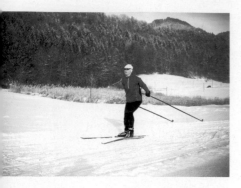

Carbohydrate loading may benefit endurance athletes, such as cross-country skiers.

Carbohydrate Loading

As you know, carbohydrate is a critical energy source to support exercise—particularly endurance-type activities—yet we have a limited capacity to store it. So it's not surprising that discovering ways to maximize carbohydrate storage has been at the forefront of sports nutrition research for many years. The practice of **carbohydrate loading,** also called *glycogen loading,* involves altering both exercise duration and carbohydrate intake to maximize the amount of muscle glycogen. **Table 14.4** provides a schedule for carbohydrate loading for an endurance athlete.

Athletes who may benefit from carbohydrate loading are those competing in marathons, ultra-marathons, long-distance swimming, cross-country skiing, and triathlons. Athletes who compete in baseball, American football, 10-kilometer runs, walking, hiking, weight lifting, and most swimming events will not gain any performance benefits from this practice, nor will people who regularly participate in moderately intense physical activities to maintain fitness.

It is important to emphasize that, even in endurance events, carbohydrate loading does not always improve performance. There are many adverse side effects of this practice, including extreme gastrointestinal distress, particularly diarrhea. We store water along with the extra glycogen in the muscles, which leaves many athletes feeling heavy and sluggish.

TABLE 14.4 Recommended Carbohydrate Loading Guidelines for Endurance Athletes

Days Prior to Event	Exercise Duration (in minutes)	Carbohydrate Content of Diet (g per kg body weight)
6	90 (at 70% max effort)	5 (moderate)
5	40 (at 70% max effort)	5 (moderate)
4	40 (at 70% max effort)	5 (moderate)
3	20 (light training)	10 (high)
2	20 (light training)	10 (high)
1	Rest	10 (high)
Day of race	Competition	Precompetition food and fluid

Source: Adapted, with permission, from M. Dunford, 2005, *Current Trends in Performance Nutrition student text*, (Champaign, IL: Human Kinetics), 23.

*Nutri-*Case

Theo

"Ever since I did that cycling test in the fitness lab, I've been watching my carbohydrates. Lately, I've been topping 500 grams of carbs a day. But now I'm beginning to wonder, am I getting enough protein? I'm starting to feel really wiped out, especially after games. We've won four out of the last five games, and I'm giving it everything I've got, but today I was really dragging myself through practice. I'm eating about 180 grams of protein a day, but I think I'm going to try one of those protein powders they sell at my gym. I guess I just feel like, when I'm competing, I need some added insurance."

Theo's weight averages about 200 lb. Given what you've learned about the role of the energy nutrients in vigorous physical activity, what do you think might be causing Theo to feel "wiped out"? Would you recommend that Theo try the protein supplement? What other strategies might be helpful for him to consider?

carbohydrate loading A process that involves altering training and carbohydrate intake so that muscle glycogen storage is maximized; also known as *glycogen loading.*

Athletes who want to try carbohydrate loading should experiment prior to competition to determine whether it is an acceptable and beneficial approach for them.

Moderate Fat Consumption Is Enough to Support Most Activities

Fat is an important energy source for both moderate physical activity and vigorous endurance training. When athletes reach a physically trained state, they are able to use more fat for energy; in other words, they become better "fat burners." This can also occur in people who are not athletes but who regularly participate in aerobic-type fitness activities. This training effect occurs for a number of reasons, including an increase in the number and activity of various enzymes involved in fat metabolism, an improved ability of the muscles to store fat, and an improved ability to extract fat from the blood for use during exercise. By using fat as a fuel, athletes can spare carbohydrate, so they can use it during prolonged, intense training or competition.

Many athletes concerned with body weight and physical appearance believe they should eat less than 15% of their total energy intake as fat, but this is inadequate for vigorous activity. Instead, a fat intake of 20% to 35% of total energy intake is generally recommended for most athletes, with less than 10% of total energy intake as saturated fat. The same recommendations are put forth for nonathletes. Fat provides not only energy but also the fat-soluble vitamins and essential fatty acids that are critical to maintaining general health. If fat consumption is too low, inadequate levels of these can eventually prove detrimental to training and performance. Athletes who have chronic disease risk factors, such as high blood lipids, high blood pressure, or unhealthful blood glucose levels, should work with their physician to adjust their intake of fat and carbohydrate according to their health risks.

Many Athletes Have Increased Protein Needs

The protein intakes suggested for active people range from 1.0 to 1.8 grams per kg body weight. Intakes at the lower end of this range are for people who exercise four to five times a week for 30 minutes or less. At the upper end are athletes who train five to seven times a week for more than an hour a day. Protein intakes as high as 1.8 to 2.0 grams per kg per day may help prevent loss of lean body mass during periods when an athlete is restricting energy to promote fat loss.[17]

Most inactive people and many athletes in the United States consume more than enough protein to support their needs. However, some athletes do not consume enough protein, including those with very low energy intakes, vegetarians or vegans who do not consume high-protein food sources, and young athletes who are growing and are not aware of their higher protein needs.

In 1995, Dr. Barry Sears published *The Zone: A Dietary Road Map*, a book that claims numerous benefits of a high-protein, low-carbohydrate diet for athletes.[18] Since that time, Sears has published more than a dozen spin-offs, all of which recommend the consumption of a 40–30–30 diet, or one composed of 40% carbohydrate, 30% fat, and 30% protein. Dr. Sears claims that high-carbohydrate diets impair athletic performance because of the unhealthful effects of insulin. These claims have not been supported by research, and, in fact, many of Dr. Sears' claims are not consistent with human physiology. The primary problem with the Zone Diet for athletes is that it is too low in both energy and carbohydrate to support training and performance.

High-quality protein sources include lean meats, poultry, fish, eggs, low-fat dairy products, legumes, and soy products. By following their personalized MyPlate food patterns, people of all fitness levels can consume more than enough protein without the use of supplements or specially formulated foods. Many athletes use protein shakes and other products in an attempt to build muscle mass and strength; some even use *ergogenic aids* to try to enhance performance. To learn more about ergogenic aids, and whether they are effective and safe, refer to the **Nutrition Myth or Fact?** on pages 582–584.

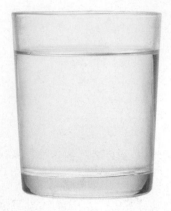

Water is essential for maintaining fluid balance and preventing dehydration.

RECAP

The type, intensity, and duration of activities a person participates in determine his or her nutrient needs. Athletes generally have higher energy needs than moderately active or sedentary people. Energy needs may range as high as 7,500 kcal per day for a male athlete in competition in a vigorous sport. Carbohydrate needs may increase for some active people. In general, athletes should consume 45% to 65% of their total energy as carbohydrate. Carbohydrate loading involves altering physical training and the diet such that the storage of muscle glycogen is maximized. Active people use more fat than carbohydrates for energy, because they experience an increase in the number and activity of the enzymes involved in fat metabolism, and they have an improved ability to store fat and extract it from the blood for use during exercise. A dietary fat intake of 20% to 35% is recommended for athletes, with less than 10% of total energy intake as saturated fat. Although protein needs are higher for athletes, most people in the United States already consume more than twice their daily needs for protein. ■

 Explain how an increase in physical activity or athletic training can affect fluid and micronutrient needs.

 Compare heat syncope, heat cramps, heat exhaustion, and heat stroke.

How Does Physical Activity Affect Fluid and Micronutrient Needs?

In this section, we review some of the basic functions of water and its role during exercise. (For a detailed discussion of fluid and electrolyte balance, see Chapter 9.) We also discuss changes in micronutrient needs to support vigorous physical activity.

Dehydration and Heat-Related Illnesses

Heat production can increase by 15 to 20 times during heavy exercise! The primary way in which this heat is dissipated is through sweating, which is also called **evaporative cooling.** When body temperature rises, more blood (which contains water) flows to the surface of the skin. In this way, heat is carried from the core of the body to the surface of the skin. By sweating, the water (and body heat) leaves our bodies, and the air around us picks up the evaporating water from our skin, cooling our bodies.

Heat illnesses occur because, when we exercise in the heat, our muscles and skin constantly compete for blood flow. When there is no longer enough blood flow to simultaneously provide adequate blood to our muscles and our skin, muscle blood flow takes priority and evaporative cooling is inhibited. Exercising in heat plus humidity is especially dangerous; whereas the heat dramatically raises body temperature, the high humidity inhibits evaporative cooling—that is, the environmental air is already so saturated with water that it is unable to absorb the water in sweat. Body temperature becomes dangerously high, and heat illness is likely.

Dehydration significantly increases our risk for heat illnesses. **Figure 14.12** identifies the symptoms of dehydration during heavy exercise.

Heat illnesses include heat syncope, heat cramps, heat exhaustion, and heat stroke:

- **Heat syncope** is dizziness that occurs when people stand for too long in the heat and the blood pools in their lower extremities. It can also occur when people stop suddenly after a race or stand rapidly from a lying position.
- **Heat cramps** are muscle spasms that occur during exercise or several hours after strenuous exercise or manual labor in the heat. They are most commonly felt in the legs, arms, or abdomen after a person cools down.
- **Heat exhaustion** and **heat stroke** occur on a continuum, with unchecked heat exhaustion leading to heat stroke. Early signs of heat exhaustion include excessive sweating, cold and clammy skin, rapid but weak pulse, weakness, nausea, dizziness, headache, and difficulty concentrating. Signs that a person is progressing to heat stroke are hot, dry skin; rapid and strong pulse; vomiting; diarrhea; a body temperature

evaporative cooling Sweating, which is the primary way in which the body dissipates heat.

heat syncope Dizziness that results from blood pooling in the lower extremities; often results from standing too long in hot weather, standing rapidly from a lying position, or stopping suddenly after physical exertion.

heat cramps Muscle spasms that occur several hours after strenuous exercise; most often occur when sweat losses and fluid intakes are high, urine volume is low, and sodium intake is inadequate.

heat exhaustion A heat illness characterized by excessive sweating, weakness, nausea, dizziness, headache, and difficulty concentrating. Unchecked, heat exhaustion can lead to heat stroke.

heat stroke A potentially fatal heat illness characterized by hot, dry skin; rapid heart rate; vomiting; diarrhea; elevated body temperature; hallucinations; and coma.

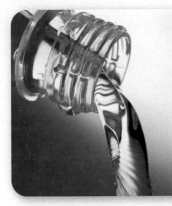
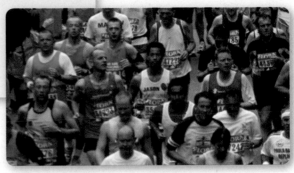

Symptoms of Dehydration During Heavy Exercise:
- Decreased exercise performance
- Increased level in perceived exertion
- Dark yellow or brown urine color
- Increased heart rate at a given exercise intensity
- Decreased appetite
- Decreased ability to concentrate
- Decreased urine output
- Fatigue and weakness
- Headache and dizziness

FIGURE 14.12 Symptoms of dehydration during heavy exercise.

greater than or equal to 104°F; hallucinations; and coma. Prompt medical care is essential to save the person's life (for more information about heat illnesses, see Chapter 9).

Guidelines for Proper Fluid Replacement

How can we prevent dehydration and heat illnesses? Obviously, adequate fluid intake is critical before, during, and after exercise. Unfortunately, our thirst mechanism cannot be relied upon to signal when we need to drink. If we rely on our feelings of thirst, we will not consume enough fluid to support exercise.

General fluid replacement recommendations are based on maintaining body weight. Athletes who are training and competing in hot environments should weigh themselves before and after the training session or event and should regain the weight lost over the subsequent 24-hour period. They should avoid losing more than 2% to 3% of body weight during exercise, as performance can be impaired with fluid losses as small as 1% of body weight.

Table 14.5 (page 580) reviews guidelines for proper fluid replacement. For activities lasting less than 1 hour, plain water is generally adequate to replace fluid losses. However, for training and competition lasting longer than 1 hour in any weather, sports beverages containing carbohydrates and electrolytes are recommended. These beverages are also recommended for people who will not drink enough water because they don't like the taste. If drinking these beverages will guarantee adequate hydration, they are appropriate to use. (For more specific information about sports beverages, see Chapter 9, page 358.)

Inadequate Micronutrient Intake Can Diminish Health and Performance

When people train vigorously for athletic events, their requirements for certain vitamins and minerals may be altered. Many highly active people do not eat enough food or a variety of foods that allows them to consume enough of these nutrients, yet it is imperative that active people do their very best to eat an adequate, varied, and balanced diet to try to meet the increased needs associated with vigorous training.

Drinking sports beverages during training or competition lasting more than 1 hour replaces fluid, carbohydrates, and electrolytes.

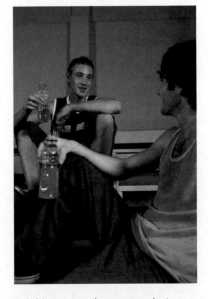

Drinking sports beverages during training or competition lasting more than 1 hour replaces fluid, carbohydrates, and electrolytes.

TABLE 14.5 Guidelines for Fluid Replacement

Activity Level	Environment	Fluid Requirements (liters per day)
Sedentary	Cool	2–3
Active	Cool	3–6
Sedentary	Warm	3–5
Active	Warm	5–10

Before Exercise or Competition
- Drink adequate fluids during the 24 hours before event; should be able to maintain body weight.
- Slowly drink about 0.17 to 0.24 fl. oz per kg body weight of water or a sports drink at least 4 hours prior to exercise or event to allow time for excretion of excess fluid prior to event.
- Slowly drink another 0.10 to 0.17 fl. oz per kg body weight about 2 hours before the event.
- Consuming beverages with sodium and/or small amounts of salted snacks at a meal will help stimulate thirst and retain fluids consumed.

During Exercise or Competition
- Drink early and regularly throughout the event to sufficiently replace all water lost through sweating.
- Amount and rate of fluid replacement depend on individual sweating rate, exercise duration, weather conditions, and opportunities to drink.
- Fluids should be cooler than the environmental temperature and flavored to enhance taste and promote fluid replacement.

During Exercise or Competition That Lasts More Than 1 Hour
- Fluid replacement beverage should contain 5–10% carbohydrate to maintain blood glucose levels; sodium and other electrolytes should be included in the beverage in amounts of 0.5–0.7 g of sodium per liter of water to replace the sodium lost by sweating.

Following Exercise or Competition
- Consume about 3 cups of fluid for each pound of body weight lost.
- Fluids after exercise should contain water to restore hydration status, carbohydrates to replenish glycogen stores, and electrolytes (for example, sodium and potassium) to speed rehydration.
- Consume enough fluid to permit regular urination and to ensure the urine color is very light or light yellow in color; drinking about 125–150% of fluid loss is usually sufficient to ensure complete rehydration.

In General
- Products that contain fructose should be limited, as these may cause gastrointestinal distress.
- Caffeine and alcohol should be avoided, as these products increase urine output and reduce fluid retention.
- Carbonated beverages should be avoided, as they reduce the desire for fluid intake due to stomach fullness.

Sources: Data adapted from Murray, R. 1997. Drink more! Advice from a world class expert. *ACSM's Health and Fitness Journal* 1:19–23; American College of Sports Medicine Position Stand. 2007. Exercise and fluid replacement. *Med. Sci. Sports Exerc.* 39(2):377–390; and Casa, D. J., L. E. Armstrong, S. K. Hillman, S. J. Montain, R. V. Reiff, B. S. E. Rich, W. O. Roberts, and J. A. Stone. 2000. National Athletic Trainers' Association position statement: fluid replacement for athletes. *J. Athlet. Train.* 35:212–224.

B-Vitamins

The B-vitamins are directly involved in energy metabolism (see Chapter 8 for full treatment of the nutrients involved in energy metabolism). There is reliable evidence that—as a population—active people may require slightly more thiamin, riboflavin, and vitamin B_6 than the current RDA because of increased production of energy in active people and inadequate dietary intake in some individuals. However, these increased needs are easily met by consuming adequate energy and plenty of fiber-rich carbohydrates. Active people at risk for poor B-vitamin status are those who consume inadequate energy or who consume mostly refined-carbohydrate foods, such as sugary drinks and snacks. Vegan athletes and active individuals may be at risk for inadequate intake of vitamin B_{12}; food sources enriched with this nutrient include soy and cereal products.

Calcium

Calcium supports proper muscle contraction and ensures bone health. Calcium intakes are inadequate for most women in the United States, including both sedentary and active women. This is most likely due to a failure to consume foods that are high in calcium, particularly dairy products. Although vigorous training does not appear to directly increase our need for calcium, we need to consume enough calcium to support bone health. If we do not, stress fractures and severe loss of bone can result.

Some female athletes suffer from a syndrome known as the *female athlete triad* (see Chapter 13.5, pages 548–549). In the female athlete triad, nutritional inadequacies cause irregularities in the menstrual cycle and hormonal disturbances that can lead to a significant loss of bone mass. Thus, for female athletes, consuming the recommended amounts of calcium is critical. For female athletes who are physically small and consume lower energy intakes, calcium supplementation may be needed to meet current recommendations.

Iron

Iron, a part of the hemoglobin molecule, is critical for the transport of oxygen in the blood to the cells and working muscles. Iron is also involved in energy production. Active individuals lose more iron in their sweat, feces, and urine than do inactive people, and endurance runners lose iron when their red blood cells break down in their feet as a result of the impact of running. Female athletes and nonathletes lose more iron than male athletes because of menstrual blood losses, and females in general tend to eat less iron in their diets. Vegetarian athletes and active people may also consume less iron. Thus, many athletes and active people are at higher risk for iron deficiency. Depending on its severity, poor iron status can impair athletic performance and the ability to maintain regular physical activity.

A phenomenon known as *sports anemia* was identified in the 1960s. Sports anemia is not true anemia but a transient decrease in iron stores that occurs at the start of an exercise program for some people, as well as in some athletes who increase their training intensity. Exercise training increases the amount of water in the blood (called *plasma volume*); however, the amount of hemoglobin does not increase until later into the training period. Thus, the iron content in the blood appears to be low but instead is falsely depressed due to increases in plasma volume. Sports anemia, since it is not true anemia, does not affect performance.

In general, it appears that physically active females are at relatively high risk of suffering from the first stage of iron depletion, in which iron stores are low. Because of this, it is suggested that blood tests of iron stores and monitoring of dietary iron intakes be part of routine healthcare for active people. In some cases, iron needs cannot be met through the diet and supplementation is necessary. Iron supplementation should be done with a physician's approval and proper medical supervision.

RECAP

Regular exercise increases fluid needs. Fluid is critical to evaporative cooling, a process by which the body regulates core body temperature. Dehydration is a serious threat during exercise in extreme heat and high humidity. Heat illnesses include heat syncope, a sensation of dizziness caused by pooling of blood in the lower extremities; heat cramps, muscle spasms that occur during or shortly after vigorous physical activity in the heat; and heat exhaustion and heat stroke, which occur on a continuum in a person whose core body temperature rises without intervention. Signs and symptoms begin as excessive sweating, nausea, and confusion and progress to dry, hot skin, vomiting, and eventually coma and, if untreated, death. Active people may need more thiamin, riboflavin, and vitamin B_6 than inactive people to adequately support energy metabolism. Exercise itself does not increase calcium needs, but most women, including active women, do not consume enough calcium. Some female athletes suffer from the female athlete triad, a condition that involves the interaction of low energy availability, low bone density, and menstrual dysfunction. Iron is critical for the transport of oxygen to working muscles and is involved in energy production. Also, active individuals lose more iron in their sweat, feces, and urine than do inactive people. As a result, many active individuals require more iron, particularly female athletes and vegetarian athletes.

Nutrition Myth OR Fact?

Are Ergogenic Aids Necessary for Active People?

Many competitive athletes and even some recreationally active people continually search for that something extra that will enhance their performance. **Ergogenic aids** are substances used to improve exercise and athletic performance. For example, dietary supplements can be classified as ergogenic aids, as can anabolic steroids and other pharmaceuticals. Interestingly, people report using ergogenic aids not only to enhance athletic performance but also to improve their physical appearance, prevent or treat injuries and diseases, and help them cope with stress. Some people even report using them because of peer pressure!

As you have learned in this chapter, adequate nutrition is critical to athletic performance and to regular physical activity, and products such as sports bars and beverages can help athletes maintain their competitive edge. However, as we will explore shortly, many ergogenic aids are not effective, some are dangerous, and most are very expensive. For the average consumer, it is virtually impossible to track the latest research findings for these products. In addition, many have not been adequately studied, and unsubstantiated claims surrounding them are rampant. How can you become a more educated consumer about ergogenic aids?

New ergogenic aids are available virtually every month. It is therefore not possible to discuss every available product here. However, a brief review of a number of currently popular ergogenic aids is provided.

Do Anabolic Products Enhance Muscle and Strength?

Many ergogenic aids are said to be **anabolic**, meaning that they build muscle and increase strength. Most anabolic substances promise to increase testosterone, which is the hormone associated with male sex characteristics and that increases muscle size and strength. Although some anabolic substances are effective, they are generally associated with harmful side effects.

Anabolic Steroids

Anabolic steroids are testosterone-based drugs known to be effective in increasing muscle size, strength, power,

Anabolic substances are often marketed to people striving to increase muscle size, but many cause harmful side effects.

and speed. They have been used extensively by strength and power athletes; however, these products are illegal in the United States, and their use is banned by all major collegiate and professional sports organizations, in addition to both the U.S. and the International Olympic Committees. Proven long-term and irreversible effects of steroid use include infertility; early closure of the plates of the long bones, resulting in permanently shortened stature; shriveled testicles, enlarged breast tissue (that can be removed only surgically), and other signs of "feminization" in men; enlarged clitoris, facial hair growth, and other signs of "masculinization" in women; increased risk for certain forms of cancer; liver damage; unhealthful changes in blood lipids; hypertension; severe acne; hair thinning or baldness; and depression, delusions, sleep disturbances, and extreme anger (so-called roid rage).

Androstenedione and Dehydroepiandrosterone

Androstenedione ("andro") and dehydroepiandrosterone (DHEA) are precursors of testosterone. Manufacturers of these products claim that taking them will increase testosterone levels and muscle strength. Androstenedione became very popular after baseball player Mark McGwire claimed he used it during the time he was breaking home run records. Contrary to popular claims, neither androstenedione nor DHEA increases testosterone levels, and early research on androstenedione has been shown to increase the risk for heart disease in men aged 35 to 65 years.[1] There are no studies that support the products' claims of improving strength and increasing muscle mass.

Gamma-Hydroxybutyric Acid

Gamma-hydroxybutyric acid, or GHB, is a central nervous system depressant. It was once promoted as an alternative to anabolic steroids for building muscle. The production and sale of GHB were never approved in the United States; however, it was illegally produced and sold on the black market as a dietary supplement. For many users, GHB caused only dizziness, tremors, or vomiting, but others experienced severe side effects, including seizures, respiratory depression, sedation, and coma. Many people were hospitalized, and some died.

In 2001, the federal government placed GHB on the controlled substances list, making its manufacture, sale, and possession illegal. A form of GHB is available by prescription for the treatment of narcolepsy, a rare sleep disorder, but extra paperwork is required by the prescribing physician, and prescriptions are closely monitored. After the ban, two similar products (gamma-butyrolactone, or GBL, and BD, or 1,4-butanediol) were marketed in its place. Both products were found to be dangerous and the FDA removed both from the market. BD is an industrial solvent and is listed on ingredient labels as tetramethylene glycol, butylene glycol, or sucol-B. Side effects include wild, aggressive behavior; nausea; incontinence; and sudden loss of consciousness.

Creatine

Creatine, or creatine phosphate, is found in meat and fish and stored in our muscles. Because cells use creatine phosphate (CP) to regenerate ATP, it is theorized that creatine supplements make more CP available to replenish ATP, which prolongs a person's ability to train and perform in short-term, explosive activities, such as weight lifting and sprinting. Between 1994 and 2015, more than 18,000 research articles, book chapters and abstracts related to creatine and exercise in humans were published. Creatine does not seem to enhance performance in aerobic-type events but may increase the work performed and amount of strength gained during resistance exercise and to enhance sprint performance in swimming, running, and cycling.

Although side effects such as dehydration, muscle cramps, and gastrointestinal disturbances have been reported with creatine use, there is very little information on how long-term use impacts health. Further research is needed to determine the effectiveness and safety of creatine use over prolonged periods of time.

What About the Claims That Some Products Optimize Fuel Use?

Certain ergogenic aids are touted as increasing energy levels and improving athletic performance by optimizing the use of fat, carbohydrate, and protein. The products reviewed here are caffeine, ephedrine, carnitine, chromium, ribose, and beta-alanine.

Ephedrine is made from the herb *Ephedra sinica* (Chinese ephedra).

Caffeine

Caffeine is a stimulant that makes us feel more alert and energetic, decreasing feelings of fatigue during exercise. In addition, caffeine has been shown to increase the use of fat as a fuel during endurance exercise, thereby sparing muscle glycogen and improving performance. Energy drinks that contain high amounts of caffeine, such as Red Bull, have become popular with athletes and many college students. These drinks should be avoided during exercise, however, because they can prompt severe dehydration due to the combination of fluid loss from exercise and increased fluid excretion from the caffeine. Research also indicates that energy drinks are associated with serious side effects in children, adolescents, and young adults, including irregularities in heart rhythm, seizures, diabetes, and mood disorders.[2] It should be recognized that caffeine is a controlled or restricted drug in the athletic world, and athletes can be banned from Olympic competition if their urine levels are too high. However, the amount of caffeine that is banned is quite high, and athletes would need to consume caffeine in pill form to reach this level. Side effects of caffeine use include increased blood pressure, increased heart rate, dizziness, insomnia, headache, and gastrointestinal distress.

Ephedrine

Ephedrine, also known as ephedra, Chinese ephedra, and *ma huang*, is a strong stimulant marketed as a weight-loss supplement and energy enhancer. In reality, many products sold as Chinese ephedra (or herbal ephedra) contain ephedrine synthesized in a laboratory and other stimulants, such as caffeine. The use of ephedra does not appear to enhance performance, but supplements containing both caffeine and ephedra have been shown to prolong the amount of exercise that can be done until exhaustion is reached. Ephedra is known to reduce body weight and body fat in sedentary women, but its impact on weight loss and body fat levels in athletes is unknown. Side effects of ephedra use include headaches, nausea, nervousness, anxiety, irregular heart rate, and high blood pressure; and at least 17 deaths have been attributed to its use. It is currently illegal to sell ephedra-containing supplements in the United States.

Carnitine

Carnitine is a compound made from amino acids and is found in the membranes of mitochondria in our cells.

ergogenic aids Substances used to improve exercise and athletic performance.

anabolic The characteristic of a substance that builds muscle and increases strength.

Carnitine helps shuttle fatty acids into the mitochondria, so that they can be used for energy. It has been proposed that exercise training depletes our cells of carnitine and that supplementation should restore carnitine levels, thereby enabling us to improve our use of fat as a fuel source. Thus, carnitine is marketed not only as a performance-enhancing substance but also as a "fat burner." Research studies of carnitine supplementation do not support these claims, as neither the transport of fatty acids nor their oxidation appears to be enhanced with supplementation. The use of carnitine supplements has not been associated with significant side effects.

Chromium

Chromium is a trace mineral that enhances insulin's action of increasing the transport of amino acids into the cell. It is found in whole-grain foods, cheese, nuts, mushrooms, and asparagus. It is theorized that many people are chromium deficient and that supplementation will enhance the uptake of amino acids into muscle cells, which will increase muscle growth and strength. Like carnitine, chromium is marketed as a fat burner, with claims that its effect on insulin stimulates the brain to decrease food intake. Chromium supplements are available as chromium picolinate and chromium nicotinate. Early studies of chromium supplementation showed promise, but more recent, better-designed studies do not support any benefit of chromium supplementation on muscle mass, muscle strength, body fat, or exercise performance.

Ribose

Ribose is a five-carbon sugar that is critical to the production of ATP. Ribose supplementation is claimed to improve athletic performance by increasing work output and by promoting a faster recovery time from vigorous training. While ribose has been shown to improve exercise tolerance in patients with heart disease, ribose supplementation appears to have no impact on athletic performance.

Beta-Alanine

Beta-alanine is a nonessential amino acid that has been identified as the limiting factor in the production of carnosine, a dipeptide composed of beta-alanine and L-histidine and synthesized in skeletal muscle. Carnosine plays a key role in the regulation of pH in the muscle and is thought to buffer acids produced during exercise, thereby enhancing a person's ability to perform short-term, high-intensity activities.[3,4] Recent evidence suggests that beta-alanine supplementation can increase muscle carnosine levels and delay the onset of muscle fatigue. Additionally, beta-alanine supplementation results in improved exercise performance during single or repeated high-intensity exercise bouts or maximal muscle contractions.[3,4] It appears that several weeks of supplementation is needed to increase muscle carnosine levels and positively affect performance.[4]

As this review indicates, many ergogenic aids fail to live up to their claims of enhancing athletic performance, strength, or body composition. And many have uncomfortable or even dangerous side effects. Be a savvy consumer. Before purchasing any ergogenic aid, do some homework to make sure you wouldn't be wasting your money or putting your health at risk by using it.

 Want to learn what the U.S. Food and Drug Administration is doing to crack down on fraudulent health claims and the companies that make them? Click on www.fda.gov and enter "fraudulent health claims" in the search box. Then select "Cracking Down on Health Fraud" to read more.

Critical Thinking Questions

- Now that you've read this *Nutrition Myth or Fact*, are you thinking of trying any ergogenic aids? If so, which one(s) and why?
- Do you feel there should be more strict regulations on the promotion and sales of ergogenic aids? Why or why not?

References

1. Broeder, C. E., J. Quindry, K. Brittingham, L. Panton, J. Thomson, S. Appakondu,…, and C. Yarlagadda. 2000. The Andro Project: physiological and hormonal influences of androstenedione supplementation in men 35 to 65 years old participating in a high-intensity resistance training program. *Arch. Intern. Med.* 160:3093–3104.
2. Seifert, S. M., J. L. Schaechter, E. R. Hershorin, and S. E. Lipshultz. 2011. Health effects of energy drinks on children, adolescents, and young adults. *Pediatrics* 127(3):511–528.
3. Artioli, G. G., B. Gualano, A. Smith, J. Stout, and A. H. Lancha, Jr. 2010. Role of β-alanine supplementation on muscle carnosine and exercise performance. *Med. Sci. Sports Exerc.* 42(6):1162–1173.
4. Derave, W., I. Everaert, S. Beeckman, and A. Baguet. 2010. Muscle carnosine metabolism and β-alanine supplementation in relation to exercise and training. *Sports Med.* 40(3):247–263.

STUDY **PLAN** MasteringNutrition™

Customize your study plan—and master your nutrition!—in the Study Area of MasteringNutrition.

TEST YOURSELF | *ANSWERS*

1 **T** Just under one-half (48%) of Americans do not get enough physical activity, and 22.9% report doing no leisure-time physical activity at all.

2 **F** Walking, water aerobics, heavy gardening, and other forms of moderate physical activity do yield significant health benefits if you engage in these activities for approximately 30 minutes a day most days of the week.

3 **F** Carbohydrate loading may help improve performance for endurance events, such as marathons and triathlons, but does not improve performance in nonendurance types of athletic events, such as a 1,500-meter run.

4 **F** Evidence indicates that adequate protein intake is critical for muscle growth, and active people have higher protein needs than inactive people. However, protein supplements are not required to support muscle growth, as most Americans consume more than adequate protein from food. In contrast, weight-bearing exercise is necessary to appropriately stress the body and increase muscle mass and strength.

5 **F** Unfortunately, our thirst mechanism cannot be relied upon to signal when we need to drink. If we rely solely on our feelings of thirst, we will not consume enough fluid to support exercise.

summary

Scan to hear an MP3 Chapter Review in MasteringNutrition.

LO 1 ■ Physical activity is defined as any movement produced by muscles that increases energy expenditure. Physical fitness is the ability to carry out daily tasks with vigor and alertness, without undue fatigue, and with ample energy to enjoy leisure-time pursuits and meet unforeseen emergencies.

■ Physical activity improves our health in two ways: it increases our fitness and reduces our risk for chronic disease. Specific health benefits of physical activity include a reduced risk for obesity, cardiovascular disease, type 2 diabetes, and osteoporosis, as well as stress management, improved sleep, and many others. Despite these benefits, nearly half of all people in the United States, including many children, are insufficiently active.

LO 2 ■ The components of fitness include cardiorespiratory fitness, musculoskeletal fitness (which includes muscular strength and muscular endurance), flexibility, and body composition. Precise categories of exercise—including aerobic exercise, resistance training, and stretching—help to build each one of these components of fitness.

LO 3 ■ A 1996 report of the U.S. Surgeon General advised engaging in at least 30 minutes of physical activity most days of the week. In contrast, a 2002 report from the Institute of

Medicine recommended 60 minutes of physical activity per day. The 2008 Physical Activity Guidelines for Americans, released by the HHS, recommended 150 minutes of moderate physical activity per week, or 75 minutes of vigorous physical activity per week, as well as twice-weekly strength training, and more activity to achieve greater health benefits. These guidelines have been supported by recent large-scale studies.

LO 4 ■ A sound fitness program begins with an assessment of your current level of fitness. It is designed to meet your personal goals, guided by the specificity principle, which states that specific actions yield specific results. A sound fitness program is varied, consistent, and enjoyable. It appropriately overloads the body, inducing muscle hypertrophy without increasing the risk of injury. It includes warm-up exercises, which prepare the body for exertion by increasing blood flow and body temperature, and a cool-down period, which helps prevent injury and may help reduce muscle soreness. Finally, a sound fitness program starts slowly and progresses gradually.

LO 5 ■ To achieve an appropriate overload for fitness, the FITT principle should be followed. *Frequency* refers to the number of activity sessions per week. For example, you might choose to walk five days a week, and lift weights and stretch twice a week.

■ *Intensity* refers to how difficult the activity is to perform. Low-intensity activity causes mild changes in breathing, heart rate, and sweating, whereas moderate and vigorous-intensity activity produces more significant increases in these three functions.

■ Your maximal heart rate, commonly calculated as 220 minus your age, is used to determine your target heart rate, which is a range of aerobic training intensity. For example, for moderate-intensity activity, your target heart range should be between 50% and 70% of your maximal heart rate.

■ *Time* refers to how long each activity session lasts. *Type* refers to the range of physical activities a person can engage in to promote health and physical fitness.

LO 6 ■ The amount of ATP stored in a muscle cell is limited and can keep a muscle active for only about 1 to 3 seconds.

■ For activities lasting about 3 to 15 seconds, creatine phosphate can be broken down in an anaerobic reaction to provide energy and support the regeneration of ATP.

■ To support activities that last from 30 seconds to 2 minutes, energy is produced from glycolysis. Glycolysis produces two ATP molecules for every glucose molecule broken down. Pyruvate is the final end product of glycolysis.

■ The further metabolism of pyruvate in the presence of adequate oxygen provides energy for activities that last from 3 minutes to 4 hours. During this aerobic process, each molecule of glucose can yield 36 to 38 ATP molecules.

■ Fat can be broken down aerobically to support activities of low intensity and long duration.

■ Amino acids can be used to make glucose to maintain our blood glucose levels during exercise and can contribute from 3% to 6% of the energy needed during exercise. Amino acids also help build and repair tissues after exercise.

LO 7 ■ Vigorous-intensity exercise requires extra energy, and male athletes typically need more energy than female athletes because of their higher muscle mass and larger body weight. Athletes engaging in competitive sports may need as little as 1,500 kcal per day to as much as 7,500 kcal per day. If an athlete is losing weight, his or her energy intake in inadequate. Athletes who are concerned with making a competitive weight or with the aesthetic demands of their sport may be at risk for insufficient energy and nutrient intakes.

■ It is generally recommended that athletes consume 45% to 65% of their total energy as carbohydrate. In addition, it is recommended that athletes consume a daily carbohydrate intake of approximately 6 to 10 g of carbohydrate per kg body weight to optimize muscle glycogen stores. To enhance glycogen storage, athletes should increase carbohydrate intake during the first 24 hours of recovery from exercise, including a food or beverage high in protein.

■ A dietary fat intake of 20% to 35% is generally recommended for athletes, with less than 10% of total energy intake as saturated fat.

■ Protein needs are higher for athletes and regularly active people, and range from 1.0 to 1.8 grams per kg body weight. However, most people in the United States already consume more than twice their daily needs for protein.

LO 8 ■ Carbohydrate loading involves altering physical training and the diet such that the storage of muscle glycogen is maximized in an attempt to enhance endurance performance. It may be beneficial for athletes competing in marathons and other endurance events, but not for swimmers, baseball players, short- and medium-distance runners, and people who participate in moderate physical activity. Adverse effects of carbohydrate loading include gastrointestinal distress and sluggishness.

LO 9 ■ Regular exercise increases our fluid needs to help cool core body temperature and prevent heat illnesses. Adequate fluid intake is critical before, during, and after exercise. For training and competition lasting longer than 1 hour in any weather, sports beverages containing carbohydrates and electrolytes are recommended.

■ Active people may need more thiamin, riboflavin, and vitamin B$_6$ than inactive people, because these vitamins are critical for energy metabolism. Most women, including active women, do not consume enough calcium. Iron is critical for the transport of oxygen to working

muscles and is involved in energy production. Also, active individuals lose more iron in their sweat, feces, and urine than do inactive people. As a result, many athletes require more iron, particularly female athletes and vegetarian athletes.

LO 10 ■ Heat illnesses include heat syncope, which is dizziness that occurs when blood pools in the extremities; heat cramps, which occur during or shortly after vigorous exercise in hot weather; and heat exhaustion and heat stroke. Heat exhaustion is the first stage in a continuum that if untreated leads to heat stroke. Signs that a person is progressing to heat stroke include hot, dry skin; vomiting; a body temperature greater than or equal to 104°F; hallucinations; and coma. Prompt medical care is essential to save the person's life. Adequate fluid intake before, during, and after exercise will help prevent heat illnesses.

review questions

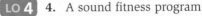

LO 1 1. Regular physical activity
a. increases our ability to carry out daily tasks with vigor and alertness, without undue fatigue.
b. reduces our risk for cancer.
c. can be an effective treatment for severe depression.
d. all of the above.

LO 2 2. The four components of physical fitness are
a. aerobic capacity, resistance, strength, and flexibility.
b. aerobic fitness, strength and tone, flexibility, and lean body mass.
c. cardiorespiratory fitness, musculoskeletal fitness, flexibility, and body composition.
d. cardiovascular fitness, respiratory fitness, musculoskeletal fitness, and chronic disease resistance.

LO 3 3. Terence is a 32-year-old software engineer. He has not been regularly active since high school, but now wants to join the walking program at work in order to improve his health. Following the 2008 Physical Activity Guidelines for Americans, Terence should walk
a. for 30 minutes most days of the week.
b. for 60 minutes a day.
c. for at least 150 minutes a week.
d. for 150 minutes a day.

LO 4 4. A sound fitness program
a. requires a preliminary assessment by a cardiopulmonary specialist.
b. begins with an initiation phase, during which you exercise at moderate intensity for at least 30 minutes a day.

c. promotes muscle atrophy.
d. includes a cool-down period to help prevent injury and muscle soreness.

LO 5 5. To achieve moderate-intensity physical activity, your target heart rate should be
a. 30% to 60% of your estimated maximal heart rate.
b. 50% to 70% of your estimated maximal heart rate.
c. 70% to 85% of your estimated maximal heart rate.
d. 80% to 95% of your estimated maximal heart rate.

LO 6 6. The amount of ATP stored in a muscle cell can keep it active for
a. about 1 to 3 seconds.
b. up to 15 seconds.
c. up to 15 minutes.
d. about 1 to 3 hours.

LO 7 7. Which of the following protein intake levels would be most appropriate, on average, for athletes who train five to seven times a week for more than an hour a day?
a. 0.8 g/kg body weight.
b. 1.0 g/kg body weight.
c. 1.8 g/kg body weight
d. 2.8 g/kg body weight.

LO 8 8. Which of the following statements about carbohydrate loading is true?
a. It supports activities across a wide range of intensities, including baseball and marathon running.
b. It concludes with 20 minutes of vigorous training and a carbohydrate intake of 20 g/kg body weight the day before the competition.

c. It involves altering both exercise duration and carbohydrate intake to maximize the amount of muscle glycogen.

d. It is consistently shown to improve endurance performance.

LO 9 9. Athletes participating in an intense competition lasting more than 1 hour should drink:

a. plain, room-temperature water.

b. a beverage containing carbohydrates and sodium and other electrolytes.

c. a beverage containing 100% fruit juice.

d. a beverage containing caffeine.

LO 10 10. Dizziness is a common symptom of

a. dehydration.

b. heat syncope.

c. heat exhaustion.

d. all of the above.

true or false?

LO 4 11. **True or false?** A sound fitness program overloads the body.

LO 5 12. **True or false?** FITT stands for frequency, intensity, time, and type of activity.

LO 7 13. **True or false?** A dietary fat intake of 15% to 25% is generally recommended for athletes.

LO 9 14. **True or false?** Sports anemia is a chronic decrease in iron stores that occurs in some athletes who have been training intensely for several months to years.

LO 10 15. **True or false?** If heat exhaustion goes unchecked, it can lead to heat stroke.

short answer

LO 3 16. Marisa and Conrad are students at the same city college. Marisa walks to and from school each morning from her home seven blocks away. Conrad lives in a suburb 12 miles away and drives to school. Marisa, an early childhood education major, covers the lunch shift, 2 hours a day, at the college's day care center, cleaning up the lunchroom and supervising the children on the playground. Conrad, an accounting major, works in his department office 2 hours a day, entering data into computer spreadsheets. On weekends, Marisa and her sister walk downtown and go shopping. Conrad goes to the movies with his friends. Neither Marisa nor Conrad participates in sports or scheduled exercise sessions. Marisa has maintained a normal, healthful weight throughout the school year, but in the same period of time, Conrad has gained several pounds. Identify at least two factors that might play a role in Marisa's and Conrad's current weights.

LO 4 17. Write a plan for a weekly activity/exercise routine that does the following:

- Meets your personal fitness goals
- Is fun for you to do

- Includes variety and consistency
- Uses all components of the FITT principle
- Includes a warm-up and cool-down period

18. Given what you have learned about Gustavo in the Nutri-Cases in previous chapters, would you advise him to begin a planned exercise program of low to moderate intensity? Why or why not? If so, what steps should he take before starting an exercise program?

19. You decide to start training for your school's annual marathon. After studying this chapter, which of the following preparation strategies would you pursue, and why?

- Use of B-vitamin supplements
- Use of creatine supplements
- Use of sports beverages
- Carbohydrate loading

LO 10 20. Explain why an athlete's risk for heat stroke is greater during training outdoors on a hot day if that athlete begins practice moderately dehydrated.

math review

LO 5 **20.** Liz is a dance major. She participates in two 90-minute dance classes each day on five days a week, plus does a 60-minute strength-training workout during her lunch break twice a week. She is a vegetarian, and her current energy intake is 1,800 kcal per day. She weighs 105 lb. After referring to Table 6.2 (Chapter 6, page 230) Liz estimates her protein intake should be 1.5 g per kg body weight, and she wants to keep her fat intake relatively low at 20% of her total daily energy intake. Based on this information, calculate how many grams of protein, fat, and carbohydrate Liz needs to consume daily to support this activity program. Does Liz's carbohydrate intake fall within the AMDR, which is 45% to 65% of total energy intake?

Answers to Review Questions and Math Review are located in the MasteringNutrition Study Area.

web links

www.heart.org
American Heart Association
The "Getting Healthy" part of this site has sections on health tools, exercise and fitness, healthy diet, lifestyle management, and more.

www.acsm.org
American College of Sports Medicine
Click on "Access Public Information" under the "Brochures and Fact Sheets" section for guidelines on healthy aerobic activity and calculating your exercise heart rate range, and under the "Newsletters" section to access the ACSM's Fit Society Page newsletter.

www.hhs.gov
U.S. Department of Health and Human Services
Review this site for multiple statistics on health, exercise, and weight, as well as information on supplements, wellness, and more.

www.win.niddk.nih.gov
Weight-Control Information Network
To find out more about healthy fitness programs log onto this site and search under "Publications" and "Weight Control."

www.ods.od.nih.gov
NIH Office of Dietary Supplements
Look on this National Institutes of Health site to learn more about the health effects of specific nutritional supplements.

www.fnic.nal.usda.gov
Food and Nutrition Information Center
Visit this site, searching on "ergogenic aids," and "sports nutrition" for links to detailed information about these topics.

www.adultfitnesstest.org
The President's Challenge Adult Fitness test
Go to this site to determine you are healthy enough to exercise by completing the American Heart Association Physical Activity Readiness Questionnaire, and then complete the test to determine your fitness level.

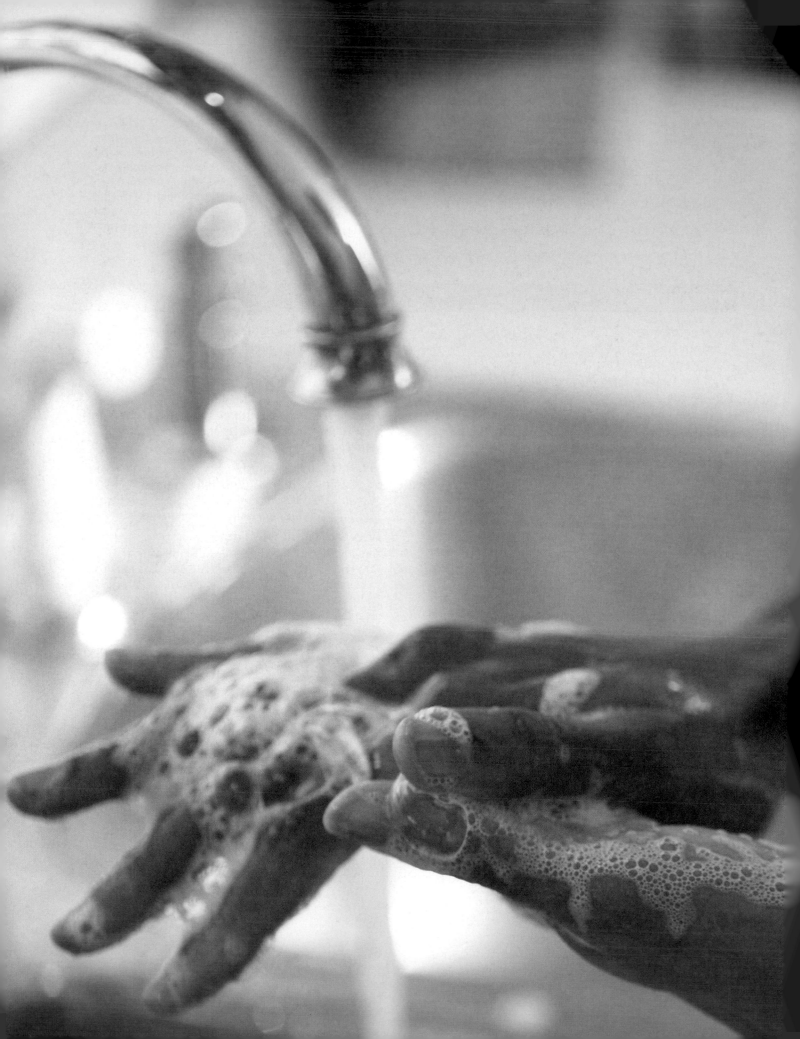

15 Food Safety and Technology: Protecting Our Food

Learning Outcomes

After studying this chapter, you should be able to:

1 Explain what foodborne illness is and why it is of concern, *pp. 592–594.*

2 Discuss the microorganisms and toxins responsible for most foodborne illnesses and deaths, *pp. 594–599.*

3 Identify four conditions that encourage the reproduction of microorganisms in food, *p. 599.*

4 Discuss strategies for preventing foodborne illness at home and while eating out, *pp. 600–605.*

5 Compare and contrast the various methods manufacturers use to preserve foods, *p. 606.*

6 Debate the safety of food additives, including the role of the GRAS list, *pp. 607–609.*

7 Identify five steps in recombinant DNA technology and the five most common reasons that crops are genetically modified in the United States, *pp. 609–611.*

8 Describe the process by which persistent organic pollutants accumulate in foods, *pp. 611–612.*

9 Discuss the potential health concerns associated with residues from heavy metals, plasticizers, dioxins, PFASs, pesticides, growth hormones, and antibiotics, *pp. 611–615.*

10 Identify the key characteristics of organic foods, and compare their nutrient and residue levels with those of foods conventionally grown, *pp. 615–617.*

MasteringNutrition™

Go online for chapter quizzes, pre-tests, interactive activities, and more!

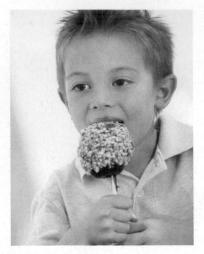

In 2014, three people died after eating caramel apples contaminated with bacteria.

LO 1 Explain what foodborne illness is and why it is of concern.

I n December, 2014, the U.S. Centers for Disease Control and Prevention (CDC) announced that 35 people across 12 states had become ill and 3 had died after eating caramel apples contaminated with a bacterium called *Listeria monocytogenes*. Early in 2015, three more people died after eating ice cream contaminated with the same bacterium. But *Listeria* is not by any means the only contaminant in our food supply. *Salmonella* bacteria are routinely found in raw poultry, eggs, meats, sprouts, melons, and other foods, and in 2014 it showed up in cucumbers sold in 29 states, causing 275 illnesses and one death. And a bacterium called *Escherichia coli* commonly resides in raw and undercooked meats: in recent years, *E. coli*–contaminated beef has caused several outbreaks of severe illness, including kidney failure and death. Moreover, these are just 3 of the 31 agents known to cause foodborne illness.[1]

How do disease-causing agents enter our food and water supplies, and how can we protect ourselves from them? What makes foods spoil, and what techniques help keep foods fresh longer? And as technologies like genetic modification or the use of pesticides increase the quantity and variety of our food supply, do they also expose us to risk? We explore these and other questions in this chapter.

What Is Foodborne Illness and Why Is It a Critical Concern?

Foodborne illness is a term used to encompass any symptom or disorder that arises from ingesting food or water contaminated with disease-causing (pathogenic) microscopic organisms (called microorganisms), their toxic secretions, or pollutants like mercury and other industrial chemicals. You probably refer to foodborne illness more commonly as *food poisoning*.

Ingestion of Contaminants Prompts Acute Illness

The human immune system has evolved to handle most cases of foodborne illness effectively. Many foodborne contaminants are killed in the mouth by first-line defenses such as the antimicrobial enzymes in saliva or the hydrochloric acid in the stomach. Any that survive these chemical assaults usually trigger acute vomiting and/or diarrhea as the gastrointestinal tract attempts to expel them. Simultaneously, the white blood cells of the immune system induce a generalized inflammatory response that causes the person to experience nausea, fatigue, fever, and muscle aches.

According to the CDC, approximately 48 million Americans—one out of every six—report experiencing foodborne illness each year.[1] Most cases are self-limiting; that is, the person's vomiting and diarrhea, though unpleasant, rid the body of the offending agent. However, depending on the status of one's health, the precise agent involved, and the "dose" ingested, symptoms can be severe. Each year, an estimated 128,000 Americans are hospitalized with foodborne illness, and 3,000 die.[1] At highest risk for hospitalization or death are people with reduced immunity. This includes the following populations:

- Developing fetuses, infants, and young children, as their immune system is immature
- Pregnant women, people who are very old, and people with a serious chronic illness, as their immune system may be compromised
- People with acquired immunodeficiency syndrome (AIDS)
- People who are receiving immune system–suppressing drugs, such as transplant recipients and cancer patients

foodborne illness An illness transmitted by food or water contaminated by a pathogenic microorganism, its toxic secretions, or a toxic chemical.

Reducing Foodborne Illness Is a Challenge

Foodborne illness has emerged as a major public health threat in recent years. One reason is that a "substantial and increasing" portion of the U.S. food supply is imported,[2]

FIGURE 15.1 Food is at risk for contamination at any of the five stages from farm to table, but following food-safety guidelines can reduce the risks.

Farms

Animals raised for meat can harbor harmful microorganisms, and crops can be contaminated with pollutants from irrigation, runoff from streams, microorganisms or toxins in soil, or pesticides. Contamination can also occur during animal slaughter or from harvesting, sorting, washing, packing, and/or storage of crops.

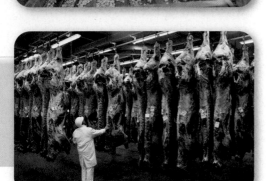

Processing

Some foods, such as produce, may go from the farm directly to the market, but most foods are processed. Processed foods may go through several steps at different facilities. At each site, people, equipment, or environments may contaminate foods. Federal safeguards, such as cleaning protocols, testing, and training, can help prevent contamination.

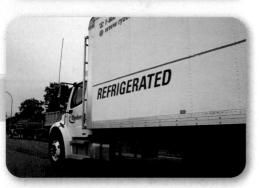

Transportation

Foods must be transported in clean, refrigerated vehicles and containers to prevent multiplication of microorganisms and microbial toxins.

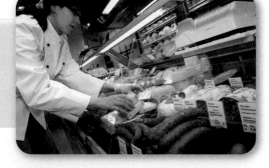

Retail

Employees of food markets and restaurants may contaminate food during storage, preparation, or service. Conditions such as inadequate refrigeration or heating may promote multiplication of microorganisms or microbial toxins. Establishments must follow FDA guidelines for food safety and pass local health inspections.

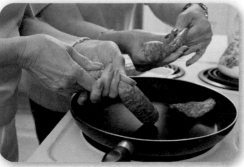

Table

Consumers may contaminate foods with unclean hands, utensils, or surfaces. They can allow the multiplication of microorganisms and microbial toxins by failing to follow the food-safety guidelines for storing, preparing, cooking, and serving foods discussed in this chapter.

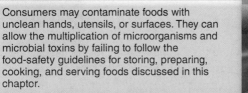

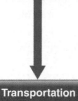

and regulation and oversight of food production may be inadequate in the country of origin. In addition, a great deal of our imported food—such as fresh produce—is consumed raw.[2] The CDC reports that contaminated produce is responsible for the greatest percentage of cases of foodborne illness, although meat and poultry are responsible for the greatest percentage of deaths.[3] However, domestic, processed foods—like the caramel apples and ice cream mentioned earlier—also can be unsafe, especially when they include a combination of ingredients from a variety of fields, feedlots, and processing facilities. These various sources can remain hidden not only to consumers, but even to the food companies using the ingredients. Contamination can occur at any point from farm to table (**Figure 15.1**, page 593), and when it does, it can be difficult to trace.

Another challenge is that federal oversight of food safety is fragmented among 15 different agencies.[2] One of the most important of these is the CDC, mentioned earlier, which monitors reports from state public health agencies for indications of outbreaks of foodborne illness and assists in investigating and controlling such outbreaks. The agencies most directly responsible for preventing foodborne illness are the Food Safety and Inspection Service (FSIS) of the United States Department of Agriculture (USDA), which oversees meats, poultry, and egg products, and the Food and Drug Administration (FDA), which oversees all other foods.[2] Moreover, the Environmental Protection Agency (EPA) monitors and regulates certain aspects of food production and water quality. Information about these agencies and how to access them appears in **Table 15.1**.

In 2009, President Barack Obama announced the creation of an interagency Food Safety Working Group to coordinate federal efforts; however, the group has not met since 2011.[2] The U.S. Congress passed into law a new food-safety bill, the Food Safety Modernization Act, in January 2011. This bill provided for increased federal inspections of food-production facilities, new regulations to prevent contamination of foods, and more robust FDA enforcement tools, including the authority to force companies to recall tainted foods. It may be too soon to judge the effectiveness of these provisions; however, the most recent food safety progress report from the CDC shows no progress in reducing foodborne illness from the six major bacterial culprits, and incidents involving two of the bacteria have actually increased.[4]

RECAP

Foodborne illness arises from the ingestion of contaminated food or water. It affects 48 million Americans a year, and about 3,000 die. Contamination can occur at any point from farm to table. Fifteen federal agencies, primarily the Centers for Disease Control and Prevention, the Food and Drug Administration, the Food Safety and Inspection Service of the United States Department of Agriculture, and the Environmental Protection Agency, play roles in monitoring and regulating food production and preservation. The Food Safety Modernization Act of 2011 increased the inspection and regulation of food production facilities by federal agencies and authorized the FDA to swiftly recall contaminated foods from the market; however, the most recent progress report from the CDC shows no reductions in foodborne illness from six major bacterial culprits. ■

LO 2 Discuss the microorganisms and toxins responsible for most foodborne illnesses and deaths.

LO 3 Identify four conditions that encourage the reproduction of microorganisms in food.

What Causes Most Foodborne Illness?

The consumption of food containing pathogenic microorganisms—those capable of causing disease—results in food infections. Food intoxications result from consuming food in which microorganisms have secreted harmful substances called **toxins.** Naturally occurring plant and marine toxins also contaminate food. Finally, chemical residues in foods, such as heavy metals, pesticides, and packaging residues, can cause illness. Residues are discussed later in this chapter.

TABLE 15.1 Government Agencies That Regulate Food Safety

Name of Agency	Year Established	Role in Food Regulations	Website
U.S. Department of Agriculture (USDA) Food Safety and Inspection Service (FSIS)	1785	Oversees safety of meat, poultry, and processed egg products; also ensures accuracy of meat and poultry labeling	www.fsis.usda.gov
U.S. Food and Drug Administration (FDA)	1862	Regulates food standards of food products (except meat, poultry, and eggs) and bottled water; regulates food labeling and enforces pesticide use as established by EPA	www.fda.gov
Centers for Disease Control and Prevention (CDC)	1946	Works with public health officials to promote and educate the public about health and safety; is able to track information needed in identifying foodborne illness outbreaks	www.cdc.gov
Environmental Protection Agency (EPA)	1970	Regulates use of pesticides and which crops they can be applied to; establishes standards for water quality	www.epa.gov

Several Types of Microorganisms Contaminate Foods

The microorganisms that most commonly cause food infections are viruses and bacteria.

Viruses Involved in Foodborne Illness

Viruses are extremely tiny noncellular agents that can survive only by infecting living cells. Just one type, norovirus, causes an average of 19–21 million infections, well over 50,000 hospitalizations, and up to 800 deaths annually in the United States.[5] In fact, norovirus is the culprit behind about 50% of all foodborne illness (**Figure 15.2**).[5]

Norovirus is so common and contagious that many people refer to it simply as "the stomach flu"; however, it is not a strain of influenza. Symptoms of infection typically come on suddenly as *gastroenteritis*, inflammation of the lining of the stomach and intestines. This causes stomach cramps as well as both vomiting and diarrhea. Because the vomiting begins abruptly, the person is likely to be in a social setting. Because it is forceful, anyone nearby is likely to become contaminated. Another characteristic that makes norovirus so contagious is that, whereas most viruses perish quickly in a dry environment, norovirus is able to survive on dry surfaces and objects, from countertops to utensils, for days or even weeks. Also, ingestion of even a few "particles" of norovirus can result in full-blown illness.[5]

toxin Any harmful substance; in microbiology, a chemical produced by a microorganism that harms tissues or causes harmful immune responses.

viruses A group of infectious agents that are much smaller than bacteria, lack independent metabolism, and are incapable of growth or reproduction outside of living cells.

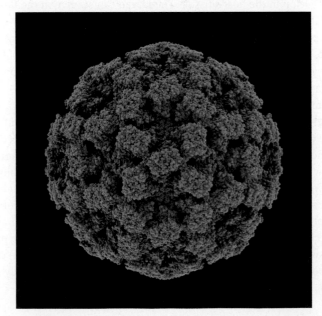

FIGURE 15.2 Norovirus is responsible for about half of all foodborne illness in the United States. Infection typically produces a mild illness; however, because it affects so many people, it is a leading cause of foodborne deaths.

To learn more about norovirus infection, including tips for prevention, go to 4- CDC at http://www2c.cdc.gov **to listen to a podcast on the topic.**

Healthcare facilities, cruise ships, college campuses, and restaurants and catered events commonly report outbreaks. The best way to prevent the spread of norovirus is to wash your hands, kitchen surfaces, and utensils with warm, soapy water. Alcohol-based hand sanitizers may be used in addition to hand-washing, but not as a substitute.[5] If you experience vomiting or diarrhea, immediately clean and disinfect all nearby surfaces and remove and wash laundry thoroughly.

Whereas norovirus is estimated to infect about 21 million Americans annually, hepatitis A virus (HAV) causes about 3,000 infections.[6] Like norovirus, HAV can be transmitted person-to-person or via contaminated food and water. The term *hepatitis* means inflammation of the liver. This causes jaundice (a yellowish skin tone), a common sign of HAV infection.[6] Typically, the symptoms of HAV infection include a mild fever, abdominal pain, and nausea and vomiting that lasts a few weeks. Rarely, in elderly patients and those with pre-existing liver disease, HAV infection can lead to liver failure and even death.

Bacteria Involved in Foodborne Illness

In contrast to viruses, **bacteria** are cellular microorganisms; however, they lack the true cell nucleus common to plant and animals cells, and they reproduce either by dividing in two or by forming reproductive spores. In contrast to our resident bacteria, which contribute to our health and functioning, pathogenic bacteria are capable of causing mild to severe disease.

Foodborne bacterial illness commonly occurs when we ingest pathogenic bacteria living in or on undercooked or raw foods or fluids. These bacteria, which often come from human or animal feces, can damage our cells and tissues either directly or by secreting a destructive toxin. Of the seven pathogens the CDC identifies as of greatest concern in causing foodborne illnesses, hospitalizations, and deaths among Americans, five are species of bacteria.[7] These are identified in **Table 15.2**. Of these, *Salmonella* is responsible for the most deaths (**Figure 15.3**).

Other Microorganisms Involved in Foodborne Illness

Parasites are microorganisms that simultaneously derive benefit from and harm their host. They are responsible for only about 2% of foodborne illnesses. The most common culprits are helminths and protozoa:

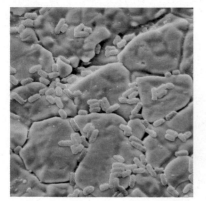

FIGURE 15.3 *Salmonella* is the second leading cause of foodborne illness, after norovirus, and the primary cause of foodborne deaths. Infection can cause fever, diarrhea, and abdominal cramps, and cells of some strains can perforate the intestines and invade the blood.

bacteria Microorganisms that lack a true nucleus and reproduce by division or by spore formation.

parasite A microorganism that simultaneously derives benefit from and harms its host.

helminth A multicellular microscopic worm.

protozoa Single-celled, mobile parasites.

fungi Plantlike, spore-forming organisms that can grow as either single cells or multicellular colonies.

prion A pathogenic form of a normal and protective protein that misfolds and becomes infectious and destructive; prions are not living cellular organisms or viruses.

- **Helminths** are multicellular worms, such as tapeworms (**Figure 15.4**), flukes, and roundworms. They reproduce by releasing their eggs into vegetation or water. Animals, including fish, then consume the contaminated matter. The eggs hatch inside their host, and larvae develop in the host's tissue. The larvae can survive in the flesh long after the host is killed for food. Thoroughly cooking beef, pork, or fish destroys the larvae. In contrast, people who eat contaminated foods either raw or undercooked consume living larvae, which then mature into adult worms in their small intestine. Some worms cause mild symptoms, such as nausea and diarrhea, but others can grow large enough to cause intestinal obstruction or even death.
- **Protozoa** are single-celled organisms. One of these, *Toxoplasma gondii*, is responsible for about 24% of deaths and 8% of hospitalizations due to foodborne illness, making it one of the CDC's top seven foodborne pathogens.[7] People typically become infected by eating undercooked, contaminated meat, or by ingesting minute amounts after handling raw meat and then failing to wash their hands. Illness is usually mild, but if a pregnant woman becomes infected, she may transmit the infection to her fetus, who may die *in utero* or suffer severe consequences after birth.[8] Another protozoan parasite common worldwide is *Giardia*, which lives in the intestines of infected animals and humans and is passed into the environment from their stools. People typically consume *Giardia* by swallowing contaminated water (in lakes, rivers, and so on) or by eating contaminated food. Infection produces a diarrheal illness, which usually resolves within 2 to 6 weeks.[9]

TABLE 15.2 Five Top Bacteria of Concern in Foodborne Illness and Deaths

Bacteria	Incubation Period	Duration	Symptoms	Foods Most Commonly Affected	Steps for Prevention
Campylobacter (several species)	1–7 days	2–10 days	Headache Diarrhea Nausea Abdominal cramps	Raw and undercooked meat, poultry, eggs Cake icing Untreated water Unpasteurized milk	Only drink pasteurized milk. Cook foods properly. Avoid cross-contamination.
Clostridium perfringens	8–22 hours	24 hours	Abdominal cramps Diarrhea Dehydration	Beef Poultry Gravies Leftovers	Cook foods thoroughly and serve hot. Refrigerate leftovers promptly. Reheat leftovers thoroughly before serving.
Listeria monocytogenes	1–42 days	Days to weeks	Fever Muscle aches Diarrhea Sometimes headache and confusion	Meats, especially hot dogs and deli meats Vegetables Dairy products, especially raw milk and soft cheeses Smoked fish	Cook foods thoroughly and serve hot. Wash produce carefully. If pregnant, do not consume deli meats, smoked fish, or products containing raw milk.
Salmonella (more than 2,300 types)	12–24 hours	4–7 days	Nausea Diarrhea Abdominal pain Chills Fever Headache	Raw or undercooked eggs, poultry, and meat Raw milk and dairy products Seafood Fruits and vegetables	Cook foods thoroughly. Avoid cross-contamination. Only drink pasteurized milk. Practice proper hand washing and sanitizing.
Staphylococcus aureus (which produces an enterotoxin)	1–6 hours	1–2 days	Sudden, severe nausea and vomiting Abdominal cramps Diarrhea may occur	Custard- or cream-filled baked goods Ham Poultry Dressings, sauces, and gravies Eggs Potato salad	Refrigerate foods. Practice proper hand washing and sanitizing.

Sources: Data from Iowa State University Extension, Food Safety 2015. *What Are the Most Common Foodborne Pathogens?* http://www.extension.iastate.edu/foodsafety/L1.7, U.S. Food and Drug Administration, Foodborne Illnesses: What You Need to Know, Updated January 29, 2015, from http://www.fda.gov/Food/FoodborneIllnessContaminants/FoodborneIllnessesNeedToKnow/default.htm; and L. H. Gould, et al., 2013. Surveillance for Foodborne Disease Outbreaks—United States, 1998–2008, *MMWR*, 62(SS02):1–34.

Fungi are plantlike, spore-forming organisms that can grow as either single cells or multicellular colonies. Three common types are yeasts, which are globular; molds, which are long and thin; and the familiar mushrooms. Very few species of fungi cause serious disease in people with healthy immune systems, and those that do cause disease in humans are not typically foodborne. In addition, unlike bacterial growth, which is invisible and often tasteless, fungal growth typically makes food look and taste so unappealing that we immediately discard it (**Figure 15.5**, page 598).

A foodborne illness in beef cattle that has had front-page exposure in recent years is mad cow disease, or *bovine spongiform encephalopathy (BSE)*. This neurologic disorder is caused by a **prion,** a proteinaceous infectious particle that is self-replicating. Prions are normal proteins of animal tissues that can misfold and become infectious. When they do, they can transform other normal proteins into abnormally shaped prions until they eventually cause illness. The human form of BSE, called *variant Creutzfeldt–Jakob Disease (vCJD),* can develop in people who consume contaminated meat or tissue. Symptoms take years to appear, but vCJD causes progressive neurological disease and is eventually fatal. Over 200 people have died from vCJD, the great majority in Europe, where it was once common practice to feed livestock with meal made from the tissues of other animals. This practice has ceased. In the United States, one person is currently infected and three people have died from vCJD, but two of these individuals are thought to have acquired the disease

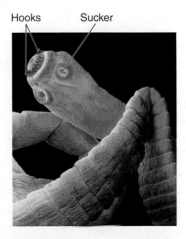

Hooks　　Sucker

FIGURE 15.4 Tapeworms have long bodies with hooks and suckers, they use to attach to a host's tissue.

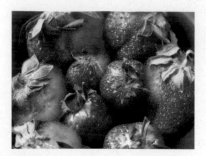

FIGURE 15.5 Molds rarely cause foodborne illness, in part because they look so unappealing that we throw the food away.

while living in the United Kingdom.[10] The United States rigorously controls the quality of animal feed and practices continual surveillance to detect BSE before an animal is approved for meat consumption.

Some Foodborne Illness Is Due to Toxins

The microorganisms just discussed cause illness by directly infecting and destroying body cells. In contrast, other bacteria and fungi secrete toxins that bind to body cells and can cause a variety of symptoms, such as diarrhea, vomiting, organ damage, convulsions, and paralysis. Toxins can be categorized depending on the type of cell they bind to; the two primary types of toxins associated with foodborne illness are neurotoxins, which damage the nervous system and can cause paralysis, and enterotoxins, which target the gastrointestinal system and generally cause severe diarrhea and vomiting.

Bacterial Toxins

One of the most common foodborne toxins is produced by the bacterium *Staphylococcus aureus* (see Table 15.2). Although the vomiting it typically provokes is severe, it is usually self-limiting. In contrast, the neurotoxin produced by the bacterium *Clostridium botulinum* is deadly. This botulism toxin blocks nerve transmission to muscle cells and causes paralysis, including of the muscles required for breathing. A common source of contamination is food from a damaged (split, pierced, or bulging) can. If you spot damaged canned goods while shopping, notify the store manager. If you inadvertently purchase food in a damaged can, or find that the container spurts liquid when you open it, throw it out immediately. *Never taste the food, as even a microscopic amount of botulism toxin can be fatal.*[11] Other common sources of *C. botulinum* are foods improperly canned at home, raw honey, oils infused with garlic or herbs, and potatoes baked in foil.

Some strains of *E. coli*, including those involved in the outbreaks mentioned at the beginning of this chapter, are particularly dangerous because they produce a toxin called *Shiga toxin*. These types are referred to as *Shiga toxin-producing E. coli*, or STEC. The most common STEC is *E. coli* O157. STECs are particularly dangerous because, in the vulnerable populations mentioned earlier, infection can result in kidney failure and, in some cases, death.

Eating spoiled fish—commonly tuna or mackerel—is unwise because the bacteria responsible for the spoilage release toxins into the fish. The result is *scombrotoxic fish poisoning*, which causes headache, vomiting, a rash, sweating, and flushing within a few minutes to 2 hours after consumption. Symptoms usually resolve within a few hours in healthy people.[12]

Fungal Toxins

Some fungi produce poisonous chemicals called *mycotoxins*. (The prefix *myco-* means "fungus.") These toxins are typically found in grains stored in moist environments. In some instances, moist conditions in the field encourage fungi to reproduce and release their toxins on the surface of growing crops. Long-term consumption of mycotoxins can cause organ damage or cancer.

A highly visible fungus that causes food intoxication is the poisonous mushroom. Most mushrooms are not toxic, but a few, such as the deathcap mushroom (*Amanita phalloides*), can be fatal. Some poisonous mushrooms are quite colorful (**Figure 15.6**), a fact that helps explain why the victims of mushroom poisoning are often children.[13]

Toxic Algae

You may have seen signs warning of a "red tide" along a stretch of coastline. Shellfish beds are closed during a red tide to protect the public from a foodborne illness called *paralytic shellfish poisoning (PSP)*.[12] Red tides are caused by the excessive production of certain species of toxic algae, whose bloom turns ocean waters purple, pink, or red. The blooms occur most commonly along the Gulf of Maine and on the Gulf Coast of Florida, but they also appear in U.S. West Coast waters. Humans don't consume these marine toxins directly;

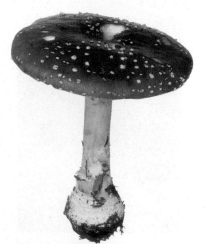

FIGURE 15.6 Some mushrooms, such as this fly agaric, contain fungal toxins that can cause illness or even death.

rather, mussels, clams, and other shellfish consume the toxic algae. When people consume the affected seafood—which typically looks, smells, and tastes normal—PSP results.[12]

Finfish can also be contaminated with toxic algae. *Ciguatoxins* are marine toxins commonly found in fish caught off the coasts of Hawaii, Puerto Rico, and other tropical regions. They are produced by algae called *dinoflagellates*, which are consumed by small fish. The toxins become progressively more concentrated as larger fish eat these small fish, and high concentrations can be present in fish such as grouper, sea bass, snapper, and a number of other large fish from tropical regions. Symptoms of ciguatoxin poisoning include nausea, vomiting, diarrhea, headache, itching, and even nightmares or hallucinations, but the illness is rarely fatal and typically resolves within a few weeks.[12]

Plant Toxins

A variety of plants contain toxins that, if consumed, can cause illness. As humans evolved, we learned to avoid such plants. However, one plant toxin is still commonly found in kitchens. Potatoes that have turned green contain the toxin *solanine*, which forms during the greening process. The green color is actually due to chlorophyll, a harmless pigment that forms when the potatoes are exposed to light. Although the production of solanine occurs simultaneously with the production of chlorophyll, the two processes are unrelated. Solanine is very toxic even in small amounts, and potatoes that appear green beneath the skin should be thrown away. Toxicity causes vomiting, diarrhea, fever, headache, and other symptoms and can progress to shock. Rarely, the poisoning can be fatal.[14]

You can avoid the greening of potatoes by storing them for only short periods in a dark cupboard or brown paper bag in a cool area. Wash the potato to expose its color, and throw it away if it has turned green.

Certain Conditions Help Microorganisms Multiply in Foods

Given the correct environmental conditions, microorganisms can thrive in many types of food. Four factors affect the survival and reproduction of food microorganisms:

- *Temperature.* Many microorganisms capable of causing human illness thrive at warm temperatures, from about 40°F to 140°F (4°C to 60°C). You can think of this range of temperatures as the **danger zone** (**Figure 15.7**). These microorganisms can be destroyed by thoroughly heating or cooking foods, and their reproduction can be slowed by refrigeration and freezing. Safe cooking and food-storage temperatures are identified later in this chapter.
- *Humidity.* Many microorganisms require a high level of moisture; thus, foods such as boxed dried pasta do not make suitable microbial homes, although cooked pasta left at room temperature would prove hospitable.
- *Acidity.* Most microorganisms have a preferred pH range in which they thrive. Pathogenic bacteria prefer a pH range from slightly acidic to neutral—about 4.6 to 7.0. However, there are exceptions. *Clostridium botulinum*, for example, thrives in alkaline environments. It cannot grow or produce its toxin in acidic environments, so the risk for botulism is decreased in citrus fruits, pickles, and tomato-based foods, whereas alkaline foods, such as fish and most vegetables, are a magnet for *C. botulinum*.
- *Oxygen content.* Many microorganisms require oxygen to function; thus, food-preservation techniques that remove oxygen, such as industrial canning and bottling, keep foods safe for consumption. In contrast, *C. botulinum* thrives in an oxygen-free environment. For this reason, the canning process heats foods to an extremely high temperature to destroy this deadly microorganism.

In addition, microorganisms need an entryway into a food. Just as our skin protects our bodies from microbial invasion, the peels, rinds, and shells of many foods seal off access to the nutrients within. Eggshells are a good example of a natural food barrier. Once such a barrier is pierced or removed, however, the food loses its primary defense against contamination. Slicing through an unwashed melon, for example, can contaminate the edible interior.

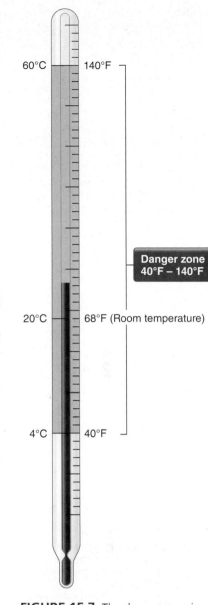

FIGURE 15.7 The danger zone is a temperature range within which many pathogenic microorganisms thrive. Notice that "room temperature" (about 68°F) is within the danger zone!

danger zone The range of temperature (about 40°F to 140°F, or 4°C to 60°C) at which many microorganisms capable of causing human disease thrive.

RECAP

Food infections result from the consumption of food containing living microorganisms, such as bacteria, whereas food intoxications result from consuming food containing toxins. Norovirus is responsible for about 50% of all cases of foodborne illness and is a leading cause of foodborne deaths. Five species of bacteria, including *Salmonella* and *Listeria*, are also among the CDC's top seven pathogens contributing to foodborne illnesses and deaths, as is *Toxoplasma gondii*, a parasite. Prions are self-replicating particles that can contaminate the tissues of animals, including cattle. *Clostridium botulinum*, "STEC" species of *E. coli*, and other bacteria can produce toxins capable of causing severe illness and even death. Mushrooms, seafood, and potatoes may also contain toxins. In order to reproduce in foods, microorganisms require a precise range of temperature, humidity, acidity, and oxygen content. ■

Nutri-Case

Theo

"I got really sick yesterday after eating lunch in the cafeteria. I had a turkey sandwich, potato salad, and a cola. A few hours later, in the middle of basketball practice, I started to shake and sweat. I felt really nauseated and barely made it to the bathroom before vomiting. Then I went back to my dorm room and crawled into bed. This morning I still feel a little sick to my stomach, and sort of weak. I asked a couple of my friends who ate in the cafeteria yesterday if they got sick, and neither of them did, but I still think it was the food. I'm going off-campus for lunch from now on!"

Do you think that Theo's illness was foodborne? If so, what food(s) do you most suspect? What do you think of his plan to go off-campus for lunch from now on?

LO 4 Discuss strategies for preventing foodborne illness at home and while eating out.

How Can You Prevent Foodborne Illness?

The United States Department of Health & Human Services' Foodsafety.gov is the nation's gateway to federal food safety information. Foodsafety.gov identifies four basic rules for food safety (**Figure 15.8**).

Clean: Wash Your Hands and Kitchen Surfaces Often

One of the easiest and most effective ways to prevent foodborne illness is to consistently wash your hands before and after handling food. Remove any rings or bracelets before you begin, because jewelry can harbor bacteria. Scrub for at least 20 seconds with a mild soap, being sure to wash underneath your fingernails and between your fingers. Rinse under warm, running water. Although you should wash dishes in hot water, it's too harsh for hand washing: It causes the surface layer of the skin to break down, increasing the risk that microorganisms will be able to penetrate your skin. Dry your hands on a clean towel or fresh paper towel.

Thoroughly wash utensils, containers, and cutting boards with soap and hot water, either in a dishwasher, or by hand, wearing gloves. You can sanitize them with a solution of 1 tablespoon of chlorine bleach to 1 gallon of water. Flood the surface with the bleach solution and allow it to air dry. Also wash countertops with soap and hot water.

Wash fruits and vegetables thoroughly under running water just before eating, cutting, or cooking them. Prewashed and bagged salad greens clearly

| CLEAN | SEPARATE | COOK | CHILL |

FIGURE 15.8 This food safety logo from Foodsafety.gov can help you remember the four steps for reducing your risk of foodborne illness.

marked as ready-to-eat do not need to be washed again. Washing fruits and vegetables with soap or detergent, or using commercial produce washes, is not recommended. Also, do not wash meat, poultry, or fish, as doing so can spread contaminants. Microorganisms in these foods will be destroyed when you thoroughly cook them.[15]

Separate: Don't Cross-Contaminate

Cross-contamination is the spread of microorganisms from one food to another. This commonly occurs when raw foods, such as chicken and vegetables, are cut using the same knife or cutting board, or stored or carried to the table on the same plate.[16] Invest in a set of cutting boards of different colors, and reserve one for fresh breads, one for produce, and one for meat, fish, and poultry.

In the refrigerator, keep raw meat, poultry, eggs, and seafood and their juices away from ready-to-eat food. Keep them wrapped in plastic on the lowest shelf of your refrigerator.

When preparing meals with a marinade, reserve some of the fresh marinade in a clean container; then add the raw ingredients to the remainder. In this way, some uncontaminated marinade will be available if needed later in the cooking process. While marinating raw food, keep it in the refrigerator.[16]

Prevent cross-contamination while food shopping. Keep raw meat, poultry, and seafood away from other foods in your cart, and make sure they're wrapped in plastic at the checkout, so their juices won't contaminate other foods. Inspect eggs before putting them in your cart. If a carton has a broken egg, bring it to the store manager. Also, watch out for unsafe practices in the store. For example, the displaying of food products such as cooked shrimp on the same bed of ice as raw seafood is not safe, nor is slicing cold cuts with the same knife used to trim raw meat. Report such practices to your local health authorities.

Chill: Store Foods in the Refrigerator or Freezer

The third rule for keeping food safe from bacteria is to promptly refrigerate or freeze it. Remember the danger zone: microorganisms that cause foodborne illness can reproduce in temperatures above 40°F. To keep them from multiplying in your food, keep it cold. Refrigeration (between 32°F and 40°F) and freezing (at or below 0°F)[17] do not kill all microorganisms, but cold temperatures diminish their ability to reproduce in quantities large enough to cause illness. Also, many naturally occurring enzymes that cause food spoilage are deactivated at cold temperatures.

Shopping for Perishable Foods

When choosing perishable foods, check the "sell by" or "best used by" date on the label. The "sell by" date indicates the last day a product can be sold and still maintain its quality during normal home storage and consumption. The "best used by" date tells you how long a product will maintain best flavor and quality before eating.[18] The "use by" date indicates the last day recommended to consume the food. No matter the type, if the stamped date has passed, don't purchase the item and notify the store manager. These foods should be promptly removed from the shelves.

When shopping for food, purchase refrigerated and frozen foods last. After you check out, get perishable foods home and into the refrigerator or freezer within 1 hour. If your trip home will be longer than an hour, take along a cooler to transport them in.

Refrigerating Foods at Home

As soon as you get home from shopping, put meats, eggs, cheeses, milk, and any other perishable foods in the refrigerator. Store meat, poultry, and seafood in the back of the refrigerator away from the door, so that they stay cold, and on the lowest shelf, so that their juices do not drip onto any other foods. If you are not going to use raw poultry, fish, or

To learn "Clean" tips for preventing foodborne illness, watch a video at http://www.foodsafety.gov/ and type in "foodborne illness" into the search bar.

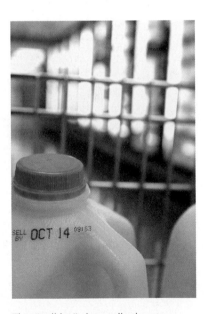

The "sell by" date tells the store how long to display the product for sale.

cross-contamination Contamination of one food by another via the unintended transfer of microorganisms through physical contact.

ground beef within 2 days of purchase, store it in the freezer. A guide for refrigerating foods is provided in **Figure 15.9**.

After a meal, refrigerate leftovers promptly—even if still hot—to discourage microbial growth. The standard rule is to refrigerate leftovers within 2 hours of serving. If the ambient temperature is 90°F or higher, such as at a picnic, foods should be refrigerated within 1 hour.[17] A larger quantity of food takes longer to cool, so divide and conquer: separate leftovers into shallow containers for quicker cooling.[17] Finally, avoid keeping leftovers for more than a few days (see Figure 15.9). If you don't plan to finish a dish within the recommended time frame, freeze it.

Freezing and Thawing Foods

The temperature in your freezer should be set at or below 0°F. Use a thermometer and check it periodically. If your electricity goes out, avoid opening the freezer until the power is restored. When the power does come back on, check the temperature. If it is at or below 40°F, or if the food contains ice crystals, the food should still be safe to eat, or refreeze.[19]

As with refrigeration, smaller packages will freeze more quickly. Rather than attempting to freeze an entire casserole, divide the food into multiple, small portions in freezer-safe containers; then freeze.

Sufficient thawing will ensure adequate cooking throughout, which is essential to preventing foodborne illness. The safest way to thaw meat, poultry, and seafood is to place the frozen package on the bottom shelf of the refrigerator, on a large plate or in a large bowl to catch its juices. It should be ready to cook within 24 hours. Never thaw frozen meat, poultry, or seafood on a kitchen counter or in a basin of warm water. Room temperatures allow the growth of bacteria on the surface of food. You can also thaw foods in your microwave, following the manufacturer's instructions. Another option is to cook the food without first thawing it. Just allow for a cooking time about 50% longer than usual.[17]

Food	Keeps for...
Uncooked hamburger	1–2 days
Uncooked roasts, steaks, and chops	3–5 days
Uncooked poultry	1–2 days
Uncooked fish	1–2 days
Cooked meats, poultry, and fish	3–4 days
Fresh eggs in shell	3–5 weeks
Hardboiled eggs	1 week
Egg, chicken, tuna, ham, and pasta salads	3–5 days
Soups or stews	3–4 days
Hot dogs and luncheon meats, unopened package	2 weeks
Hot dogs, opened package	1 week
Luncheon meats, opened package	3–5 days

Safe zone
32°F – 40°F

FIGURE 15.9 While it's important to keep a well-stocked refrigerator, it's also important to know how long foods will keep.

Source: Data from U.S. Department of Agriculture, Food Safety and Inspection Service. May, 2010. Food Safety Information. Refrigeration and Food Safety. http://www.fsis.usda.gov/shared/PDF/Refrigeration_and_Food_Safety.pdf

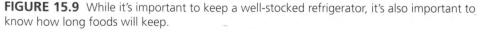

Dealing with Molds in Refrigerated Foods

Some molds like cool temperatures. Mold spores are common in the atmosphere, and they randomly land on food in open containers. If the temperature and acidity of the food are hospitable, they will grow.

If the surface of a small portion of a firm, solid food, such as hard cheese, becomes moldy, it is generally safe to cut off that section down to about an inch and eat the unspoiled portion. However, if soft cheese, sour cream, tomato sauce, a leftover casserole, or another soft or fluid product becomes moldy, discard it entirely, as foods with a high moisture content may be contaminated below the surface.[20]

Cook: Heat Foods Thoroughly

Thoroughly cooking food is a sure way to kill the intestinal worms discussed earlier and many other microorganisms. Color and texture are unreliable indicators of safety. Use a food thermometer to ensure that you have cooked food to a safe minimum internal temperature to destroy any harmful bacteria. The minimum temperatures vary for the type of food:[21]

- Beef, pork, veal, lamb steaks, roasts, and chops: 145°F with a 3-minute rest time before serving
- Fish: 145°F
- Ground beef: 160°F
- Egg dishes: 160°F
- Poultry, whole, pieces, and ground: 165°F

Place the thermometer in the thickest part of the food, away from bone, fat, or gristle. See the **Highlight** box on page 604 for tips about grilling and barbequing foods.

> To learn how to use a food thermometer, watch the video at http://www.foodsafety.gov/ titled *Cook*.

Microwave cooking is convenient, but you need to be sure your food is thoroughly and evenly cooked and that there are no cold spots in the food where bacteria can thrive. For best results, cover food, stir often, and rotate for even cooking. Raw and semi-raw (such as marinated or partly cooked) fish delicacies, including sushi and sashimi, may be tempting, but their safety cannot be guaranteed. Always cook fish thoroughly. When done, fish should be opaque and flake easily with a fork. If you're wondering how sushi restaurants can guarantee the safety of their food, the short answer is they can't. All fish to be used for sushi must be frozen using a method that effectively kills any parasites that are in the fish, but it does not necessarily kill bacteria or viruses. Another myth is that hot sauce can kill microbes in raw foods. It can't.

You may have fond memories of licking cake or brownie batter off a spoon when you were a kid, but such practices are no longer considered safe. That's because most cake batter contains raw eggs, one of the most common sources of *Salmonella*. Cook eggs until they are firm.

Protect Yourself from Toxins in Foods

Killing microorganisms with heat is an important step in keeping food safe, but it won't protect you against their toxins. That's because many toxins are unaffected by heat and are capable of causing severe illness even when the microorganisms that produced them have been destroyed.

For example, let's say you prepare a casserole for a team picnic. Too bad you forget to wash your hands before serving it to your teammates, because you contaminate the casserole with the bacterium *Staphylococcus aureus*, which is commonly found on skin. You and your friends go off and play soccer, leaving the food in the sun, and a few hours later you take the rest of the casserole home. At supper, you heat the leftovers thoroughly, thinking that this will kill any bacteria that multiplied while it was left out. That night you experience nausea, severe vomiting, and abdominal pain. What happened? While your food

Food-Safety Tips for Your Next Barbecue

It's the end of the term and you and your friends are planning a lakeside barbecue to celebrate! Here are some tips from the Center for Food Safety and Applied Nutrition at the U.S. Food and Drug Administration for preventing foodborne illness at any outdoor gathering.

- **Wash your hands, utensils, and food-preparation surfaces.** Even in outdoor settings, food safety begins with hand washing. Take along a water jug, some soap, and paper towels or a box of moist, disposable towelettes. Keep all utensils and platters clean when preparing foods.

- **Keep foods cold—and separate—during transport.** Use small coolers with ice or frozen gel packs to keep food at or below 40°F. Put beverages in one cooler, washed fruits and vegetables and containers of potato salad in another, and wrapped, frozen meat, poultry, and seafood in another. Keep coolers in the air-conditioned passenger compartment of your car, rather than in a hot trunk.

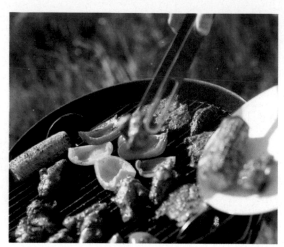

At a barbecue, it's essential to heat foods to the proper temperature.

- **Grill foods thoroughly.** Use a food thermometer to be sure the food has reached an adequate internal temperature before serving. Hamburgers should reach 160°F and chicken at least 165°F.

- **Avoid contaminating cooked foods.** When taking food from the grill to the table, never use the same platter or utensils that previously held raw meat or seafood!

- **Keep hot foods hot.** Keep grilled food hot until it is served by moving it to the side of the grill, just away from the coals, so that it stays at or above 140°F. If grilled food isn't going to be eaten right away, wrap it well and place it in an insulated container.

- **Keep cold foods cold.** Cold foods, such as chicken salad, should be kept in a bowl of ice during your barbecue. Drain off water as the ice melts and replace the ice frequently. Don't let any perishable food sit out longer than 2 hours. In temperatures above 90°F, don't let food sit out for more than 1 hour.

Source: Data from U.S. Food and Drug Administration. 2014, July 2. Barbecue Basics: Tips to Prevent Foodborne Illness. http://www.fda.gov/forconsumers/ucm094562.htm

---

was left out, *Staphylococcus* multiplied in the casserole and produced a toxin (**Figure 15.10**). When you reheated the food, you killed the microorganisms, but their toxin was unaffected by the heat. When you then ate the food, the toxin made you sick.

Be Choosy When Eating Out—Close to Home or Far Away

When choosing a place to eat out, avoid restaurants that don't look clean. Grimy tabletops and dirty restrooms indicate indifference to hygiene. On the other hand, the cleanliness of areas used by the public doesn't guarantee that the kitchen is clean. That is why health inspections are important. Public health inspectors randomly visit and inspect the food-preparation areas of all businesses that serve food, whether eaten in or taken out. When in doubt, check the inspection results posted in the restaurant.

Another way to protect yourself when dining out is by ordering foods to be cooked thoroughly. If you order a hamburger and it arrives pink in the middle, or scrambled eggs and they arrive runny, send the food back to be cooked thoroughly. If you order potato, egg, tuna, or chicken salad or a dish with a cream sauce, and it arrives looking somewhat congealed or simply less than fresh, it may have been left out too long. Send it back.

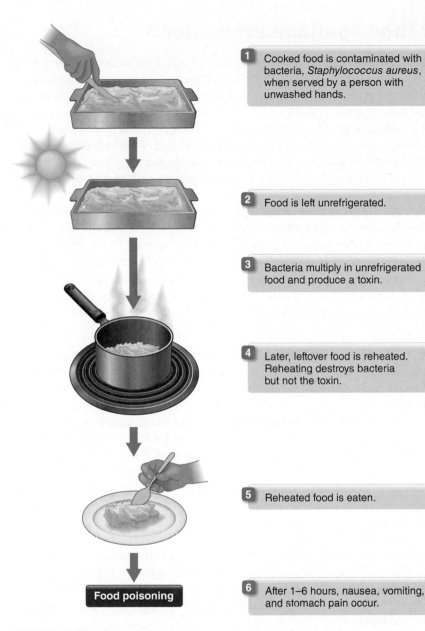

1. Cooked food is contaminated with bacteria, *Staphylococcus aureus*, when served by a person with unwashed hands.

2. Food is left unrefrigerated.

3. Bacteria multiply in unrefrigerated food and produce a toxin.

4. Later, leftover food is reheated. Reheating destroys bacteria but not the toxin.

5. Reheated food is eaten.

Food poisoning

6. After 1–6 hours, nausea, vomiting, and stomach pain occur.

FIGURE 15.10 Food contamination can occur long after the microorganism itself has been destroyed.

When planning a trip, tell your physician your travel plans and ask about vaccinations you need or any medications you should take along in case you get sick. Pack a waterless antibacterial hand cleanser and use it frequently. When dining, choose cooked foods and bottled and canned beverages or tea or coffee made with boiling water (see Chapter 3). All raw food has the potential for contamination.

RECAP

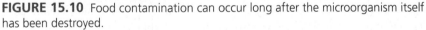

Foodborne illness can be prevented at home by following four tips: (1) Clean: wash your hands and kitchen surfaces often. (2) Separate: isolate foods to prevent cross-contamination. (3) Chill: store foods in the refrigerator or freezer (4) Cook: heat foods long enough and at the correct temperatures to ensure proper cooking. When eating out, avoid restaurants that don't look clean, and ask that all food be cooked thoroughly. ∎

LO 5 Compare and contrast the various methods manufacturers use to preserve foods.

How Is Food Spoilage Prevented?

Any food that has been harvested and that people aren't ready to eat must be preserved in some way or, before long, it will degrade enzymatically and become home to a variety of microorganisms. Even processed foods—foods that are manipulated mechanically or chemically—have the potential to spoil.

The most ancient methods of preserving foods are salting, sugaring, drying, and smoking, all of which draw the water out of plant or animal cells. By dehydrating the food, these methods make it inhospitable to microorganisms and dramatically slow the action of enzymes that would otherwise degrade the food. We still use many of these methods today to preserve and prepare foods and meats, such as salted or smoked fish ham.

Natural methods of cooling have also been used for centuries, including storing foods in underground cellars, caves, running streams, and even "cold pantries"—north-facing rooms of the house that were kept dark and unheated, often stocked with ice. The forerunner of the modern refrigerator—the miniature icehouse, or icebox—was developed in the early 1800s, and in cities and towns a local iceman would make rounds delivering ice to homes.

More recently, technological advances have helped food producers preserve the integrity of their products for months and even years between harvesting and consumption:

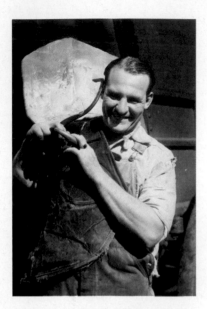

Before the modern refrigerator, an "iceman" would deliver ice to homes and businesses.

pasteurization A form of sterilization using high temperatures for short periods of time.

irradiation A sterilization process in which food is exposed to gamma rays or high-energy electron beams to kill microorganisms. Irradiation does not impart any radiation to the food being treated.

- *Canning.* Developed in the late 1700s, canning involves washing and blanching food, placing it in cans, siphoning out the air, sealing the cans, and then heating them to a very high temperature. Canned food has an average shelf life of at least 2 years from the date of purchase.
- *Pasteurization.* The technique called **pasteurization** exposes a beverage or other food to heat high enough to destroy microorganisms, but for a short enough period of time that the taste and quality of the food are not affected. For example, in flash pasteurization, milk or other liquids are heated to 162°F (72°C) for 15 seconds.
- *Aseptic packaging.* You probably know aseptic packaging best as "juice boxes." Food and beverages are first heated, then cooled, then placed in sterile containers. The process uses less energy and materials than traditional canning, and the average shelf life is about 6 months.
- *Modified atmosphere packaging.* In this process, the oxygen in a package of food is replaced with an inert gas, such as nitrogen or carbon dioxide. This prevents a number of chemical reactions that spoil food, and it slows the growth of bacteria that require oxygen. The process can be used with a variety of foods, including meats, fish, vegetables, and fruits.
- *High-pressure processing.* In this technique, the food to be preserved is subjected to an extremely high pressure, which inactivates most bacteria while retaining the food's quality and freshness.
- *Irradiation.* The **irradiation** process exposes foods to gamma rays from radioactive metals. Energy from the rays penetrates food and its packaging, killing or disabling microorganisms in the food. The process does not cause foods to become radioactive! A few nutrients, including thiamin and vitamins A, E, and K, are lost, but these losses are also incurred in conventional processing and preparation. Although irradiated food has been shown to be safe, the FDA requires that all irradiated foods be labeled with a Radura symbol and a caution against irradiating the food again (**Figure 15.11**).

FIGURE 15.11 The U.S. Food and Drug Administration requires the Radura—the international symbol of irradiated food—to be displayed on all irradiated food sold in the United States.

RECAP

Salting, sugaring, drying, smoking, and cooling have been used for centuries to preserve food. Canning, pasteurization, irradiation, and several packaging techniques are used to preserve a variety of foods during shipping, as well as on grocer and consumer shelves.

What Are Food Additives, and Are They Safe?

LO 6 Debate the safety of food additives, including the role of the GRAS list.

Have you ever picked up a loaf of bread and started reading its ingredients? You'd expect to see flour, yeast, water, and some sugar, but what are all those other items? They are collectively called *food additives*, and they are in almost every processed food. **Food additives** are not foods in themselves but, rather, natural or synthetic chemicals added to foods to enhance them in some way. More than 3,000 different food additives are currently used in the United States. **Table 15.3** (page 608) identifies only a few of the most common.

Food Additives Include Nutrients and Preservatives

Vitamins and minerals are added to foods as nutrients and as preservatives. Vitamin E is usually added to fat-based products to keep them from going rancid, and vitamin C is used as an antioxidant in many foods. Iodine is added to table salt to help decrease the incidence of goiter, a condition that causes the thyroid gland to enlarge. Vitamin D is added to milk, and calcium is added to soy milk, rice milk, almond milk, and some juices to help preserve healthy bone. Folate is added to cereals, breads, and other foods to help prevent neural tube defects, a type of birth defect associated with low folate intake. Many cereals and breads are also fortified with iron.

The following two preservatives have raised health concerns:

- *Sulfites*. A small segment of the population is sensitive to sulfites, preservatives used in many beers and wines and some other processed foods. These people can experience asthma, headaches, or other symptoms after eating food containing the offending preservatives.
- *Nitrites*. Commonly used to preserve processed meats, nitrites can be converted to nitrosamines during the cooking process. Nitrosamines have been found to be carcinogenic in animals, so the FDA has required all foods with nitrites to contain additional antioxidants to decrease the formation of nitrosamines.

Other Food Additives Include Flavorings, Colorings, and Other Agents

Flavoring agents are used to replace the natural flavors lost during food processing. In contrast, *flavor enhancers* have little or no flavor of their own but accentuate the natural flavor of foods. One of the most common flavor enhancers is monosodium glutamate (MSG). In some people, MSG causes symptoms such as headaches, difficulty breathing, and heart palpitations.

Common food *colorings* include beet juice, which imparts a red color; beta-carotene, which gives a yellow color; and caramel, which adds brown color. The coloring tartrazine (FD&C Yellow #5) causes an allergic reaction in some people, and its use must be indicated on the product packaging.

Texturizers are added to foods to improve their texture. *Emulsifiers* help keep fats evenly dispersed within foods. *Stabilizers* give foods "body" and help them maintain a desired texture or color. *Humectants* keep foods such as marshmallows, chewing gum, and shredded coconut moist and stretchy. *Desiccants* prevent the absorption of moisture from the air; for example, they are used to prevent table salt from forming clumps.[22]

Nutrition MILESTONE

In **1859**, French chemist and microbiologist Louis Pasteur boiled a meat broth in a flask that had a long, slender, curved neck that allowed air, but not dust, access to the broth. The flask remained free of contamination by microorganisms. However, when the neck of the flask was changed so that dust could enter, the broth quickly became contaminated. This experiment disproved a belief held for 2,000 years that life could arise spontaneously from inanimate matter. Just 3 years later, in 1862, Pasteur showed that the growth of microorganisms is responsible for spoiling beverages such as beer, wine, and milk. He heated milk to a very high temperature, theorizing that the heat would kill any microorganisms present. The experiment was a success, and the technique, called pasteurization, bears his name.

food additive A substance or mixture of substances intentionally put into food to enhance its appearance, safety, palatability, and quality.

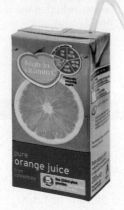

Aseptic packaging allows foods to be stored unrefrigerated for several months without spoilage.

TABLE 15.3 Examples of Common Food Additives

Food Additive	Foods Found In
Coloring Agents	
Beet extract	Beverages, candies, ice cream
Beta-carotene	Beverages, sauces, soups, baked goods, candies, macaroni and cheese mixes
Caramel	Beverages, sauces, soups, baked goods
Tartrazine	Beverages, cakes and cookies, ice cream
Preservatives	
Alpha-tocopherol (vitamin E)	Vegetable oils
Ascorbic acid (vitamin C)	Breakfast cereals, cured meats, fruit drinks
BHA	Breakfast cereals, chewing gum, oils, potato chips
BHT	Breakfast cereals, chewing gum, oils, potato chips
Calcium proprionate/sodium proprionate	Bread, cakes, pies, rolls
EDTA	Beverages, canned shellfish, margarine, mayonnaise, processed fruits and vegetables, sandwich spreads
Propyl gallate	Mayonnaise, chewing gum, chicken soup base, vegetable oils, meat products, potato products, fruits, ice cream
Sodium benzoate	Carbonated beverages, fruit juice, pickles, preserves
Sodium chloride (salt)	Most processed foods
Sodium nitrate/sodium nitrite	Bacon, corned beef, lunch meats, smoked fish
Sorbic acid/potassium sorbate	Cakes, cheese, dried fruits, jellies, syrups, wine
Sulfites (sodium bisulfite, sulfur dioxide)	Dried fruits, processed potatoes, wine
Texturizers, Emulsifiers, and Stabilizers	
Calcium chloride	Canned fruits and vegetables
Carageenan/pectin	Ice cream, chocolate milk, soy milk, frostings, jams, jellies, cheese, salad dressings, sour cream, puddings, syrups
Cellulose gum/guar gum/gum arabic/locust gum/xanthan gum	Soups and sauces, gravies, sour cream, ricotta cheese, ice cream, syrups
Gelatin	Desserts, canned meats
Lecithin	Mayonnaise, ice cream
Humectants	
Glycerin	Chewing gum, marshmallows, shredded coconut
Propylene glycol	Chewing gum, gummy candies

Are Food Additives Safe?

Federal legislation was passed in 1958 to regulate food additives. The Delaney Clause, also enacted in 1958, states, "No additive may be permitted in any amount if tests show that it produces cancer when fed to man or animals or by other appropriate tests." Before a new additive can be used in food, the producer of the additive must demonstrate its safety to the FDA by submitting data on its reasonable safety. The FDA determines the additive's safety based on these data.

Also in 1958, the U.S. Congress recognized that many substances added to foods would not require this type of formal review by the FDA prior to marketing and use, as their safety had already been established through long-term use or because their safety had been recognized by qualified experts through scientific studies. These substances are exempt from the more stringent testing criteria for new food additives and are referred to as substances that are **Generally Recognized as Safe (GRAS).** The GRAS list identifies substances that either have been tested and determined by the FDA to be safe and approved for use in the food industry or are deemed safe as a result of consensus among experts qualified by scientific training and experience.

In 1985, the FDA established the Adverse Reaction Monitoring System (ARMS). Under this system, the FDA investigates complaints from consumers, physicians, and food companies about food additives. The GRAS list is not static; in 2015, for example, the FDA determined that partially hydrogenated oils (PHOs), the main source of *trans* fatty acids in the U.S. diet, are no longer GRAS. Food companies were given until June, 2018, to comply, after which time they will no longer be allowed to produce foods containing PHOs.

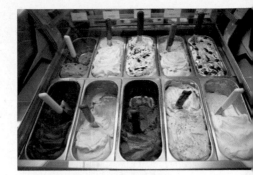

Many foods, such as ice cream, contain colorings.

RECAP

Food additives are chemicals intentionally added to foods to enhance their color, flavor, texture, nutrient density, moisture level, or shelf life. Although there is continuing controversy over food additives in the United States, the FDA regulates additives used in our food supply and considers safe those it approves. ◼

How Is Genetic Modification Used in Food Production?

In **genetic modification,** also referred to as *genetic engineering*, the genetic material, or DNA, of an organism is altered to bring about specific changes in its seeds or offspring. Selective breeding is one example of genetic modification; for example, Brahman cattle, which have poor-quality meat but high resistance to heat and humidity, are bred with English shorthorn cattle, which have good meat but low resistance to heat and humidity. The outcome of this selective breeding process is Santa Gertrudis cattle, which have the desired characteristics of higher-quality meat and resistance to heat and humidity. Although selective breeding is effective and has helped increase crop yields and improve the quality and quantity of our food supply, it is a relatively slow and imprecise process, because a great deal of trial and error typically occurs before the desired characteristics are achieved.

Advances in biotechnology have moved genetic modification beyond selective breeding. These advances include the manipulation of the DNA of living cells of one organism to produce the desired characteristics of a different organism. Called **recombinant DNA technology,** the process commonly begins when scientists isolate from an animal, a plant, or a microbial cell a particular segment of DNA—one or more genes—that codes for a protein conferring a desirable trait, such as salt tolerance in tomato plants (**Figure 15.12**). Scientists then splice the DNA into a "host cell," usually a microorganism. The cell is cultured to produce many copies—a *gene library*—of the beneficial gene. Then, many scientists can readily obtain the gene to modify other organisms that lack the desired trait—for example, traditional tomato plants. The modified DNA causes the plant's cells to

LO 7 Identify five steps in recombinant DNA technology and the five most common reasons that crops are genetically modified in the United States.

Generally Recognized as Safe (GRAS) A list established by Congress to identify substances used in foods that are generally recognized as safe based on a history of long-term use or on the consensus of qualified research experts.

genetic modification The process of changing an organism by manipulating its genetic material.

recombinant DNA technology A type of genetic modification in which scientists combine DNA from different sources to produce a transgenic organism that expresses a desired trait.

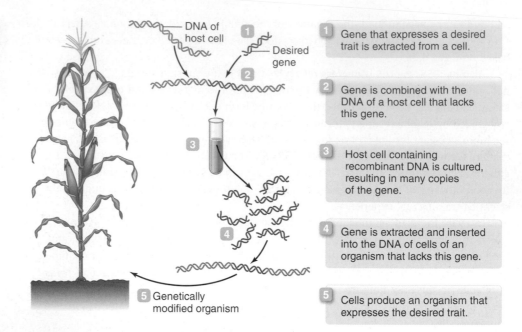

1. Gene that expresses a desired trait is extracted from a cell.

2. Gene is combined with the DNA of a host cell that lacks this gene.

3. Host cell containing recombinant DNA is cultured, resulting in many copies of the gene.

4. Gene is extracted and inserted into the DNA of cells of an organism that lacks this gene.

5. Cells produce an organism that expresses the desired trait.

FIGURE 15.12 Recombinant DNA technology involves producing plants and other organisms that contain modified DNA, which enables them to express desirable traits that are not present in the original organism.

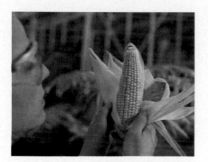

Corn is one of the most widely cultivated genetically modified crops.

build the protein of interest, and the plant expresses the desired trait. The term *genetically modified organism* (*GMO*) refers to any organism in which the DNA has been altered using recombinant DNA technology.

Cultivation of GMO food crops began in 1996. In the United States, the most common genetic modification in food crops induces tolerance to herbicides, chemicals that kill weeds. Herbicide-tolerant crops (HT GMOs) can be sprayed liberally with chemicals that previously would have destroyed the crops themselves.[23] The second most common genetic modification induces insect resistance by inserting the gene from the soil bacterium Bt (*Bacillus thuringiensis*). The Bt gene codes for the assembly of a protein that is toxic to specific insects, protecting the plant throughout its lifespan.[23] Genetic modification can also increase a plant's resistance to disease or make crops more tolerant of challenging environmental conditions such as drought or poor soil. Another use is to increase the nutritional value of a crop. Researchers have modified soybeans and canola, for instance, to increase their content of monounsaturated fatty acids, and a beta-carotene enriched rice called Golden Rice is currently under development.

Since 1996, an increasing number and quantity of food crops have been genetically modified. The most common are corn and soybeans. The USDA reports that, in 2014, 89% of all corn crops and 94% of all soybean crops grown in the United States were HT GMOs, and a great majority of these crops were Bt modified as well.[23] As the use of genetic modification increases, however, some environmental scientists and public health experts have become increasingly concerned about evidence of its risks to the surrounding ecology and even to human health. For more information on this controversy, see the **Nutrition Myth or Fact?** essay at the end of this chapter.

RECAP

In genetic modification, the genetic material, or DNA, of an organism is altered to enhance certain qualities. The process is called recombinant DNA technology, and begins when scientists isolate from an animal, a plant, or a microbial cell a particular segment of DNA—one or more genes—that codes for a protein conferring a desirable trait. In U.S. agriculture, genetic modification is most often used to induce herbicide tolerance and insect resistance. It may also be used to boost a crop's protection from disease or ability to grow in challenging conditions. It is sometimes used to increase nutrients in the resulting food. As the use of genetic modification increases, evidence of its environmental and health risks is increasing as well. ■

How Do Residues Harm Our Food Supply?

Food **residues** are chemicals that remain in foods despite cleaning and processing. Residues of global concern include persistent organic pollutants, pesticides, and the hormones and antibiotics used in animals. The health concerns related to residues include nerve damage, disorders of the reproductive system, cancer, and the development of antibiotic-resistant pathogenic bacteria.

LO 8 Describe the process by which persistent organic pollutants accumulate in foods.

LO 9 Discuss the potential health concerns associated with residues from heavy metals, plasticizers, dioxins, PFASs, pesticides, growth hormones, and antibiotics.

Persistent Organic Pollutants Can Cause Illness

Some chemicals released into the atmosphere as a result of industry, agriculture, automobile emissions, and improper waste disposal can persist in soil or water for years or even decades. These chemicals, collectively referred to as **persistent organic pollutants (POPs),** can travel thousands of miles in gases or as airborne particles, in rain, snow, rivers, and oceans, eventually entering the food supply through the soil or water.[24] If a pollutant gets into the soil, a plant can absorb the chemical into its structure and pass it on as part of the food chain. Animals can also absorb the pollutant into their tissues or consume it when feeding on plants growing in the polluted soil. Fat-soluble pollutants are especially problematic, as they tend to accumulate in the animal's body tissues in ever-greater concentrations as they move up the food chain. This process is called **biomagnification.** The POPs are then absorbed by humans when the animal is used as a food source (**Figure 15.13**, page 612).

POP residues have been found in virtually all categories of foods, including baked goods, fruit, vegetables, meat, poultry, fish, and dairy products. Significant levels have been detected all over the Earth, even in pristine regions of the Arctic thousands of miles from any known source.[24]

Health Risks of POPs

POPs are a health concern because of their range of harmful effects on the body. Some are neurotoxins. Many others are carcinogens. Still others act as *endocrine disruptors*, chemicals thought to interfere with the body's endocrine glands and their production of hormones. As you know, hormones play roles in a vast number of body processes, but endocrine disruptors are particularly associated with developmental problems, reproductive system disorders, nerve disorders, and impaired immune function.[27] They disrupt normal body processes by blocking the binding sites for natural hormones on body cells; mimicking natural hormones and thereby augmenting their actions; or altering the synthesis or metabolism of natural hormones.[27]

Some pesticides leave residues that qualify as POPs. These include DDT, a pesticide banned in phases between 1969 and 1972 but still present in the environment.[24] DDT and certain other pesticides can act as neurotoxins, carcinogens, and endocrine disruptors. Pesticides are discussed shortly.

residues Chemicals that remain in foods despite cleaning and processing.

persistent organic pollutants (POPs) Chemicals released as a result of human activity into the environment, where they persist for years or decades.

biomagnification The process by which persistent organic pollutants become more concentrated in animal tissues as they move from one creature to another through the food chain.

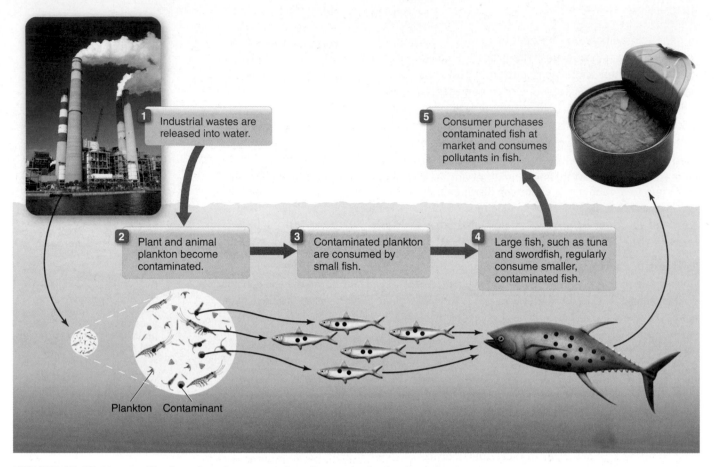

FIGURE 15.13 Biomagnification of persistent organic pollutants in the food supply.

Heavy Metals

Mercury, a naturally occurring heavy metal element, is found in soil, rocks, and water. It is also released into the air by pulp and paper processing and the burning of garbage and fossil fuels. As mercury falls from the air, it finds its way to streams, rivers, lakes, and the ocean, where it accumulates. Fish absorb mercury as they feed on aquatic organisms, and this mercury is passed on to us when we consume the fish. As mercury accumulates in the body, it has a toxic effect on the nervous system, prompting memory loss and mood swings, as well as impaired vision, hearing, speech, and movement.[25]

Large predatory fish, such as swordfish, shark, king mackerel, and tilefish, tend to contain the highest levels of mercury.[25] Because mercury is especially toxic to the developing nervous system of fetuses and growing children, pregnant and breastfeeding women and young children are advised to entirely avoid eating these types of fish. Canned light tuna, salmon, cod, pollock, sole, shrimp, mussels, and scallops do not contain high levels of mercury and are safe to consume; however, the FDA and EPA recommend that pregnant women and young children eat no more than two servings (12 oz) per week of low-mercury fish.[25]

Lead is another heavy metal of concern. It can be found naturally in the soil, water, and air, but also occurs as industrial waste from leaded gasoline, lead-based paints, and lead-soldered cans, now outlawed but decomposing in landfills. Older homes may have

For a portable guide to safe seafood consumption, visit the Natural Resources Defense Council at www.nrdc.org. In the search bar, type "mercury in fish wallet card" and click on the link.

high levels of lead paint dust, or the lead paint may be peeling in chips, which young children may put it their mouths. Some old ceramic mugs and other dishes are fired with lead-based glaze, allowing residues to build up in foods. No amount of lead is safe. Exposure can cause decreased IQ, serious learning and behavioral disorders, and hearing impairment in children and decreased fertility, nerve disorders, and cardiovascular and kidney disease in adults.[26]

Plasticizers

Chemicals added to paint, varnish, cements, and plastics to increase their workability are collectively known as plasticizers. Two plasticizers found in plastic food containers can leach into foods and act as endocrine disruptors. A chemical called *bisphenol A (BPA)* is routinely used in the linings of canned foods and in some plastic food packaging. BPA is a form of synthetic estrogen, a female reproductive hormone, and research has linked it to genital abnormalities, breast and prostate cancer, miscarriage, reduced sperm count, hypertension[27] and heart disease, and even diabetes.[28] *Phthalates* are a large group of plasticizers that are found in plastic food packaging, shampoos, carpeting and vinyl flooring, pesticides, and many other products. They're also found in dairy products, meats, and drinking water. Phthalates have been linked to reproductive-system and developmental disorders, especially in male infants, shortened pregnancy, and reduced sperm quality in men.[28,29]

Here are some recommendations for consumers who want to limit their exposure to BPA and phthalates:[30]

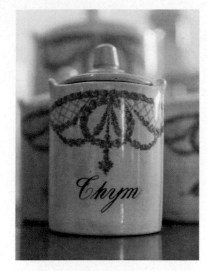

Antique porcelain is often coated with lead-based glaze.

- Reduce your consumption of canned foods.
- Avoid purchasing food in plastic containers with the recycling codes 3 or 7. These plastics may contain BPA or phthalates.
- Do not microwave foods in these containers or use them to hold hot foods or beverages. They are more likely to leach endocrine disruptors when they become heated.
- Whenever possible, choose glass, porcelain, or stainless steel containers.

Dioxins

Dioxins are both carcinogens and endocrine disruptors. These industrial pollutants are typically formed as a result of combustion processes, such as waste incineration or the burning of wood, coal, or oil. Dioxins enter the soil and can persist in the environment for many years. There is concern that long-term exposure to dioxins can result in an increased risk for cancer, heart disease, diabetes, reproductive system disorders, and other disorders.[31] Because dioxins easily accumulate in the fatty tissues of animals, most dioxin exposure in humans occurs through dietary intake of animal fats.[31] To reduce your exposure to dioxins, eat meat less frequently, trim the fat from the meats you consume, and avoid fatty meats. Choose nonfat milk and yogurt, and low-fat cheeses, and replace butter with plant oils.

Polyfluorinated Chemicals

Concern has also been increasing about persistent residues from poly- and perfluoroalkyl substances (PFASs) that degrade very slowly and have been found all over the globe, including in the tissues of animals and humans. PFASs are used to limit leaking and staining in many commercial products, including pizza boxes, fast food wrappers, and microwave popcorn bags. They have been associated with organ damage, cancer, endocrine disorders, and other health problems.

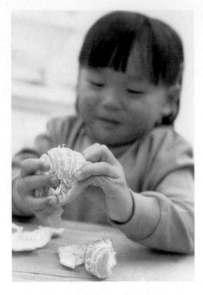

Peeling a fruit reduces its level of pesticide residue; however, you should still scrub fruits before peeling.

Pesticides Protect Against Crop Losses—But at a Cost

Pesticides are a family of chemicals used in both fields and farm storage areas to decrease the destruction and crop losses caused by weeds, animals, insects, and fungi and other microorganisms. They increase overall crop yield and allow for greater crop diversity. The three most common types of pesticides used in food production are

- *herbicides*, which are used to control weeds and other unwanted plant growth;
- *insecticides*, which are used to control insects that can infest crops; and
- *fungicides*, which are used to control plant-destroying fungal growth.

Some pesticides used today have a low impact on the environment and are not considered harmful to human health. These include **biopesticides,** which are species-specific and work to suppress a pest's population, not eliminate it. For example, pheromones are a biopesticide that disrupts insect mating by attracting males into traps. Biopesticides also do not leave residues on crops—most degrade rapidly and are easily washed away with water.

In contrast, pesticides made from petroleum-based products can persist in the environment, polluting soils, water, plants, and animals. They can also harm agricultural workers and consumers, acting as neurotoxins, carcinogens, and endocrine disruptors. In 2015, the World Health Organization's International Agency for Research on Cancer classified the herbicide glyphosate (commonly known as Roundup) and the insecticides malathion and diazinon as probable carcinogens.[32] Moreover, the 2014 update of the Agricultural Health Study, a joint effort of the National Cancer Institute, EPA, and other federal agencies, found a link between certain pesticides and an increased risk for an aggressive form of prostate cancer.[33] In 2012, the American Academy of Pediatrics published a report describing the harmful effects of pesticides on children, including pediatric cancers, decreased cognitive function, and behavioral problems, and recommending that families strictly limit their exposure.[34]

The EPA is responsible for regulating the labeling, sale, distribution, use, and disposal of all pesticides in the United States. Before a pesticide can be accepted by the EPA for use, it must be determined that it performs its intended function with minimal impact to the environment. Once the EPA has certified a pesticide, states can set their own regulations for its use. The EPA offers the following strategies for reducing your level of exposure to pesticides.[35]

- Wash and scrub all fresh fruits and vegetables thoroughly under running water.
- Peel fruits and vegetables whenever possible, and discard the outer leaves of leafy vegetables, such as cabbage and lettuce. Trim the excess fat from meat and remove the skin from poultry and fish because some pesticide residues collect in the fat.
- Eat a variety of foods from various sources, as this can reduce the risk of exposure to a single pesticide.

You can also reduce your exposure to pesticides by choosing organic foods, as discussed shortly.

Growth Hormones and Antibiotics Are Used in Animals

Introduced in the U.S. food supply in 1994, **recombinant bovine growth hormone (rBGH)** is a genetically engineered growth hormone. It is used in beef herds to induce animals to grow more muscle tissue and less fat. It is also injected into a third of U.S. dairy cows to increase milk output.

Although the FDA has allowed the use of rBGH in the United States, both Canada and the European Union have banned its use for two reasons:

- The available evidence shows an increased risk for mastitis (inflamed udders), in dairy cows injected with rBGH.[36] Farmers treat mastitis with antibiotics, promoting the development of strains of pathogenic bacteria that are resistant to antibiotics.

pesticides Chemicals used either in the field or in storage to decrease destruction and crop losses by weeds, predators, or disease.

biopesticides Primarily insecticides, these chemicals use natural methods to reduce damage to crops.

recombinant bovine growth hormone (rBGH) A genetically engineered hormone injected into dairy cows to enhance their milk output.

- The milk of cows receiving rBGH has higher levels of a hormone called insulin-like growth factor (IGF-1). This hormone can pass into the bloodstream of humans who drink milk from cows that receive rBGH, and some studies have suggested that an elevated level of IGF-1 in humans may increase the risk for certain cancers. However, the evidence from these studies is inconclusive.[36]

The American Cancer Society suggests that more research is needed to help better appraise these health risks. In the meantime, consumer concerns about rBGH have caused a decline in rBGH injection in cows to below 20%.[36]

Antibiotics are also routinely given to animals raised for food. For example, they are added to the feed of swine to reduce the number of disease outbreaks in overcrowded pork-production facilities. Many researchers are concerned that cows, pigs, chickens, and other animals treated with antibiotics are becoming significant reservoirs for the development of virulent antibiotic-resistant strains of bacteria—so-called "superbugs." Recent federal testing of supermarket meats found that 39% of chicken products, 55% of ground beef, 69% of pork, and 81% of ground turkey harbored significant amounts of superbug bacteria.[37] A particularly dangerous superbug, methicillin-resistant *Staphylococcus aureus* (MRSA), is commonly resident in swine, and about 2% of the U.S. population has been infected.[38] This superbug cannot be killed with common antibiotics, including methicillin, penicillin, and amoxicillin. Infection with MRSA can cause symptoms ranging from a fever and skin rash to widespread invasion of tissues, including the bloodstream. MRSA blood infections are sometimes fatal.[38]

Because of concerns about the risk of antibiotic use in animals promoting the spread of antibiotic-resistant infections in humans, in 2013, the FDA began implementing voluntary restrictions to phase out the use of certain antibiotics in food production. They are no longer allowed to increase an animal's growth, but are still allowed for prevention and treatment of disease.

You can reduce your exposure to growth hormones and antibiotics by choosing organic eggs, milk, yogurt, and cheeses and by eating free-range meat from animals raised without the use of these chemicals. You can also reduce your risk by eating vegetarian and vegan meals more often.

The resistant strain of bacteria responsible for methicillin-resistant *Staphylococcus aureus* (MRSA).

RECAP

Foodborne persistent organic pollutants (POPs) of greatest concern include the heavy metals mercury and lead, plasticizers, dioxins, and PFASs. Pesticides are used to prevent or reduce food crop losses; however, they too can persist in the environment. POPs and some pesticides can act as neurotoxins, carcinogens, or endocrine disruptors; therefore, it is essential to take action to reduce your exposure. The use of recombinant bovine growth hormone (rBGH) has been associated with harm to dairy cows and a possible risk for cancer in humans; however, the research on rBGH is currently inconclusive. The use of—and residues from—antibiotics in animals raised for food increases the U.S. population's risk for antibiotic-resistant infections. ■

Are Organic Foods Worth the Cost?

LO 10 Identify the key characteristics of organic foods, and compare their nutrient and residue levels with those of foods conventionally grown.

In the population boom that followed the end of World War II, the demand for food increased dramatically. The American chemical industry helped increase agricultural production by providing a variety of new fertilizers and pesticides, including an insecticide called DDT, which began poisoning not just insects but also fish and birds from the time it was first released for agricultural use in 1945. Then, in 1962, marine biologist Rachel Carson published *Silent Spring*, a book in which she described the harmful effects of DDT and other synthetic pesticides. The book's title referred to the effect of pesticides on songbirds, whose extinction would someday lead to a "silent spring." Scientists found Carson's research convincing, and readers flocked to her cause, creating a small but ever-growing demand for organic food.

The USDA defines the term *organic* as crops, livestock, and multiple-ingredient foods that are produced in a way that protects natural resources, conserves biodiversity, and uses only approved substances. Specifically, organic producers cannot use: irradiation, sewage sludge, synthetic fertilizers, prohibited pesticides, GMOs, growth hormones, or antibiotics. Animals must be fed 100% organic feed and have access to the outdoors.[39]

Between 1990 and 2013, sales of organic products in the United States skyrocketed from $1 billion to over $35 billion.[40] A recent national survey indicates that 81% of United States families purchase organic foods at least sometimes; however, 51% of families said that the higher cost of these foods was one factor limiting their organic purchases. In fact, families who regularly purchase organic foods spend an average of $15 a week more on groceries than families who don't buy organic items.[40] So it's reasonable to ask: Are organic foods worth the cost?

To Be Labeled Organic, Foods Must Meet Federal Standards

In 2002, the National Organic Program (NOP) of the USDA established organic standards that provide uniform definitions for all organic products. Any product claiming to be organic must comply with the following definitions:

- *100% organic:* products containing only organically produced ingredients, excluding water and salt
- *Organic:* products containing 95% organically produced ingredients by weight, excluding water and salt, with the remaining ingredients consisting of those products not commercially available in organic form
- *Made with organic ingredients:* a product containing more than 70% organic ingredients

If a processed product contains less than 70% organically produced ingredients, those products cannot use the term *organic* in the principal display panel, but ingredients that are organically produced can be specified on the ingredients statement on the information panel. Products that are "100% organic" and "organic" may display the USDA organic seal (**Figure 15.14**).

Farms certified as organic must pass an inspection by a government-approved certifier, who verifies that the farmer is following all USDA organic standards.[39] Organic farming methods are strict and require farmers to find natural alternatives to many common problems, such as weeds and insects. Contrary to common belief, organic farmers can use pesticides as a final option for pest control when all other methods have failed or are known to be ineffective, but they are restricted to a limited number that have been approved for use. Organic farmers emphasize the use of renewable resources and the conservation of soil and water. Once a crop is harvested, a winter crop (usually a legume) is planted to help fix nitrogen in the soil and decrease erosion, which also lessens the need for fertilizers.

Organic meat, poultry, eggs, and dairy products come from animals fed only organic feed, and if the animals become ill, they are removed from the others until well again. None of these animals are given growth hormones or antibiotics to increase their size or ability to produce milk.

Organic Foods Are Safer but Not Necessarily More Nutritious

Over the past few decades, hundreds of studies have attempted to compare the nutrient levels of organic foods to those of foods conventionally grown. The results have been inconclusive. For example, two large review studies published in 2011 and 2012 reached opposite conclusions on this issue, one finding consistently higher levels of nutrients in organic produce, and the other finding no nutritional advantage.[41,42] Then, in 2013, a national study found 62% more omega-3 fatty acids in organic milk as compared to conventional milk,[43] and in 2014, a comprehensive review concluded that organically grown produce does have a higher level of antioxidant nutrients and phytochemicals.[44]

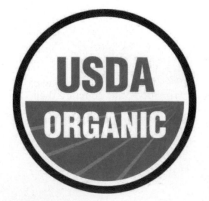

FIGURE 15.14 The USDA organic seal identifies foods that are at least 95% organic.

Many people choose organic foods because of concerns about their exposure to pesticide residues, and indeed, two of the studies just mentioned found that organically produced foods were about 30% less likely to be contaminated with detectable pesticide residues or antibiotic-resistant bacteria.[42,44] In addition, researchers for the American Academy of Pediatrics recently reviewed all available evidence on organic foods and concluded that "Organic diets have been convincingly demonstrated to expose consumers to fewer pesticides associated with human disease."[45]

Do you think organic foods are worth the extra cost? If you do, but you're on a budget, a smart strategy is to spend more for organic when the alternative—the conventionally grown version—is likely to retain a high pesticide residue. **Table 15.4** identifies the foods that the Environmental Working Group advises should be your priority organic purchases. If your food budget is limited, spend your money on the organically grown versions of these foods. The table also identifies the fifteen foods that tend to be lowest in pesticide residues. You can feel confident purchasing conventional versions of these.

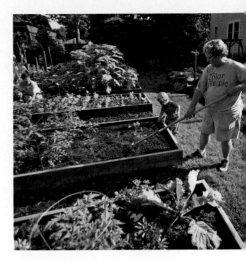

Modified farming techniques, such as using raised beds, enable urban and suburban residents to grow their own fruits and vegetables.

RECAP

The USDA regulates organic farming standards and inspects and certifies farms that follow all USDA organic standards. Organic producers cannot use: irradiation, sewage sludge, synthetic fertilizers, prohibited pesticides, GMOs, growth hormones, or antibiotics. Animals must be fed 100% organic feed, and have access to the outdoors. Products bearing the USDA organic seal contain at least 95% organically produced ingredients by weight, excluding water and salt, with the remaining ingredients consisting of those products not commercially available in organic form. Studies of the nutritional benefits of organic versus conventionally grown foods have been inconclusive; however, organic foods have been shown to be lower in pesticide residues and antibiotic-resistant bacteria. ◼

TABLE 15.4 The Environmental Working Group's 2015 Shopper's Guide to Pesticides in Produce

The Dirty Dozen + Buy these organic	The Clean Fifteen Lowest in Pesticides
Apples	Asparagus
Celery	Avocados
Cherry tomatoes	Cabbage
Cucumbers	Cantaloupe
Grapes	Cauliflower
Nectarines	Eggplant
Peaches	Grapefruit
Potatoes	Kiwi
Snap peas	Mangoes
Spinach	Onions
Strawberries	Papayas
Sweet bell peppers	Pineapples
+ Hot peppers	Sweet corn
+ Kale	Sweet peas (frozen)
+ Collard greens	Sweet potatoes

+Although they don't make the "Dirty Dozen" list, these foods are commonly contaminated with residues particularly toxic to the nervous system.
Source: Environmental Working Group. 2015. EWG's Shopper's Guide to Pesticides in Produce. http://www.ewg.org/foodnews/

Nutrition Myth OR Fact?

Genetically Modified Organisms: A Blessing or a Curse?

Current advances in biotechnology have opened the door to one of the most controversial topics in food science: genetically modified organisms (GMOs). GM foods—foods containing modified genes—are also known as biotech foods and transgenic foods. Since their introduction in 1994, hundreds of GM foods have been incorporated into our global market. In 2014, nearly 450 million acres of GM crops were grown in 28 countries worldwide.[1]

Benefits Cited for GM Foods

Many agricultural experts support GM foods, citing numerous benefits resulting from the application of this technology:[1–4]

- GM crops grow faster and have average yields 22% higher than conventional crops. Crops have been engineered for drought-tolerance, salt-tolerance, and other characteristics that enable them to thrive in challenging climates.

- The global adoption of GM crops has decreased chemical pesticide use overall by 37%.

- Cultivation of GM crops has had other environmentally responsible outcomes, as well. These include conservation of water due largely to the development of drought-tolerant species of corn, reduced use of energy and emission of greenhouse gases because of reduced need for ploughing and pesticide spraying, and soil conservation due to higher productivity on arable land.

- GM crops can be produced with enhanced taste and nutritional quality, as well as attributes such as improved digestibility and lower levels of carcinogens.

- Farmer profits have increased by an average of 50% in both developed and developing countries, on both corporate and family farms, the majority owned by resource-poor farmers.

- Food security for countries struggling with food insecurity and starvation has increased, due to the increased income of small farmers, higher crop yields, and production of GM food crops with greater resistance to challenging environmental conditions.

Potential Risks of GM Foods

Despite these benefits, there is significant opposition to genetic engineering. Detractors cite a wide range of concerns related to health risks, environmental hazards, and economic instability.

Health Risks

In 2014, the World Health Organization (WHO) identified three primary health concerns of GM foods:[5]

- *Allergenicity.* Theoretically, the transfer of genes from organisms with commonly allergenic proteins—such as fractions of wheat or soy—to nonallergenic organisms

could occur. This could prompt allergic reactions in susceptible individuals who consume the food, unaware that it now contains the allergen. However, evaluations of GM foods by the Food and Agricultural Organization (FAO) of the United Nations, as well as the WHO, have not found allergic effects from GM foods currently on the market.

- *Antimicrobial properties.* It is possible that consumption of GM foods containing antibiotic-resistance genes could harm human body cells or the beneficial microbial flora in the GI tract. Although the WHO encourages the use of gene transfer techniques that do not involve antibiotic-resistance genes, the risk remains.

- *Indirect effects on food safety.* Genes have migrated from GM crops to conventional food crops some distance away (e.g., via wind, birds, or insects), and some farmers have deliberately mixed GM and traditional seeds in the same planting. Cases have been reported in which genes from GM crops approved for animal or industrial use were detected in products intended for human consumption. Several countries have adopted strategies to prevent such mixing, including clear separation of GM and conventional fields; however, a considerable amount of research suggests that it remains a concern.[4]

In addition, in 2015, the International Agency for Research on Cancer (IARC), an agency of the WHO, classified the herbicide glyphosate, commercially known as Roundup, and the herbicide in greatest use in GM crops, as a probable carcinogen. The IARC linked glyphosate specifically to an increased risk for non-Hodgkin lymphoma,[6] a cancer that killed nearly 19,000 Americans in 2014, making it the eighth leading cause of cancer death.[7]

Environmental Risks

Environmental scientists have become increasingly concerned about the effects of GM crops on local and global ecologies. We focus on three such concerns here.

- *Loss of biodiversity.* As already noted, unintentional transfer of genes from one crop to another has occurred. Several studies of Mexican maize (corn) over the last fifteen years, for example, have yielded evidence of transgenes in maize crops thought to be both indigenous and organic.[4] And in 2013, an unapproved HT GMO wheat was found on an Oregon farm; to date, researchers have been unable to determine how the contamination occurred.[8] But even the intentional planting of GM crops at the scale now occurring may be reducing species diversity. Still, research into this effect has been inconclusive, and proponents of GMOs point to the fact that, by increasing yield per acre, GM crops reduce the loss of natural habitat to agricultural use, thereby helping to preserve biodiversity.[9]

- *Generation of superweeds.* There is no question that the adoption of HT GMOs—and the liberal application of glyphosate—has led to the generation of *superweeds*; that is, weeds that have evolved a tolerance to herbicides.[4,10] The International Survey of Herbicide-Resistant Weeds has now identified 245 species of superweeds resistant to 156 different herbicides. These weeds have appeared in 66 countries, including in 22 states in the United States.[10] Superweeds can grow faster, taller, and tougher than typical weeds, requiring farmers to apply more toxic pesticides, not only to the weeds themselves, but to the soil prior to planting. In 2014, the EPA released new regulations on pesticide producers to combat the problem of superweeds, but environmental advocacy groups say they do not go far enough to address the crisis.

■ *Threats to other species.* Ecologists have associated the rise in GM crops to the decline in populations of certain species of birds, insects, and other creatures. One of the most commonly cited examples is the 80% decline in the size of the population of monarch butterflies since 1999. Although climate change and other factors almost certainly contribute, researchers point out that the butterfly larvae feed on milkweed, which has greatly declined in agricultural fields in the Midwest coincident with the increased use of glyphosate in conjunction with increased planting of HT GMO corn and soybeans.[11]

Economic Instability

Critics charge that GMOs have introduced the potential for only a few food companies, including Monsanto, the world's largest agricultural biotechnology corporation, to control the majority of world food production. For example, the seed industry has become increasingly dominated by Monsanto, which has bought up smaller seed companies, impeding competition and leading to increased seed prices.

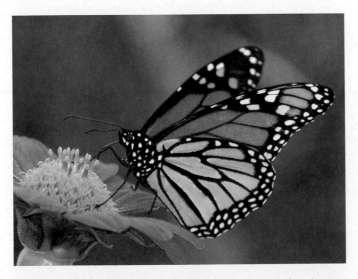

The increased use of glyphosate on HT GMO corn and soybeans has been associated with an 80% decline in the population of monarch butterflies.

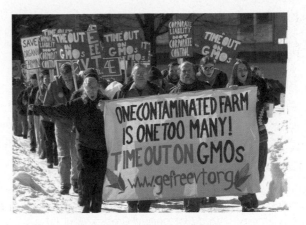

Many people oppose the genetic engineering of foods for environmental, health, or economic reasons.

Regulation of GM Foods

Many who oppose genetic engineering—and some who do not—agree that all GM foods should be labeled, so that consumers know what they are purchasing. The European Union (EU) has long required that GM foods be clearly labeled as such. Not only foods produced for human consumption, but all animal feed products that contain GMOs must be labeled. In addition, any foods that are produced from GM ingredients must be clearly labeled, even if the final food product does not contain the DNA or protein of the original GMO. In contrast, as of 2015, the US Food and Drug Administration did not require such labeling. Thus, the only way for consumers to avoid GM foods is to purchase organic.

The European Union (EU) has other strict regulations regarding GMOs as well. These include mechanisms for tracking GMO products through production and distribution and for monitoring effects on the environment. Currently, only an insect-resistant GM corn is grown commercially in the EU, although in 2015, the EU granted individual countries authority to negotiate directly with biotech firms as long as they adhere to strict risk assessment and monitoring.

Globally, most nations, including the United States, perform rigorous assessments of the quality and safety of GM foods.[5] As the WHO notes, similar evaluations are generally not performed for conventional foods. Thus, although consumers may believe that conventional foods are safe, this is not necessarily the case. As you have read in this chapter, contamination by microorganisms, toxins, and residues can make non-GMO food unsafe as well. The WHO recommends, therefore, that the safety of individual GM foods be assessed on a case-by-case basis, and does not take a specific position on the safety of all GM foods.

The year 2014 marked the 20th anniversary of the introduction of GM foods into the marketplace. As more and more of the world's food supply depends on GM crops, the need for rigorous research into their risks, and the development of effective safeguards to reduce those risks, continues to grow as well.

Critical Thinking Questions

- Do you support the growth of GM crops, both within the United States and around the world? Why or why not?

- Do you think that genetically modified foods should be clearly labeled for consumers?

- Do you have any reservations about buying and consuming genetically modified foods? If so, what are they, and why?

References

1. International Service for the Acquisition of Agri-Biotech Applications (ISAAA). 2014. *Global Status of Commercialized Biotech/GM Crops: 2014*. ISAAA Brief No. 49-2014: Executive summary. Ithaca, NY: ISAAA. www.isaaa.org/resources/publications/briefs/49/executivesummary/default.asp

2. Klumper, W., and M. Qaim. 2014. A meta-analysis of the impacts of genetically modified crops. *PLOS One*, e111629. doi:10.1371/journal.pone.0111629

3. Kathage, J., and M. Qaim. 2012. Economic impacts and impact dynamics of Bt (*Bacillus thuringiensis*) cotton in India. *Proc. Natl. Acad. Sci.* 109:11652–11656. doi: 10.1073/pnas.1203647109

4. Gilbert, N. 2013. Case studies: a hard look at GM crops. *Nature* 497:7447. Available at http://www.nature.com/news/case-studies-a-hard-look-at-gm-crops-1.12907

5. WHO. 2014, May. *Frequently asked questions on genetically modified foods*. Retrieved from World Health Organization, http://www.who.int/foodsafety/areas_work/food-technology/Frequently_asked_questions_on_gm_foods.pdf?ua=1

6. International Agency for Research on Cancer. 2015, March 20. IARC Monographs Volume 112: Evaluation of five organophosphate insecticides and herbicides. http://www.iarc.fr/en/media-centre/iarcnews/pdf/MonographVolume112.pdf

7. National Cancer Institute. 2015. SEER Stat Fact Sheets: Non-Hodgkin Lymphoma. http://seer.cancer.gov/statfacts/html/nhl.html

8. Bjerga, A. 2013, May 29. Monsanto Modified Wheat Not Approved by USDA Found in Field. *Bloomberg News*. Available at http://www.bloomberg.com/news/articles/2013-05-29/monsanto-modified-wheat-unapproved-by-usda-found-in-oregon-field

9. Carpenter, J. E. 2011. Impact of GM crops on biodiversity. *GM Crops* 2(1):7–23. Available at http://www.tandfonline.com/doi/pdf/10.4161/gmcr.2.1.15086

10. Heap, I. 2015. The International Survey of Herbicide Resistant Weeds. Available at www.weedscience.org

11. Pleasants, J. M, and K. S. Oberhauser. 2012. Effect on milkweed/monarchs: Insect Conservation and Diversity. doi: 10.1111/j.1752-4598.2012.00196. Available at http://www.mlmp.org/results/findings/Pleasants_and_Oberhauser_2012_milkweed_loss_in_ag_fields.pdf

STUDY **PLAN** MasteringNutrition™

Customize your study plan—and master your nutrition!— in the Study Area of MasteringNutrition.

TEST YOURSELF | ANSWERS

1 (F) Foodborne illness actually sickens about 48 million Americans each year, and about 3,000 die.

2 (F) Most cases of foodborne illness are caused by just one species of virus, called norovirus. Bacteria also commonly cause foodborne illness.

3 (F) Freezing destroys some microorganisms but only inhibits the ability of other microorganisms to reproduce. When the food is thawed, these cold-tolerant microorganisms resume reproduction.

4 (T) Although genetic modification can also improve a crop's nutritional profile or yield, nearly all GM seeds marketed to U.S. farmers are modified for pest management.

5 (T) Although some studies have found higher levels of certain vitamins, essential fatty acids, and antioxidant phytochemicals in organic foods, there are not enough studies published on this topic to state with confidence that organic foods are consistently more nutritious than nonorganic foods.

summary

Scan to hear an MP3 Chapter Review in MasteringNutrition.

LO 1 ▪ Foodborne illness results from the consumption of food or water containing living pathogenic microorganisms, their toxic secretions, or pollutants like mercury and other industrial chemicals.

▪ Approximately 48 million Americans experience foodborne illness each year, and approximately 3,000 die as a result.

▪ The body has several defense mechanisms, such as saliva, stomach acid, vomiting, diarrhea, and the inflammatory response, that help rid us of offending microorganisms and toxins. People with reduced immunity, such as pregnant women, infants and young children, older adults, and people with HIV, cancer, or certain other diseases, are at increased risk for hospitalization or death due to foodborne illness.

▪ Whether imported or domestic, processed, or consumed raw, food can become contaminated at any point from farm to table. Another challenge to food safety is the fragmentation of our system of federal oversight. The most recent CDC report showed no reduction in foodborne illness from six major bacterial culprits.

LO 2 ▪ About 50% of all cases of foodborne illnesses due to known agents are caused by a single species of virus called norovirus. *Salmonella* is the most common bacterium involved in foodborne illness and the leading cause of fatal infections. Other top bacterial culprits are *Campylobacter, Clostridium perfringens, Listeria monocytogenes,* and *Staphylococcus aureus.* The parasite *Toxoplasma gondii* is also on the CDC's list of top seven contributors to foodborne illnesses and deaths.

▪ Many species of bacteria produce toxins. One of the most common is produced by *S. aureus.* Of all foodborne toxins, the botulism toxin, produced by the bacterium *Clostridium botulinum,* is the most deadly. The Shiga toxin, produced by strains of bacteria known as Shiga toxin-producing *E. coli* (STEC), is also very dangerous and can cause death.

▪ Other common foodborne toxins include mycotoxins produced by fungi; toxic algae in fish and shellfish; and plant toxins such as solanine in potatoes.

LO 3 ▪ In order to reproduce in foods, microbes require a precise range of temperature, from 40°F to 140°F, known as the danger zone. Foodborne microbes also require moisture (humidity), and have a preferred pH range, typically from neutral to slightly acidic. Finally, many microbes require oxygen to function. A rare exception to two of these rules is *C. botulinum,* which thrives in an alkaline, oxygen-free environment.

LO 4 ▪ You can prevent foodborne illness at home by following these tips: Clean: wash your hands and kitchen surfaces often. Wash produce thoroughly. Do not wash meat, poultry, or seafood. Separate: isolate foods to prevent cross-contamination. Watch especially that the juices of meat, poultry, seafood, and raw eggs does not contact cooked food, fresh bread, salad, or any other ready-to-eat food. Chill: refrigerate or freeze perishable foods, including leftovers. Do not leave food at room temperature for more than two hours, and if the environmental temperature is high, refrigerate foods within one hour. Cook: heat foods long enough and at the required temperature to ensure proper cooking. Use a food thermometer to ensure that the internal temperature is high enough to kill any bacteria or parasites that may be present.

▪ Protect yourself from toxins in foods by refrigerating leftovers promptly, and by strictly avoiding any food from a split, pierced, or bulging can.

▪ When eating out, avoid establishments that don't look clean. Order meats cooked well done, and send back eggs that look runny and prepared salads and foods with sauces that look congealed or otherwise spoiled.

LO 5 ▪ Ancient methods of preserving foods include salting, sugaring, drying, smoking, and cooling. These are all still used today.

▪ Modern food preservation techniques include canning and pasteurization, which expose foods to high heat, and special packaging, including aseptic packaging, modified atmosphere packaging, and high-pressure processing. The process of irradiation exposes foods to gamma rays from radioactive metals. Chemical preservatives, including vitamin C and vitamin E, are also commonly added to foods.

LO 6 ■ Food additives are natural or synthetic ingredients added to foods during processing to enhance them in some way. They include flavorings, colorings, nutrients, texturizers, and others.

■ The FDA reviews data on the safety of food additives and determines their safety prior to use in foods. The GRAS list identifies several hundred substances "generally recognized as safe" that are exempt from testing. These additives have either been extensively tested in the past and found to be safe and approved for use in the food industry, or are deemed safe as a result of consensus among experts qualified by scientific training and experience.

LO 7 ■ Genetic modification is the process of changing an organism by manipulating its genetic material. The technique uses recombinant DNA technology, in which scientists identify a gene conferring a desirable trait and extract it from the organism; combine it with the DNA of a host cell (usually a bacterium); culture the host cell, producing many copies; extract the gene and insert it into the target organism (such as corn); and grow the modified crop.

■ In the United States, genetic modification is used primarily to confer herbicide tolerance. The second most common goal is insect resistance. Genetic modification is also used to enhance a crop's protection from disease, its ability to grow in challenging conditions, or its nutrient concentration.

LO 8 ■ Persistent organic pollutants (POPs) are chemicals released into the atmosphere as a result of industry, agriculture, automobile emissions, and improper waste disposal. Plants, animals, and fish absorb the chemicals from contaminated soil or water and pass them on as part of the food chain.

■ In the process of biomagnification, POPs become more concentrated in animal tissues as they move from smaller to larger predators through the food chain. Humans can then consume high concentrations of POPs when they eat the meat, poultry, or fish of affected animals.

LO 9 ■ Large predatory fish, such as swordfish, shark, king mackerel, and tilefish, tend to contain high levels of mercury, which is toxic to the nervous system. Lead may be found in the paint in older homes and in industrial wastes. Exposure can cause decreased IQ, learning and behavioral disorders, and hearing impairment in children, and decreased fertility, nerve disorders, and cardiovascular and kidney disease in adults.

■ Plasticizers, dioxins, and PFASs are chemical residues found worldwide, including in animals and humans. Plasticizers and PFASs are used in food packaging. These three POPs have been associated with an increased risk for endocrine dysfunction, certain cancers, and neurological and other disorders.

■ Although pesticides prevent or reduce crop losses, some are toxic and can persist in the environment. In agricultural workers and consumers, pesticide residues may act as neurotoxins, carcinogens, and endocrine disruptors. The EPA regulates their use.

■ Recombinant bovine growth hormone (rBGH) is injected into beef and dairy cows to increase their yield. Although this hormone is known to be harmful to cattle, the research into human health effects is inconclusive.

■ Cows, pigs, and chickens administered antibiotics have become significant reservoirs for the development of antibiotic-resistant strains of bacteria, such as MRSA. The FDA has imposed a voluntary ban on the use of antibiotics to increase growth. They now may be used only for the prevention and treatment of disease.

LO 10 ■ Organic crops, livestock, and multiple-ingredient foods are produced in a way that protects natural resources, conserves biodiversity, and uses only approved substances. Organic producers cannot use: irradiation, sewage sludge, synthetic fertilizers, prohibited pesticides, GMOs, growth hormones, or antibiotics. Animals must be fed 100% organic feed, and have access to the outdoors.

■ Organic Standards in 2002 established uniform definitions for all organic products sold in the United States. Products bearing the USDA's organic seal contain 95% organically produced ingredients by weight, excluding water and salt, with the remaining ingredients consisting of those products not commercially available in organic form.

■ Research is inconclusive on the question of whether or not organically grown foods are more nutritious than foods conventionally grown; however, organic foods have been shown to have lower residues of pesticides and antibiotics.

To further your understanding, go online and apply what you've learned to real-life case studies that will help you master the content!

review questions

LO 1 1. One reason that foodborne illness has become a serious public health concern in the United States is that
a. an estimated 4.8 million Americans experience foodborne illness each year, and about 300 die.
b. Americans are eating more and more processed foods containing potentially toxic levels of food additives.
c. federal oversight of food safety is fragmented among 15 different agencies.
d. the most recent progress report from the Food Safety Working Group indicates that no progress has recently been made in reducing foodborne illness.

LO 2 2. Among the CDC's top seven microorganisms responsible for foodborne illness,
a. six are species of bacteria.
b. *Salmonella* is responsible for the greatest number of illnesses.
c. Shiga toxin-producing *E. coli* is responsible for the most deaths.
d. *Toxoplasma gondii* is the only species of protozoa.

LO 3 3. The majority of foodborne microorganisms reproduce most successfully
a. between 40°F and 140°F.
b. in dry conditions.
c. in alkaline conditions.
d. in an anaerobic environment.

LO 4 4. During a 4th of July barbecue on a hot afternoon, a family enjoys grilled fish, potato salad, and coleslaw. Leftovers of these foods should be safe to eat later on as long as they are brought back indoors and refrigerated
a. immediately after serving.
b. within a maximum of 30 minutes after serving.
c. within a maximum of 1 hour after serving.
d. within a maximum of 2 hours after serving.

LO 5 5. A food preservation technique in which the oxygen in a food is replaced with an inert gas is
a. aseptic packaging.
b. modified atmosphere packaging.
c. high-pressure processing.
d. irradiation.

LO 6 6. Food additives that have raised health concerns include
a. sodium chloride and beta-carotene.
b. sulfites and nitrites.
c. alpha-tocopheral and ascorbic acid.
d. all of the above.

LO 7 7. The most common reason that crops in the United States are genetically modified is to
a. confer tolerance to herbicides.
b. protect them from disease.
c. enable them to grow in challenging environmental conditions.
d. boost their concentration of nutrients.

LO 8 8. Which of the following best describes how biomagnification occurs?
a. Conventional fertilizers and pesticides are sprayed onto food crops.
b. Industrial pollutants initiate DNA mutations that lead to cancer.
c. Animal wastes contaminate soils where food crops are grown.
d. Industrial contaminants become more concentrated in animal tissues as they move up the food chain.

LO 9 9. Residues from heavy metals, plasticizers, dioxins, PFASs, and certain pesticides pose a threat to public health because
a. they confer antibiotic resistance to livestock.
b. they cause allergies, asthma, and migraine headaches.
c. they can act as neurotoxins, carcinogens, or endocrine disruptors.
d. they can cause nausea, severe vomiting, and diarrhea.

LO 10 10. Foods that are labeled 100% organic
a. contain only organically produced ingredients, excluding water and salt.
b. may display the EPA's organic seal.
c. were produced without the use of pesticides.
d. contain foods from plant sources only.

true or false?

LO 2 11. **True or false?** A bacterium that commonly contaminates deli meats, smoked fish, and soft cheeses is *Listeria monocytogenes*.

LO 4 12. **True or false?** An important food-safety strategy is to wash meat, poultry, and fish under running water before cooking.

LO 5 13. **True or false?** Irradiation makes foods radioactive.

LO 9 14. **True or false?** The FDA has imposed a voluntary ban on the use of recombinant bovine growth hormone (rBGH) to increase the amount and quality of meat in beef herds and milk production in dairy cows. It can now be used only for prevention and treatment of disease.

LO 10 **15.** **True or false?** In the United States, farms certified as organic are allowed to use pesticides under certain conditions.

short answer

LO 4 **16.** Your sister Joy, who attends a culinary arts school, is visiting you for dinner. You want to impress her, so you've decided to make chicken marsala. You begin that afternoon by removing two chicken breasts from the freezer and putting them in a bowl in the refrigerator to thaw. Then you go shopping for fresh salad ingredients. When you get home from the market, you take the chicken breasts from the refrigerator and set them on a clean cutting board. You then take the lettuce, red pepper, and scallions you just bought, put them in a colander, and rinse them. Next, you slice them with a clean knife on your marble countertop and toss them together in a salad. You put the chicken breasts in a frying pan and cook them until they lose their pink color. In a separate pan, you prepare the sauce. Finally, using a clean knife, you slice some freshly baked bread on the countertop. You then wash the knives and the cutting board you used for the chicken. Joy arrives and admires your skill in cooking. Later that night, you both wake up vomiting. Identify at least two aspects of your food preparation that might have contributed to your illness.

LO 5 **17.** Pickling is a food-preservation technique that involves soaking foods, such as cucumbers, in a solution containing vinegar (acetic acid). Why is pickling effective in preventing food spoilage?

LO 9 **18.** Steven and Dante go to a convenience store after a tennis match, looking for something to quench their thirst. Steven chooses a national brand of pasteurized orange juice, and Dante chooses a bottle of locally produced, organic, unpasteurized apple juice. Steven points out to Dante that his juice is not pasteurized, but Dante shrugs and says, "I'm more afraid of the pesticides they used on the oranges in your juice than I am of microorganisms in mine!" Which juice would you choose, and why?

19. In the 1950s and 1960s in Minamata, Japan, more than 100 cases of a similar illness were recorded: patients, many of whom were infants or young children, suffered irreversible damage to the nervous system. A total of 46 people died. Adults with the disease and mothers of afflicted young children had one thing in common: they had frequently eaten fish caught in Minamata Bay. What do you think might have been the cause of this illness? Using key words from this description, research the event on the Internet and identify the culprit(s).

LO 10 **20.** A box of macaroni and cheese has the words *Certified Organic* on the front and displays the USDA organic seal. The following ingredients are listed on the side: organic durum semolina pasta (organic durum semolina, water), organic cheddar cheese (organic cultured pasteurized milk, salt, enzymes), whey, salt. Is this food 100% organic? Why or why not? Does it contain any food additives? If so, identify them.

math review

LO 4 **21.** Below are the proper cooking temperatures for meat, poultry, and fish from the USDA. Use the formula to convert each from Fahrenheit to Celsius. Round off. Show your work!

(°Fahrenheit − 32) × 5/9 = (°Celsius)

Example: (90°F − 32) × 5/9 = (°Celsius)

90 − 32 = 58

58 × 5/9 = 32°C

- Beef, pork, veal, lamb steaks, roasts, and chops 145°F with a 3-minute rest time before serving; fish 145°F

- Ground beef and egg dishes 160°F

- Poultry, whole, pieces, and ground 165°F

Answers to Review Questions can be found online in the MasteringNutrition Study Area.

web links

www.foodsafety.gov

Foodsafety.gov

Use this website as a gateway to a range of government food safety information; it contains updates, safety reports, help with reporting illnesses and product complaints, news on foodborne pathogens, and more.

www.cdc.gov/foodsafety/index.html

CDC Food Safety Homepage

This section of the larger CDC website focuses on issues specifically related to food safety, with a range of informational resources.

www.fsis.usda.gov/food_safety_education/ index.asp

USDA Food Safety and Inspection Service

The Food Safety and Inspection Service area of the larger USDA website is designed to educate the public about safe food handling practices, and reduce the risks from foodborne illnesses through a variety of tools, resources, and links to related topic areas.

www.epa.gov/pesticides

US Environmental Protection Agency: Pesticides

This site provides information on agricultural and home-use pesticides, pesticide-related health and safety issues, environmental effects, and government regulation of pesticide types and uses.

www.ams.usda.gov

USDA National Organic Program

Click on "National Organic Program" to get to the web page describing the NOP's standards and labeling program, consumer information, and publications.

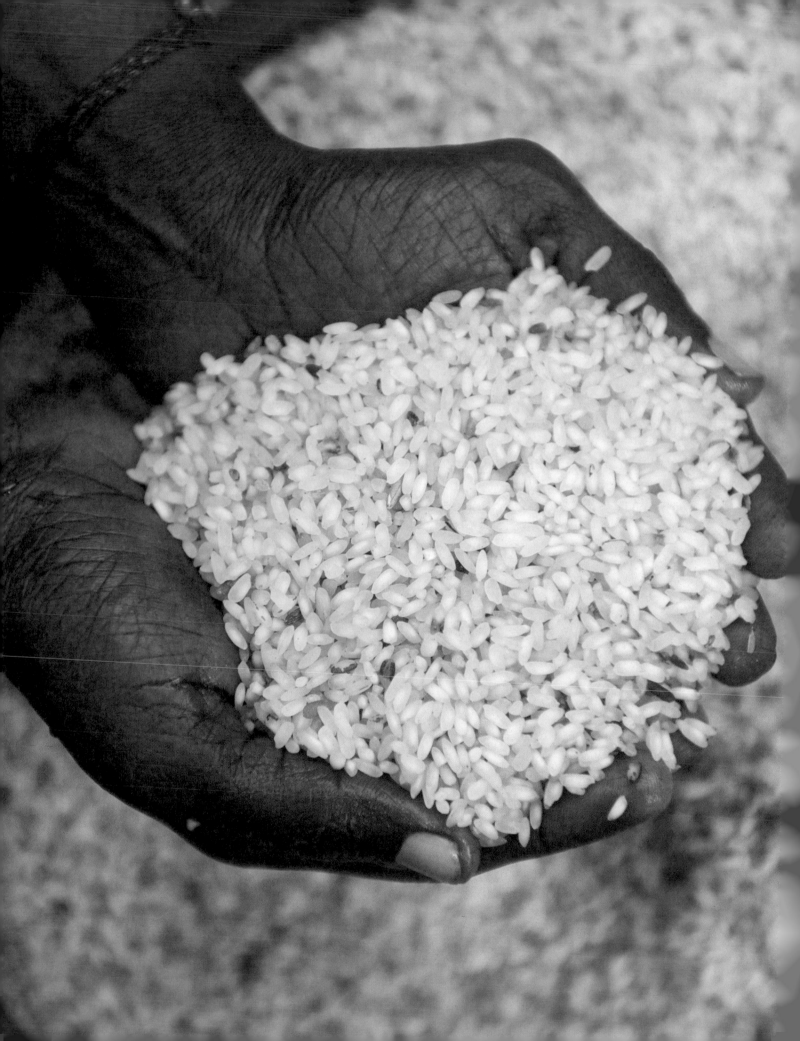

16 Food Equity, Sustainability, and Quality: The Challenge of "Good" Food

Learning Outcomes

After studying this chapter, you should be able to:

1 Compare and contrast levels of food insecurity globally and in the United States, *pp. 628–630.*

2 Discuss several ways in which human behavior contributes to food insecurity, *pp. 630–632.*

3 Explain what climate change is and how it is affecting the world's food supply, *pp. 632–633.*

4 Describe the health and societal problems associated with undernourishment, *pp. 633–635.*

5 Explain how obesity can result from limited access to nourishing food, *pp. 635–638.*

6 Identify inequities in agricultural and food-service labor, and their effects on workers and the consumers they serve, *pp. 638–639.*

7 Discuss the effects of industrial agriculture on food security and the environment, *pp. 639–641.*

8 Explain how the food industry has influenced the quality and diversity of our food supply, *p. 641.*

9 Discuss international, governmental, philanthropic, corporate, and local initiatives aimed at increasing the world's supply of and access to "good" food, *pp. 642–644.*

10 Identify several steps you can take to promote production of and access to "good" food, *pp. 645–646.*

TEST YOURSELF

True or False?

1 Because of insufficient money or other resources, people in more than 5% of U.S. households go without food. **T** *or* **F**

2 A person can be both obese and undernourished. **T** *or* **F**

3 In the United States, as compared to workers in other industries, a farm worker has nearly twice the risk of dying from an on-the-job injury. **T** *or* **F**

4 More than half of cash revenues for all U.S. farmers come from just two crops, corn and soybeans. **T** *or* **F**

5 Methane, a greenhouse gas emitted during livestock production, has nearly double the atmospheric warming effect of carbon dioxide. **T** *or* **F**

Test Yourself answers are located in the Study Plan.

MasteringNutrition™

Go online for chapter quizzes, pre-tests, interactive activities, and more!

Hailey knows she should eat more fresh fruits and vegetables, but she doesn't have a car, and the nearest grocery store is several miles away, over busy roads without sidewalks. Besides, she tells herself, even if she took the bus there, she wouldn't be able to afford fresh produce. The few dollars in her purse have to last until the end of the month. So she walks two blocks to a corner store where she purchases a steamed hot dog and a large bag of corn chips.

What is "good" food? Although a farmer, chef, and public health expert would likely propose very different definitions, in this chapter, we define "good" food as nutrient-dense food that is equitably and sustainably produced, distributed, and sold. That might sound like a tall order, but such foods do exist. The challenge is to make them in large enough quantities to feed the world, and make sure that consumers have the ability and the desire to obtain them.[1]

We begin this chapter by looking at two issues of food equity: **food insecurity,** which is unreliable access to a sufficient supply of nourishing food, and inequities in agricultural and food-service employment. We then discuss the effects of our food production system on our environment and on the quality and diversity of our food supply. Finally, we'll look at some ways that nations and organizations are meeting the challenge of "good" food, and how you can help.

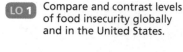

LO 1 Compare and contrast levels of food insecurity globally and in the United States.

How Prevalent Is Food Insecurity?

In Namibia, a nation in southern Africa, more than 35% of the population is undernourished.[2] Forty-six out of every 1,000 Namibian infants die before reaching their first birthday, and among those who survive to age 5, 18% are underweight. Average life expectancy is 52 years.[3] Across the globe in the United States, infant mortality is only 6 per 1,000, and in low-income counties, instead of being undernourished, over 14% of children age 2 to 4 are obese.[3,4] Average life expectancy is now over 78 years; however, the average life expectancy in the wealthiest U.S. counties is 85 years for women and 81 years for men, whereas in the poorest U.S. counties, those numbers drop to 73 years for women and 64 years for men.[5]

Although a variety of factors contribute to disparities in infant mortality, body weight, and life expectancy, a population's diet is one of the most important. Globally, the greatest health disparities are found between populations that are impoverished and those with a dependable supply of nourishing food. As the above comparisons illustrate, however, these disparities exist not only between poor and wealthy nations, but also between poor and wealthy counties within the United States. Are food distribution and access equitable? Let's have a look.

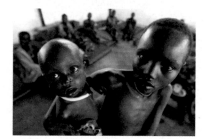

Hunger and malnutrition are still experienced by many people around the world today.

About 795 Million People Worldwide Are Hungry

The Food and Agricultural Organization of the United Nations (FAO) estimates that about one in nine people in the world is chronically undernourished, and 98% of these people live in developing nations.[6] Although this is a disturbing statistic, it represents considerable progress: in 1990, over 1 billion people were undernourished. Then, in September of 2000, the United Nations (UN) and heads of state from around the world committed to a coordinated effort to reduce poverty. Using 1990 as a baseline, they set eight Millennium Development Goals, the first of which was to halve by the year 2015 the proportion of the world's people who suffer from hunger. Significant progress was made toward this goal: The share of undernourished people in the global population fell from 18.6% in 1990–92 to 10.9% in 2014–16, a reduction of nearly 45%.[6]

Still, hunger is endemic to many nations of the world (**Figure 16.1**). About 64% of the world's hungry people live in Asia, and sub-Saharan Africa—the region with the highest prevalence of hungry people—23%—accounts for almost 28%.[6] Closer to home, at least 10% of people in some regions of Central and South America are undernourished, and in Haiti, the prevalence is greater than 50%.

To read the FAO's 2015 report of The State of Food Insecurity in the World, visit www.fao.org/.

food insecurity Unreliable access to a sufficient supply of nourishing food.

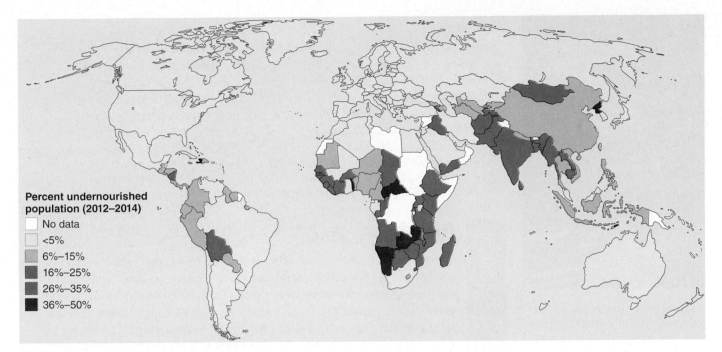

FIGURE 16.1 Although people throughout the world—including in North America—are undernourished, Asia and sub-Saharan Africa have the greatest prevalence of undernourishment overall. *Source:* Food and Agricultural Organization of the United Nations (FAO). 2014. FAO Hunger Map 2014. Available at http://www.fao.org/fileadmin/templates/ess/foodsecurity/poster_web_001_WFS.jpg

Over 17 Million American Households Are Food Insecure

Although the United States is one of the top 20 richest countries in the world,[3] many of our poorest citizens go hungry. As shown in **Figure 16.2,** the Economic Research Service of the U.S. Department of Agriculture (USDA) estimates that 14.3% of U.S. households (about 17.5 million households) experienced food insecurity in 2013.[7] This means that, at times during the year, members of these households were uncertain of having, or unable to acquire, enough food to meet their needs, because they had insufficient money or other resources for food.[7]

Of these 17.5 million households, 6.8 million had *very low food security,* meaning that in over 5% of U.S. households, one or more members had to reduce not only the quality, variety, or desirability of their food choices, but also the amount they were able to eat.[7] In other words, people in these homes, at times, were hungry. How do "households" translate into human beings? In 2013, nearly 13 million Americans, including 765,000 children (1% of U.S. children), experienced very low food security.[7]

Those at higher risk for food insecurity are households with incomes below 185% of the official U.S. poverty threshold (which was $23,634 for a family of four in 2013), families consisting of single mothers or single fathers and their children, African American households, and Hispanic households.[7] Among geographic regions of the United States, the South has the highest prevalence of food insecurity, and the Northeast the lowest.

Sometimes physical, psychological, or social factors contribute to food insecurity among Americans. For instance, people with chronic diseases or disabilities may lose paid work hours due to illness, have to accept lower-wage jobs, or have medical expenses that limit money for food. Depression, addiction to alcohol or other substances, and other psychological disorders can similarly limit productivity and reduce income. Divorce frequently leads to financial stressors, especially for women, who may be unable to collect alimony or child support payments and may have jobs that do not provide an income sufficient to provide fully for the family's needs.

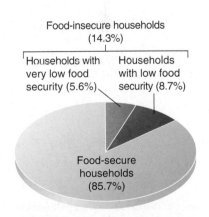

FIGURE 16.2 Prevalence of food insecurity and very low food security in U.S. households, 2013. *Source:* Economic Research Service. 2015, January 12. *Food Security Status of U.S. Households in 2013.* United States Department of Agriculture. Available at http://www.ers.usda.gov/topics/food-nutrition-assistance/food-security-in-the-us/key-statistics-graphics.aspx#verylow

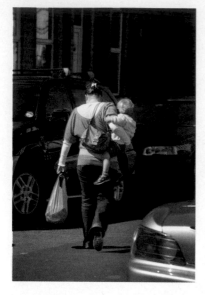

Single parents face unique economic challenges that can leave them and their children vulnerable to food insecurity.

RECAP

Health disparities exist between poor and wealthy nations, and between poor and wealthy regions within the same nation. Food insecurity, which is unreliable access to a sufficient supply of nourishing food, contributes to health disparities. Although significant progress has been made toward the Millennium Development Goal to halve the 1990 prevalence of global hunger by the year 2015, about 795 million people, or one in nine people in the world, is still chronically undernourished. More than 14% of U.S. households experienced food insecurity in 2013, and nearly 13 million Americans, including about 1% of all U.S. children, had very low food security. Low-income families and families headed by a single parent are among those with the highest rates of food insecurity. ■

Judy

Nutri-Case

"I never seem to be able to make ends meet. I keep hoping next month will be different, but rent and utilities eat up most of my paycheck, so when something unexpected happens, I'm short. Last week, my car broke down and I'm way behind on my credit card payments. Today, a collections guy called and said that, if I didn't pay at least $100 right away, they'd take me to court. When I got off the phone, I started to cry, and Hannah asked me what was wrong. When I told her how bad the money situation is, she thought we might qualify for food stamps. I have a full-time job, so I don't think we'll qualify, but even if we do, I wonder if it'll help much."

In 2015, the federal minimum wage was $7.25 an hour. As a nurse's aide, Judy earns $9 an hour, or $1,560 a month. She is eligible for the Supplemental Nutrition Assistance Program (food stamps). Are you surprised that someone making almost 25% more than the minimum wage, and working full-time, qualifies for food assistance?

Before you're too certain that Judy's eligibility will solve her problems, consider that the average SNAP allotment in 2015 was $127.90 per person per month, or about $30 per week.* If you had just $30 to keep yourself fed for a week, what would you buy?

Take this challenge one step further and follow the example of some U.S. college students to raise local awareness of food insecurity: For 1 week, restrict yourself to just $30 for all your food purchases. Let your campus newspaper and local media outlets know what you're doing, and ask readers to make donations to local food banks.

*Congressional Budget Office. 2015, March. Supplemental Nutrition Assistance Program March 2015 Baseline. http://www.cbo.gov/sites/default/files/cbofiles/attachments/44211-2015-03-SNAP.pdf

---

LO 2 Discuss several ways in which human behavior contributes to food insecurity.

LO 3 Explain what climate change is and how it is affecting the world's food supply.

Why Don't All People Have Access to Nourishing Food?

Weather events and human activity can result in a food supply that is inadequate to support the needs of all of the people in a particular place. Moreover, a recent and ongoing concern is the effect of climate change on the global food supply.

Acute Food Shortages Are Often Caused by Weather Events and Wars

famine A severe food shortage affecting a large percentage of the population in a limited geographic area at a particular time.

A **famine** is a severe food shortage affecting a large percentage of the population in a limited geographic area at a particular time. Famines have occurred throughout human history and typically result from a combination of factors, including weather events and human miscalculations. For example, an estimated 20–43 million people died in the so-called great famine in China from 1958 to 1961 when disastrous government land-use policies, combined with both floods and droughts, dramatically limited crop yields. When a population is already living in extreme poverty, even a minor climate event can have dire consequences. In 2014, for example, lower-than-average rainfall in Pakistan's Thar desert led to the deaths of almost 500 people. Other natural disasters that can quickly destroy crops are tsunamis, high winds, hurricanes, frosts, pest infestations, and plant diseases.

Wars can induce acute food shortages when they interfere with planting or harvest times, when they destroy standing crops, or when populations are forced to flee. Since the civil war in Syria began in 2011, for example, there have been numerous reports of starvation, either because of insufficient funds for food relief to refugees or as a deliberate tactic of oppression.

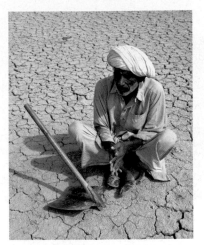

An Indian farmer inspects what is left of his crop during a drought.

The Major Cause of Chronic Hunger Is Unequal Distribution of Food

The world produces enough food to meet everyone's needs. Even developing nations currently produce about 2,600 kcal per person per day. Worldwide, the leading cause of longstanding hunger in a region is unequal distribution of this adequate food supply, largely because of poverty.[8] The most at-risk populations are the rural poor. Lacking sufficient land to grow their own foods, the rural poor must work for others to earn money to buy food, but because they live in rural areas, employment opportunities are limited.

Unequal distribution also occurs because of cultural biases. In many countries, limited food is distributed first to men and boys and only secondarily to women and girls. In such situations, pregnant women and growing girls are the most vulnerable because of their increased needs. Food distribution to the elderly is sometimes also limited, particularly in developing countries where nutrition services are primarily directed toward pregnant and lactating women, infants, and young children. Access to food also can differ by ethnicity and religion. For example, officials in authority may order that food aid be distributed preferentially to areas where their own ethnic group dominates.

Overpopulation Contributes to Chronic Food Shortages

Experts estimate that, in the year 1000 BCE, the world population was about 50 million people. Over the next 2,000 years, by the year 1000, it had multiplied only five-fold to about 250 million. Yet by the year 2000, global population had skyrocketed to 6 billion; by the end of 2011, it had passed 7 billion; and by 2026, it is projected to reach 8 billion.[9] Can the Earth sustain this many inhabitants?

An area is said to experience **overpopulation** when its resources are insufficient to support the number of people living there. In parts of the world with fertile land and adequate rainfall or irrigation systems to support abundant harvests, food shortages rarely happen. However, in more arid climates, especially in areas with high birthrates and poor access to imported foods, seasonal and chronic food shortages are common. Of course, resources other than food may become depleted in overpopulated areas. Water, clean air, safe housing, jobs, health care, quality education, and many other resources can be insufficient for the population's needs.

Is the world already overpopulated? Or will it soon become so? No one can answer these questions with absolute certainty, because we cannot predict how advances in technology will affect our depletion of the Earth's natural resources or our ability to produce more food with fewer resources. However, reducing the demand for food within a region by slowing population growth is one way of improving an area's food supply, and one of the most effective methods of reducing birthrates is to improve the education of women and girls.[10] Their increased earning potential, access to information about contraception, and better health practices lead to smaller, healthier, more economically stable families. Other methods of improving an area's food supply are to increase food production and to import foods into the area.

overpopulation Condition in which a region's available resources are insufficient to support the number of people living there.

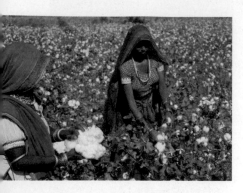

Cotton is a cash crop that farmers often grow instead of local food crops.

Local Conditions Can Contribute to Chronic Hunger

Agricultural practices, lack of infrastructure, and the burden of disease can also contribute to hunger in regions around the world.

Agricultural Practices

Some traditional farming practices have the potential to destroy useable land. Deforestation by burning or any other means and overgrazing pastures and croplands destroy the trees and grass roots that preserve soils from wind and water erosion. Growing the same crop year after year on the same plot of ground can deplete the soil of nutrients and reduce crop yield. Use of agricultural land for **cash crops,** such as cotton, coffee, and tobacco, may replace land use for local food crops, or food crops such as corn and soybeans may be diverted to industrial uses. Also harmful is the practice of growing food for livestock, which compared to food crops feed far fewer people for the resources used. We compare the environmental costs of livestock versus food crops later in this chapter.

Lack of Infrastructure

Exacerbating the scarcity of food production in some areas is a lack of infrastructure. For example, many developing countries lack roads and transportation into rural areas. This limits available food to whatever can be produced locally. In addition, lack of electricity and refrigeration can limit storage of perishable foods before they can be used.

Water management is another aspect of infrastructure that influences nutrition. In dry areas, irrigation can improve food production, but it must be managed carefully to avoid increasing the numbers of mosquitoes, intestinal parasites, and other pests, which can spread infectious diseases. The provision of safe drinking water and sewage systems is another aspect of water management that helps prevent disease.

Impact of Disease

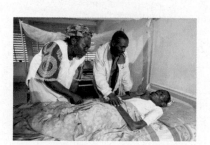

HIV/AIDS is most severe in undernourished populations, especially in Africa.

Disease and lack of healthcare resources to fight disease reduce the work capacity of individuals, and this in turn reduces their ability to ward off poverty and malnutrition. This economic phenomenon is demonstrated by the AIDS epidemic. In 2014, the World Health Organization (WHO) reported that there were 35 million people living with HIV. About 1.5 million people died from AIDS in 2013.[11] HIV is most likely to affect young, sexually active adults who are the primary wage earners in their families. Thus, their illness or death can orphan and impoverish their children, as well as create populations in which children and the elderly predominate.

Climate Change Threatens Global Food Security

cash crops Crops grown to be sold rather than eaten, such as cotton or tobacco.

global warming The increase of about 1.4°F (0.8°C) in temperature that has occurred near the Earth's surface over the past century.

climate change Any significant change in the measures of climate—such as temperature, precipitation, or wind patterns—that occurs over several decades or longer.

Global warming is the general term used for the increase of about 1.4°F (0.8°C) in temperature that has occurred near the Earth's surface over the past century.[12] The great majority of climate scientists agree that it has been caused by human activities that have released large amounts of carbon dioxide and other heat-trapping *greenhouse gases* into the atmosphere.[12] Global warming is, in turn, the most significant factor contributing to **climate change,** which the U.S. Environmental Protection Agency (EPA) defines as any significant change in the measures of climate—such as temperature, precipitation, or wind patterns—that occurs over several decades or longer.[13] A 2015 analysis, for example, attributed 75% of heat extremes and 18% of precipitation extremes to global warming.[14]

The United Nations' Intergovernmental Panel on Climate Change (IPCC) reports that global warming and climate change are affecting global food security in a number of ways:[15]

- Reduced crop yields. Higher average temperatures and elevations in greenhouse gases have reduced crop yields in many regions of the world.
- Crop destruction. Heat waves, droughts, tornados, hurricanes, and floods have all destroyed standing crops outright. In 2014, for example, California experienced its

worst drought on record, following several years of drought, and causing losses in excess of $1 billion. Crops have also been destroyed by emerging varieties of pests such as fungal species that thrive in higher heat and humidity.

■ Impacts on seafood availability. Climate change is reducing the abundance and distribution of seafood in tropical and temperate regions.

In contrast, very northern and southern latitudes of the globe have seen some minimal benefits from warmer temperatures. However, negative impacts of climate trends have been more common.[15] Moreover, a 2015 analysis found that food security is becoming increasingly susceptible to the effects of climate change and population growth.[16]

RECAP

The world produces enough food to meet everyone's needs. Famines are widespread, severe food shortages that can result in starvation and death. They are most commonly caused by natural disasters or wars. Worldwide, the leading cause of longstanding hunger in a region is unequal distribution of an adequate food supply, largely because of poverty. Chronic food shortages can be influenced by regional overpopulation. Education of women and girls is an effective method of reducing birthrates. Poor agricultural practices, lack of infrastructure, and the burden of disease also contribute to chronic food shortages. Climate change reduces crop yields, destroys crops, and changes availability of seafood. ■

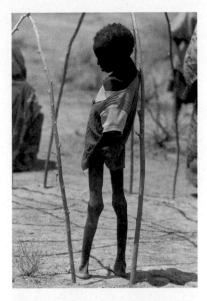

Wasting (extreme thinness) and stunting (short stature for age) are commonly seen in undernourished children.

What Problems Result from Limited Access to Nourishing Food?

 Describe the health and societal problems associated with undernourishment.

 Explain how obesity can result from limited access to nourishing food.

Limited access to nourishing foods promotes nutritional imbalance. That is, an individual may be unable to consume adequate energy to maintain weight and physiologic functioning; or the individual may consume enough energy, but experience deficiencies of one or more nutrients. In some cases, especially in wealthier nations, limited access to nourishing foods can actually promote simultaneous obesity and deficiency—in an individual who has an excessive intake of high-energy, nutrient-poor foods.

Low Energy Intake Promotes Wasting, Stunting, and Mortality

At least 17.3 million children worldwide suffer from **severe acute malnutrition (SAM),** a condition in which energy intake is so inadequate that the child experiences **wasting,** a very low body-weight-for-height.[17] This is a conservative estimate; that is, experts believe that the figure could be as much as 8 times higher.[17] Typically, these children also experience **stunted growth;** they are shorter than expected for their age. Stunting occurs when energy intake or specific nutrients are inadequate to sustain normal linear growth. In some impoverished communities, the great majority of residents are very short and small; thus, community members may not perceive their stunted growth as unusual or recognize it as a sign of chronic undernourishment.

SAM also dramatically increases a population's rate of **maternal mortality** (deaths of a woman during pregnancy, childbirth, or in the immediate postpartal period) and **infant mortality** (the death of infants between birth and 1 year). For example, the infant mortality rate in industrialized countries of Western Europe ranges from about 2 to 5 per 1,000, whereas in Afghanistan, Mali, and Somalia, three of the world's poorest countries, the infant mortality rate is more than 100 per 1,000.[3]

Many of the deaths associated with SAM occur as a result of decreased resistance to infection. Even mild underweight is estimated to double a child's risk for death from infection.[10] Protein and many micronutrients are essential to an effective immune response; therefore, infections occur more frequently and take longer to resolve. These prolonged infections exacerbate malnutrition by decreasing appetite, causing vomiting and diarrhea,

severe acute malnutrition (SAM) A state of severe energy deficit defined as a weight for height more than 3 standard deviations below the mean, or the presence of nutrition-related edema.

wasting A physical condition of very low body-weight-for-height or extreme thinness.

stunted growth A condition of shorter stature than expected for chronological age, often defined as 2 or more standard deviations below the mean reference value.

maternal mortality A population's rate of deaths of a woman during pregnancy, childbirth, or in the immediate postpartal period.

infant mortality A population's rate of death of infants between birth and 1 year of age.

producing weight loss, and further weakening the immune system. A vicious cycle of malnutrition, infection, worsening malnutrition, and increased vulnerability to infection develops. **Figure 16.3** summarizes the effects of SAM throughout the lifecycle.

Micronutrient Deficiencies Lead to Preventable Diseases

In impoverished countries, micronutrient deficiencies are major public health concerns. These are some of the most severe:

- Iron deficiency is the most common micronutrient deficiency in the world.[19] Although it occurs in both males and females of all ages, it is more prevalent in pregnant women and young children because of the demands of fetal and childhood growth. Iron-deficiency anemia contributes to 20% of maternal deaths.

- Prenatal iodine intake is particularly important for fetal brain development, and severe iodine deficiency is the single largest cause of preventable mental impairment worldwide. Nearly a third of the world's population is iodine deficient.[20] Iodine-deficiency disorders have largely been eliminated in areas of the world with access to iodized salt or oil and areas where iodine is added to irrigation water.

- Vitamin A deficiency is the leading cause of blindness in children.[19] An estimated 250 million children worldwide are vitamin A deficient. In addition, because of greater vulnerability to severe infection, these children are at high risk for death. The WHO and other global health agencies provide vitamin A supplements, promote breastfeeding, and support family and community vegetable gardens. These efforts have reduced mortality by 23%.[19]

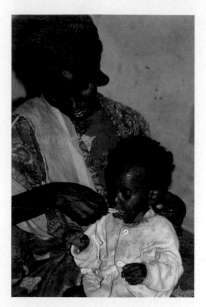

In developing nations, providing vitamin A supplements twice a year to children under age 5 has significantly reduced mortality.

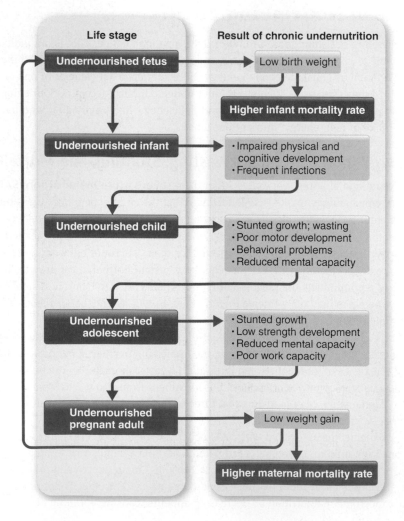

FIGURE 16.3 Acute and long-term effects of chronic undernourishment throughout the life cycle.

Life stage	Result of chronic undernutrition
Undernourished fetus	Low birth weight
	Higher infant mortality rate
Undernourished infant	• Impaired physical and cognitive development • Frequent infections
Undernourished child	• Stunted growth; wasting • Poor motor development • Behavioral problems • Reduced mental capacity
Undernourished adolescent	• Stunted growth • Low strength development • Reduced mental capacity • Poor work capacity
Undernourished pregnant adult	Low weight gain
	Higher maternal mortality rate

Undernourishment Promotes Socioeconomic Problems

Undernourishment has long been known to diminish work capacity. In addition to iodine, vitamin B_{12}, folate, certain essential fatty acids, and many other nutrients contribute to the development and maintenance of a healthy nervous system; thus, undernourishment—especially during fetal development, infancy, and early childhood—can permanently reduce cognitive functioning and an individual's ability to contribute to a nation's economic progress. Similarly, the vision loss caused by vitamin A deficiency can severely limit an individual's work capacity.

Inadequate energy intake and micronutrient deficiency can also prompt debilitating weakness, which is especially detrimental when manual labor is the main source of income. The reduced earning capacity of poor, undernourished adults often regenerates a cycle of poverty onto the next generation. Iron-deficiency anemia is particularly debilitating because of iron's role in oxygen transport. Because iron deficiency is a problem among women of childbearing age in both developed and developing countries, it is a global drain on work capacity and productivity.

Limited Access to Nourishing Food Can Promote Obesity

Throughout the world, the prevalence of obesity is increasing at an alarming rate and, along with it, obesity-related chronic diseases. The WHO estimates that the worldwide prevalence of obesity more than doubled between 1980 and 2014. Currently, 1.9 billion people worldwide are overweight, and 600 million of these are obese. Moreover, overweight and obesity are now linked to more deaths worldwide than underweight.[21]

Obesity used to be considered a disease of affluence, but in recent decades, public health researchers have observed an increasing prevalence of obesity in impoverished communities. If food is still scarce in many developing nations, how has the global rate of obesity more than doubled? And if an individual is poor and undernourished, how could he or she also be obese? Let's explore these two paradoxes.

The Nutrition Paradox

The **nutrition paradox** is characterized by the coexistence of stunting and overweight/obesity within the same region, the same household, and even the same person. People born in developing nations who were undernourished when young are likely to be short (due to growth stunting) but experience rapid weight gain when their country transitions out of poverty. The nutrition paradox is especially common in China, India, Mexico, and South America. In Colombia, for example, 5% of households have both an overweight or obese mother and a stunted child, and in Ecuador, researchers found that 2.8% of children nationwide exhibited both stunting and overweight or obesity.[22,23]

The WHO identifies two key factors behind the nutrition paradox in transitioning nations:[21]

- *A trend toward decreased physical activity* due to the increasingly sedentary nature of many forms of work, changing modes of transportation, and increasing urbanization
- *A global shift in diet toward increased intake of energy-dense foods* that are high in saturated fats and added sugars but low in micronutrients and fiber

In effect, all nations have been exposed to a nutritional transition over the past 30 years, as international food companies have made processed, energy-dense foods available at lower cost to more people worldwide.

The Poverty–Obesity Paradox

Could poverty be an independent risk factor for obesity? Even among established (non-immigrant) populations in developed nations, some research has suggested a **poverty–obesity paradox** in which obesity is more prevalent in low-income populations. In the United States, for example, studies following children over time have found that a reduction in family income

nutrition paradox The coexistence of aspects of both stunting and overweight/obesity within the same region, household, family, or person.

poverty–obesity paradox The high prevalence of obesity in low-income populations.

during early childhood increases the child's risk for becoming overweight or obese, whereas a shift to a higher family income increases the likelihood of weight loss.[24,25] Some researchers have also observed a so-called *hunger–obesity paradox*, in which low-income people are obese while also deficient in one or more nutrients, and in some cases even hungry. For example, the studies in Columbia and Ecuador cited earlier found an increased prevalence of iron-deficiency anemia in impoverished households whose members were also overweight or obese.

What factors could explain these associations? Research is inconclusive, but several hypotheses are being studied. One of the most common proposes that low-income people purchase energy-dense foods with longer shelf lives, such as vegetable oils, sugar, refined flour, snack foods, soft drinks, and canned goods, because they are less expensive than perishable foods such as meats, fish, milk, and fresh fruits and vegetables. Choosing such inexpensive, shelf-stable foods may be an important money-saving strategy especially for the rural poor. However, healthful eating doesn't always have to be expensive. To learn more, check out the *Highlight: Does It Cost More to Eat Right?*

HIGHLIGHT

Does It Cost More to Eat Right?

The shelves of American supermarkets are filled with an abundance of healthful food options: organic meats and produce, exotic fish, out-of-season fresh fruits and vegetables that are flown in from warmer climates, whole-grain breads and cereals, and low-fat and low-sodium options of traditional foods. With all of this choice, it would seem easy for anyone to consume healthful foods throughout the year. But a closer look at the prices of these foods suggests that, for many, they simply are not affordable. This raises the question "Does eating right have to be expensive?"

The truth is, some of the lowest-cost foods currently available in stores are also some of the most nutritious. These include beans, lentils, and other legumes; fresh fruits in season; many common vegetables, such as broccoli, carrots, sweet potatoes, summer and winter squashes, and onions; eggs; brown rice and plain oats; low-cost brands of whole-grains breads; cooking oils high in mono- and polyunsaturated fats; and frozen as well as canned fruits and vegetables, which are generally just as nutritious as fresh options. Thus, people can still eat healthfully on a tight budget.

Here are some more tips to help you save money when shopping for healthful foods:

- Buy whole grains, such as cereals, brown rice, and pastas in bulk—they store well for longer periods and provide a good base for meals and snacks.

- Buy frozen vegetables on sale and stock up—these are just as healthful as fresh vegetables, require less preparation, and are typically cheaper.

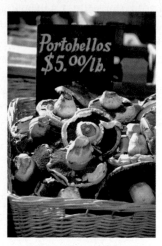

Some specialty foods (such as organic or imported products) can be expensive, but lower-cost alternatives can be just as nutritious.

- If lower-sodium options of canned beans and other vegetables are more expensive, buy the less expensive regular option and drain the juice from the vegetables before cooking.

- Consume leaner meats and in smaller amounts—by eating less, you'll not only save money but reduce your total intake of energy and fat while still obtaining the nutrients that support good health.

- Choose frozen fish or canned salmon or tuna packed in water as an alternative to fresh fish.

- Avoid frozen or dehydrated prepared meals. They are usually expensive; high in sodium, saturated fats, and energy; and low in fiber and important nutrients.

- Buy generic or store brands of foods—be careful to check the labels to ensure that the foods are similar in nutrient value to the higher-priced options.

- Cut coupons from local newspapers and magazines, and watch the sale circulars, so that you can stock up on healthful foods you can store.

- Consider cooking more meals at home; you'll have more control over what goes into your meals and you'll be able to cook larger amounts and freeze leftovers for future meals.

As you can see, eating healthfully does not have to be expensive. However, it helps to become a savvy consumer by reading food labels, comparing prices, and gaining the skills and confidence to cook at home.

A second hypothesis suggests that low-income people select cheap, energy-dense foods for their higher satiety value. Individuals with limited money to spend are likely to prefer foods that help them to feel full for a longer period of time.

Third, low-income people's high rates of obesity may reflect their environment. Many obese people live in so-called **food deserts,** defined by the USDA as geographic areas where people lack access to fresh, healthy, and affordable food.[26] Rural food deserts may have no access to any foods, whereas inner-city food deserts may be served only by fast food restaurants and convenience stores that offer few healthy options. For example, 30% of the residents of Detroit, Michigan receive food assistance from the federal government's Supplemental Nutrition Assistance Program (SNAP), commonly referred to as food stamps. Yet 92% of Detroit retailers accepting food stamps offer few or no fresh fruits or vegetables.[27] The USDA's Economic Research Service estimates that 23.5 million people live in food deserts.[26] More than half of those people (13.5 million) are low-income. Living in a food desert might limit not only options for nourishing food but also options for physical activity; that is, a neighborhood that is separated from the nearest supermarket by freeways is also likely to have low walkability.[28]

Fourth, the link between obesity and poverty might be explained in part by stress. That is, the stress of having insufficient resources to meet day-to-day expenses results in chronic release of stress hormones—such as cortisol—that slow metabolism and increase appetite, while simultaneously prompting short-sighted decision-making.[29,30] Moreover, some research suggests that self-control itself is a limited resource. People who must continually make difficult economic decisions may "deplete" their ability to make thoughtful, healthful decisions around eating.[28] Thus, the person may be more likely to overeat or eat empty-Calorie "comfort foods." A recent study also suggests that sugar may be particularly appealing to people experiencing chronic stress: Sugar consumption appears to trigger a negative feedback loop that "turns off" the stress response, prompting a measurable decrease in cortisol levels. In other words, for people under stress, sugar may be calming.[31]

In summary, then, although not all factors contributing to the coincidence of poverty and obesity are entirely clear, there is now substantial evidence of a global burden of overweight and obesity among the poor.

Fetal Undernourishment Can Lead to Adult Obesity

Finally, poor nutritional status in the mother can affect her offspring not only *in utero* but also throughout childhood and even into adulthood. The "fetal origins theory" (also called the theory of "developmental origins of adult health and disease") states that biological adjustments to poor maternal nutrition made by a malnourished fetus as its organs are developing may help the child during times of food shortages, but make the child susceptible to obesity and chronic disease when food is plentiful. For example, when a mother is malnourished during the pregnancy, her baby will tend to have a low birth weight but be relatively fat. This can occur because the fetal body has preserved fat tissue as a source of energy for growth of the brain, but at the expense of less muscle tissue. The imbalance results in metabolic disease later in life; there is now significant evidence supporting this hypothesis (see Chapter 17, pages 697–699, for a more detailed discussion).

These effects can also be passed on to future generations when affected girls of the current generation grow up and start their own families. For this reason, immigrants to richer nations and the poor in developing nations may need four or more generations of improved conditions to overcome all past risks for short stature and overweight.

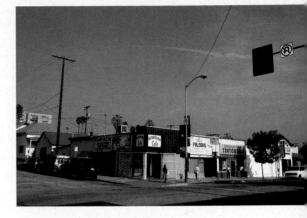

"Food deserts" are geographic areas where people lack access to affordable, nutritious food, typically because of an absence of grocery stores.

Do you live in a food desert? Go to the USDA site, http://ams.usda.gov/ and type in "food desert" in the search box to find out!

food desert A geographic area where people lack access to fresh, healthy, and affordable food.

RECAP

The most serious manifestation of undernourishment is severe acute malnutrition (SAM), which is characterized by wasting and stunting. Populations that are undernourished have increased rates of infant, childhood, and maternal mortality, and lower life expectancy, in part because of increased susceptibility to infection. Micronutrient deficiency diseases include iron-deficiency anemia, brain damage, and other disorders associated with iodine deficiency, and vitamin-A-deficiency-induced blindness. Undernourished people also have low work capacity. Obesity is a global public health concern. Lack of physical activity and increased access to nutrient-poor, high-Calorie foods have contributed to a nutrition paradox, whereby growth stunting and overweight/obesity are found in the same community, family, or individual. The poverty–obesity paradox—the increased prevalence of obesity in low-income populations— may be due to the lower cost, increased shelf life, and increased satiety value of empty-Calorie foods; the prevalence of food deserts; and the stresses of poverty. The theory called *fetal origins of adult disease* suggests that fetal undernourishment contributes to obesity and chronic disease in adulthood.

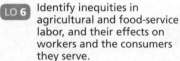 Identify inequities in agricultural and food-service labor, and their effects on workers and the consumers they serve.

Is Our Food Equitably Produced and Sold?

Most people consider fresh fruits and vegetables good food, but if we're defining "good" as equitably produced and sold, then much of the produce we eat each day doesn't qualify. A recent report from the Rockefeller Foundation calls the working conditions in America's agricultural and food service industries "grossly inequitable."[32] Why?

Farm Labor Is Dangerous and Poorly Paid

Throughout the U.S. labor market, in retail, industry, and even white-collar professions such as college teaching, more and more businesses are hiring "contingent workers." These positions typically offer little job security; no healthcare insurance, accrued sick- or vacation-leave, or retirement benefits; and low wages. This trend is nowhere more clearly seen than in agriculture, where about 20% of the workforce is contingent, up from 14% in the early 1990s.[33] Often referred to as "migrant workers" because they move from one region to another with changing harvest times, agricultural contingent workers also face hazardous conditions in the field. Consider these statistics:[32–35]

■ The average annual income for a contingent U.S. farm worker is $10,000–12,500. Large farms are required to pay minimum wage, but small farms are not, and a majority of contingent farm workers live below the poverty line.
■ Under federal law, young people aged 16 years and older are allowed to work on farms during school hours, and children aged 12 years and older may work on farms after school and on weekends with parental permission.
■ Farm workers are not entitled to breaks for rest or meals mandated for other U.S. workers by the Fair Labor Standards Act (FLSA).
■ Only 17% have any form of healthcare insurance and few have paid sick leave.
■ Agriculture ranks as one of the most dangerous industries, with a fatality rate 7 times higher than the average for all workers in private industry. On average, more than 100 youths (under age 20) die each year from farm-labor injuries. Deaths are most commonly due to tractor overturns and other traumatic injuries and heat stroke.
■ Long-term exposure to pesticides, crop dusts, and excessive UV radiation causes lung disease and cancer, and constant bending and stooping causes musculoskeletal injury.
■ Contingent farm worker housing is often overcrowded and substandard, with some units lacking electricity, toilets, and running water.

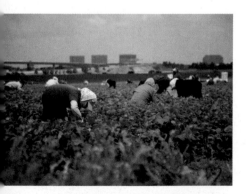

Contingent farm workers are inadequately compensated for their labor, receive few benefits, and have high rates of occupational injury and disease.

Food Service Work Maintains the "Working Poor"

Conditions are only marginally better for the over 4 million food and beverage service workers in the United States.[36] Although the median hourly wage is $8.84, many work at or below the minimum wage, and in many states, workers who earn more than $30 a month in tips may lawfully be paid just $2.13 an hour.[36] Thus, it's not surprising that, like farm workers, a majority of food service workers live below the poverty line, accounting for many of America's "working poor."

Low wages in the food service industry affect everyone. Nearly 30% of food service workers receive Medicaid, and 14% receive SNAP benefits.[32] In essence, this means that the average American taxpayer is subsidizing fast-food chains and other food-service corporations, "making up the difference" in the inadequate wages they pay their employees. This situation has recently led cities and states across the United States to reexamine their minimum wage laws; in 2015, Seattle, Washington led the way by increasing its minimum wage to $15 an hour.

Many food service workers also have no paid sick leave. These workers are likely to show up for work even when ill with an infectious disease. You've learned (in Chapter 15) that the leading culprit in foodborne illness is norovirus, and the primary way that norovirus spreads is through infected food service workers. Foodborne illness is also a risk when farm workers don't receive paid sick leave. Farm workers infected with norovirus, hepatitis A virus, *Salmonella enteriditis,* and other foodborne microbes can contaminate produce during harvesting, and meat during processing.

Inequities in food security and labor can be discouraging and even distressing. Later in this chapter (pages 645–646) we'll explore some ways you can help promote the equitable production, distribution, and sale of food.

RECAP

Working conditions in America's agricultural and food service industries are inequitable. Contingent farm workers are inadequately paid, receive few benefits considered standard in other industries, and face much greater risks for occupational injury, chronic disease, and workplace fatality. A majority of farm and food service workers live below the poverty line. Many food service workers receive Medicaid and SNAP benefits funded by all Americans. The majority of agricultural and food service workers also lack paid time off for illness, and therefore are likely to work even when they risk contaminating foods during harvesting, production, preparation, and service.

What Factors Influence the Sustainability and Quality of Our Food Supply?

LO 7 Discuss the effects of industrial agriculture on food security and the environment.

LO 8 Explain how the food industry has influenced the quality and diversity of our food supply.

Sustainability is the ability to satisfy humanity's basic needs now and in the future without undermining the natural resource base and environmental quality on which life depends. Whereas some people view sustainability as a lofty but impractical ideal, others point out that it's a necessary condition of human survival. That's because sustainable practices can reduce pollution of our air, soil, and water and preserve resources for future generations. Is our current system of food production sustainable? Let's begin with some history.

Industrial Agriculture Has Increased Food Security but Threatens Our Environment

Like other modern wars, World War II led to innovations in industrial technology, engineering, and chemistry. After the war ended, these innovations were directed toward agriculture, specifically toward increasing worldwide food production to meet the food

sustainability The ability to meet or satisfy basic economic, social, and security needs now and in the future without undermining the natural resource base and environmental quality on which life depends.

needs of a dramatically increasing postwar population. Together, the new technologies and practices became known as the **Green Revolution,** a massive program that has led to improved seed quality, fertilizers, pesticides, and farming techniques, which have boosted crop yields throughout the world. As part of the Green Revolution, for example, new **high-yield varieties** (HYVs) of grain were produced by cross-breeding plants and selecting for the most desirable traits. The first HYVs were rice and wheat, but now corn, beans, and many other crops are HYVs.

Industrial techniques were also applied to livestock production. As the total number of livestock and poultry farms with small numbers of animals declined, fewer but much larger operations increased. Between 1964 and 2012, for example, the number of farms raising cattle declined from over 2 million to just 26,500.[37,38] Cattle, pigs, and chickens are now increasingly raised in huge and crowded *confined animal feeding operations* (CAFOs) where their movement is restricted and they are fattened with high-energy feed often containing growth hormones and—until recently banned in the United States by the Food and Drug Administration—growth-promoting antibiotics.

These increases in food crop and animal production have vastly increased the global food supply and improved nutrition for millions of formerly undernourished people. This improvement in global nutrition—and the millions of lives it has saved—is important to bear in mind as we consider the environmental costs it has incurred. These include the following:

- Loss of topsoil due to erosion from heavy tilling, from extensive planting of row crops such as corn and soybeans, and from run-off due to irrigation
- Pollution of soils from salt build-up due to excessive irrigation, leading to abandonment of formerly productive land
- Depletion of fossil fuels
- Depletion of ground water supplies from irrigation techniques requiring heavy water consumption, and pollution of water from pesticide residues, animal waste, and other run-off
- Development of insecticide-resistant species of insects and herbicide-resistant varieties of weeds resulting from intensified use of agrochemical products
- Increased release of greenhouse gases from increasingly mechanized production and from methane released from animals in CAFOs

Beef production is a particular concern. Research data point to the inefficiency of eating meat from grain-fed cattle instead of eating the grains themselves, including in terms of the resources required and the level of greenhouse gas emissions generated. For corn-fed animals, for example, the efficiency of converting grain Calories to meat and dairy Calories ranges from roughly 3% to 40%, meaning that, on average, a crop capable of sustaining four to five people per acre will sustain only one person.[39] Livestock production also leads to deforestation, as forests are cut down to clear land for grazing or for production of animal feed. The contribution of meat consumption to global warming and resource depletion is discussed in the ***Nutrition Myth or Fact?*** essay on page 647.

Monopolization of Agriculture Reduces Food Diversity

Industrial agriculture has also reduced **food diversity**—that is, the variety of different species of food crops available. Beginning in the 1960s, revisions of the federal Agricultural Adjustment Act, commonly called the "farm bill," provided financial incentives for America's farmers to grow single crops on a massive scale. The number of small farms dwindled, and the remaining industrial operations focused on increasing their production of the few subsidized crops, especially corn, soybeans, wheat, and rice. These few crops then began to monopolize the food supply. Because no subsidies were paid for production of fresh fruits and vegetables, their availability and variety plummeted, and they became more expensive.

As a result of this monopolization, the average American diet lost its variety. As you know, variety is a key component of a healthful diet: different species of fruits, vegetables, and whole grains provide different combinations of nutrients, fiber, and phytochemicals that support our health. Moreover, variety reduces the vulnerability of crops to pests; in

Green Revolution The tremendous increase in global productivity between 1944 and 2000 due to selective cross-breeding or hybridization to produce high-yield grains and industrial farming techniques.

high-yield varieties Semi-dwarf varieties of plants that are unlikely to fall over in wind and heavy rains and thus can carry larger amounts of seeds, greatly increasing the yield per acre.

food diversity The variety of different species of food crops available.

contrast, "monoculture" farming requires the use of larger quantities of stronger pesticides. Similarly, because growing the same crop year after year depletes the soil of natural plant nutrients, monocultures require the application of heavy doses of synthetic fertilizers. Finally, different plants respond differently to variations in temperature, rainfall, and other climate conditions. Thus, agricultural variety decreases a region's vulnerability to dramatic food shortages during heat waves, droughts, or other climate events.

The loss of food diversity is not limited to the United States. A 2014 study found that, worldwide, over the past 50 years, national food supplies have become increasingly similar, based on a dwindling number of crop plants, and as a result, global food security is threatened.[40]

The Food Industry Influences America's Diet

When the preliminary report on the *2015 Dietary Guidelines for Americans* was released early in 2015, it proposed to include in the final Guidelines a recommendation that Americans consume less red meat and processed meat. In response, meat industry lobbyists sprang into action, meeting with officials at the USDA and the Department of Health and Human Services (HHS) to request that the 2015 Guidelines recommend that Americans eat lean meats. This attempt to influence the American diet is not an isolated incident: In 2014, the livestock industry donated almost $1.7 million to congressional candidates' election campaigns.[41] Nor is it limited to meat. Consider the following:

- The U.S. dairy industry donated $1.6 million to 2014 congressional campaigns.[41] Meanwhile, the USDA sponsors a program that collects funds from dairy farmers that are used to promote consumption of milk, cheese, and yogurt.[42]
- Crop production and processing lobbies contributed more than $8 million to politicians during the 2014 congressional election campaign.[41]
- Between 2010 and 2015, Coca-Cola spent $118 million to fund public health and nutrition organizations and experts.
- In 2014, the American Beverage Association spent over $11 million to convince voters in San Francisco and Berkeley, California to reject proposed taxes on sugary drinks. The tax was defeated in San Francisco but was passed in Berkeley.
- Also in 2014, the Grocery Manufacturers Association and a number of other food industry groups sued to stop the state of Vermont from requiring labeling of foods made with GM ingredients. In 2015, a federal judge allowed the Vermont law to stand.
- The Yale Rudd Center for Food Policy and Obesity reports that, in 2013, the fast-food industry spent over $4.6 billion to advertise their products, a figure which is more than 12 times higher than the costs for advertising spent on fruits, vegetables, milk, and bottled water combined.[43]

Marion Nestle, PhD, MPH, and professor of nutrition at New York University, points out that the bottom line is simple: The U.S. food industry produces about twice as many Calories per capita per year than Americans require; thus, to continue to make a profit, the industry must encourage consumers to overeat.[44]

RECAP

Sustainability is the ability to satisfy humanity's basic needs now and in the future without undermining the natural resource base and environmental quality on which life depends. The Green Revolution, a set of innovations in agricultural technologies and practices, has vastly increased the global food supply. Its environmental costs include depletion and pollution of soils and water, the evolution of pesticide-resistant insects and weeds, and increased emissions of greenhouse gases. Industrial agriculture has also reduced food diversity and increased the vulnerability of our food supply to pests and climate events. The food industry spends billions of dollars annually on lobbying efforts, campaign contributions, legal challenges, advertising, and other efforts to influence America's diet. ■

What Initiatives Are Addressing the Challenges of "Good" Food?

By now it should be clear that everyone, from world leaders to food-industry executives to farmers to consumers, plays a role in addressing the complex and interconnected challenges of ensuring everyone's access to "good" food. Here, we address large-scale efforts to promote food security and sustainability. We'll discuss what you can do as an individual in the section that follows.

Global, National, and Local Initiatives Increase Access to Nourishing Food

Long-term solutions are critical to achieve and maintain global and regional food security. The UN acknowledges the efforts of "the international community, national governments, civil society, and the private sector" to eradicate global poverty and ensure universal access to ample, nourishing food.[45] Here, we discuss some of these efforts.

International Programs

One of the most effective ways to improve the health and nutrition of children worldwide is to encourage breastfeeding. Breast milk not only provides optimal nutrition for healthy growth of the newborn but also contains antibodies that protect against infections. Moreover, infants who are breastfed exclusively are not exposed to the contaminants that may be present in local water and foods. In 1991, WHO and UNICEF initiated the Baby Friendly Hospital Initiative to increase breastfeeding rates worldwide. Under this initiative, new mothers are educated about the benefits of breast milk, and are encouraged to breastfeed exclusively for the first 6 months of the child's life and as part of the child's daily diet until the child is at least 2 years old.

Breastfeeding is one step among many that can significantly reduce a child's risk for infectious disease. Another important step is vitamin A supplementation. Because vitamin A can be stored in the body's fat tissues, one high-strength vitamin A supplement given every 6 months can prevent deficiency and significantly reduce a child's risk for death from infectious disease. As part of an international Micronutrient Initiative (MI), the WHO and several other national and international organizations collaborate to provide twice-yearly vitamin A supplements to children in developing countries. The MI also promotes children's intake of iron, zinc, iodine, and folic acid, all of which are also important to the immune system. In addition, programs for deworming and mosquito control combat not only helminth and malarial infection but also their accompanying iron deficiency.

During famines or other acute food shortages, for example as a result of natural disasters and wars, the United Nations World Food Programme delivers food and other emergency aid. It also helps communities develop new technologies and practices to reduce chronic food shortages and increase resilience in the face of challenging climate conditions. The United States and other nations also donate food and other emergency aid independently.

In addition, many international organizations help improve food security by assisting communities and families to produce their own foods. For example, both USAID and the Peace Corps have agricultural education programs, the World Bank provides loans to fund small business ventures, and many nonprofit and nongovernmental organizations (NGOs) support community and family farms and gardens.

National and Local Programs

In the United States, several USDA programs help low-income citizens acquire food over extended periods of time. Among these are the Supplemental Nutrition Assistance Program, mentioned earlier, which provides an allotment to low-income individuals of all ages to purchase food. In addition, the Special Supplemental Nutrition Program for Women, Infants,

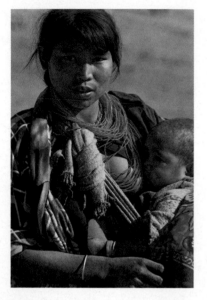

Breastfeeding is highly recommended worldwide.

To find out more about the World Food Programme's goal to eliminate hunger—and how you can help—go to www.wfp .org **and click on the link to the** *WFP and Zero Hunger* **video.**

and Children (WIC) helps pregnant women and children to age 5; the National School Lunch and National School Breakfast Programs provide low-income schoolchildren with free or low-cost meals; and the Summer Food Service Program provides meals to low-income children during the summer months.

The USDA's Commodity Supplemental Food Program distributes surplus foods to charitable agencies for distribution to low-income adults at least 60 years of age. The available items are typically limited to shelf-stable foods: canned fruits, vegetables, meats, and fish; dry beans, pasta, and rice and other grains; ready-to-eat cereals; peanut butter; and instant dry milk. Thus, the program is meant to supplement the fresh foods purchased by the individual.

Both federal health agencies and local governments can provide financial incentives to encourage markets selling fresh produce and other healthful foods to move into low-income areas, or to encourage stores already serving the area to offer more healthful foods. The CDC's Healthy Corner Stores initiative, for example, is helping communities from Philadelphia to Sacramento to invest in corner stores to increase city residents' access to healthy foods such as fresh produce. In addition, a new "urban agriculture" movement is helping to decrease the number of food deserts. Across the United States, city governments are changing zoning codes to encourage the cultivation of vegetable gardens on rooftops, in abandoned parking lots, and even as part of the landscaping on municipal properties.

The United States also has a broad network of local soup kitchens and food pantries that provide meals and food items to needy families. They are supported by volunteers, individual donations, and food contributions from local grocery stores and restaurants.

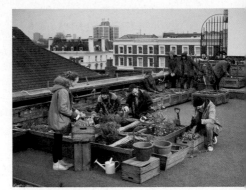

Eagle Street Rooftop Farm is a 6,000-square foot organic vegetable garden located on top of a warehouse in Brooklyn, New York.

Sustainable Agriculture Reduces Environmental Impact and Increases Food Diversity

In response to the environmental problems and loss of food diversity associated with industrial agriculture, a new global movement toward **sustainable agriculture** has evolved. The goal of sustainable agriculture is to develop local, site-specific farming methods that improve soil conservation, crop yields, food security, and food diversity in a sustainable manner. For example, soil erosion can be controlled by **crop rotation,** by terracing sloped land for the cultivation of crops, and by tillage that minimizes disturbance to the topsoil. Organic farming is one method of sustainable agriculture, because to be certified organic, farms must commit to sustainable agricultural practices, including avoiding the use of synthetic fertilizers and toxic and persistent pesticides. Organic meats are produced without the use of antibiotics and hormones for animal growth. Sustainable agriculture also promotes the use of otherwise unusable plants for high-quality animal feed, recycles animal wastes for fertilizers and fuel, and practices humane treatment of animals.

The sustainable agriculture movement has led to an increase in family farms and a variety of farming programs, some of which you probably recognize:

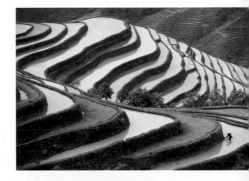

Terracing sloped land to avoid soil erosion is one practice of sustainable agriculture.

- *Family farms.* For three decades, the number of farms in the United States has been decreasing, from 2.48 million in 1982 to 2.11 million in 2012.[38] However, since 2007, the number of small farms (1 to 9 acres) has not declined, and in some states, mainly in New England and the Southwest, they have increased. Some small farmers are taking advantage of programs offering land at reduced prices, community support, and mentoring. Many of these small farms are dedicated to organic farming, crop diversity, and other practices of sustainable agriculture.
- *Community supported agriculture (CSA).* In CSA programs, a farmer sells a certain number of "shares" to the public. Shares typically consist of a box of produce from the farm on a regular basis, such as once weekly throughout the growing season. Farmers get cash early on, as well as guaranteed buyers. Consumers get fresh, locally grown food. Together, farmers and consumers develop ongoing relationships as they share the bounty in a good year, and the losses when weather extremes or blight reduces yield. Although there is no national database on CSA programs, the organization LocalHarvest lists thousands.[46]

sustainable agriculture Term referring to techniques of food production that preserve the environment indefinitely.

crop rotation The practice of alternating crops in a particular field to prevent nutrient depletion and erosion of the soil and to help with control of crop-specific pests.

Find a farmers' market near you! Go to the USDA's Farmers' Market Search page at http://ams.usda.gov. Click on "Farmers Markets and Local Food Marketing," then choose "Find a Farmers Market."

- *Farmers' markets.* There are now more than 8,000 farmers' markets in the United States, more than four times the number when the USDA began compiling these data in 1994.[47] With the help of the USDA, many farmers markets are now able to accept SNAP benefits for payment. Thus, farmers' markets are helping to increase everyone's access to nourishing food.

- *School gardens.* The School Garden Association of America was founded in 1910, and during World Wars I and II, school gardening became part of the war effort; however, in the postwar decades, school gardens dwindled. Recently, school garden programs have been increasing across the United States. In addition to promoting student acceptance of fruits and vegetables, school garden programs teach valuable lessons in nutrition, agriculture, and even cooking. In many schools, cafeterias incorporate the foods into the school lunch menu.

- *Slow food.* Experts in sustainable agriculture and public health are increasingly challenging our loss of food quality and diversity by advocating "slow food"; that is, nutritious, fresh food produced in ways that preserve biodiversity, sustain the environment, ensure animal welfare, and are affordable by all while respecting the dignity of labor from field to fork.[48] Slow food, to the extent possible, is locally grown, a term that typically refers to food grown within a few hundred miles of the consumer. Consuming local food limits energy use and greenhouse gas emissions from transportation (so-called "food miles"). Also, because these foods move much more quickly from farm to table, they tend to be fresher, retaining more of their micronutrients. In cold climates, of course, growing and storing a healthful variety of local food from fall through spring is difficult if not impractical, using more energy than transporting foods from warmer climates.

Business and Philanthropic Initiatives Are Promoting "Good" Food

Many individuals and venture capital firms are now investing in food technologies dedicated to increasing food security and preserving human health and the environment. Howard Buffett, son of investor Warren Buffett, is supporting no-till farming, crop rotation, and other techniques of sustainable agriculture to help relieve food insecurity in Africa, whereas philanthropist Bill Gates is supporting companies producing vegan versions of chicken, eggs, and other high-protein foods. Other investors are funding indoor agricultural growing systems that do not require soil, food-waste recycling programs, crop monitoring systems that identify specific pests and reduce the random use of pesticides, and services that bring fresh produce from local farms directly to consumers' doors.

Whereas many smaller natural-food companies have long made "good" food part of their company identity, only recently has this goal moved into corporate America. In the past few years, Walmart, Kellog, McDonald's, and several other corporations have begun to partner with local growers to promote sustainable agriculture, and in 2015, both Walmart and McDonald's announced that they would modestly increase the wages they pay their employees.

RECAP

Programs encouraging breastfeeding and providing micronutrient supplementation can significantly improve children's nutrition and reduce their risk for infectious disease. The World Food Programme and other efforts provide emergency food aid and support for investments in long-term food security. In the United States, the Supplemental Nutrition Assistance Program, the Commodity Supplemental Food Program, the Healthy Corner Stores initiative, and many other national and local programs help increase access for low-income Americans to nourishing food. The goal of sustainable agriculture is to develop local, site-specific farming methods that improve soil conservation, crop yields, food security, and food diversity in a sustainable manner. Some of its more visible familiar efforts are organic farming, farmers markets, school gardens, and slow food. Individual investors and corporations are beginning to support or implement initiatives aimed at increasing the equity, sustainability, and quality of America's food. ■

What Can You Do to Promote "Good" Food?

LO 10 Identify several steps you can take to promote production of and access to "good" food.

A national debate about food safety and food politics began in the early 1990s in response to incidents of fatal foodborne illness, America's rising obesity rate, and increasing concerns about GM foods, pesticide residues, and the effects of agriculture on global warming. A series of investigative news articles, books, and films explored not only the health risks but also the environmental and social costs of contemporary methods of food production. Advocates for public health, animal welfare, farmland preservation, the rights of farm workers, and environmental quality all came together in a common cause. The food movement was born. Under its umbrella are thousands of local to global initiatives in which millions of ordinary consumers are involved. Here, we review a few simple actions you can take to join them.

Support Food Security

Have you ever wondered whether efforts you make locally can help feed people thousands of miles away? Let's take a look.

Eating just the Calories you need to maintain a healthy weight leaves more of the global harvest for others and will also likely reduce your use of medical resources. So to raise your consciousness about the physical experience of hunger, try turning off your cell phone and other devices and keeping silent during each meal for a day, so that you can more fully appreciate the food you're eating and reflect on those who are hungry. Also check in with your body before and as you eat: are you really hungry, and if so, how much and what type of food does your body really need right now?

Try to stay aware of how much food you throw away, and ask yourself why. Do you put more food on your plate than you can eat? Do you allow foods stored in your refrigerator to spoil?

Join a community garden or shared farming program, with the goal of donating a portion of your produce each week to a local food pantry. While you're there, consider volunteering to help!

Donate to or raise money for one of the international agencies that work to relieve global hunger. Or join other students fighting food insecurity in the United States by becoming a member of the National Student Campaign Against Hunger and Homelessness. See the **Web Links** for websites.

Get the word out! If you find an organization whose goals you share, recommend them on your social networking page. Or send a short article about the organization's work to your campus news site, with suggestions about how other students can support their work.

Purchase Fair Trade Goods

The **fair trade** movement was born in response to the exploitation of farm laborers around the world. It began decades ago in North America and Europe but is now a global effort that depends on support from consumers worldwide to purchase fruits, vegetables, coffee, tea, cocoa, wine, and many other products that display the Fair Trade Certified logo [49] (**Figure 16.4**). Fair trade empowers farm laborers to demand living wages and humane treatment. It also reduces child labor and increases children's access to education, because parents earning higher wages are able to allow their children to leave the fields and attend school. Profits from fair trade purchases also support the building of schools and health clinics, provide funds to help farmers adopt sustainable agricultural practices, and provide financial assistance to women so they can set up small businesses.[49]

The choices you make when you shop can contribute to food equity, because your purchases influence local and global markets. To support equitable production worldwide, purchase Fair Trade goods whenever possible, whether at your grocery store or shopping online. The Fair Trade USA website has a handy shopping guide where you can check out what's available, from hundreds of brands of coffee to chocolate, produce, and even fair trade clothing!

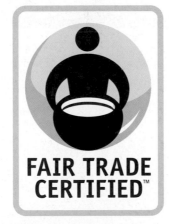

FIGURE 16.4 The Fair Trade Certified logo guarantees that the product has been produced equitably without exploitation of workers or the environment.

fair trade A trading partnership promoting equity in international trading relationships and contributing to sustainable development by securing the rights of marginalized producers and workers.

Choose Foods That Are Healthful for You and the Environment

Any grocery store manager will tell you that your purchases influence the types of foods that are manufactured and sold. In our global economy, your food choices can even influence the types of foods that are imported. So to the extent that you can:

- Buy organic foods to reduce the use of synthetic pesticides and fertilizers.
- Buy produce from a local farmer's market to encourage greater local availability of fresh foods. This reduces the costs and resources devoted to distribution, transportation, and storage of foods.
- Choose whole or less processed versions of packaged foods. This encourages their increased production and saves energy.
- Does your grocery store display candy and other junk foods at children's eye level—for example, beside the check-out line? If so, complain to the store manager.
- Both when you're shopping and when you're eating out, avoid empty-Calorie foods and beverages to discourage their profitability.
- When you eat at a fast-food restaurant, ask for information about the nutritional value of their menu items. Analyze the information. If you see aspects that concern you, take a few minutes to send the company an email sharing your concerns and asking for improved recipes.

The amount of meat you eat also affects the environment and the global food supply, because the production of plant-based foods uses fewer natural resources and releases fewer greenhouse gases than the production of animal-based foods. To promote reduced meat consumption on campus, talk with your food services manager about sponsoring "Meatless Mondays." See the *Web Links* for a link to the Meatless Monday website, where you can download a *Meatless Monday Goes to College* toolkit. For more information on the link between meat production and climate change, see the **Nutrition Myth or Fact?** essay beginning on the following page.

You know that physical activity is important in maintaining health, but walking, biking, and taking public transportation also limits your consumption of nonrenewable fossil fuels and the emission of greenhouse gases. When it's time to purchase a car, research your options and choose the one with the best fuel economy.

As Francis Moore Lappe, author of the groundbreaking *Diet for a Small Planet*, explains, the food movement encourages us to think with an "eco-mind," refusing to accept scarcity, oppression, pollution, and depletion of natural resources in the name of production and profit. By promoting the values of equity, sustainability, and quality, the food movement encourages us to make choices in ways that can change our world.[50]

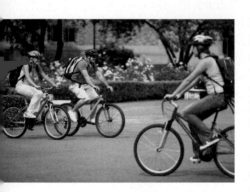

Bicycling is a healthful option that helps limit the use of fossil fuels.

RECAP

The food movement refers to advocacy for public health, animal welfare, farmland preservation, the rights of farm workers, and environmental quality in relation to food production, marketing, and consumption. Increasing your awareness of your own food cues and food waste can help motivate you to make choices that reduce your use of resources. Consider donating to or volunteering for a food relief organization. Make fair trade purchases whenever possible, and when you're shopping for food, eating at your campus dining hall, or eating out, choose and request healthful foods. Consider eating vegetarian meals at least one day a week, and walk, bike, or take public transportation as often as possible. ■

Meat Consumption and Climate Change: Tofu to the Rescue?

The surge in the world's population has been accompanied by the growth of livestock production. Over the last five decades, while the human population roughly doubled, the number of domestic animals roughly tripled.[1] Increased livestock production and meat consumption has been observed throughout the world, but has been particularly notable in nations like China and India transitioning out of poverty. In the United States, we consumed 25.5 billion pounds of beef in 2013.[2] Why is this a concern?

Meat production, particularly the production of beef, is a major contributor to global warming and climate change, releasing much higher levels of several potent greenhouse gases (GHGs) than are emitted from the production of pork, poultry, eggs, dairy foods, and especially plants. It also degrades more land and uses more of the Earth's limited freshwater supplies than the production of non-meat animal proteins and plant proteins. Let's look at the data.

Beef Production Releases More GHG Emissions

According to the Food and Agricultural Organization of the United Nations, globally, livestock production generates 18% of the greenhouse gases (GHGs) responsible for global warming.[3] Some studies cite a slightly lower percentage and others, such as a 2009 study from researchers at the World Watch Institute, suggest that the percentage is dramatically higher—51%.[4] The GHGs generated by livestock production include not only carbon dioxide (CO_2), but methane (CH_4). As the EPA explains, livestock such as cattle, buffalo, sheep, and goats produce large amounts of CH_4 as part of their normal digestive process (belching and flatulence). Also, CH_4 is produced from the animals' stored manure. Globally, the agriculture sector is the primary source of CH_4 emissions. Pound for pound, the comparative impact of CH_4 on climate change is 25 times greater than that of CO_2 over a 100-year period.[5]

Another emission of concern in beef production is reactive nitrogen (Nr). This gas has approximately 300 times the global warming potential of carbon dioxide and is the major contributor to the depletion of the Earth's ozone layer.[1] Moreover, Nr can easily relocate from soil to water to air, producing smog and acid rain, and damaging crops, seafood, and non-food species, decreasing biodiversity overall.

So precisely how different are emissions from beef consumption versus non-meat foods and food crops? Of the many different studies that have tackled this question over the past 20 years, one of the most recent is a 2014 analysis conducted by an international team of scientists and published in the *Proceedings of the National Academy of Sciences*.[6] They found that beef production releases 5 times more GHGs and 6 times more Nr emissions than the average of four non-meat animal foods (pork, poultry, eggs, and dairy), and

11 times more GHGs and 19 times more Nr than the average of three plant foods (wheat, potatoes, and rice). **Figure 16.5** compares the costs of beef to plant production per 1,000 kcal consumed.

Rather than disputing this research, the Cattlemen's Beef Board and National Cattlemen's Beef Association website offers a different perspective.[7] Citing the EPA's home page, they state that GHGs released by U.S. beef production represent a small portion of all U.S. GHG emissions—about

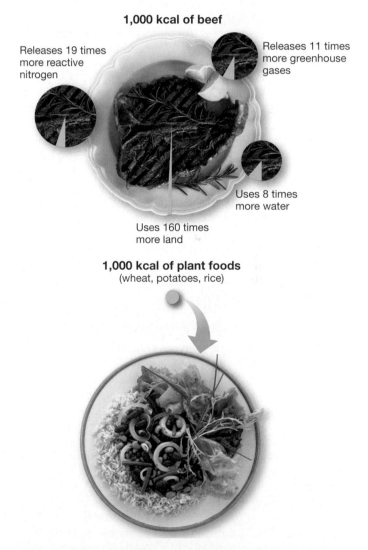

1,000 kcal of beef

Releases 19 times more reactive nitrogen

Releases 11 times more greenhouse gases

Uses 8 times more water

Uses 160 times more land

1,000 kcal of plant foods
(wheat, potatoes, rice)

FIGURE 16.5 Comparison of resource use and emissions for beef versus plant foods. *Data from*: Eshel, G., A. Shepon, T. Makov, and R. Milo. 2014. Land, irrigation water, greenhouse gas, and reactive nitrogen burdens of meat, eggs, and dairy production in the United States. *PNAS* 111(33):11996–12001. doi: 10.1073/pnas.1402183111

3%, versus 26% for transportation. Still, comparing cows to cars may be more distracting than helpful. We choose what to eat several times a day, and each of these choices can either contribute to or help mitigate climate change.

Beef Production Depletes More Natural Resources

In addition to being a major source of greenhouse gas emissions, livestock production contributes to land degradation, using 30% of the earth's land surface for pasture or feed production.[8] Deforestation for agriculture and industry began to increase in the 1970s. The Brazilian Amazon region, for example, has lost nearly 20% of its plant mass since the early 1980s, the majority for cattle grazing.[9] This loss has global effects, as it reduces the capture of greenhouse gases performed by plants during photosynthesis. Livestock's presence in vast tracts of land and its demand for feed crops also have contributed significantly to a reduction in biodiversity and a decline in ecosystems. The analysis mentioned earlier found that beef production uses 28 times more land than non-meat animal foods and 160 times more land than plant foods.[6]

Another environmental concern is the effect of livestock production on the global water supply. Beef production uses 11 times more water than non-meat animal foods and 8 times more water than plant foods.[6] Moreover, animal waste, antibiotics, and hormones can run off into neighboring streams, rivers, and lakes and into nearly irrigation fields used to produce crops for human consumption.

Again, the beef industry website avoids challenging this data directly but offers additional considerations. It states that more than two-thirds of the land used for grazing cattle in the United States is not suitable for raising crops, and that "cattle serve a valuable role in the ecosystem by converting plants humans cannot consume into a nutrient-dense food." It also reports that beef production today requires 12% less water than was used in the 1970s.[7]

You Can Reduce Your Consumption of Beef

Although some individuals choose vegetarianism to protect the environment, it is not practical or realistic to expect every human around the world to adopt this lifestyle. Animal products provide important nutrients: the beef industry website points out that a 3-ounce serving of beef supplies 51% of the Daily Value (DV) for protein, 38% of the DV for zinc, and 14% of the DV for iron.[7] Many people living in poverty depend on small amounts of dairy, eggs, poultry, pork, and meat in their diet to preserve their health.

Still, if most Americans were to reduce their consumption of meat even modestly, the change would have a powerful collective impact. A 2014 study of the contribution of a variety of 2,000 kcal diets to climate change found that meat-eating releases almost twice the GHGs of a vegetarian diet and well over twice the GHGs of a vegan diet. The study concluded that, "reducing the intake of meat and other animal based products can make a valuable contribution to climate change mitigation."[10] Moreover, as we noted earlier in this chapter, replacing meat with plant proteins would improve food

security because, Calorie for Calorie, growing crops for human consumption rather than conversion to meat is much more efficient.

If we were to reduce our meat consumption significantly, we might even be able to return to the system of small family farming, which is more environmentally friendly. When animals are raised on smaller farms and/or allowed to range freely, they consume grass, crop wastes, and scraps recycled from the kitchen, which is an efficient means of utilizing food sources that humans do not consume. What's more, the waste produced by these animals can be used for fertilizer and fuel.

As researchers debate the precise extent of environmental harm attributable to meat consumption, one thing is clear: You can help reduce the damage, starting with your next meal.

Critical Thinking Questions

- Given the accelerated pace of climate change, as well as land and water degradation, do we have an ethical responsibility to others with whom we share the planet, especially children, to reduce our consumption of meat?
- What adverse impact might reducing meat consumption have on farmers and ranchers? Would this be greater or worse than the impact of climate change?
- Could some sectors of the food industry actually benefit from reduced meat consumption? Explain.
- Would eating less meat be practical for you? More healthful? More or less expensive? Why or why not?

References

1. Aneja, V. P., W. H. Schlesinger, J. W. Erisman, S. N. Behera, M. Sharma, and W. Battye. 2012. Reactive nitrogen emissions from crop and livestock farming in India. *Atmos. Environ.* 4:7 92–103. Available at http://www.meas.ncsu.edu/airquality/pubs/pdfs/157.pdf
2. U.S. Department of Agriculture (USDA). 2014, December 29. Cattle & Beef: Statistics & Information. Available at http://www.ers.usda.gov/topics/animal-products/cattle-beef/statistics-information.aspx
3. Food and Agricultural Organization of the United Nations. 2015. The Role of Livestock in Climate Change. Accessed May 1, 2015. Available at http://www.fao.org/agriculture/lead/themes0/climate/en/
4. Goodland, R. and J. Anhang. 2009. Livestock and Climate Change. *World Watch*, November/December 2009. Available at http://www.worldwatch.org/files/pdf/Livestock%20and%20Climate%20Change.pdf
5. U.S. Environmental Protection Agency (EPA). 2015. Overview of Greenhouse Gases. April 14, 2015. Available at http://epa.gov/climatechange/ghgemissions/gases/ch4.html
6. Eshel, G., A. Shepon, T. Makov, and R. Milo. 2014. Land, irrigation water, greenhouse gas, and reactive nitrogen burdens of meat, eggs, and dairy production in the United States. *PNAS.* 111(33):11996–12001. doi: 10.1073/pnas.1402183111
7. Cattlemen's Beef Board and National Cattlemen's Beef Association. 2015. Explore Beef. http://www.explorebeef.org/environment.aspx

8. Havlik, P, H. Valin, M. Herroro, M. Obersteiner, E. Schmid, M. C. Rufino,..., and A. Notenbaert. 2014. Climate change mitigation through livestock system transitions. *PNAS*. 111(10): 3709–3714. doi: 10.1073/pnas.1308044111 Available at http://www.pnas.org/content/111/10/3709.long

9. Stokes, S., M. Lowe, and S. Zoubek. 2014. *Deforestation and the Brazilian Beef Value Chain*. Datu Research on behalf of the Environmental Defense Fund. Available

at http://www.daturesearch.com/wp-content/uploads/Brazilian-Beef-Final_Optimized1.pdf

10. Scarborough, P., P. N. Appleby, A. Mizdrak, A. D. M. Briggs, R. C. Travis, K. E. Bradbury, and T. J. Key. 2014. Dietary greenhouse gas emissions of meat-eaters, fish-eaters, vegetarians and vegans in the UK. *Clim Change*. 125(2):179–192. Available at http://www.ncbi.nlm.nih.gov/pmc/articles/PMC4372775/

STUDY **PLAN** MasteringNutrition™

Customize your study plan—and master your nutrition!—in the Study Area of MasteringNutrition.

TEST YOURSELF | ANSWERS

1 **T** In 2013, the most recent year for which data is available, 5.6% of U.S. households experienced very low food security, meaning that at least some members of those households reduced food intake because of insufficient money or other resources.

2 **T** Many obese people consume a diet excessive in "empty Calories" from saturated fats and added sugars, but deficient in one or more micronutrients.

3 **F** The occupational fatality rate for U.S. farm workers is seven times higher than the average for workers in other industries.

4 **T** Corn and soybeans together make up more than half of all cash revenues earned by American farmers. In contrast, all other vegetables, fruits, and nuts make up less than 22% of farm revenues and wheat makes up 7%. Hay and cotton are also sizeable U.S. crops.

5 **F** Methane emissions are 23 times more potent greenhouse gases than carbon dioxide. In the United States, beef production alone is responsible for 18% of all methane emissions.

summary

 Scan to hear an MP3 Chapter Review in MasteringNutrition.

LO 1 ■ Health disparities exist between poor and wealthy nations and between poor and wealthy regions within the same nation. For example, average life expectancy in some of the world's poorest countries lags about a quarter-century behind that of the United States; however, within the United States, average life expectancy in the poorest counties is more than a dozen years behind that of the wealthiest counties. Food insecurity, which is unreliable access to a sufficient supply of nourishing food, contributes to health disparities.

■ About one in nine people worldwide, or about 795 million people, are chronically undernourished. However, this represents an overall reduction of almost 45% in global hunger since 1990.

- More than 14% of American households experienced food insecurity in 2013, and more than 5% experienced very low food security, meaning that members of the household periodically had to reduce their intake of food. Nearly 13 million Americans, including 765,000 children, had very low food security in 2013. Households at greatest risk for food insecurity are those with incomes below 185% of the official U.S. poverty threshold, singe-parent households, African American households, and Hispanic American households.

LO 2
- Famines are widespread, acute, severe food shortages that can result in starvation and death. They are most commonly caused by natural disasters, but human behaviors, such as harmful agricultural policies or wars, often contribute.

- The world produces enough food to meet everyone's needs. Worldwide, the leading cause of longstanding hunger in a region is unequal distribution of an adequate food supply, largely because of poverty. Chronic food shortages may also reflect regional overpopulation. Education of women and girls is an effective method of reducing birthrates. Poor agricultural practices, lack of infrastructure, and the burden of diseases such as HIV/AIDS also can significantly affect a region's local economy and food availability.

LO 3
- Global warming, the increase of about 1.4°F (0.8°C) in temperature that has occurred near the Earth's surface over the past century, is the main driver of climate change, a persistent change in temperatures, precipitation, and other climate conditions over several decades or longer.

- Global warming and climate change have reduced crop yields, destroyed crops outright as a result of weather events and emerging species of heat-tolerant pests, and reduced the abundance and distribution of seafood in tropical and temperature regions.

LO 4
- The most extreme manifestation of undernourishment is severe acute malnutrition (SAM), a condition characterized by wasting, a very low body-weight-to-height ratio, and often stunted growth. SAM also increases a population's rate of maternal, infant, and childhood mortality, often because of increased susceptibility to infection.

- The micronutrient deficiencies most common in impoverished populations include iron deficiency, which causes anemia; iodine deficiency,

which causes numerous disorders, including mental impairment; and vitamin A deficiency, which causes blindness and increases the risk for death.

- Undernourishment also promotes socioeconomic problems because it decreases work capacity.

LO 5
- About 600 million people worldwide are obese. The nutrition paradox, the coexistence of stunting and overweight/obesity within the same region, the same household, and even the same person, is thought to be due to decreased physical activity along with increased intake of energy-dense food as a region transitions out of poverty.

- The high prevalence of obesity in low-income populations is referred to as the poverty–obesity paradox. Factors thought to contribute to this paradox include preferential purchase of energy-dense, shelf-stable foods that have a higher satiety value; reduced access to food among low-income residents of so-called food deserts; and the physiologic and psychological effects of stress on impoverished populations.

- According to the *fetal origins of adult disease* theory, undernourishment *in utero* can lead to overweight, obesity, and obesity-related chronic diseases in childhood and adulthood.

LO 6
- Inequities in agriculture keep farm workers impoverished and increase their risk for occupational injury, chronic diseases such as lung disease and cancer, and workplace fatality.

- The low hourly wages and poor benefits in the food service industry keep a majority of workers living below the poverty line. Many receive Medicaid and SNAP benefits.

- Lack of paid time off for illness in both agricultural and food service work increases the probability that workers with infectious illnesses will contaminate foods during harvesting, production, preparation, or service.

LO 7
- Sustainability is the ability to satisfy humanity's basic needs now and in the future without undermining the natural resource base and environmental quality on which life depends. The Green Revolution, a set of innovations in agricultural technologies and practices, has vastly increased global food security.

- Environmental costs of industrial agriculture include depletion and pollution of soils and water, the evolution of pesticide-resistant insects and weeds, and increased emissions of greenhouse gases. Meat production is inefficient in terms of resource use and greenhouse gas emissions for Calories produced.

LO 8
■ Industrial agriculture has increasingly focused on monocultures, mainly corn, soybeans, wheat, and rice. This practice has reduced global food diversity and increased the vulnerability of our food supply to pests and climate events.

■ The U.S. food industry produces about twice as many Calories per capita per year than Americans require. It spends billions of dollars annually on lobbying efforts, campaign contributions, legal challenges, advertising, and other efforts to influence the content, quality, and diversity of America's diet.

LO 9
■ The World Health Organization's support of breastfeeding and micronutrient supplementation and the World Food Programme's provision of emergency food aid are just a few examples of many international efforts to improve food security. In the United States, federal food programs include the Supplemental Nutrition Assistance Program, the National School Breakfast and Lunch Programs, and many others.

■ In municipalities across the United States, new zoning laws are encouraging community

and rooftop gardens and financial incentives are encouraging markets selling affordable, nourishing foods to serve urban food deserts.

■ Sustainable agriculture develops site-specific farming methods that improve soil conservation, crop yields, food security, and food diversity in a sustainable manner. Some manifestations of sustainable agriculture in recent decades have been an increase in organic farms, family farms, community supported agriculture, farmers markets, school gardens, and the "slow food" and "local food" initiatives.

■ Private investors and corporations are beginning to support "good" food by supporting the development of high-protein plant foods, local growers, and increased wages for workers.

LO 10
■ You can support food security by consuming only what your body needs, reducing food waste, joining a community garden, donating to a food pantry or other food-relief organization, or volunteering. Within your budget, you can commit to purchasing fair trade goods, organic foods, and local foods. You can also purchase less processed foods, and when cooking at home or eating out, prepare or choose healthful meals, and vegetarian meals more often. Finally, you can walk, bike, or take public transportation whenever possible.

review questions

LO 1 1. The majority of the world's hungry people live in
a. Asia.
b. South Africa.
c. sub-Saharan Africa.
d. the developed world.

LO 2 2. The leading cause of longstanding hunger in a region is
a. famine.
b. war.
c. unequal distribution of food, largely because of poverty.
d. overpopulation.

LO 3 3. Which of the following qualifies as an example of climate change?
a. In 2011 in Japan, an earthquake and resulting tsunami killed over 15,800 people.
b. In June, 2015 in Pakistan, a sustained a heat wave killed over one thousand people.

c. Worldwide, the probability of extreme heat events has been five times higher over the past 60 years than prior to the Industrial Age.
d. In 2013, United States greenhouse gas emissions totaled 6,673 million metric tons of carbon dioxide equivalents.

LO 4 4. Deficiency of vitamin A can
a. increase an individual's risk for infection.
b. lead to blindness.
c. decrease an individual's work capacity.
d. all of the above.

LO 5 5. In the United States, a food desert is
a. typically located in a suburb.
b. by definition also served by fast-food restaurants and convenience stores.
c. by definition also inhabited almost exclusively by low-income populations.
d. a geographic area where people lack access to fresh, healthy, and affordable food.

LO 6 6. Which of the following statements about farm and food service labor is true?

   a. In many states in the United States, farm and food service workers may lawfully be paid just $2.13 an hour.
   b. The majority of farm and food service workers live below the poverty line.
   c. On average, nearly 100 workers die each year from farm-labor injuries.
   d. All of the above are true.

LO 7 7. Which of the following statements about the Green Revolution is true?

   a. It has increased global production of organic foods.
   b. It has dramatically increased food security throughout South America, Asia, and Africa.
   c. It has ended the loss of topsoil that had been common with traditional farming methods.
   d. It has reduced the depletion and pollution of ground water.

LO 8 8. Which of the following statements about the food industry is true?

   a. The only crop that U.S. farmers receive subsidies to grow is corn.
   b. The food industry spends about $4.6 billion a year on advertising.

   c. The U.S. food industry produces about twice as many Calories per capita per year than Americans require.
   d. All of the above are true.

LO 9 9. Of the following federal programs, which provides food assistance to low-income individuals of all ages?

   a. the Supplemental Nutrition Assistance Program
   b. the Special Supplemental Nutrition Program for Women, Infants, and Children
   c. the Commodity Supplemental Food Program
   d. all of the above

LO 10 10. Which of the following purchases would optimally support food equity, sustainability, and quality?

   a. a fair trade certified t-shirt
   b. a cup of hot apple cider you buy at a farmer's market
   c. a certified organic beef burger on a whole-grain bun from an organic foods restaurant
   d. a pint of strawberries you pick yourself at an organic farm

true or false?

LO 1 11. **True or false?** Adults over age 65 years are at greatest risk for food insecurity in the United States.

LO 5 12. **True or false?** The high prevalence of obesity in low-income populations is called the nutrition paradox.

LO 6 13. **True or false?** The blackberries on your morning cereal could have been harvested by a 12-year-old.

LO 7 14. **True or false?** Loss of crop diversity increases the vulnerability of crops to pests and climate events.

LO 9 15. **True or false?** Crop rotation and terracing are farming methods used in sustainable agriculture.

short answer

LO 2 16. Why might programs to improve the education of women also improve a nation's food/population ratio?

LO 4 17. Jeanette is a healthcare provider in a free clinic in an impoverished area of India. She is 5′8″ tall. Explain why she is not surprised to hear the patients who come to the clinic refer to her as a giant.

LO 5 18. José grew up in a slum in Mexico City, but his brilliance in school earned him recognition and a patron who funded his education. Now in

medical school in the United States, he plans to return to Mexico as a pediatrician and specialize in the treatment of children with type 2 diabetes. Explain why José might be drawn to work with this population.

LO 8 19. Identify four ways that the food industry attempts to influence America's diet.

LO 9 20. Explain why breastfeeding is effective in reducing a population's rate of common childhood infections.

math question

LO 6 **21.** In the Rodgers family, Steve works 40 hours a week, all year, at a fast-food restaurant. He earns the federal minimum wage of $7.25. He has one week of paid vacation a year. Steve and his wife, Diane, have struggled to make ends meet since the birth of their son, now 5 months old, so Diane has decided to return to work at the same fast-food restaurant where her husband works. They have decided to stagger their schedules in order to avoid the cost of daycare for their son. The federal poverty threshold in 2015 was $20,090 for a family of three. Answer these questions: Are Steve, Diane, and their son currently living above, at, or below the federal poverty line? If Diane were to return to work 40 hours a week, would the family be characterized as at increased risk for food insecurity? Why or why not?

Answers to Review Questions can be found online in the MasteringNutrition Study Area.

web links

www.care.org
Care
Since 1945, this organization has been working to relieve hunger and improve economic conditions around the world.

www.freefromhunger.org
Freedom from Hunger
Visit this site to learn about an established international development organization, founded in 1946, that works toward sustainable self-help against chronic hunger and poverty.

www.heifer.org
Heifer International
Visit this site to learn how you can give a cow, some rabbits, or a flock of chickens to a community in a developing country, so that they are better able to provide food for themselves.

www.studentsagainsthunger.org
National Student Campaign Against Hunger and Homelessness
Visit this site to learn what students like you are doing to fight hunger, as well as how you can get involved.

www.unicef.org/nutrition
United Nations Children's Fund
Visit this site to learn about international concerns affecting the world's children, including nutrient deficiencies and hunger.

www.who.int/nutrition/en
World Health Organization Nutrition
Visit this site to learn about global malnutrition, micronutrient deficiencies, and the nutrition transition.

www.fooddemocracynow.org
Food Democracy Now
Visit this grassroots community dedicated to building a sustainable, equitable food system.

www.slowfoodusa.org/
Slow Food USA
Slow Food links the pleasure of growing, preparing, and consuming food with commitment to our communities and environment. Visit this site to learn more about the slow food movement and get involved.

www.fairtradeusa.org
Fair Trade USA
Visit this website to find out why "Every Purchase Matters!"

www.meatlessmonday.com/
Meatless Monday
This website offers information on the environmental and health benefits of going meatless one day a week, as well as recipes for vegetarian meals and a toolkit to promote Meatless Mondays on your campus.

www2.epa.gov/learn-issues/green-living
Environmental Protection Agency's Sustainability Tips
This site offers a wide variety of tips and tools to help you reduce your environmental footprint.

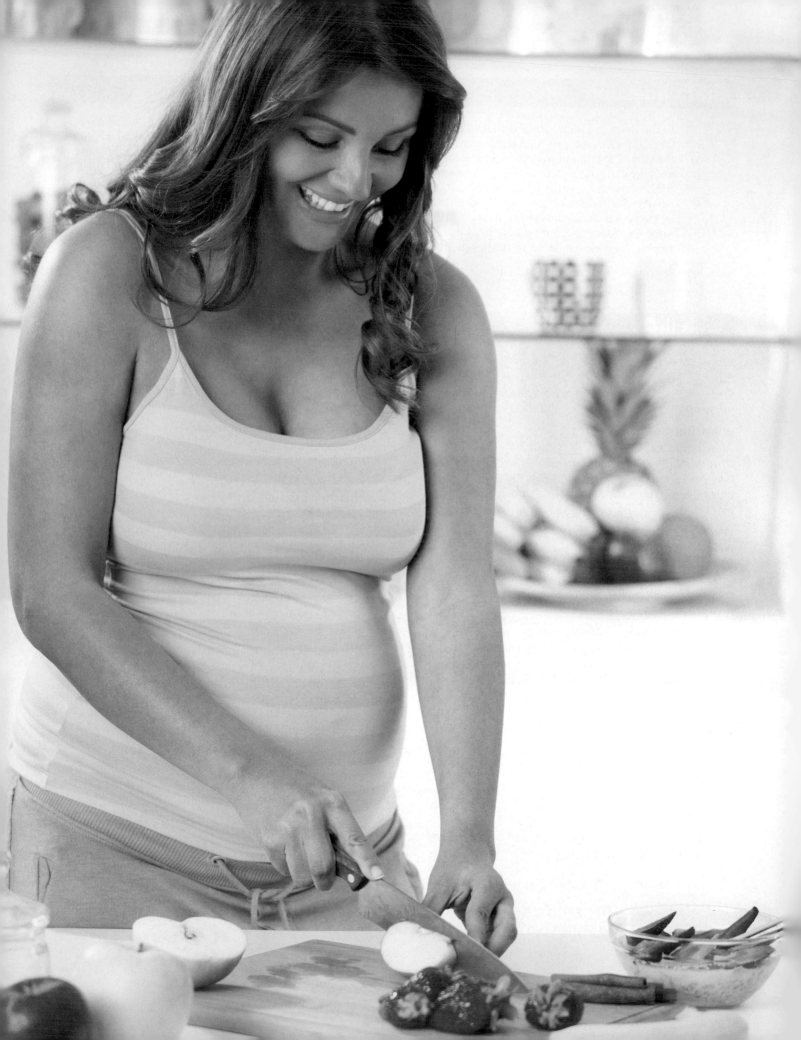

17 Nutrition Through the Life Cycle: Pregnancy and the First Year of Life

Learning Outcomes

After studying this chapter, you should be able to:

1 Discuss several reasons that maintaining a nutritious diet is important for a woman of childbearing age even prior to conception, *pp. 656–657.*

2 Explain the interrelationships of fetal development, physiologic changes in the pregnant woman, and increasing nutrient requirements during the course of a pregnancy, *pp. 657–661.*

3 Identify the ranges of optimal weight gain for pregnant women, and the implications of too little or too much weight gain during pregnancy for both the mother and the developing baby, *pp. 661–663.*

4 Identify the macronutrient and micronutrient needs of pregnant women, including for supplements and fluids, *pp. 663–669.*

5 Discuss the key nutrition-related disorders of pregnancy, and the influence of maternal age on pregnancy, *pp. 670–675.*

6 Discuss the effects of exercise, caffeine, artificial sweeteners, alcohol, tobacco, illicit drugs, and medications and supplements on the pregnant woman and her fetus, *pp. 675–678.*

7 Describe the physiologic aspects of lactation, and identify the key nutrient recommendations for and needs of breastfeeding women, *pp. 678–682.*

8 Summarize the advantages and challenges of breastfeeding, *pp. 682–686.*

9 Describe an infant's growth patterns and nutrient needs, and the nutrient profile of different types of infant formula, *pp. 687–692.*

10 Discuss several nutrient-related concerns for infants, *pp. 692–696.*

TEST YOURSELF

True or False?

1 A pregnant woman needs to consume twice as many Calories as she did prior to the pregnancy. **T** *or* **F**

2 Very few pregnant women actually experience morning sickness, food cravings, or food aversions. **T** *or* **F**

3 Breast-fed infants tend to have fewer infections and allergies than formula-fed infants. **T** *or* **F**

4 When a breastfeeding woman drinks caffeinated beverages, such as coffee, the caffeine enters her breast milk. **T** *or* **F**

5 Most infants begin to require solid foods by about 3 months (12 weeks) of age. **T** *or* **F**

Test Yourself answers are located in the Study Plan.

MasteringNutrition™

Go online for chapter quizzes, pre-tests, interactive activities, and more!

A n active, curious 2-year-old, Tomas brings joy and laughter to his parents and family. That wasn't always the case, however. Tomas weighed just over 3 lb 5 oz at birth—about half of what an average full-term newborn weighs. Even today, Tomas is still small for his age and continues to struggle with his coordination and speech. Although the United States has an extensive and expensive healthcare system, the rate of low-birth-weight babies remains at 8%.[1] Moreover, our infant mortality rate—the number of deaths of infants before their first birthday—is now just over 6 infant deaths for every 1,000 live births, higher than that of many other developed countries, including most European countries.[2]

What contributes to these troubling statistics? What are the short- and long-term effects of low birth weight on developing children? And what role does prenatal diet play in determining other aspects of a child's health and well-being?

At no developmental stage is nutrition more crucial than from conception through the end of the first year of life. An individual's ability to reach his or her peak physical and intellectual potential in adulthood is partly determined by the nutrition received during this life stage. Public health officials view pregnancy-related nutrition as so important to the health of the nation that several *Healthy People 2020* objectives are specific to prenatal and postnatal nutrition.[3] These objectives will be identified throughout this chapter as we explore how adequate nutrition supports fetal development, maintains a pregnant woman's health, contributes to lactation, and supports an infant's growth and health.

LO 1 Discuss several reasons that maintaining a nutritious diet is important for a woman of childbearing age even prior to conception.

During conception, a sperm fertilizes an egg, creating a zygote.

conception The uniting of an ovum (egg) and sperm to create a fertilized egg, or zygote; also called *fertilization.*

Why Is Nutrition Important Before Conception?

Several factors make adequate nutrition important even before **conception,** the point at which a woman's ovum (egg) is fertilized with a man's sperm. First, some problems related to nutrient deficiency develop extremely early in the pregnancy, typically before the mother even realizes she is pregnant. An adequate and varied preconception diet reduces the risk for such problems, providing "insurance" during those first few weeks of pregnancy.

For example, failure of the spinal cord to close results in *neural tube defects;* these defects are closely related to inadequate folate status during the first few weeks after conception. For this reason, all women capable of becoming pregnant are encouraged to consume 400 μg of folic acid from fortified foods such as cereals or supplements daily, in addition to natural sources of folate from a varied, healthful diet. This recommendation should be followed by all women of childbearing age whether or not they plan to become pregnant.

Second, adopting a healthful diet and lifestyle prior to conception requires women to avoid alcohol, illegal drugs, tobacco, and other known *teratogens* (substances that cause birth defects). Women should also consult their healthcare provider about their consumption of caffeine, medications, herbs, and supplements; and if they smoke, they should attempt to quit.

Third, a healthful diet and appropriate levels of physical activity can help women achieve and maintain an optimal body weight prior to pregnancy. Women with a prepregnancy body mass index (BMI) between 19.8 and 26 have the best chance of an uncomplicated pregnancy and delivery, with low risk for negative outcomes, such as prolonged labor and cesarean section. As we will discuss in greater detail shortly, women with a BMI below or above this range prior to conception are at greater risk for pregnancy-related complications. Moreover, women who are obese are at increased risk for a disorder called polycystic ovarian syndrome (PCOS), which can result in infertility.

Finally, maintaining a balanced and nourishing diet before conception reduces a woman's risk of developing a nutrition-related disorder of pregnancy, such as gestational diabetes and gestational hypertension. Although genetic and metabolic abnormalities are beyond the woman's control, following a healthful diet prior to conception is something a woman can do to help her fetus develop into a healthy baby.

A man's nutrition and lifestyle prior to conception is important as well. Malnutrition, such as severe zinc deficiency, contributes to abnormalities in sperm. Calcium, vitamin D, folic acid, and dietary antioxidants such as vitamin C have also been linked to improved sperm health and male fertility. In contrast, high saturated fat diets, obesity, and diabetes have been linked to impaired male fertility. Both sperm number and *motility* (ability to move) are reduced by alcohol consumption, as well as the use of certain prescription and illegal drugs. Moreover, smoking is known to damage sperm and reduce male fertility.

RECAP

Conception is the point at which a woman's ovum (egg) is fertilized with a man's sperm. A healthful diet prior to conception is essential for four reasons. First, it helps to prevent certain nutrient-deficiency disorders that develop extremely early in the pregnancy, typically before the woman even realizes she is pregnant. These include, for example, neural tube defects, which are closely related to inadequate folate status during the first few weeks after conception. Second, it establishes a practice of limiting or entirely avoiding the intake of substances could harm the fetus. Third, it can help the woman achieve and maintain a body mass index (BMI) between 19.8 and 26.0, which is considered optimal prior to pregnancy. Fourth, it can help prevent the development of gestational diabetes and other nutrition-related disorders of pregnancy. A man's preconception diet is also important. Certain micronutrients are essential to healthy sperm and male fertility, and obesity, obesity-related diseases, and substance abuse can reduce fertility.

> Watch how the cell divides, travels, and implants in the uterus during the first few days after conception at http://www.nlm.nih.gov/.

How Does Nutrition Support Fetal Development?

A balanced, nourishing diet throughout pregnancy provides the nutrients needed to support fetal growth and development without depriving the mother of nutrients she needs to maintain her own health. It also minimizes the risks of excess energy intake. A full-term pregnancy, also called the period of **gestation,** lasts 38 to 42 weeks and is divided into three **trimesters,** with each trimester lasting about 13 to 14 weeks.

> **LO 2** Explain the interrelationships of fetal development, physiologic changes in the pregnant woman, and increasing nutrient requirements during the course of a pregnancy.

> **LO 3** Identify the ranges of optimal weight gain for pregnant women, and the implications of too little or too much weight gain during pregnancy for both the mother and the developing baby.

The First Trimester Is Characterized by Cell Multiplication and Tissue Differentiation

About once each month, a nonpregnant woman of childbearing age experiences *ovulation,* the release of an ovum (egg cell) from an ovary. The ovum is then drawn into the uterine (fallopian) tube. The first trimester (approximately weeks 1 through 13) begins when the ovum and sperm unite to form a single, fertilized cell called a **zygote.** As the zygote travels through the uterine tube, it further divides into a ball of 12 to 16 cells, which at about day 4, arrives in the uterus (**Figure 17.1**, page 658). By day 10, the inner portion of the zygote, called the *blastocyst,* implants into the uterine lining. The outer portion becomes part of the placenta, which is discussed shortly.

Further cell growth, multiplication, and differentiation occur, resulting in the formation of an **embryo.** Over the next 6 weeks, embryonic tissues fold into a primitive, tubelike structure with limb buds, organs, and facial features recognizable as human (**Figure 17.2**, page 658). It isn't surprising, then, that the embryo is most vulnerable to teratogens during this time. Not only alcohol and illegal drugs but also prescription and over-the-counter medications, megadoses of supplements such as vitamin A, certain herbs, viruses, cigarette smoking, infection, and radiation can interfere with embryonic development and cause birth defects. Moreover, significant nutrient deficiencies during this time can lead to irreversible

gestation The period of intrauterine development from conception to birth.

trimester Any one of three stages of pregnancy, each lasting approximately 13 to 14 weeks.

zygote A fertilized egg (ovum) consisting of a single cell.

embryo The human growth and developmental stage lasting from the third week to the end of the eighth week after fertilization.

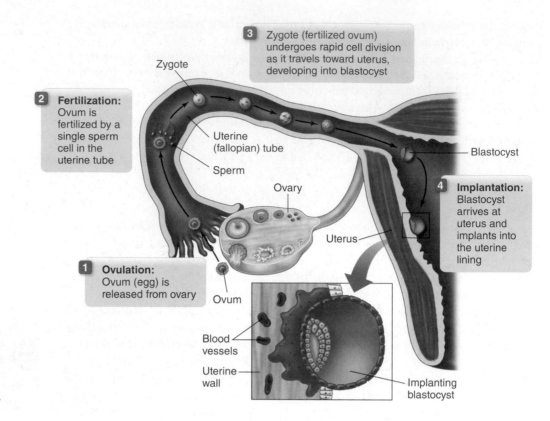

FIGURE 17.1 Ovulation, conception, and implantation.

spontaneous abortion The natural termination of a pregnancy and expulsion of pregnancy tissues because of a genetic, developmental, or physiologic abnormality that is so severe that the pregnancy cannot be maintained; also called *miscarriage*.

placenta A pregnancy-specific organ formed from both maternal and embryonic tissues. It is responsible for oxygen, nutrient, and waste exchange between mother and fetus.

structural or functional damage. In some cases, the damage is so severe that the pregnancy is naturally terminated in a **spontaneous abortion** (*miscarriage*), which occurs most often in the first trimester.

During the first weeks of pregnancy, the embryo obtains its nutrients from cells lining the uterus. But by the fourth week, a primitive **placenta** has formed in the uterus from both embryonic and maternal tissue. Within a few more weeks, the placenta will be a fully functioning organ through which the mother will provide nutrients and remove fetal wastes (**Figure 17.3**).

By the end of the embryonic stage, about 8 weeks postconception, the embryo's tissues and organs have differentiated dramatically. A primitive skeleton, including fingers and toes, has formed. Muscles have begun to develop in the trunk and limbs, and some movement is now possible. A primitive heart has also formed and begun to beat, and the digestive

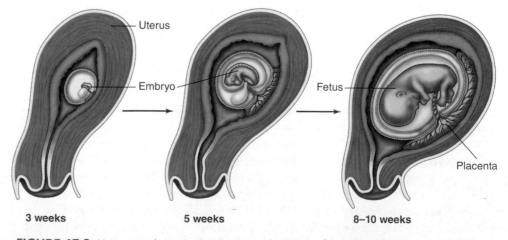

3 weeks   **5 weeks**   **8–10 weeks**

FIGURE 17.2 Human embryonic development during the first 10 weeks. Organ systems are most vulnerable to teratogens during this time, when cells are dividing and differentiating.

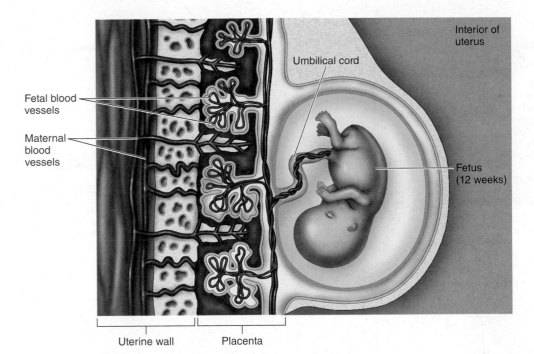

Interior of
uterus

Umbilical cord

Fetal blood
vessels

Maternal
blood
vessels

Fetus
(12 weeks)

Uterine wall   Placenta

FIGURE 17.3 Placental development. The placenta is formed from both embryonic and maternal tissues. When the placenta is fully functional, fetal blood vessels and maternal blood vessels are intimately intertwined, allowing the exchange of nutrients and wastes between the two. The mother transfers nutrients and oxygen to the fetus, and the fetus transfers wastes to the mother for disposal.

system is differentiating into distinct organs (stomach, liver, and so forth). The brain and cranial nerves have differentiated, and the head has a mouth, eyespots with eyelids, and primitive ears.

The third month of pregnancy marks the transition from embryo to **fetus.** The fetus requires abundant nutrients from the mother's body to support its dramatic growth during this period. The placenta is now a fully functioning, mature organ and can provide these nutrients. It is connected to the fetal circulatory system via the **umbilical cord,** an extension of fetal blood vessels emerging from the fetus's navel (called the *umbilicus*). Blood rich in oxygen and nutrients flows through the placenta and into the umbilical vein (see Figure 17.3). Once inside the fetus's body, the blood travels to the fetal liver and heart. Wastes are excreted in blood returning from the fetus to the placenta via the umbilical arteries. Although many people think there is a mixing of blood from the fetus and the mother, the two blood supplies remain separate; the placenta is the "go-between" that allows the transfer of nutrients and wastes.

During the Second and Third Trimesters, Most Growth Occurs

During the second trimester (approximately weeks 14 through 27 of pregnancy), the fetus continues to grow and mature (**Figure 17.4**, page 660). At the beginning of the second trimester, the fetus is about 3 inches long and weighs about 1.5 lb. By the end, it is generally more than 12 inches long and weighs more than 2 lb. Its ears begin to hear, its eyes can open and close and react to light, and it can suck its thumb. Some babies born prematurely in the last weeks of the second trimester survive with intensive **neonatal** care.

The third trimester (approximately week 28 to birth) is a time of remarkable growth for the fetus. During 3 short months, the fetus gains nearly half its body length and three-quarters of its body weight! At the time of birth, an average baby is approximately 18 to 22 inches long and about 7.5 lb in weight (see Figure 17.4). Brain growth (which continues to be rapid for the first 2 years of life) is also quite remarkable, and the lungs

fetus The human growth and developmental stage lasting from the beginning of the ninth week after conception to birth.

umbilical cord The cord containing arteries and veins that connects the baby (from the navel) to the mother via the placenta.

neonatal Referring to a newborn.

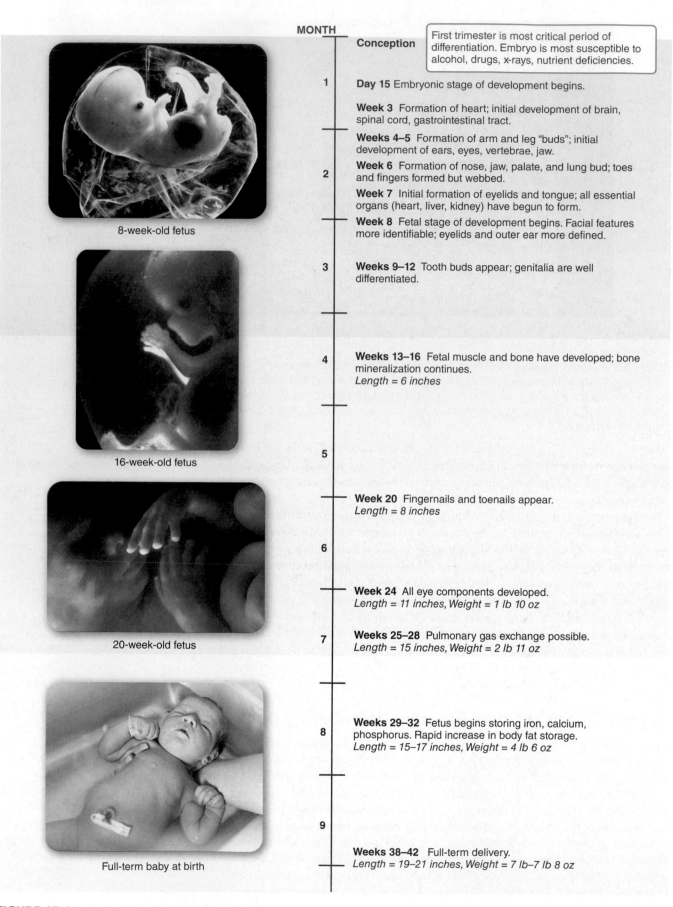

MONTH

Conception

> First trimester is most critical period of differentiation. Embryo is most susceptible to alcohol, drugs, x-rays, nutrient deficiencies.

8-week-old fetus

1 **Day 15** Embryonic stage of development begins.

Week 3 Formation of heart; initial development of brain, spinal cord, gastrointestinal tract.

Weeks 4–5 Formation of arm and leg "buds"; initial development of ears, eyes, vertebrae, jaw.

2 **Week 6** Formation of nose, jaw, palate, and lung bud; toes and fingers formed but webbed.

Week 7 Initial formation of eyelids and tongue; all essential organs (heart, liver, kidney) have begun to form.

Week 8 Fetal stage of development begins. Facial features more identifiable; eyelids and outer ear more defined.

3 **Weeks 9–12** Tooth buds appear; genitalia are well differentiated.

16-week-old fetus

4 **Weeks 13–16** Fetal muscle and bone have developed; bone mineralization continues.
Length = 6 inches

5

Week 20 Fingernails and toenails appear.
Length = 8 inches

20-week-old fetus

6

Week 24 All eye components developed.
Length = 11 inches, Weight = 1 lb 10 oz

7 **Weeks 25–28** Pulmonary gas exchange possible.
Length = 15 inches, Weight = 2 lb 11 oz

8 **Weeks 29–32** Fetus begins storing iron, calcium, phosphorus. Rapid increase in body fat storage.
Length = 15–17 inches, Weight = 4 lb 6 oz

Full-term baby at birth

9

Weeks 38–42 Full-term delivery.
Length = 19–21 inches, Weight = 7 lb–7 lb 8 oz

FIGURE 17.4 A timeline of embryonic and fetal development.

become fully mature. Because of the intense growth and maturation of the fetus during the third trimester, it remains very important that the mother eat an adequate and balanced diet.

Appropriate Weight Gain Is Essential

An adequate, nourishing diet is one of the most important modifiable variables increasing the chances for birth of a mature newborn. Proper nutrition also increases the likelihood that the newborn's weight will be appropriate for his or her gestational age. Generally, a birth weight of at least 5.5 lb is considered a marker of a successful pregnancy.

An undernourished mother is likely to give birth to a **low-birth-weight** infant who is at increased risk for infection, learning disabilities, impaired physical development, and death in the first year of life, as well as many health complications later in life (**Figure 17.5**).[4] Many low-birth-weight infants are born **preterm**—that is, before 38 weeks of gestation. Others are born at term but weigh less than would be expected for their gestational age; this condition is called **small for gestational age (SGA).** Although nutrition is not the only factor contributing to maturity and birth weight, its role cannot be overstated.

Recommendations for weight gain vary according to a woman's weight *before* she became pregnant and whether the pregnancy is singleton (one fetus) or multiple (two or more fetuses). As you can see in **Table 17.1** (page 662), the average recommended weight gain for women of normal prepregnancy weight is 25 to 35 lb; underweight women should gain a little more than this amount, and overweight and obese women should gain somewhat less.[5] Adolescents should follow the same recommendations as those for adults. Women of normal prepregnancy weight who are pregnant with twins are advised to gain 37 to 54 lb.[5]

Women who have a low prepregnancy BMI (< 18.5) or gain too little weight during their pregnancy increase their risk of having a preterm or low-birth-weight baby and of dangerously depleting their own nutrient reserves. Gaining *too much* weight during pregnancy or being overweight (BMI ≥ 25) or obese (BMI ≥ 30) prior to conception is also risky—and much more common. Excessive prepregnancy weight or prenatal weight gain increases the risk that the fetus will be large for his or her gestational age. **Large for gestational age (LGA)** babies have an increased risk for trauma during vaginal delivery and for cesarean birth. Also, children born to overweight or obese mothers

low birth weight An infant weight of less than 5.5 lb at birth.

preterm The birth of a baby prior to 38 weeks of gestation.

small for gestational age (SGA) A birth weight that falls below the 10th percentile for gestational age.

large for gestational age (LGA) A birth weight that falls above the 90th percentile for gestational age.

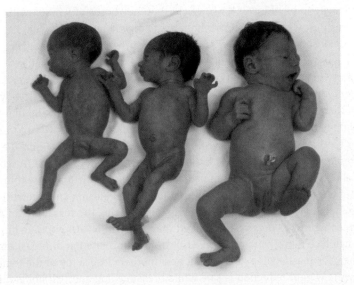

FIGURE 17.5 A healthy 2-day-old infant (right) compared to two low-birth-weight infants.

TABLE 17.1 Recommended Weight Gain for Women During Pregnancy

Prepregnancy Weight Status	Body Mass Index (kg/m²)	Recommended Total Weight Gain (lb)
Normal	18.5–24.9	25–35
Underweight	<18.5	28–40
Overweight	25.0–29.9	15–25
Obese	≥30.0	11–20

Source: Rasmussen, K. M., and A. L. Yaktine, eds. 2009. *Weight Gain During Pregnancy: Reexamining the Guidelines*. Institute of Medicine; National Research Council. Washington, DC: National Academy Press.

have higher rates of childhood obesity and metabolic abnormalities.[6] A high birth weight has also been linked to increased risk for adolescent obesity. In addition, the more weight gained during pregnancy, the more difficult it is for the mother to return to her prepregnancy weight and the more likely it is that her weight gain will be permanent. This weight retention can become especially problematic if the woman has two or more children; the extra weight also increases her long-term risk for type 2 diabetes and hypertension. One goal of *Healthy People 2020* is to increase the proportion of mothers who achieve a recommended weight gain during their pregnancies, thus avoiding excessive and inadequate weight gains.[3]

In addition to the amount of weight, the *pattern* of weight gain is important. During the first trimester, a woman of normal weight should gain no more than 3 to 5 lb. During the second and third trimesters, an average of about 1 lb a week is considered healthful for normal-weight women. For overweight women, a gain of 0.6 lb/week is considered appropriate, and obese women are advised to gain no more than 0.5 lb/week.[5] Some researchers suggest that these guidelines for overweight and obese women are too generous, especially when you consider that 60% of overweight and 25% of obese women exceed the guidelines.[7] In fact, some healthcare practitioners are starting to encourage otherwise healthy overweight or obese women not to gain any weight during pregnancy and, if carefully supervised, actually to lose a few pounds. If weight gain is excessive within a single week, month, or trimester, the woman should attempt to slow the rate of weight gain. On the other hand, if a woman has not gained sufficient weight in the early months of her pregnancy, she should gradually increase her energy and nutrient intake. The newborns of women who lose weight during the first trimester—due to severe nausea and vomiting, for example—are likely to be of lower birth weight than newborns of women with appropriate weight gain. In short, weight gain throughout pregnancy should be slow and steady.

In a society obsessed with thinness, it is easy for pregnant women to worry about weight gain. Focusing on the quality of food consumed, rather than the quantity, can help women feel more in control. In addition, following a physician-approved exercise program helps pregnant women maintain a positive body image and prevent excessive weight gain. A pregnant woman may also feel less anxious about her weight gain if she understands how that weight is distributed. Of the total weight gained in pregnancy, 10 to 12 lb are accounted for by the fetus itself, the amniotic fluid, and the placenta (**Figure 17.6**). Another 3 to 4 lb represents an increase of 40% to 50% in maternal blood volume. A woman can expect to be about 10 to 12 lb lighter immediately after giving birth and, within about 2 weeks, another 5 to 8 lb lighter because of fluid loss (from plasma and interstitial fluid).

After the first 2 weeks following the infant's birth, losing the remainder of pregnancy weight requires that more energy be expended than is taken in. Appropriate physical activity can help women lose those extra pounds. Also, because production of breast milk requires significant energy, breastfeeding helps many new mothers lose some of the remaining weight. Moderate weight reduction is safe while breastfeeding and will not compromise the weight gain of the nursing infant.

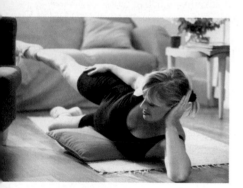

Following a physician-approved exercise program helps pregnant women maintain a positive body image and prevent excess weight gain.

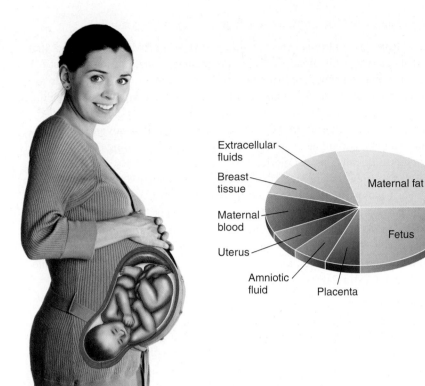

FIGURE 17.6 The weight gained during pregnancy is distributed between the mother's own tissues and the pregnancy-specific tissues.

RECAP

A full-term pregnancy lasts from 38 to 42 weeks and is traditionally divided into trimesters lasting 13 to 14 weeks. During the first trimester, cells differentiate and divide rapidly to form the various tissues of the human body. The fetus is especially susceptible to nutrient deficiencies, toxicities, and teratogens during this time. The second and third trimesters are characterized by continued growth and maturation. Nutrition is important before and throughout pregnancy to support fetal development without depleting the mother's reserves. An adequate, nourishing diet increases the chance that a baby will be born after 37 weeks and will weigh at least 5.5 lb. Sufficient Calories should be consumed so that a pregnant woman gains an appropriate amount of weight, typically 25 to 35 lb, to ensure adequate growth of the fetus. The Calories consumed during pregnancy should be nutrient-dense, so that both the mother and the fetus obtain the nutrients they need from food. ■

What Are a Pregnant Woman's Nutrient Needs?

LO 4 Identify the macronutrient and micronutrient needs of pregnant women, including for supplements and fluids.

The requirements for nearly all nutrients increase during pregnancy to accommodate the growth and development of the fetus without depriving the mother of the nutrients she needs to maintain her own health. Although most women do need supplemental iron, they can usually meet their increased needs for other nutrients by carefully selecting foods high in nutrient density. The Choose MyPlate.gov website provides a useful tool that reinforces the concepts of adequacy, balance, and variety in food choices; it also suggests food patterns for pregnant women. See the Web Links at the end of this chapter.

Macronutrients Provide Energy and Build Tissues

In pregnancy, macronutrients provide necessary energy for building tissue. They are also the very building blocks for the fetus, as well as for the mother's pregnancy-associated tissues.

Energy

Given what you've learned about pregnancy weight gain, you've probably figured out that energy requirements increase only modestly during pregnancy. In fact, during the first trimester, a woman should consume approximately the same number of Calories daily as during her nonpregnant days. Instead of eating more, she should attempt to maximize the nutrient density of what she eats. For example, drinking low-fat milk or calcium-fortified soy milk is preferable to drinking soft drinks. Low-fat milk and fortified soy milk provide valuable protein, vitamins, and minerals to feed the fetus's rapidly dividing cells, whereas soft drinks provide nutritionally empty Calories.

During the last two trimesters of pregnancy, energy needs increase by about 350 to 450 kcal/day. For a woman normally consuming 2,000 kcal/day, an extra 400 kcal represents only a 20% increase in energy intake, a goal that can be met more easily than many pregnant women realize. For example, one cup of low-fat yogurt and a graham cracker with jam is about 400 kcal. At the same time, some vitamin and mineral needs increase by as much as 50%—so again, the key for getting adequate micronutrients while not consuming too many extra Calories is choosing nutrient-dense foods.

Protein

During pregnancy, protein needs increase to about 1.1 grams per day per kilogram body weight over the entire 9-month period.[8] This is an increase of 25 g of protein per day. One half of a turkey (2 oz) and cheese (1 oz) sandwich would provide the extra 25 g of protein. For a pregnant woman weighing approximately 142 lb, the total recommended intake would average 71 g per day. Keep in mind that many women already eat this much protein each day, especially in the United States. Dairy products, meats, fish, poultry, eggs, and soy products are all rich sources of protein, as are legumes, nuts, and seeds. Still, it can be challenging for vegetarian and vegan women to meet their increased protein needs. To try designing a protein-rich snack for a vegetarian mother-to-be, see the **You Do the Math** box.

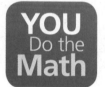

Planning a Protein-Packed Snack

Earlier in this chapter we pointed out that, during the last two trimesters of pregnancy, a woman's energy needs increase by about 350 to 450 kcal/day. At the same time, a pregnant woman's need for protein increases by 25 g per day. To help you appreciate how important it is for pregnant women to choose nutrient-dense foods, here's a two-part challenge:

Part 1. Annabelle is 6 months pregnant with her first child. She is an ovo-lacto vegetarian. Before she was pregnant, she never ate a mid-afternoon snack at work. Now, she eats a snack consisting of one slice of whole-wheat bread topped with 2 tablespoons of peanut butter, along with an 8-ounce carton of calcium-fortified orange juice. Let's see if this snack fulfills her need for extra Calories, as well as her increased protein needs.

1. List each food item, the kcal and the g protein provided:

One slice whole-wheat bread:	110 kcal	5 g protein
2 tablespoons peanut butter:	190 kcal	8 g protein
8 ounces orange juice:	110 kcal	2 g protein

2. Calculate the total kcal in this snack: 110 + 190 + 110 = **410.**

3. Does the snack meet her increased energy needs? Yes

4. Calculate the total g protein in this snack: 5 + 8 + 2 = 15.

5. Does the snack meet her increased protein needs? No. This snack meets 60% of Annabelle's increased protein needs: 15/25 = 0.60. She could increase the protein content of her snack by choosing a different beverage, such as milk or soy milk. Alternatively, she could decide to increase the amount of protein in other meals she eats during the day.

Part 2. Now it's your turn. Design a mid-afternoon snack for Annabelle that would meet but not exceed her needs for both increased Calories and increased protein.

Answers will vary according to individual inputs.

Carbohydrate

Pregnant women are advised to aim for a carbohydrate intake of at least 175 g per day.[8] All pregnant women should be counseled on the potential hazards of very-low-carbohydrate diets. Glucose is the primary metabolic fuel of the developing fetus; thus, pregnant women need to consume healthful sources of carbohydrate throughout the day. The recommended intake will also prevent ketosis (discussed in detail in Chapter 4, page 126) and help maintain normal blood glucose levels. Additional carbohydrate may be needed to support daily physical activity.

The recommendation of 175 g is easily met by consuming a balanced diet. The majority of carbohydrate intake should come from whole foods, such as whole-grain breads and cereals, brown rice, fruits, vegetables, and legumes. Not only are these carbohydrate-rich foods good sources of micronutrients, such as the B-vitamins, but they also contain a lot of fiber, which can help prevent constipation. Fiber-rich foods contribute to one's sense of fullness and can be an advantage to women who need to be careful not to gain too much weight.

Fat

The guideline for the percentage of daily Calories that comes from fat does not change during pregnancy.[8] Pregnant women should be aware that, because new tissues and cells are being built, adequate consumption of dietary fat is even more important than in the nonpregnant state.

Consumption of the right kinds of fats is important. Like anyone else, pregnant women should limit their intakes of saturated and *trans* fats because of their negative impact on cardiovascular health(as discussed in Chapter 5). Poly- and monounsaturated fats should be chosen whenever possible. The omega-3 polyunsaturated fatty acid *docosahexaenoic acid (DHA)* has been found to be linked to enhanced brain and eye development. Because the fetal brain grows dramatically during the third trimester, DHA is especially important in the maternal diet. Good sources of DHA are oily fish, such as anchovies, mackerel, salmon, and sardines. It is also found in lower amounts in tuna, chicken, and eggs (some eggs are DHA-enhanced by feeding hens a DHA-rich diet).

Pregnant women should be aware of the potential for mercury contamination in certain types of fish, as even a limited intake of mercury during pregnancy can impair a fetus's developing nervous system. Pregnant women should avoid large fish, such as swordfish, shark, tilefish, and king mackerel, and should limit their intake of white (albacore) tuna to 6 ounces per week.[9] Other than these specific limitations, however, pregnant women are strongly advised to eat 8 to 12 oz of most other types of fish per week, including salmon, tilapia, cod, catfish, light canned tuna and shrimp.[10] Eating 2 to 3 servings of fish per week will provide nutrients that are important for fetal development.

Micronutrients Support Increased Energy Needs and Tissue Growth

The need for micronutrients increases during pregnancy because of the expansion of the mother's blood supply and growth of the uterus, placenta, breasts, body fat, and the fetus itself. In addition, the increased need for energy during pregnancy correlates with an increased need for micronutrients involved in the metabolism of macronutrients. Discussions about the micronutrients most critical during pregnancy follow. Refer to **Table 17.2** (page 666) for an overview of the changes in micronutrient needs with pregnancy.

Folate

Since folate is necessary for cell division, it is logical that, during a time when both maternal and fetal cells are dividing rapidly, the requirement for this vitamin would be increased. Adequate folate is especially critical during the first 28 days after conception, when it is

TABLE 17.2 Changes in Nutrient Recommendations with Pregnancy for Adult Women

Micronutrient	Prepregnancy	Pregnancy	% Increase
Folate	400 µg/day	600 µg/day	50
Vitamin B$_{12}$	2.4 µg/day	2.6 µg/day	8
Vitamin C	75 mg/day	85 mg/day	13
Vitamin A	700 µg/day	770 µg/day	10
Iron	18 mg/day	27 mg/day	50
Zinc	8 mg/day	11 mg/day	38
Iodine	150 µg/day	220 µg/day	47

neural tube Embryonic tissue that forms a tube, which eventually becomes the brain and spinal cord.

spina bifida An embryonic neural tube defect that occurs when the spinal vertebrae fail to completely enclose the spinal cord, allowing it to protrude.

anencephaly A fatal neural tube defect in which there is partial absence of brain tissue, most likely caused by failure of the neural tube to close.

required for the formation and closure of the **neural tube,** an embryonic structure that eventually becomes the brain and spinal cord. Folate deficiency is associated with neural tube defects, such as **spina bifida** (**Figure 17.7**) and **anencephaly,** a fatal defect in which there is partial absence of brain tissue. Adequate folate intake does not guarantee normal neural tube development, as the precise cause of neural tube defects is unknown, and in some cases there is a genetic component. It is estimated, however, that up to 70% of all neural tube defects could be prevented by simply improving maternal intake of folic acid or folate.[11] One goal of *Healthy People 2020* is to reduce the occurrence of spina bifida and other neural tube defects by ensuring women in their childbearing years consume at least 400 µg of folic acid from fortified foods or dietary supplements.[3]

So, to reduce the risk for neural tube defects, all women capable of becoming pregnant are encouraged to consume 400 µg of folic acid per day from supplements, fortified foods, or both in addition to a variety of foods naturally high in folates. The emphasis on obtaining folic acid from supplements and fortified foods is due to the higher bioavailability of these sources. Of course, folate remains very important even after the neural tube has closed. The RDA for folate for pregnant women is therefore 600 µg/day, a full 50% increase over the RDA for a nonpregnant female.[12] A deficiency of folate during pregnancy can result in macrocytic anemia (a condition in which blood cells do not mature properly) and has been associated with low birth weight, preterm delivery, and failure of the fetus to grow properly. Sources of food folate include orange juice; green, leafy vegetables (such as spinach and broccoli); and lentils. For more than two decades, the Food and Drug Administration (FDA)

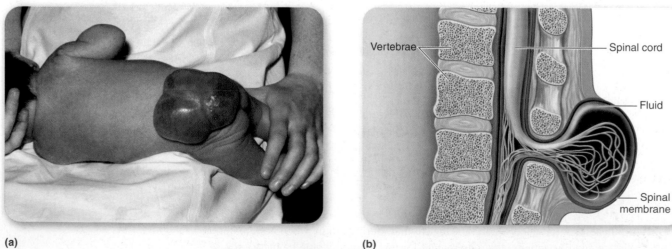

(a)

(b)

FIGURE 17.7 Spina bifida, a common neural tube defect. **(a)** An external view of an infant with spina bifida. **(b)** An internal view of the protruding spinal membrane and fluid-filled sac.

has mandated that all enriched grain products, such as cereals, breads, and pastas, be fortified with folic acid; thus, including these foods, ideally as whole grains, in the daily diet can further increase folate intake.

Vitamin B$_{12}$

Vitamin B$_{12}$ (cobalamin) is vital during pregnancy, because it regenerates the active form of folate. Not surprisingly, deficiencies of vitamin B$_{12}$ can also result in macrocytic anemia, yet the RDA for vitamin B$_{12}$ for pregnant women is only 2.6 µg/day, a mere 8% increase over the RDA of 2.4 µg/day for nonpregnant women.[12] How can this be? One reason is that, during pregnancy, absorption of vitamin B$_{12}$ is more efficient. The required amount of vitamin B$_{12}$ can easily be obtained from animal food sources, such as meats, dairy products, and eggs. However, deficiencies have been observed in women who have followed a vegan diet for several years; these deficiencies have also been observed in the infants of some mothers who follow a vegan diet. Fortified foods or supplementation provides these women with the needed amounts of vitamin B$_{12}$.

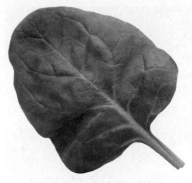

Spinach is an excellent source of folate.

Vitamin C

Because blood plasma volume increases during pregnancy, and because vitamin C is being transferred to the fetus, the concentration of vitamin C in maternal blood usually decreases. Vitamin C deficiency during pregnancy has been associated with an increased risk for premature birth and other complications. The RDA for vitamin C during pregnancy is increased by a little more than 10% over the RDA for nonpregnant women (from 75 mg to 85 mg per day for adult pregnant women, 80 mg per day for pregnant adolescents). Women who smoke during pregnancy should consume even higher levels of vitamin C, because smoking lowers both serum and amniotic fluid levels. Many foods are rich sources of vitamin C, such as citrus fruits and juices, peppers, and numerous other fruits and vegetables.

Vitamin A

Vitamin A needs increase during pregnancy by about 10%, to 770 µg per day for adult pregnant women and 750 µg per day for pregnant adolescents.[13] Vitamin A deficiency during pregnancy has been linked to an increased risk for low birth weight, growth problems, and preterm delivery. However, excess preformed vitamin A exerts teratogenic effects. Consumption of excessive preformed vitamin A, particularly during the first trimester, increases the risk for birth of an infant with craniofacial malformations, including cleft lip or palate; heart defects; and abnormalities of the central nervous system.[13] A well-balanced diet supplies sufficient vitamin A, so supplementation during pregnancy is not recommended. Note that provitamin A, in the form of beta-carotene (which is converted to vitamin A in the body), has not been associated with birth defects.

Vitamin D

Despite the role of vitamin D in calcium absorption, the RDA for this nutrient does not increase during pregnancy. According to the Institute of Medicine, the amount of vitamin D transferred from the mother to the fetus is relatively small and does not appear to negatively affect maternal vitamin D status.[14] Pregnant women who receive adequate exposure to sunlight do not need vitamin D supplements. However, pregnant women with darkly pigmented skin and/or limited sun exposure who do not regularly drink milk will benefit from vitamin D supplementation. It has been estimated that almost 30% of dark-skinned pregnant women living in the northeastern United States are in a state of vitamin D deficiency, which may result in impaired fetal growth, preeclampsia, placental infections, preterm birth, and increased risk for type 1 diabetes later in the offspring's life.[15] Most prenatal vitamin supplements contain 10 µg/day of vitamin D, which is considered safe and acceptable, although some researchers view that level as inadequate for maintaining normal serum levels of vitamin D.[14] Because vitamin D is fat soluble, pregnant women should avoid consuming excessive vitamin D from supplements, as toxicity can cause developmental disability in the newborn.

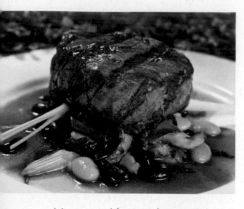

Meats provide complete protein, which is essential for building and maintaining both maternal and fetal tissues.

Calcium

Growth of the fetal skeleton requires as much as 30 g of calcium, most during the last trimester. However, the RDA for calcium does not change during pregnancy; it remains at 1,300 mg/day for pregnant adolescents (14–18 years) and 1,000 mg/day for adult pregnant women (19–50 years).[14] Why is there no increase? First, pregnant women absorb dietary calcium more efficiently than do nonpregnant women, assuming adequate vitamin D status. Second, the extra demand for calcium has not been found to cause permanent demineralization of the mother's bones or to increase fracture risk; thus, there is no justification for recommending higher intakes. Sources of calcium include milk, calcium-fortified soy milk and other milk substitutes, calcium-fortified juices, yogurt and cheese, fortified breakfast cereals, tofu, and a variety of green, leafy vegetables.

Iron

Recall (from Chapter 12) the importance of iron in the formation of red blood cells, which transport oxygen throughout the body. During pregnancy, the demand for red blood cells increases to accommodate the needs of the expanded maternal blood volume, growing uterus, placenta, and fetus itself. Thus, more iron is needed. Fetal demand for iron increases even further during the last trimester, when the fetus stores iron in the liver for use during the first few months of life. This iron storage is protective, because breast milk is low in iron. While recognizing that iron supplements are routinely prescribed to pregnant women, women who are pregnant or capable of becoming pregnant should routinely eat foods high in heme iron, such as meat, fish, and poultry, and/or to consume iron-rich plant foods, such as legumes, or iron-fortified foods with vitamin C–rich foods.

Severely inadequate iron intake has the potential to harm the fetus, resulting in an increased rate of low birth weight, preterm birth, stillbirth, and death of the newborn in the first weeks after birth. However, in most cases, the iron-deprived fetus builds adequate stores by "robbing" maternal iron, resulting in iron-deficiency anemia in the mother. During pregnancy, maternal iron deficiency causes extreme paleness and exhaustion, but at birth it endangers the mother's life: anemic women are more likely to die during or shortly after childbirth, because they are less able to tolerate blood loss and fight infection. One goal of *Healthy People 2020* is to reduce iron deficiency among pregnant females.[3]

The RDA for iron during pregnancy is 27 mg per day, compared to 18 mg per day for nonpregnant women and 15 mg per day for nonpregnant adolescents.[13] This represents a 50% to 80% increase, despite the fact that iron loss is minimized during pregnancy because menstruation ceases. Typically, women of childbearing age have poor iron stores, and the demands of pregnancy are likely to produce a deficiency. To ensure adequate iron stores during pregnancy, an iron supplement (as part of, or separate from, a total prenatal supplement) is routinely prescribed during the last two trimesters. Vitamin C enhances iron absorption, as do dietary sources of heme iron; however, substances in coffee, tea, milk, bran, and oxalate-rich foods decrease absorption. Therefore, many healthcare providers recommend taking iron supplements with foods high in vitamin C and/or heme iron.

Zinc

The RDA for zinc for adult pregnant women increases by about 38% over the RDA for nonpregnant adult women, from 8 mg per day to 11 mg per day, and the RDA increases from 9 mg per day to 12 mg per day for pregnant adolescents.[13] Because zinc has critical roles in DNA, RNA, and protein synthesis, it is extremely important that adequate zinc status be maintained during pregnancy to ensure proper growth and development of both maternal and fetal tissues. Inadequate zinc can lead to fetal malformations, premature birth, decreased birth size, and extended labor. The absorption of zinc from supplements may be inhibited by high intakes of nonheme iron, such as those found in iron supplements, when these two minerals are taken together.[16] However, when food sources of iron and zinc are consumed within one meal, absorption of zinc is not affected, largely because the amount of iron in the meal is not high enough to block zinc uptake. Good dietary sources of zinc include red meats, shellfish, and fortified cereals.

Sodium and Iodine

During pregnancy, the AI for sodium is the same as for a nonpregnant adult woman, or 1,500 mg (1.5 g) per day.[17] Although too much sodium is associated with fluid retention and bloating, as well as high blood pressure, increased body fluids are a normal and necessary part of pregnancy, so some sodium is needed to maintain fluid balance.

Iodine needs increase significantly during pregnancy, but the RDA of 220 µg per day is easy to achieve by using a modest amount of iodized salt (sodium chloride) during cooking. Sprinkling salt onto food at the table is unnecessary; a balanced, healthful diet will provide all the iodine needed during pregnancy.

Do Pregnant Women Need Supplements?

Prenatal multivitamin/mineral supplements are not strictly necessary during pregnancy, but most healthcare providers recommend them. Meeting all the nutrient needs would otherwise take careful and somewhat complex dietary planning. Prenatal supplements are especially good insurance for vegans, adolescents, and others whose diets might normally be low in one or more micronutrients. It is important that pregnant women understand, however, that supplements are to be taken *in addition to*, not as a substitute for, a nutrient-rich diet.

Fluid Needs of Pregnant Women Increase

Fluid plays many vital roles during pregnancy. It allows for the necessary increase in the mother's blood volume, acts as a lubricant, aids in regulating body temperature, and is necessary for many metabolic reactions. Fluid that the mother consumes also helps maintain the **amniotic fluid** that surrounds, cushions, and protects the fetus in the uterus. The AI for total fluid intake, which includes drinking water, beverages, and food, is 3 liters per day (about 12.7 cups). This recommendation includes approximately 2.3 liters (10 cups) of fluid as total beverages, including drinking water.[17]

Drinking adequate fluid helps combat two common discomforts of pregnancy: fluid retention and, possibly, constipation. Drinking lots of fluids (and going to the bathroom as soon as the need is felt) will also help prevent **urinary tract infections,** which are common in pregnancy. Fluids also combat dehydration, which can develop if a woman with morning sickness has frequent bouts of vomiting. For these women, fluids such as soups, juices, and sports beverages are usually well tolerated and can help prevent dehydration.

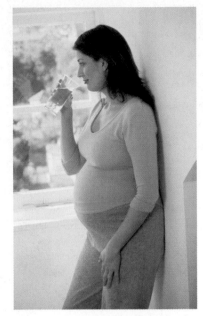

It's important that pregnant women drink about 10 cups of fluid a day.

RECAP

During the last two trimesters of pregnancy, energy needs increase by about 350 to 450 kcal/day. Protein needs increase by an average of about 25 g per day, to about 71 g per day in a woman weighing about 142 lb. Pregnant women need at least 175 g of carbohydrate per day, and should avoid low-carbohydrate diets. Dietary fats provide the building blocks for new cells and tissues, but should be mostly unsaturated fats, particularly DHA, which is linked to enhanced brain and eye development. Pregnant women can consume DHA in fatty fish, but should avoid fish high in mercury. Folate deficiency has been associated with neural tube defects, and all women capable of becoming pregnant are encouraged to consume 400 µg of folic acid per day. Vitamin A supplementation during pregnancy is not recommended, because excessive amounts can be teratogenic. In contrast, iron supplementation is typically prescribed during the second and third trimesters, because women of childbearing age have poor iron stores, and the demands of pregnancy are likely to produce a deficiency, which can be harmful to both mother and fetus. Most healthcare providers recommend prenatal multivitamin/mineral supplements for pregnant women to ensure that sufficient micronutrients are consumed. Fluid provides for increased maternal blood volume and amniotic fluid. ■

amniotic fluid The watery fluid within the innermost membrane of the sac containing the fetus. It cushions and protects the growing fetus.

urinary tract infection A bacterial infection affecting any portion of the urinary tract, but most commonly affecting the bladder or the urethra, the tube leading from the bladder to the body exterior.

LO 5 Discuss the key nutrition-related disorders of pregnancy, and the influence of maternal age on pregnancy.

LO 6 Discuss the effects of exercise, caffeine, artificial sweeteners, alcohol, tobacco, illicit drugs, and medications and supplements on the pregnant woman and her fetus.

What Are Some Common Nutrition-Related Concerns of Pregnancy?

Pregnancy-related conditions involving a particular nutrient, such as iron-deficiency anemia, have already been discussed. The following sections describe some of the most common discomforts and disorders of pregnant women that are related to their general nutrition.

Some Disorders of Pregnancy Are Related to Nutrition

Pregnancy is a normal life stage for the great majority of women; however, it can bring a range of disorders, from temporary conditions such as morning sickness to life-threatening emergencies such as eclampsia.

Morning Sickness

Morning sickness, or *nausea and vomiting of pregnancy (NVP)*, occurs in up to 80% of pregnant women during the first trimester.[18] It can vary from occasional, mild queasiness to constant nausea with bouts of vomiting. In truth, "morning sickness" is not an appropriate name because the nausea and vomiting can begin at any time of the day and may last all day. NVP usually resolves by week 12 to 16 and the mother and fetus do not suffer lasting harm. However, some women experience such frequent vomiting that it becomes a serious medical condition, requiring hospitalization or in-home intravenous (IV) therapy. There is no cure for morning sickness. However, here are some practical tips for reducing the severity:

- Eat small, frequent meals and snacks throughout the day. An empty stomach can trigger nausea.
- Consume most of the day's fluids between meals. Frozen ice pops, watermelon, gelatin desserts, and mild broths are often well-tolerated sources of fluid.
- Keep snacks such as crackers at the bedside to ease nighttime queasiness or to eat before rising.
- Take prenatal supplements at a time of day when vomiting is least likely.
- Avoid sights, sounds, smells, and tastes that bring on or worsen queasiness. Cold or room-temperature foods are often better tolerated than hot foods.
- For some women, alternative therapies, such as acupuncture, acupressure wrist bands, biofeedback, meditation, and hypnosis, help. Always check with your healthcare provider to ensure that the therapy you are using is safe and does not interact with other medications or supplements.

Cravings and Aversions

It seems as if nothing is more stereotypical about pregnancy than the image of a frazzled husband getting up in the middle of the night to run to the convenience store to get his pregnant wife some pickles and ice cream. This image, although humorous, is far from reality. Although some women have specific cravings, most crave a particular type of food (such as "something sweet" or "something salty") rather than a particular food.

Why do pregnant women crave certain tastes? Does a desire for salty foods mean that the woman is experiencing a sodium deficit? Although there may be some truth to the assertion that we crave what we need, scientific evidence for this claim is lacking.

Most cravings are, of course, for edible substances. But a surprising number of pregnant women crave nonfoods, such as laundry starch, chalk, and clay. This craving, called **pica,** may result in nutritional or health problems for the mother and fetus and is the subject of the *Highlight* on the next page.

Food aversions are also common during pregnancy and may originate from social, cultural, or religious beliefs. In some cultures, for example, women traditionally avoid shellfish ("it causes allergies") or duck ("child will be born with webbed feet"). Such aversions and taboos are often strongly woven into the family's belief system.

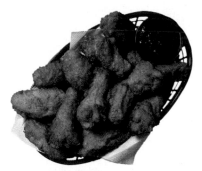

Deep-fried foods are often unappealing to pregnant women.

morning sickness A condition characterized by varying degrees of nausea and vomiting associated with pregnancy, most commonly in the first trimester.

pica An abnormal craving to eat various nonfood substances, such as clay, chalk, or soap.

The Danger of Nonfood Cravings

A few weeks after she learned she was pregnant, Darlene started feeling "funny." She experienced bouts of nausea lasting several hours every day, and her appetite seemed to disappear. At the grocery store, she wandered through the aisles with an empty cart, confused about what foods she should be eating and unable to find anything that appealed to her. Eventually, she'd return home with a few small items—and a large bag of ice. At the assembly plant where she worked, she took cupfuls of ice from the soda machine and ate it throughout the day. Each weekend, she went through more than a boxful of popsicles to "settle her stomach."

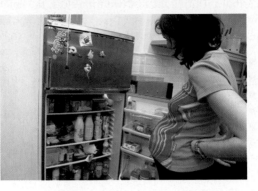

Pica is the condition of craving nonfood substances, such as dirt, chalk, pebbles, or soap.

At Darlene's next checkup, her nurse became concerned because she had lost weight. Darlene was too embarrassed to admit to that the only thing she wanted to eat was ice.

Some people believe that pregnant women with unusual cravings are intuitively seeking out nutrients their bodies need. Arguing against this theory is the phenomenon of *pica*—the craving and persistent consumption of nonfood material—which can occur during pregnancy. Pica is not the same as the common cravings for out-of-the-ordinary foods that many women experience while pregnant. A woman with pica may crave ice, clay, dirt, chalk, coffee grounds, baking soda, laundry starch, hair, burnt matches, stones, charcoal, mothballs, toothpaste, soap, rocks, and many other nonfood items, including even feces.[1] The cause of these cravings for nonfood substances of little or no nutritional value is not known; however, it is more common among children and among people with developmental disabilities.[2] Underlying biochemical disorders, lower socioeconomic status, and family stress have been implicated as possible causes, as have cultural factors. For example, in the United States, pica is more common among pregnant African American women than women from other racial or ethnic groups; among refugees and recent immigrants versus nonimmigrants; and among lower-socioeconomic groups compared to higher ones.[2-4] Nutrient deficiencies have also been associated with pica, although it is not at all clear that nutrient deficiencies cause it. In fact, inhibition of nutrient absorption caused by the ingestion of clay and other substances can produce nutrient deficiencies.

Whatever the cause, pica is often dangerous. Excessive consumption of ice can lead to inadequate weight gain in pregnancy if the ice substitutes for food. Ingestion of clay, starch, and other materials can not only inhibit absorption of nutrients but may also cause constipation, intestinal blockage, and even excessive weight gain. Women with pica are at greater risk for high exposure to lead, as well as to other toxic substances, which can impair the neurodevelopment of the fetus and increase the risk for pregnancy-related complications.[4] In addition, ingestion of certain substances, such as talcum powder, can lead to severe weight loss and lung disease.

Some pregnant women with pica are able to find foods they can substitute for the craved nonfood items—for instance, peanut butter instead of clay, or nonfat powdered milk instead of starch. If a woman experiences pica, she should talk with her healthcare provider immediately to identify strategies to avoid eating dangerous substances and instead consume healthful foods that will support optimal growth and development of her fetus. In addition, women consuming dirt, clay, or paint should be tested for blood lead levels to minimize risk for fetal lead exposure.[4] Pica should not be viewed as "weird" or "awful"—it is a potentially dangerous condition that should be addressed in a sensitive and caring manner. In this way, pregnant women with pica will be more likely to be open and honest with their healthcare providers about their cravings, opening the door for appropriate support.

References

1. Uher, R., and M. Rutter. 2012. Classification of feeding and eating disorders: review of evidence and proposals for ICD-11. *World Psychiatry* 11: 80–92.
2. Mishori, R., and C. McHale. 2014. Pica: an age-old eating disorder that's often missed. *J Fam Pract* 63: E1–E4.
3. Corbett, R. W., and K. M. Kolasa. 2014. Pica and weight gain in pregnancy. *Nutr Today* 49: 101–108.
4. Thihalolipavan, S., B. M Candalla, and J. Ehrlich. 2012. Examining pica in NYC pregnant women with elevated blood lead levels. *Matern. Child Health J.* 17(1): 49–55. doi:10.1007/s10995-012-0947-5

Gastroesophageal Reflux

Gastroesophageal reflux, also termed *heartburn,* is common during pregnancy. Pregnancy-related hormones relax lower esophageal smooth muscle, increasing the incidence of heartburn. During the last two trimesters, the enlarging uterus pushes up on the stomach, compounding the problem. Practical tips for minimizing heartburn during pregnancy include the following:

- Avoid excessive weight gain.
- Eat small, frequent meals and chew food slowly.
- Don't wear tight clothing.
- Wait for at least 1 hour after eating before lying down.
- Sleep with your head elevated.
- Ask your healthcare provider to recommend an antacid that is safe for use during pregnancy.

Constipation

Hormone production during pregnancy causes the smooth muscles to relax, including the muscles of the large intestine, slowing colonic movement of food residue. Pressure exerted by the growing uterus on the colon can slow movement even further, making elimination difficult. Practical hints that may help a woman avoid constipation include the following:

- Include 25 to 35 g of fiber in the daily diet, concentrating on fresh fruits and vegetables, dried fruits, legumes, and whole grains.
- Keep fluid intake high as fiber intake increases. Drink plenty of water and eat water-rich fruits and vegetables, such as melons, citrus, and lettuce.
- Keep physically active, as exercise is one of many factors that help increase motility of the large intestine.

Pregnant women should use over-the-counter fiber supplements only as a last resort and should not use any laxative product without first discussing it with their healthcare provider.

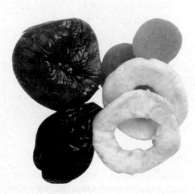

Consuming foods high in fiber, such as dried fruits, may reduce the chances of constipation.

Gestational Diabetes

Gestational diabetes, diagnosed in up to 10% of all U.S. pregnancies[19], is usually a temporary condition in which a pregnant woman is unable to produce sufficient insulin or becomes insulin resistant, and thus develops elevated levels of blood glucose. Fortunately, gestational diabetes has no ill effects on either the mother or the fetus if blood glucose levels are strictly controlled through diet, physical activity, and/or medication. Screening for gestational diabetes is routine for almost all healthcare practitioners and is necessary because several of the symptoms, which include frequent urination, fatigue, and an increase in thirst and appetite, mimic what is seen in a normal pregnancy. If poorly controlled or untreated, gestational diabetes can result in a baby who is too large as a result of receiving too much glucose across the placenta during fetal life. Infants who are overly large are at risk for early birth and trauma during vaginal birth, and often need to be born by cesarean section. There is also evidence that exposing a fetus to maternal diabetes significantly increases the risk for overweight and metabolic disorders, including diabetes, later in life.[20]

Women who are obese, who are age 35 years or older, who have a family history of diabetes, and who are of Native American, African American, or Hispanic origin have a greater risk of developing gestational diabetes, as do women who previously delivered a large-for-gestational-age infant. In addition, women with gestational diabetes are seven times more likely to develop type 2 diabetes 5 to 10 years after delivery.[19] As with any type of diabetes, attention to diet, weight control, and physical activity reduces the risk for gestational diabetes.

gestational diabetes Insufficient insulin production or insulin resistance that results in consistently high blood glucose levels, specifically during pregnancy; the condition typically resolves after birth occurs.

Nutri-*Case*

Hannah

"In my nutrition class, I learned that having a mother with diabetes increases my risk for diabetes, too. That helps me understand my risk, but it doesn't tell me what to do about it."

Is Hannah destined to develop type 2 diabetes? Why or why not? What factors increase her risk, and what can she do to reduce her blood glucose levels and avoid the disease? (Review Chapter 4 if necessary.)

Hypertensive Disorders in Pregnancy

About 8% of United States and up to 15% of global pregnancies are complicated by some form of hypertension, or high blood pressure, yet it accounts for almost 16% of pregnancy-related deaths in industrialized nations, such as the United States.[21] The term *hypertensive disorders in pregnancy* encompasses several different conditions. A woman who develops high blood pressure, with no other signs or symptoms, during the pregnancy is said to have *gestational hypertension.* **Preeclampsia** is characterized by a sudden increase in maternal blood pressure during pregnancy with the presence of swelling, excessive and rapid weight gain unrelated to food intake, and protein in the urine. If left untreated, it can progress to *eclampsia,* a medical emergency characterized by seizures and kidney failure and, if untreated, fetal and/or maternal death.

No one knows exactly what causes the various hypertensive disorders in pregnancy, but the risk is increased in women who are pregnant for the first time, adolescents, over age 35, African American, diabetic, smokers, or low-income. The risk is also increased for women who have a family or personal history of eclampsia. In addition, the rate of preeclampsia is three times higher in overweight and obese women compared to women of normal weight.[22]

Management of preeclampsia focuses mainly on blood pressure control. Typical treatment includes bed rest and medical oversight. Ultimately, the only thing that will cure the condition is childbirth. Today, with good prenatal care, gestational hypertension is nearly always detected early and can be appropriately managed, and prospects for both mother and fetus are usually very good. In nearly all women without prior chronic high blood pressure, blood pressure returns to normal within about a day or so after the birth, although recent studies suggest that women with preeclampsia are at greater risk for cardiovascular disease later in life.

Foodborne Illness

Pregnancy alters a woman's immune system in a way that leaves her more vulnerable to infectious diseases, including foodborne illness. A developing fetus is also at high risk. The bacterium *Listeria monocytogenes,* which causes **listeriosis,** is of particular concern to a pregnant woman and her fetus. Listeriosis is the third leading cause of death from foodborne illness, and 90% of people who contract the disease are in highly vulnerable groups, including pregnant women. In the fetus, listeriosis can result in severe infection that triggers miscarriage or premature birth.[23]

To reduce their risk for listeriosis, pregnant women should avoid unpasteurized milk and soft cheeses such as brie, feta, Camembert, and Mexican-style cheeses (called *queso blanco* or *queso fresco*), unless the label specifically states the product is made with pasteurized milk. They should also avoid refrigerated, smoked seafood such as salmon (lox) and refrigerated meat spreads. Hot dogs should not be consumed unless they are steaming hot, and cold cuts and other deli meats should be entirely avoided unless part of a thoroughly cooked dish. Melons should be scrubbed under running water and dried before

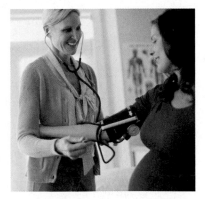

Pregnant women should have their blood pressure measured to screen for pregnancy-related hypertension.

 To learn more about preeclampsia, and how it can affect the fetus, watch this short video from the National Library of Medicine at http://www.nlm.nih.gov/.

preeclampsia High blood pressure that is pregnancy-specific and accompanied by protein in the urine, edema, and unexpected weight gain.

Listeriosis Potentially fatal foodborne illness caused by infection with the bacterium *Listeria monocytogenes.*

cutting, and should be refrigerated promptly. Pregnant women should also avoid raw or partially cooked eggs, raw or undercooked meat/fish/poultry, unpasteurized juices, and raw sprouts.[24,25]

Pregnant women should follow safe food-handling practices to ensure a healthy pregnancy outcome(see Chapter 15). When eating out, pregnant women should ask that their food be thoroughly cooked and served very hot. If taking restaurant meal leftovers home, make sure the food is brought right home and promptly refrigerated.

Maternal Age Can Affect Pregnancy

Both adolescents and older women have unique concerns of pregnancy. Some of these are related to diet and body weight.

Throughout the adolescent years, girls' bodies are still changing and growing. Peak bone mass has not yet been reached, and full physical stature may not have been attained; thus, pregnant adolescents have higher needs for bone-related nutrients, such as calcium, phosphorus, and magnesium. Teens also commonly begin pregnancy in an iron-deficient state and, so, have an increased iron need. Teens are also more likely to be underweight than are young adult women, and they are more likely to fail to gain adequate weight during pregnancy. In addition, many adolescents have not established healthful nutritional patterns. Thus, adhering to a diet that provides the appropriate level of energy to meet the adolescent's own needs as well as those of her fetus can be a challenge. At the same time, higher rates of prenatal alcohol use, smoking, and drug use also contribute to higher rates of preterm births, low-birth-weight babies, and other complications.

Many pregnant adolescents delay or fail to seek prenatal care. This is especially unfortunate because, in the adolescent age group, prenatal care is the most significant factor in pregnancy outcome. With regular prenatal care and close attention to proper nutrition and other healthful behaviors, the likelihood of a positive outcome for both the adolescent mother and the infant is similar to that for older mothers and their infants.

In 2013, the adolescent birthrate dropped to 26.5 births for every 1,000 U.S. women aged 15–19.[26] Although this is the lowest teen birth-rate since the 1940s, it is also among the highest of all industrialized nations. One of the goals of *Healthy People 2020* is to reduce pregnancies among adolescent females.[3]

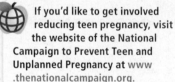

If you'd like to get involved reducing teen pregnancy, visit the website of the National Campaign to Prevent Teen and Unplanned Pregnancy at www.thenationalcampaign.org.

Although there is no strict definition of an "older" pregnant woman, many healthcare researchers use age 35 as a cut-off point.[27] More and more U.S. women are delaying pregnancy: the rate of first births at age 35 to 39 was only 1.7 per 1,000 women in 1973 but rose to 11.0 in 2012.[28] Older pregnant women on average have higher incomes and more education than women in younger groups, and these factors can help them maintain a healthy pregnancy. Nevertheless, pregnancy in older women does have unique risks. First, fertility begins to decline in most women in their early 30s, and as a woman ages, pregnancy is more likely to end in miscarriage or stillbirth. As a woman's ova mature, the risk for certain chromosomal birth defects such as Down syndrome rises. Also, after age 35, pregnant women are at increased risk for gestational diabetes and hypertension.[29,30] Thus, older pregnant women need to avoid excessive weight gain, and should be extra vigilant when planning their meals and snacks. Older women are also more likely to have twins or even triplets, and therefore to have increased total nutrient needs. Despite these risks, the majority of pregnancies in women over age 35 have the best possible outcome: a healthy baby![30]

A Careful Vegetarian Diet Is Safe During Pregnancy

A recent review of maternal and birth outcomes among pregnant vegetarians/vegans reported no evidence of increased risk for severe complications of pregnancy or birth defects.[31] With the possible exception of iron and zinc, vegetarian women who consume dairy products and eggs (lacto-ovo-vegetarians) have no nutritional challenges beyond those encountered by every pregnant woman. Since vegetarians do not consume fish, they can consume adequate DHA by purchasing eggs that have been enriched with DHA.

In contrast, women who are totally vegetarian (vegan) need to be more vigilant than usual about their intake of nutrients that are derived primarily or wholly from animal products. These include vitamin D (unless regularly exposed to sunlight throughout the pregnancy), vitamin B_6, vitamin B_{12}, calcium, iron, and zinc as well as DHA. Pregnant vegans can add algae-based products to their diet or decide to use a DHA-rich omega-3 oil supplement. Supplements can also provide the other nutrients low or absent in a vegan diet. A regular prenatal supplement will fully meet the vitamin, iron, and zinc needs of a vegan woman but does not fulfill calcium needs, so a separate calcium supplement, or consumption of calcium-fortified soy milk or orange juice, is usually required.

Exercise Is Recommended for Most Pregnant Women

Physical activity during pregnancy is recommended for all women experiencing normal pregnancies.[32-34] Women who rarely, if ever, exercised before becoming pregnant and overweight and obese women can benefit greatly from increased activity but should begin slowly and progress gradually under the guidance of their healthcare provider. Women should avoid exercising outdoors when it is hot and humid and should always maintain appropriate fluid intake. Exercise during pregnancy benefits both mother and fetus in the following ways:

- Reduces maternal risk for gestational diabetes and preeclampsia
- Helps prevent excessive prenatal weight and body fat gain
- Improves maternal mood, energy level, and sleep patterns
- Enhances maternal posture, balance, muscle tone, strength, and endurance
- Reduces maternal lower back pain and shortens the duration of active labor
- Lowers the risk for preterm birth and large-for-gestational age infants

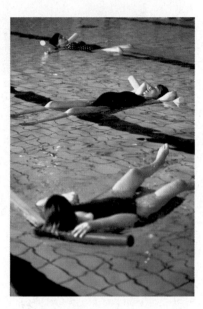

During pregnancy, women should adjust their physical activity to comfortable, low-impact exercise.

Women should select exercises that engage large muscle groups in a continuous manner, including a combination of moderate-intensity aerobic activity (brisk walking, leisurely swimming, dancing), vigorous-intensity aerobic activity (very brisk walking, swimming at a moderate-to-hard pace, cycling on a stationary bike, indoor rowing), and muscle-strengthening activities. Moderate activity is often described as one during which it is still possible to carry on a normal conversation; vigorous activity produces sweating, noticeable increases in breathing rate and depth, and an inability to converse normally. The more vigorous the activity, the less total time is needed to reap its benefits: 6.5 hours/week of brisk walking versus fewer than 3 hours/week of stationary cycling.

Recommendations for muscle-strengthening exercise during pregnancy are straightforward:

- Choose lighter weights and more repetitions.
- Opt for resistance bands over free weights, which might accidentally hit or fall on the abdomen.
- Don't lift weights while lying on your back, which might compress a major blood vessel and restrict blood flow to the fetus.
- Avoid moves that require sudden movements or might place you off balance, such as lunges or twists.
- Pay attention to your body's signals!

What about yoga and Pilates? Both offer classes tailored to pregnant women, adapting certain exercises to accommodate the body's changing center of gravity and increased joint flexibility. Activities that strengthen body core, abdominals, and pelvic floor or Kegel muscles make for an easier pregnancy and delivery. See **Table 17.3** (page 676) for a sample program of physical activity for a pregnant woman.

Pregnant women should avoid activities such as horseback riding, scuba diving, water or snow skiing, hockey, gymnastics, and soccer. They need to stay hydrated, especially in hot and humid weather, and dress comfortably. If symptoms of stress, such as dizziness,

 Watch a slideshow on exercise during and after pregnancy: Go to www.webmd.com. In the Search box, type "slideshow pregnancy fitness" and select **Slideshow: Pregnancy Fitness: Your Best Moves Before Baby Arrives.**

TABLE 17.3 Exercise Plan for Pregnant Women

Day of the Week	Warm-Up	Aerobic Activity	Muscle Strengthening	Cool-Down
Monday	5–10 min	30–45 min, moderate-intensity activity (leisurely lap swimming)		5 min
Tuesday	5–10 min		30 min light weights, high repetitions; upper and lower body	5 min
Wednesday	5–10 min	30 min vigorous activity (indoor cycling or rowing)		5 min
Thursday	5–10 min		45 min yoga, Pilates, or other core exercises	5 min
Friday	5–10 min	30–45 min moderate-intensity activity (outdoor hike, flat or gentle slope)		5 min
Saturday	5–10 min		30 min light weights, high repetitions; upper and lower body	5 min

Note: Women with established prepregnancy exercise routines should aim for the higher duration; women who rarely/never exercised before pregnancy should start with short durations of low-intensity activity and gradually build endurance.

shortness of breath, chest pain, vaginal bleeding or leakage, or uterine contractions, occur, all physical activity should stop and a healthcare provider contacted immediately.

Many Substances Can Harm the Fetus

Anything a pregnant woman takes into her body has the potential to reach and affect her fetus; however, certain substances are of particular concern.

Caffeine

Caffeine, a stimulant found in coffee, tea, soft drinks, and some foods, crosses the placenta and thus reaches the fetus, whose ability to metabolize caffeine is limited. In addition, the rate at which caffeine is metabolized by pregnant women greatly decreases in late pregnancy.[35] Although several U.S. health organizations advise pregnant women to limit their daily caffeine intake to 200 mg or less[35], recent evidence suggests that an intake as low as 100 mg per day may increase risk of miscarriage, stillbirth, preterm birth, and low birth weight.[36] It is sensible, then, for pregnant women to limit their daily caffeine intake to no more than one cup of coffee or its equivalent until more research is available. See Appendix E "Foods Containing Caffeine" for a list of common sources of caffeine.

Another reason for avoiding coffee and caffeinated soft drinks during pregnancy is that they can make one feel full and, if sweetened, provide considerable Calories. If a pregnant woman retains a very strong desire for coffee, she might try a low- or nonfat decaf café latte, known to Latinas as *café con leche*, which offers a healthier nutrient profile than just coffee alone.

Artificial (Non-Nutritive) Sweeteners

While there is very limited research on the safety of artificial sweeteners during pregnancy, the FDA[24] and Health Canada[37] have provided some guidance. The FDA recognizes sucralose (Splenda) and rebaudioside A (Stevia) as safe, including for pregnant women. The FDA describes aspartame (Equal, NutraSweet) and acesulfame potassium (Sunett) as "safe to use in moderation" during pregnancy. In contrast, Saccharin (Sweet'n Low) is known to cross the placenta and may accumulate in fetal tissues; thus, its use by pregnant women is not appropriate. Health Canada recommends that pregnant women who wish to use artificial sweeteners do so "in moderation."[37]

Alcohol

Alcohol is a known teratogen that readily crosses the placenta and accumulates in the fetal bloodstream. The immature fetal liver cannot readily metabolize alcohol, and its presence in fetal blood and tissues is associated with a variety of birth defects. These effects are dose dependent: the more the mother drinks, the greater the potential harm to the fetus.

The term *fetal alcohol spectrum disorders (FASD)* encompasses a range of complications that can develop when a pregnant woman consumes alcohol.[38] Drinking more than three to four drinks per day during pregnancy can result in the birth of a baby with *fetal alcohol syndrome (FAS)*, the most severe form of FASD. (For details on FAS and FASD, see Chapter 4.5, page 161.) These infants have a high mortality rate, and those who do survive suffer from malformations of the face, limbs, heart, and nervous system and typically face lifelong emotional, behavioral, social, and learning problems. Another form of FASD, *alcohol-related neurodevelopmental disorder (ARND)*, is a more subtle set of alcohol-related abnormalities. These include developmental and behavioral problems (for example, hyperactivity, attention deficit disorder, and impaired cognition).[39]

In addition to FASD, frequent drinking (more than seven drinks per week) or occasional binge drinking (more than four to five drinks on one occasion) during pregnancy can increase the risk for miscarriage, complications during delivery, low birth weight, neonatal asphyxia, and intrauterine growth retardation.

Although some pregnant women do have the occasional alcoholic drink with no apparent ill effects, there is no level of alcohol consumption known to be safe.[35] The best advice regarding alcohol during pregnancy is to abstain, if not from before conception then as soon as pregnancy is suspected. As with other critical national health concerns, *Healthy People 2020* directly addresses this issue with the stated goals of increasing abstinence from alcohol among pregnant women and reducing the incidence of FAS.[3]

Tobacco

Despite the well-known consequences of cigarette smoking and the growing social stigma associated with smoking during pregnancy, 14% of U.S. pregnant women smoke, and the rate is even higher among adolescents.[40,41]

Maternal smoking exposes the fetus to toxins such as lead, cadmium, cyanide, nicotine, and carbon monoxide. Fetal blood flow is reduced, which limits the delivery of oxygen and nutrients, resulting in impaired fetal growth and development. Maternal smoking greatly increases risk for miscarriage, stillbirth, placental abnormalities, intrauterine growth retardation, preterm delivery, and low birth weight.[40–43] Rates of sudden infant death syndrome, overall neonatal mortality (within the first 28 days of life), respiratory illnesses, risk for cleft lip or cleft palate, and allergies are higher in the infants and children of smokers compared to nonsmokers. Women who smoked while pregnant had more than double the risk of stillbirth compared to nonsmokers; exposure to second-hand smoke also increased risk of stillbirth.[43]

Healthy People 2020 has the goal of increasing the number of women who stop smoking during their first trimester and stay off cigarettes for the duration of their pregnancy.[3] Smoking cessation is a highly effective and inexpensive lifestyle change that dramatically improves both maternal and fetal health.

Illegal, Prescription, and Over-the-Counter Drugs and Supplements

Despite the fact that illegal drug use during pregnancy is unquestionably harmful to the fetus, nearly 5% of U.S. pregnant women between the ages of 15 and 44 years report having

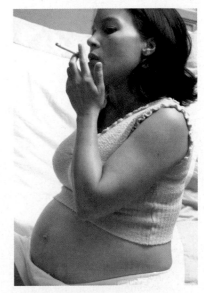

Maternal smoking is extremely harmful to the developing fetus.

used illicit drugs and as many as 20% of pregnant women abuse prescription drugs.[44] Most drugs pass through the placenta into the fetal blood, where they accumulate in fetal tissues and organs, including the liver and brain.

Drugs such as marijuana, cocaine, heroin, ecstasy, opiates, and amphetamines all pose similar risks: impaired placental blood flow (thus, reduced transfer of oxygen and nutrients to the fetus) and higher rates of stillbirths, low birth weight, premature delivery, placental defects, and miscarriage. Newborns suffer signs of withdrawal, including tremors, excessive crying, sleeplessness, and poor feeding. Even after several years, children born to women who used illicit drugs or abused prescription drugs during pregnancy are at greater risk for developmental delays, impaired learning, and behavioral problems. As more states act to legalize medical and recreational marijuana, public health officials fear an increase in poor pregnancy outcomes.

All women are strongly advised to stop taking illegal drugs *before* becoming pregnant. There is no safe level of use for illegal drugs during pregnancy nor is legalized use of marijuana considered safe for pregnancy women.

Over 90% of pregnant women use prescription or over-the-counter (OTC) medication, however few actually consult with their healthcare provider.[45] The FDA provides safety data related to use of many medications during pregnancy and lactation, although many OTC drugs are not safety rated and the FDA website is not always appropriately updated. In general, pregnant women are advised to always consult with their healthcare provider when considering using any medication, and to use the lowest dose possible for the shortest time. Women are also advised to avoid medication use during the first trimester if at all possible.

In addition, although many pregnant women view herbal supplements as "natural" and thus safe, they should consult their healthcare provider before using them. Herbal supplements are not evaluated for safety by the FDA, and research into their safety and effectiveness is inadequate.[46] Ginger, chamomile, and peppermint are commonly used during pregnancy to ease nausea and vomiting, and cranberry therapies are used for urinary tract infection. However, there are concerns that some herbal products, including *yerba mate* herbal tea (which is high in caffeine), St. John's wort infusion, and licorice root, may increase the risk for miscarriage, premature birth, and/or fetal distress.[46]

RECAP

About half of all pregnant women experience morning sickness, and many crave or feel aversions to specific types of foods. Gastroesophageal reflux and constipation in pregnancy are related to hormonal relaxation of smooth muscle. Gestational diabetes and hypertensive disorders can seriously affect maternal and fetal well-being. Pregnant women are at increased vulnerability to foodborne illness, especially from *Listeria monocytogenes*. The nutrient needs of pregnant adolescents are so high that adequate nourishment becomes difficult. Older pregnant women are at increased risk for gestational diabetes and hypertension. Women who follow a vegan diet usually need to consume multivitamin and mineral supplements, plus supplemental calcium, during pregnancy. Exercise (provided the mother has no contraindications) can enhance the health of a pregnant woman. Caffeine intake should be limited to no more than one cup of coffee a day. Some artificial sweeteners are considered safe during pregnancy, but others should be limited or avoided. Use of alcohol, tobacco, and illegal drugs should be completely avoided during pregnancy, and use of any medications and supplements should be discussed with the woman's healthcare provider. ■

LO 7 Describe the physiologic aspects of lactation, and identify the key nutrient recommendations for and needs of breastfeeding women.

How Does Nutrition Support Lactation?

Throughout most of human history, infants have thrived on only one food: breast milk. As early as 1867, however, synthetic milk substitutes became available. During the first half of the 20th century, commercially prepared infant formulas slowly began to replace breast milk as many women's preferred feeding method. Aggressive marketing campaigns promoting formula as more nutritious than breast milk convinced many families, even in developing nations, to switch. Soon formula-feeding became a status symbol, proof of a family's wealth and modern thinking.

In the 1970s, this trend began to reverse with a renewed appreciation for the natural simplicity of breastfeeding. At the same time, several international organizations, including the World Health Organization, UNICEF, and La Leche League, began to promote the nutritional, immunologic, financial, and emotional advantages of breastfeeding and developed programs to encourage and support breastfeeding worldwide.

These efforts have paid off. According to a 2014 report, almost 80% of U.S. newborns started breastfeeding, an all-time high, and nearly 50% of mothers were still partially or exclusively breastfeeding their babies at 6 months of age, as were 27% at 12 months.[47] Worldwide, slightly more than half of all women breastfeed *exclusively* for at least 6 months; however, this value is significantly lower in the United States, where only 19% of children are breast-fed exclusively at 6 months of age.[47] One goal of *Healthy People 2020* is to increase early postpartum breastfeeding to 82% of U.S. mothers, with 60% of women still breastfeeding at 6 months and 34% at 12 months postpartum.[3] Although U.S. mothers have nearly achieved the early postpartum goal, they still fall well below the 6- and 12-month goals.

Lactation Is Maintained by Hormones and Infant Suckling

Lactation, the production of breast milk, is a process that is set in motion during pregnancy in response to several hormones. Once established, lactation can be sustained as long as the mammary glands continue to receive the proper stimuli.

The Body Prepares During Pregnancy

Throughout pregnancy, the placenta produces the hormones estrogen and progesterone. In addition to performing various functions to maintain the pregnancy, these hormones physically prepare the breasts for lactation. The breasts increase in size, and milk-producing glands (alveoli) and milk ducts are formed (**Figure 17.8**). Toward the end of pregnancy, the hormone *prolactin* increases. Prolactin is released by the anterior pituitary gland and is responsible for milk synthesis. However, estrogen and progesterone suppress the effects of prolactin during pregnancy.

Production of Colostrum

By the time a pregnancy has come to full term, the level of prolactin is about ten times higher than it was at the beginning of pregnancy. At birth, the suppressive effect of estrogen and progesterone ends, and prolactin is free to stimulate milk production. The first substance to be released from the breasts for intake by the newborn is **colostrum,** sometimes called premilk or first milk. It is thick, yellowish in color, and rich in protein, and it includes antibodies that help protect the newborn from infection. It is also relatively high in vitamins and minerals. Colostrum also contains a factor that fosters the growth of beneficial bacteria in the infant's gastrointestinal (GI) tract. These bacteria in turn prevent the growth of other, potentially harmful bacteria. Finally, colostrum has a laxative effect in infants, helping the infant to expel *meconium,* the sticky "first stool." Within 2 to 4 days, colostrum is fully replaced by mature milk. Mature breast milk contains protein, fat, and carbohydrate (as the sugar lactose).

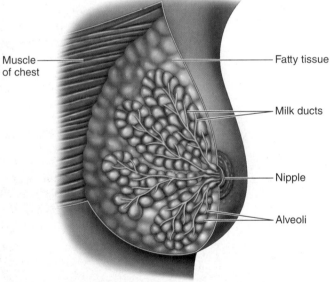

Muscle of chest — Fatty tissue — Milk ducts — Nipple — Alveoli

FIGURE 17.8 Anatomy of the breast. During pregnancy, estrogen and progesterone secreted by the placenta foster the preparation of breast tissue for lactation. This process includes breast enlargement and development of the milk-producing glands, or alveoli.

lactation The production of breast milk.

colostrum The first fluid made and secreted by the breasts from late in pregnancy to about a week after birth. It is rich in immune factors and protein.

Milk Production

Continued, sustained breast milk production depends entirely on infant suckling (or a similar stimulus, such as a mechanical pump or manual expression of breast milk). Infant suckling stimulates the continued production of prolactin, which in turn stimulates more milk production. The longer and more vigorous the feeding, the more milk will be produced. Thus, even twins and triplets can be successfully breastfed.

Prolactin allows for milk to be produced, but that milk has to move through the milk ducts to the nipple in order to reach the baby's mouth. The hormone responsible for this "let-down" of milk is *oxytocin*. Like prolactin, oxytocin is produced by the pituitary gland, and its production is dependent on the suckling stimulus at the beginning of a feeding (**Figure 17.9**). This response usually occurs within 10 to 30 seconds but can be inhibited by stress. Finding a relaxed environment in which to breastfeed is therefore important. Many women experience let-down in response to other cues, such as hearing a baby cry or even thinking about their infant.

Breastfeeding Women Have High Nutrient Needs

You might be surprised to learn that breastfeeding requires even more energy and nutrients than pregnancy! This is because breast milk has to supply an adequate amount of all the nutrients an infant needs to grow and develop.

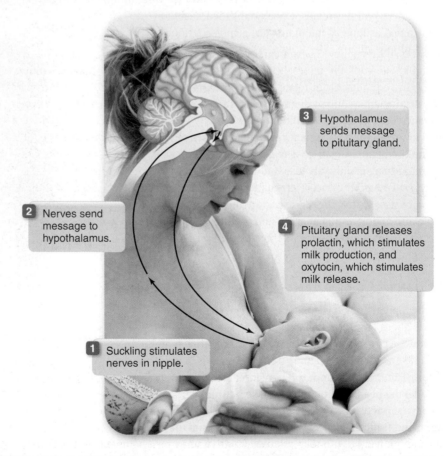

3 Hypothalamus sends message to pituitary gland.

2 Nerves send message to hypothalamus.

4 Pituitary gland releases prolactin, which stimulates milk production, and oxytocin, which stimulates milk release.

1 Suckling stimulates nerves in nipple.

FIGURE 17.9 Sustained milk production depends on the mother–child interaction during breastfeeding, specifically the suckling of the infant. Suckling stimulates the continued production of prolactin, which is responsible for milk production, and oxytocin, which is responsible for the let-down response.

Energy and Macronutrient Recommendations

It is estimated that milk production requires about 700 to 800 kcal/day. It is generally recommended that lactating women aged 19 years and above consume 330 kcal/day above their prepregnancy energy needs during the first 6 months of breastfeeding and 400 additional kcal/day during the second 6 months.[8] This additional energy is sufficient to support adequate milk production. At the same time, the remaining energy deficit will assist in the gradual loss of excess body weight gained during pregnancy. It is critical that lactating women avoid severe energy restriction, as this practice can result in decreased milk production.

The weight loss that occurs during breastfeeding should be gradual, approximately 1 to 4 lb per month. Moderate aerobic exercise (45 min/day, 5 days/week) does not affect breast milk volume or composition, nor does it reduce infant growth. There are, however, some very active women who may lose too much weight during breastfeeding and must either increase their energy intake or reduce their activity level to maintain health and milk production.

A lactating woman's needs for carbohydrate and protein increase over pregnancy requirements. Increases of 15 to 20 g of protein per day and 80 g of carbohydrate per day above prepregnancy requirements are recommended.[8] Women who breastfeed also need good dietary sources of DHA to support the rapid brain growth that occurs during the first 3 months of life. The DHA in the mother's diet is incorporated into the breast milk, to the benefit of the infant.

Micronutrient Recommendations

Micronutrient requirements for several vitamins and minerals increase over the requirements of pregnancy. These include vitamins A, C, E, riboflavin, vitamin B_{12}, biotin, and choline and the minerals copper, chromium, manganese, iodine, selenium, and zinc. The requirement for folate during lactation is 500 µg/day, which is decreased from the 600 µg/day required during pregnancy but is higher than prepregnancy needs (400 µg/day).[12]

Requirements for iron decrease significantly during lactation, to a mere 9 mg/day. This is because iron is not a significant component of breast milk, and breastfeeding usually suppresses menstruation for at least a few months, minimizing iron losses.[13]

Calcium is a significant component of breast milk; however, as in pregnancy, calcium absorption is enhanced during lactation, and urinary loss of calcium is decreased. In addition, some calcium appears to come from the demineralization of the mother's bones, and increased dietary calcium does not prevent this. Thus, the recommended intake for calcium for a lactating woman 19 years or older is unchanged from pregnancy and nonpregnant guidelines: 1,000 mg/day. Because of their own continuing growth, however, teen mothers (14–18 years) who are breastfeeding should continue to consume 1,300 mg/day.[14] Typically, if calcium intake is adequate, a woman's bone density returns to normal shortly after lactation ends.

Do Breastfeeding Women Need Supplements?

If a breastfeeding woman appropriately increases her energy intake, and does so with nutrient-dense foods, her nutrient needs can usually be met without supplements. The USDA's ChooseMyPlate.gov website provides recommendations for food choices for women who are breastfeeding their infants (see Web Links at the end of this chapter). However, there is nothing wrong with taking a basic multivitamin, as long as it is not considered a substitute for proper nutrition. Lactating women should consume omega-3 fatty acids either in fish, DHA-enriched eggs, or in supplements to increase breast milk levels of DHA. Women who do not consume dairy products should monitor their calcium intake carefully and may need supplements.

Fluid Recommendations

Because extra fluid is expended with every feeding, lactating women need to consume about an extra quart (about 1 liter) of fluid per day. The AI for total water is 3.8 liters per day for breastfeeding women, including about 13 cups of beverages.[17] This extra fluid enhances milk production and reduces the risk for dehydration. Many women report that, within a minute or two of beginning to nurse their baby, they become intensely thirsty. To prevent this thirst and achieve the recommended fluid intake, women are encouraged to drink a nutritious beverage (water, juice, milk, and so forth) each time they nurse their baby. However, women should avoid drinking hot beverages while nursing, because accidental spills could burn the infant.

RECAP

Lactation is the result of the coordinated effort of several hormones. Breasts are prepared for lactation during pregnancy, and infant suckling provides the stimulus that sustains the production of prolactin and oxytocin needed to maintain the milk supply. It is recommended that lactating women consume extra energy above prepregnancy guidelines, including increased protein, certain vitamins and minerals, and fluids. The requirements for folate and iron decrease from pregnancy levels, while the requirement for calcium remains the same. Lactating women need to consume about an extra quart (about 1 liter) of fluid per day. If nutrient intake is inadequate, milk production will decline and the woman will produce a smaller volume of breast milk. ∎

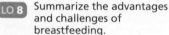

LO 8 Summarize the advantages and challenges of breastfeeding.

What Are Some Advantages and Challenges of Breastfeeding?

Breastfeeding is recognized as the preferred method of infant feeding because of the immediate and long-term nutritional value and health benefits of human milk.[48] However, the technique does require patience and practice, and teaching from an experienced mother or a certified lactation consultant is important. The CDC recommends that breastfeeding support be provided by healthcare providers, trained lactation specialists, peer support groups, the workplace, childcare facilities, and legal protections.[49] La Leche League International is an advocacy group for breastfeeding: its website (included in the Web Links), publications, and local meetings are all valuable resources for breastfeeding mothers and their families. Some U.S. hospitals, designated as "Baby Friendly," have adopted policies that enhance lactation success, and the recently enacted Affordable Care Act requires employers to provide "reasonable break time" and a private place "other than a bathroom" for women to pump their breast milk.[50,51]

Breast Milk Is Nutritionally Superior to Infant Formula

For help with breastfeeding, listen to the free podcasts at http://www.llli.org. Click on the resources tab.

As adept as formula manufacturers have been at simulating components of breast milk, an exact replica has never been produced. The amount and types of proteins in breast milk are ideally suited to the human infant. The main protein in breast milk, lactalbumin, is easily digested in infants' immature GI tracts, reducing the risk for gastric distress. Other proteins in breast milk bind iron and prevent the growth of harmful bacteria that require iron. Antibodies from the mother are additional proteins that help prevent infection while the infant's immune system is still immature. Certain proteins in human milk improve the absorption of iron; this is important because breast milk is low in iron. Cow's milk contains too much protein for infants, and the types of protein in cow's milk are harder for the infant to digest.

The primary carbohydrate in breast milk is lactose; its galactose component is important in nervous system development. Lactose provides energy and prevents ketosis in the infant, promotes the growth of beneficial bacteria, and increases the absorption of calcium. Breast milk has more lactose than cow's milk.

The amounts and types of fat in breast milk are ideally suited to the human infant. DHA and arachidonic acid (ARA) are fatty acids that have been shown to be essential for the growth and development of the infant's nervous system and for development of the retina of the eyes. Until 2002, these fatty acids were omitted from commercial infant formulas in the United States, although they were available in formulas in other parts of the world. Interestingly, the concentration of DHA in breast milk varies considerably, is sensitive to maternal diet, and is highest in women who consume large quantities of fish during pregnancy and/or lactation.[52]

The fat content of breast milk, which is higher than that of whole cow's milk, changes according to the gestational age of the infant and during the course of every feeding. The milk that is initially released (called *foremilk*) is watery and low in fat, somewhat like skim milk. This milk is thought to satisfy the infant's initial thirst. Because of their small size, infants are at risk for dehydration, which is one reason feedings must be consistent and frequent. As the feeding progresses, the milk acquires more fat and becomes more like whole milk. Finally, the very last 5% or so of the milk produced during a feeding (called the *hindmilk*) is very high in fat, similar to cream. This milk is thought to satiate the infant. It is important to let infants suckle for at least 20 minutes at each feeding, so that they get this hindmilk. Breast milk is also relatively high in cholesterol, which supports the rapid growth and development of the brain and nervous system.

In terms of micronutrients, breast milk is a good source of readily absorbed calcium and magnesium. It is low in iron, but the iron it does contain is easily absorbed. Because healthy full-term infants store iron in preparation for the first few months of life, most experts agree that their iron needs can be met by breast milk alone for the first 6 months, after which iron-rich foods are needed. Although breast milk has some vitamin D, the American Academy of Pediatrics recommends that all breast-fed infants be provided with a vitamin D supplement.

Breast milk composition continues to change as the infant grows and develops. Because of this ability to change as the baby changes, breast milk alone is entirely sufficient to sustain infant growth for the first 6 months of life. Throughout the next 6 months of infancy, as solid foods are gradually introduced, breast milk remains the baby's primary source of superior-quality nutrition. The American Academy of Pediatrics encourages exclusive breastfeeding (no food or other source of sustenance) for the first 6 months of life, continuing breastfeeding for at least the first year of life and, if acceptable within the family unit, into the second year of life.[53]

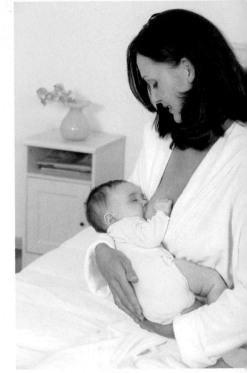

Breastfeeding has important benefits for both the mother and the infant.

Breastfeeding Has Many Other Benefits for the Infant and Mother

In addition to its nutritional advantages, breast milk provides a variety of other healthful compounds, and breastfeeding itself has physiologic, emotional, and financial benefits.

Protection from Infections, Allergies, and Residues

Immune factors from the mother, including antibodies and immune cells, are passed directly from the mother to the newborn through breast milk. These factors provide important disease protection for the infant while its immune system is still immature. It has been shown that breast-fed infants have a lower incidence of respiratory tract, GI tract, and ear infections than formula-fed infants.[53] Even a few weeks of breastfeeding is beneficial, but the longer a child is breastfed, the greater the level of passive immunity from the mother.

In addition, breast milk is nonallergenic, and breastfeeding is associated with a reduced risk for allergies during childhood and adulthood. Breast-fed babies also have a decreased chance of developing diabetes, overweight and obesity, hypercholesterolemia, and chronic digestive disorders.[48,53]

Exclusively breast-fed infants are also protected from exposure to known and unknown contaminants and residues that may be found in baby bottles and cans of infant formulas. Recent concerns have centered on bisphenol A (BPA), a toxic chemical that has been found in a few brands of reusable bottles and formulas. In 2012, the FDA banned the use of BPA in all baby bottles and toddler's cups (also known as sippy cups).[54]

Physiologic Benefits for the Mother

Breastfeeding also has physiologic benefits for the mother. In the first few hours and days after childbirth, breastfeeding prompts uterine contractions that quicken the return of the uterus to prepregnancy size and reduce bleeding. Many women also find that breastfeeding helps them lose the weight they gained during pregnancy, particularly if it continues for more than 6 months. In addition, breastfeeding appears to be associated with a decreased risk for breast cancer and possibly osteoporosis.[55] Breastfeeding also suppresses ovulation, lengthening the time between pregnancies and giving a mother's body the chance to recover before she conceives again. This benefit can be life-saving for malnourished women living in countries that discourage or outlaw the use of contraceptives. Ovulation may not cease completely, however, so it is still possible to become pregnant while breastfeeding. Healthcare providers typically recommend the use of additional birth control methods while breastfeeding to avoid another conception too soon to allow a mother's body to recover from the earlier pregnancy.

Mother–Infant Bonding

Breastfeeding is among the most intimate of human interactions. Ideally, it is a quiet time away from distractions when mother and baby begin to develop an enduring bond of affection known as *attachment*. Breastfeeding enhances attachment by providing the opportunity for frequent, direct skin-to-skin contact, which stimulates the baby's sense of touch and is a primary means of communication. The cuddling and intense eye contact that occur during breastfeeding begin to teach the mother and baby about the other's behavioral cues. Breastfeeding also reassures the mother that she is providing the best possible nutrition for her baby. Healthcare providers recommend that hospitals permit continuous rooming-in of breast-fed infants throughout the day and night to enhance the initiation and continuation of breastfeeding.[51]

Undoubtedly, bottle-feeding does not preclude parent–infant attachment! As long as attention is paid to closeness, cuddling, and skin contact, bottle-feeding can foster bonding as well. Fathers and other family members can participate in infant feeding using a bottle of stored breast milk as soon as breastfeeding has become well established. That way, the infant will not be confused by the artificial nipple. Fathers and other family members can also bond with the infant when bathing and/or dressing them, as well as through everyday cuddling and play.

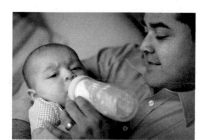

Fathers and siblings can bond with infants through bottle-feeding.

Convenience and Cost

Breast milk is always ready, clean, at the right temperature, and available on demand, whenever and wherever it's needed. In the middle of the night, when the baby wakes up hungry, a breastfeeding mother can respond almost instantaneously, and both are soon back to sleep. In contrast, formula-feeding is a time-consuming process: parents have to continually wash and sterilize bottles, and each batch of formula must be mixed and heated to the proper temperature.

In addition, breastfeeding costs nothing other than the price of a modest amount of additional food for the mother. In contrast, formula can be expensive, plus there are costs for bottles and other supplies, and energy for washing and sterilization. Breastfeeding is also environmentally responsible, using no external energy and generating no greenhouse gas emissions or environmental wastes.

Physical, Social, and Emotional Concerns Can Make Breastfeeding Challenging

For some women and infants, breastfeeding is easy from the very first day. Others experience some initial difficulty, but with support from an experienced nurse, lactation consultant, or volunteer mother from La Leche League, the experience becomes successful and pleasurable. Some families, however, encounter difficulties that make formula-feeding their best choice, temporarily or permanently.

Effects of Drugs and Other Substances on Breast Milk

Many substances, including prescription and over-the-counter medications, pass into breast milk. Breastfeeding mothers should inform their physician that they are breastfeeding. If a safe and effective form of the necessary medication cannot be found, the mother will have to avoid breastfeeding while she is taking the drug. During this time, she can pump and discard her breast milk, so that her milk supply will be adequate when she resumes breastfeeding.

Caffeine, alcohol, nicotine, and illicit drugs also enter breast milk. Caffeine, nicotine, and other stimulant drugs can make the baby agitated and fussy and can disturb infant sleep patterns. Breastfeeding women should reduce their caffeine intake to no more than the equivalent of two or three cups of coffee per day and avoid caffeine intake within 2 hours prior to nursing their infant. They should also quit smoking and avoid the use of illicit drugs. Alcohol can make the baby sleepy, depress the central nervous system, and slow motor development, in addition to inhibiting the mother's milk supply. Breastfeeding women should abstain from alcohol in the early stages of lactation, since it easily passes into the breast milk and infants 0–3 months of age metabolize alcohol at a rate half that of adults. It takes about 2 to 3 hours for the alcohol from a single serving of beer or wine to be eliminated from the body, so it is possible for breastfeeding women to plan ahead and coordinate moderate alcohol intake with their breastfeeding schedule.

Environmental contaminants, including pesticides, industrial solvents, and heavy metals such as lead and mercury, can pass into breast milk when breastfeeding mothers are exposed to these chemicals. Mothers can limit their infants' exposure to these harmful substances by controlling their environment. Fresh fruits and vegetables should be thoroughly washed and peeled to minimize exposure to pesticides and fertilizer residues. Exposure to solvents, paints, gasoline fumes, furniture strippers, and similar products should also be limited. Even with some exposure to these environmental contaminants, United States and international health agencies all agree that the benefits of breastfeeding almost always outweigh potential concerns.

Food components that pass into the breast milk may seem innocuous; however, some substances, such as those found in garlic, onions, peppers, broccoli, and cabbage, are distasteful enough to the infant to prevent proper feeding. Some babies have allergic reactions to foods the mother has eaten, such as wheat, cow's milk, eggs, or citrus, and suffer gastrointestinal upset, diaper rash, or another reaction. The offending foods must then be identified and avoided.

Effects of Maternal HIV Infection and Obesity

HIV, the virus that causes AIDS, can be transmitted from mother to baby through breast milk. Thus, HIV-positive women in the United States and Canada are encouraged to feed their infants formula. This recommendation does not apply to all women worldwide, however, because the low cost and sanitary nature of breast milk, as compared to the high cost and potential for waterborne diseases with formula-feeding, often make exclusive breastfeeding the best choice for HIV-infected women in developing countries.[56]

There is strong evidence that maternal obesity significantly reduces the rate of successful breastfeeding.[57] Fewer obese women plan to breastfeed and fewer actually initiate breastfeeding compared to normal weight women. Among those obese women who do breastfeed, they do so for shorter durations and produce a less adequate supply of milk. Obese women report more difficulties, such as cracked nipples and difficulty initiating breastfeeding, and are more likely to feel uncomfortable breastfeeding in front of others. These findings are particularly troubling because breastfeeding helps a woman lose some of her pregnancy weight, and has been shown to reduce the risk of overweight and obesity in the child, whereas children of obese mothers are, on average, at increased risk for overweight and obesity later in life.

Employment Challenges

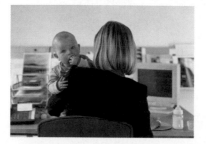

Working moms can be discouraged from—or supported in—breastfeeding in a variety of ways.

Breast milk is absorbed more readily than formula, making more frequent feedings necessary. Newborns commonly require breastfeeding every 1 to 3 hours versus every 2 to 4 hours for formula-feeding. Mothers who are exclusively breastfeeding and return to work within the first 6 months after the baby's birth must leave several bottles of pumped breast milk for others to feed the baby in their absence each day. This means that working women have to pump their breasts to express the breast milk during the work day. This can be a challenge in companies that do not provide the time, space, and privacy required, a scenario most often seen in low-paying jobs. As previously noted, the Affordable Care Act of 2010 sets specific standards under the Fair Labor Standards Act that support breastfeeding workers, although employers with fewer than 50 employees may request an exemption.[50]

Work-related travel is also a concern: if the mother needs to be away from home for longer than 24 to 48 hours, she can typically pump and freeze enough breast milk for others to give the baby in her absence. Understandably, many women cite returning to work as the reason they switch to formula-feeding.

Some working women successfully combine breastfeeding with formula-feeding. For example, a woman might breastfeed in the morning before she leaves for work, as soon as she returns home, and again at bedtime. Other feedings are formula given by the infant's father or a childcare provider. Women who choose this approach usually find that their bodies adapt quickly and produce ample milk for the remaining breastfeedings.

Social Concerns

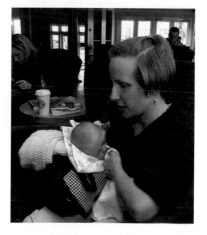

Although breastfeeding in public is a much more common practice today than in the past, some people still consider it inappropriate.

In North America, women have at times been insulted or otherwise harassed for breastfeeding in public. Over the past decade, however, both social customs and state laws have become more accommodating and supportive of nursing mothers. Some states have passed legislation preserving a woman's right to breastfeed in public. Advocacy groups and greater social and cultural awareness have also contributed to a more forgiving climate for women to breastfeed. When women feel free (and legally protected) to do so, the baby's feeding schedule becomes much less confining.

RECAP

Breastfeeding provides many benefits to both mother and newborn, including superior nutrition, heightened immunity, protection from residues, a reduction in the mother's postpartal bleeding and body weight, and suppression of ovulation. It also promotes mother–infant bonding, is convenient, and has no cost except for a small amount of extra food for the mother. However, breastfeeding may not be the best option for every family. A mother may need to use a medication that enters the breast milk and makes it unsafe for consumption. Women with HIV can pass the virus to the infant in breast milk, and obesity may reduce the milk supply. A mother's job may interfere with the baby's requirement for frequent feedings. The mother may also feel uncomfortable or be harassed when breastfeeding in public.

What Are an Infant's Nutrient Needs?

LO 9 Describe an infant's growth patterns and nutrient needs, and the nutrient profile of different types of infant formula.

Most first-time parents are amazed at how rapidly their infant grows and develops. Optimal nutrition is extremely important during the first year, as the baby's organs and systems continue to develop and mature and as the baby grows physically and acquires new skills.

During the first year of an infant's life, breast milk remains the food of choice; however, iron-fortified formula is an acceptable substitute for parents deciding that breastfeeding is not an option. After approximately 6 months, most infants are ready for *complementary* foods, such as baby cereals and strained meats, which provide key nutrients and introduce the infant to new tastes and textures. An infant who is lovingly and consistently fed when hungry will feel secure and well cared for. A relaxed, consistent feeding relationship between parent and child fosters a positive and healthy outlook toward food. In many ways, an infant's diet "sets the stage" for future health and development.

Nutrition Fuels Infant Growth and Activity

In the first year of life, an infant generally grows about 10 inches in length and triples in weight—a growth rate more rapid than will ever occur again. To support this phenomenal growth, energy needs per unit body weight are also the highest they will ever be, approximately triple that of adults. Energy needs are also very high, because the basal metabolic rates of babies are high (**Figure 17.10**). This is in part because the body surface area of a baby is large compared to its body size, increasing its loss of body heat. Still, the limited physical activity of a baby keeps total energy expenditure relatively low.

For the first few months of life, an infant's activities consist mainly of eating and sleeping. As the first year progresses, the range of activities gradually expands to include rolling over, sitting up, crawling, standing, and finally taking the first few wobbly steps. As shown in Figure 17.10, the relative need for energy to support growth slows during the second 6 months of life, just as activity begins to increase.

Growth charts—one set for girls and one set for boys—are routinely used by healthcare providers and parents to track growth. They are available from the Centers for Disease Control and Prevention (CDC) free of charge. An example of one for boys and one for girls is provided in Appendix F "Stature-for-Age Charts." Charts for children birth to 36 months assess length-for-age, weight-for-age, and weight-for-length, all expressed as percentiles. If an infant is in the 90th percentile for length, he or she is longer than 89% of U.S. infants of that age and gender and thus is considered very long. If an infant is in the 10th percentile for weight, only 10% of U.S. infants of the same age and gender weigh less than he or she does, so that baby can be viewed as relatively underweight compared to other infants. Although every infant is unique, in general, healthcare providers look for a close correlation between length and weight rankings. In other words, an infant who is in the 60th percentile for length is usually in about the 50th to 70th percentile for weight. A child in the 50th percentile for length but the 10th percentile for weight may be malnourished. Consistency over time is also a consideration: for example, an infant who suddenly drops well below his or her established profile for weight might be underfed or ill. The CDC has also developed BMI-for-age charts for children over 24 months of age.

Although growth charts are effective tools for assessing an infant's nutrition status, there are some limitations. For example, it is important to consider the physical stature of the baby's parents. If both parents are tall, you would expect the infant to remain close to the upper percentiles for length. Exclusively breast-fed infants often track at a lower percentile weight-for-age compared to formula-fed infants, although no differences in length-for-age or head circumference are noted. Families need to know that this slower rate of weight gain has not been associated with any negative outcomes. Indeed, many healthcare providers believe that the slower growth rate of breast-fed infants should be considered the norm, not the exception, because formula-feeding is a relatively recent cultural phenomenon.

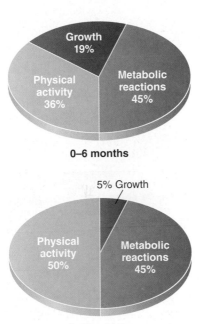

FIGURE 17.10 Energy expenditure during infancy. During the first 6 months of life, infants expend more energy to support growth and less energy on physical activity than in the second 6 months of life.

The growth of the brain is more rapid during the first year than at any other time, and infants' heads are typically large in proportion to the rest of their bodies, approximately one-fourth of their total length. Pediatricians use head circumference as an additional tool for the assessment of growth and nutritional status; CDC growth charts for head-circumference-for-age are available for infants and toddlers birth to 36 months of age. After around 18 months of age, the rate of brain growth slows, and gradually the body "catches up" to head size, resulting in body proportions that are closer to those of a child.

As infants grow and develop, their proportions of muscle, fat, and bone evolve. Body fat, as a percentage of total body weight, increases after birth and peaks around 9 months of age. Muscle tissue increases slowly but steadily, and body calcium, a marker for skeletal growth, more than doubles during the first year of life.[14] Body water, as a percentage of total body weight, is highest in newborns and gradually decreases through and beyond early childhood.[17]

Infants Have Unique Nutrient Needs

Three characteristics of infants combine to make their nutritional needs unique. These are (1) their high energy needs per unit body weight to support rapid growth, (2) their immature GI tract and kidneys, and (3) their small size.

Macronutrient Needs of Infants

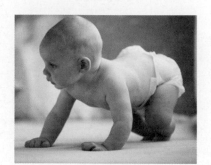

The proportions of muscle, fat, and bone in the bodies of infants change as they grow and become more active.

An infant needs to consume about 40 to 50 kcal/lb of body weight per day, with newborns at the higher end of the range and infants 6 to 12 months old at the lower end. This amounts to about 600 (girls) to 650 (boys) kcal/day at around 6 months of age.[8] Although providing this much energy may seem difficult, breast milk and commercial formulas are energy dense, providing about 650 kcal/L of fluid.[8] When complementary (solid) foods are introduced, they provide even more energy in addition to the breast milk or formula.

Infants are not small versions of adults; they are growing rapidly compared to the typically stable adult phase of life. The proportions of macronutrients they require differ from adult proportions, as do the types of food they can tolerate. It is generally agreed that about 40% to 50% of an infant's energy intake should come from fat during the first year of life and that fat intakes below this level can be harmful before the age of 2 years. Given the high energy needs of infants, it makes sense to take advantage of the energy density of fat (9 kcal/g). Breast milk and commercial formulas are both high in fat (about 50% of total energy).

Breast milk is an excellent source of the fatty acids arachidonic acid (AA) and docosahexaenoic acid (DHA), although levels of DHA vary widely with the mother's diet. Both of these fats are thought to support the rapid growth and development of the brain and entire nervous system, including the retina of the eye, that occurs in the first 1 to 2 years of life. Many formula manufacturers are now adding AA and DHA to their products.

The recommended carbohydrate intake for infants 0 to 6 months of age, 60 g/day, is based on the lactose content of human milk.[8] The carbohydrate AI for older infants 7 to 12 months of age reflects the intake of human milk and complementary foods, and is set at 95 g/day.

The recommended intake of protein for infants 0 to 6 months of age is about 1.5 g/kg body weight per day.[8] Again, this value is based on the protein content of human milk. Formula-fed infants typically consume higher amounts of protein compared to breast-fed infants; however, the proteins in commercial formulas are less efficiently digested and absorbed. The protein guideline for infants 7 to 12 months of age is 1.1 g/kg body weight per day.[8] Recall (from Chapter 6) that the adult RDA for protein is 0.8 g/day. The relatively higher intake for infants is to accommodate their rapid growth. However, no more than 20% of an infant's daily energy requirement should come from protein. Immature infant kidneys are not able to process and excrete the excess amine groups from higher-protein diets. Breast milk and commercial formulas both provide adequate total protein and appropriate essential amino acids to support growth and development.

Micronutrient Needs of Infants

An infant's micronutrient needs are also high to accommodate rapid growth and development. Fortunately, breast milk and commercial formulas provide most of the micronutrients needed for infant growth and development, with some special considerations.

First, all infants are routinely given an injection of vitamin K shortly after birth. This provides vitamin K until the infant's intestine can develop its own healthful bacteria, which provide vitamin K thereafter.

Second, although breast milk and commercial formulas provide most of the vitamins and minerals infants need, breast milk is low in vitamin D, and deficiencies of this nutrient have been detected in breast-fed infants with dark skin and in those with limited sunlight exposure. Breast-fed infants and those consuming less than 1 L of vitamin D–fortified formula should be prescribed a supplement containing vitamin D.[58]

Breast-fed infants also require additional iron beginning no later than 6 months of age, because the infant's iron stores become depleted and breast milk is a poor source of iron. Iron is extremely important for cognitive development and prevention of iron-deficiency anemia. Puréed meats and infant rice cereal fortified with iron can serve as excellent sources of absorbable iron. Only if breast-fed infants are not yet consuming these iron-rich foods is there the need for iron supplements.

Fluoride is important for strong tooth development, but fluoride supplementation is not recommended during the first 6 months of life. Depending on the fluoride content of the household water supply, breast-fed infants over the age of 6 months may need a fluoride supplement. Most brands of bottled water have low levels of fluoride, and many home water treatment systems remove fluoride. On the other hand, fluoride toxicity may be a risk for infants simultaneously exposed to fluoridated toothpaste and rinses, fluoridated water, and fluoride supplements.

The breast milk of a vegan mother may be low in vitamin B_{12}. A supplement of this vitamin should be given to the baby.

For formula-fed infants, the need for supplementation depends on the formula composition and other factors. Many formulas are already fortified with iron, for example; thus, no additional iron supplement is necessary. If the baby is getting adequate vitamin D through either the ingestion of at least 1 liter of vitamin D–fortified formula or via regular sun exposure, an extra supplement may not be necessary.

If a supplement is given, careful consideration should be given to dose. The supplement should be formulated specifically for infants, and the recommended daily dose should not be exceeded. High doses of micronutrients can be dangerous. For example, too much iron can be fatal, and too much fluoride can cause mottling, pitting, and staining of the teeth. Excessive vitamin D can cause abnormally high levels of serum calcium and calcification of soft tissues, such as the kidney.

Fluid Recommendations for Infants

Fluid is critical for everyone, but for infants the balance is more delicate for two reasons. First, they proportionally lose more water through evaporation from the skin surface area than adults. Second, their kidneys are immature and unable to concentrate urine. Hence, they are at even greater risk for dehydration. An infant needs about 2 oz of fluid per pound of body weight, and either breast milk or formula is almost always adequate in providing this amount. Experts recently confirmed that "infants exclusively fed human milk do not require supplemental water."[17] This is true for infants living in hot and humid climates as well as more moderate environments. Parents can be reassured that their infant's fluid intake is appropriate if the infant produces six to eight wet diapers per day.

Certain conditions, such as diarrhea, vomiting, fever, or extreme hot weather, can accelerate fluid loss. In these instances, supplemental fluid, ideally as water or an infant

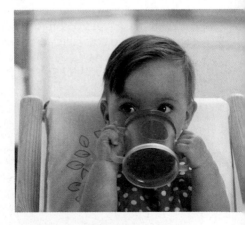

Infants are at high risk for dehydration and should be offered water and other nutritious beverages on a regular basis.

Nutrition
MILESTONE

The practice of "hand feeding" infants with animal milk and/or grain-based mixtures is documented going as far back as 2000 BC. These mixtures, however, were so incompatible with infant nutritional needs that as many as 90% or more of "formula-fed" infants died, up through the early 1800s. It wasn't until the nutrient differences between cow's and human milk were understood that successful infant formulas were developed. Justus von Liebig is credited with developing and marketing the first commercial powdered infant formula in

1867
. Made from cow's milk, wheat, malt flour, and potassium bicarbonate, it quickly became a popular option for well-to-do families. By 1883, 27 brands of this or similar infant formulas were available.

In the United States, the first federal regulations related to infant formulas were established in 1941. In 1951, concentrated liquid formulas were introduced, followed by the marketing of iron-fortified formulas in 1959. In the 1960s, manufacturers modified their protein sources to create whey-dominant formulas, and formulas made with highly digestible isolated soy protein became widely available. More recently, as the science of infant feeding has advanced, formula manufacturers have improved vitamin and mineral levels and have added components such as DHA and taurine. Infant formulas have also been enhanced through the addition of *probiotics,* which are certain types of live bacteria known to be beneficial to health. With these types of improvements, infants who are fed commercial formulas today can sustain growth and development that are nearly on par with breast-fed infants.

electrolyte formula, may be needed, but should be given only under the advice of a physician. Generally, it is advised that supplemental fluids not exceed 4 oz per day. Parents should avoid giving infants sugar water, fruit juices, or sweetened beverages in a bottle, especially at bedtime, as the practice can cause decay of developing teeth.

Infant Formula Is a Nutritious Alternative to Breast Milk

If breastfeeding is not feasible, several types of commercial formulas provide nutritious alternatives. In the United States, as many as 80% to 85% of infants are fed commercial formula by the age of 1 year. Formula manufacturers must comply with federal standards for minimum and maximum levels for 29 nutrients. Although most formula manufacturers try to mimic the nutritional value of breast milk, these formulas still cannot completely duplicate the immune factors, enzymes, and other unique components of human milk.

Most formulas are based on cow's milk that is modified to make it more appropriate for infants. The amount of total protein is reduced and levels of milk proteins are altered in order to mirror the types of proteins in breast milk. In addition, the product is heated to denature the proteins and make them more digestible. The naturally occurring lactose may be supplemented with sucrose to provide adequate carbohydrate. Vegetable oils and/or microbiologically produced fatty acids replace the naturally occurring butterfat. Vitamins and minerals are added to meet national standards. Recently, some manufacturers have added compounds such as taurine, carnitine, and the fatty acids AA and DHA to more closely mimic the nutrient profile of breast milk. This chapter's *Nutrition Label Activity* gives you the opportunity to review some of these ingredients.

Soy-based formulas are effective alternatives for infants who are lactose intolerant (although this is rare in infants). While soy formulas may also be used with infants who cannot tolerate the proteins in cow's milk–based formulas, many infants who are allergic to cow's milk protein are also allergic to soy protein. Soy formulas will satisfy the requirements of families who are strict vegans. However, soy-based formulas are not without controversy. Because soy contains isoflavones, or plant forms of estrogens, there is some concern over the effects these compounds have on growing infants. Currently, it is believed that soy formulas are safe, but they should only be used when breast milk or cow's milk–based formulas are contraindicated. Soy-based formulas are not the same as soy milk, which is not suitable for infant feeding.

Finally, there are specialized formulas for specific medical conditions. Some contain proteins that have been predigested, for example, or have nutrient compositions designed to accommodate certain genetic abnormalities. Others have been developed to meet the unique nutritional needs of preterm infants. Many of these specialized or medical formulas are available only through a physician.

Commercial formulas provide infants with a nutritious alternative to breast milk. Cow's milk, including fresh, evaporated, condensed, and dried milks, should not be introduced to infants until after 1 year of age. Cow's milk is too high in protein, the protein is difficult to digest, and the poor digestibility may contribute to gastrointestinal bleeding. In addition, cow's milk has too much sodium, too little iron, and a poor balance of other vitamins and minerals. Goat's milk is also inappropriate for infants and should not be used as a substitute for breast milk or formula.

Reading Infant Food Labels

Imagine that you are a new parent shopping for infant formula. **Figure 17.11** shows the label from a typical can of formula. As you can see, the ingredients list is long and has many technical terms. Even well-informed parents would probably be stumped by many of them. Fortunately, with the information you learned in previous chapters, you can probably answer the following questions:

- One of the ingredients listed is a modified form of *whey protein concentrate*. What common food is the source of *whey*?

- The second ingredient listed is *lactose*. Is lactose a form of protein, fat, or carbohydrate? Why is lactose important for infants?

- The front label states the formula has added DHA (docosahexaenoic acid). Is DHA a form of protein, fat, or carbohydrate? Why is this nutrient thought to be important for infants?

The label also claims that this formula is "Our closest formula to mature breast milk." Can you think of some differences between breast milk and this formula that still exist? Also, look at the list of nutrients on the back label. You'll notice that there is no "% Daily Value" column, which you see on most food labels. Next time you are at the grocery store, look at other baby food items, such as baby cereal or puréed fruits. Do their labels simply list the nutrient content, or is the "% Daily Value" column used? Why do you think infant formula has a different label format?

Let's say you are feeding a 6-month-old infant who needs about 500 kcal/day. Using the information from the nutrition section of the label, you can calculate the number of fluid ounces of formula the baby needs (this assumes that no cereal or other foods are eaten):

There are 100 kcal per 5 fl. oz:

$$100 \text{ kcal} \div 5 \text{ fl. oz} = 20 \text{ kcal/fl. oz}$$

$$500 \text{ kcal} \div 20 \text{ kcal/fl. oz} = 25 \text{ fl. oz of formula per day to}$$
meet this baby's energy needs

A 6-month-old infant needs about 210 mg calcium per day. Based on an intake of 25 fl. oz of formula per day, as just calculated, you can use the label nutrition information to calculate the amount of calcium that is provided:

There are 78 mg calcium per 5 fl. oz serving of formula:

$$78 \text{ mg} \div 5 \text{ fl. oz} = 15.6 \text{ mg calcium per fl. oz}$$

$$15.6 \text{ mg calcium per fl. oz} \times 25 \text{ fl. oz} = 390 \text{ mg}$$
calcium per day

You can see that the infant's need for calcium is easily met by the formula alone.

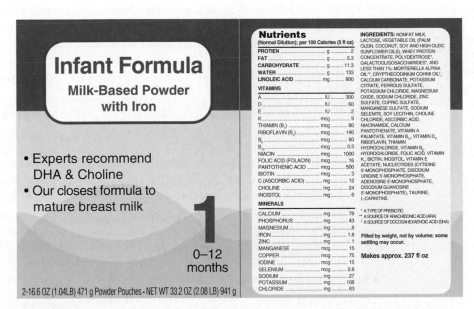

FIGURE 17.11 An infant formula label. Notice that there is a long list of ingredients and no % Daily Value.

RECAP

Infancy is characterized by the most rapid rate of growth a human being will ever experience, and an infant's energy needs are correspondingly high. Assessment of the infant's growth pattern can provide important clues to his or her nutritional state. Three characteristics of infants combine to make their nutritional needs unique. These are (1) their high energy needs—40 to 50 kcal/lb—to support their rapid growth, (2) their immature GI tract and kidneys, and (3) their small size. Breast milk is the ideal infant food for the first 6 months of life; iron-fortified infant formula also provides the necessary nutrients. DRIs for infants are based on the nutrients in breast milk. About 40% to 50% of an infant's energy intake should come from fat, and no more than 20% from protein. All infants are routinely given an injection of vitamin K shortly after birth. Vitamin D supplements are recommended for exclusively breast-fed infants; iron and fluoride supplements may be prescribed for infants older than 6 months of age. Infants of vegan mothers are typically given supplemental vitamin B_{12}. Infants lose more body fluid through evaporation, and their kidneys are immature and unable to concentrate urine; thus, they have an increased risk for dehydration. An infant needs about 2 oz of fluid per pound of body weight. Commercial formulas provide infants with a nutritious alternative to breast milk. Most are based on cow's milk that has been modified to mimic the nutritional profile of breast milk.

LO 10 Discuss several nutrient-related concerns for infants.

What Are Some Common Nutrition-Related Concerns of Infancy?

Nutrition is one of the primary concerns of new parents. Many are uncertain when to begin offering solid foods, and what to offer. Moreover, as infants begin to take in a variety of foods, they may begin to experience allergic reactions or other disorders or feeding challenges.

Infants Begin to Need Solid Foods Around 6 Months of Age

As the result of declining nutrient stores, particularly iron, and continued growth, infants begin to need complementary, or solid, foods at around 6 months of age (Table 17.4). As previously noted, the American Academy of Pediatrics recommends exclusive breastfeeding for the first 6 months of life, but also recognizes that there is no evidence of significant harm if complementary foods are offered no earlier than 4 months of age.

TABLE 17.4 Guidelines for the Introduction of Foods to Infants

Guideline	Explanation
Introduce single-item foods, one at a time, at 3- to 5-day intervals. Avoid multigrain cereals and mixed dishes.	This makes it easier to identify possible food allergies.
Start with foods that provide key nutrients, such as iron-fortified infant cereals and puréed meats.	Iron and zinc are the most common nutrient deficiencies in infants. Meat provides both.
One hundred percent undiluted fruit juices should not be introduced until the infant is at least 6 months of age. When introduced, limit to 4 to 6 oz/day and vary the types of juice offered.	High juice intake displaces calcium- and protein-rich breast milk and formula. Many popular juices, such as apple juice, offer limited nutritional value.
Do not introduce cow's milk until the infant is at least 1 year old. When introduced, provide whole milk, not reduced-fat milk.	The nutrient profile of cow's milk is not optimal to meet the needs of the growing infant. Healthy 1-year-olds need the energy provided by whole milk.
Introduce a variety of foods by the age of 1 year.	Variety and diversity in foods improve nutrient intake; stimulate the senses of taste, odor, and touch; and positively influence future eating habits.

One factor limiting an infant's ability to take solid foods is the *extrusion reflex*. During infant feeding, the suckling response depends on a particular movement of the tongue that draws liquid out of the breast or bottle. But when solid foods are introduced with a spoon, this tongue movement (the extrusion reflex), causes the baby to push most of the food back out of the mouth. The extrusion reflex begins to lessen around 4 to 5 months of age.

Another factor is muscle development. To minimize the risk for choking, the infant must have gained muscular control of the head and neck and must be able to sit up (with or without support).

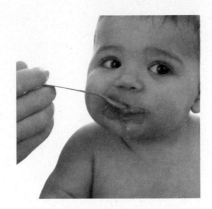

The extrusion reflex will push solid food out of an infant's mouth.

Still another part of being ready for solid foods is sufficient maturity of the digestive and urinary systems. Infants can digest and absorb lactose from birth; however, the ability to digest starch does not fully develop until the age of 3 to 4 months. If an infant is fed cereal, for example, before he or she can digest the starch, diarrhea and discomfort may develop. In addition, early introduction of solid foods can lead to improper absorption of intact, undigested proteins, setting the stage for allergies. Finally, the kidneys must have matured, so that they are better able to process nitrogen wastes from proteins and concentrate urine.

The need for solid foods is also related to nutrient needs. At about 6 months of age, infant iron stores become depleted; thus, puréed meats or iron-fortified infant cereals are often the first foods introduced. Rice cereal rarely provokes an allergic response and is easy to digest. If all goes well after a few days with the first food, another single-grain cereal (other than wheat, which is highly allergenic) or a vitamin C–rich strained vegetable or fruit can be introduced.

Commercial baby foods are convenient and are typically made without added salt; some are made only with organic ingredients. Dessert items and dinner-type foods are not recommended, because they contain added sugars and starches. Parents can use an inexpensive food grinder to prepare homemade baby foods that are inexpensive and reflect the cultural diversity of the family.

Throughout the first year, solid foods should only supplement, not substitute for, breast milk or iron-fortified formula. Infants still need the nutrient density and energy that breast milk and formula provide.

The following foods should never be offered to an infant:

- *Foods that could cause choking.* Foods such as grapes, raisins, hot dogs, cheese sticks, nuts, popcorn, and hard candies cannot be chewed adequately by infants and can cause choking.
- *Corn syrup and honey.* These may contain spores of the bacterium *Clostridium botulinum*. These spores can germinate and grow into active bacteria in the immature GI tract of infants, where they produce a potent toxin that can, in severe cases, be fatal. Children older than 1 year can safely consume these substances, however, because the beneficial bacteria in their GI tract has reached levels sufficient to competitively inhibit any *C. botulinum* bacteria.
- *Goat's milk.* Goat's milk is notoriously low in many nutrients that infants need, such as folate, vitamin C, vitamin D, and iron.
- *Cow's milk.* For children under 1 year, cow's milk is too concentrated in minerals and protein and contains too few carbohydrates to meet infant energy needs. Infants can begin to consume whole cow's milk after the age of 1 year. Infants and toddlers should not be given reduced-fat cow's milk before the age of 2 years, as it does not contain enough fat and is too high in mineral content for the kidneys to handle effectively. Infants should not be given evaporated milk or sweetened condensed milk.
- *Large quantities of fruit juices.* Fruit juices are poorly absorbed in the infant GI tract, causing diarrhea if consumed in excess. Large quantities of fruit juice can make an infant feel full and reject breast milk or formula at feeding time, reducing intake of essential nutrients. Many fruit juices are also high in sugar. Breast milk, infant formula, and plain water will effectively quench an infant's thirst.

- *Too much salt and sugar.* Infant foods should not be seasoned with salt or other seasonings or sweetened. Cookies, cakes, and other excessively sweet, processed foods also should be avoided.
- *Too much breast milk or formula.* As nutritious as breast milk and formula are, once infants reach the age of 6 months, solid foods should be introduced gradually. Six months of age is a critical time, as that is when a baby's iron stores begin to be depleted. In addition, infants are physically and psychologically ready to incorporate solid foods at this time, and solid foods can help appease their increasing appetites. Between 6 months and the time of weaning (from breast or bottle), solid foods should gradually make up an increasing proportion of the infant's diet. Overreliance on breast milk or formula, to the exclusion or displacement of iron-rich foods, can result in a condition known as *milk anemia.*

Some Infants Develop Disorders or Distress Related to Food and Feeding

Many foods have the potential to stimulate an allergic reaction or gastrointestinal distress. Feedings can also be frustrating for parents if the child is not growing properly, develops anemia, or has feeding challenges.

Allergies

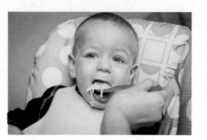

Early introduction of solid foods may play a role in the development of food allergies, especially if infants are introduced to highly allergenic foods early on.

Breastfeeding reduces the risk for allergy development, as does delaying the introduction of solid foods until the age of 6 months. One of the most common allergies in infants is to the proteins in cow's milk–based formulas. Egg whites, peanuts, soy, and wheat are other common triggers to allergic reactions. Every food should be introduced in isolation, so that any allergic reaction can be identified and the particular food avoided.

Symptoms of an allergic reaction vary but may include gastrointestinal distress such as diarrhea or vomiting, rashes or hives, runny nose or sneezing, or even difficulty breathing. Peanut allergy is the leading cause of fatal food reactions in a pediatric population. While many infants who are allergic to cow's milk, wheat, soy, and eggs develop a tolerance for them, very few infants allergic to peanuts are able to outgrow the allergy.[59]

Colic

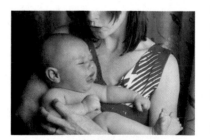

Colicky babies will cry for no apparent reason, even if they otherwise appear well nourished and happy.

Perhaps nothing is more frustrating to new parents than the relentless crying spells of some infants, typically referred to as **colic.** In this condition, newborns and young infants who appear happy, healthy, and well nourished suddenly begin to cry or even shriek and continue no matter what their caregiver does to console them. The spells tend to occur at the same time of day, typically late in the afternoon or early in the evening, and often occur daily for a period of several weeks. Crying may last for hours at a time. Overstimulation of the nervous system, feeding too rapidly, swallowing of air, and intestinal gas pain are considered possible culprits, but the precise cause is unknown.

As with allergies, if a colicky infant is breastfed, breastfeeding should be continued, but the mother should try to determine whether eating certain foods seems to prompt crying and, if so, eliminate the offending food(s) from her diet. Avoidance of spicy or other strongly flavored foods may also help. Formula-fed infants may benefit from a change in type of formula. In the worst cases of colic, a physician may prescribe medication. Fortunately, most cases disappear spontaneously, possibly because of maturity of the GI tract, around 3 months of age.

Gastroesophageal Reflux

colic A condition of unconsolable infant crying of unknown origin that can last for hours at a time.

The regurgitation, or reflux, of stomach contents into the esophagus often results in the all too familiar "spitting up" of young infants. Particularly common in preterm infants, gastroesophageal reflux occurs in about 3% of newborns. Typically, as the GI tract matures within the first 12 months of life, this condition resolves. Caretakers should avoid overfeeding the infant, keep the infant upright after each feeding, and watch for choking or gagging.

Failure to Thrive

At times, seemingly healthy infants reach an inappropriate plateau or decline in their growth. Pediatric healthcare providers describe **failure to thrive (FTT)** as a condition in which, in the absence of disease or physical abnormalities, the infant's weight or weight-for-height is below the 3rd percentile, or the infant has fallen more than two percentile lines on the NCHS growth charts after a previously stable pattern of growth. Acute malnutrition often results in *wasting*, or low weight-for-height, and chronic malnutrition typically produces growth *stunting*, in which the child has low height-for-age.

Psychosocial factors that increase the risk for FTT include poverty, inadequate knowledge, extreme nutritional beliefs, social isolation, domestic violence, and/or substance abuse. If not corrected in a timely manner, FTT may result in developmental, motor, and cognitive delays typically associated with infants in developing nations.

Anemia

As previously noted, full-term infants are born with sufficient iron stores to last for approximately the first 6 months of life. In older infants and toddlers, however, iron is the mineral most likely to be deficient. Iron-deficiency anemia causes pallor, lethargy, and impaired growth. Iron-fortified formula is a good source for formula-fed infants. Some pediatricians prescribe a supplement containing iron especially formulated for infants. Iron for older infants is typically supplied by iron-fortified rice cereal or puréed meats. Overconsumption of cow's milk remains a common cause of anemia among U.S. infants and children.

Dehydration

Whether the cause is diarrhea, vomiting, prolonged fever, or inadequate fluid intake, dehydration is extremely dangerous to infants and if left untreated can quickly result in death. (The factors behind infants' increased risk for dehydration were discussed earlier in this chapter on page 689.) Treatment includes providing fluids, a task that is difficult if vomiting is occurring. In some cases, the physician may recommend giving a pediatric electrolyte product (beverage or frozen pop), readily available at most grocery and drug stores, on a temporary basis. In more severe cases, hospitalization may be necessary. If possible, breastfeeding should continue throughout an illness. A physician or other healthcare provider should be consulted on decisions related to the use of formula and solid foods.

Feeding Challenges in Special Populations

Feeding problems are common among children born with physical abnormalities such as *cleft lip* or *cleft palate* (**Figure 17.12,** page 696), infants with genetic or inborn errors of metabolism, and those with developmental delays. In many cases, occupational and speech therapists, registered dietitians, and other health professionals provide the family with the necessary skills and knowledge to ensure the nutritional health and well-being of their children.

While most infants born with cleft lip alone have few feeding problems, babies born with cleft palate can't create enough suction to withdraw milk from the breast or bottle. Specialized bottles and nipples are available that can provide the infant with formula or breast milk that has been expressed. While there is no firm consensus, many doctors consider the best age range to surgically repair cleft palate to be between approximately 5 and 15 months of age, or earlier. Cleft lip and cleft palate often occur together.

failure to thrive (FTT) A condition in which an infant's weight gain and growth are far below typical levels for age and previous patterns of growth, for reasons that are unclear or unexplained.

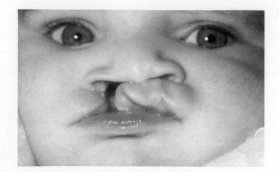

FIGURE 17.12 This baby has a condition known as unilateral cleft lip, also sometimes called *hare lip*. Cleft lip results from failure of the tissues of a fetus's face and mouth to fuse properly during the second and third months of pregnancy. Cleft lip is closely related to the condition of cleft palate, and the two often occur together.

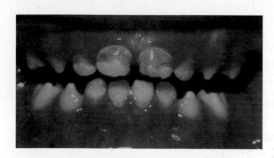

FIGURE 17.13 Leaving a baby alone with a bottle can result in the tooth decay of nursing bottle syndrome.

Infants with inborn errors of metabolism may have neuromuscular disorders that decrease their muscular strength, endurance, and coordination and contribute to a slow pace of feeding, difficulty swallowing and/or chewing, and poor head control. Some infants with developmental delays demonstrate poor lip closure, abnormal gag reflex, tongue thrust, or hypersensitivity to temperature or texture. Each infant requires careful evaluation by a pediatric dietitian and feeding team to develop an individualized feeding plan.

Nursing Bottle Syndrome

Infants should never be left alone with a bottle, whether lying down or sitting up. As infants manipulate the nipple of the bottle, the high-carbohydrate fluid (whether breast milk, formula, or fruit juice) drips out, coming into prolonged contact with the developing teeth. This high-carbohydrate fluid provides an optimal food source for the bacteria that are the underlying cause of dental caries (cavities). Severe tooth decay can result (**Figure 17.13**). Encouraging the use of a cup around the age of 8 months helps prevent nursing bottle syndrome, as does weaning the baby from a bottle entirely by the age of 15 to 18 months. In addition, infants' gum tissue and emerging teeth should be gently cleaned with a wash cloth to minimize bacterial growth and increase acceptance of a toothbrush when introduced.

Lead Poisoning

Lead is especially toxic to infants and children, because their brains and central nervous systems are still developing. Lead poisoning can result in decreased mental capacity, behavioral problems, anemia, impaired growth, impaired hearing, and other problems. Unfortunately, lead in old pipes and lead paint can still be found in older homes and buildings. Measures to reduce lead exposure include the following:

- Allowing tap water to run for a minute or so before use, to clear the pipes of any lead-contaminated water
- Using only cold tap water for drinking, cooking, and infant formula preparation, as hot tap water is more likely to leach lead
- Professionally removing lead-based paint or painting it over with latex paint

RECAP

Solid foods can gradually be introduced into an infant's diet at 4 to 6 months of age, beginning with puréed meats or iron-fortified rice cereal (or other nonwheat cereals), then moving to single-item vegetables and fruits. Parents should carefully select and prepare the foods to be given to their infants, avoiding those that represent a choking hazard and limiting high-sugar foods and beverages. Solid foods expand the infant's exposure to tastes and textures and represent an important developmental milestone. Risk for food allergies can be reduced by delaying the introduction of solid foods until the infant is at least 6 months of age. Infants with colic or gastroesophageal reflux present special challenges, but both conditions generally improve over time. Infants who present with failure to thrive require close monitoring by healthcare providers, as do infants experiencing anemia or dehydration. Anemia is easily prevented through the use of iron-fortified formulas and cereals. Families need the support and guidance of healthcare professionals when feeding infants with birth defects, metabolic disorders, or developmental delays. Nursing bottle syndrome is characterized by dental caries in infants left lying down or sitting up with a bottle containing any carbohydrate-containing fluid. Lead poisoning can result in cognitive, behavioral, and other problems. ■

Nutrition
Myth OR Fact?

The Fetal Environment: Does it Leave a Lasting Impression?

Would you be surprised to learn that your risk of developing obesity and certain chronic diseases as an adult might have been influenced by what happened even before you were born? Research suggests that the fetal environment, including the mother's nutritional status, influences the risks for obesity and chronic diseases later in life. This relationship is often described as the "fetal origins of adult disease" (FOAD) hypothesis.

How Does Fetal Exposure to Famine Influence Adult Health?

Some of the earliest research into the fetal origins theory investigated the health of adults born during or shortly after the 1944 Netherlands famine. During World War II, the Dutch population had been relatively well nourished until October 1944, when the Germans embargoed all food transport. At the same time, an unusually early and harsh winter set in. As a result, a severe famine hit the western Netherlands and energy intakes were as low as 500 kcal/day. In May 1945, with the liberation of the country, food supplies were restored and dietary intake rapidly normalized. Luckily for scientists, the Dutch maintained an excellent system of healthcare records, providing important data on pregnancy outcomes and the health of the offspring over the next 60 years. Similar data have been collected and analyzed for the offspring of families subjected to the German invasion of the British Channel Islands and the subsequent famine conditions in 1944–1945[1] and survivors of the famine that affected much of China's population from 1959 through 1961.[2]

Not surprisingly, among these diverse populations, exposure to famine lowered maternal weight gains and infant birth weights. What was surprising, however, was the long-term impact of the famine as the babies progressed through adulthood.[3] Specifically, exposure to famine resulted in a much higher risk among the offspring for obesity, coronary heart disease, HTN, metabolic syndrome, and abnormal serum lipid profile during adulthood.[3,4] The consequences of fetal exposure to malnutrition, and childhood starvation, are often lifelong.

Why, you might wonder, would low pregnancy weight gain and low birth weight lead to an increased risk for obesity and other diseases some 50 years later? While there are many theories, most relate to a process referred to as *fetal adaptation*.[4] This occurs when a fetus is exposed to a harmful environment, such as maternal starvation or malnutrition, and goes into survival mode. Hormone production and enzyme activity shift in favor of energy storage, and the size and functioning of organs such as the liver, kidneys, and pancreas are affected. There may even be changes in the activation—and thus the expression—of certain genes. Although these adaptations help the fetus survive the harmful prenatal environment, they may contribute to the development of chronic diseases over the life span.

The results of other "natural experiments" suggest that the effects of the prenatal environment on adult health depend heavily on the precise circumstances. For example, Leningrad (now St. Petersburg) was under siege by the Germans during World War II for over 2½ years, and as a result the population experienced starvation. And yet, adults who were born during this period did not have the same increased disease risks as found in those exposed, *in utero*, to the Dutch famine.[5] How could this be, since the Leningrad babies were exposed to conditions far worse than those experienced by the Dutch babies? Researchers theorize that the impact of fetal exposure to malnutrition is actually worsened if followed by high nutrient intakes and rapid weight gain shortly after birth.[5] This was a key difference between the Netherlands and Leningrad famines: once the Dutch embargo was lifted, the population returned to a nourishing, adequate diet. This allowed the underweight infants to experience rapid weight gain and catch-up growth during their first year of life (**Figure 17.14**, page 698). In contrast, the Leningrad infants who survived into adulthood may have continued to be underfed throughout infancy and even into toddlerhood. Rapid catch-up growth in the postnatal period is associated with severe increases in blood pressure and other chronic diseases during adulthood.

More recently, people born during weather- and war-related famines in Africa and other parts of the world have provided researchers with additional information on the impact of the fetal environment on adult health/disease outcomes. Researchers in Israel are pressing for a similar evaluation of the adult health outcomes of children born during or surviving the famines of the Holocaust.[6]

In addition to famine, deficiencies of specific micronutrients may have long-term consequences.[7] For example, evidence suggests that poor maternal intake of calcium increases risk for HTN in adult offspring. Moreover, poor maternal folate status has been linked

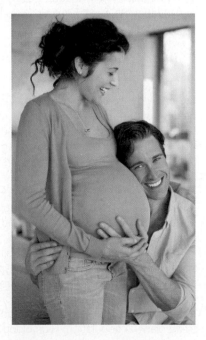

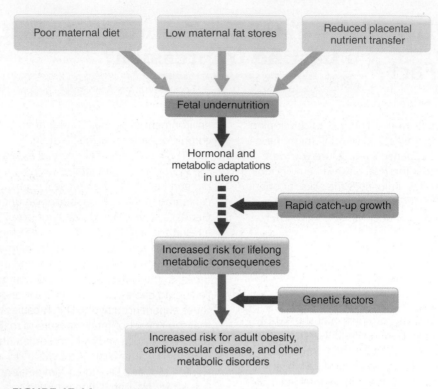

FIGURE 17.14 Fetal adaptation to undernutrition can lead to a variety of diseases in childhood and throughout adulthood.

not only to neural tube defects in the newborn, but also to early signs of atherosclerosis and increased mortality. The offspring of women with low prenatal vitamin B_{12} and high folate status demonstrated greater insulin resistance and higher abdominal fat as early as 6 years of age, putting them at higher risk for type 2 diabetes later in life. Low vitamin D status in pregnant women led to reduced bone density in their children.[8] Research with rats has revealed other links between micronutrient deficiencies and adult health.[7] Thus, fetal stressors that influence adult health include not only starvation and inadequate energy but also specific micronutrient deficiencies.

Could Exposure to Excessive Nutrients Also Be Harmful?

Strong evidence also links maternal dietary excesses to poor health outcomes in adult offspring. Maternal obesity has been linked to an increased risk for childhood and adult obesity[9,10] and to changes in the "programming" of the fetal brain, resulting in altered feeding behaviors. Maternal obesity is also linked to a higher risk for birth defects, many of which have lifelong implications for health.[11] Population studies have also reported an association between high birth weight, common in infants born to obese women, and an increased risk for breast cancer in adulthood.

Maternal diabetes and its high-glucose environment has been shown to increase the risk for type 2 diabetes, overweight, excess adiposity, and metabolic syndrome in adult offspring.[4,12–14] Children of diabetic women are up to eight times more likely to develop type 2 diabetes or pre-diabetes as adults compared to the general population. High blood levels of triglycerides,

abdominal obesity, and hypertension are other examples of adult-onset disorders associated with maternal diabetes.

Prenatal exposure to excessive levels of certain individual nutrients may also have lifelong implications. A high maternal intake of *trans* and/or saturated fatty acids, for example, is associated with increased risk for CVD, HTN, and type 2 diabetes in the offspring.[15] Scientists are also investigating the possible effects of high maternal intake of sodium on risk for hypertension in adult offspring. In short, research suggests that there are lifelong consequences to any type of nutrient imbalance during pregnancy, including total energy deficit, single nutrient deficiency, or energy or nutrient excess.

What About Alcohol, Tobacco, and Other Toxic Agents?

You've already learned of the lifelong impact of fetal alcohol syndrome, resulting from exposure to high maternal blood alcohol levels. In addition, maternal smoking has been shown to negatively impact the long-term health of the offspring, increasing their risk for congenital heart defects, childhood allergies and respiratory diseases, adult-onset hypertension, childhood behavioral problems, and cleft lip and palate.[16,17]

We've discussed lead exposure during infancy, but maternal exposure to lead is also harmful, increasing the risk for preterm birth and reduced birth weight, head circumference, and length.[18] Prenatal lead exposure also increases the risk for developmental delays, behavioral and learning problems, and hearing loss.[19] Maternal exposure to mercury can result in irreversible damage to the baby's nervous system, as well as hearing and vision problems.[20]

What's the Bottom Line?

If your mother experienced some type of nutritional, metabolic, or environmental stress during pregnancy, you certainly are not doomed to suffer from one or more of the health problems mentioned here. That's because most research reports on large groups of people, not individuals. Moreover, it calculates increases in risk for—or susceptibility to—certain conditions, but it does not and cannot predict health outcomes for individuals.

Any type of fetal programming that develops as a result of the fetal environment is just one factor in your personal wellness. A much more significant influence is your own lifestyle, especially your personal food choices, dietary patterns, activity habits, alcohol intake, and smoking.

Critical Thinking Questions

■ In most states, pregnant women can be arrested for child abuse if, at the time of their delivery, they are found to have cocaine, heroin, or other illegal drugs in their system. Do you think similar laws should be enacted for pregnant women with alcohol or nicotine in their blood? Why or why not?

■ If you were a member of a women's healthcare team, would you advise an obese client to avoid known pregnancy risks by deferring pregnancy until she was able to bring her weight and blood glucose level down to a recommended range? Why or why not? If you went forward with the advice, how would you present it?

References

1. Ellison, G. T. H. The health in later life of channel islanders exposed to the 1940–1945 occupation and Siege. In: Humney, L. H., and A. Vaiserman, eds. *Early Life Nutrition and Adult Health and Development.* Hauppauge, NY: Nova Publishers Inc; 2013.
2. Li, Y., Y. He, L. Qi, V. W. Jaddoe, E. J. Feskens, X. Yang, G. Ma, and F. B. Hu. 2010. Exposure to the Chinese famine in early life and the risk of hyperglycemia and type 2 diabetes in adulthood. *Diabetes* 59:2400–2406.
3. Lumey, L. H., and F. W. A. van Poppel. 2013. The Dutch Famine of 1944–1945 as a human laboratory: changes in the early life environment and adult health. In: Humney, L. H., and A. Vaiserman, eds. *Early Life Nutrition and Adult Health and Development.* Hauppauge, NY: Nova Publishers Inc; 2013.
4. Langley-Evans, S. C. 2015. Nutrition in early life and the programming of adult disease: a review. *J Human Nutrition and Dietetics* 28(Suppl 1): 1–14.
5. Stanner, S. A., and J. S. Yudkin. 2001. Fetal programming and the Leningrad siege study. *Twin Research* 4: 287–292.
6. Keinan-Boker, L. 2014. "The mothers have eaten unripe grapes and the children's teeth are set on edge": the potential inter-generational effects of the Holocaust on chronic morbidity in Holocaust survivors' offspring. *Israel J Health Policy Research* 3: 11–17.
7. Vanhees, K., I. G. C. Vonhögen, F. J. van Schooten, and R. W. L. Godschalk. 2014. You are what you eat, and so are your children: the impact of micronutrients on the epigenetic programming of offspring. *Cell Mol Life Sci* 71: 271–285.
8. Javaid, M. K., S. R. Crozier, N. C. Harvey, C. R. Gale, E. M. Dennison, B. J. Boucher,…, and Princess Anne Hospital Study Group. 2006. Maternal vitamin D status during pregnancy and childhood bone mass at age 9 years: a longitudinal study. *Lancet* 367(9504): 36–43.
9. Keane, E., R. Layte, J. Harrington, P. M. Kearney, and U. Perry. 2012. Measured parental weight status and familial socio-economic status correlates with childhood overweight and obesity at age 9. *PLoS One* 7:e43503.
10. Schellong, K., S. Schuylz, T. Harder, and A. Plagemann. 2012. Birth weight and long-term overweight risk: systematic review and meta-analysis including 643,902 persons from 66 studies and 26 countries globally. *PLoS One* 7:e47776.
11. Weedn, A. E., B. S. Mosley, M. A. Cleves, D. K. Waller, M. A. Canfield, A. Correa, C. A. Hobbs, and the National Birth Defects Prevention Study. 2014. Maternal reporting of prenatal ultrasounds among women in the National Birth Defects Prevention Study. *Birth Defects Research (Part A)* 100: 4–12,
12. Van Kijk, S. J., P. L. Malloy, H. Varinln, J. L. Morrison, B. S. Muhlhausler, and members of EpiSCOPE. 2015. Epigenetics and human obesity. *International J Obesity* 39: 85–97.
13. Garcia-Vargas, L., S. S. Addison, R. Nistala, D. Kurukulasuriya, and J. R. Sowers. 2012. Gestational diabetes and the offspring: implications in the development of the cardiorenal metabolic syndrome in offspring. *Cardiorenal Med.* 2: 134–142.
14. Nielsen, G. L., C. Dethlefsen, S. Lundbye-Christensen, J. F. Pedersen, L. Mølsted-Pedersen, and M. W. Gillman. 2012. Adiposity in 277 young adult male offspring of women with diabetes compared with controls: a Danish population-based cohort study. *Acta Obstetricia et Gynecologica Scandinavica* 91: 838–843.
15. Mennitti, L. V., J. L. Oliveira, C. A. Morais, D. Estadella, L. M. Oyama, C. M. Oller do Nascimento, and L. P. Pisani. 2015. Type of fatty acids in maternal diets during pregnancy and/or lactation and metabolic consequences of the offspring. *J Nutr Biochem* 26: 99–111.
16. Sullivan, P. M., L. A. Dervan, S. Reiger, S. Buddhe, and S. M. Schwartz. 2015. Risk of congenital heart defects in the offspring of smoking: a population-based study. *J Pediatrics* 166: 801–804.
17. Dixon, M. J., M. L. Marazita, T. H. Beaty, and J. C. Murray. 2011. Cleft lip and palate: understanding genetic and environmental influences. *Nature Reviews: Genetics.* 12: 167–178.
18. Taylor, C. M. J. Golding, and A. M. Emond. 2015. Adverse effects of maternal lead levels on birth outcomes in the ALSPAC study: a prospective birth cohort study. *BJOG: An International Journal of Obstetrics & Gynaecology* 122: 322–328.
19. March of Dimes. 2014. Your Baby's Environment: Lead and your baby. Available at http://www.marchofdimes.org/baby/lead-and-your-baby.aspx. Accessed May 2015.
20. March of Dimes. 2014. Staying safe: mercury and pregnancy. Available at http://www.marchofdimes.org/pregnancy/mercury.aspx. Accessed May 2015.

STUDY **PLAN** MasteringNutrition™

Customize your study plan—and master your nutrition!—in the Study Area of MasteringNutrition.

summary

Scan to hear an MP3 Chapter Review in **MasteringNutrition.**

LO 1 ■ A healthful diet is important before conception, the point at which a woman's ovum is fertilized by a man's sperm, for four reasons: First, it can build nutrient stores and prevent deficiency during the early weeks of pregnancy, when critical stages of cell division, tissue differentiation, and organ development occur. For example, adequate intake of maternal folate supports complete closure of the embryonic neural tube. Second, maintaining a healthful diet establishes a practice of limiting the intake of substances such as caffeine that can be harmful to the fetus, as well as teratogenic substances such as alcohol and illicit drugs. Third, a healthful diet and regular physical activity help a woman achieve and maintain a body mass index between 19.8 and 26.0, which is considered optimal prior to pregnancy. Fourth, it can help

prevent the development of nutrition-related disorders of pregnancy.

■ Preconception nutrition is also important to men. Certain micronutrients help maintain sperm health and motility, and obesity and substance abuse both reduce male fertility.

LO 2 ■ A plentiful, nourishing diet is important throughout pregnancy to provide the nutrients needed to support fetal development without depriving the mother of nutrients she needs to maintain her own health.

■ A normal pregnancy progresses over the course of 38 to 42 weeks. This time is divided into three trimesters of 13 to 14 weeks. Each trimester is associated with particular developmental phases of the embryo/fetus.

■ Over the first 8 weeks of pregnancy, the zygote divides repeatedly to form an embryo, the tissues of which form and fold into a primitive, tubelike structure with limb buds, organs, and facial features. The embryo is most vulnerable to teratogens as well as nutrient deficiencies (especially folate deficiency) during this time. The second and third trimesters are characterized by growth of the fetus, and increased energy intake is essential to support this growth.

LO 3 ■ Pregnant women of normal weight should consume adequate energy to gain 25 to 35 lb during pregnancy. Women who are underweight should gain slightly more, and women who are overweight or obese should gain less.

■ Gaining too little weight during pregnancy increases the risk for a preterm or low-birth-weight baby. Gaining too much weight increases the risk for a baby that is large for gestational age, as well as the risk that the mother will be unable to lose the weight and will develop a type 2 diabetes or hypertension.

LO 4 ■ During the second and third trimesters of pregnancy, the woman needs to consume an average of 350 to 450 additional kcal/day. Protein needs increase to 1.1 g/kg of body weight, which averages about 25 g additional protein per day. A carbohydrate intake of at least 175 g/day is important because glucose is the primary metabolic fuel of the developing fetus. Fat intake recommendations do not change during pregnancy. Unsaturated fatty acids are healthful sources of energy and help build new cells and tissues; DHA is important for fetal brain and eye development, and can be obtained from fatty fish, chicken, and DHA-enhanced eggs.

■ Pregnant women need to be especially careful to consume adequate amounts of folate, vitamin B$_{12}$, vitamin C, vitamin D, calcium, iron, and zinc. An iron supplement is commonly prescribed, as is a multivitamin/mineral prenatal supplement, to ensure adequate intake of these nutrients. Supplemental vitamin A should be avoided because excessive preformed vitamin A can be teratogenic.

■ Fluid requirements during pregnancy increase to about 2.3 liters (about 10 cups) of beverages, including water, daily to support the increased maternal blood volume and amniotic fluid.

LO 5 ■ Many pregnant women experience nausea and/or vomiting during pregnancy, and many crave or feel aversions to specific types of foods and nonfood substances.

■ Gastroesophageal reflux and constipation in pregnancy are related to the relaxation of smooth muscle caused by certain pregnancy-related hormones.

■ Gestational diabetes and gestational hypertension are nutrition-related disorders that can seriously affect maternal and fetal health. Preeclampsia is gestational hypertension accompanied by edema, weight gain, and protein in the urine. It can progress to life-threatening eclampsia if not effectively managed.

■ Listeriosis is a potentially fatal foodborne illness of particular concern during pregnancy, when the immune system response against the bacterium is less effective. Pregnant women should avoid unpasteurized milk and soft cheeses made with unpasteurized milk, as well as cold cuts, refrigerated smoked salmon, and several other foods.

■ The bodies of adolescents are still growing and developing; thus, their nutrient needs during pregnancy are higher than those of older pregnant women. Pregnancy after age 35 carries certain risks, such as an increased prevalence of gestational diabetes, hypertension, twins, and triplets; however, the majority of older women have healthy pregnancies and healthy babies.

■ A carefully planned vegetarian or vegan diet is safe for pregnant women; however, supplemental iron, zinc, calcium, and certain vitamins are typically prescribed.

LO 6 ■ Exercise is safe and healthful for most pregnant women. Regular exercise helps prevent excessive weight gain, reduces the risk for gestational diabetes and hypertension, improves mood, energy, and muscle tone, and shortens the duration of labor.

■ Caffeine intake during pregnancy may increase the risk of stillbirth, miscarriage, preterm birth, and low birth weight. Intake should be limited to below 100 mg/day, an amount in no more than one cup of coffee. Some artificial sweeteners are safe, but others should be limited or avoided.

■ Alcohol, tobacco, and illicit drugs are harmful to the developing fetus and should not be used in any amount during pregnancy. Alcohol is a known teratogen and smoking exposes the fetus to toxins and reduces fetal blood flow and therefore delivery of oxygen and nutrients. Pregnant women should discuss with their healthcare provider any prescription and over-the-counter medications and dietary supplements they are taking or plan to take.

LO 7 ■ Successful breastfeeding requires the coordination of several hormones, including estrogen, progesterone, prolactin, and oxytocin. These hormones govern the preparation of the breasts, as well as actual milk production and the let-down response.

- The first fluid secreted from the breasts in late pregnancy and immediately after childbirth is colostrum, which is rich in immune factors and protein. Mature milk production begins about 2 to 4 days after birth and is sustained by infant suckling.

- Breastfeeding women require more energy than they needed during pregnancy. Protein and carbohydrate needs increase, as do requirements for several micronutrients and fluid. Intake of DHA continues to be essential to support the newborn's developing brain. An overall nutritious diet with plentiful fluids is important in maintaining milk quality and quantity, as well as preserving the mother's health.

LO 8 - Breast milk is nutritionally superior to infant formula. The amount and types of protein are easily digested in the infant's immature GI tract, and boost the infant's absorption of iron. The amounts and types of carbohydrates and fats, including DHA and ARA, are ideally suited to the infant's needs. The ratio of fat and water changes within a single feeding, initially satisfying an infant's thirst and then satisfying hunger. Breast milk also supplies micronutrients. Overall, it is entirely sufficient to sustain an infant for the first 6 months of life.

- Breast milk also provides immune factors that protect the infant from infections and allergies, and infants who exclusively breastfeed are protected from exposure to contaminants and residues in baby bottles and in packages of formula. Women who breastfeed may find it easier to lose the weight they gained in pregnancy, and ovulation is delayed, giving their body time to recover before another pregnancy. Breastfeeding also promotes maternal-infant bonding, is convenient, and has a much lower cost than formula feeding.

- Breastfeeding exclusively for the first 6 months of a baby's life is recommended by North American and international healthcare organizations. Women are also encouraged to continue breastfeeding for at least the next 6 months, and into the second year if acceptable to the family.

- Challenges that might be encountered with breastfeeding include the effect of medications on breast milk, and contamination of the mother's milk with substances such as caffeine, alcohol, nicotine, illicit drugs, and toxins in the environment. In addition, women who are HIV-positive may transmit HIV to their breastfeeding infant, and obesity may reduce a mother's milk supply as well as her comfort with breastfeeding.

- Mothers may also face scheduling conflicts and other challenges when they return to work, and have social concerns about breastfeeding in public.

LO 9 - Infants are characterized by their extremely rapid growth—about 10 inches in length and tripling in weight—and brain development, which is more rapid during the first year than at any other time.

- Physicians use length and weight measurements as the main tools for assessing an infant's nutritional status.

- Infants need to consume about 40 to 50 kcal/lb of body weight per day. In addition to this high energy requirement, the immaturity of their GI tract and kidneys and their overall small size make their nutritional needs unique. About 40% to 50% of an infant's energy intake should come from fat, and no more than 20% from protein. The rest should be carbohydrate. Intake of the fatty acids AA and DHA is important to support growth and development of the nervous system, including the brain itself and the retina of the eyes.

- Micronutrient needs can largely be met through breast milk or infant formula; however, all infants are given an injection of vitamin K after birth; breast-fed infants are typically prescribed a vitamin D supplement, and iron after 6 months of age. Fluoride is sometimes prescribed after 6 months of age, and breast-fed babies of vegan mothers may need supplemental vitamin B_{12}. Infants lose more body fluid through evaporation, and their kidneys are immature and unable to concentrate urine; thus, they have an increased risk for dehydration. They need about 2 oz of fluid per pound of body weight, and either breast milk or formula is almost always adequate in providing this amount. Most infant formulas are based on cow's milk that has been modified and fortified to produce a fluid with a nutritional profile as close as possible to that of breast milk.

LO 10 - Breast milk or formula is entirely sufficient for the first 6 months of life. Solid food should not be introduced until the extrusion reflex begins to lessen, around 4 to 5 months of age, the infant has gained muscular control of the head and neck and the ability to sit upright, and the digestive and urinary systems have matured. After that, solid foods can be introduced (for example, puréed meat or rice cereal fortified with iron) and expanded gradually, with breast milk or formula remaining very important throughout the first year.

- Infants should never be offered foods that could cause choking, either corn syrup or honey, goat's milk, cow's milk, large quantities of fruit juice, or sweets or salty foods.

- Infants need to be monitored carefully for appropriate growth, a marker of nutrient adequacy, and daily for appropriate number of wet diapers to assess hydration.

- Nutrition-related concerns arise for infants as they are gradually introduced to solid foods. Risk for food allergies can be reduced by delaying the introduction of solid foods until the infant is at least 6 months of age. Infants with colic

or gastroesophageal reflux present special challenges, but both conditions generally improve over time. Infants who present with failure to thrive require close monitoring by healthcare providers, as do infants experiencing anemia or dehydration. Anemia is easily prevented by feeding iron-fortified formulas and cereals, strained meats, or supplements, but dehydration may result from an infectious disease and may require feeding with a special electrolyte solution or hospitalization. Infants with special medical needs such as cleft lip or palate benefit from the support of a pediatric dietitian and other feeding professionals. To avoid nursing bottle syndrome, infants should not be left alone with a bottle. Exposure to lead, a neurotoxin, must be avoided.

To further your understanding, go online and apply what you've learned to real-life case studies that will help you master the content!

review questions

LO 1 **1.** Folate deficiency in the first weeks after conception has been linked with an increased risk for which of the following problems in the newborn?

a. FASD
b. neural tube defects
c. large for gestational age
d. all of the above

LO 2 **2.** The period of pregnancy during which Calorie needs are highest to support fetal growth is

a. the embryonic period (conception through week 8).
b. the first 5 weeks of the fetal period (weeks 9 through 13).
c. the second trimester.
d. the third trimester.

LO 3 **3.** A pregnancy weight gain of 28 to 40 lb is recommended for

a. all women.
b. women who begin their pregnancy underweight.
c. women who begin their pregnancy at a normal weight.
d. women who begin their pregnancy overweight or obese.

LO 4 **4.** The RDA for pregnant women is increased over the RDA for nonpregnant women for

a. protein
b. vitamin D
c. calcium
d. all of the above

LO 5 **5.** Preeclampsia is

a. likely to be diagnosed in a pregnant woman with high blood pressure but no other signs or symptoms.
b. a medical emergency characterized by seizures and kidney failure.
c. more common in overweight and obese women compared to women of normal weight.
d. managed by exercise and a reduced Calorie diet.

LO 6 **6.** Which of the following is considered safe for most pregnant women?

a. exercise
b. drinking no more than two cups of brewed coffee a day
c. using the artificial sweetener saccharin in moderation
d. none of the above

LO 7 **7.** Which of the following hormones is responsible for the let-down response?

a. progesterone
b. estrogen
c. oxytocin
d. prolactin

LO 8 **8.** Which of the following is an advantage of breastfeeding?

a. Breastfeeding boosts fertility.
b. Breast milk provides all of the nourishment an infant needs for the first year of life.
c. Breastfeeding can help the mother more easily lose the weight she gained during pregnancy.
d. All of the above are advantages of breastfeeding.

LO 9 9. Which of the following nutrients should be added to the diet of breast-fed infants when they are around 6 months of age?
   a. the fatty acids AA and DHA
   b. vitamin K
   c. vitamin D
   d. iron

LO 10 10. Which of the following would be the most appropriate food to offer an infant who is 9 months old?
   a. Cream of Wheat cereal
   b. whole cow's milk
   c. small fruits such as grapes and raisins
   d. puréed peas

true or false?

LO 2 11. **True or false?** Exposure to teratogens and nutrient deficiencies is most likely to cause developmental errors and birth defects when it occurs during the third trimester of pregnancy.

LO 5 12. **True or false?** If gestational diabetes is not well controlled, the fetus may not receive enough glucose and is at high risk for low birth weight.

LO 6 13. **True or false?** Alcohol easily passes from the mother's bloodstream into fetal blood and, in breastfeeding women, into the breast milk.

LO 7 14. **True or false?** Infant suckling is a critical component of successful and continued lactation.

LO 9 15. **True or false?** Growth is a key indicator of adequate infant nutrition.

short answer

LO 4 16. Your cousin, who is pregnant with her first child, tells you that her physician prescribed supplemental iron tablets for her but that she decided not to take them. "You know me," she says, "I'm a natural food nut! I'm absolutely certain that my careful diet is providing all the nutrients my baby needs!" Is it possible that your cousin is partly right and partly wrong? Explain.

LO 5 17. You are a registered dietitian in a public health clinic. A pregnant 15-year-old is referred to you for nutrition-related counseling and services. Identify at least three topics that you would discuss with this client.

LO 8 18. Identify five advantages and five disadvantages of breastfeeding. Can you think of others?

LO 9 19. You are on a picnic with your sister at a park, who drapes a shawl over her shoulders and breastfeeds her 11-month-old son. A woman walking by stops and says, "Isn't that child getting too old for that?" What information could you share with the woman in response to her question?

LO 10 20. You visit your neighbors one afternoon to congratulate them on the birth of their daughter, Katie. While you are there, 2-week-old Katie suddenly starts crying as if she is in terrible pain. "Oh, no," Katie's dad says to his wife. "Here we go again!" He turns to you and explains, "She's been like this every afternoon for the past week, and it goes on until sunset. I just wish we could figure out what we're doing wrong." What would you say?

Math Review

LO 9 21. Mature breast milk averages about 700 kcal per liter, with 35 g of fat and 9 g of protein. Calculate the % of kcal from fat and protein. How do these values compare to those recommended for a healthy young adult? Why are the nutrient proportions of breast milk appropriate for infants?

Answers to Review Questions and Math Review can be found online in the MasteringNutrition Study Area.

web links

www.aap.org
American Academy of Pediatrics
Visit this website for information on infants' and children's health. Clinical information as well as guidelines for parents and caregivers can be found. Searches can be performed for topics such as "neural tube defects" and "infant formulas."

www.choosemyplate.gov/pregnancy-breastfeeding
ChooseMyPlate Plans for Pregnant and Breastfeeding Women
This website is designed for pregnant and breastfeeding women and provides meal plans that can be personalized to address the needs of women who are pregnant or breastfeeding.

www.fnic.nal.usda.gov
Food and Nutrition Information Center of the USDA
Click on "Lifecycle Nutrition." This page provides links to topics on pregnancy, breastfeeding, and infant nutrition.

www.marchofdimes.com
March of Dimes
Click on "Pregnancy" and "Baby" to find links on nutrition during pregnancy, breastfeeding, and baby care.

www.llli.org
La Leche League
This site provides information about breastfeeding; search or browse to find multiple articles on the health effects of breastfeeding for mother and infant.

www.nofas.org
National Organization on Fetal Alcohol Syndrome
This site provides news and information relating to fetal alcohol syndrome.

www.helppregnantsmokersquit.org
National Partnership to Help Pregnant Smokers Quit
This is a site created to educate healthcare providers and smokers about the dangers of smoking while pregnant and to provide tools to help pregnant smokers quit.

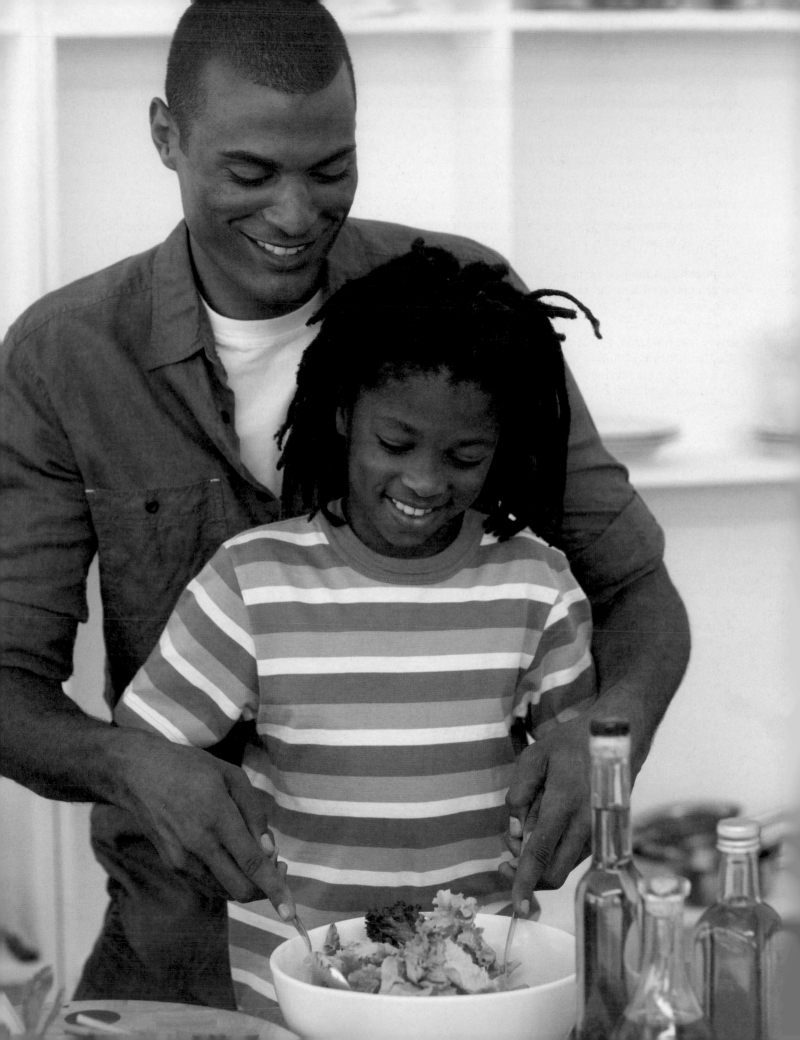

18 Nutrition Through the Life Cycle: Childhood and Adolescence

Learning Outcomes

After studying this chapter, you should be able to:

1 Describe the key nutrient needs of toddlers, *pp. 708–711.*

2 Discuss strategies for encouraging toddlers to eat nutritious foods and the suitability of vegetarian diets for toddlers, *pp. 712–715.*

3 Identify the growth and activity patterns and specific nutrient needs of preschool and school-age children, *pp. 715–719.*

4 Discuss food choices, food insecurity, and other nutritional concerns affecting children, *pp. 719–721.*

5 Explain how school attendance and school lunch programs affect children's nutrition and health, *pp. 721–724.*

6 Describe the key nutrient needs of adolescents, taking into account their psychosocial development and growth and activity patterns, *pp. 724–726.*

7 Discuss food choices, disordered eating patterns, and other nutritional concerns affecting adolescents, *pp. 726–729.*

8 Describe the health problems associated with pediatric obesity and the etiology of the problem, *pp. 729–731.*

9 Discuss the dietary and activity options for preventing childhood obesity, including the roles of the family and school, *pp. 731–732.*

10 Identify a range of options for treating moderate and severe obesity in children, *pp. 732–735.*

TEST YOURSELF

True or False?

1 After their first birthday, all children should be fed nonfat milk products to reduce their risk for obesity. **T** *or* **F**

2 The nutrient needs of boys do not differ from those of girls for the first 8 or 9 years of life. **T** *or* **F**

3 Millions of American children live in households without a dependable supply of food. **T** *or* **F**

4 Adolescents experience an average 10% to 15% increase in height during the pubertal years. **T** *or* **F**

5 More than 5 out of every 100 U.S. children and youth aged 2 to 19 years is severely obese. **T** *or* **F**

Test Yourself answers are located in the Study Plan.

MasteringNutrition™

Go online for chapter quizzes, pre-tests, interactive activities, and more!

Christina is a happy 7-year-old who loves school, her kitten, and TV. According to her mother, Christina never "grew out" of her baby fat and, because she is often teased by other children, rarely goes outside to play. Her school's 30-minute physical education classes twice a week provide the only real exercise Christina gets. Six weeks ago, at the start of the school year, the school nurse sent home a note explaining that Christina's weight and height ratio indicated she is obese. Following up on the nurse's advice, Christina and her mom visited a local clinic specializing in pediatrics and found out that Christina has hypertension, high triglycerides, high total and LDL cholesterol, low HDL cholesterol, and type 2 diabetes. "How can my baby have diabetes?" asked her mom. "My dad didn't get it until he was almost 60 years old and I didn't get it until I was 42." Unfortunately, Christina is one of a growing number of children under the age of 10 who are diagnosed with what used to be regarded as adult diseases. Why are more and more children developing these diseases at such young ages? How can families, healthcare providers, school personnel, and society as a whole work together to improve the health of America's children?

This chapter will help answer these and related questions. Although most topics are discussed within specific age groupings (toddlers, children, and adolescents), the chapter closes with an in-depth review of pediatric obesity, which affects children of all ages.

LO 1 Describe the key nutrient needs of toddlers.

What Are a Toddler's Nutrient Needs?

When babies celebrate their first birthday, they transition out of infancy and into the active world of toddlers. Personality and behavioral changes introduce potential conflict into mealtimes, and parents who have been accustomed to making all decisions about their baby's diet must now begin to consider the child's preferences, while still ensuring they retain responsibility for their child's health and well-being. In addition, toddlers attending day care may be exposed to foods that are more or less nutritious than the foods served at home. These and other circumstances sometimes make it challenging to meet a toddler's nutrient needs.

As Activity Expands, More Energy Is Needed

The rapid growth rate of infancy begins to slow during toddlerhood, the second and third years of life. A toddler will grow a total of about 5.5 to 7.5 inches and gain an average of 9 to 11 pounds. Toddlers expend more energy in order to fuel their increasing levels of activity as they explore their expanding world and develop new skills. They progress from taking a few wobbly steps to running, jumping, and climbing with confidence, and they begin to dress, feed, and toilet themselves. Thus, their diet should provide an appropriate quantity and quality of nutrients to fuel their growth and activity. Refer to **Table 18.1** for specific nutrient recommendations.

Although the energy requirement per kilogram of body weight for toddlers is just slightly less than for infants, total energy requirements are higher because toddlers are larger and much more active than infants. The estimated energy requirement (EER) varies according to a toddler's age, body weight, and level of activity.

Although there is currently insufficient evidence available to set a recommended daily allowance (RDA) for fat for toddlers, healthy toddlers of appropriate body weight need to consume 30% to 40% of their total daily energy intake as fat.[1] That's because fat provides a concentrated source of energy in a relatively small amount of food, and this is important for toddlers, especially those who are fussy eaters or have little appetite. Fats, especially the unsaturated fatty acids AA and DHA, remain necessary during the toddler years to support the continuously developing nervous system.

Toddlers' protein needs increase modestly, because they weigh more than infants and are still growing rapidly. The RDA for protein for toddlers is 1.1 g/kg body weight per day,

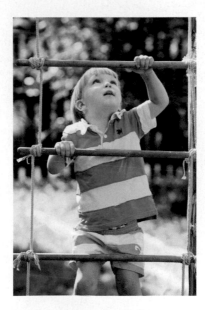

Toddlers expend significant amounts of energy actively exploring their world.

TABLE 18.1 Nutrient Recommendations for Children and Adolescents

Nutrient	Children Age 1–3 Years	Children Age 4–8 Years	Children Age 9–13 Years	Adolescents Age 14–18 Years
Fat	No RDA	No RDA	No RDA	No RDA
Protein	1.10 g/kg body weight per day	0.95 g/kg body weight per day	0.95 g/kg body weight per day	0.85 g/kg body weight per day
Carbohydrate	130 g/day	130 g/day	130 g/day	130 g/day
Vitamin A	300 µg/day	400 µg/day	600 µg/day	Boys = 900 µg/day Girls = 700 µg/day
Vitamin C	15 mg/day	25 mg/day	45 mg/day	Boys = 75 mg/day Girls = 65 mg/day
Vitamin E	6 mg/day	7 mg/day	11 mg/day	15 mg/day
Calcium	500 mg/day	800 mg/day	1,300 mg/day	1,300 mg/day
Iron	7 mg/day	10 mg/day	8 mg/day	Boys = 11 mg/day Girls = 15 mg/day
Zinc	3 mg/day	5 mg/day	8 mg/day	Boys = 11 mg/day Girls = 9 mg/day
Fluid	1.3 L/day	1.7 L/day	Boys = 2.4 L/day Girls = 2.1 L/day	Boys = 3.3 L/day Girls = 2.3 L/day

or approximately 13 g of protein daily.[1] Recall that two cups of milk alone provide 16 g of protein; thus, most toddlers have little trouble meeting their protein needs.

The RDA for carbohydrate for toddlers is 130 g/day, and carbohydrate intake should be about 45% to 65% of total energy intake.[1] As is the case for older children and adults, most of the carbohydrates eaten should be complex, and refined carbohydrates from high-fat/high-energy foods, such as cookies and candy, should be kept to a minimum. Fruits and 100% fruit juices are nutritious sources of simple carbohydrates that can also be included in a toddler's diet. Keep in mind, however, that too much fruit juice can displace other foods and nutrients and can cause diarrhea. If consumed at bedtime or between meals, the sugars in fruit juice may also contribute to tooth decay. The American Academy of Pediatrics (AAP) recommends that the intake of fruit juice be limited to 4 to 6 fl. oz per day for children 1 to 6 years of age.[2]

Adequate fiber is important for toddlers to maintain regularity. The adequate intake (AI) is 14 g of fiber per 1,000 kcal of energy, or, based on the average energy intake of this age group, 19 g/day.[1] Unfortunately, dietary fiber intake is inadequate in most U.S. children.[3] Whole-grain cereals, fresh fruits and vegetables, and whole-grain breads are healthful choices for toddlers' meals and snacks. Too much fiber, however, can inhibit the absorption of several nutrients, such as iron and zinc; harm toddlers' small digestive tracts; and cause them to feel too full to consume adequate nutrients.

Determining the macronutrient requirements of toddlers can be challenging. See the **You Do the Math** box (page 710) for analysis of the macronutrient levels in one toddler's daily diet.

Toddlers' Micronutrient Needs Increase

As toddlers grow, their micronutrient needs increase. Of particular concern with toddlers are adequate intakes of the micronutrients associated with fruits and vegetables. In addition, vitamin D, calcium, and iron have been identified as "priority nutrients" for children aged 2 to 4 years.

Vitamin D intake, which often decreases in toddlers, is closely linked to milk consumption. The American Academy of Pediatrics recommends vitamin D supplements for

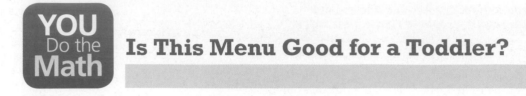

Is This Menu Good for a Toddler?

A dedicated mother and father want to provide the best nutrition for their young son, Ethan, who is now 18 months old and has just been completely weaned from breast milk. Ethan weighs about 26 lb (11.8 kg). Following is a typical day's menu for Ethan. Grams of protein, fat, and carbohydrate are given for each food. The day's total energy intake is 1,168 kcal. Calculate the percentage of Ethan's Calories that come from protein, fat, and carbohydrate (numbers may not add up to exactly 100% because of rounding). Where are Ethan's parents doing well, and where could they use some advice for improvement?

Meal	Foods	Protein (g)	Fat (g)	Carbo-hydrate (g)
Breakfast	Oatmeal (½ cup, cooked)	2.5	1.5	13.5
	Brown sugar (1 tsp.)	0	0	4
	Milk (1%, 4 fl. oz)	4	1.25	5.5
	Grape juice (4 fl. oz)	0	0	20
Midmorning Snack	Banana slices (1 small banana)	0	0	16
	Yogurt (nonfat fruit-flavored, 3 fl. oz)	5.5	0	15.5
	Orange juice (4 fl. oz)	1	0	13
Lunch	Whole-wheat bread (1 slice)	1.5	0.5	10
	Peanut butter (1 tbsp.)	4	8	3.5
	Strawberry jam (1 tbsp.)	0	0	13
	Carrots (cooked, 1/8 cup)	0	0	2
	Applesauce (sweetened, ¼ cup)	0	0	12
	Milk (1%, 4 fl. oz)	4	1.25	5.5
Afternoon Snack	Bagel (½)	3	1	20
	American cheese product (1 slice)	3	5	1
	Water	0	0	0
Dinner	Scrambled egg (1)	11	5	1
	Baby food spinach (3 oz)	2	0.5	5.5
	Whole-wheat toast (1 slice)	1.5	0.5	10
	Mandarin orange slices (¼ cup)	0.5	0	10
	Milk (1%, 4 fl. oz)	4	1.25	5.5

Note: This activity focuses on the macronutrients. It does not ask you to consider Ethan's intake of micronutrients or fluids.

There is a total of 47.5 g protein in Ethan's menu:

47.5 g × 4 kcal/g = 190 kcal

190 kcal protein/1,168 total kcal × 100 = 16% protein

There is a total of 25.75 g fat in Ethan's menu:

25.75 g × 9 kcal/g = 232 kcal

232 kcal fat/1,168 total kcal × 100 = 20% fat

There is a total of 186.5 g carbohydrate in Ethan's menu:

186.5 g × 4 cal/g = 746 kcal

746 kcal carbohydrate/1,168 total kcal × 100

= 64% carbohydrate

Ethan's parents are doing very well at offering a wide range of foods from various food groups; they are especially doing well with fruits and vegetables. Also, according to his EER, Ethan requires about 970 kcal/day, and he is consuming 1,168 kcal/day, thus meeting his energy needs.

Ethan's total carbohydrate intake for the day is 186.5 g, which is higher than the RDA of 130 g per day; however, this value falls within the recommended 45% to 65% of total energy intake that should come from carbohydrates. Thus, high carbohydrate intake is adequate to meet his energy needs.

However, Ethan is being offered far more than enough protein. The DRI for protein for toddlers is about 13 g per day, and Ethan is being offered more than three times that much!

It is also readily apparent that Ethan is being offered too little fat for his age. Toddlers need at least 30% to 40% of their total energy intake from fat, and Ethan is only consuming about 20% of his Calories from fat. He should be drinking whole milk, not 1% milk. He should occasionally be offered higher-fat foods, such as cheese for his snacks or macaroni and cheese for a meal. Yogurt is a healthful choice, but it shouldn't be nonfat at Ethan's age.

In conclusion, Ethan's parents should be commended for offering a variety of nutritious foods but should be counseled that a little more fat is critical for toddlers' growth and development. Some of the energy currently being consumed as protein and carbohydrate should be shifted to fat.

all children who consume less than 1 liter of vitamin D–fortified dairy products each day—a group that includes the majority of U.S. children.[4] Vitamin D–fortified soy milk and other milk alternatives, in adequate amounts, are also acceptable.

Calcium is necessary to promote optimal bone mass through early adulthood. For toddlers 1 to 3 years, the RDA for calcium is 700 mg/day.[5] Dairy products are excellent sources of calcium. When a child reaches the age of 1 year, whole cow's milk can be given; however, reduced-fat milk (2% or less) should *not* be given until age 2. If dairy products are not feasible, calcium-fortified orange juice and milk alternatives can supply calcium, or children's calcium supplements can be given. Toddlers generally cannot consume enough food to be able to depend on alternate calcium sources, such as dark-green vegetables.

Iron-deficiency anemia is the most common nutrient deficiency in young children in the United States and around the world. Iron-deficiency anemia can affect a child's energy level, attention span, and ability to learn. The RDA for iron for toddlers is 7 mg/day.[6] Good sources of well-absorbed heme iron include lean meats, fish, and poultry; nonheme iron is provided by egg yolks, legumes, greens, and fortified foods such as breakfast cereals. When toddlers consume nonheme sources of iron, such as beans or greens, a rich source of vitamin C at the same meal will enhance the absorption of iron from these sources.

Toddlers can be well nourished by consuming a balanced, varied diet. But given their typically erratic eating habits, the child's healthcare provider may recommend a multivitamin/multimineral supplement as a precaution against deficiencies. The toddler's physician or dentist may also prescribe a fluoride supplement if the community water supply is not fluoridated. Supplements should also be considered for children in vegan families, children from families who cannot afford adequate amounts of nourishing foods, children with certain medical conditions or dietary restrictions, and very picky or erratic eaters.

As with other age groups, many children between the ages of 2 and 5 years use supplements, with little risk of excessive intakes.[8] As always, if a supplement is given, it should be formulated especially for toddlers and the recommended dose should not be exceeded. A supplement should not contain more than 100% of the Daily Value of any nutrient per dose.

Adequate Fluid Is Critical

Toddlers lose less fluid from evaporation than infants, and their more mature kidneys are able to concentrate urine, conserving the body's fluid. However, as toddlers become active, they start to lose significant fluid through sweat, especially in hot weather. Parents need to make sure an active toddler is drinking adequately. The recommended fluid intake for toddlers is listed in Table 18.1 and includes about 4 cups as beverages, including water.[7] Suggested beverages include plain water, milk, calcium-fortified beverages. In addition, children should consume a variety of nutritious foods high in water content, such as vegetables and fruits.

RECAP

Between their first and third birthdays, toddlers gain an average of 9 to 11 pounds and become much more active. Their energy requirement varies with age, body weight, and level of activity. Toddlers should consume 30% to 40% of their total daily energy intake as fat. Until age 2, they should drink whole milk, not reduced-fat milk. The RDA for protein for toddlers is 1.1 g/kg body weight per day, and the RDA for carbohydrates is 130 g/day. The AI for fiber for toddlers is 14 g per 1,000 kcal of energy, an intake level most toddlers do not achieve. Priority micronutrients for toddlers are vitamin D, calcium, and iron. Milk, yogurt, cheese, and many milk alternatives provide vitamin D and calcium. Toddlers need 7 mg of iron daily. Toddlers eating a healthful diet do not need supplements; however, any supplement given should be formulated for toddlers. An average intake of about four cups of water and other beverages is essential. ■

What Are Some Common Nutrition-Related Concerns of Toddlerhood?

LO 2 Discuss strategies for encouraging toddlers to eat nutritious foods and the suitability of vegetarian diets for toddlers.

Parents of toddlers are commonly concerned about their child's food preferences and eating behaviors. However, offering a range of developmentally appropriate, nutritious, and fun-food choices and introducing new foods gradually can help.

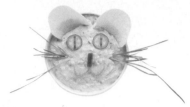

Most toddlers are delighted by food prepared in a "fun" way.

Food Choices Should Be Appropriate, Nutritious, and Fun

Parents and pediatricians have long known that toddlers tend to be choosy about what they eat. Some avoid entire foods groups, such as all meats or vegetables. Others refuse all but one or two favorite foods (such as peanut butter on crackers) for several days or longer. Still others eat in extremely small amounts, seemingly satisfied by a single slice of apple or two bites of toast. These behaviors frustrate and worry many parents, but in fact, as long as a variety of healthful food is available, most normal-weight toddlers are able to match their food intake with their needs. A toddler will most likely make up for one day's nutrient or energy deficiency later in the week. Food should never be "forced" on a child, as doing so sets the stage for eating and control issues later in life.

Toddlers' stomachs are still very small, and they cannot consume all of the energy they need in three meals. They need small meals, interspersed with nutritious snacks, every 2 to 3 hours. A successful technique is to create a snack tray filled with small portions of nutritious food choices, such as one-third of a banana, a few small strips of cheese, and two whole-grain crackers, and leave it within reach of the child's play area. The child can then "graze" on these healthful foods while he or she plays. Limiting their food alternatives can also be effective in helping toddlers eat nutritiously. For example, parents can say, "It's snack time! Would you like apples and cheese, or bananas and yogurt?"

Even at mealtime, portion sizes should be small. One tablespoon of a food for each year of age constitutes a serving throughout the toddler and preschool years (**Figure 18.1**). Realistic portion sizes can give toddlers a sense of accomplishment when they "eat it all up" and reduce parents' fears that their child is not eating enough.

Foods prepared for toddlers should be developmentally appropriate. Nuts, cubed cheese, raw carrots, grapes, raisins, and cherry tomatoes are difficult for a toddler to chew and pose a choking hazard. Foods should be soft and sliced into strips or wedges that are easy for children to grasp. As a child develops more teeth and becomes more coordinated, the foods offered can become more varied.

Foods prepared for toddlers should also be fun. Parents can use cookie cutters to turn a peanut-butter sandwich into a pumpkin face, or arrange cooked peas or carrot slices to create a smiling face on top of mashed potatoes. Juice and yogurt can be frozen into popsicles or blended into milkshakes.

Though certainly not necessary, several food companies now market "toddler foods" geared specifically to their developmental stage. The **_Nutrition Label Activity_** provides the opportunity to compare labeling practices for toddler and adult foods.

FIGURE 18.1 Portion sizes for toddlers and preschoolers are much smaller than for older children. Use the following guideline: 1 tablespoon of the food for each year of age equals one serving. For example, the meal shown here—2 tablespoons of brown rice, 2 tablespoons of soft, mashed beans, and 2 tablespoons of chopped tomatoes—is appropriate for a 2-year-old toddler.

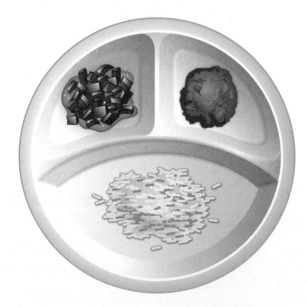

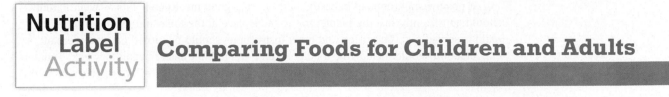

Comparing Foods for Children and Adults

Parents who purchase packaged foods for their toddlers often check the label for information on the food's ingredients and nutrient values. Many of these parents may not realize that the FDA and USDA have specific label requirements for products made for children under age 2; for example, the Nutrition Facts panel cannot list the amount of saturated fat or cholesterol, or the Calories from fat. This is to avoid the impression that fat is bad for young children.

Compare the Nutrition Facts panels of the "chicken noodle dinner" for children under age 2 and the adult chicken noodle meal (**Figure 18.2**). What other differences do you see between the two? Compare the ingredient lists. What are the most

prevalent ingredients in each food? Does the toddler food contain any of the food additives listed in the adult product? Why do you believe there is a difference? Also, how do the serving sizes and age-appropriate Daily Values compare?

You should also be aware that foods for children under 2 years of age cannot be labeled with nutrient claims ("low-fat") or health claims that often appear on food labels. Labels of foods for children under the age of 2 years are, however, allowed to make statements such as "Provides 100% of the Daily Value for vitamin C." They can also describe the product as *unsweetened* or *unsalted*, because those terms describe taste features more than nutrient value.

Nutrition Facts

Serving Size	1 Pack
Servings Per Container	

Amount Per Serving	
Calories	70
Total Fat	2.5g
Trans Fat	0g
Sodium	45mg
Potassium	130mg
Total Carbohydrate	9g
Dietary Fiber	1g
Sugars 2g	3g
Protein	2g

% Daily Value (DV)	
Protein	9 %
Vitamin A	170 % (100% from beta carotene)
Vitamin C	0 %
Calcium	2 %
Iron	2 %

INGREDIENTS: CARROTS, WATER, PEAS, COOKED ENRICHED EGG NOODLES (WATER, [DURUM WHEAT FLOUR, EGGS, NIACIN, FERROUS SULFATE, THIAMIN MONONITRATE, RIBOFLAVIN, FOLIC ACID]), GROUND CHICKEN, WHOLE GRAIN BROWN RICE FLOUR, CANOLA OIL, ONION POWDER.

(a)

Nutrition Facts

Serving Size 2/3 cup mix (60g) Makes 1 cup prepared
Servings Per Container 2

Amount Per Serving	**Mix**	**Prepared as Directed**
Calories	220	260
Calories from Fat	30	80

	% Daily Value**	
Total Fat 3.5g*	**5%**	**13%**
Saturated Fat 1g	**4%**	**10%**
Trans Fat 0g		
Cholesterol 50mg	**17%**	**17%**
Sodium 860mg	**36%**	**38%**
Total Carbohydrate 40mg	**13%**	**13%**
Dietary Fiber 2g	**6%**	**6%**
Sugars 2g		
Protein 8g		

Vitamin A	6%	10%
Vitamin C	10%	10%
Calcium	2%	2%
Iron	10%	10%
Thiamin	30%	30%
Riboflavin	15%	15%
Niacin	15%	15%
Folate	25%	25%

*Amount in Mix. 1/2 tbsp. of margarine add 40 calories, 5g fat (1g saturated), and 50mg sodium.

**Percent Daily Values are based on a 2,000 calorie diet. Your daily values may be higher or lower depending on your calorie needs.

	Calories:	2,000	2,500
Total Fat	Less than	65g	80g
Sat. Fat	Less than	20g	25g
Cholesterol	Less than	300mg	300mg
Sodium	Less than	2,400mg	2,400mg
Total Carbohydrate		300g	375g
Dietary Fiber		25g	30g

INGREDIENTS: ENRICHED EGG NOODLES (WHEAT FLOUR, EGGS, NIACIN, FERROUS SULFATE, THIAMIN MONONITRATE, RIBOFLAVIN, FOLIC ACID), CORN STARCH, SALT, CORN SYRUP*, ONION*, MALTODEXTRIN, CHICKEN FAT*, CHICKEN BROTH*, NATURAL FLAVORS, HYDROLYZED PROTEIN (SOY, CORN), AUTOLYZED YEAST EXTRACT, BELL PEPPER*, GARLIC*, PARTIALLY HYDROGENATED SOYBEAN OIL, PARSLEY*, SPICES (INCLUDING PAPRIKA), XANTHAN AND GUAR GUMS, GUM ARABIC, WHEY, SODIUM CASEINATE, DISODIUM PHOSPHATE, DISODIUM INOSINATE, DISODIUM GUANYLATE, ANNATTO AND OLEORESIN TURMERIC (FOR COLOR).
*DEHYDRATED
CONTAINS: EGG, WHEAT, SOY, MILK

(b)

FIGURE 18.2 Label guidelines for foods targeting children under the age of 2 differ from the guidelines for foods for older children and adults. **(a)** Label from "chicken noodle dinner" for children under age 2. **(b)** Label from a chicken noodle meal for older children and adults.

A positive environment helps toddlers develop good mealtime habits as well. Parents should consistently seat the toddler in the same place at the table and make sure that the child is served first. Television and other distractions should be turned off, and pleasant conversation should include the toddler, even if the toddler hasn't begun to speak. Toddlers should not be forced to sit still until they finish every bite, as they still have short attention spans.

Introduce New Foods Gradually

New foods should be introduced gradually throughout toddlerhood. As during infancy, wheat, peanuts, cow's milk, soy, citrus, egg whites, and seafood remain common food allergens. New foods should be presented one at a time, and the toddler should be monitored for allergic reactions for a week before another new food is introduced. To prevent the development of food allergies, even foods that are established in the diet should be rotated rather than served every day.

Most toddlers are leery of new foods, spicy foods, hot (temperature) foods, mixed foods such as casseroles, and foods with strange textures. A helpful rule is to encourage the child to eat at least one bite of a new food: if the child does not want the rest, nothing negative should be said, and the child should be praised just for the willingness to try. The same food should be reintroduced a few weeks later. Eventually, after as many as 10–15 attempts, the child might accept the food. Some foods, however, won't be accepted until well into adulthood as tastes expand and develop. Parents should never bribe with food—for example, promising dessert if the child finishes her squash. Bribing teaches children that food can be used to reward and manipulate. Instead, parents should try to positively reinforce good behaviors—for example, "Wow! You ate every bite of your squash! That's going to help you grow big and strong!"

Role modeling is important because toddlers mimic older children and adults: if they see their parents enjoying a variety of healthful foods, toddlers will be likely to do so as well. Adults have a significant impact on the nutritional quality of their children's choices.[9]

Finally, toddlers are more likely to eat food they help prepare. Encourage them to assist in the preparation of simple foods, such as helping to pour a bowl of cereal, stir yogurt, or arrange raw vegetables on a plate.

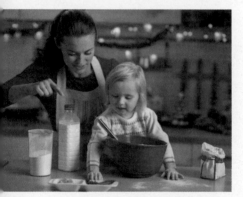

Parents are important role models for toddlers.

Vegetarian Diets Should Be Planned with Care

Lacto-ovo-vegetarian diets, in which eggs and dairy foods are included, are increasingly popular and can be as wholesome as an omnivorous diet.[10] However, because meat, poultry, and fish are important sources of zinc and heme iron, the most bioavailable form of iron, vegetarian families must be careful to include enough zinc and iron from other sources in their child's diet and maximize the absorbability of those minerals through use of leavened whole grains and addition of vitamin C rich foods and beverages at meals.[11]

In contrast, a vegan diet, in which no foods of animal origin are consumed, poses several potential nutritional risks for toddlers:

- *Protein*: Vegan diets can be too low in protein for toddlers, who need protein for growth and increasing activity. Few toddlers can consume enough legumes and whole grains to provide sufficient protein. The high-fiber content of these foods quickly produces a sense of fullness for the toddler, decreasing total food intake.
- *Calcium, iron, and zinc*: Calcium is a concern because of the avoidance in a vegan diet of milk, yogurt, and cheese. Many milk alternatives are fortified with calcium, but supplementation may be advised. Iron and zinc are also commonly low in vegan diets, as just discussed, and may need to be provided by fortified cereals, legumes, and possibly supplements.[11]

- *Vitamins D and B$_{12}$*: Both vitamins are typically lower in vegan diets. Some cereals and milk alternatives are now fortified with these vitamins; however, some toddlers may still need supplements.
- *Fiber*: Vegan diets often contain a higher amount of fiber than is recommended for toddlers, resulting in lowered absorption of iron and zinc, as well as a premature sense of fullness or satiety at mealtimes.

Although the practice of feeding a vegan diet to infants and young children is somewhat controversial, vegan children demonstrate appropriate growth, comparable with that of nonvegetarian children.[12] With proper planning, parents can successfully provide a healthful vegan diet.

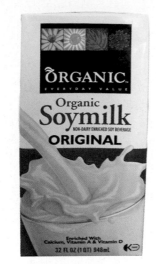

Enriched and fortified foods, such as fortified soy milk, provide important nutrient supplementation that should be included in vegan diets given to toddlers.

RECAP

Toddlers' eating behaviors are erratic and their stomachs small, so small portions of nutritious foods, offered frequently, are appropriate. Firm foods that could present a choking hazard must be avoided. New foods should be introduced one at a time, and parents should continue to monitor for allergic reactions. If the child refuses a new food, parents should not respond negatively but should offer it again at a later date. When possible, food should be prepared in a fun way, and distractions such as television should be avoided at mealtimes. Role modeling by parents, access to ample healthful foods, and participation in meal preparation can help toddlers make nutritious choices. Vegan diets can be a safe and healthful for toddlers if parents are knowledgeable and carefully plan meals that avoid potential deficiencies of calcium, iron, zinc, vitamin D, and vitamin B$_{12}$. ■

What Are a Child's Nutrient Needs?

LO 3 Identify the growth and activity patterns and specific nutrient needs of preschool and school-age children.

Children develop increased language fluency, improved decision-making skills, and greater physical coordination and dexterity as they progress through the preschool and school-age years. The nutrient requirements and nutrition issues of importance to children are discussed in this section.

Childhood Growth and Activity Boosts Energy-Nutrient Needs

Total energy requirements continue to increase throughout childhood because of increasing body size. Children at this stage of development experience a slow and steady rate of growth, averaging 2 to 4 inches per year, until the rapid growth of adolescence begins.

Activity levels among children vary dramatically—some love sports, dance, and other physical activity, whereas some prefer quieter activities, such as reading and drawing. Television, computer use, and electronic games often tempt children into a sedentary lifestyle. All children can be encouraged to have fun using their muscles in various ways that suit their interests. Activity-based interactive DVD games can be an excellent option for children who must remain indoors for extended periods of time.

The EER varies according to a child's age, body weight, and level of activity.[1] Parents should provide diets that support normal growth and appropriate physical activity while minimizing risk for excess weight gain.

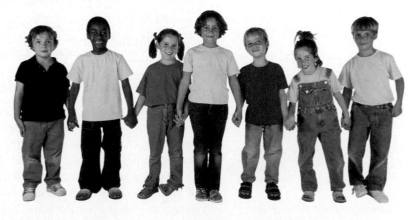

School-age children grow an average of 2 to 3 inches per year.

Three-year-olds have the same set of nutrient recommendations that apply to toddlers (see Table 18.1). From age 4 through 8, the values for most nutrients increase. Until age 9, the nutrient needs of young boys do not differ significantly from those of girls; because of this, the DRI values for macronutrients, fiber, and micronutrients are grouped together for boys and girls aged 4 to 8 years. The onset of sexual maturation, however, has a dramatic effect on the nutrient needs of children. Boys' and girls' bodies develop differently in response to gender-specific hormones. Because the process of sexual maturation begins subtly between the ages of 8 and 9, the DRI values are separately defined for boys and girls beginning at age 9[1,5–7] (see Table 18.1).

Fat

Although dietary fat remains a key macronutrient in the preschool years, as a child ages, total fat should gradually be reduced to a level closer to that of an adult, around 25% to 35% of total energy.[1] One easy way to start reducing dietary fat is to limit intake of fried foods, high-fat protein sources such as hot dogs, baked goods, and high-fat snacks. This is also a good time to transition to lower-fat dairy products, such as 2% or 1% milk, low-fat yogurt, and low-fat mozzarella cheese sticks. A diet providing fewer than 25% of Calories from fat is not recommended for children, as they are still growing, developing, and maturing. In fact, unless a child is overweight or has specific health concerns, parents should avoid putting too much emphasis on fat restriction during this age span. Impressionable and peer-influenced children may be prone to categorizing foods as "good" or "bad." This may lead to skewed views of food and inappropriate dietary restrictions.

Carbohydrate

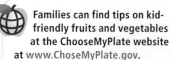

Families can find tips on kid-friendly fruits and vegetables at the ChooseMyPlate website at www.ChoseMyPlate.gov.

The RDA for carbohydrate for children is 130 g/day, which is about 45% to 65% of total daily energy intake.[1] Complex carbohydrates from whole grains, fruits, vegetables, and legumes should be emphasized. Simple sugars should come from fruits and 100% fruit juices, with foods high in refined sugars, such as cakes, cookies, and candies, saved for occasional indulgences. The AI for fiber for children is 14 g/1,000 kcal, which can be met by the consumption of fresh fruits, vegetables, legumes, and whole grains.[1] As is the case with toddlers, too much fiber can be detrimental, because it can make a child feel full and can interfere with adequate food intake and lower the absorption of certain nutrients, such as iron and zinc.

Protein

Total need for protein (shown in Table 18.1) increases for children because of their larger size, even though their growth rate has slowed. The RDA for protein is 0.95 g/kg body weight per day.[1] This protein requirement is easily met by portions such as one chicken drumstick and two glasses of milk or ½ cup of pinto beans, 1 oz of cheese, and half a peanut butter sandwich. Lean meats, poultry, fish, lower-fat dairy products, soy-based foods, and legumes are nutritious sources of protein that can be provided to children of all ages.

Micronutrient Recommendations for Children Increase

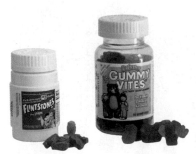

Children's multivitamins often appear in shapes or bright colors.

The need for most micronutrients increases slightly for children up to age 8 because of their increasing size. A sharper increase occurs during the transition years approaching adolescence; this increase is due to the impending adolescent growth spurt and the early phases of sexual maturation. Children who fail to consume the recommended amount of fruits and vegetables each day may become deficient in vitamins A, C, and E. Offering fruits and fresh vegetables as snacks as well as during mealtimes can increase intakes of these vitamins as well as fiber and potassium, two priority nutrients found lacking in the diets of low-income children.

The RDA for calcium is 1,000 mg/day for children aged 4 to 8 years and 1,300 mg/day for children aged 9 to 13 years.[5] Because peak bone mass is achieved in the late teens or early 20, childhood and adolescence are critical times to ensure adequate deposition of bone tissue. Inadequate calcium intake during childhood and adolescence leads to poor bone health and potentially osteoporosis in later years. Milk, yogurt, cheese, fortified milk alternatives, and fortified fruit juices are child-friendly and convenient sources of calcium. However, nearly 60% of U.S. children consume fewer than two servings of dairy per day.[13] This low intake is related to "milk displacement," when children stop drinking milk in favor of soda, punch, energy drinks, and sport drinks. As a result of lower milk/dairy intakes, children's diets are lower in calcium, protein, vitamin D, and magnesium.

The RDAs for children aged 4 to 8 years for iron and zinc increase slightly to 10 mg/day and 5 mg/day, respectively.[6] The RDA for iron drops to 8 mg/day for boys and girls aged 9 to 13 years. These recommendations are based on the assumption that most girls do not begin menstruation until after age 13.[6] Mild-flavored, tender cuts of meat and poultry are readily accepted by most children, and legumes offer a fiber-rich, fat-free alternative that will also add iron and zinc to the diet. Refer again to Table 18.1 for a review of the micronutrient needs of children.

If there is any concern that a child's nutrient needs are not being met for any reason, such as missed meals or inadequate family resources, age-specific vitamin and mineral supplements may help correct any deficit. Fluoride supplements, for example, if not available through a municipal water supply, may be needed to deter the development of dental caries, which develop when bacteria in the mouth feed on carbohydrates deposited on teeth. As a result of metabolizing the carbohydrates, the bacteria secrete acids that begin to erode tooth enamel, leading to tooth decay. Dental caries can also be prevented by limiting between-meal sweets, especially jelly beans, caramels, and others that stick to teeth. Frequent brushing helps eliminate the sugars on teeth, as well as the bacteria that feed on them.

Children Need Five to Eight Cups of Fluid per Day

The fluid recommendations for children are summarized in Table 18.1 and average about five to eight cups of beverages per day, including water.[7] The exact amount of fluid needed varies according to the child's level of physical activity and weather conditions. At this point in their lives, children are mostly in control of their own fluid intake. However, as they become more active during school, in sports, and while playing, young children in particular may need reminders to drink in order to stay properly hydrated, especially if the weather is hot.

Most, if not all, of the beverages offered should be free of caffeine and added sugars. An unfortunate trend in school-age children is increasing consumption of energy drinks and sweetened coffee drinks, which contain both caffeine and added sugars.[14] These drinks have a variety of negative effects on children's physical and psychological health and academic success. For example, a recent study of over 1,600 middle school students found that those who report consuming energy drinks were 66% more likely to be at risk for hyperactivity and inattention.[15] The American Academy of Pediatrics reports that energy drinks and sweetened coffee drinks can prompt heart rate irregularities, high blood pressure, hyperactivity, anxiety, and increased blood glucose in children, and states that these beverages have no place in children's diets.[14]

The U.S. Department of Agriculture (USDA) has produced a Daily Food Plan for preschoolers to guide parents in choosing nourishing meals and snacks for young children (**Figure 18.3**, page 718). This plan meets the nutrient requirements for preschoolers that have been discussed in this section.

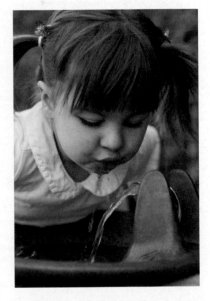

Fluid intake is important for young children, who may become so involved in their play that they ignore the sensation of thirst.

Healthy Eating *for Preschoolers* Daily Food Plan

Use this Plan as a general guide.

● These food plans are based on average needs. Do not be concerned if your child does not eat the exact amounts suggested. Your child may need more or less than average. For example, food needs increase during growth spurts.

● Children's appetites vary from day to day. Some days they may eat less than these amounts; other days they may want more. Offer these amounts and let your child decide how much to eat.

Food group	2 year olds	3 year olds	4 and 5 year olds	What counts as:
Fruits	1 cup	1 - 1½ cups	1 - 1½ cups	½ cup of fruit? ½ cup mashed, sliced, or chopped fruit ½ cup 100% fruit juice ½ medium banana 4-5 large strawberries
Vegetables	1 cup	1½ cups	1½ - 2 cups	½ cup of veggies? ½ cup mashed, sliced, or chopped vegetables 1 cup raw leafy greens ½ cup vegetable juice 1 small ear of corn
Grains Make half your grains whole	3 ounces	4 - 5 ounces	4 - 5 ounces	1 ounce of grains? 1 slice bread 1 cup ready-to-eat cereal flakes ½ cup cooked rice or pasta 1 tortilla (6" across)
Protein Foods	2 ounces	3 - 4 ounces	3 - 5 ounces	1 ounce of protein foods? 1 ounce cooked meat, poultry, or seafood 1 egg 1 Tablespoon peanut butter ¼ cup cooked beans or peas (kidney, pinto, lentils)
Dairy Choose low-fat or fat-free	2 cups	2 cups	2½ cups	½ cup of dairy? ½ cup milk 4 ounces yogurt ¾ ounce cheese 1 string cheese

Some foods are easy for your child to choke on while eating. Skip hard, small, whole foods, such as popcorn, nuts, seeds, and hard candy. Cut up foods such as hot dogs, grapes, and raw carrots into pieces smaller than the size of your child's throat—about the size of a nickel.

There are many ways to divide the Daily Food Plan into meals and snacks. View the "Meal and Snack Patterns and Ideas" to see how these amounts might look on your preschooler's plate at www.choosemyplate.gov/preschoolers.html.

FIGURE 18.3 The MyPlate Daily Food Plan provides families with an easy-to-use guide to healthful meals. (*Source:* United States Department of Agriculture Food and Nutrition Service)

RECAP

Children have a slower growth rate than toddlers, yet their larger body size and greater level of physical activity increase their total energy and nutrient needs. Children need a lower percentage of energy from fat than toddlers but slightly more than adults. Like toddlers, they need a minimum of 130 g/day of carbohydrate, and their RDA for protein is 0.95 g/kg body weight per day. Micronutrients of concern in children who do not consume enough fruits and vegetables are vitamins A, C, and E. Calcium requirements increase to 1,000 mg/day for ages 4–8 and 1,300 beginning at age 9. Iron and zinc may be deficient in children who do not eat meat, poultry, or fish. Fluoride supplements may be helpful in preventing dental caries in children who do not drink fluoridated water. Among highly active children, fluid intake should be monitored and encouraged. Beverages should include plain water, low-fat milk, and dilute 100% fruit juice. Beverages with caffeine and added sugars should not be part of children's diets.

What Are Some Common Nutrition-Related Concerns of Childhood?

LO 4 Discuss food choices, food insecurity, and other nutritional concerns affecting children.

New concerns about food choices arise during childhood. In addition, many children are at risk for iron-deficiency anemia. Food insecurity is also a significant challenge for many of America's children. Finally, pediatric obesity is a critical concern continuing into adolescence, and is discussed in more detail at the end of this chapter.

Parents Can Model Nutritious Food Choices

Peer pressure can be extremely difficult for both parents and their children to deal with during this stage of life. Most children want to feel that they "belong" and will mirror the actions of children they view as popular. Some children have their own spending money, and most are very susceptible to TV and other messages encouraging unhealthful food choices. Children also spend more time visiting friends and eating more meals and snacks without their parents' supervision. The impact of this increasing autonomy on the health of children can be profound.

As children approach puberty, appearance and body image play increasingly important roles in food choices by both girls and boys. These concerns are not necessarily detrimental to health, particularly if they result in children making more healthful food choices, such as eating more whole grains, fruits, and vegetables. However, it is important for children to understand that being thin does not guarantee health, popularity, or happiness and that a healthy body image includes accepting our own individual body type and recognizing that we can be physically fit and healthy at a variety of weights, shapes, and sizes. Excessive concern with thinness can lead children to experiment with fad diets, food restriction, and other behaviors that can result in undernutrition and perhaps even trigger a clinical eating disorder.

Parents remain important role models and must continue to take responsibility for the healthfulness of foods provided to their children. Parents and children can work together to find compromises by planning and talking about healthful foods and a healthful diet overall. Families who plan, prepare, and eat meals together are more successful at promoting good food choices. In fact, research has consistently shown an association between family meal preparation and consumption and better diet quality and healthier body weight among children.[16] Moreover, family meals encourage shared conversations that help family members connect. A recent systematic review has found that frequent family meals reduce the risk for disordered eating, substance abuse, and depression.[17] The "Eat Better, Eat Together" nutrition education program promotes family mealtime (**Figure 18.4**). Parents should continue to demonstrate healthy eating and physical activity patterns to maintain a consistent message to their children.

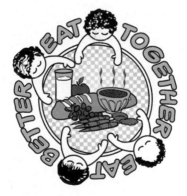

FIGURE 18.4 "Eat Better, Eat Together" promotes family mealtimes as a way to improve children's diets. (*Source*: Figure from Washington State University Extension.)

 Visit the Food & Nutrition page for kids at BAM! Body and Mind!, a program from the CDC at http://www.cdc.gov.

Iron-Deficiency Anemia Affects Many Children

Despite the best efforts of public health nutritionists and other healthcare providers, iron-deficiency anemia remains a significant problem for many children.[18] Rates of iron-deficiency anemia are higher among children from Mexican American and low-income families, emphasizing the need to evaluate each child in light of his or her family's unique risk factors. Meat, poultry, and fish provide well-absorbed sources of heme iron, and child-friendly foods such as iron-fortified cereals, dried fruits, and legumes can provide additional iron. Children who have very poor appetites or erratic eating habits may need to use an iron-containing supplement, although parents must provide careful supervision because of iron's high potential for childhood toxicity.

If left untreated, iron deficiency with or without anemia can lead to behavioral, cognitive, and motor deficits, developmental delays, and impaired immune response. In those children exposed to lead, iron deficiency increases the rate of lead absorption and severity of lead toxicity. Iron-deficiency anemia reduces a child's energy level and contributes to passivity and lethargy. The cognitive and behavioral consequences of iron deficiency in young children can be long-standing, making prevention a critical goal. Early detection through dietary assessments and simple blood tests, followed by effective treatment, ensures all children will enter school healthy and ready to learn.

Millions of American Children Experience Food Insecurity and Hunger

Although most children in the United States grow up with an abundant and healthful supply of food, 16 million American children are faced with food insecurity and hunger.[19] As you've learned (in Chapter 16), food insecurity occurs when a household is not able to ensure a consistent, dependable supply of safe and nutritious food. Overall, as many as one in every five children experience food insecurity, although rates vary widely from state to state and even from county to county.[19] For example, over 28% of households in one northern Arizona county experience food insecurity whereas half that percentage in a neighboring county suffer the same fate.[19] One in four African-American and Latino households are food insecure, compared to one in ten Caucasian households. These statistics are definitely at odds with America's image as "the land of plenty."

The effects of food insecurity and hunger can be very harmful to children.[20,21] Without an adequate breakfast, they will not be able to concentrate or pay attention to their parents, teachers, or other caretakers. Impaired nutrient status can blunt children's immune responses, making them more susceptible to common childhood illnesses and school absences. Increased rates of hospitalizations have been linked to food insecurity. Children's psychosocial health is also affected by food insecurity: rates of anxiety and suicide are increased with food insecurity. Many, but not all, studies find a link between child food insecurity and obesity or overweight.[21] Finally, maternal depression is more common within food-insecure households, creating an environment that often leads to poor mental health outcomes in the child.

Options for families facing food insecurity include a number of government and privately funded programs, including school breakfast and lunch programs, the Special Supplemental Nutrition Program for Women, Infants and Children (WIC), and the Supplemental Nutrition Assistance Program (SNAP, commonly known as the Food Stamp program). Families who face economic difficulties should be referred to public health or social service agencies and encouraged to apply for available nutrition benefits. Private and faith-based food pantries and kitchens can provide a narrow range of foods for a limited period of time but cannot be relied on to meet the nutritional needs of children and their families over an extended period of time.

RECAP

Peer pressure has a strong influence on nutritional choices in school-age children, and body-image concerns arise in both boys and girls as they approach the adolescent years. Parents can encourage healthful eating and act as role models. Sharing family meals improves nutrition and body weight, and can help family members connect. Iron deficiency anemia is a common problem among children, and can lead to severe behavioral, learning, and motor deficits. Overall, as many as one in five U.S. children experiences food insecurity, about 16 million children in all. Families facing economic challenges can be assisted by a number of government and privately funded programs.

How Does School Attendance Affect Children's Nutrition?

LO 5 Explain how school attendance and school lunch programs affect children's nutrition and health.

School attendance can affect a child's nutrition in several ways, both negatively and positively.

School Attendance Can Reduce Intake of Nourishing Foods

Hectic schedules and long bus or car rides cause many children to minimize or skip breakfast completely. School-age children who don't eat breakfast may not get a chance to eat until lunch. If the entire morning is spent in a state of hunger, children are more likely to do poorly on schoolwork, have decreased attention spans, and have more behavioral problems than their peers who do eat breakfast. In fact, you might have heard that breakfast is the most important meal of the day. Is this really true? Read the *Highlight* on page 722 and find out.

Another consequence of attending school is that, with no one monitoring what they eat, children do not always consume adequate amounts of nourishing food. If they buy a school lunch, they might not like the foods being served, or their peers might influence them to skip certain foods. Nutritious homemade lunches may be left uneaten or traded for less nutritious fare. Many children rush through lunch in order to spend more time on the playground. Some schools send students to the playground first, allowing the children time to burn off their pent-up energy as well as build their hunger and thirst.[22]

Finally, some schools continue to accept revenues from food companies in exchange for the right to advertise and sell their products to children. Although increasing numbers of states and school districts are strictly limiting or banning sales of foods low in nutrient density during the school day, some schools still provide vending machines filled with snacks that are high in empty Calories.

School Attendance Can Boost Children's Access to Nourishing Foods

Two federally funded food programs help increase all U.S. public school children's access to nourishing food. These are the School Breakfast Program (SBP) and the National School

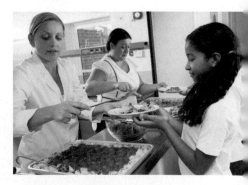

School-age children may receive a standard school lunch, but many choose less healthful foods when given the opportunity.

HIGHLIGHT

Is Breakfast the Most Important Meal of the Day?

You've heard the saying that breakfast is the most important meal of the day, but that's just a myth—isn't it? As long as you eat a nutritious lunch and dinner, why should skipping breakfast matter?

Actually, research has confirmed the importance of a healthful breakfast, especially a high protein meal.[1,2] Most studies highlight one or more of three health benefits: improved academic performance and mental functioning; improved nutritional intake and/or status overall; achievement and maintenance of a more healthful weight. Some studies, however, report little or no change in certain measures of academic achievement with breakfast consumption.[3] Let's examine the evidence.

The word *breakfast* was initially used as a verb meaning "to break the fast"—that is, to end the hours of fasting that naturally occur while we sleep. When we fast, our bodies break down stored nutrients to provide energy. First, cells break down glycogen stores in the liver and muscle tissues, using the newly released glucose for energy. These stores last about 12 hours. But people who skip breakfast typically go without food for much longer than that: if they finish dinner around 7:00 PM and don't eat again until noon the next day, they are fasting for 17 hours! Long before this point, essentially all stored glycogen is used up, and the body has turned to fatty acids and amino acids as fuel sources.

If you're like most people, when your blood glucose is low, not only are you hungry but you also may feel weak, shaky, and irritable and have poor concentration. So it wouldn't be surprising if children and teens who skip breakfast didn't function as well as their breakfast-eating peers. Recent research generally, but not always, supports this hypothesis. Here are some specific findings:[1]

■ Missing breakfast and experiencing hunger impair students' ability to learn and overall cognitive performance. In students who are poorly nourished overall, eating a school breakfast positively impacts mathematics grades. Regular consumption of breakfast is associated with improved academic performance. Students who skip breakfast demonstrate reduced attention span, poor "on task" performance, and more behavioral problems, than students who consume breakfast at home or at school.

■ As part of an "in-class breakfast" program, breakfast decreases tardiness, improves school attendance, and increases participation in the breakfast program.[4]

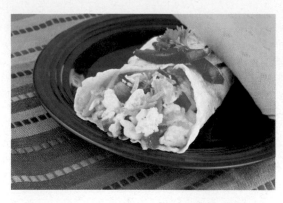

Breakfast doesn't have to be boring! A breakfast burrito with scrambled eggs, low-fat cheese, and vegetables wrapped in a whole-grain tortilla provides energy and nutrients to start your day off right.

What about the claims for improved nutritional status and body weight? Studies have found the following:

■ Skipping breakfast often leads to lower daily intakes of key nutrients. Nutrients such as protein, vitamins A and C, calcium, and iron that are not consumed during breakfast are not replaced at later meals.[5]

■ Eating a protein-rich, high fiber, and/or low glycemic-load breakfast decreases hunger and increases satiety, although subsequent caloric intake does not always decline. Studies report an association between breakfast consumption and lower body fat and/or body weight.[3]

Although research has generally linked breakfast with many positive outcomes, fewer than half of eligible students participate in the free/reduced price School Breakfast Program.[6] Many schools have improved participation with in-class breakfast service and by involving students in the planning of the menus and meal service. Whether breakfast is truly "the most important meal of the day" or not, it certainly provides multiple benefits.

References

1. Adolphus, K., C. L. Lawton, and L. Dye. 2013. The effects of breakfast on behavior and academic performance in children and adolescents. *Front. Hum. Neurosci.* 7:425. doi:10.3389/frhum.2013.00425.
2. Leidy, H. J., L. C. Ortinau, S. M. Douglas, and H. A. Hoertel. 2013. Beneficial effects of a higher-protein breakfast on the appetitive, hormonal, and neural signals controlling energy intake regulation in overweight/obese, "breakfast-skipping," late-adolescent girls. *Am. J. Clin. Nutr.* 97:677–688.
3. Adolphus, K., C. L. Lawton, and L. Dye. 2015. The relationship between habitual breakfast consumption frequency and academic performance in British adolescents. *Front Publ. Health.* Available at http://dx.doi.org/10.3389/fpubh.2015.00068.
4. Anzman-Frasca, S., H. C. Djang, M. M. Halmo, P. R. Dolan, and C. D. Economos. 2015. Estimating impacts of a breakfast in the classroom program on school outcomes. *JAMA Pediatr.* 169:71–77.
5. Affenito, S. G., D. Thompson, A. Dorazio, A. M. Albertson, A. Loew, and N. M. Holschuh. 2013. Ready-to-eat cereal consumption and the School Breakfast Program: relationship to nutrient intake and weight. *J. School Health* 83:28–35.
6. Bailey-Davis, L., A. Virus, T. A. McCoy, A. Wojtanowski, S. S. Vander Veur, and G. D. Foster. 2013. Middle school student and parent perceptions of government-sponsored free school breakfast and consumption: a qualitative inquiry in an urban school. *J. Acad. Nutr. Diet* 113:251–257.

Lunch Program (NSLP). The USDA's Food and Nutrition Service administers both programs, providing funding to states to establish local nonprofit breakfast and lunch services. Meals for all students are subsidized and thus inexpensive; however, students in families with incomes at or below 185% of the federal poverty level qualify for reduced-price or free meals.

In addition, the USDA encourages schools to offer "in-class breakfast," which is free to all students, removing any stigma associated with cafeteria-based breakfast programs. These breakfasts help children optimize their nutrient intake, avoid the behavioral and learning problems associated with hunger in the classroom, and have the potential to improve math and reading achievement, particularly among low-performing students.[23]

The impact of the SBP and NSLP on children's diets is enormous: 99% of public schools participate, serving over 32 million children.[24] On the surface, it would appear that school meals improve children's diets, because they are required to meet the nutritional standards of the 2010 Healthy, Hunger-Free Kids Act (HHFKA):

- Students must be offered both fruits and vegetables every day and must SELECT at least one serving for the school to be reimbursed for the meal. In addition, dark green and red/orange vegetables and legumes must be offered each week.
- Milk must be fat-free or low-fat.
- All grains must be whole-grain-rich, unless a school has requested an exemption (available through 2016).
- Calories, averaged over a week, and portion sizes must be appropriate for the age of the children being served.
- Saturated and *trans* fats must be reduced to specified levels.

In addition, vending machines and other sources of competitive food on school campuses must meet specific nutrient guidelines. Finally, those schools that are able to improve their meals get additional federal funding.

While these regulations represent the first major enhancement of nutritional standards in over 15 years, some caution remains. The actual amount of nutrients a student gets depends on what the student actually *selects* and *eats*. So a child might eat a slice of whole-wheat cheese pizza and low-fat milk but skip an apple and carrot sticks. Keep in mind also that children can still bring high-fat and high-sugar snacks and beverages from home or trade with classmates who bring them.

The good news is that many schools are working to ensure a more healthful food environment. School districts are required, for example, to develop wellness policies that address nutrition. In many schools, this increased attention has resulted in the installation of salad bars, baked potato bars, and soup stations to entice students into more healthful choices. Many schools now cultivate gardens on school grounds or even on the school rooftop where children help grow the vegetables that will be used in their lunches. The USDA has developed several programs to encourage children to adopt healthy lifestyles, for example by supplying schools with less common fruits and vegetables that children might not otherwise have the chance to try.

As nutritionists, school foodservice directors, educators, and parents continue to work together to improve the school meal programs, efforts will focus on increasing the use and consumption of fruits, vegetables, and whole grains in order to meet students' nutrient needs while minimizing their risk for hunger and obesity.

Nutrition MILESTONE

In **1853**, the Children's Aid Society of New York began serving meals to students attending its vocational school. It took another 50 years, however, before *penny lunches* were begun in one Philadelphia school. The practice quickly spread to eight others. By 1910, Boston, Cleveland, St. Louis, Cincinnati, Chicago, and Milwaukee were offering meals to elementary and high school students. By the 1920s, many boards of education had recognized their responsibility to feed children, "train them in sane habits of eating, and teach them to choose wisely what food they buy." During the Great Depression in the 1930s, the number of malnourished children exploded, and many school lunch programs were funded by state and city governments.

It wasn't until 1946 that President Harry Truman initiated the National School Lunch Program, prompted in part by the large numbers of young men reporting for World War II military duty in a malnourished state. The federal legislation served multiple purposes: to ensure national security, to safeguard the health and well-being of the nation's children, and to encourage the domestic consumption of nutritious agricultural commodities and other food. In 1966, President Lyndon Johnson expanded the initiative by including more options for school breakfast programs, followed in 1968 by a further expansion into a Summer Meals Program. The Federal School Lunch and Breakfast Program currently serves 2.3 billion breakfasts and 5 billion lunches per year, two-thirds of which are free or reduced-price.

RECAP

Children who skip breakfast are more likely to do poorly on schoolwork, have decreased attention spans, and have more behavioral problems. The USDA's Food and Nutrition Service administers funding for the School Breakfast Program and National School Lunch Program, and sets nutritional standards designed to improve children's nutrient intake. These programs make school meals affordable for all children, and reduced-price or free to children of low-income families. Not all children take full advantage of the programs; they may, for example, eat the entrée but skip the carrot sticks and apple. Increasing numbers of states and school districts are strictly limiting or banning sales of competitive foods from kiosks and vending machines, unless these foods meet nutritional standards. Schools are also required to develop wellness policies that address nutrition. ∎

LO 6 Describe the key nutrient needs of adolescents, taking into account their psychosocial development and growth and activity patterns.

What Are an Adolescent's Nutrient Needs?

The adolescent years are typically defined as beginning with the onset of **puberty,** the period in life in which secondary sexual characteristics develop and there is the capacity for reproducing. Adolescence continues through age 18.

Adolescence Is a Period of Dramatic Change

Adolescence is a period when emotions and behaviors often seem unpredictable and confusing. It is characterized by increasing independence as the adolescent establishes a personal sense of identity and works toward greater self-reliance. Adolescents may, for example, decide to follow a vegetarian or vegan diet as a means of setting themselves apart from the family unit. Whereas younger adolescents tend to be self-centered, living for the present, older teens typically focus on defining their role in life. All teens deal with their emerging sexuality, and many experiment with risky lifestyle choices—such as drugs, alcohol, or cigarettes—that lie outside their traditional cultural or social boundaries. During this developmental phase, they may be less responsive to parental guidance and attempts to improve their diet and activity patterns. Most adolescents, of course, successfully navigate the challenges of this life stage and mature into self-reliant, healthy adults.

Growth during adolescence is primarily driven by hormonal changes, including increased levels of testosterone for boys and estrogen for girls. Both boys and girls experience growth spurts, or periods of accelerated growth, during later childhood and adolescence. Growth spurts for girls tend to begin around 10 to 11 years of age, and growth spurts for boys begin around 12 to 13 years of age. These growth spurts lead to an average 20% to 25% increase in height during the pubertal years. During an average 1-year spurt, girls tend to grow 3.5 inches and boys tend to grow 4 inches. The average girl reaches almost full height by the onset of menstruation (called **menarche**). Boys typically experience continual growth throughout adolescence, and some even grow slightly taller during early adulthood.

Skeletal growth ceases once closure of the *epiphyseal plates* occurs (**Figure 18.5**). The **epiphyseal plates** are plates of cartilage located toward the end of the long bones (that is, the bones of the arms and legs) that provide for growth in length. In some circumstances, such as malnutrition or use of anabolic steroids, the epiphyseal plates can close early in adolescents and result in a failure to reach full stature.

Weight and body composition also change dramatically during adolescence. Weight gain is extremely variable during this time and reflects the adolescent's energy intake, physical activity level, and genetics. The average weight gained by girls and boys during these years is 35 and 45 lb, respectively. The weight gained by girls and boys is dramatically different in terms of its composition. Girls tend to gain significantly more body fat than boys, with this fat accumulating around the buttocks, hips, breasts, thighs, and upper arms. Although many girls are uncomfortable or embarrassed by these changes, they are a natural result of

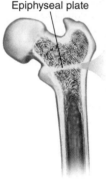

Epiphyseal plate

Bone growth occurs at epiphyseal plate

Long bone

FIGURE 18.5 Skeletal growth ceases once closure of the epiphyseal plates occurs.

puberty The period in life in which secondary sexual characteristics develop and the body becomes biologically capable of reproduction.

menarche The onset of menstruation, or the menstrual period.

epiphyseal plates Plates of cartilage located toward the end of long bones that provide for growth in the length of long bones.

maturation. Boys gain significantly more muscle mass than girls, and they experience an increase in muscle definition. Other changes that occur with sexual maturation include a deepening of the voice in boys and the growth of pubic hair in both boys and girls.

The physical activity levels of adolescents are also highly variable. Many are physically active in sports, dance, or other organized activities, whereas others become more interested in intellectual or artistic pursuits. This variability in activity levels of adolescents results in highly individual energy needs. Although the rapid growth and sexual maturation that occur during puberty require a significant amount of energy, adolescence is often a time in which overweight begins.

Adolescents' Nutrient Needs Reflect Their Rapid Growth

The nutrient needs of adolescents are influenced by rapid growth, weight gain, and sexual maturation, in addition to the demands of physical activity.

Energy and Macronutrient Recommendations

Adequate energy intake is necessary to maintain adolescents' health, support their dramatic growth and maturation, and fuel their physical activity. Because of these competing demands, the energy needs of adolescents can be quite high. The EER for this life stage is based on the adolescent's age, physical activity level, weight, and height.[1]

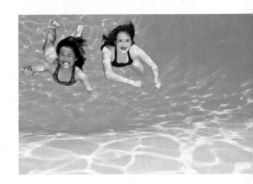

Because of rapid growth and the active lifestyle of many adolescents, their energy needs can be quite high.

As with the younger age groups, there is no RDA for fat for adolescents.[1] However, adolescents are at risk for the same chronic diseases as adults, including obesity, type 2 diabetes, and cardiovascular disease; thus, it is recommended that they consume 25% to 35% of total energy from fat, no more than 10% of total energy from saturated fat, and no *trans* fat.

The RDA for carbohydrate for adolescents is 130 g/day.[1] As with adults, this amount of carbohydrate covers what is needed to supply adequate glucose to the brain, but it does not cover the amount of carbohydrate needed to support daily activities. Thus, it is recommended that adolescents consume more than the RDA, or about 45% to 65% of their total energy as carbohydrate, the majority from fiber-rich sources. The AI for fiber for adolescent girls is 26 g/day and for adolescent boys is 38 g/day. These levels are virtually the same as for adult women and men.[1]

The RDA for protein for adolescents, at 0.85 g protein per kilogram of body weight per day, is similar to that of adults, which is 0.80 g per kilogram body weight.[1] This amount is assumed to be sufficient to support health and to cover the additional needs of growth and development during the adolescent stage. As with adults, most U.S. adolescents consume protein in amounts that far exceed the RDA.

Micronutrient Recommendations

Micronutrients of particular concern for adolescents include calcium, iron, and vitamin A. Adequate calcium intake is critical to achieve peak bone density, and the RDA for calcium for adolescents 14–18 years of age is 1,300 mg/day.[5] This amount of calcium can be difficult for many adolescents to consume, because the quality of foods they select is often less than optimal to meet their nutrient needs. To achieve this level of calcium intake, adolescents need to eat at least four servings of dairy foods or calcium-fortified products daily. Green, leafy vegetables and legumes also provide calcium, although the per-serving amount and bioavailability may be lower than in dairy and calcium-fortified foods.

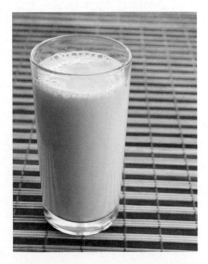

Adequate calcium intake during adolescence is necessary to achieve peak bone mass, in addition to other critical body and cell functions.

The iron needs of adolescents are relatively high; this is because iron is lost during menstruation in girls and is required to support the increased blood volume and growth of muscle mass in both girls and boys. The RDA for iron for girls is 15 mg/day and for boys is 11 mg/day.[6] If energy intake is adequate and adolescents consume heme-iron food sources, such as meat, poultry, and fish, each day, they should be able to meet the RDA for iron. However, some young people adopt a vegetarian lifestyle during this life stage, or they consume foods that have limited nutrient density. Both of these situations can prevent adolescents from meeting the RDA for iron.

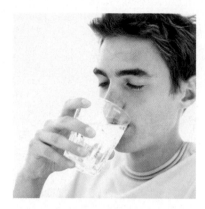

Check out the Best Bones Forever site for recipes and other resources for bone health at http://www.bestbonesforever.org

Adolescents have higher fluid needs than younger children.

Vitamin A is critical to support the rapid growth and development that occurs during adolescence. The RDA for vitamin A is 900 μg per day for boys and 700 μg per day for girls,[6] which can be met by consuming five to nine servings of fruits and vegetables each day. As with iron and calcium, meeting the RDA for vitamin A can be a challenging goal in this age group due to their potential to make less healthful food choices.

If an adolescent is unable or unwilling to eat adequate amounts of nutrient-dense foods, then a multivitamin and mineral supplement that provides no more than 100% of the Daily Value for the micronutrients can be beneficial as a safety net. As with younger children and adults, a supplement should not be considered a substitute for a balanced, healthful diet.

Fluid Recommendations

The fluid needs of adolescents are higher than those for children because of their higher physical activity levels and the extensive growth and development that occur during this phase of life. The recommended daily fluid intakes for adolescents are summarized in Table 18.1 and average about 11 cups of beverages, including water, for boys and 10 cups for girls.[7] Boys are generally more active than girls and have more lean tissue; thus, they require a higher fluid intake to maintain fluid balance. Very active adolescents who are exercising in the heat may have higher fluid needs than the AI, and these individuals should be encouraged to drink often to quench their thirst and avoid dehydration.

RECAP

Adolescents experience rapid increases in height, weight, and lean body mass and fat mass. Adequate energy is needed to support growth, maturation, and physical activity. Fat intake should be 25% to 35% of total energy, and carbohydrate intake should be 45% to 65% of total energy intake. The RDA for protein for adolescents is 0.85 g protein per kilogram of body weight per day. The RDA for calcium is 1,300 mg/day to optimize bone growth and to achieve peak bone density. This level of calcium intake can be challenging for teens to meet. Iron needs are increased to support increased blood volume and muscle mass and to replace the iron lost in menstruation in girls. Vitamin A is critical to support growth and development. Adolescent boys need about 11 cups of beverages and girls about 10 cups a day. ■

LO 7 Discuss food choices, disordered eating patterns, and other nutritional concerns affecting adolescents.

What Are Some Common Nutrition-Related Concerns of Adolescence?

Even while still living in their parents' home, adolescents make many if not most of their own food choices, and their selections may not always be high in nutrient density, or might reflect a preoccupation with weight and body image that could contribute to disordered eating. Acne is also a common concern, and some teens experiment with tobacco, alcohol, and illegal drugs.

Most Adolescents Choose Their Own Foods

Adolescents make many of their own food choices and buy a significant amount of the foods they consume. Although parents can still be effective role models, adolescents are generally strongly influenced by their peers, mass media, personal preferences, and their own developing sense of what foods make up an adequate diet.

Areas of particular concern in the adolescent diet are the lack of vegetables, fruits, and whole grains. Many teens eat on the run, skip meals, and select fast foods and convenience foods, because they are inexpensive and accessible, and taste good. Excessive weight gain may begin during this period, especially in teens who are sedentary or only lightly active. Parents, caretakers, and school foodservice programs can capitalize on adolescents' preferences for pizza, burgers, spaghetti, and sandwiches by providing more healthful meat and cheese alternatives, whole-grain breads, and plenty of appealing vegetable-based side-dishes. In addition, keeping healthful snacks, such as fruits and vegetables, that are already cleaned and prepared in easy-to-eat pieces may encourage adolescents to consume more of

Nutri-Case

Liz

"High school was really hard for me. Because dance took up such a big part of my life, I just didn't make a lot of friends. When I looked at the popular girls, I always noticed how slender they all were. So I started skipping lunch and eating less at dinner. This went on until I went to an audition for a production of *The Nutcracker*. I wanted so badly to be chosen, but I was feeling so spaced out—I guess from hunger—that before I knew what had happened, I was on the floor! I sprained my ankle and didn't get a chance to dance at all that year. So that's why, as I've been preparing for my audition with the City Ballet, I've been making myself eat at least 1,000 Calories a day. The audition is tomorrow, and I'm not going to end up on the floor this time!"

Do you, or does someone you know, equate body weight with popularity? Why are adolescents prone to this type of thinking? Or are they? If Liz succeeds in getting into the City Ballet, what health risks might she face? How could she reduce these risks?

these foods as between-meal snacks. Teens should also be encouraged to consume adequate milk and other calcium-enriched beverages.

Many teens move out of their family home when they attend college or get their first full-time job. One question these teens commonly have is how to stock their kitchen. The nearby *Highlight* (page 728) identifies staples to keep on hand for healthful snacks and meals.

Disordered Eating Is a Common Concern of Adolescence

An initially healthful concern about body image and weight can turn into a dangerous obsession during this emotionally challenging life stage. Clinical eating disorders frequently begin during adolescence and can occur in boys as well as girls. Warning signs include rapid and excessive weight loss, a preoccupation with weight and body image, habitual bathroom visits after meals, and signs of frequent vomiting or laxative use.

There is increasing evidence that parental eating habits and attitudes strongly influence the eating practices of their children.[25,26] Parental pressure to eat (aimed at the child) increases the risk of disordered eating as do the parents' own food-restriction practices. Early dieting (before age 11 years) is more common among girls whose mother or father encouraged them to diet.[26] Rather than promoting dieting for weight loss, alternative approaches such as family-wide physical activity, child–parent sharing of food shopping and preparation tasks, and an emphasis on increasing healthful foods versus restriction of foods appear more effective with adolescents trying to achieve a healthful weight. (Disordered eating is discussed *In Depth* on pages 540–550.)

Adolescent Acne Is Not Known to Be Linked to Diet

Acne flare-ups plague many adolescents. Acne is an inflammation of the sebaceous (oil) glands associated with hair follicles. These glands produce an oily secretion, called *sebum*, that normally flows out onto the skin surface, keeping skin soft and moist and repelling microbes. In acne, excessive sebum collects in and plugs up hair follicles. "Blackheads" occur when follicles are exposed to air, and the top layer of sebum oxidizes. They are not caused by dirt! "Whiteheads" are collections of sebum in follicles not exposed to air.

The hormonal changes that occur during puberty are largely responsible for the sudden appearance of acne in many adolescents. Emotional stress, genetic factors, and personal hygiene are most likely secondary contributors.

What about foods? For decades, the potential links between the intakes of chocolate, fried foods, fatty foods, sweets, and other foods and the occurrence of acne have been widely debated, but there is no conclusive evidence that food choices influence acne. A recent review study, for example, found that the role of chocolate remains controversial.[27]

HIGHLIGHT

On Your Own: Stocking Your First Kitchen

Many teens move out of the house around age 18 or 19 and settle into apartments, college or university housing, or shared housing. One question teens often have is how to stock their first kitchen. What basic foods—or staples—do they need to always have on hand, so that they can quickly and easily assemble healthful meals and snacks? The following checklist includes the foods that many Americans consider staples. It can be modified to include items that are staples in non-Western cultures and to address vegetarian, vegan, low-fat, low-sodium, and other diets. By stocking healthful foods like the ones listed here, you should be able to quickly prepare healthful meals every day!

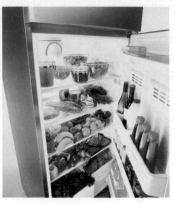

Keep Your Refrigerator Stocked with the Following:

Low-fat or skim milk and/or soy milk
Calcium-enriched 100% juice
Hard cheeses
Yogurt
Eggs
Lean deli meats
Tofu
Hummus, peanut butter, low-fat cream cheese, and/or other perishable spreads
2- to 3-day supply of dark-green lettuce and other salad fixings or ready-to-eat salads
2- to 3-day supply of other veggies
2- to 3-day supply of fresh fruits
Low-fat salad dressings, mustards, salsas, and so forth
Whole-grain breads, rolls, bagels, pizza crusts (or store these in the freezer)
Tortillas: corn, whole-wheat flour; whole-wheat pita bread

Stock Your Freezer with the Following:

Individual portions of chicken breast, extra-lean ground beef, pork loin chops, fish fillets, veggie (black bean) "burgers" or soy alternatives
Lower-fat frozen entrées ("boost" with salad, whole-grain roll, and extra veggies)
Frozen veggies (no sauce)
Frozen cheese or veggie pizza ("boost" with added mushrooms, green peppers, and so forth)

Stock Your Kitchen Cupboards with the Following:

Potatoes, sweet potatoes, onions, garlic, and so forth, as desired
Canned or vacuum-packed tuna, salmon, crab (in water, not oil)
Canned low/no-sodium veggies: corn, tomatoes, mushrooms, and so forth
Canned low/no-sodium legumes: black beans, refried beans, pinto/kidney beans, garbanzo beans
Canned soups that are low in sodium and fat and high in fiber—read the Nutrition Facts panels
Dried beans and/or lentils, if desired
Pasta and rice, preferably whole-grain; barley, couscous, tabouli
Jars of tomato-based pasta sauces
Canned fruit in juice
Dried fruits, including golden raisins, dried cranberries, apricots, cherries, plums (prunes)
Nuts, including peanuts, almonds, walnuts, and so forth
Whole-grain ready-to-eat cereals for breakfast and snacking; whole-grain cooked cereals, such as oatmeal
Whole-grain, lower-fat crackers
Pretzels, low-fat tortilla/corn chips, low/no-fat microwave popcorn
Salt, pepper, balsamic vinegar, soy sauce, other condiments and spices as desired
Olive oil, canola oil, and so forth, as desired

On the other hand, a healthful diet, rich in fruits, vegetables, whole grains, and lean meats, can provide vitamin A, vitamin C, zinc, and other nutrients to optimize skin health and maintain an effective immune system. In addition, this dietary pattern can be described as having a low glycemic load, which has been linked to a reduced occurrence and severity of adolescent acne.[28,29,30]

Prescription medications, including the vitamin A derivative 13-*cis*-retinoic acid, also known as isotretinoin (trade name Accutane), effectively control severe forms of acne. Neither Accutane nor any other prescription vitamin A derivative should be used by women who are pregnant, are planning a pregnancy, or may become pregnant. Accutane is a known teratogen, causing severe fetal malformations. The teratogenic effect is so serious that the U.S. Food and Drug Administration (FDA) requires all women of childbearing age who use Accutane to register in a risk management program, iPLEDGE, to ensure that pregnancies do not occur while under treatment. Incidentally, vitamin A taken in supplement form is not effective in acne treatment and, due to its own risk for toxicity, should not be used in amounts that exceed 100% of the Daily Value.

Substance Abuse Has Nutritional Implications

Adolescents are naturally curious, and many are open to experimenting with tobacco, alcohol, and illegal drugs. Cigarette smoking diminishes appetite and can interfere with nutrient metabolism. In fact, it is often used by adolescents to achieve or maintain a low body weight.[31] Other effects of smoking on young people include the following:

- Addiction to nicotine and continuation as adult smoker
- Reduced rate of lung growth
- Impaired athletic performance and endurance
- Shortness of breath
- Early signs of cardiovascular disease
- Increased risk for lung cancer and several other cancers as adults

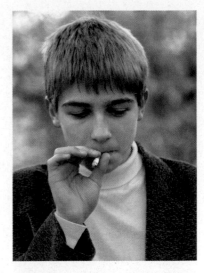

Cigarette smoking can interfere with nutrient metabolism.

Among adolescents, smoking is also associated with an increased incidence of participation in other risky behaviors, such as abuse of alcohol and other drugs, fighting, and having unprotected sex. There is also a link between pediatric/adolescent smoking and early onset of depression.[32]

Alcohol and drug use can start at early ages, even in school-age children. Among 8th, 10th, and 12th graders, alcohol intake was reported by 11%, 28%, and 42%, respectively, of students.[33] Increased levels of adult drinking and higher prevalence of bars is associated with greater teen drinking. The primary cause of death among high school–age youth is a motor-vehicle accident; while the rate of adolescent drinking and driving has dropped by more than 50% over the past 15 years, those who do drink and drive are 17 times more likely to die in a motor-vehicle accident compared to a teen who has not been drinking.[33] Alcohol can also interfere with proper nutrient absorption and metabolism, and it can take the place of foods in an adolescent's diet; these adverse effects of alcohol put adolescents at risk for various nutrient deficiencies. Alcohol consumption and use of many illegal drugs are also associated with "the munchies," a feeling of food craving that usually results in the intake of large quantities of high-fat, high-sugar, nutrient-poor foods. This behavior can result in overweight or obesity, and it increases the risk for nutrient imbalance. Teens who use drugs and alcohol are typically in poor physical condition, are either underweight or overweight, have poor appetites, and perform poorly in school.

RECAP

Adolescents' food choices are influenced by peer pressure, media, and personal preferences; however, parents remain role models. Teens often select fast foods and high-fat/high-energy snack foods in place of whole grains, fruits, and vegetables. Adolescents with lower levels of physical activity may therefore experience overweight for the first time during this period. On the other hand, a preoccupation with weight and body image may lead to disordered eating behaviors. Evidence of a dietary link to adolescent acne is not conclusive, but a low glycemic-load diet may reduce occurrence and severity. Cigarette smoking, in addition to increasing the smoker's risk for cardiovascular disease, many cancers, and several other diseases, diminishes appetite and can interfere with nutrient metabolism. Alcohol can also interfere with proper nutrient absorption and metabolism, and increases the risk of traumatic injury. Use of illegal drugs is also a concern for this age group. ■

What Makes Pediatric Obesity Harmful, and Why Does It Occur?

LO 8 Describe the health problems associated with pediatric obesity and the etiology of the problem.

Although the prevalence of obesity has stabilized for U.S. children and adolescents since 2007, rates remain unacceptably high.[34] Currently, about 32% of children and youth aged 2 to 19 years are classified as overweight, while about 17% are classified as obese. The Centers for Disease Control and Prevention (CDC) classifies children as obese whose BMI is

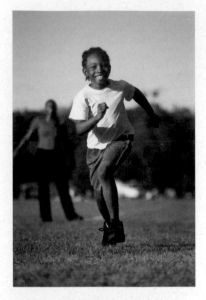

Active, healthy-weight children are less likely to become overweight adults.

at or above the 95th percentile; that is, their BMI is higher than that of 95% of U.S. children of the same age and gender who made up the reference group at the time these charts were developed. Recently, the CDC added two new categories to describe severe obesity among children and adolescents:[34]

- Class 2 obesity is a BMI greater than or equal to 120% of the 95th percentile or a BMI greater than or equal to 35; 5.9% of U.S. children meet the criteria for class 2 obesity.
- Class 3 obesity is a BMI greater than or equal to 140% of the 95th percentile or a BMI greater than or equal to 40; 2.1% of U.S. children meet the criteria for class 3 obesity.

Unfortunately, rates of class 2 and class 3 obesity have increased over the past 5 years, particularly among girls.[34]

Believe it or not, overweight and obesity can occur as early as the toddler years: over 20% of children 2 to 5 years of age are classified as overweight, while over 8% are already categorized as obese.[34] In the toddler years, even those children above the 80th percentile for weight should be monitored. Preschoolers, school-age children, and adolescents also, of course, need to be monitored for overweight and obesity. Parents should not be offended if the child's pediatrician, school nurse, or other healthcare provider expresses concern over the child's weight status; early intervention is critical to prevent lifelong obesity. The National Institutes of Health (NIH) now also recommends universal screening of serum lipids and blood pressure during childhood.[35]

Pediatric Obesity Leads to Serious Health Problems

We may feel shocked at the sight of an obese preschooler, but children's health experts point out that we should be more concerned by what we don't see. Even in early childhood, significant overweight can exacerbate asthma, cause sleep apnea, and lead to musculoskeletal disorders, impairing a child's mobility. Fatty liver is diagnosed in one-third of obese children, and can cause inflammation and scarring that compromises liver functioning. Moreover, increasing numbers of obese children are experiencing high blood lipids, high blood pressure, type 2 diabetes, metabolic syndrome, and other medical problems.[36,37] Many of these metabolic disorders are more prevalent in overweight and obese African-American, Mexican-American, and Native American children and adolescents. Class 2 and 3 obesity are more strongly associated with metabolic abnormalities than less severe obesity.[34,38]

Pediatric obesity is also associated with intense teasing, low self-esteem, social isolation, and depression. A recent study of patients in a pediatric weight management program, for example, found that 43% had psychosocial stressors, 18% were at risk for clinical depression, and 11% screened positive for urgent mental health problems.[39]

It is estimated that about 70% of obese children maintain their higher weight as adults; thus, preventing childhood obesity is crucial for children's long-term health and well-being. Reduction in the prevalence of pediatric obesity in the United States can be accomplished only through an aggressive, comprehensive, nationwide health campaign.

Pediatric Obesity Is Multifactorial

As with adults (see Chapter 13), obesity in children results from a complex interaction among genetic, environmental, and sociocultural factors. A child's weight or BMI is closely related to parental weight or BMI: children with one overweight or obese parent are twice as likely to be overweight as those with no overweight or obese parent, whereas children in families where both those parents are overweight or obese are nearly four times as likely to be overweight. Genetic risk factors, however, can be overcome through a coordinated effort involving families, healthcare providers, schools, and communities.[40]

Lower parental education and income are associated with increased risk for pediatric obesity, as are environmental factors such as access to playgrounds, safe bicycle/walking paths, and grocery stores with a full range of healthful foods. Cultural influences, particularly among recent immigrant families, may also exert a strong influence on risk for childhood obesity.

RECAP

The Centers for Disease Control and Prevention (CDC) classifies children as obese whose BMI is at or above the 95th percentile. Class 2 and 3 obesity are more severe. Currently 17% of U.S. children age 2 to 19 are classified as obese: 9% are moderately obese and another 8% are severely obese. Obesity is an important concern for children of all ages, their families, and their communities, because it is associated with an increased risk of fatty liver disease, metabolic syndrome, depression, and many other health problems. Moreover, about 70% of obese children maintain their higher weight as adults. Like obesity in adults, pediatric obesity is multifactorial.

Can Pediatric Obesity Be Prevented or Treated?

LO 9 Discuss the dietary and activity options for preventing childhood obesity, including the roles of the family and school.

LO 10 Identify a range of options for treating moderate and severe obesity in children.

Although pediatric obesity is multifactorial, eating and drinking fewer Calories and increasing physical activity are first steps in prevention and treatment. Medications and surgery are available to help children who are severely obese.

A Healthful Diet Can Help Prevent Pediatric Obesity

The family and the school play key roles in encouraging healthful eating habits in the fight against pediatric obesity.

The Role of the Family in Healthful Eating

Children typically mimic their parents, especially at the younger ages, so rather than singling out overweight children and placing them on restrictive diets, experts encourage family-wide improvements in food choices, mealtime habits, and other behaviors. Parental consumption of sugary drinks and foods high in saturated fats, eating at fast-food restaurants, eating in front of the television, and other "obesogenic" behaviors certainly influence childhood obesity. Parents who are able to modify their own eating behaviors are better prepared to support the efforts of their children.[41] On the other hand, children whose parents are overly restrictive about food actually lose less weight or gain more weight compared to parents who demonstrate more flexibility.

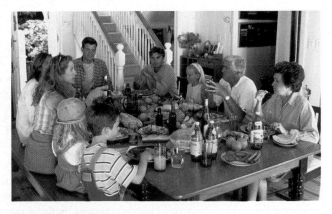

Parents should ensure that families take part in shared meals regularly.

Parents should encourage children to eat a healthful breakfast every morning, and sit down to a shared family meal each evening, as regularly as possible. Children should be invited to participate in food shopping, meal preparation, and clean-up, with age-appropriate tasks. Meals, especially dinner, should offer a colorful variety of foods, with the emphasis on green, yellow, orange, and red vegetables and deep-brown grains. If available foods are healthful, children can be free to choose among them and will gain confidence in their ability to make good food choices (self-efficacy). Also, we noted earlier that shared family meals have been associated with a reduced prevalence of obesity.

Parents should strive to provide consistently nutritious snacks, and retain control over the purchasing and preparation of snack foods until older children and teens are responsible and knowledgeable enough to make healthful decisions. Parents can keep a selection of fruits, vegetables, whole-grain products, and low-fat dairy foods readily available as healthful alternatives to high-fat, high-sugar snacks (positive parenting). For active children who frequently eat on the run, parents can keep a supply of nonperishable snacks, such as low-calorie granola bars, a mix of dried fruits, nuts, and whole-grain cereal bits, along with kid-friendly fruits, such as apples, bananas, and oranges, to grab as everyone dashes out the door.

Whenever possible, parents should minimize the number of meals eaten in restaurants, especially fast-food franchises. When families do eat out, parents should share large portion sizes and order grilled, broiled, or baked foods instead of fried foods and encourage other family members to do the same.

Many children and adolescents resent parental oversight and involvement in their weight-control program. Parents should not allow the dinner table or kitchen to turn into a war zone; instead, they should model healthful eating behaviors, provide a diverse array of healthful foods, and encourage healthful lifestyle choices, including physical activity. Even if a child's weight stabilizes rather than declines, parents should praise the absence of additional weight gain as a positive step.

> Download a free cookbook chock-full of healthy, kid-friendly recipes from the National Heart, Lung and Blood Institute at www.nhlbi.nih.gov. Type in "healthy family meals" into the search bar to begin!

The Role of the School in Healthful Eating

As previously noted, the National School Lunch Program is designed to limit the amount of total Calories, saturated and *trans* fat, and sugar served to students. Several states now ban vending machines at elementary and middle schools; efforts at high schools have generally been less successful. Consistent and repeated school-based messages on good nutrition can reinforce the efforts of parents and healthcare providers.

Many school districts have embraced "garden-based learning," an educational strategy aimed at improving student's learning and social skills, as well as their intakes of fresh produce and physical activity.[42] Children are encouraged to apply what they have learned in math, science, health, geography, and other subjects. Research has shown that children who are actively involved in growing fruits and vegetables are more likely to accept unfamiliar foods, increase their total fruit and vegetable consumption, and understand the links between dietary choices and health.

Some, but not all, research suggests that consumption of cereal as part of the School Breakfast Program is associated with improved BMI, possibly due to the higher fiber and protein intakes and the low fat profile of the meal.[43]

An Active Lifestyle Can Help Prevent Pediatric Obesity

Increased energy expenditure through increased physical activity is essential for successful weight management among children. The Institute of Medicine recommends that children participate in aerobic physical activity and exercise for at least an hour each day, a goal that as few as 10% of adolescents actually meet.[1] The Physical Activity Guidelines for Americans also advise bone- and muscle-strengthening activities at least 3 days each week.[44] For younger children, this can be divided into two or three shorter sessions, allowing them to regroup, recoup, and refocus between activity sessions. Older children should be able to be active for an hour without stopping. Obese children are more likely to engage in physical activities that are noncompetitive, fun, and structured in a way that allows them to proceed at their own pace. Children should be exposed to a variety of activities, so that they move different muscles, play at various intensities, avoid boredom, and find out what they like and don't like to do (**Table 18.2**).

The Role of the Family in Physical Activity

As with healthful eating, parental and adult role models are vital in any effort to increase the physical activity level of children and adolescents. When parents and children are active together, healthful activity patterns are established early. To encourage activity throughout the day, parents should plan shared activities, such as ball games, bicycle rides, hikes, and skating outings. In addition, community organizations, such as the YMCA and municipal recreational centers have supervised youth-oriented weight-training programs, climbing walls, skateboard parks, and other nontraditional activity options that are typically open to the whole family. Community-based organizations such as the YMCA, Boys & Girls

TABLE 18.2 Examples of Physical Activities for Children and Adolescents

Type of Physical Activity	Age Group: Children	Age Group: Adolescents
Moderate-intensity aerobic	<ul><li>Active recreation, such as hiking, skateboarding, rollerblading</li><li>Bicycle riding</li><li>Brisk walking</li></ul>	<ul><li>Active recreation, such as canoeing, hiking, skateboarding, rollerblading</li><li>Brisk walking</li><li>Bicycle riding (stationary or road bike)</li><li>Housework and yard work, such as sweeping or pushing a lawn mower</li><li>Games that require catching and throwing, such as baseball and softball</li></ul>
Vigorous-intensity aerobic	<ul><li>Active games involving running and chasing, such as tag</li><li>Bicycle riding</li><li>Jumping rope</li><li>Martial arts, such as karate</li><li>Running</li><li>Sports such as soccer, ice or field hockey, basketball, swimming, tennis</li><li>Cross-country skiing</li></ul>	<ul><li>Active games involving running and chasing, such as flag football</li><li>Bicycle riding</li><li>Jumping rope</li><li>Martial arts, such as karate</li><li>Running</li><li>Sports such as soccer, ice or field hockey, basketball, swimming, tennis</li><li>Vigorous dancing</li><li>Cross-country skiing</li></ul>
Muscle-strengthening	<ul><li>Games such as tug-of-war</li><li>Modified push-ups (with knees on the floor)</li><li>Resistance exercises using body weight or resistance bands</li><li>Rope or tree climbing</li><li>Sit-ups (curl-ups or crunches)</li><li>Swinging on playground equipment/bars</li></ul>	<ul><li>Games such as tug-of-war</li><li>Push-ups and pull-ups</li><li>Resistance exercises with exercise bands, weight machines, hand-held weights</li><li>Climbing wall</li><li>Sit-ups (curl-ups or crunches)</li></ul>
Bone-strengthening	<ul><li>Games such as hopscotch</li><li>Hopping, skipping, jumping</li><li>Jumping rope</li><li>Running</li><li>Sports such as gymnastics, basketball, volleyball, tennis</li></ul>	<ul><li>Hopping, skipping, jumping</li><li>Jumping rope</li><li>Running</li><li>Sports such as gymnastics, basketball, volleyball, tennis</li></ul>

Note: Some activities, such as bicycling, can be moderate or vigorous intensity, depending upon level of effort.
Source: 2008 Physical Activity Guidelines for Americans, from U.S. Department of Health and Human Services.

Clubs, Girls on the Run, and similar programs can boost physical activity in children and adolescents when parents are at work or not available.

In the past, children played freely outdoors and even kept active indoors in times of bad weather. In recent years, however, multiple factors have prompted childhood activities to become increasingly sedentary. One factor is the availability and attraction of sedentary entertainment technologies, including television, video games, computer games, and smart phones. The American Academy of Pediatrics recommends no media use for children younger than 2 years[45] and no more than 2 hours per day of TV viewing for preschoolers. Children who watch more TV and have higher total screen time are at increased risk for obesity. Too much screen time can interfere with the acquisition of physical skills and can hinder children's use of their own imaginations, dampening creativity. Moreover, increased screen time is associated with increased risk of overweight and obesity and impaired sleep quality and duration.[46,47] Some researchers, however, are looking to turn the appeal of smart phones into motivation for physical activity.[48] Through various text messages, teens can set activity goals, increase their sense of autonomy, and improve their self-competence.

Another factor contributing to low levels of physical activity among America's youth relates to community design and infrastructure, also known as the "built environment." A family living in a neighborhood with adequate and well-maintained sidewalks, safe parks and open spaces, well-designed bike paths, and a high "walkability score" (less need to drive everywhere) have more opportunities for physical activity.[49,50] In some communities, safety concerns may cause working parents to forbid their children, when they are home alone

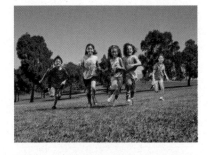

Encouraging physical play with friends is a good way to combat childhood obesity.

after school, to venture out of the house. If this is the case, the family may consider investing in electronic game systems that offer virtual tennis, step aerobics, dancing, and other active simulations or work with other families and community agencies to offer safe, well-supervised activities during after-school, evening, and weekend hours.

By increasing their physical activity, some overweight or obese children are able to gradually "catch up" to their weight as they grow taller without severely restricting their food (and thus nutrient) intake. Increased activity also helps children acquire motor skills and muscle strength, establish good sleep patterns, and develop self-esteem as they feel themselves becoming faster, stronger, and more skilled. Regular physical activity also optimizes bone mass, strengthens muscles, enhances cardiovascular and respiratory function, and lowers emotional stress in obese children.

The Role of the School in Physical Activity

As academic standards increase across the country, many schools are reducing or eliminating physical education classes and, in elementary schools, recess periods. Budget cuts have also led to the reduction or elimination of after-school physical activity programs, including school sports programs. Unfortunately, these decisions are short-sighted, because daily physical activity not only helps regulate body weight but also improves academic performance, self-efficacy, and sleep quality. Researchers have noted that, when children have the opportunity to take part in recess, classroom behavior improves, children are more attentive to their teachers, and students are more focused on assigned tasks.

Parents, healthcare providers, and other community members can join forces to work with local school boards to optimize opportunities for physical activity in the schools. A program called *We Can!* (Ways to Enhance Children's Activity & Nutrition), a collaboration of several national health and government agencies, provides resources for parents, healthcare providers, schools, and communities, so that they can develop their own local physical activity and nutrition programs. *We Can!* is just one of many programs schools can use in developing their own action plans. Other schools are offering after-school clubs that promote moderate to vigorous physical activity through a rotating menu of activity options.[51] Daily physical education in schools, continued funding for team, club, and individual sports, and noncompetitive physical activity options outside of schools can help reduce the prevalence of obesity among U.S. children and adolescents, helping to reverse what has been an alarming health trend for the past 30 years.

Pediatric Obesity Does Respond to Treatment

Although not well publicized, treatment of obese children and adolescents can be successful. It may take several attempts and, in some cases, "success" might be defined as no further weight gain (supporting normal increases in height, but not weight), but healthcare providers now have clearly defined treatment options.[52-55] These are often prescribed according to a staging system.[52]

Stage 1 incorporates lifestyle modifications to improve dietary intake while decreasing energy intake, and to increase physical activity while decreasing sedentary behaviors. It also includes behavioral therapy for the child or adolescent and his or her family.

Stage 2 personalizes the intervention with the addition of consultations with a Registered Dietitian Nutritionist, more specific behavioral goals (e.g., "at least 60 minutes/day of physical activity" vs. "be more active"), the adoption of self-monitoring, and monthly visits with the primary healthcare provider. Ideally, the entire family remains actively engaged and treatment goals account for the specific home and community environments of the child or adolescent.

Stage 3 expands the care team to include a member devoted to the behavioral health of the child or adolescent and family and an exercise specialist. The child or adolescent visits with a healthcare provider weekly.

These initial three stages are all focused on lifestyle and behavioral changes and, more recently, have been enhanced through the use of smart phone applications and text messages.[56] Although they can be effective in overweight and moderately obese children and

Watch *The Weight of the Nation for Kids*, an HBO documentary series sponsored by the National Institutes of Health. Go to www.nichd.nih.gov and press the "News & Media" tab. Go to the "Spotlights" section and choose the video to begin.

adolescents, these interventions often fail to achieve the desired health outcomes in those who are severely obese.

The most intensive and costly interventions—pharmacotherapy and surgery—occur in Stage 4. While continuing lifestyle changes and behavioral modification, the child or adolescent may be started on the prescription medication orlistat (trade name Xenical), which is the only weight-loss medication approved by the FDA for pediatric use. The patient must be 12 years of age or older.[57] Orlistat reduces fat absorption by inhibiting the action of lipase, but average weight loss is modest (about 3 to 7 pounds).

In addition, the FDA has approved the drug metformin for patients age 10 and older with type 2 diabetes to reduce blood glucose. Metformin has not been approved for weight loss; however, research has shown that it modestly reduces body weight in children as young as 6 years of age.[58,59]

In contrast to the modest effectiveness of drug therapy, **bariatric surgery,** or weight loss surgery (from the Greek root *bar-*, meaning "weight"), typically leads to the most significant weight loss and improvement in health in severely obese children and adolescents.[60] While bariatric surgery is expensive and frequently risky, a growing number of pediatricians are embracing it as the best solution to severe obesity. It is usually reserved for adults and older teens, but in rare cases is performed in children as young as age 11. This treatment option will be discussed in more detail in this chapter's *Nutrition Myth or Fact?* essay immediately following the Study Plan.

RECAP

Instead of placing obese children on restrictive diets, pediatricians encourage family-wide improvements in food choices, mealtime habits, and other behaviors. For example, parents and children should share family meals, cooked at home whenever possible, and should talk during the meal rather than watching television. Schools play an important role in providing nutritious breakfasts and lunches, and some schools are incorporating gardening and cooking into their curricula. Children should participate in aerobic physical activity and exercise for at least an hour each day, and should engage in strength training at least 3 days a week. To promote activity throughout the day, parents should encourage shared activities such as ball games and walks, and strictly limit children's screen time. School budget cuts and an emphasis on academics have reduced children's access to opportunities for physical activity both during the school day and after school; however, programs such as *We Can!* are helping schools develop physical activity programs for students. Treatment of obese children and adolescents through diet, exercise, and behavioral therapy that includes family counseling can be successful, and these interventions are key to the first three stages of pediatric obesity treatment. Stage 4 treatment for older children and teens may include the prescription medication orlistat. However, a growing number of pediatricians are embracing bariatric surgery as the best solution to severe obesity. ■

bariatric surgery Procedure in which the stomach and often the small intestine are surgically altered to induce weight loss.

Nutrition Myth OR Fact?

Bariatric Surgery for Adolescents: Is It the Answer?

Approximately 7% of U.S. adolescents fall into the newly defined categories of "class 2" and "class 3" obesity, representing the most severe forms of this disease.[1] While overall rates of pediatric obesity seem to be plateauing, rates of severe obesity continue to increase. Adolescent morbid obesity is associated with an 80% chance of adult severe obesity and high rates of medical complications, including type 2 diabetes, metabolic syndrome, hypertension, nonalcoholic fatty liver disease, hyperlipidemia, sleep apnea, and musculoskeletal injuries, as well as psychosocial disorders such as depression, anxiety, suicidal thoughts, and low self-esteem.[2,3] While prevention of obesity and severe obesity is ideal, effective prevention on a wide scale remains difficult to achieve. As a result, bariatric surgery is becoming a more common treatment approach.[1–5] Given the risks of any surgical procedure and the irreversible nature of some forms of bariatric surgery, is this intervention appropriate for adolescents?

What Are the Procedures and Protocols?

Bariatric surgery procedures are illustrated in Chapter 13. The three most common bariatric surgery procedures for adolescents are as follows:[6]

■ Gastric banding restricts food intake, is reversible, and does not interfere with normal digestion and absorption. However the weight loss results are more modest than those achieved via other methods, and it does not fully resolve the metabolic abnormalities associated with morbid obesity.

■ Gastric bypass is more invasive, drastically altering GI tract structure and absorptive functions. It requires lifelong vitamin and mineral supplementation, and has a higher rate of complications. However, it also results in much greater weight loss, up to 87% of excess body weight, is FDA approved for adolescents, and effectively improves or fully resolves many of the metabolic and psychological abnormalities associated with severe obesity.[6]

■ Laparoscopic (or vertical) sleeve gastrectomy involves surgical removal of about 85% of the stomach, yet the rest of the GI tract remains unaltered, retaining normal digestive and absorptive functions. This technique, gaining in popularity for adolescents, results in an intermediate level of weight loss, resolves many of the metabolic abnormalities seen with severe obesity, and has few reported complications.[6]

   While it is hard to accurately estimate how many adolescents undergo bariatric surgery each year, its frequency is increasing. National and international organizations have established guidelines and best practices on the appropriate use of bariatric surgery in adolescents. Eligibility requirements for adolescents commonly include the following:[4]

■ *Minimum age.* Eighteen years is the most common minimum age, although patient ages as young as 11, 13, and 15 years are cited in at least one set of guidelines. Some criteria are based on developmental (Tanner) stage, rather than chronological age.

■ *Minimum BMI.* The minimum is 40 kg/m² or 35 kg/m²; the presence of comorbidities is often included.

■ *Attainment of final or near-final adult height*

■ *History of 6 or more months of targeted weight loss efforts.* Previous lifestyle and behavioral efforts must have been proven ineffective in achieving significant weight loss before embarking on this course of action.

■ *Demonstrated commitment to and understanding of all pre- and postoperative requirements.* Candidates must agree to regular follow-up for at least 1 year,

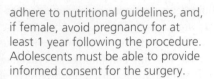

Bariatric surgery is becoming a more common treatment for severely obese adolescents.

adhere to nutritional guidelines, and, if female, avoid pregnancy for at least 1 year following the procedure. Adolescents must be able to provide informed consent for the surgery.

■ *Supportive family environment.* A supportive and involved family is a key aspect contributing to successful bariatric surgery for adolescents.

Adolescents who are pregnant or breastfeeding, abuse alcohol or drugs, have an eating disorder or other psychiatric disorder, have significant cognitive disabilities, or are diagnosed with certain medical conditions are not considered appropriate candidates for bariatric surgery.[4]

What Are the Adverse Effects and Long-Term Outcomes?

Bariatric surgery prompts a variety of physiologic responses, ranging from unpleasant to life-threatening. In adolescents, it is most commonly associated with surgical complications, such as bleeding and infection. Death, either during the surgery or in the post-operative period, is a possibility with any serious surgery. In those having the banding procedure, the band itself might slip out of place, erode, or even deflate. "Dumping" syndrome is a complication of gastric bypass, leading to nausea, cramps, vomiting, and severe diarrhea due to rapid gastric emptying. Long-term nutrient deficiencies, especially iron deficiency, are also possible complications faced by adolescents undergoing bariatric surgery.

   Data on long-term outcomes for bariatric surgery in adolescents are limited but growing. One study followed adolescents up to 5 years after their procedure. Short-term complications were rarely reported, and there were no deaths among the 345 patients.[7] Most studies have reported high rates of resolution of previous medical conditions, including type 2 diabetes, hyperlipidemia, hypertension, sleep apnea, gastroesophageal reflux, and arthritic musculoskeletal symptoms. Quality of life often greatly improves following bariatric surgery, and psychological disorders are often improved or resolved.[4] From a purely financial perspective, there is not enough data to evaluate the cost-effectiveness of adolescent bariatric surgery.[8]

   There is no doubt that pediatric morbid obesity results in significant and often long-lasting medical, psychological, and social impairments. Lifestyle interventions, including nutrition, physical activity, and behavioral components, are inexpensive and low/no risk. Bariatric surgery is expensive and often irreversible, side effects are unpleasant to life-threatening, complications do occur, and adolescents may not have the maturity to make an informed decision. However, the surgery can promote significant long-term weight loss and resolution of type 2 diabetes and other severe chronic diseases, as well as psychological disorders. Therefore, candidates and their families need to consider the risks and benefits in consultation with their healthcare team before making a decision about weight-loss treatment with bariatric surgery.

Critical Thinking Questions

■ What is your opinion of a 15-year-old boy's request to "go under the knife" because he is tired of trying to diet and hates to exercise? How much effort is "enough" when looking at failure through lifestyle interventions for morbid obesity?

■ For our society, is adolescent bariatric surgery a good investment in terms of the health of the nation? What kind of information would you need in order to make a strong argument one way or the other?

References

1. Wickham, E. P. III, and M. D. DeBoer. 2015. Evaluation and treatment of severe obesity in childhood. *Clin. Pediatr.* doi:10.1177/0009922814565886. Available at http://cpj.sagepub.com/content/early/2015/01/06/000992281456586.full (Accessed July 2015).

2. Brei, M. N., and S. Mudd. 2014. Current guidelines for weight loss surgery in adolescents: a review of the literature. *J. Ped. Health. Care* 28:288–294.

3. Michalsky, M. P., T. H. Inge, S. Teich, I. Eneli, R. Miller, M. L. Brandt, and Teen-LABS Consortium. 2014. Adolescent bariatric surgery program characteristics: the Teen Longitudinal Assessment of Bariatric surgery (Teen-LAB) study experience. *Semin. Pediatr. Surg.* 23:5–10.

4. Fitzgerald, D. A., and L. Baur. 2014. Bariatric surgery for severely obese adolescents. *Pediatr. Respir. Rev.* 15:227–230.

5. Oberbach, A., J. Neuhaus, T. Inge, K. Kirsch, N. Schlichting, S. Blüher, Y. Kullnick, J. Kugler, S. Baumann, and H. Till. 2014. Bariatric surgery in severely obese adolescents improves major comorbidities including hyperuricemia. *Metabolism.* 63:242–249.

6. Zitsman, J. L., T. H. Inge, K. W. Reichard, A. F. Browne, C. M. Harmon, and M. P. Michalsky. 2014. Pediatric and adolescent obesity: management, options for surgery, and outcomes. *J. Pediatr. Surg.* 49:491–494.

7. Lennerz, B. S., M. Wabitsch, H. Lippert, S. Wolff, C. Knoll, R. Weiner, T. Manger, W. Kiess, and C. Stroh. 2014. Bariatric surgery in adolescents and young adults—safety and effectiveness in a cohort of 345 patients. *Int. J. Obes.* 38:334–340.

8. Woolford, S. J., S. J. Clark, B. J. Sallinen, J. D. Geiger, and G. L. Freed. 2012. Bariatric surgery decision making challenges: the stability of teens' decisions and the treatment failure paradox. *Pediatr. Surg. Int.* 28:455–460.

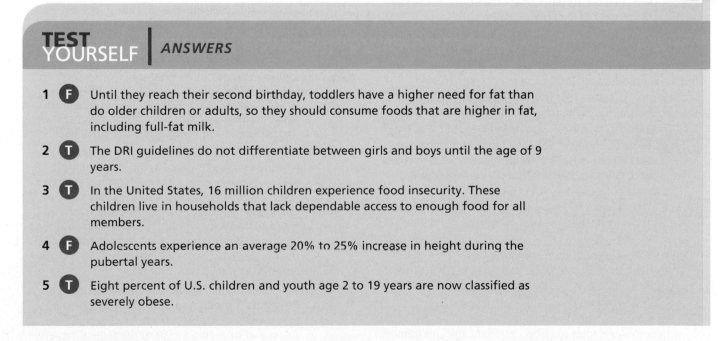

STUDY **PLAN** MasteringNutrition™

Customize your study plan—and master your nutrition!—in the Study Area of MasteringNutrition.

TEST YOURSELF | *ANSWERS*

1 **F** Until they reach their second birthday, toddlers have a higher need for fat than do older children or adults, so they should consume foods that are higher in fat, including full-fat milk.

2 **T** The DRI guidelines do not differentiate between girls and boys until the age of 9 years.

3 **T** In the United States, 16 million children experience food insecurity. These children live in households that lack dependable access to enough food for all members.

4 **F** Adolescents experience an average 20% to 25% increase in height during the pubertal years.

5 **T** Eight percent of U.S. children and youth age 2 to 19 years are now classified as severely obese.

summary

Scan to hear an MP3 Chapter Review in **MasteringNutrition**.

LO 1

- Toddlers grow more slowly than infants but are far more active. They require small, frequent, nutritious snacks and meals, and food should be soft and cut in small pieces, so that it is easy to chew and swallow.

- For toddlers and young children, a serving of food equals 1 tablespoon for each year of age. For example, 3 tablespoons of yogurt is a full serving for a 3-year-old child.

- Energy, fat, and protein requirements are higher for toddlers than for infants. Many toddlers will not eat vegetables, so micronutrients of concern include vitamins A, C, and E.

- Until age 2, toddlers should drink whole milk rather than reduced-fat milk to meet calcium requirements. Iron deficiency is a concern in the toddler years and can be minimized by the consumption of foods naturally high in iron and iron-fortified foods.

LO 2

- Toddlers' eating behaviors are typically erratic, and this should not be a concern for parents as long as the child has access to nourishing, age appropriate foods. Because of their small stomach, toddlers need small, frequent meals and snacks. Choking continues to be a risk at this age, and firm foods such as cheese cubes, grapes, hot dogs, and nuts should be avoided. Parents should still introduce new foods one at a time, monitoring the child for allergic reactions. Offering a new food several times, and praising the child for trying it, can help children expand the variety of their diet.

- Older toddlers should be given age-appropriate tasks to help prepare and serve meals, and distractions such as television during mealtimes should be avoided.

- Ovo-lacto-vegetarian diets are safe and healthful for toddlers as long as their needs for iron and zinc are met. Vegan diets can also be healthful as long as parents are aware of the many challenges they present, including potential deficiencies for protein, iron, calcium, zinc, vitamin D, and vitamin B$_{12}$.

LO 3

- School-age children grow 2 to 4 inches a year, and can be very active. Thus, their energy needs can be high.

- School-age children should eat 25% to 35% of their total energy as fat and 45% to 65% of their total energy as carbohydrate. The RDA for protein is 0.95 g/kg body weight per day.

- Children who do not consume adequate fruits and vegetables may become deficient in vitamins

A, C, and E. Calcium needs increase as children mature, to 1,000 mg/day for ages 4–8 and 1,300 beginning at age 9. Consuming adequate calcium to support the development of peak bone mass is a primary concern. Supplemental iron and zinc may be advised in children who do not eat meat, poultry, or fish, and fluoride supplements may be prescribed for children whose drinking water supply is not fluoridated.

- Children should drink five to eight cups of beverages a day. Their intake should include beverages free of caffeine and added sugars, such as water and low-fat milk. Energy drinks and sweetened coffee drinks are associated with numerous health problems and should be entirely avoided.

LO 4

- School-age children are more independent than toddlers and can make more of their own food choices. They may also begin to become concerned about their body image, and may eat inappropriately to maintain a thin appearance and gain popularity.

- Family meals have been associated with better diet quality and healthier body weight among children, as well as a reduced risk for disordered eating, substance abuse, and depression.

- Although iron needs decrease slightly in childhood, iron-deficiency anemia occurs in some children. Healthful food choices and, if appropriate, use of an iron supplement can prevent the fatigue, illness, and impaired learning that often accompany childhood iron deficiency.

- As many as 1 in 5 U.S. children, or about 16 million children, experiences food insecurity. Families experiencing food insecurity should be referred to appropriate government and social service agencies; short-term solutions such as utilizing food pantries must be supplemented with long-term, multidimensional support.

LO 5

- Many school-age children skip breakfast, a practice which can reduce their attention span and performance in school. Many children do not choose healthful foods during school lunch. Peer pressure and popularity are strong influences on food choices.

- The USDA's Food and Nutrition Service administers funding for the School Breakfast and National School Lunch Programs. The meals provided must meet strict federal nutrition guidelines, including for levels of saturated and *trans* fats and sugar, but the foods that children choose to eat at school, both during and outside the lunch break, can be high in empty Calories and low in nutrients.

- The School Breakfast and National School Lunch Programs' funding provides reduced-cost or free meals for students from families with an income at or below 185% of the federal poverty threshold. The funding also keeps the meals inexpensive for all students.

LO 6
- Puberty is the period in life in which secondary sexual characteristics develop and the physical capability to reproduce begins. Puberty results in rapid increases in height, weight, lean body mass, and fat mass. Adolescent growth spurts lead to an average 20% to 25% increase in height, and an average gain of 35 pounds for girls and 45 pounds for boys.

- Because of their rapid growth, energy needs for adolescents can be quite high, especially for adolescents who participate in sports. However, adolescence can also be a time when excessive weight gain begins.

- Fat intake should be 25% to 35% of total energy, and carbohydrate intake should be 45% to 65% of total energy intake. Fiber-rich carbohydrates are essential to meet the AI for fiber, which is 26 g/day for girls and 38 g/day for boys. Adolescents need 0.85 g protein per kilogram of body weight per day.

- Adequate calcium intake is critical to achieve peak bone density during adolescence. The RDA for calcium is 1,300 mg/day, a level higher than that for young children or adults. The RDA for iron is 11 mg/day for boys and 15 mg/day for girls. This level of iron intake supports increased blood volume and muscle mass in boys and girls, and replaces the iron lost in menstruation in girls. Vitamin A is critical to support tissue growth and development.

- Adolescent boys need about 11 cups of beverages daily, and girls need about 10 cups.

LO 7
- Although parents remain role models, adolescents are also influenced in their food choices by peer pressure, media, and personal preferences. Many adolescents replace whole grains, fruits, and vegetables with fast foods and high-fat/high-energy snack foods, placing themselves at risk for nutrient deficiencies as well as weight gain. On the other hand, many teens become preoccupied with maintaining a slender weight and begin to engage in disordered eating.

- Although there is no conclusive evidence linking dietary choices and adolescent acne, a high-glycemic-load diet might increase the prevalence and severity, whereas a low-glycemic-load diet might offer some protection. Substance abuse is a common concern among adolescents. Cigarette smoking and use of alcohol can interfere with nutrient metabolism, and increase the risk for certain cancers, and alcohol abuse is strongly linked to traumatic injury.

LO 8
- Obesity can begin to develop at any time from toddlerhood through adolescence. Currently, 32% of U.S. children and youth age 2 to 19 are overweight, and 17% are classified as obese.

- Pediatric obesity can exacerbate asthma; cause sleep apnea, musculoskeletal disorders, and fatty liver disease; and is associated with an increased risk for hypertension, type 2 diabetes, metabolic syndrome, depression, and other serious health problems. About 70% of obese children maintain their higher weight as adults.

- Obesity in children, as in adults, is multifactorial, resulting from a complex interaction of genetic, environmental, and sociocultural factors.

LO 9
- Families, schools, and communities can play important roles in encouraging smart food choices and increased physical activity. Families should make every attempt to share food shopping, preparation, serving, and family meals, sharing conversation and keeping the television off. Eating out should be avoided as much as possible. Parents should provide nutritious snacks.

- Nearly all public schools in the United States participate in the USDA's School Breakfast Program and National School Lunch Program. In addition, many school districts have embraced "garden-based learning," in which children grow their own produce, which is then used for cafeteria meals.

- Children should engage in an hour of aerobic activity each day, and strength-training at least 3 days a week. Parents should plan family physical activities such as hikes or bike rides, and encourage their children's participation in school sports. Budget cuts and an emphasis on academic success have caused many schools to reduce physical education classes, yet physical activity is associated with improved attention span and learning. Programs such as *We Can!* are helping schools develop physical activity programs for students.

LO 10
- Pediatric obesity treatment is commonly approached in stages. Stage 1 incorporates lifestyle modifications and behavioral therapy. Stages 2 and 3 continue these options, but with greater frequency and intensity, and typically with the involvement of additional nutrition or exercise specialists. Stage 4 may incorporate medication or surgery.

- The only FDA-approved medication for weight loss in pediatric patients (age 12 and older) is orlistat. Weight loss on this drug is only modest. More and more pediatricians are turning to bariatric surgery for their severely obese pediatric patients.

To further your understanding, go online and apply what you've learned to real-life case studies that will help you master the content!

review questions

LO 1 1. Toddlers need

  a. about 0.7 gram of protein per kilogram of body weight per day.
  b. about 70 grams of carbohydrate per day.
  c. about 7 mg of iron per day.
  d. about 7 cups of beverages per day.

LO 2 2. Which of the following breakfasts would be most appropriate to serve a 22-month-old child?

  a. 1 cup of oatmeal with 1 cup of skim milk and 2 tablespoons of mashed pineapple.
  b. 2 tablespoons of plain full-fat yogurt, 2 tablespoons of applesauce, 2 tablespoons of iron-fortified cooked cereal, and ½ cup of calcium-fortified orange juice.
  c. ½ cup of iron-fortified cooked cereal, ½ cup of cubed pineapple, and ½ cup of low-fat milk.
  d. two small link sausages cut in 1-inch pieces, two scrambled eggs, two slices of whole-wheat toast, two cherry tomatoes, and 1 cup of whole milk.

LO 3 3. Carbohydrate should make up what percentage of total energy for school-age children?

  a. 25% to 35%
  b. 35% to 45%
  c. 45% to 65%
  d. 55% to 75%

LO 4 4. Which of the following is a common nutrition-related concern for school-age children?

  a. inappropriately low fat intake
  b. food insecurity
  c. botulism
  d. vegetarian diets

LO 5 5. Which of the following statements about the School Breakfast Program and the National School Lunch Program is true?

  a. Under these programs, students must be offered both fruits and vegetables every day.
  b. Vending machines and other sources of competitive food are not allowed in schools participating in these programs.
  c. Under these programs, all children from food-insecure households qualify for free or reduced-cost meals.
  d. All of the above are true.

LO 6 6. The RDA for calcium for adolescents is

  a. less than that for young children.
  b. less than that for adults.

  c. less than that for pregnant adults.
  d. greater than that for young children, adults, and pregnant adults.

LO 7 7. Which of the following statements about cigarette smoking is true?

  a. Cigarette smoking can interfere with the metabolism of nutrients.
  b. Cigarette smoking commonly causes food cravings, such as "getting the munchies."
  c. The iPLEDGE program from the National Institutes of Health encourages adolescents to stop smoking.
  d. All of these statements are true.

LO 8 8. Which of the following statements about pediatric obesity is true?

  a. About 32% of U.S. children aged 2 to 19 years are classified as obese.
  b. Pediatric obesity increases a child's risk for liver disease and type 2 diabetes.
  c. Children whose parents are both overweight and obese are twice as likely to be overweight as those with no overweight or obese parent.
  d. Although toddlers may indeed be overweight, clinicians do not classify toddlers as obese.

LO 9 9. It's Saturday. What would be the most healthful option for the parents of 10-year-old Lyra and 8-year-old Lyla?

  a. Treat themselves and their daughters to a restaurant meal.
  b. Encourage their daughters to go out and play while they stay inside and clean the house.
  c. Take Lyra to a 30-minute skating lesson, and Lyla to a 30-minute session of karate.
  d. Take a one-hour hike together on a nearby trail popular with families.

LO 10 10. Kabir is only 7 years old, but he is severely obese (class 3) and has already developed type 2 diabetes. Fortunately, Kabir's family has excellent healthcare insurance and access to pediatric weight-loss specialists. Which of the following options would Kabir's healthcare team be most likely to include as part of his treatment plan?

  a. regular sessions with an exercise specialist
  b. the prescription drug orlistat
  c. the prescription drug metformin
  d. bariatric surgery

true or false?

LO 1 11. **True or false?** Toddlers need 30% to 40% of their total energy intake as fat.

LO 2 12. **True or false?** Toddlers are too young to understand and be influenced by the examples of their parents.

LO 5 13. **True or false?** Participation in the School Breakfast and National School Lunch Programs limits students' consumption of saturated and trans fats and sugar, and increases their intake of fruits and vegetables.

LO 6 14. **True or false?** Weight gain during adolescence is expected and healthful.

LO 9 15. **True or false?** National guidelines advise that all children and adolescents get 30 minutes of aerobic physical activity 3 to 4 days each week.

short answer

LO 2 16. Explain why a toddler in a vegan family might be at risk for protein deficiency.

LO 3 17. Imagine that you are taking care of four 5-year-old children for an afternoon. Design a menu for the children's lunch that is nutritious and that will be fun for them to eat.

LO 6 18. Imagine that you plan meals for a high school cafeteria. Design a menu with three lunch choices that are nutritious and that are likely to be popular with teens.

LO 7 19. Your classmate Lydia is a bit eccentric. An engineering major, she spends an average of 6

hours a day at her computer, drinking diet colas and eating pretzels. She is unusually slender, even though she admits to getting no regular exercise. Your university is in upstate New York, and Lydia is from Vermont. If you were a registered dietitian (RD) and Lydia were your client, what nutrition-related health concern(s) might you discuss with her? Identify *at least* three elements in Lydia's story that are known risk factors for the health problem(s) you identify.

LO 9 20. Identify some advantages and disadvantages of modern technology (such as television, smart phones, and computers) in terms of its impact on lifestyle and nutrition.

math review

LO 6 21. Your 16-year-old sister is following a vegan diet. Her RDA for calcium is 1,300 mg/day. If she ate a salad with two cups of raw spinach (115 mg calcium/cup), 2 ounces of firm tofu cubes

(50 mg/oz), and ¾ cup of calcium-fortified orange juice (300 mg/cup), would she meet one-third of her calcium RDA?

Answers to Review Questions and Math Review can be found online in the MasteringNutrition Study Area.

web links

http://www.nhlbi.nih.gov/health/educational/wecan/
We Can!
We Can! (Ways to Enhance Children's Activity & Nutrition) provides materials for families, schools, and healthcare providers to help children increase their physical activity, make healthy food choices, and achieve a healthy weight.

www.girlsontherun.org
Girls on the Run
Find out how to volunteer with a local chapter, or start a new one, to encourage young girls toward lifelong physical and emotional health.

http://www.vrg.org/family/kidsindex.htm
Vegetarian Resource Group
Visit the Vegetarian Resource Group's special section for teens and kids, and find information, videos, recipes, and guides for vegetarian and vegan diets.

www.choosemyplate.gov/kids/index.html
USDA MyPlate—Kid's Place
Games, videos and more for kids, recipes and more for families!

www.fns.usda.gov
USDA Food & Nutrition Services
Read about government programs to provide food to all ages, including school meal programs, the Child and Adult Care Food Program, and the Women, Infants, and Children program.

www.eatright.org
Academy of Nutrition and Dietetics
Visit this website to learn about healthy eating habits for all stages of life.

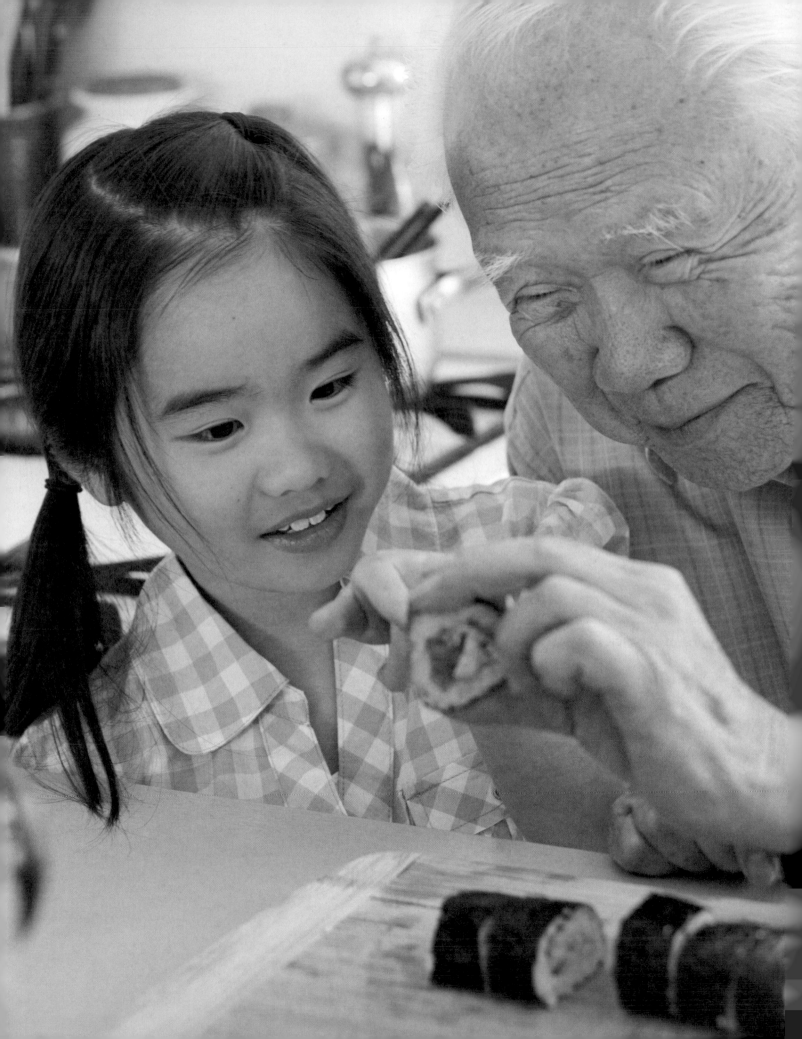

19 Nutrition Through the Life Cycle: The Later Years

Learning Objectives

After studying this chapter, you should be able to:

1 Describe the demographic changes related to the aging of America, *pp. 744–745.*

2 Summarize the programmed and error theories of human aging, *pp. 745–747.*

3 Identify several lifestyle choices that influence the rate at which we age, *pp. 747.*

4 Describe the most common physiologic changes that occur as we age, *pp. 748–752.*

5 Compare and contrast the requirements for energy and macronutrients among older adults versus younger adults, *pp. 752–753.*

6 Discuss micronutrient and fluid requirements for older adults and the benefits and risks of micronutrient supplements, *pp. 754–757.*

7 Identify and describe the range of nutrition-related concerns that threaten the health of older adults, *pp. 758–762.*

8 Describe potential interactions between certain medications and certain foods and nutrients, *pp. 762–763.*

9 Identify the social factors that can affect the nutrition of older adults, *pp. 764–765.*

10 Discuss the various community services and nutrition programs available to U.S. elderly, *pp. 765–767.*

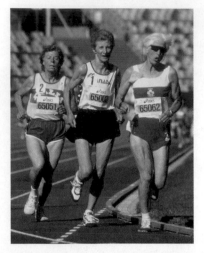

With the help of a nutritious diet and regular activity, many aging adults can remain highly active in their later years.

 LO 1 Describe the demographic changes related to the aging of America.

When Loretta finally retired from her job as a public school teacher at age 68, she looked forward to taking things a little easier. Then her daughter, Tina, a captain in the U.S. Army, was deployed overseas, leaving Tina's son, Chase, in his grandparents' care. Shortly after he moved in, Chase showed a budding interest in learning how to cook, so Loretta decided to enroll in a basic nutrition course at her local community college as a way to support Chase's new interest. When she arrived on campus, she was delighted to find that some of her fellow students were older than she was! Across the United States, colleges and universities are reporting a surge in the enrollment of older adults, some in their 80s and 90s. Many of these older students are fulfilling a lifelong dream of obtaining a college degree, whereas others, like Loretta, are taking classes for personal enrichment.

As our population continues to age, and seniors benefit from improvements in lifestyle and healthcare, life as an older adult now offers as many opportunities as challenges. Decades of research confirms the importance of a nutritious diet and regular physical activity in helping prevent or delay the onset of chronic disease, enhance productivity, and improve quality of life as we age. What are the unique nutritional needs and concerns of older adults? How can diet and lifestyle affect the aging process? These and other questions will be addressed in this chapter.

What Are the Demographics of Aging?

Before we discuss the nutrient needs and concerns of older adults, let's take a quick look at the statistics related to this population.

The American Population Is Aging

The U.S. population is getting older each year. It is estimated that in 2015, about 15% of the U.S. population was aged 65 and older, representing about 48 million people. By the year 2030, the elderly will account for nearly 21% of Americans or about 74 million. About 56% of older adults are female, a pattern that is expected to continue into the next few decades.[1] **Figure 19.1** illustrates the changing demographics of U.S. elderly.

The racial and ethnic profile of U.S. elderly continues to reflect the demographics of the country as a whole. Currently, about 20% of Americans over age 65 are minorities.[2] By the

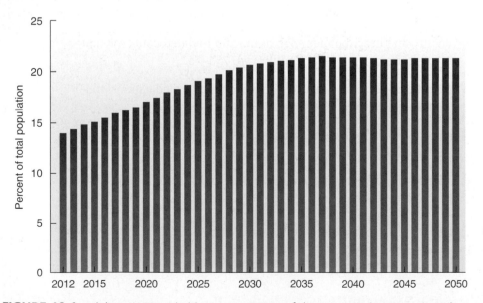

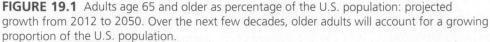

FIGURE 19.1 Adults age 65 and older as percentage of the U.S. population: projected growth from 2012 to 2050. Over the next few decades, older adults will account for a growing proportion of the U.S. population.

year 2050, it is estimated that nearly 40% of U.S. elderly will be racial and ethnic minorities. Much of the increase will come from an increase in the older Hispanic population.

Those 85 years and over, known as the "very elderly," currently represent the fastest-growing U.S. population subgroup, projected to increase from just over 6 million in 2015 to 9 million by the year 2030.[1] The number of *centenarians*, persons over the age of 100 years, and *supercentenarians*, over 110 years, continues to grow as well. In 2015, there were over 72,000 centenarians in the United States, a number that is expected to double by the year 2030![1] Most centenarians are female (83%), and 94% are between the ages of 100 and 104 years, with about 300 attaining supercentenarian status.[3]

Life Expectancy Is Increasing

U.S. **life expectancy,** or the expected number of years remaining in one's life, was about 47 years at birth in the year 1900. It has increased dramatically during the past century largely because of vaccination and other medical advances, better nutrition, and improved sanitation. It has now reached 78.8 years at birth for the population overall, or 76 years for males and 81 years for females.[4] Life expectancy for minority populations, however, is as much as 6 years less than for Caucasians, and U.S. life expectancy overall is below that of many other high-income countries.[5]

Life span is the age to which the longest-living member of the species has lived. Individual claims of longevity are very difficult to authenticate;[6] however, Madame Jeanne Calment, born in France in 1875, lived to the age of 122 and is generally viewed as achieving the oldest age in the world. Although some researchers have sought ways of extending human life span (see the *Nutrition Myth or Fact?* essay on energy-restricted diets at the end of this chapter), most agree that a life span beyond 125 to 130 years is unlikely.

For most older adults, the goal is not to live as long as possible but to live a life free of disability and disease for as long as possible. This concept of healthy longevity is often referred to as *active life expectancy,* or *health-related quality of life (HRQOL).* By most measures, the HRQOL of older Americans is improving. Older Americans are now healthier, more socially and physically active, and less likely to be confined to bed or have functional limitations than older adults living several decades ago. Many are choosing to work well beyond traditional retirement age, and increasing numbers are using the same technologies as their children and grandchildren.

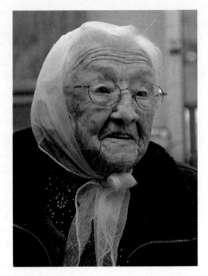

Centenarians represent the future of U.S. elderly.

 How many more years can you expect to live? Find out by using the Social Security Administration's life expectancy calculator at http://www .socialsecurity.gov/.

life expectancy The expected number of years remaining in one's life; typically stated from the time of birth. Children born in the United States in 2012 can expect to live, on average, 78.8 years.

life span The highest age reached by any member of a species; currently, the human life span is 122 years.

programmed theories of aging Aging is biologically determined, following a predictable pattern of physiologic changes, although the timing may vary from one person to another.

RECAP

In 2015, about 15% of the U.S. population was aged 65 and older, representing about 48 million people. The percentage of the population aged 65 and older is expected to increase in the coming years. Those 85 years and over represent the fastest growing population subgroup, and centenarians, persons over the age of 100 years, are a growing subgroup as well. About 300 Americans have reached supercentenarian status. U.S. life expectancy, the expected number of years remaining in one's life, reached 78.8 years for those born in the year 2012, or 76 years for males and 81 years for females. Life span is the age to which the longest-living member of the species has lived. The human life span is currently considered 122 years. ■

Why Do We Age?

Aging occurs at the molecular, cellular, and tissue levels. Although the process is natural and inevitable, much of the underlying physiology remains unknown; however, gerontologists agree that lifestyle choices influence the rate at which aging occurs.

Two Theories Attempt to Explain Aging

Theories attempting to explain the mechanisms of aging can be categorized into two lines of research (**Table 19.1**, page 746). First are the **programmed theories of aging,** proposing

LO 2 Summarize the programmed and error theories of human aging.

LO 3 Identify several lifestyle choices that influence the rate at which we age.

TABLE 19.1 Theories of Aging

Model	Description	Nutrition Interface
Programmed Theories of Aging	Aging follows a biologically driven time line, similar to that of adolescence.	None evident
Hayflick theory of aging	Cells have a limited reproductive life span. Each time a cell divides, the telomeres at the ends of its chromosomes shorten; thus, cells can divide only so many times.	None evident
Theory of programmed longevity	Aging occurs when certain genes are turned on or off; the activation or suppression of these genes then triggers age-related loss of function.	Indirectly, a diet rich in antioxidants, such as vitamins C and E, could lower free-radical damage to DNA.
Endocrine theory of aging	Senescence is due to hormonal changes, such as declines in growth hormone, DHEA, estrogen, and/or testosterone.	None directly evident
Immunologic theory of aging	Aging is linked to loss of immune system activity and/or an increase in autoimmune diseases.	Indirectly, adequate protein, zinc, iron, and vitamins A, C, and E help preserve immune function.
Error Theories of Aging	Senescence occurs as a result of cell and tissue damage caused largely by environmental insults.	Several theoretical benefits of nutrient adequacy or supplementation
Wear-and-tear theory	Over time, cells simply wear out and eventually die. The greater the exposure to toxins and stressors, the more rapid the rate of decline.	Protein, zinc, and vitamins A and C could theoretically delay the aging process by improving cellular repair and recovery.
Cross-linkage theory	Abnormal cross-linkages of proteins, such as collagen, damage cells and tissues, impairing the function of organs.	Glycosylation, the abnormal attachment of glucose to proteins, can be limited by controlling blood glucose levels. Adequate intakes of vitamin C, selenium, and copper may reduce other types of protein cross-linkages.
Free-radical theory	Senescence is due to the cumulative damage caused by various free radicals.	Diets and/or supplements rich in vitamins C and E, selenium, and antioxidant phytochemicals may limit the cellular accumulation of free radicals.
Rate-of-living theory	In general, the higher the species' average basal metabolic rate (BMR), the shorter its life span.	Theoretically, energy restriction would lower BMR and prolong life (see the **Nutrition Myth or Fact?** on pages 767–769).

that aging follows a biologically driven time line, similar to that of adolescence. For example, there is no doubt that genes exert tremendous influence on the aging process. Siblings of centenarians are four times more likely to live into their 90s than others. Researchers have even found a genetic mutation dubbed the "I'm Not Dead Yet" gene, which prolongs the life span of certain laboratory animals. Moreover, each time a cell divides, telomeres—regions of DNA at the very end of chromosomes—shorten. Telomeres that have shortened past a certain point are no longer able to divide. The cell becomes inactive, or dies. That said, researchers are still investigating the relationship between telomere length and aging.

The second category consists of the **error theories of aging,** which argue that aging occurs as a result of cell and tissue damage caused largely by environmental insults. These mechanisms include the following:

- As cells age, cell membrane function declines, allowing waste products to accumulate within the cell and decreasing normal uptake of nutrients and oxygen.
- Oxidative stress, as a result of the progressive accumulation of free radicals, is known to damage DNA and various cell proteins.
- Cellular aging has also been linked to a progressive failure in DNA repair. Throughout the life cycle, human DNA is subjected to various insults, including free radicals, toxins, and random coding errors. Normally, the cell detects and repairs damaged DNA. With aging, however, the repair process becomes less efficient, leading to abnormal protein synthesis.
- Finally, **glycosylation,** an abnormal attachment of glucose to proteins, results in loss of protein structure and function. As a result, lung tissue, blood vessels, and tendons become rigid and inflexible.

error theories of aging Aging is a cumulative process determined largely by exposure to environmental insults; the fewer the environmental insults, the slower the aging process.

glycosylation The addition of glucose to blood and tissue proteins; typically impairs protein structure and function.

Changes identified by the error theories of aging are directly or indirectly linked to nutrient or energy status. Thus, consumption of adequate levels of antioxidant nutrients could theoretically delay some of these changes while lifelong control of blood glucose levels would minimize abnormal glycosylation.

In truth, the programmed and error theories of aging are not mutually exclusive: it is likely that aging stems from a complex interplay of the factors identified in Table 19.1.

Some Lifestyle Factors Accelerate Aging

The way we live greatly influences the way we age. Whereas chronologic age is immovable, **biologic age** can be greatly influenced by personal choices. One of the most significant of these is smoking. In addition to causing a variety of cancers, smoking or exposure to secondhand smoke accelerates the aging process; inhalation of the variety of toxins found in smoke impairs lung function, damages the cardiovascular system, increases the risk for osteoporosis, and impairs taste and odor perception. Smoking also causes premature facial wrinkling and impairs dental health. Older adults should be reminded that it is never too late to quit; improvements in taste perception, physical endurance, and lung function can be detected within weeks of smoking cessation.

Excessive consumption of alcohol also speeds up the aging process by interfering with nutrient intake and utilization, injuring the liver, increasing risk for osteoporosis, and contributing to accidental injuries and deaths (see the In Depth coverage of alcohol, pages 152–163). These effects are cumulative over the years, so the earlier the alcohol abuse begins, the greater the damage to body systems.

Sunlight exposure is the primary risk factor for age-related discoloration and thinning of the skin, as well as skin cancer. Most healthcare providers recommend that, after an initial 20 minutes of sun exposure to allow for skin production of vitamin D, people apply sunscreen in order to limit sun-induced skin damage.

As you learned (in Chapter 13), obesity is not solely a matter of poor lifestyle choices. However, eating a nutritious, lower-energy diet and engaging in regular physical activity are choices within an individual's control that do promote a healthy weight. This is important, because obesity accelerates aging, in part because of its association with excessive blood glucose, which promotes glycosylation and prompts complications that seem to mimic the aging process. Obesity also accelerates age-related declines in cardiovascular health, speeds up the deterioration of joints, and increases the risk for certain cancers and numerous other disorders.[7]

Lack of physical activity in older adults accelerates loss of muscle mass and bone density, increases risk for falls, and is associated with significant mobility disability (inability to walk on one's own), all of which greatly reduces the ability to live independently and maintain a high quality of life during later life.[8] Physical inactivity also increases risk of depression and contributes to loss of cognitive function in older adults, even among older adults already experiencing mild cognitive impairment.[9]

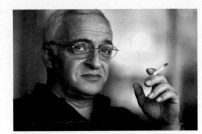

Older adults who smoke should remember that it's never too late to quit, and significant health improvements can manifest within weeks of quitting.

RECAP

Much of the underlying physiology of aging remains unknown; however, two lines of research dominate. The programmed theories of aging propose that aging follows a biologically driven time line determined, to a great extent, by the DNA we inherit from our parents and by the normal and inevitable shortening of telomeres at the ends of chromosomes each time a cell divides. In contrast, the error theories of aging argue that aging occurs as a result of cell and tissue damage caused largely by environmental insults that reduce cell membrane function, promote oxidative stress, inhibit DNA repair, and promote glycosylation, an abnormal attachment of glucose to body proteins. Factors that strongly accelerate biological aging include smoking, excessive consumption of alcohol, excessive exposure to sunlight, obesity, and lack of physical activity.

biologic age Physiologic age as determined by health and functional status; often estimated by scored questionnaires.

LO 4 Describe the most common physiologic changes that occur as we age.

How Do We Age?

Some age-related changes, such as thinning of hair, don't affect body functioning. Others, such as loss of bone density and muscle tissue, clearly do. **Senescence** is a term encompassing the age-related processes that increase risk for disability, disease, and death. If the following discussion of senescence seems disturbing or depressing, remember that the changes described are at least partly within an individual's control. For instance, some of the decrease seen in bone and muscle mass is due to low physical activity levels. Older adults who regularly participate in strengthening exercises and aerobic-type activities reduce their risks for low bone mass and muscle atrophy, which in turn reduces their risk for falls.

Sensory Perception Declines

Odor, taste, and visual perception, which are closely linked to appetite, all decline with age. As they do, an older adult's food intake and nutritional status can decline as well.

More than half of elderly adults and up to 80% of those age 80 years and up experience significant loss of olfactory (odor) perception. This condition is more common than loss of taste perception, although "successfully aged" older adults experience less of a decline.[10] The enjoyment of food relies heavily on the sense of smell: think of your own response to the aroma of bread baking in the oven. Older adults who cannot adequately appreciate the appealing aromas of food may be unable to fully enjoy the foods offered within the meal. Loss of olfaction also restricts the ability to detect spoiled food, increasing the risk for food poisoning.[11] Although often a simple consequence of aging, loss of odor perception can also be caused by zinc deficiency or can occur as a side effect of medication. If this is the case, a zinc supplement or change of medication may be a simple solution.

With increasing age, taste perception dims as well. This is one reason older adults seem to add so much salt to their foods or complain about the blandness of their foods. The ability to perceive sweetness and sourness also declines, but to a lesser extent.[12] Some elderly experience **dysgeusia,** or abnormal taste perception, which can be caused by disease or medication use.

Loss of visual acuity has unexpected consequences for the nutritional health of the elderly. Many older adults have difficulty reading food labels, including nutrient information. Driving skills decline, limiting the ability of some older Americans to acquire healthy, affordable foods. Older adults with vision loss may not be able to see the temperature knobs on stoves or the controls on microwave ovens and may therefore choose cold meals, such as sandwiches, rather than meals that require heating. The visual appeal of a colorful, attractively arranged plate of food is also lost to visually impaired elderly, further reducing their desire to eat healthful meals.

Friends and family members can help older adults adjust to these sensory losses by encouraging appropriate food selections and preparation techniques. Flavor enhancers such as herbs and spices, meat concentrates, and sauces can increase the desirability of otherwise bland foods. Visual enhancements such as brightly colored garnishes and an array of different shapes on the plate can also make meals more appealing.

Gastrointestinal Function Changes

Significant changes in the mouth and gastrointestinal tract occur with aging. Some of these changes have the potential to increase the risk for nutrient deficiency.

With increasing age, salivary production declines. In older adults with **xerostomia,** teeth are more susceptible to decay, chewing and swallowing become more difficult, and taste perception declines.[13] Risk for fungal infections, such as candidiasis, increases. A diet rich in moist foods, including fruits and vegetables, sauces or gravies on meats, and high-fluid desserts such as puddings, is well tolerated by older adults with xerostomia. In the most severe cases, older adults can use an artificial saliva, which is sprayed into the mouth.

As people age, their ability to smell foods often declines.

senescence The progressive deterioration of bodily functions over time, resulting in increased risk for disability, disease, and death.

dysgeusia Abnormal taste perception.

xerostomia Dry mouth due to decreased saliva production.

Some older adults, including those with Parkinson's disease, experience **dysphagia** (difficulty swallowing foods). Smooth, thick foods, such as cream soups, are easy to swallow, but foods with mixed textures, such as gelatin with fruit pieces, should be avoided. Milkshakes and other thick beverages are better tolerated than thin liquids. Dysphagia requires professional assessment and treatment, drawing on the expertise of an occupational therapist, a physician, and a dietitian. If not accurately diagnosed and treated, dysphagia can lead to malnutrition, inappropriate weight loss, aspiration of food or fluid into the lungs, and pneumonia.

Older adults are at risk for reduced gastric secretion of hydrochloric acid (HCl), intrinsic factor, pepsin, and mucus. HCl and intrinsic factor are secreted by the parietal cells of the gastric glands. **Achlorhydria,** a severe reduction in HCl production, limits the absorption of minerals, such as calcium, iron, and zinc, and food sources of folic acid and vitamin B_{12}. Lack of intrinsic factor reduces the absorption of vitamin B_{12} and leads to pernicious anemia (see Chapter 12, page 485). These elderly, therefore, benefit from vitamin B_{12} supplements and/or injections. Older adults may also experience a delay in gastric emptying, resulting in a prolonged sense of fullness and a reduced appetite. Although this may be viewed as a positive factor in people who are overweight or obese, it can lead to inappropriate weight loss.

There is increasing evidence that the gut microbiota of the elderly differs from that of younger adults, with important health implications.[14] Microbes in the gut digest fibers; produce short-chain fatty acids, which provide anti-inflammatory effects; and reduce the ability of pathogenic microorganisms to flourish. Age-related changes in dietary patterns, medication usage, and other lifestyle factors contribute to a reduction in the biodiversity of gut microbiota, a decrease in protective bacteria, and an increase in pathogenic bacteria. The onset of the "aging gut" appears to be highly individualized and difficult to predict. The potential consequences, however, are clear: an increased inflammatory state, decreased immune functioning of the intestinal tract, and impaired functioning of the gut mucosal cells.

Recent research suggests that age-related changes in the release of appetite-regulating gut hormones may contribute to a condition known as "anorexia of aging." Many elderly people report feeling less hunger and an increased sense of satiety, both of which contribute to inappropriately low food intake. Some studies suggest that the release of anorexigenic or satiety-inducing hormones such as cholecystokinin (CCK) is increased, and that of hunger-inducing ghrelin is decreased. These alterations would shift the regulation of appetite such that food intake would decline.

Compared to younger adults, the healthy elderly demonstrate no significant loss in digestive enzyme activity, the ability to absorb nutrients, or intestinal motility. Therefore, healthy elderly people generally digest and absorb protein, fat, and carbohydrate as efficiently as younger adults. The one exception is the digestion of lactose: only about 30% of older adults retain an "adequate" level of lactase enzyme activity. Thus, many older adults need to restrict their fluid milk intake to ½-cup servings, use lactose-reduced milk or lactase enzyme supplements, or eliminate milk from their diet entirely. To meet their need for calcium, older adults can also consume calcium-fortified milk alternatives and fruit juices; fortified breakfast cereals; calcium-enriched tofu; and leafy green vegetables.

Body Composition Changes

With aging, body fat increases and muscle mass declines. It has been estimated that women and men lose 20% to 25% of their lean body mass, respectively, as they age from 30 to 70 years. Decreased production of certain hormones, including testosterone and growth hormone, and chronic diseases contribute to this loss of muscle, as do poor diet and an inactive lifestyle. In a large sample of U.S. older (60 years and above) adults, 35% of women and 75% of men were diagnosed with **sarcopenia,** an age-related, progressive loss of muscle mass, strength, and function.[15] Many adults with sarcopenia are so weak that they

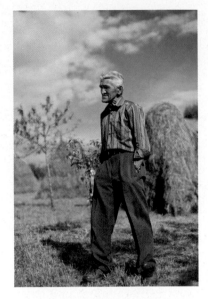

A variety of gastrointestinal and other physiologic changes can lead to weight loss in older adults.

dysphagia Abnormal swallowing.

achlorhydria Severely reduced hydrochloric acid secretion by the parietal cells of the stomach.

sarcopenia Age-related, progressive loss of muscle mass, muscle strength, and muscle function.

are unable to rise from a seated position, climb stairs, or carry a bag of groceries. Sarcopenia has also been found to increase risk of death in older adults.[15] Along with adequate dietary intake, regular physical activity, including strength or resistance training, can help older adults maintain their muscle mass and strength, delaying or preventing the need for institutionalization.

Body fat increases from young adulthood through middle age, peaking at approximately 55 to 65 years of age. Females experience a sharper increase in percent body fat compared to males. At the same time, body fat shifts from subcutaneous stores, just below the skin, to internal or visceral fat stores. This shift, which tends to be more pronounced in males, coincides with an increased risk for heart disease, diabetes, and metabolic syndrome[16] as well as functional impairments and all-cause mortality. Maintaining an appropriate energy intake and remaining physically active can help keep body fat, particularly abdominal fat, to a healthful level.

An increasing number of elderly are at risk for **sarcopenic obesity,** which is strongly associated with atherosclerosis, insulin resistance, and metabolic syndrome, as well as frailty, disability, and inability to perform normal activities of daily living.[17] While total body weight and body fat are increased in these persons, their underlying muscle mass and strength are not adequate in amount or functionality to support normal mobility and health. An increased protein intake (up to 1.5 g/kg/d for malnourished and at-risk older adults) and daily physical activity could minimize or reverse sarcopenic obesity.[17]

Bone mineral density declines with age and may eventually drop to the critical fracture zone. Among older women, the onset of menopause leads to a sudden and dramatic loss of bone due to the lack of estrogen (**Figure 19.2**). Although less dramatic, elderly males also experience loss of bone, due in part to decreasing levels of testosterone. (The nutrients recognized as essential to optimal bone health are identified in Chapter 11.) As noted in the nearby *Highlight*, seniors can help to preserve their bone health by engaging in regular weight-bearing activity well into their 90s and beyond.

Changes in Tissues and Organs Reduce Functioning

sarcopenic obesity A condition in which increased body weight and body fat mass coexist with inappropriately low muscle mass and strength.

Aged organs are less adaptable to environmental or physiologic stressors. Young adults, for example, readily adapt to varying fluid and sodium intakes because of the kidney's ability to maintain fluid balance. With increasing age, however, the kidneys lose their ability to concentrate waste products, leading to an increase in urine output and greater risk for dehydration. The aging liver is less efficient at breaking down drugs and alcohol, and

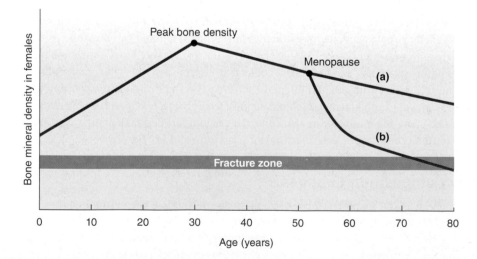

FIGURE 19.2 Bone mineral density in women tends to decline with aging. **(a)** A healthful lifestyle, an optimal diet, physical activity, and possible use of medication slow loss of bone. **(b)** The rapid loss of estrogen with menopause can cause a decrease in bone density and increased risk for bone fracture for women who do not adhere to a regimen of healthful lifestyle, diet, physical activity, and possibly medication.

HIGHLIGHT

Seniors on the Move

Relatively few older adults participate in regular leisure-time physical activity. Yet, for a minor investment of time and energy, older adults reap benefits worth literally thousands of dollars in reduced healthcare costs. A regular program of physical activity lowers the risk for heart disease, hypertension, type 2 diabetes, obesity, certain cancers, depression, mobility disability, and cognitive impairment.[1-3] The complications of arthritis can also be reduced with appropriate exercise, as can the risk for falls, bone fractures, and functional impairment. A recent study concluded that increased physical activity in elderly men was as beneficial as smoking cessation in reducing mortality.[4]

Older adults should plan an activity program that includes four basic types of exercises:

- **Flexibility exercises.** These activities set the stage for other forms of exercise by stretching the muscles and improving range of motion. Gentle arm swings, ankle circles, and torso twists are examples of moves that can slowly increase flexibility while sitting in a chair, standing, or even while in a shallow pool. Ideally, older adults should stretch every day of the week.

- **Balance exercises.** Balance is important in reducing the risk for falls. Older adults should also have confidence in their ability to maintain balance before starting strength or endurance exercises. Toe raises, side leg raises, and rear leg swings are examples of balance activities; tai chi is another popular way to improve balance. Older adults should practice balance activities daily.

- **Strength or resistance training.** This type of activity can increase muscle mass and strength as well as enhance bone density, preserving the ability of older adults to maintain an independent lifestyle. Gains in muscle strength also improve balance and provide the foundation for endurance exercise.

- **Endurance or aerobic exercise.** Activities should be low impact to protect aging bones and joints, including brisk walking, bicycle riding, swimming, and dancing in order to increase heart rate and improve cardiorespiratory function.

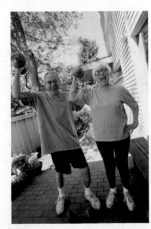

The recommendations of the 2008 Physical Activity Guidelines (see Chapter 14) for frequency and duration of activity apply.

Some seniors are vulnerable to exercise-related complications, such as dehydration, heat stress, fractures, or falls. Exercise rooms should offer appropriate temperature, ventilation and lighting, and supervised warm-up and cool-down periods should be incorporated into each activity. A thorough medical exam is advised prior to the start of programmed exercise.

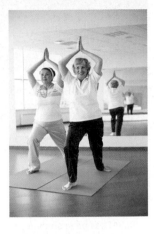

In addition to the benefits of purposeful exercise, there is growing evidence that nonexercise physical activity such as housework and gardening improves blood lipid profile, reduces blood insulin and glucose levels, and lowers the risk of metabolic syndrome, as well as reducing all-cause mortality.[5,6] The greater the time spent in sedentary behavior, the higher the risk of disability and disease.[7]

In short, for older adults, the benefits of regular physical activity, as vigorous as possible, almost always far outweigh potential risks, and promote a longer, happier life!

References

1. Taylor, D. 2014. Physical activity is medicine for older adults. *Postgrad. Med.* 90:26–32.
2. Fiatarone, S. M. A., N. Gates, N. Saigal, G. C. Wilson, J. Meiklejohn, H. Brodaty,..., and M. Valenzuela. 2014. The study of Mental and Resistance Training (SMART) study—resistance training and/or cognitive training in mild cognitive impairment: a randomized, double-blind, double-sham controlled trial. *J. Am. Med. Dir. Assoc.* 15:873–880.
3. Lee, I-M., E. J. Shiroma, F. Lobelo, P. Puska, S. N. Blair, P. T. Katzmarzyk, for the Lancet Physical Activity Series Working Group. 2012. Effect of physical inactivity on major non-communicable diseases worldwide: an analysis of burden of disease and life expectancy. *The Lancet* 380:219–229.
4. Holme, I., and S. A. Anderssen. 2015. Increases in physical activity is as important as smoking cessation for reduction in total mortality in elderly men: 12 years of follow-up of the Oslo II study. *Brit. J. Sports Med.* 49:743–748.
5. Ekblom-Bak, E., B. Ekblom, M. Vikström, U. de Faire, and M. L. Hellénius. 2014. The importance of non-exercise physical activity for cardiovascular health and longevity. *Brit. J. Sports Med.* 48:233–238.
6. Hamer, M., C. de Oliveira, and P. Demakakos. 2014. Non-exercise physical activity and survival: English Longitudinal Study of Aging. *Am. J. Prev. Med.* 47:452–460.
7. Blodgett, J., O. Theou, S. Kirkland, P. Andreou, and K. Rockwood. 2015. The association between sedentary behavior, moderate-vigorous physical activity and frailty in NHANES cohorts. *Maturitas* 80:187–191.

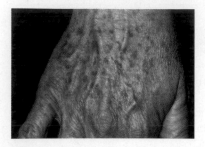

Lifelong exposure to sunlight can lead to discoloration and thinning of the skin in old age.

Since 1958, the National Institute on Aging's Baltimore Longitudinal Study on Aging (BLSA) has been studying what happens as we age. Watch a 7-minute video introduction to the BLSA at https://www.blsa.nih.gov/.

the aging heart lacks the endurance to sustain a sudden increase in physical activity. The pancreas is less precise in regulating blood glucose levels, and bladder control may decline with aging. In most instances, older adults can adapt to these age-related changes through minor lifestyle adjustments, such as eating meals and snacks on a regular basis and ensuring an adequate fluid intake.

As a result of abnormal protein cross-linkages, connective tissues and blood vessels become increasingly stiff. Joint pain, elevated blood pressure, and impaired blood flow are typical consequences. The skin of older adults can become thin, dry, and fragile. Bruises and skin tears are very common and are slow to heal. The growth of nails slows and hair loss is common among elderly males and females. Although some of these consequences are simply cosmetic and represent no disease risk, the skin's tendency to bruise and tear may increase the risk for infection. A diet rich in vitamins C and A, zinc, copper, and protein may reduce the severity of bruising in some elderly.

The number of neurons in the brain decreases with age, impairing memory, reflexes, coordination, and learning ability. Whereas some believe that dementia is an inevitable part of the aging process, this is not true. As we discuss shortly, a healthful diet, regular physical activity, social interaction, intellectual stimulation, and other lifestyle choices can promote cognitive functioning.

RECAP

With aging, sensory perception declines. A diminished or altered ability to smell, taste, and properly see foods—such as dysgeusia, abnormal taste perception—can lead to reduced food intake and malnourishment. Xerostomia, a dry mouth due to decreased production of saliva, can also reduce food intake or contribute to dysphagia, difficulty in swallowing. Older adults are also at risk for achlorhydria, reduced gastric secretion of hydrochloric acid, and for insufficient production of intrinsic factor and delayed gastric emptying. These can affect nutrient status. The "aging gut" may also be characterized by reduced biodiversity of gut microbiota, hormonal changes that contribute to the "anorexia of aging," and lactose intolerance. Body composition changes include loss of muscle mass and bone density, and increased fat mass along with a shift in fat tissue from subcutaneous to visceral stores. Body tissues and organs can lose functional capacity and become less tolerant of stressors. These age-related changes influence the nutritional needs of older adults and their ability to consume a healthful diet. ∎

LO 5 Compare and contrast the requirements for energy and macronutrients among older adults versus younger adults.

LO 6 Discuss micronutrient and fluid requirements for older adults and the benefits and risks of micronutrient supplements.

What Are an Older Adult's Nutrient Needs?

The requirements for many nutrients are the same for older adults as for young and middle-aged adults. A few nutrient requirements increase, and a few are actually lower. **Table 19.2** identifies those recommendations that change with age, as well as the physiologic reason behind these changes.

Older Adults Have Lower Energy Needs

The energy needs of older adults are lower than those of younger adults, because loss of muscle mass and lean tissue results in a lower basal metabolic rate, and most older adults have a less physically active lifestyle. It is estimated that total daily energy expenditure decreases approximately 10 kcal each year for men and 7 kcal each year for women ages 19 and older. This means that a woman who needed 2,000 kcal at age 20 needs just 1,650 kcal at age 70. Some of this decrease in energy expenditure is in response to age-related decreases in muscle mass, but some of the decrease can be delayed or minimized by staying physically active.

Because their total daily energy needs are lower, older adults need to pay particularly close attention to consuming a diet high in nutrient-dense foods but not too high in energy

TABLE 19.2 Nutrition Recommendations That Change with Increased Age

Changes in Nutrient Recommendations	Rationale for Changes
Increased need for vitamin D from 600 IU/day for adults up to age 70, to 800 IU/day for adults over 70	■ Decreased bone density ■ Decreased ability to synthesize vitamin D in the skin
Increased need for calcium from 1,000 mg/day for all adults up to age 51 and males 51–70 years of age to 1,200 mg/day for females 51 years of age and older and males over age 70 years	■ Decreased absorption of dietary calcium ■ Decreased bone density (earlier onset in women)
Decreased need for fiber from 38 g/day for males up to age 51 to 30 g/day for males 51 and older; decreases for females are from 25 g/day for females up to age 51 to 21 g/day for females 51 and older	■ Decreased energy intake
Increased need for vitamin B_6 in both males and females from 1.3 mg/day up to age 51 to 1.7 mg/day in males and 1.5 mg/day in females age 51 and older; need for vitamin B_{12} *from fortified foods or supplements,* as opposed to foods of animal origin	■ Increased need for these vitamins to maintain blood levels adequate to reduce homocysteine levels and to optimize immune function ■ Lower levels of stomach acid ■ Decreased absorption of food B_{12} from gastrointestinal tract
Decreased need for iron for females, from 18 mg/day up to age 51 to 8 mg/day for females 51 and older; no change in 8 mg/day iron recommendations for males	■ Cessation of menstruation in women; some loss of muscle and lean tissue in men and women

in order to avoid weight gain. The USDA MyPlate model can be adapted to reflect the needs of older adults and help guide their food choices (**Figure 19.3**, page 754).

Macronutrient Recommendations Are Similar for Adults of All Ages

Because there is no evidence identifying a minimal amount of dietary fat needed to maintain health, there is no RDA for total fat intake for adults.[18] However, to reduce the risk for heart disease and other chronic diseases, it is recommended that total fat intake remain within 20% to 35% of total daily energy intake, with no more than 10% of total energy intake coming from saturated fat. Dietary sources of *trans* fatty acids should be kept to a minimum.

The RDA for carbohydrate for adults of all ages is 130 g/day, an amount sufficient to support glucose utilization by the brain.[18] There is no evidence to indicate what percentage of carbohydrate should come from sugars or starches. However, it is recommended that older individuals consume a diet that contains no more than 25% of total energy intake as sugars.[18]

The fiber recommendations are slightly lower for older adults than for younger adults, because older adults consume less energy. After age 50, 30 g of fiber per day for men and 21 g per day for women is assumed sufficient to reduce the risks for constipation and diverticular disease, maintain healthful blood levels of glucose and lipids, and provide good sources of nutrient-dense, low-energy foods.[18]

The RDA for protein is also the same for adults of all ages: 0.8 g of protein per kilogram of body weight per day.[18] Many researchers argue for a higher protein allowance of up to 1.2 g/kg/day for older adults in order to optimize protein status and, in combination with physical activity, blunt age-related losses in muscle mass and function.[19–21] Protein is also important for maintaining immunity, enhancing wound healing and disease recovery, and helping prevent excessive loss of bone. Protein-rich foods are important sources of vitamins and minerals that are typically low in the diets of older adults, including iron, zinc, and certain B-vitamins. There is growing evidence of the importance of the distribution of protein throughout the day.[22,23] Instead of consuming most of their daily protein intake at dinner, older adults may benefit from consuming at least 20 g protein at each meal.[22]

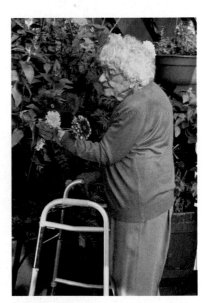

A less physically active lifestyle leads to lower total energy requirements in older adults.

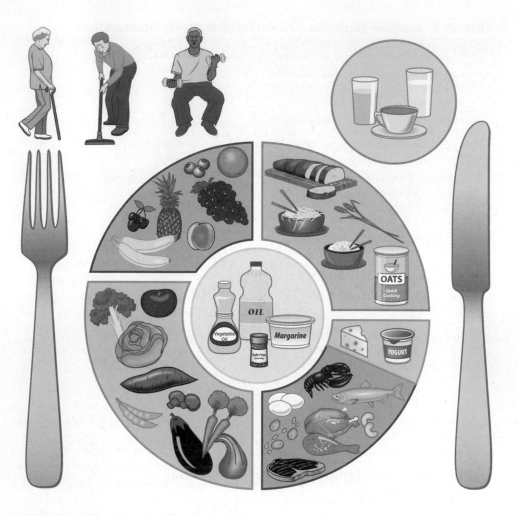

FIGURE 19.3 This adaptation of the USDA MyPlate illustrates healthful food and fluid choices for older adults.

Some Micronutrient Recommendations Vary for Older Adults

The vitamins and minerals of particular concern for older adults are identified in Table 19.2.

Vitamin D and Calcium

Adequate vitamin D status is critical for preventing or minimizing the consequences of osteoporosis among older adults as well as optimizing immunity, the cardiovascular system, muscle and pancreatic function, and possibly even mental health.[24,25] A deficiency of this nutrient is associated with increased risk for cognitive impairment, falls, and overall mortality. The requirement for vitamin D is higher than for younger adults because of an age-related reduction in the production of vitamin D in the skin and a decrease in the absorption of dietary vitamin D.[25] An increasing number of older adults are at risk for vitamin D deficiency because they are institutionalized and are not exposed to adequate amounts of sunlight. Older adults living in the community are also at risk for vitamin D deficiency due to the widespread use of sunscreen.

The RDA for calcium is higher for all adults over the age of 70 years and for women aged 51 to 70 years compared to younger adults. The calcium requirement increases at an earlier age for women compared to men due to the earlier onset of bone loss, typically at the onset of menopause.[26]

It is critical that older adults consume foods that are high in calcium and vitamin D and, when needed, use supplements providing both nutrients in appropriate amounts and under the guidance of a healthcare provider.

Iron and Zinc

Iron needs decrease with aging as a result of reduced muscle mass in both men and women and the cessation of menstruation in women. The decreased need for iron in older men is not significant enough to change the recommendations for iron intake in this group; thus, the RDA for iron is the same for older men as for younger, 8 mg/day. The RDA for iron in older women is also 8 mg/day, but this represents a significant decrease from the 18 mg/day RDA for younger women.[27]

Although zinc recommendations are the same for all adults, zinc is especially critical for optimizing immune function and wound healing in older adults. Intakes of both zinc and iron can be inadequate in older adults if they do not regularly eat red meats, poultry, and/or fish. These foods are relatively expensive, and older adults on a limited income may not be able to afford to eat them regularly. Also, the loss of teeth or use of dentures may increase the difficulty of chewing meats. Although legumes such as black or pinto beans also provide zinc and iron, they are absorbed at a much lower rate. Finally, age-related impairments in absorption and transport of these minerals can contribute to a deficient state.

Vitamins C and E

The recommendations for vitamin C and vitamin E intakes are the same as for younger adults; however, researchers continue to investigate the potential benefits of dietary or supplemental vitamin C in lowering the risk for hypertension, impaired physical performance, and other age-related health problems.[28] Vitamin E also continues to be evaluated for its potential to reduce risk for bone fractures[29], cataracts[30], age-related macular degeneration, and other forms of oxidative stress.

B-Vitamins

Vitamin B_6 recommendations are slightly higher for adults age 51 and older.[31] The increased requirement is based on data indicating that more vitamin B_6 is required to maintain normal vitamin B_6 status as we age. These higher amounts appear necessary to reduce homocysteine levels and optimize attentiveness and cognition, as well as decrease risk for depression.

The RDA for vitamin B_{12} is the same for younger and older adults; however, up to 30% of older adults experience atrophic gastritis and cannot absorb enough vitamin B_{12} from foods. It is therefore recommended that older adults consume foods that are fortified with vitamin B_{12} or take B_{12} supplements, because the vitamin B_{12} in these products is absorbed more readily.[31] As many as 40% of older adults are deficient in vitamin B_{12}, with the highest incidence among institutionalized elderly. It has been recommended that all older adults admitted for psychiatric and/or cognitive disorders be screened for vitamin B_{12} deficiency.[32]

Vitamin A

Vitamin A requirements are the same for adults of all ages; however, older adults should be careful not to consume more than the RDA, as absorption of vitamin A is actually greater in older adults. The consequences of vitamin A toxicity in the elderly can be significant: liver damage, neurologic problems, and increased risk for hip fracture.[27] Consuming foods high in beta-carotene or other carotenoids is safe and does not lead to vitamin A toxicity. In fact, increased intakes of lutein and zeaxanthin, two common carotenoids, reduce risk for late-onset age-related macular degeneration.[33]

Do Older Adults Need Micronutrient Supplements?

A variety of factors may limit an older adult's ability to eat healthfully. Limited financial resources may prevent some older people from buying nutrient-dense foods on a regular basis; others may experience reduced appetite, social isolation, inability to prepare foods, or illnesses that limit nutrient absorption and metabolism. Older women are at greater risk for inadequate micronutrient intake compared to older men, likely due to their smaller food intake. Thus, many older adults do benefit from taking a multivitamin/multimineral (MVMM) supplement that contains no more than the RDA for each nutrient. Healthcare providers typically encourage use of these supplements under the following conditions:

- When the amount and/or variety of food is so restricted that nutrient intake is probably deficient

- If the older adult eats fewer than two meals per day or limits food choices because of dental problems
- Whenever there are lifestyle or functional limitations that prevent adequate food intake
- If the older adult suffers from depression, dementia, social isolation, or extreme poverty
- If the older adult has a disease that impairs nutrient status or that could be relieved by nutrient supplementation
- If the older adult has osteoporosis, gastrointestinal diseases, or anemia

Additional single-nutrient supplements, especially for vitamin B_{12}, may also be prescribed. In establishing the DRI for vitamin B_{12} for men and women over the age of 50 years, the Institute of Medicine stated, "It is advisable for most of this amount to be obtained by consuming foods fortified with B_{12} or a B_{12} containing supplement."[31] This is the first time that the Institute of Medicine specifically acknowledged and supported the use of a nutrient supplement as an adjunct to a healthful diet. Many healthcare providers also recommend routine use of calcium and vitamin D supplements.

High-potency single-nutrient supplements can pose risks to the elderly. Older adults are more vulnerable to high-potency vitamin A supplements than younger adults, especially if they abuse alcohol. Vitamin D is also extremely toxic at high levels of intake, and megadoses of vitamin C can produce diarrhea and cramping. Inappropriate supplementation with iron leads to its accumulation in the liver, pancreas, and other soft tissues, particularly in middle-aged and older men and has been associated with an increased mortality rate.[34] In short, older adults should avoid high-potency single-nutrient supplements unless they have been prescribed. The nearby *Highlight* explains the formulation of commercial MVMM supplements designed specifically for older adults.

Fluid Recommendations Are the Same for All Adults

The AI for fluid is the same for all adults.[35] Men should consume 3.7 L (about 15.5 cups) of total water per day, which includes 3.0 L (about 13 cups) as total beverages, including drinking water. Women should consume 2.7 L (about 12.7 cups) of total water per day, which includes 2.2 L (about 9 cups) as total beverages, including drinking water.

In general, the elderly do not perceive thirst as effectively as do younger adults. In addition, their kidneys have a reduced ability to concentrate waste products, leading to an increase in urine output. Also, some older adults intentionally limit their beverage intake because they have urinary incontinence or do not want to be awakened for nighttime urination, often because their mobility is limited, making it difficult to reach the bathroom. Thus, older adults are at increased risk for chronic dehydration and hypernatremia (elevated blood sodium levels).[35] Chronic dehydration increases the risk for kidney stones, urinary tract infection, dizziness and falls, and various aspects of cognition and mood. Therefore, it is important for incontinent adults to seek treatment, and for all older adults to drink adequate amounts of fluids. Older adults may need visual and/or verbal reminders in order to maintain adequate fluid intake, such as providing two thermos bottles that must be consumed by the end of the day.

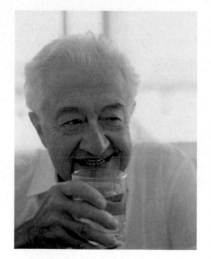

Older adults need the same amount of fluid as other adults.

RECAP

Older adults have lower energy needs due to their loss of lean tissue and lower physical activity levels. They should consume 20% to 35% of total energy as fat and 45% to 65% as carbohydrate. Their RDA for carbohydrate remains the same as for younger adults. The RDA for protein is also the same as for younger adults, although some research suggests the need for higher intakes of up to 1.2 g/kg/day to preserve muscle mass and function. Micronutrients of concern for older adults include calcium, zinc, vitamin D, and vitamins B_6 and B_{12}. Older adults should not consume more than the RDA for vitamin A because it can readily reach toxic levels. Many older adults benefit from taking a multivitamin/multimineral supplement; however, single-nutrient supplements should be avoided unless prescribed by their healthcare provider. A reduced thirst mechanism makes older adults at increased risk for chronic dehydration and hypernatremia, so ample fluid intake should be encouraged.

HIGHLIGHT

Supplements for Seniors

Older adults looking for a "simple" multivitamin–multimineral (MVMM) supplement have dozens of options, including products formulated specifically for seniors. How do these senior ("silver") products differ from other MVMM products? Are they actually better for seniors or just a marketing ploy?

Although every product line has its own formulation, a side-by-side comparison of the nutrients in one typical "adult" MVMM supplement with those in a "senior" MVMM product from the same manufacturer reveals very few differences. Of the 33 nutrients in the adult product, 2 (iron and tin) are omitted from the senior supplement, 1 (vitamin K) is provided at a lower dosage, 3 (calcium and vitamins E and B_6) are included at slightly higher levels, and 1 (vitamin B_{12}) is four times higher. Why?

Although the DRI for vitamin E does not change for males or females aged 19 to 70 years or above, there is good evidence that older adults are often in a state of "oxidative stress." Chronic inflammation, as occurs with arthritis and other conditions, is more common among older adults than younger populations and may increase the need for antioxidants, such as vitamin E. In addition, as previously discussed, there is preliminary, but inconsistent, research supporting the use of vitamin E in lowering the risk for age-associated eye disorders and dementia. Knowing that vitamin E has a relatively low risk for toxicity, the small increase provided in the senior supplement certainly poses no harm.

As with vitamin E, the DRI for vitamin K does not change with increased age. Why, then, does the senior supplement provide a lower dose? Persons on anticoagulant drugs, many of them elderly, are advised to tightly regulate vitamin K intake. By minimizing the amount of vitamin K in the senior supplement, there is less risk for a negative drug–nutrient interaction among seniors taking both the MVMM supplement and anticoagulant drugs. Some physicians might consider even 13% of the vitamin K Daily Value to be too much, so it would be important for each senior to check with his or her doctor before using a MVMM with any vitamin K.

Although the senior supplement provides about 40 mg more calcium than the more general adult product,

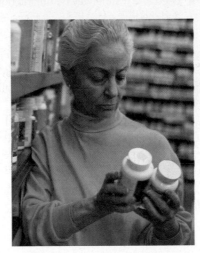
Many supplements are targeted for the elderly.

that amount does not go very far toward satisfying the DRI guideline of an additional 200 mg of calcium per day for adults 51 years and above. Calcium is too "bulky" for most MVMM supplements, so all adults, regardless of their stage of life, should ask their healthcare provider whether or not they should take a specific calcium supplement (possibly one with vitamin D and/or vitamin K).

The DRI for vitamin B_6 for adults 51 years and older is slightly higher than that for younger adults, and the senior supplement reflects that increase by providing 50% more vitamin B_6 than the MVMM product targeting the general adult population. This higher intake may provide additional protection against elevated serum homocysteine, a possible risk factor for heart disease.

As discussed earlier, many adults over the age of 50 years poorly absorb vitamin B_{12} from food sources. Older adults are advised to consume foods that are fortified with vitamin B_{12} or supplements, because the vitamin B_{12} in these sources is absorbed more readily than the vitamin B_{12} in food. Although the DRI recommends a change in the *source* of vitamin B_{12} rather than in the *amount,* the higher dosage in the senior supplement poses no harm.

What about the omission of iron from the senior supplement? Certainly, iron is a nutrient essential for good health; why would a manufacturer totally omit it from the product? A woman's need for iron decreases dramatically after menopause; most women can easily meet that need from food alone. In addition, risk for iron overload increases with age, particularly in older men; thus, eliminating iron from senior supplements actually lowers the risk for inappropriate iron loading. If an older adult has a specific need for supplemental iron—for example, following significant blood loss—his or her physician can recommend an iron-only supplement. Tin is the other mineral eliminated from the senior product; because tin has no Daily Value or DRI, there is no strong justification for including it in the senior supplement.

In summary, when consumed with a well-balanced diet, senior supplements can help older adults obtain the appropriate amounts of the micronutrients they need.

Gustavo

*Nutri-*Case

"I don't believe in taking vitamins. If you eat good food, you get everything you need and it's the way nature intended it. My daughter kept nagging at my wife and me to start taking B-vitamins. She said when people get to be our age, they have problems with their nerves if they don't. I didn't fall for it, but my wife did, and then her doctor told her she needed calcium pills and vitamin D too. The kitchen counter is starting to look like a medicine chest! You know what I think? I think this whole vitamin thing is just a hoax to get you to empty your wallet."

Would you support Gustavo's decision to avoid taking a B-vitamin supplement? Given what you have learned in previous Nutri-Cases about Gustavo's wife, would you support or oppose her taking a B-vitamin, calcium, or vitamin D supplement? Explain your choices.

LO 7 Identify and describe the range of nutrition-related concerns that threaten the health of older adults.

LO 8 Describe potential interactions between certain medications and certain foods and nutrients.

What Nutrition-Related Concerns Threaten the Health of Older Adults?

In this section, we discuss several common nutrition-related concerns of older adults. As we explore each concern, we will attempt to answer two questions: (1) What, if any, nutrient concerns develop as a result of a specific medical disorder? (2) What, if any, effect does nutritional status have on the risk of developing that disorder?

Both Obesity and Underweight Are Serious Concerns

In the United States, over 37% of older adults are classified as obese. It is predicted that the rate of geriatric obesity will climb over the next few decades as a result of the higher rate of obesity in young and middle-aged adults. The elderly population as a whole has a high risk for heart disease, hypertension, type 2 diabetes, and cancer, and these diseases are more prevalent in older adults who are overweight or obese. Obesity increases the severity and consequences of osteoarthritis, limits the mobility of elderly adults, and is associated with functional declines in activities of daily living and cognition.

Although some healthcare providers may question the necessity or value of attempting weight loss in obese older adults, even moderate weight loss can improve metabolic and functional status.[36] It should therefore be encouraged in obese elderly who suffer from metabolic or functional complications. Older adults diagnosed with sarcopenic obesity need ongoing medical oversight if weight-loss efforts are undertaken. For all overweight or obese elderly, the goals are the same: clinically significant weight loss that minimizes muscle and bone loss. The interventions for obese elderly are similar to those for younger and middle-aged adults: lifestyle interventions, including the adoption of dietary modifications to achieve a modest energy deficit while retaining adequate nutrient intakes; gradual and medically appropriate initiation of physical activity to preserve lean body mass and bone mineral density; and culturally appropriate behavior modification. In those cases where medications contribute to inappropriate weight gain, it may be possible to find an effective alternative medication that does not cause weight gain.

There are very few research studies on the effectiveness of anti-obesity drugs in the elderly. Bariatric (weight-loss) surgery has been studied in older adults, who account for 10% of bariatric surgery patients at academic centers.[37] A recent follow-up of gastric banding bariatric surgery patients 70 years and older reported no admissions to intensive care and no 30-day hospital readmissions, suggesting few if any serious complications.[38] Moreover, between 30% and 35% of these patients demonstrated modest clinical improvements in blood pressure, blood lipid profile, lower back pain, and type 2 diabetes. Despite the known risks of surgical interventions among the elderly, there is general consensus that older adults should not be denied bariatric surgery only on the basis of their age.[39]

Mortality rates are higher in adults who are underweight (BMI below 18.5) compared to people who are overweight (BMI 25.0 to 29.9). Significantly underweight older adults have fewer protein reserves to call upon during periods of catabolic stress, such as after surgery or after trauma, and are more susceptible to infection. Inappropriate weight loss suggests inadequate intake of both energy and nutrients. Chronic deficiencies of protein, vitamins, and minerals leave older adults at risk for poor wound healing and a depressed immune response. It is estimated that inappropriately low body weight occurs in as many as 25% of community living seniors, 62% of hospitalized seniors, and 85% of older adults in nursing homes.

Because underweight is so risky for elders, geriatric weight loss is an important healthcare concern. Gerontologists have identified nine "Ds" that account for most cases of inappropriate geriatric weight loss, most by reducing energy intake (**Figure 19.4**). They include drugs that decrease appetite, as well as several eating impairments. Depression, which is common after the death of family members and friends or when adult children move out of the area, also contributes to reduced food intake. Treatment of inappropriate weight loss in the elderly is often a complex and lengthy process, relying on behavioral, medical, and psychological interventions.

In summary, any of the nine Ds can promote underweight, nutrient deficiencies, and frailty, significantly increasing the risk for serious illnesses, injuries, and death. The multifaceted approaches used to prevent and treat geriatric weight loss reflect the complexity of this concern.

Millions of Older Adults Have Osteoporosis or Osteoarthritis

More than 10 million Americans have osteoporosis; another 43 million are estimated to have low bone mass, a predictor of osteoporosis.[40] Among women, osteoporosis is typically diagnosed within a few years of menopause as estrogen levels sharply decline. Due in part

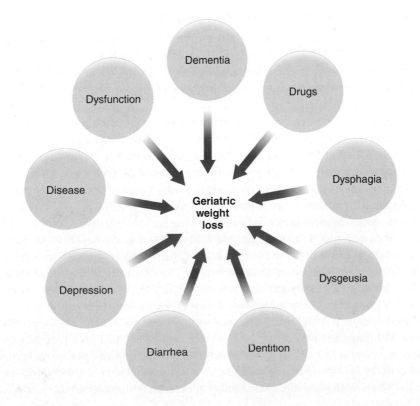

FIGURE 19.4 The nine Ds of geriatric weight loss: many factors contribute to inappropriate food intake in the elderly.

to a higher peak bone density, the onset in males is usually delayed until their 70s or 80s and is linked to declining testosterone levels, steroid therapy, and alcohol abuse. Men with osteoporosis are less likely than women to be diagnosed or treated, although the medical community is now more aware of and responsive to the problem in men. Osteoporosis results in 1.5 million fractures each year.[41]

Many options are available for the treatment of osteoporosis, including a combination of dietary interventions, strength or resistance training, falls prevention programs, and medications.[42] While calcium and vitamin D are typically associated with bone health, many other vitamins and minerals, protein, and total energy are important in sustaining bone density and structure.

Osteoarthritis (OA) is one of the most prevalent chronic diseases among the elderly. It is a disease of "wear and tear" in which protective tissues at the ends of articulating bones degrade, leaving bone grinding on bone.[43] The disease can affect one or multiple joints, cause pain on a daily or intermittent basis, and limit range of motion of one or more joints.

People with OA who are overweight or obese are strongly advised to lose weight. All people with OA should participate in water exercise, which is gentle on joints, or other prescribed forms of physical activity. Pain medications and anti-inflammatory drugs may be prescribed. In extreme cases, hip or knee replacement surgery is required to reestablish normal mobility and function.

Constipation Is a Common Concern

Although constipation is four to eight times more common in older adults than in younger adults, elderly who are healthy and physically active are not necessarily at greater risk. Certain medications, chronic diseases, laxative abuse, low levels of physical activity and possibly low fiber and fluid intakes contribute to risk for constipation, as does immobility. Initial treatment usually revolves around dietary intervention: increased fluid intake and an emphasis on insoluble fiber from foods, such as wheat bran. However, medication may be necessary, especially in patients with underlying disease. Use of laxatives by older adults should be monitored by a healthcare provider.

Dental Health Is Important for Adequate Nutrition

Diet and nutritional status play important roles in the maintenance of dental health in the elderly.[44] Dietary habits linked to improved dental health include consumption of fresh fruits and vegetables, whole grain breads and cereals, high-quality proteins such as meats, cheese, fish, and legumes, and use of sugarless gum after meals and snacks. In contrast, sugary snacks like cookies and cakes, sticky foods such as raisins or caramels, and frequent consumption of sugary drinks are all associated with increased risk of dental decay. Deficiencies of calcium, vitamin D, protein, vitamin C, and the B-vitamins also impair dental health. As described earlier, saliva production decreases with age, increasing the risk for dental decay. In addition, diabetes and cardiovascular disease, both more common in older versus younger adults, contribute to poor dental health. Older adults should be counseled on the importance of a healthful diet in maintaining good oral health.

Despite great advances in dental health over the past several decades, about 33% of U.S. elderly have untreated dental caries, 40% have periodontal (gum) disease, and 25% have no natural teeth.[44] Adults with dentures have diets of poorer nutrient quality and less satisfaction with their meals. Denture wearers also demonstrate more food avoidance (avoiding, for example, meats and firm vegetables and fruits), in part because they have difficulty chewing them. Older adults with dental problems can select soft, protein-rich foods, such as eggs, peanut butter, cheese, yogurt, ground meat, fish, and well-cooked legumes. Red meats and poultry can be stewed or cooked in liquid for a long period of time. Oatmeal and other whole-grain cooked cereals can provide needed fiber, as do berries, canned corn, bananas, and ripened melons. Shredded and minced raw vegetables can be added to dishes. With planning, older adults with oral health problems can maintain a varied, healthful diet.

Many Vision Disorders Are Related to Aging

More than 1.75 million U.S. adults suffer from age-related **macular degeneration (AMD)**, the leading cause of blindness in U.S. elderly.[45] The *macula* is the central part of the retina, and it is responsible for central vision and the ability to see details. A person with macular degeneration loses the ability to see small print, small objects, and facial features. Objects seem to fade or disappear, straight lines or edges appear wavy, and the ability to read standard printed material is lost (**Figure 19.5a**). Macular degeneration does not affect peripheral vision. There is no known cure. Although the specific cause of the disease remains unknown, a family history of AMD increases risk, as do lifestyle practices such as excessive sunlight exposure and smoking. Consumption of a diet high in green, leafy vegetables and fish may lower risk of AMD, along with regular exercise and maintenance of normal blood cholesterol levels.[46]

A **cataract** is an area of cloudiness on the *lens,* the portion of the eye through which entering light is focused. This impairs vision (Figure 19.5b). People with cataracts have a very difficult time seeing in bright light; for instance, they see halos around lights, glare, and scattering of light. Having cataracts also impairs the ability to adjust from darkness to bright light. It is estimated that more than half of adults over the age of 65 years have some cataract development. Cataracts can be treated with surgery. As with macular degeneration, certain lifestyle habits, including dietary patterns, impact the risk for this disease.

Recent research suggests, but does not definitively prove, that consumption of certain nutrients and phytochemicals may slow the progress of these two degenerative eye diseases.[46] Several, but not all, studies have shown beneficial effects of vitamins C and E on cataract formation,[47,48] and some suggest a benefit from the phytochemicals lutein and zeaxanthin.[49] These are found in colorful fruits and vegetables, nuts, and whole grains. In addition, the results of two large studies on age-related eye disease (AREDS 1 and 2) suggest that supplementation with these nutrients and phytochemicals may help delay the progression of cataracts and AMD.[49]

Age-Related Cognitive Impairment Is Not Inevitable

Dementia is a decline in brain functioning that typically affects memory, thinking, language, judgment, and behavior. Its most common and severe form is Alzheimer's disease (AD), a progressive degeneration of neurons in the brain. About one in nine older Americans has AD. Nearly 65% of Americans with AD are women, largely because they live longer than men. AD is the sixth leading cause of death in the United States.[50]

Recently, dietary guidelines were developed to help reduce the risk of late-life onset of AD:[51]

- Minimize the intake of saturated and *trans* fats and prioritize the intake of legumes and other vegetables, fruits, and whole grains over meats and dairy products
- Consume vitamin E from healthful food sources (nuts, seeds, green leafy vegetables, and whole grains) instead of supplements
- Include vitamin B$_{12}$ fortified foods or B$_{12}$ supplements in the daily diet
- If using MVMM supplements, select those without added iron or copper (unless advised by a healthcare provider to take iron supplements)
- There is also strong evidence that physical activity and fitness can blunt the loss of brain "gray matter" (associated with cognitive function) in older adults[52] and, specifically, reduce the risk of AD in older adults.[53]

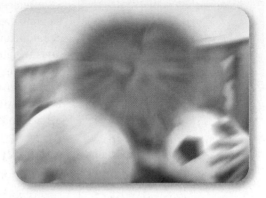
(a)

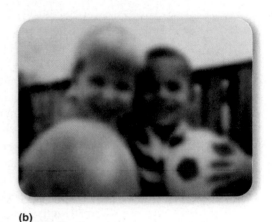
(b)

FIGURE 19.5 These photos simulate two forms of vision loss common in older adults. **(a)** Macular degeneration results in a loss of central vision. **(b)** Cataracts impair vision across the visual field. (*Sources*: Data from National Eye Institute, National Institutes of Health. November 2003. Photos, Images, and Videos. Ref. no. EDSO5. https://nei.nih.gov/photo/amd; and National Eye Institute, National Institutes of Health. November 2003. Photos, Images, and Videos. Ref. no. EDSO3. https://nei.nih.gov/photo/cataract.)

 To learn more about the changes that take place in the brain of someone with AD, watch this short video from the National Institute on Aging at **www.nia.nih.gov/.**

macular degeneration A vision disorder caused by deterioration of the central portion of the retina and marked by loss or distortion of the central field of vision.

cataract A damaged portion of the eye's lens, which causes cloudiness that impairs vision.

dementia A decline in brain function.

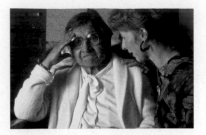

Many people with dementia have difficulty eating adequate portions of healthful food and require help to sustain sufficient energy intake.

Dementia is one of the nine Ds associated with geriatric weight loss. Many people with dementia and other forms of cognitive decline simply refuse to eat. Also, AD can trigger agitation and pacing, increasing energy expenditure. As the disease progresses, the person loses the ability to manipulate utensils and eventually even to swallow.

Helping people with dementia eat adequately can be challenging. Finger foods, such as cut-up fruit, cheese, or meat, vegetable slices, and small pieces of bread, can be eaten without utensils. Between-meal snacks and liquid nutritional supplements can also improve dietary intake. MVMM supplements may also be necessary.

Poor Nutrition Increases the Risk for Pressure Ulcers

Pressure ulcers, also known as bedsores or pressure sores, are more common among older versus younger adults. Risk factors include prolonged immobilization, poor nutrition, obesity, and bowel incontinence.[54] Persons with diabetes, circulatory disorders, and dementia are also at higher risk. Older adults who maintain adequate body weight (neither obese nor underweight), protein status, and level of hydration are at lower risk for pressure ulcers. Liquid nutritional supplements may also prove beneficial in the prevention of this condition.[55]

Once pressure ulcers occur, effective treatment will require the support of a multidisciplinary team of healthcare providers including the physician, nurse, registered dietitian/nutritionist (RDN), and others. The RDN can consult national and international guidelines for the treatment of pressure ulcers.[55] Whether the older adult is treated at home or in an institutionalized setting, proper nutrition is a critically important aspect of their care.

Interactions between Medications and Nutrition Can Be Harmful

Although the elderly account for less than 15% of the U.S. population, they are responsible for over 30% of all spending on prescription medication.[56] **Polypharmacy,** concurrent use of 5 or more medications, and *excessive polypharmacy,* concurrent use of 10 or more medications, are much more likely to occur in older adults compared to young or middle-aged adults. Within a given year, adults between the ages of 65 and 69 years use an average of 14 prescription medications while those between the ages of 80 and 84 years average 18 different prescription medications.[57] As life expectancy increases and medical management of chronic diseases improves, both of these conditions are likely to become more prevalent.

Effects of Medications on Nutrition

Prescription and over-the-counter drugs interact not only with each other but also with nutrients (**Table 19.3**).[58] Some medications increase or decrease food intake, either directly or indirectly. For example, many medications impact neural or hormonal regulation of food intake, whereas others lead to nausea or vomiting or result in decreased production of saliva. The taste, aftertaste, and/or odor of oral medications may be so unpleasant that they reduce appetite. Some drugs cause visual impairment, lead to abnormal motor control, or alter cognition, all of which have the potential to interfere with food acquisition and preparation.

Numerous drugs are known to alter nutrient digestion and absorption. Acid blockers (also termed acid reducers) decrease the absorption of several micronutrients, including vitamin B_{12}, calcium, magnesium, and iron. Long-term antibiotic therapy can lead to diarrhea and generalized malabsorption, as well as malabsorption of calcium specifically. Other drugs may block uptake of other minerals and vitamins.

Many drugs negatively affect the activation or metabolism of nutrients such as vitamin D, folate, and vitamin B_6, contributing to secondary nutrient deficiencies even when nutrient intake is adequate. Several types of anti-epileptic drugs interfere with the activation of dietary vitamin D, leading to impaired bone health. Other medications, including many diuretics, increase the kidneys' excretion of potassium or other nutrients, increasing the risk of deficiency.[59]

polypharmacy The concurrent use of five or more medications.

TABLE 19.3 Examples of Common Drug–Nutrient Interactions

Category of Drug	Common Nutrient/Food Interactions
Antacids	May decrease the absorption of iron, calcium, folate, vitamin B_{12}
Antibiotics	May reduce the absorption of calcium, fat-soluble vitamins; reduce the production of vitamin K by gut bacteria; iron supplementation can reduce drug absorption
Anticonvulsants	Interfere with the activation of vitamin D
Anticoagulants ("blood thinners")	Oppose the clotting activity of vitamin K; vitamin E magnifies effect
Antidepressants	May cause weight gain as a result of increased appetite
Antiretroviral agents (treatment of HIV/AIDS)	Reduce the absorption of most nutrients
Aspirin	Decrease blood folate levels; increase loss of iron due to gastric bleeding
Diuretics	Some types may increase urinary loss of potassium, sodium, calcium, magnesium; others cause retention of potassium and other electrolytes
Laxatives	Increase fecal excretion of dietary fat, fat-soluble vitamins, calcium, other minerals

Effects of Nutritional Status or Dietary Intake on Medications

The activity of a specific drug is often influenced by nutritional status, including obesity, protein deficiency, and fluid status. Excessive fat tissue, for example, may alter the distribution of certain drugs in the body. In other cases, micronutrient status or intake alters drug metabolism, such as the rate at which the drug is broken down. For example, older adults taking the blood-thinning (anticoagulant) drug warfarin (Coumadin) should avoid consuming excess vitamin E, as vitamin E magnifies the effects of this drug. Both ibuprofen (Advil or Motrin) and acetaminophen (Tylenol) are commonly prescribed for muscle, joint, and headache pain, but taking these drugs with alcohol increases the risk for liver damage and bleeding, so alcohol should not be consumed with these medications. Consumption of iron supplements often reduces the absorption of certain antibiotics, and vitamin C deficiency prolongs the effect of pentobarbital.[58]

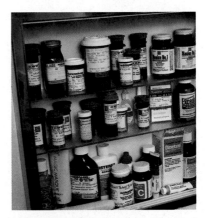

Medications taken by older adults can interact with nutrients.

Some medications, including those known to trigger gastrointestinal distress, should be taken before or between meals whereas others are best absorbed and/or utilized when taken with meals. Meals high in fat or fiber will slow gastric emptying. By prolonging drug exposure to HCl, this in turn can reduce drug activity, or even increase drug activity if the medication dissolves more rapidly in the gastric fluid.

Foods as diverse as grapefruit juice, spinach, salami, and aged cheeses are known to react negatively with specific drugs. Certain nutrient and herbal supplements have the ability to alter the activity of drug-metabolizing enzymes, leading to blood drug levels that are either below or above the desired therapeutic level.

A final consideration relates to medication administration for people with dysphagia, which is common in older adults with Parkinson's disease, stroke, dementia, and multiple sclerosis.[60] Many caregivers crush the patient's tablets or capsules and administer the medication mixed into a thick beverage or a soft food such as yogurt or pudding. It has been shown that this approach can increase or decrease the rate of drug absorption, the rate at which the crushed pill dissolves, and the blood concentration (thus therapeutic effect) of a given medication.

Since it is impossible to describe or predict all possible food/drug combinations, it is very important to stay informed on current guidelines for specific drug–food interactions.[58] All older adults should be counseled on the potential for drug–food, drug–nutrient, and drug–supplement interactions.

RECAP

Obesity and underweight threaten the health of older adults. The "nine Ds" are nine factors (such as dysphagia and depression) that contribute to geriatric weight loss. Osteoporosis increases the risk of fractures in older adults, and osteoarthritis causes joint pain that limits mobility. Dental problems such as gum disease can affect nutrition. Adequate intake of antioxidants may provide some benefit in slowing the progression of the age-related vision disorders, macular degeneration and cataracts. Dementia is not inevitable with aging, and a nourishing diet and regular physical activity may reduce the risk. Poor nutrition increases an older adult's vulnerability to pressure ulcers, and nutritional interventions are important in treatment. An older adult's nutritional status and food intake can influence the effectiveness of certain medications. Many of the drugs used by the elderly have the potential to contribute to nutrient deficiencies.

∎

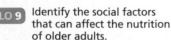 **LO 9** Identify the social factors that can affect the nutrition of older adults.

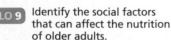 **LO 10** Discuss the various community services and nutrition programs available to U.S. elderly.

What Social Concerns Affect the Nutrition of Older Adults?

We have explored the physical conditions that affect an older adult's nutritional status and needs, but social factors play a role as well. These include elder abuse and neglect, food insecurity, and social isolation.

Many Older Adults Experience Elder Abuse and Neglect

It has been estimated that up to 1 in 10 U.S. elderly are abused by their spouses, children, neighbors, or paid caretakers each year.[61] Elder abuse can be physical, sexual, emotional, financial, neglectful, or unintentional. Denial of healthful food and adequate fluids falls within the scope of elder abuse and neglect. Although it can be difficult to detect, possible signs of such abuse include fear of the caregiver, anxiety, increased depression, and a desire for death. Home-bound elderly people who are abused or neglected may demonstrate new health problems, unexplained weight loss, dehydration and malnutrition, poor personal hygiene, and unexplained or suspicious physical injuries. Older adults without a trusted relative or friend may need to turn to a healthcare provider, court representative, or social service agency for protection and advice. Every state and local municipality has laws against elder abuse and can offer assistance if abuse or neglect is suspected. More information is available from the National Center on Elder Abuse (www.ncea.aoa.gov).

Food Insecurity Affects over 4 Million Older Americans

Food insecurity occurs when a family or individual is not able to ensure a consistent, dependable supply of safe and nutritious food. "Very low food security" is a more severe economic state in which there is reduced food intake and disruption of normal eating patterns. The overall rate of U.S. food insecurity is 14.3%, which is over 49 million Americans.[62] Over 4 million older Americans, or 8.7% of U.S. households with older adults and 9% of older adults living alone, experience food insecurity. At greatest risk are African American, Hispanic, and other minority elderly; those living in the southern United States; and those living with one or more grandchildren. Other predictors of food insecurity include being widowed/divorced/single, having low educational attainment, no private insurance coverage, and concurrent depression.[63]

Older adults cope with food insecurity in several ways. Some make use of federal or local food assistance programs, such as the Supplemental Nutrition Assessment Program (formerly termed the *Food Stamp Program*), discussed shortly. A small number turn to food banks or food pantries for short-term assistance. Older adults can be embarrassed by their inability to provide for themselves and may resort to stealing food or going without adequate food.

The most common cause of food insecurity among older adults is poverty. Older adults in poverty often live in areas with few or no supermarkets, may not be able to afford transportation to buy healthful food, and may fear leaving their homes to shop for groceries. Their homes may lack working refrigerators and/or stoves, limiting the types of foods that can be bought, stored, and prepared. Many low-income elderly are forced to decide whether to spend their limited income on medications or food. Purchasing healthful food often leads to medication underuse, yet purchasing medications can leave little money for food.[64]

Adults with food insecurity, including older adults, consume fewer fruits, vegetables, and dairy products compared to food secure adults.[65] Healthcare and social service providers should carefully probe for information on the ability of low-income elders to afford an adequate and healthful food supply. They should refer at-risk older adults to appropriate community services for immediate and long-term assistance.

Social Isolation Increases Health Risks

Older adults may become socially isolated for many reasons. Retirement severs social ties in the workplace. Those who are restricted to bed or wheelchairs, have impaired walking, or are in poor health are prone to isolation even if they live in a household with others. The death of a spouse can precipitate isolation, especially among those who have also lost siblings and friends. Among older adults with language barriers, isolation can occur as bilingual children move out of the household. Loss of a driver's license, or lack of funds for adequate transportation, also increase the risk for isolation. Even if government-funded vans or buses are available for the elderly, transportation may be limited to weekdays and certain hours of the day.

Social isolation increases the risk for substance abuse and depression, as well as malnutrition. Isolated older adults are at high risk for victimization, such as telephone scams, and premature institutionalization. Social service agencies are critical in both urban and rural communities to ensure that older adults are not forgotten within their homes.

Community Services Can Help Meet the Nutritional Needs of Older Adults

As the American population continues to age, greater demands are placed on social service agencies. This section identifies several programs available for older adults in need.

Community Nutrition Programs for Older Adults

The federal government has developed an extensive network of food and nutrition services for older Americans. Some are open to people of all ages. Many are coordinated with state or local governments and community organizations. They include the following:

- *Supplemental Nutrition Assistance Program (SNAP):* This U.S. Department of Agriculture (USDA) program, formerly known as the *Food Stamp Program,* provides food assistance for low-income households. Participants are provided with a monthly allotment, typically as a prepaid debit card. There are very few restrictions on the foods that can be purchased under this plan. Fewer than 10% of all SNAP participants are elderly; of those, 80% are older adults living alone.[66]

Nutrition
MILESTONE

When nutritionists think of malnutrition, most immediately visualize an undernourished infant or child. It wasn't until the 1980s that geriatric malnutrition was recognized as a significant problem within the United States and across the globe.

In **1991**, researchers in France, Switzerland, and the United States began collaborating to develop a valid tool to assess the nutritional status of the elderly. The result was the Mini Nutritional Assessment (MNA), which remains the "gold standard." The MNA is composed of only 18 questions but takes at least 10–15 minutes to complete, and it must be administered by a healthcare professional. In the 1990s, the American Dietetic Association (now known as the Academy of Nutrition and Dietetics), the American Academy of Family Physicians, and the National Council on Aging developed a shorter, self-administered nutrition questionnaire known by its acronym DETERMINE. Since then, other screening tools have been developed, each with its own strengths and disadvantages, but all with the potential to identify elderly, whether living in their own homes, in a care center, or in the hospital, who are at risk for malnutrition. The problem of geriatric malnutrition cannot be addressed unless it is first appropriately identified.

■ *Senior Farmers' Market Nutrition Program:* This program is designed to provide fresh, unprocessed, locally grown fruits, vegetables, herbs, and honey from farmers' markets, community-supported agriculture (CSA) programs, and roadside stands. Low-income seniors are given coupons, in total amounts ranging from $20 to $50 per year, to be redeemed for eligible foods. In 2013, nearly 850,000 low-income seniors participated, getting fresh produce from over 20,000 farmers across the country.[67]

■ *Child and Adult Care Program:* This program provides healthy meals and snacks to older and functionally impaired adults in qualified adult day-care settings. Relatively small, this program serves about 120,000 seniors.

■ *Commodity Supplemental Food Program:* This USDA program distributes to low-income older adults commodity foods purchased by the USDA, including fresh and canned fruits and legumes and other vegetables; cereals and other grains; canned and frozen meats, poultry, and fish; and even dairy products. Unlike SNAP, however, this program is not intended to provide a complete array of foods. The program serves about 600,000 individuals.

■ *Nutrition Services Incentive Program:* The Administration on Aging provides cash and commodity foods to state agencies for meals for senior citizens. There is no income criteria; any person 60 years or above (plus his or her spouse, even if younger) can take part. Targeted recruitment efforts focus on older adults who are low income, from a racial/ethnic minority group, living in a rural community, at risk of institutionalization, and have limited English language skills. Although free, participants are encouraged to contribute what they can to cover meal costs. Lunch meals, designed to provide one-third of the RDA for key nutrients, are served at senior centers, churches, and other sites. Some provide "bag dinners" for evening meals, and others send home meals on Fridays for weekend use. Meals also can be delivered to the homes of qualified elders through the Meals on Wheels Association of America. This program serves over 900,000 meals a day throughout the United States.

■ *The Emergency Food Assistance Program:* The USDA distributes commodity foods to state agencies for use by food banks, food pantries, and soup kitchens. Each state or agency establishes eligibility criteria, if any. The elderly are more likely to use the services of food banks and local food pantries, avoiding soup kitchens.

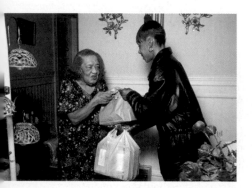

For home-bound disabled and older adults, community programs such as Meals on Wheels provide nourishing, balanced meals as well as vital social contact.

In addition, nongovernmental nonprofit groups continue to supplement government programs. In 2013, for example, a total of 7 million older adults were served by Feeding America, the largest charitable food assistance organization in the United States.[68]

Participation in these programs improves the dietary quality and nutrient intakes of older adults. Unfortunately, many programs have long waiting lists and are unable to meet current demands. As the number of elderly adults grows, the demand and need for these essential services will continue to increase.

Serving Minority Elderly

It is predicted that by 2020 nearly 25% of U.S. elderly will be classified as racial or ethnic minorities. Hispanics have a life expectancy of almost 81 years, 3 years higher than that of whites and almost 8 years longer than African Americans.[69] The changing profile of the U.S. elderly population will require adaptations in current medical and social service interventions. For example, as compared to non-Hispanic whites, Hispanics have higher rates of diabetes; African Americans experience greater rates of stroke, kidney failure, and high blood pressure; and Native Americans are at higher risk for diabetes, obesity, and alcohol abuse. Immigrants from around the world represent additional challenges for healthcare providers. To meet the needs of minority elderly, nutrition professionals must develop an awareness of the cultures they serve, maintain flexibility in the foods/meals provided or prescribed, and work toward effective communication.

End-of-Life Care

Advances in medical care can prolong the lives of seriously ill persons, resulting in challenging legal and ethical issues. Healthcare providers must be well informed on end-of-life issues, including the provision of food and fluids, in order to help elderly clients and families make difficult decisions that honor the client's personal wishes.[70] Ideally, advance directives, such as a living will and a durable power of attorney for healthcare, are available to guide decision-making.

The legalities surrounding end-of-life care are in continual flux as courts and legislative bodies enact, and then modify, decisions on enteral nutrition (tube feeding), hydration, and other nutritional issues. Religious and cultural considerations often overlay legal issues, contributing to their complexity.

Healthcare providers, with agreement from the patient and/or appropriate legal authority, can provide **palliative care** to terminally ill individuals. The goal of palliative care is primarily to minimize patient discomfort, offer social and spiritual support, and extend assistance to family and friends. Individuals who are facing imminent death rarely express hunger and have little or no thirst. If requested, specific foods or fluids are provided, even if they have no nutritional value, to comfort the patient. **Hospice** organizations are growing in number and availability and can provide palliative care to terminally ill individuals, either in their own homes or in a care facility.

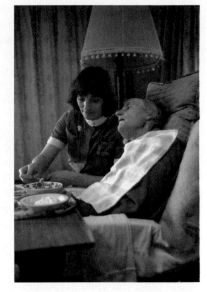

End-of-life care can be provided to elderly people who are terminally ill.

RECAP

As many as 10% of older adults are estimated to experience abuse or neglect, including deprivation of nourishing food. Nearly 9% of U.S. elderly experience food insecurity. Retirement, disease, disability, death of a spouse, lack of transportation, and language barriers increase the risk for social isolation, which in turn increases the risk for malnutrition. Many social service agencies and programs exist to help older Americans with nutritional needs. These include the Supplemental Nutrition Assistance Program (SNAP), the Nutrition Services Incentives Program, and many others, which can improve the dietary quality and nutrient intakes of older adults. Minority elderly populations may have higher rates of certain nutrition-related disorders such as type 2 diabetes. The need for culturally appropriate nutrition counseling may therefore increase. As older adults face end-of-life decisions, healthcare providers must be ready to assist them and their families with difficult decisions related to the provision of food and fluid. ■

palliative care Patient care aimed at reducing an individual's pain and discomfort without attempting to treat or cure.

hospice Supportive care provided to individuals at end-of-life; a program providing such care.

Nutrition Myth OR Fact?

Can We Live Longer in Good Health by Eating a Low-Energy Diet?

Throughout human history, legends have told of a "fountain of youth," which reverses decades of aging in anyone who drinks its waters. Although no one believes such tales any longer, modern equivalents persist: consider anti-aging diets, supplements, cosmetics, and spa treatments. If you were to read that you could live in good health to age 100 by eating about a quarter less than the average energy intake for your gender, level of activity, and height, would you do it? Or would you assume that this is just a fairy tale too? What other actions could you take right now to live longer in good health? Let's find out.

Does Calorie Restriction Increase Life Span?

A practice known as *Calorie restriction (CR)* has been getting a great deal of press for some time. CR involves eating 20% to 30% fewer Calories than would be typical for your gender,

age, body composition, and level of activity, while still getting enough nutrients to keep your body functioning in good health.

The earliest research to show that CR could significantly extend the life span of rats was conducted in 1935.[1] Since then, research has expanded to nonhuman primates, such as monkeys, and, within the past decade, to humans. The results of these largely preliminary and often uncontrolled studies suggest that CR can improve certain metabolic measures of health in humans and, thus, might be able to extend the human life span.[2]

How might CR prolong life span? Although not fully understood, the reduction in metabolic rate that occurs with restricted caloric intake results in a much lower production of free radicals, which in turn reduces oxidative damage and inflammatory processes throughout the body, possibly lowering chronic disease risk and prolonging life. Several, but not all, human studies also show that CR improves insulin sensitivity and decreases blood glucose, LDL- and total cholesterol, and blood pressure, thereby reducing the risk for heart disease, stroke, and type 2 diabetes. There is also evidence that CR can alter gene expression in ways that delay the onset of age-related physiological changes and lower the risk for cancer and other diseases.[3]

It is important to emphasize that animals and human participants in experimental studies of CR are fed highly nutritious diets. Human situations such as starvation, anorexia nervosa, and extreme fad dieting, in which both energy and nutrient intakes are severely restricted, do not result in prolonged life and health but are actually associated with an increased risk for premature death.

It's also essential to understand that the benefits of CR are thought to correlate to the age at which the program begins. The later in life the CR protocol is started, the lower the expected benefit.

What Are the Challenges of Calorie Restriction?

Although the benefits listed in the previous section appear promising, the research supporting these benefits in humans is only preliminary. Research that can precisely study CR in humans might never be conducted because of logistical and ethical concerns. There are also ethical concerns related to the risk for malnutrition and, in women, the potential for harmful in-utero "programming," as previously described (in Chapter 17).

In the absence of high-quality, controlled human studies, several CR groups, including the "CRONies" (Caloric

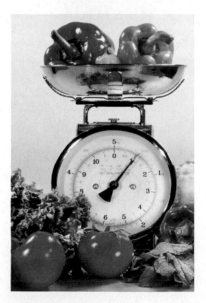

All foods must be carefully measured and weighed in a Calorie-restricted diet.

Restriction with Optimal Nutrition), have provided researchers with some data. Most of the CRONies are males in their late thirties to mid-fifties. One report indicated that most CRONies had followed the CR diet for about 10 years and had reduced their Caloric intake by about 30%. Overall, members reported improved blood lipids and the other health benefits listed earlier. Still, researchers lack specific data on how well free-living adults actually follow the rigid and extensive demands of CR protocols.

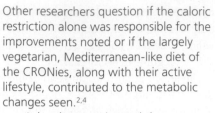

Maintaining a Calorically restricted diet that is also highly nutritious requires significant meal planning and preparation.

Other researchers question if the caloric restriction alone was responsible for the improvements noted or if the largely vegetarian, Mediterranean-like diet of the CRONies, along with their active lifestyle, contributed to the metabolic changes seen.[2,4]

It has been estimated that, on average, humans would need to restrict their typical energy intake by at least 20% for 40 years or more in order to gain an addition 4–5 years of healthy living. If you normally eat about 2,000 kcal/day, a 20% reduction would result in an energy intake of about 1,600 kcal per day. Moreover, the diet would have to be of very high nutrient density, and you would have to maintain it every day for a lifetime.

Those who follow the CR program report several side effects including constant hunger, frequently feeling cold, and a loss of libido (sex drive). Also, the long-term effects of the diet are not known. There is concern that, if initiated in early adulthood, CR might reduce bone density or lead to inappropriate loss of muscle mass. And because the production of female reproductive hormones is linked to a certain level of body fat, CR could impair a woman's fertility. Interestingly, as noted earlier, most of the members of the CRONies are males.

Are There Alternatives to Calorie Restriction?

A number of researchers have begun to question the long-term effectiveness and biological plausibility of CR.[4–6] A possible alternative is the practice of *intermittent fasting (IF)*, also known as every-other-day-feeding (EODF) or alternate-day fasting (ADF).[2,4,7] This approach, which does not reduce average energy intake but simply alters the pattern of food intake, has also been shown, in animals, to prolong life span. Some human studies on IF have reported improvements in a range of metabolic measures of health, including insulin and glucose status, blood lipid levels, and blood pressure.

Additionally, some researchers have proposed that the lower and largely plant protein intake of CR drives some of the metabolic improvements. Even without caloric restrictions, vegan diets are known to lower blood pressure, LDL cholesterol, triglycerides, and fasting glucose levels.[2] Most people would find it easier to simply reduce their total protein intake and/or convert to a largely vegan diet compared to cutting caloric intake by 30% for the rest of their lives. Finally, other research suggests that combining a healthful diet with exercise could decrease inflammation and oxidative stress without the need for CR.[4]

If CR doesn't interest you, is there anything else you can do to increase your chances of living a long and healthful life? The Centers for Disease Control and Prevention (CDC) reminds us that chronic disease is responsible for 7 of every

10 deaths of Americans. Just four behaviors, all within your control, are largely responsible for most chronic diseases:

- Lack of physical activity
- Poor nutrition, including excessive Caloric intake
- Tobacco use
- Excessive consumption of alcohol

So if you want to live a longer, healthier life, the following health habits are less extreme than CR and have no potential risks:

- Engage in at least 30 minutes of moderate or vigorous physical activity most days of the week.
- Consume a diet based on the 2015 *Dietary Guidelines for Americans*, the Mediterranean diet, or a vegan/vegetarian diet, and achieve and maintain a healthful weight.
- If you smoke or use any other form of tobacco, stop. If you don't, don't start.
- If you drink alcohol, do so only in moderation, meaning no more than two drinks per day for men and one drink per day for women.

Critical Thinking Questions

- Given the pros and cons presented here, would you be willing to make the sacrifices necessary to follow a Calorie-restricted diet, even though you couldn't be sure that it would prolong your life? Why or why not?

- If research were to eventually show that CR substantially improves health and prolongs life, would you support recommending it on a large-scale basis? Explain your reasoning.

References

1. McCay, C. M., M. F. Crowell, and L. A. Maynard. 1935. The effect of retarded growth upon the length of the life span and upon the ultimate body size. *J. Nutr.* 10:63–79.
2. Rizza, W., N. Veronese, and L. Fontana. 2014. What are the roles of calorie restriction and diet quality in promoting healthy longevity? *Age. Res. Rev.* 13:38–45.
3. Gilmore, L. A., E. Ravussin, and L. M. Redman. 2015. Anti-aging effects of nutritional modification: the state of the science on caloric restriction. In: Bales, C. W. et al., eds. *Handbook of Clinical Nutrition and Aging.* New York, NY: Springer Science & Business Media.
4. Chrysohoou, C., and C. Stefanadis. 2013. Longevity and diet. Myth or pragmatism? *Maturitas* 76:303–307.
5. Sohal, R. S., and M. J. Forster. 2014. Caloric restriction and the aging process: a critique. *Free Rad. Biol. Med.* 73:366–382.
6. Varady, K. A. 2012. Alternate day fasting: effects on body weight and chronic disease risk in humans. In: McCue, M. D., ed. *Comparative Physiology of Fasting, Starvation and Food Limitation.* Berlin: Springer-Verlag.
7. De Cabo, R., D. Carmona-Gutierrez, M. Bernier, M. N. Hall, and F. Madeo. 2014. The search for antiaging interventions: from elixirs to fasting regimens. Cell 157:1515–1526.

STUDY **PLAN** MasteringNutrition™

Customize your study plan—and master your nutrition!—in the Study Area of MasteringNutrition.

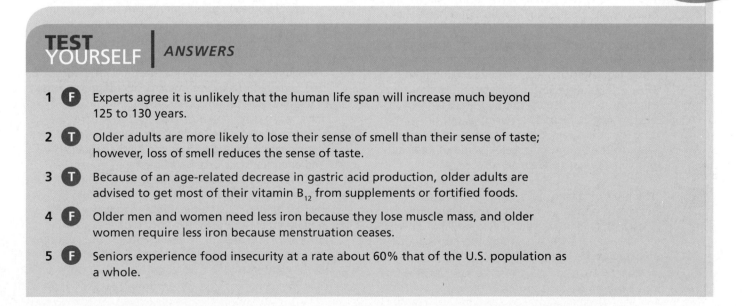

TEST YOURSELF | *ANSWERS*

1 **F** Experts agree it is unlikely that the human life span will increase much beyond 125 to 130 years.

2 **T** Older adults are more likely to lose their sense of smell than their sense of taste; however, loss of smell reduces the sense of taste.

3 **T** Because of an age-related decrease in gastric acid production, older adults are advised to get most of their vitamin B_{12} from supplements or fortified foods.

4 **F** Older men and women need less iron because they lose muscle mass, and older women require less iron because menstruation ceases.

5 **F** Seniors experience food insecurity at a rate about 60% that of the U.S. population as a whole.

summary

Scan to hear an MP3 Chapter Review in **MasteringNutrition**.

LO 1 ▪ The U.S. population is aging at an unprecedented rate. About 15% of Americans are now age 65 or older. Average life expectancy at birth in 2012 was 78.8 years: over 76 years for males and 81 years for females. The very elderly, 85 and above, are the fastest-growing segment of the U.S. population; the numbers of centenarians (100 or older) and supercentenarians (over age 110) also continue to climb.

▪ The human life span, the age to which the oldest human being is known to have lived, is considered 122 years. Experts agree that the human life span is unlikely to increase by more than a few years.

LO 2 ▪ Although much of the underlying physiology of aging remains unknown, two lines of research dominate gerontology. These are not mutually exclusive.

▪ The programmed theories of aging explain aging as a process largely determined by an individual's genetic inheritance (DNA) along with the inevitable shortening of telomeres at the ends of chromosomes each time a cell divides.

▪ The error theories of aging explain aging largely as a result of cell and tissue damage originating from the environment. These include a decline in cell membrane function, oxidative stress, failure of DNA repair, and glycosylation, an abnormal attachment of glucose to proteins.

LO 3 ▪ Scientists are researching the impact of a variety of lifestyle choices on aging. It is well known that smoking accelerates the physical and functional losses associated with aging and greatly increases the risk of premature death. Excessive alcohol intake, excessive sun exposure, and a sedentary lifestyle also greatly accelerate the aging process. Obesity is multifactorial; however, lifestyle choices, including consumption of excessive energy and inadequate levels of physical activity, contribute. Obesity promotes metabolic, cardiovascular, musculoskeletal, and other health problems that accelerate aging.

LO 4 ▪ The physiologic changes of aging include sensory declines, such as diminished or altered senses of smell and taste, and vision loss. These deficits, along with xerostomia (dry mouth) due to decreased saliva production, and dysphagia (difficulty swallowing) can reduce food intake and promote malnourishment.

▪ Achlorhydria (reduced HCl secretion), insufficient secretion of intrinsic factor, and delayed gastric emptying can reduce nutrient absorption and nutritional status. Loss of diversity of gut microbiota, hormonal changes that contribute to the "anorexia of aging," and lactose intolerance can also affect nutritional status.

▪ Typical body composition changes include a decline in muscle mass, increased fat mass, and a shift in fat from subcutaneous to the visceral stores. Decreased bone density is also common. Body organs lose functional capacity. These changes influence the nutritional needs of older adults and their ability to consume a healthful diet.

LO 5 ▪ Older adults need less energy, as well as less fiber. The AMDR for the macronutrients remains the same as for younger adults.

▪ The RDAs for carbohydrates and proteins remain the same for adults of all ages; however, some research suggests the need for higher intakes—up to 1.2 g/kg/day—of protein in order to preserve muscle mass and function.

LO 6 ▪ Micronutrients of concern for older adults include calcium, zinc, vitamin D, and vitamins B_6 and B_{12}. Iron needs for women decrease as menstruation ceases. Vitamin A absorption is increased in older adults and can accumulate in body tissues to toxic levels; thus, intake higher than the RDA should be avoided.

▪ Appropriate use of a multivitamin–multimineral supplement can enhance the nutritional status of older adults; however, certain high-dose, single-nutrient supplements can be dangerous unless prescribed. Calcium and vitamins B_{12} and D are single-nutrient supplements commonly prescribed for older adults.

▪ Older adults have a reduced thirst mechanism and are at risk for chronic dehydration, so ample fluid intake should be encouraged.

LO 7 ▪ Obesity is an increasing concern among older adults, contributing to cardiovascular and metabolic disease, some types of cancer, and other disorders. Geriatric underweight is also a significant concern, as it increases an individual's vulnerability to infection and other health problems. The "nine Ds" are nine factors, including dementia, drugs, and so forth, that increase an individual's risk for geriatric weight loss.

- Nutritional status influences an older adult's risk for osteoporosis, which increases the risk for fractures. Osteoarthritis is one of the most common chronic diseases in older adults, and occurs as protective tissues covering the ends of bones at joints degrade.

- Dental problems, including dental caries and gum disease, can affect nutrition. Constipation is common among older adults with limited mobility, and can occur as a side effect of certain medications. The progression of two age-related vision problems, macular degeneration and cataracts, may possibly be slowed by adequate consumption of antioxidant nutrients and phytochemicals.

- Alzheimer's disease, the most common form of dementia, is the sixth leading cause of death in the United States. A progressive, degenerative disease, it affects nutritional status as well as memory and other aspects of cognition. Pressure ulcers are more likely to develop in older adults with poor nutritional status. At the same time, a nutrient-dense diet is important in promoting healing.

LO 8
- Polypharmacy, the concurrent use of five or more medications, is common among older adults. Many drugs are known to alter nutrient digestion and absorption, to affect the sense of taste or smell, or to cause anorexia, nausea, or other symptoms that affect food intake and can contribute to nutrient deficiencies.

- An older adult's nutritional status, nutrient intake, and food intake also can alter the effects of certain medications. For example, vitamin E magnifies the blood-thinning effect of the drug warfarin; alcohol and the over-the-counter pain relievers, acetaminophen and ibuprofen, can interact to promote liver damage; and presence of food in the GI tract can influence medication release and activity.

LO 9
- As many as 1 in 10 older Americans experiences elder abuse or neglect. These elderly may demonstrate unexplained weight loss, dehydration, and malnutrition.

- Food insecurity affects about 8.7% of U.S. households with an older adult, and 9% of older adults living alone. The most common cause is poverty.

- Retirement, the death of family members and friends, and illness and immobility all increase the risk for social isolation, which in turn increases the risk for malnutrition.

LO 10
- The USDA's Supplemental Nutrition Assistance Program (SNAP) provides funds to low-income Americans to purchase food. The Commodity Supplemental Food Program distributes to older adults a variety of USDA-purchased foods. The Nutrition Services Incentives Program provides cash and commodity foods to state agencies for meals for senior citizens. These are only a few of the various programs available to help meet the nutritional needs of older Americans. Demands on these programs increase as the population ages.

- Minority elderly populations may have higher rates of certain nutrition-related disorders such as type 2 diabetes. The need for culturally appropriate nutrition counseling may therefore increase.

- As older adults face end-of-life decisions, healthcare providers must be ready to assist them and their families with difficult decisions related to the provision of food and fluid.

To further your understanding, go online and apply what you've learned to real-life case studies that will help you master the content!

review questions

LO 1
1. Currently, the human life span is
   a. 74.2 years.
   b. 78.8 years.
   c. 114 years.
   d. 122 years.

LO 2
2. According to the error theories of aging, which of the following conditions results in the defective protein cross-linkages and loss of tissue structure and function associated with aging?
   a. xerostomia
   b. macular degeneration
   c. glycosylation
   d. achlorhydria

LO 3
3. Which of the following lifestyle choices is most strongly associated with premature aging and premature death?
   a. smoking
   b. alcohol consumption
   c. excessive energy intake
   d. a sedentary lifestyle

LO 4 4. Abnormal taste perception is clinically known as

a. dysgeusia.
b. dysphagia.
c. dyspnea.
d. dysmorphia.

LO 5 5. Current research suggests that, compared to younger adults, older adults have an increased need for

a. energy.
b. fat.
c. carbohydrate.
d. protein.

LO 6 6. As compared to the RDA for younger adults, the RDA for older adults is increased for which of the following micronutrients?

a. vitamin B_{12}
b. vitamin D
c. vitamin A
d. iron

LO 7 7. Antioxidant supplements have shown promise in some studies for delaying the progression of

a. osteoporosis.
b. macular degeneration.
c. Alzheimer's disease.
d. all of the above.

LO 8 8. Which of the following statements about antibiotic medications is true?

a. Consumption of iron supplements can reduce the absorption of certain antibiotics.
b. Consumption of yogurt and other probiotic foods and supplements should be avoided when taking antibiotics.
c. Vitamin E supplementation should be avoided by people who are taking antibiotic medications, because of concerns about an increased risk for bleeding.
d. All of the above are true.

LO 9 9. A very elderly couple walk to the local senior center every Monday morning, when the center provides day-old baked goods from local stores to seniors free of charge. The spouses are very affectionate and caring of each other, are dressed in clean, if worn, clothes, and are well groomed. However, both are severely underweight. Which of the following factors is most likely to be contributing to their underweight?

a. immobility
b. elder abuse or neglect
c. food insecurity
d. social isolation

LO 10 10. Providing cookies and lemonade to a terminally ill patient is an example of

a. long-term care.
b. geriatric care.
c. palliative care.
d. inappropriate care.

true or false?

LO 2 11. **True or false?** According to programmed theories of aging, nutrition has little, if any, direct impact on aging.

LO 4 12. **True or false?** Percentage of body fat typically continues to increase throughout an individual's life span.

LO 6 13. **True or false?** Older adults should obtain the DRI for vitamin B_{12} by consuming whole foods, not supplements.

LO 7 14. **True or false?** Mortality rates are higher in underweight elderly than in overweight elderly.

LO 10 15. **True or false?** The Nutrition Services Incentives Program serves any person of any income age 60 years or above.

short answer

LO 4 16. Identify four nutrient deficiencies that may arise from decreased production of gastric acid in older adults.

LO 6 17. Identify several factors that increase the risk for dehydration in older adults.

LO 7 18. Margaret is 68 years old. Her BMI is 32.0. She suffers from osteoarthritis. After conducting a thorough physical examination, Margaret's physician prescribes a weight-loss diet and approves her for a supervised program of swimming three times weekly. Explain why.

LO 8 **19.** Arthur has dysphagia. His wife crushes his mid-afternoon medications and stirs them into a milkshake she has made by blending full-fat milk and vanilla ice cream. Explain why this manner of medication administration, unless approved by Arthur's physician, is not advised.

LO 9 **20.** State two reasons a recent elderly immigrant from Southeast Asia may experience nutrient deficiencies after the death of her husband.

math review

LO 6 **21.** While helping her 72-year-old grandmother put away groceries, Kristina notices several new supplement bottles. One is a single-nutrient vitamin A supplement, which provides 3,333 µg/dose. Another is a special "Healthy Skin Formula," which also contains vitamin A, at 1,500 µg/dose. The third is a multivitamin–multimineral supplement that provides 2,200 µg of vitamin A/dose. When Kristina asks about these new products, her grandmother explains that she read something online that said vitamin A made your skin look younger. So, her grandmother takes each of the three supplements every day to make her wrinkles go away faster! If Kristina's grandmother takes one dose of each of the three supplements per day, what percentage of the RDA does she consume? Of the UL? Do you see any potential problems with this level of intake?

Answers to Review Questions and Math Review can be found online in the MasteringNutrition Study Area.

web links

www.aoa.gov
Administration on Aging
Follow legislative updates on this website for information related to Congregate Meal and Meals on Wheels programs. Also provided are resources on Alzheimer's disease, elder rights and resources, housing, and elder nutrition.

www.cdc.gov
Centers for Disease Control and Prevention
Select "Health Promotion" and choose topics such as "Aging & Elderly Health" for accurate information on the health of America's seniors.

www.fns.usda.gov/fns
Food & Nutrition Service, U.S. Department of Agriculture

This site provides information on federal programs for low-income elderly, such as the Nutrition Services Incentive Program.

www.nia.nih.gov
National Institute on Aging
The National Institute on Aging provides information about how older adults can benefit from physical activity and good diet.

www.nihseniorhealth.gov
National Institutes of Health: Senior Health
This web-based resource, displayed in large print, was developed specifically for older adults and offers up-to-date information on popular health topics for older Americans.

Appendices

Appendix A
Metabolism Pathways and Biochemical Structures

When learning about the science of nutrition, it is important to understand basic principles of metabolism and to know the molecular structures of important nutrients and molecules. Chapter 8 of this text provides a detailed discussion of the major metabolic processes that occur within the body. This appendix provides additional information and detail on several metabolism pathways and biochemical structures of importance. Red arrows indicate catabolic reactions.

Metabolism Pathways

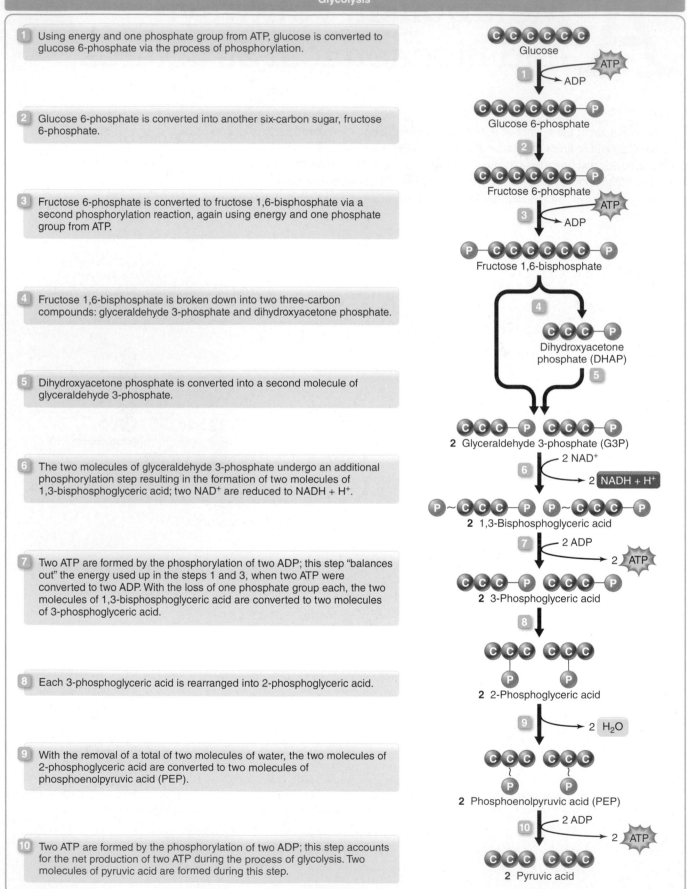

1. Using energy and one phosphate group from ATP, glucose is converted to glucose 6-phosphate via the process of phosphorylation.

2. Glucose 6-phosphate is converted into another six-carbon sugar, fructose 6-phosphate.

3. Fructose 6-phosphate is converted to fructose 1,6-bisphosphate via a second phosphorylation reaction, again using energy and one phosphate group from ATP.

4. Fructose 1,6-bisphosphate is broken down into two three-carbon compounds: glyceraldehyde 3-phosphate and dihydroxyacetone phosphate.

5. Dihydroxyacetone phosphate is converted into a second molecule of glyceraldehyde 3-phosphate.

6. The two molecules of glyceraldehyde 3-phosphate undergo an additional phosphorylation step resulting in the formation of two molecules of 1,3-bisphosphoglyceric acid; two NAD^+ are reduced to $NADH + H^+$.

7. Two ATP are formed by the phosphorylation of two ADP; this step "balances out" the energy used up in the steps 1 and 3, when two ATP were converted to two ADP. With the loss of one phosphate group each, the two molecules of 1,3-bisphosphoglyceric acid are converted to two molecules of 3-phosphoglyceric acid.

8. Each 3-phosphoglyceric acid is rearranged into 2-phosphoglyceric acid.

9. With the removal of a total of two molecules of water, the two molecules of 2-phosphoglyceric acid are converted to two molecules of phosphoenolpyruvic acid (PEP).

10. Two ATP are formed by the phosphorylation of two ADP; this step accounts for the net production of two ATP during the process of glycolysis. Two molecules of pyruvic acid are formed during this step.

FIGURE A.1 Glycolysis.

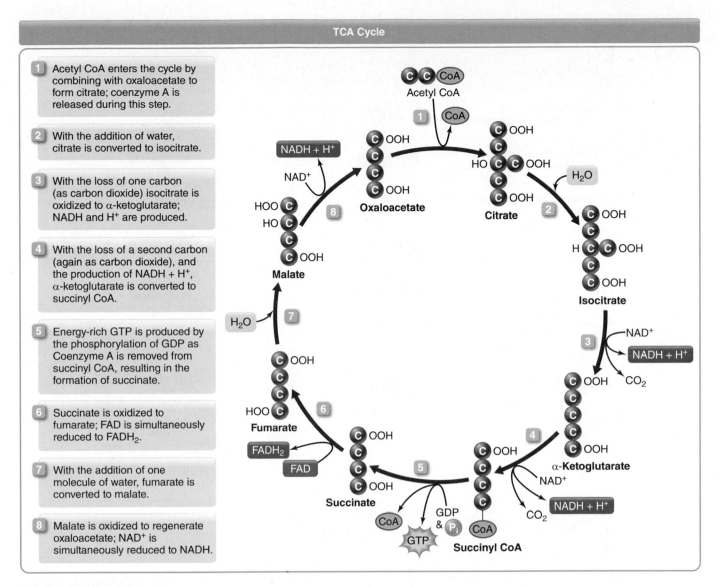

TCA Cycle

1 Acetyl CoA enters the cycle by combining with oxaloacetate to form citrate; coenzyme A is released during this step.

2 With the addition of water, citrate is converted to isocitrate.

3 With the loss of one carbon (as carbon dioxide) isocitrate is oxidized to α-ketoglutarate; NADH and H⁺ are produced.

4 With the loss of a second carbon (again as carbon dioxide), and the production of NADH + H⁺, α-ketoglutarate is converted to succinyl CoA.

5 Energy-rich GTP is produced by the phosphorylation of GDP as Coenzyme A is removed from succinyl CoA, resulting in the formation of succinate.

6 Succinate is oxidized to fumarate; FAD is simultaneously reduced to FADH₂.

7 With the addition of one molecule of water, fumarate is converted to malate.

8 Malate is oxidized to regenerate oxaloacetate; NAD⁺ is simultaneously reduced to NADH.

FIGURE A.2 TCA cycle.

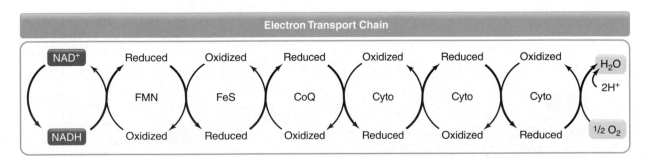

Electron Transport Chain

FIGURE A.3 Electron transport chain. ATP is released at various points in the electron transport chain as electrons are passed from one molecule to another. The process, termed *oxidative phosphorylation*, occurs within the electron transport chain.

Net Energy Production for Glucose Oxidation

	Metabolic reaction	Reaction by-product	Number used	Number produced	Net usage/ production
Glycolysis	Glucose ⟶ Fructose 1,6-bisphosphate	ATP	2		−2 ATP
	Glyceraldehyde 3-phosphate ⟶ 1,3-Bisphosphoglyceric acid	NADH + H⁺		2	2 NADH + H⁺ via electron transport chain
	1,3-Bisphosphoglyceric acid ⟶ Pyruvic acid	ATP		4	4 ATP
Intermediate step	Pyruvic acid ⟶ Acetyl CoA	NADH + H⁺		2	2 NADH + H⁺ via electron transport chain
TCA cycle	Isocitrate ⟶ Succinyl CoA	NADH + H⁺		4	4 NADH + H⁺ via electron transport chain
	Succinyl CoA ⟶ Succinate	GTP		2	2 GTP
	Succinate ⟶ Fumarate	FADH₂		2	2 FADH₂ via electron transport chain
	Malate ⟶ Oxaloacetate	NADH + H⁺		2	2 NADH + H⁺ via electron transport chain

(a) Sources of energy use and production during glucose oxidation

Reaction by-product	Number produced	Number of ATP produced per product	Net usage/ production
ATP	4 − 2 = 2	1	2 x 1 = 2 ATP
NADH + H⁺ (from glycolysis)	2	2 to 3	2 x 2 = 4 or 2 x 3 = 6 ATP
NADH + H⁺ (from TCA cycle)	8	3	8 x 3 = 24 ATP
GTP	2	1	2 x 1 = 2 ATP
FADH₂ (via electron transport chain)	2	2	2 x 2 = 4 ATP

Balance of energy from the oxidation of one unit of glucose

36 to 38 ATP

(b) Energy balance sheet for glucose oxidation

FIGURE A.4 Net energy production for glucose oxidation.

Fatty Acid Oxidation

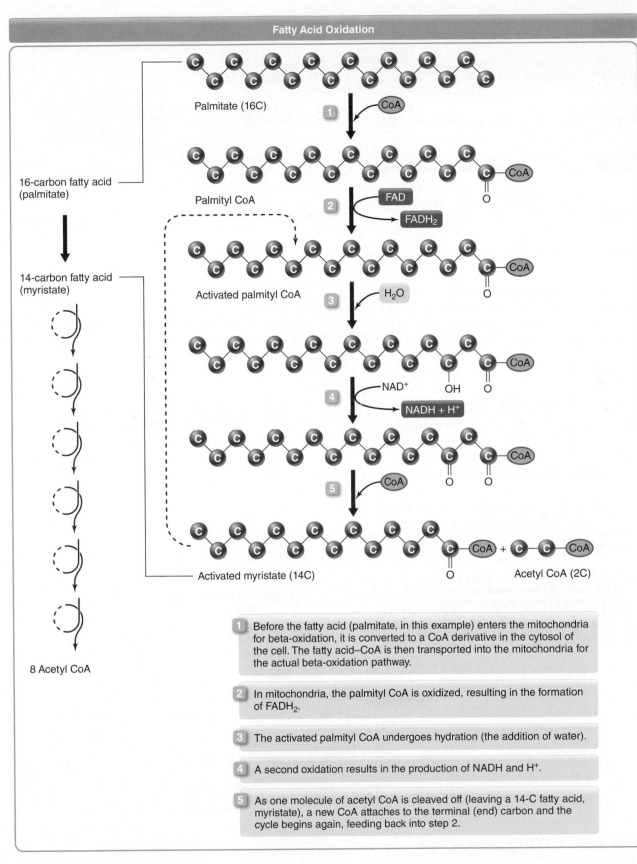

16-carbon fatty acid (palmitate)

14-carbon fatty acid (myristate)

8 Acetyl CoA

Palmitate (16C)

① CoA

Palmityl CoA

② FAD → FADH$_2$

Activated palmityl CoA

③ H$_2$O

④ NAD$^+$ → NADH + H$^+$ OH

⑤ CoA

Activated myristate (14C)

Acetyl CoA (2C)

① Before the fatty acid (palmitate, in this example) enters the mitochondria for beta-oxidation, it is converted to a CoA derivative in the cytosol of the cell. The fatty acid–CoA is then transported into the mitochondria for the actual beta-oxidation pathway.

② In mitochondria, the palmityl CoA is oxidized, resulting in the formation of FADH$_2$.

③ The activated palmityl CoA undergoes hydration (the addition of water).

④ A second oxidation results in the production of NADH and H$^+$.

⑤ As one molecule of acetyl CoA is cleaved off (leaving a 14-C fatty acid, myristate), a new CoA attaches to the terminal (end) carbon and the cycle begins again, feeding back into step 2.

FIGURE A.5 Fatty acid oxidation.

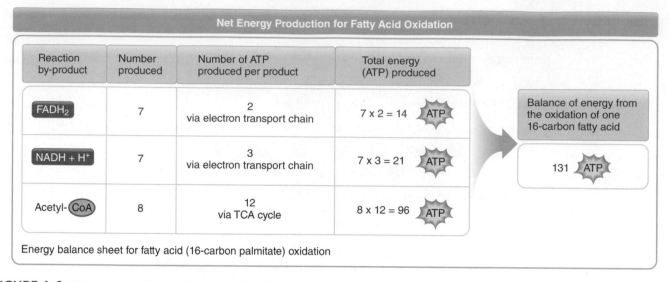

Energy balance sheet for fatty acid (16-carbon palmitate) oxidation

FIGURE A.6 Net energy production for fatty acid oxidation (16-carbon palmitate). With each sequential cleavage of the two-carbon acetyl CoA, one FADH$_2$ (which yields 2 ATP when oxidized by the electron transport chain) and one NADH (which yields 3 ATP when oxidized by the electron transport chain) are produced. Each molecule of acetyl CoA yields 12 ATP when metabolized through the TCA cycle. The complete oxidation of palmitate yields 7 FADH$_2$ (14 ATP), 7 NADH (21 ATP), and 8 acetyl CoA (96 ATP), for a grand total of 131 ATP.

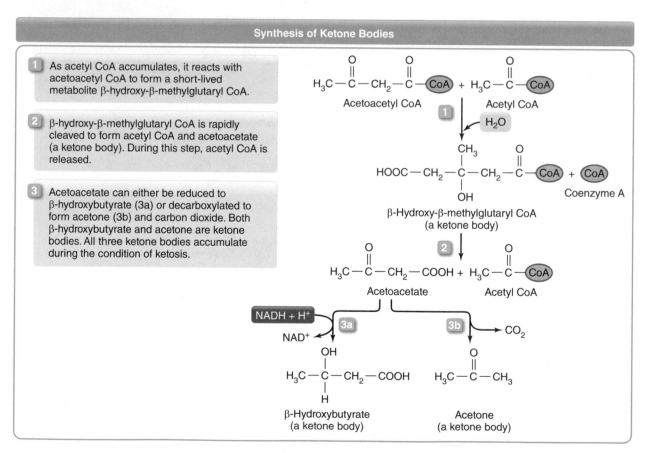

FIGURE A.7 The synthesis of ketone bodies.

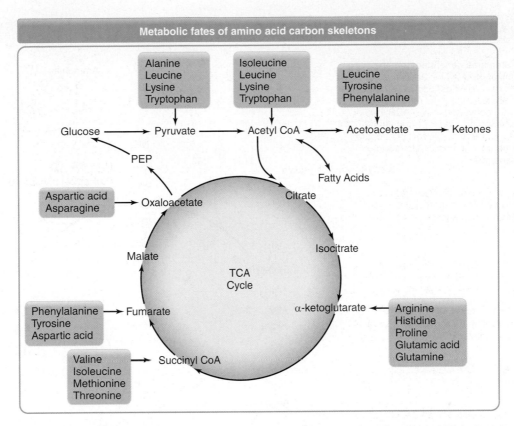

FIGURE A.8 The metabolic fates of amino acid carbon skeletons. After the deamination of amino acids, their carbon skeletons feed into various metabolic pathways. Glucogenic amino acids can be converted into pyruvate and/or intermediates of the TCA cycle, which can ultimately feed into glucose synthesis. Ketogenic amino acids can be converted into acetyl CoA, which then feeds into the synthesis of fatty acids. Some amino acids have more than one metabolic pathway available.

Urea Cycle

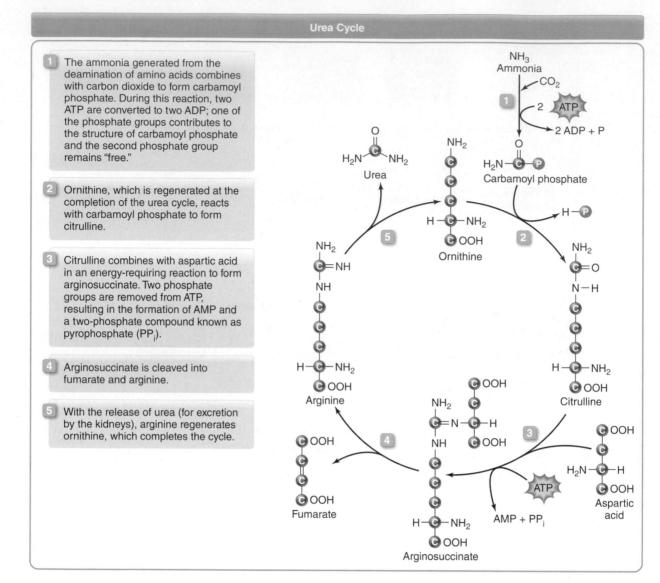

1. The ammonia generated from the deamination of amino acids combines with carbon dioxide to form carbamoyl phosphate. During this reaction, two ATP are converted to two ADP; one of the phosphate groups contributes to the structure of carbamoyl phosphate and the second phosphate group remains "free."

2. Ornithine, which is regenerated at the completion of the urea cycle, reacts with carbamoyl phosphate to form citrulline.

3. Citrulline combines with aspartic acid in an energy-requiring reaction to form arginosuccinate. Two phosphate groups are removed from ATP, resulting in the formation of AMP and a two-phosphate compound known as pyrophosphate (PP_i).

4. Arginosuccinate is cleaved into fumarate and arginine.

5. With the release of urea (for excretion by the kidneys), arginine regenerates ornithine, which completes the cycle.

FIGURE A.9 Urea cycle.

Ethanol Metabolism

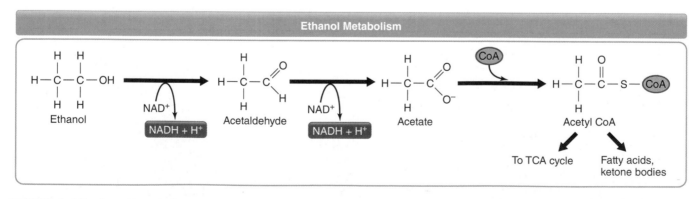

FIGURE A.10 Ethanol metabolism.

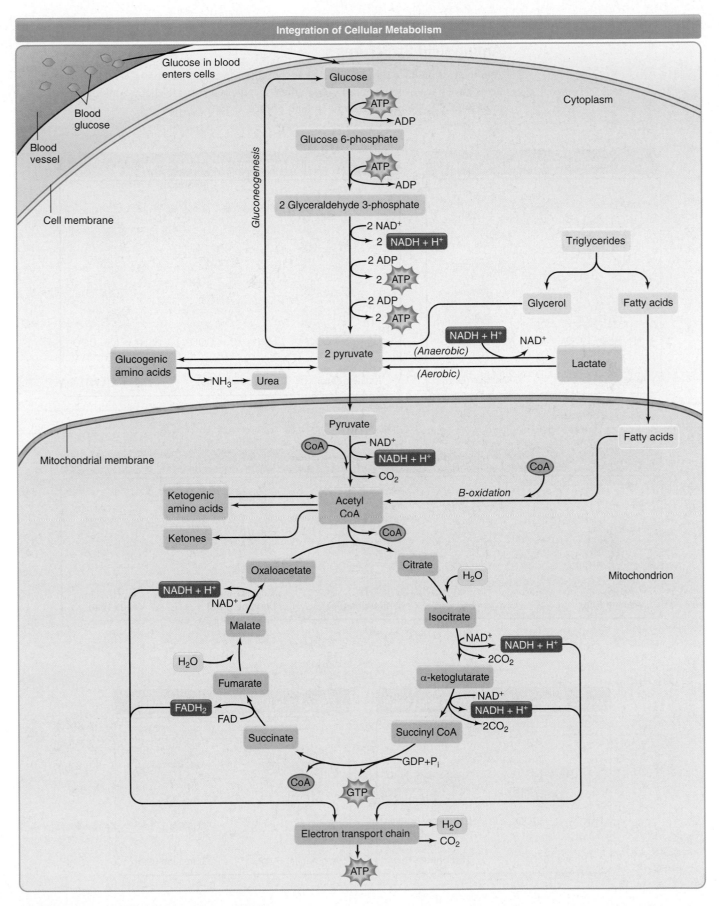

FIGURE A.11 Integration of cellular metabolism.

Biochemical Structures

Amino Acid Structures

Amino acids all have the same basic core but differ in their side chains. The following amino acids have been classified according to their specific type of side chain. Amino acids that are essential to humans are noted in bold print.

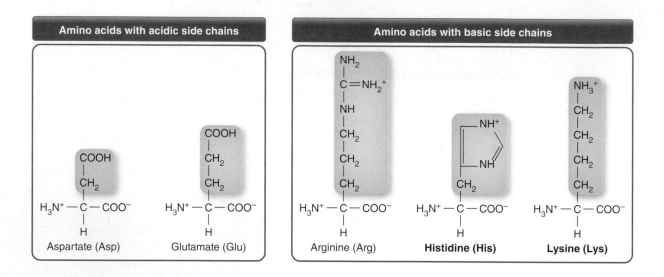

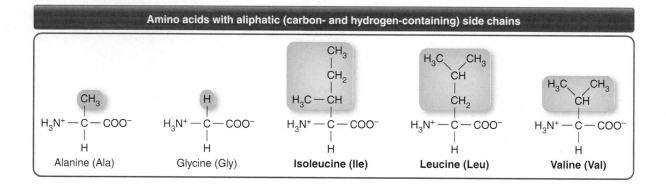

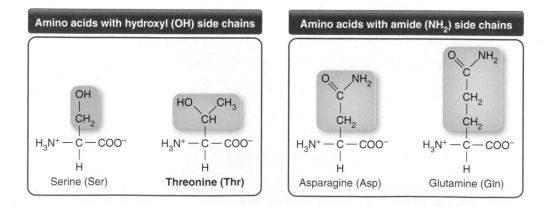

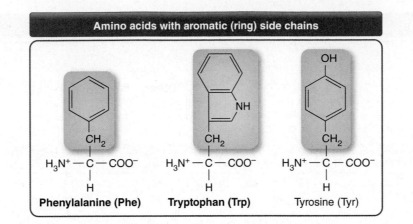

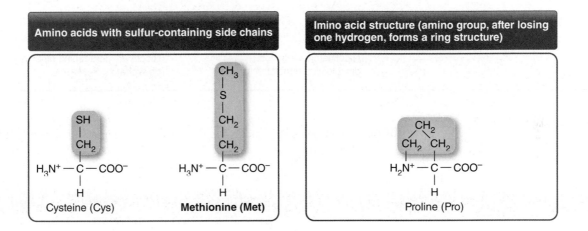

Vitamin Structures and Coenzyme Derivatives

Many vitamins have common names (for example, vitamin C, vitamin E) as well as scientific designations (for example, ascorbic acid, α-tocopherol). Most vitamins are found in more than one chemical form. Many of the vitamins illustrated here have an active coenzyme form; review both the vitamin and the coenzyme structures and see if you can locate the "core vitamin" structure within each of the coenzymes. The vitamins found in foods or supplements are not always in the precise chemical form needed for metabolic activity, and therefore the body often has to modify the vitamin in one way or another. For example, many of the B-vitamins are phosphorylated, meaning they have a phosphate group attached.

Water-Soluble Vitamins

Niacin has two forms: nicotinic acid and nicotinamide. Both forms can be converted into the coenzymes nicotinamide adenine dinucleotide (NAD^+) and nicotinamide adenine dinucleotide phosphate ($NADP^+$).

Niacin

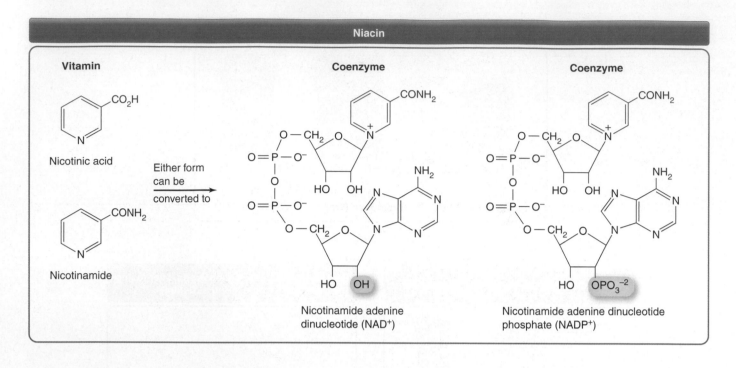

Riboflavin can be converted into the coenzymes flavin adenine dinucleotide (FAD) and flavin mononucleotide (FMN).

Riboflavin

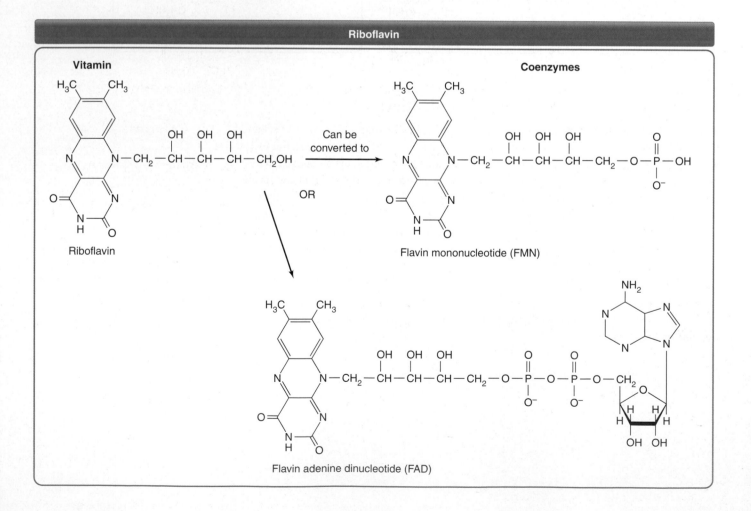

Thiamin can be converted into the coenzyme thiamin pyrophosphate (TPP).

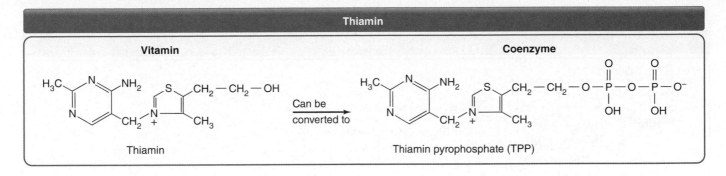

Vitamin B_6 includes the forms pyridoxine, pyridoxal, and pyridoxamine. The two common coenzymes derived from vitamin B_6 are pyridoxal 5′ phosphate (PLP) and pyridoxamine 5′ phosphate (PNP).

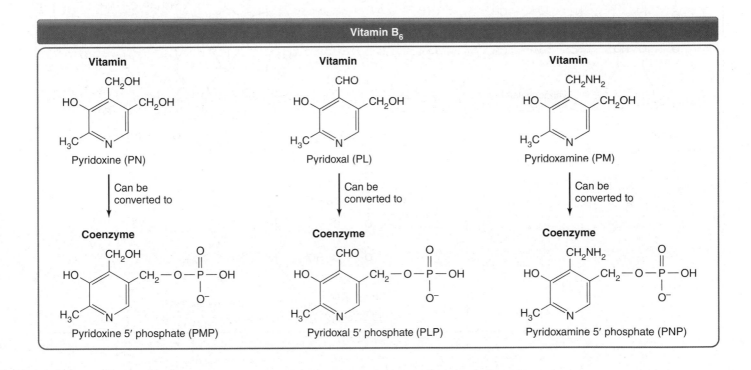

Two forms of vitamin B$_{12}$ are cyanocobalamin and methylcobalamin.

Vitamin B$_{12}$

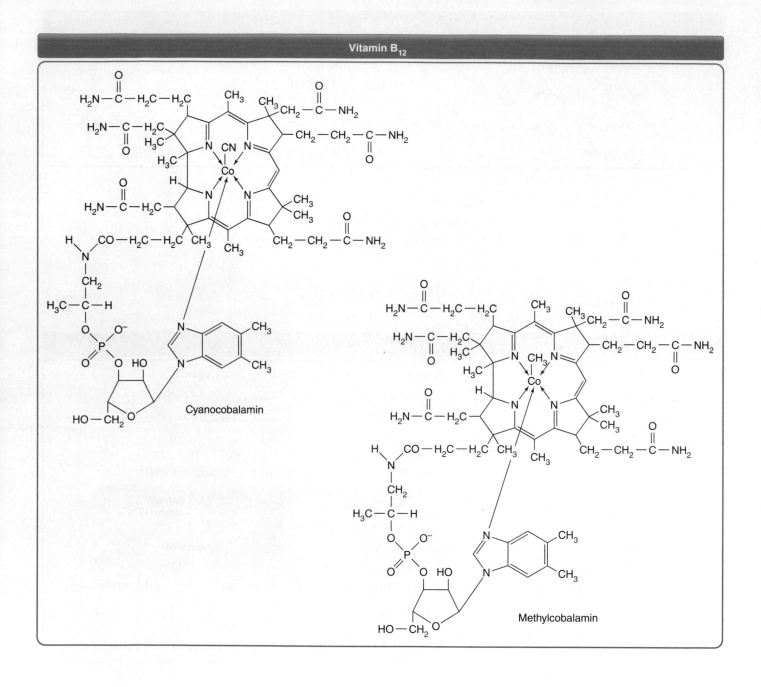

Cyanocobalamin

Methylcobalamin

Folic acid is one specific chemical form of folate. This vitamin can be converted into several coenzymes, including tetrahydrafolic acid.

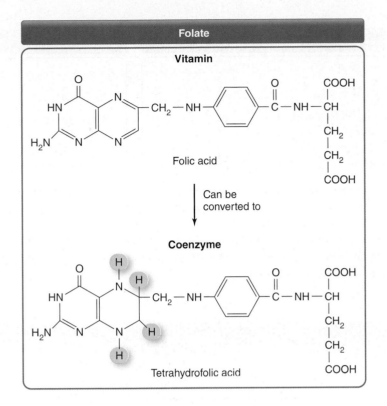

Pantothenic acid is a component of Coenzyme A (CoA).

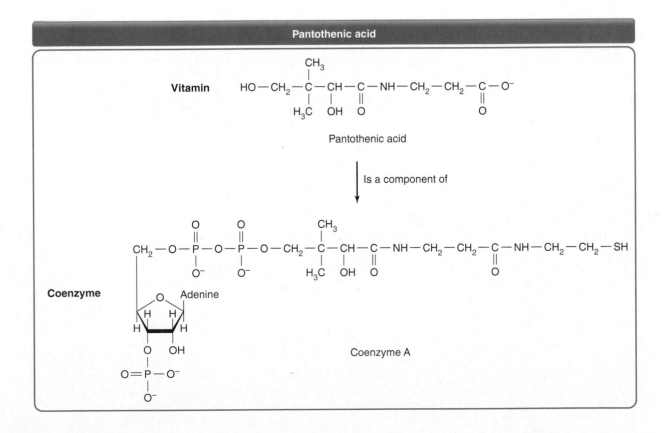

Biotin binds to several different metabolic enzymes. Choline serves as a methyl donor and as a precursor of acetylcholine and phospholipids.

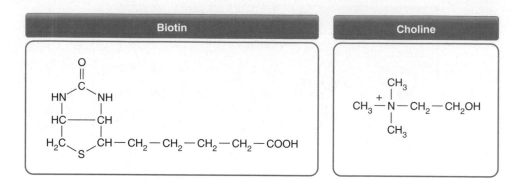

The two forms of vitamin C (ascorbic acid and dehydroascorbic acid) are readily interconverted as two hydrogens are lost through the oxidation of ascorbic acid or gained through the reduction of dehydroascorbic acid.

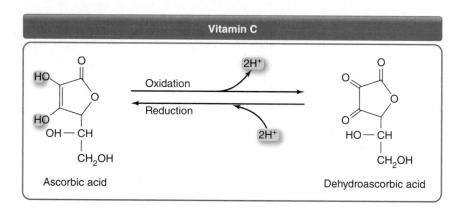

Fat-Soluble Vitamins

Vitamin A exists as an alcohol (retinol), an aldehyde (retinal), and an acid (retinoic acid). Beta-carotene is a common and highly potent precursor that can be converted into vitamin A by the body.

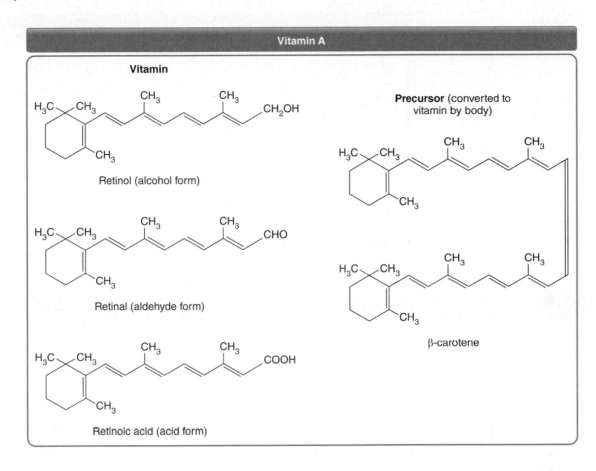

Vitamin A

Retinol (alcohol form)

Retinal (aldehyde form)

Retinoic acid (acid form)

Precursor (converted to vitamin by body)

β-carotene

Vitamin D as cholecalciferol must be activated by two hydroxylation reactions (the addition of one OH group at each step) to form the active form of the vitamin, calcitriol (also called $1,25\ (OH)_2D$).

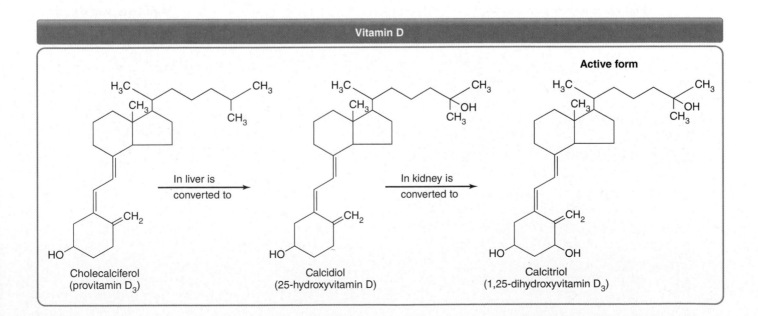

Vitamin D

Cholecalciferol (provitamin D_3)

In liver is converted to

Calcidiol (25-hydroxyvitamin D)

In kidney is converted to

Active form

Calcitriol (1,25-dihydroxyvitamin D_3)

α-tocopherol is the most active form of vitamin E; the number and location of the methyl (CH₃) groups attached to the ring structure distinguish the four unique forms of the tocopherols.

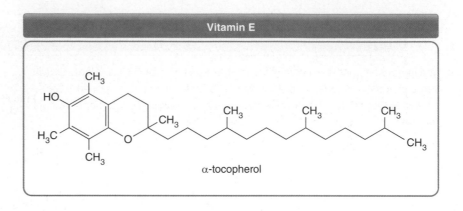

Vitamin E

α-tocopherol

Vitamin K can be derived from plant sources (phylloquinones) and bacterial synthesis (menaquinones). A synthetic form of vitamin K (menadione) is also available.

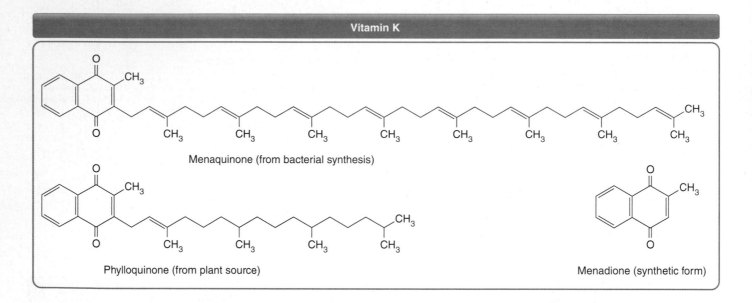

Vitamin K

Menaquinone (from bacterial synthesis)

Phylloquinone (from plant source)

Menadione (synthetic form)

Appendix

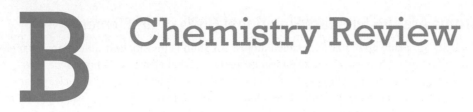 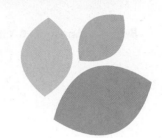

B Chemistry Review

A basic grasp of chemistry is necessary for the introductory nutrition student. You may have taken a chemistry course at your college or in high school; this appendix can help you review concepts about atoms, molecules, pH, chemical reactions, and energy that you have learned previously.

All Matter Consists of Elements

Matter is anything that has mass and occupies space. All matter is composed of elements. An element is a fundamental (pure) form of matter that cannot be broken down to a simpler form. Aluminum and iron are elements, and so are oxygen and hydrogen. There are just over 100 known elements, and together they account for all matter on earth. The periodic table of elements arranges all the elements into groups according to their similar properties (**Figure B.1**).

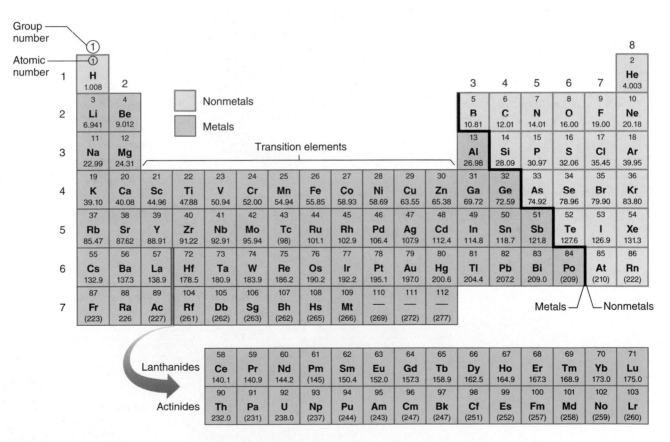

FIGURE B.1 The periodic table shows all known elements in order of increasing atomic number.

Atoms Are the Smallest Functional Units of an Element

Elements are made up of particles called atoms. An atom is the smallest unit of any element that still retains the physical and chemical properties of that element. Although we now know that atoms can be split apart under unusual circumstances (such as a nuclear reaction), atoms are the smallest units of matter that can take part in chemical reactions. So, for all practical purposes, atoms are the smallest functional units of matter.

Even the largest atoms are so small that we can see them only with specialized microscopes. Chemists can also infer what they look like from studying their physical properties (**Figure B.2**).

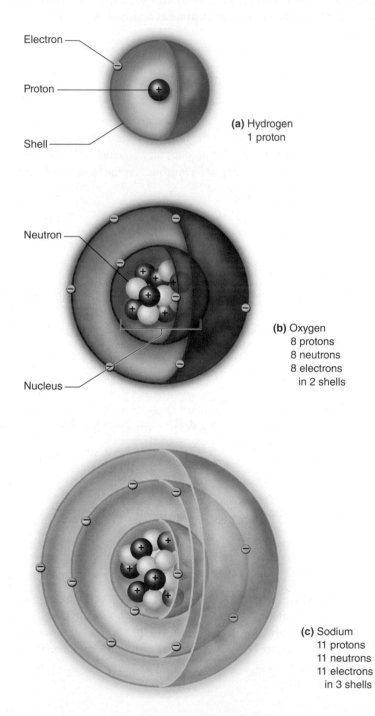

FIGURE B.2 The structure of atoms. Atoms consist of a nucleus, comprised of positively charged protons and neutral neutrons, surrounded by spherical shells of negatively charged electrons.

The central core of an atom is called the *nucleus.* The nucleus is made of positively charged particles called *protons* and a nearly equal number of neutral particles called *neutrons,* all tightly bound together. An exception is the smallest atom, hydrogen, whose nucleus consists of only a single proton. Smaller negatively charged particles called *electrons* orbit the nucleus. Because electrons are constantly moving, their precise position at any one time is unknown. You may think of electrons as occupying one or more spherical clouds of negative charge around the nucleus called *shells.* Each shell can accommodate only a certain number of electrons. The first shell, the one closest to the nucleus, can hold two electrons, the second can accommodate eight, and the third shell (if there is one) can contain even more. Each type of atom has a unique number of electrons. Under most circumstances the number of electrons equals the number of protons, and, as a result, the entire atom is electrically neutral.

Protons and neutrons have about the same mass, and both have much more mass than electrons. (Over 99.9% of an atom's mass is due to the protons and neutrons in its nucleus.)

In the periodic table and in chemical equations, atoms are designated by one- or two-letter symbols taken from English or Latin. For example, oxygen is designated by the letter O, nitrogen by N, sodium by Na (from the Latin word for sodium, *natrium*), and potassium by K (from the Latin *kalium*). A subscript numeral following the symbol indicates the numbers of atoms of that element. For example, the chemical formula O_2 represents two atoms of oxygen linked together, the most stable form of elemental oxygen.

In addition to a symbol, atoms have an *atomic number,* which represents the characteristic number of protons in the nucleus, and an *atomic mass* (or mass number), which is generally fairly close to the total number of neutrons and protons.

Isotopes Have a Different Number of Neutrons

Although all the atoms of a particular element have the same number of protons, the number of neutrons can vary slightly. Atoms with either more or fewer neutrons than the usual number for that element are called *isotopes.* Isotopes of an element have the same atomic number as the more common atoms but a different atomic mass. For example, elemental carbon typically consists of atoms with six protons and six neutrons, for an atomic mass of 12. The isotope of carbon known as carbon-14 has an atomic mass of 14 because it has two extra neutrons.

Isotopes are always identified by a superscript mass number preceding the symbol. For instance, the carbon-14 isotope is designated ^{14}C. The superscript mass number of the most common elemental form of carbon is generally omitted because it is understood to be 12.

Many isotopes are unstable. Such isotopes are called *radioisotopes* because they tend to give off energy (in the form of radiation) and particles until they reach a more stable state. The radiation emitted by radioisotopes can be dangerous to living organisms because the energy can damage tissues.

Atoms Combine to Form Molecules

A *molecule* is a stable association between two or more atoms. For example, a molecule of water consists of two atoms of hydrogen plus one atom of oxygen (written as H_2O). A molecule of ordinary table salt (written as NaCl) consists of one atom of sodium (Na) plus one atom of chlorine (Cl). A molecule of hydrogen gas (written as H_2) consists of two atoms of hydrogen. In order to understand *why* atoms join together to form molecules, we need to know more about energy.

Energy Fuels the Body's Activities

Energy is the capacity to do work, or the capacity to cause some change in matter. Joining atoms is one type of work, and breaking up molecules is another—and both require energy. Stored energy that is not actually performing any work at the moment is called *potential energy* because it has the *potential* to make things happen. Energy that is actually *doing* work—that is, energy in motion—is called *kinetic energy*.

Potential energy is stored in the bonds that hold atoms together in all matter, both living and nonliving. The body takes advantage of this general principle of chemistry by using certain molecules to store energy for its own use. When the chemical bonds of these energy-storage molecules are broken, potential energy becomes kinetic energy. The body relies on this energy to power "work" such as breathing, moving, and digesting food.

Matter is most stable when it is at the *lowest possible energy level,* that is, when it contains the least potential energy. This fact has important implications for the formation of molecules, because even single atoms contain energy.

Electrons Have Potential Energy

Recall that electrons carry a negative charge, whereas protons within the nucleus have a positive charge. Electrons are attracted to the positively charged nucleus and repelled by each other. As a result of these opposing attractive and repulsive forces, each electron occupies a specific shell around the nucleus. Each shell corresponds to a specific level of electron potential energy, and each shell farther out represents a potential energy level higher than the preceding one. When an electron moves to a shell closer to the nucleus, it loses energy. In order to move to a shell that is farther from the nucleus, the electron must absorb energy.

Chemical Bonds Link Atoms to Form Molecules

A key concept in chemistry is that *atoms are most stable when their outermost occupied electron shell is completely filled.* An atom whose outermost electron shell is not normally filled tends to interact with one or more other atoms in a way that fills its outermost shell. Such interactions generally cause the atoms to be bound to each other by attractive forces called *chemical bonds.* The three principal types of chemical bonds are called covalent, ionic, and hydrogen bonds.

Covalent Bonds Involve Sharing Electrons

One way that an atom can fill its outermost shell is by sharing a pair of electrons with another atom. An electron-sharing bond between atoms is called a *covalent bond* (**Figure B.3**). Covalent bonds between atoms are among the strongest chemical bonds in nature; they are so strong that they rarely break apart. In structural formulas, a covalent bond is depicted as a line drawn between two atoms.

Hydrogen gas offers an example of how a covalent (electron-sharing) bond fills the outermost shells of two atoms. Each of the two hydrogen atoms has just one electron in the first shell, which can accommodate two electrons. When joined together by a covalent bond (forming H_2, a gas), each atom has, in effect, a "full" first shell of two electrons. As a result, H_2 gas is more stable than the same two hydrogen atoms by themselves. The sharing of one pair of electrons, as in H_2, is called a *single* bond.

Oxygen gas is another example of covalent bonding. An oxygen atom has eight electrons: Two of these fill the first electron shell, and the remaining six occupy the second electron shell (which can accommodate eight). Two oxygen atoms may join to form a molecule of oxygen gas by sharing two pairs of electrons, thus completing the outer shells of both atoms. When two pairs of electrons are shared, the bond is called a *double bond*. In structural formulas, double bonds are indicated by two parallel lines.

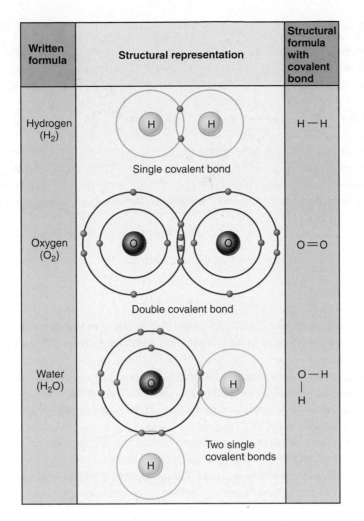

Written formula	Structural representation	Structural formula with covalent bond
Hydrogen (H₂)	Single covalent bond	H—H
Oxygen (O₂)	Double covalent bond	O=O
Water (H₂O)	Two single covalent bonds	O—H | H

FIGURE B.3 Covalent bonds. Sharing pairs of electrons is a way for an atom to fill its outermost shell.

A molecule of water forms from one oxygen and two hydrogen atoms because this combination completely fills the outermost shells of both hydrogen and oxygen. The prevalence of water on earth follows from the simple rule described earlier: Matter is most stable when it contains the least potential energy. That is, both hydrogen and oxygen are more stable when together (as H₂O) than when they are independent atoms.

Ionic Bonds Occur Between Oppositely Charged Ions

A second way that atoms can fill their outer shell of electrons is to give up electrons completely (if they have only one or two electrons in their outermost shell) or to take electrons from other atoms (if they need one or two to fill their outermost shell). Such a loss (or gain) of electrons gives the atom a net charge, because now there are fewer (or more) negatively charged electrons than positively charged protons in the nucleus. The net charge is positive ($+$) for each electron lost and negative ($-$) for each electron gained.

An electrically charged atom or molecule is called an ion. Examples of ions are sodium (Na^+), chloride (Cl^-), calcium (Ca^{2+}), and hydrogen phosphate (HPO_4^-). Note that ions can have a shortage or surplus of more than one electron (for example, Ca^{2+} has lost two electrons). A positively charged ion is called a *cation*; a negatively charged ion is called an *anion*.

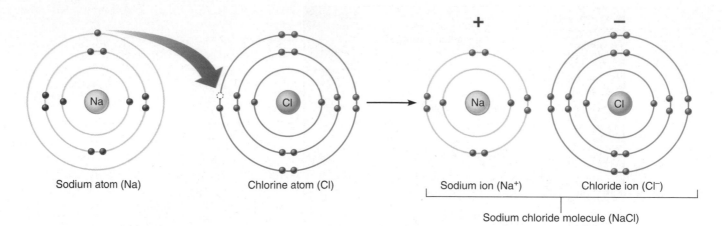

Sodium atom (Na)   Chlorine atom (Cl)   Sodium ion (Na⁺)   Chloride ion (Cl⁻)

Sodium chloride molecule (NaCl)

FIGURE B.4 Ionic bonds. Electrically charged ions form when an atom gives up or gains electrons. The oppositely charged ions are attracted to each other, forming an ionic bond.

Ever heard the expression "opposites attract"? It should come as no surprise that oppositely charged ions are attracted to each other. This attractive force is called an *ionic bond* (**Figure B.4**).

In aqueous (watery) solutions, where ionic bonds are not as strong as covalent bonds, ions tend to dissociate (break away) from each other relatively easily. In the human body, for example, almost all of the sodium is in the form of Na^+, and most of the chlorine is in its ionized form, *called chloride* (Cl^-).

When positive and negative ions are united by ionic bonds, they are called *ionic compounds*. The physical and chemical properties of an ionic compound such as NaCl are very different from those of the original elements. For example, the original elements of NaCl are sodium, a soft, shiny metal, and chlorine, a yellow-green poisonous gas. Yet, as positive and negative ions, they form table salt, a white, crystalline substance that is common in our diet. In ionic compounds, the attraction between the ions is very strong, which makes the melting points of ionic compounds high, often greater than 300°C. For example, the melting point of NaCl is 800°C. At room temperature, ionic compounds are solids.

The structure of an ionic solid depends on the arrangement of the ions. In a crystal of NaCl, which has a cubic shape, the larger Cl^- ions are packed close together in a lattice structure. The smaller Na^+ ions occupy the holes between the Cl^- ions.

Ions in aqueous solutions are sometimes called *electrolytes* because solutions of water containing ions are good conductors of electricity. Cells can control the movement of certain ions, creating electrical forces essential to the functioning of nerves, muscles, and other living tissues.

Weak Hydrogen Bonds Form Between Polar Molecules

A third type of attraction occurs between molecules that do not have a net charge. Glance back at the water molecule in Figure C.3 and note that the two hydrogen atoms are found not at opposite ends of the water molecule but fairly close together. Although the oxygen atom and the two hydrogen atoms share electrons, the sharing is unequal. The shared electrons in a water molecule actually spend slightly more of their time near the oxygen atom than near the hydrogen atoms because the oxygen atom attracts electrons more strongly than do the hydrogen atoms. Although the water molecule is neutral overall, the uneven sharing gives the oxygen end a partial negative charge and the hydrogen end a partial positive charge.

Molecules such as water that are electrically neutral overall but still have partially charged ends, or *poles*, are called *polar* molecules. According to the principle that opposites attract, polar molecules arrange themselves so that the negative pole of one molecule is oriented toward (attracted by) the positive pole of another molecule. The weak attractive

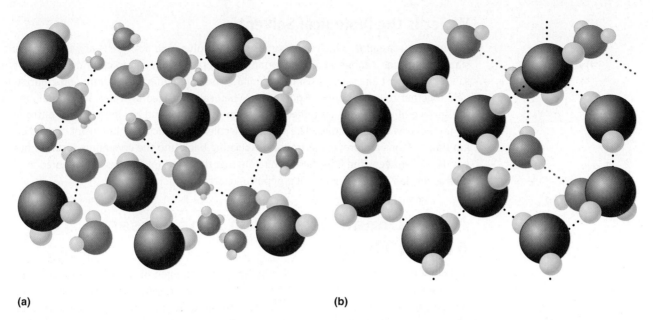

(a)   **(b)**

FIGURE B.5 Hydrogen bonds. **(a)** In water, weak hydrogen bonds continually form, break, and re-form between hydrogen and oxygen atoms of adjacent water molecules. **(b)** Ice is a solid because stable hydrogen bonds form between each water molecule and four of its neighbors.

force between oppositely charged regions of polar molecules that contain covalently bonded hydrogen is called a *hydrogen bond* **(FIGURE B.5)**.

Hydrogen bonds between water molecules in liquid water are so weak that they continually break and re-form, allowing water to flow. When water becomes cold enough to freeze, each water molecule forms four stable, unchanging hydrogen bonds with its neighbors. When water is vaporized (becomes a gas), the hydrogen bonds are broken and stay broken as long as the water is in the gas phase.

Hydrogen bonds are important in biological molecules. They provide the force that gives proteins their three-dimensional shape, and they keep the two strands of the DNA molecule together.

Table B.1 summarizes covalent, ionic, and hydrogen bonds.

The Body Depends on Water

No molecule is more essential to life than water. Indeed, it accounts for between 50% and 70% of body weight. The following properties of water are especially important to the body: water molecules are polar, water is a liquid at body temperature, and water can absorb and hold heat energy.

These properties make water an ideal solvent and an important factor in temperature regulation, as discussed in Chapter 9.

Table B.1 Summary of the Three Types of Chemical Bonds

Type	Strength	Description	Examples
Covalent bond	Strong	A bond in which the sharing of electrons between atoms results in each atom having a maximally filled outermost shell of electrons	The bonds between hydrogen and oxygen in a molecule of water
Ionic bond	Moderate	The bond between two oppositely charged ions (atoms or molecules that were formed by the permanent transfer of one or more electrons)	The bond between Na^+ and Cl^- in salt
Hydrogen bond	Weak	The bond between oppositely charged regions of molecules that contain covalently bonded hydrogen atoms	The bonds between molecules of water

Water Is the Biological Solvent

A *solvent* is a liquid in which other substances dissolve, and a *solute* is any dissolved substance. Consider a common and important solid: crystals of sodium chloride (NaCl), or table salt. Crystals of table salt consist of a regular, repeating pattern of sodium and chloride ions held together by ionic bonds (**Figure B.6**). When salt is placed in water, individual ions at the surface of the crystal are pulled away from the crystal and are immediately surrounded by the polar water molecules. The water molecules form such a tight cluster around each ion that the ions are prevented from reassociating back into the crystalline form. In other words, water keeps the ions dissolved. Note that the water molecules are oriented around ions according to the principle that opposite charges attract.

Acids Donate Hydrogen Ions; Bases Accept Them

Although the covalent bonds between hydrogen and oxygen in water are strong and thus are rarely broken, it can happen. When it does, the electron from one hydrogen atom is transferred to the oxygen atom completely, and the water molecule breaks into two ions—a *hydrogen ion* (H^+) and a *hydroxide ion* (OH^-).

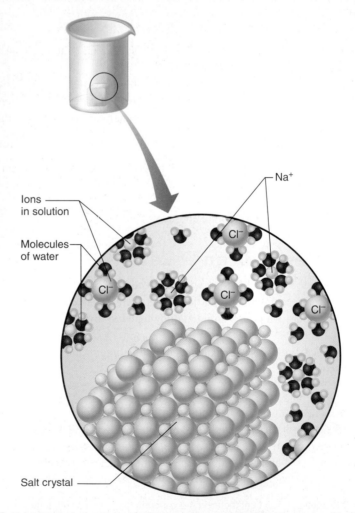

Ions in solution

Na⁺

Cl⁻

Cl⁻

Molecules of water

Cl⁻

Cl⁻

Salt crystal

FIGURE B.6 How water keeps ions in solution. The slightly negative ends of polar water molecules are attracted to positive ions, whereas the slightly positive ends of water molecules are attracted to negative ions. The water molecules pull the ions away from the crystal and prevent them from reassociating with each other.

In pure water, only a very few molecules of water are dissociated (broken apart) into H^+ and OH^- at any one time. However, there are other sources of hydrogen ions in aqueous solutions. An *acid* is any molecule that can donate (give up) an H^+. When added to pure water, acids produce an *acidic* solution, one with a higher H^+ concentration than that of pure water. (By definition, an aqueous solution with the same H^+ concentration as that of pure water is a *neutral* solution.) Common acidic solutions are vinegar, carbonated beverages, and orange juice. Conversely, a *base* is any molecule that can accept (combine with) an H^+. When added to pure water, bases produce a basic or *alkaline* solution, one with a lower H^+ concentration than that of pure water. Common alkaline solutions include baking soda in water, detergents, and drain cleaner.

Because acids and bases have opposite effects on the H^+ concentration of solutions, they are said to neutralize each other.

The pH Scale Expresses Hydrogen Ion Concentration

Scientists use the pH scale to indicate the acidity or alkalinity of a solution. The *pH scale* is a measure of the hydrogen ion concentration of a solution. The scale ranges from 0 to 14, with the pH of pure water defined as a pH of 7.0, the neutral point. A pH of 7 corresponds to a hydrogen ion concentration of 10^{-7} moles/liter (a *mole* is a term used by chemists to indicate a certain number of atoms, ions, or molecules). An *acidic* solution has a pH of *less* than 7, whereas a *basic* solution has a pH of *greater* than 7. Each whole-number change in pH represents a tenfold change in the hydrogen ion concentration in the opposite direction. For example, an acidic solution with a pH of 6 has an H^+ concentration of 10^{-6} moles/liter (ten times greater than pure water), whereas an alkaline solution with a pH of 8 has an H^+ concentration of 10^{-8} moles/liter (1/10 that of water). Figure 3.7 on page 85 shows the pH scale and indicates the pH values of some common substances and foods.

The pH of blood is 7.4, just slightly more alkaline than neutral water. The hydrogen ion concentration of blood plasma is low relative to other ions (the hydrogen ion concentration of blood plasma is less than one-*millionth* that of sodium ions, for example). It is important to maintain homeostasis of this low concentration of hydrogen ions in the body because hydrogen ions are small, mobile, positively charged, and highly reactive. Hydrogen ions tend to displace other positive ions in molecules, and this displacement then alters molecular structures and changes the ability of the molecule to function properly.

Changes in the pH of body fluids can affect how molecules are transported across the cell membrane and how rapidly certain chemical reactions occur. pH changes may even alter the shapes of proteins that are structural elements of the cell. In other words, a change in the hydrogen ion concentration can be dangerous because it alters the body's metabolism and threatens homeostasis.

Buffers Minimize Changes in pH

A *buffer* is any substance that tends to minimize the changes in pH that might otherwise occur when an acid or base is added to a solution. Buffers are essential to the body's ability to maintain homeostasis of pH in body fluids.

In biological solutions such as blood or urine, buffers are present as *pairs* of related molecules that have opposite effects. One molecule of the pair is the acid form of the molecule (capable of donating an H^+), and the other is the base form (capable of accepting an H^+). When an acid is added and the number of H^+ ions increases, the base form of the buffer pair will accept some of the H^+, minimizing the fall in pH that might otherwise occur. Conversely, when a base is added that might take up too many H^+ ions, the acid form of the buffer pair will release additional H^+ and thus minimize the rise in pH. Buffer pairs are like absorbent sponges that can pick up excess water and then can be wrung out to release water when necessary.

One of the most important buffer pairs in body fluids such as blood is bicarbonate (HCO_3^-, the base form) and carbonic acid (H_2CO_3, the acid form). When blood becomes too acidic, bicarbonate accepts excess H^+ according to the following reaction:

$$HCO_3^- + H^+ \rightarrow H_2CO_3$$

When blood becomes too alkaline, carbonic acid donates H^+ by the reverse reaction:

$$HCO_3^- + H^+ \leftarrow H_2CO_3$$

In a biological solution such as blood, bicarbonate and carbonic acid take up and release H^+ all the time. Ultimately, a chemical *equilibrium* is reached in which the rates of the two chemical reactions are the same, as represented by the following combined equation:

$$HCO_3^- + H^+ \leftrightarrow H_2CO_3$$

When excess acid is produced, the combined equation shifts to the right as the bicarbonate combines with the H^+. The reverse is true for alkalinity.

There are many other buffers in the body. The more buffers that are present in a body fluid, the more stable the pH will be.

The Organic Molecules

Organic molecules are molecules that contain carbon and other elements held together by covalent bonds. The name "organic" came about at a time when scientists believed that all organic molecules were created only by living organisms and all "inorganic" molecules came from nonliving matter. Today scientists know that organic molecules can be synthesized in the laboratory under the right conditions.

Carbon Is the Common Building Block of Organic Molecules

Carbon is the common building block of all organic molecules because of the many ways that it can form strong covalent bonds with other atoms. Carbon has six electrons, two in the first shell and four in the second. Because carbon is most stable when its second shell is filled with eight electrons, *its natural tendency is to form four covalent bonds with other molecules*. This makes carbon an ideal structural component, one that can branch in a multitude of directions.

Using the chemist's convention that a line between the chemical symbols of atoms represents a pair of shared electrons in a covalent bond, **Figure B.7** shows some of the many structural possibilities for carbon. Carbon can form covalent bonds with hydrogen, nitrogen, oxygen, or another carbon. It can form double covalent bonds with oxygen or another carbon. It can even form five- or six-membered carbon rings, with or without double bonds between carbons.

In addition to their complexity, there is almost no limit to the size of organic molecules derived from carbon. Some, called *macromolecules* (from the Greek *makros*, long), consist of thousands or even millions of smaller molecules. Protein and glycogen are two examples of macromolecules.

Chemical Reactions

In a chemical reaction, original substances (reactants) are changed to new substances (products) with different physical properties and different compositions. All of the atoms of the original reactants are found in the products. However, some of the bonds between the atoms in the reactants have been broken and new bonds have formed between different combinations of atoms to produce the products. For example, when you light a gas burner, the molecules of methane gas (CH_4) react with oxygen (O_2) in the air to produce CO_2, H_2O, and heat.

In another chemical reaction, when an antacid tablet is placed in water, as the sodium bicarbonate ($NaHCO_3$) and citric acid ($C_6H_8O_7$) in the tablet react, bubbles of carbon dioxide

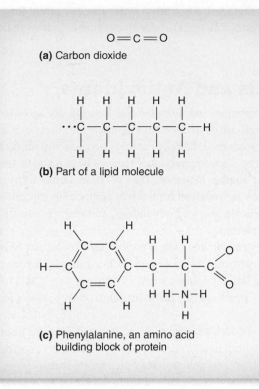

FIGURE B.7 Examples of the structural diversity of carbon. **(a)** In carbon dioxide, a carbon atom forms two covalent bonds with each oxygen atom. **(b)** Lipid molecules contain long chains of carbon atoms covalently bound to hydrogen. **(c)** Carbon is the backbone of the amino acid phenylalanine.

(CO_2) gas appear. In both these chemical reactions, new properties can be observed. These clues tell you that a chemical reaction has taken place.

Oxidation and Reduction Reactions

In every oxidation–reduction reaction (abbreviated redox), electrons are transferred from one substance to another. If one substance loses electrons, another substance must gain an equal number of electrons. Oxidation is defined as the *loss* of electrons; reduction is the *gain* of electrons. Every time a reaction involves an oxidation and a reduction, the number of electrons lost is equal to the number of electrons gained. The following is an example of oxidation and reduction:

$$Zn \rightarrow Zn^{2+} + 2^{e-} \text{ Oxidation of Zn}$$
$$Cu^{2+} + 2^{e-} \rightarrow Cu \text{ Reduction of } Cu^{2+}$$

Enzymes Facilitate Biochemical Reactions

An *enzyme* is a protein that functions as a biological *catalyst*. A catalyst is a substance that speeds up the rate of a chemical reaction without being altered or consumed by the reaction. Enzymes help biochemical reactions to occur, but they do not change the final result of the reaction. That is, they can only speed reactions that would have happened anyway, although much more slowly. A chemical reaction that could take hours by itself might take place in minutes or seconds in the presence of an enzyme.

Without help from thousands of enzymes, most biochemical reactions in our cells would occur too slowly to sustain life. Each enzyme facilitates a particular chemical reaction or group of reactions. Some enzymes break molecules apart; others join molecules together. Enzymes serve as catalysts because, as proteins, they can change shape. The ability to change shape allows them to bind to other molecules and orient them so that they may interact. Figure 6.12 on page 225 depicts how an enzyme facilitates bonding between two compounds.

Free Radicals and Antioxidants

Oxygen free radicals, sometimes simply called free radicals, are an especially unstable class of molecules. Free radicals are oxygen-containing molecules that have an unpaired electron in their outer shell. They are exceptionally unstable because any unpaired electron has a very high potential energy. Consequently, free radicals have a strong tendency to oxidize (remove electrons from) another molecule. They set in motion a destructive cascade of events in which electrons are removed from stable compounds, producing still more unstable compounds. Free radicals damage body tissues, and many scientists believe that they contribute to the aging process.

One of the most destructive free radical molecules is molecular oxygen with an extra electron (O_2^-), called superoxide. Other important free radicals include peroxide (H_2O_2) and hydroxyl (OH). The latter is formed when a hydroxide ion (OH^-) loses an electron. Please refer to Figure 10.3 on page 382 for more detail on free radical formation in the cell membrane.

Some free radicals are accidentally produced in small amounts during the normal process of energy transfer within living cells. Exposure to chemicals, radiation, ultraviolet light, cigarette smoke, alcohol, and air pollution may also create them.

We now know that certain enzymes and nutrients called antioxidants are the body's natural defense against oxygen free radicals. Antioxidants prevent oxidation either by preventing the formation of free radicals in the first place or by inactivating them quickly before they can damage other molecules. Important antioxidants include vitamin E, vitamin C, beta-carotene, and an enzyme called superoxide dismutase.

Dehydration Synthesis and Hydrolysis

Macromolecules are built (synthesized) within the cell itself. In a process known as *dehydration synthesis* (also called *condensation*), smaller molecules called subunits are joined together by covalent bonds, like pearls on a string. The name of the process accurately describes what is happening, for each time a subunit is added, the equivalent of a water molecule is removed ("dehydration"). The subunits needed to synthesize macromolecules come from the foods you eat and from the biochemical reactions in your body that break other large molecules down to smaller ones.

The synthesis of macromolecules from smaller molecules requires energy. That is one reason why we need energy to survive and grow. It is no accident that children seem to eat enormous amounts of food. Growing children require energy to make the macromolecules necessary to create new cell membranes, muscle fibers, and other body tissues.

Organic macromolecules are broken down by a process called *hydrolysis*. During hydrolysis, the equivalent of a water molecule is added each time a covalent bond between single subunits in the chain is broken. Note that hydrolysis is essentially the reverse of dehydration synthesis, and thus it should not surprise you that the breakdown of macromolecules releases energy that was stored as potential energy in the covalent bonds between atoms. Hydrolysis of energy-storage molecules is how the body obtains much of its energy. Hydrolysis is also used to break down molecules of food during digestion, to recycle materials so that they can be used again, and to get rid of substances that are no longer needed by the body. Figure 7.4 on page 256 provides an overview of dehydration synthesis and hydrolysis.

Appendix

C Anatomy and Physiology Review

The Cell

Whereas atoms are the smallest units of matter and make up both living and nonliving things, cells are the smallest units of life. That is, cells can grow, reproduce themselves, and perform certain basic functions, such as taking in nutrients, transmitting impulses, producing chemicals, and excreting wastes. The human body is composed of billions of cells that are constantly replacing themselves, destroying worn or damaged cells, and manufacturing new ones. To support this constant demand for new cells, we need a ready supply of nutrient molecules, such as simple sugars, amino acids, and fatty acids, to serve as building blocks. These building blocks are the molecules that come from the breakdown of foods. All cells, whether of the skin, bones, or brain, are made of the same basic molecules of amino acids, sugars, and fatty acids that are also the main components of the foods we eat.

Cells Are Encased in a Functional Membrane

Cells are encased in a membrane called the cell membrane, or *plasma membrane* (**Figure C.1**). This membrane is the outer covering of the cell and defines the cell's boundaries. It encloses the cell's contents and acts as a gatekeeper, either allowing or denying the entry and exit of molecules such as nutrients and wastes.

Cell membranes are composed of two layers, called the *lipid bilayer*, because each layer is made of molecules called *phospholipids*. Phospholipids consist of a long lipid "tail" bound to a round phospholipid "head." The phosphate head interacts with water, whereas the lipid tail repels water. In the cell membrane, the lipid tails of each layer face each other, forming the membrane interior, whereas the phosphate heads face either the extracellular environment or the cell's interior. Located throughout the membrane are molecules of another lipid, cholesterol, which helps keep the membrane flexible. The membrane also contains various proteins, which assist in transport of nutrients and other substances across the cell membrane and in the manufacture of certain chemicals.

Cells Contain Organelles That Support Life

Enclosed within the cell membrane is a liquid called cytoplasm and a variety of organelles (see **Figure C.1**). These tiny structures accomplish some surprisingly sophisticated functions. A brief review of some of them and their functions related to nutrition is as follows:

- **Nucleus.** The nucleus is where our genetic information is located, in the form of deoxyribonucleic acid (DNA). The cell nucleus is darkly colored because DNA is a huge molecule that is tightly packed within it. A cell's DNA contains the instructions that the cell uses to make certain proteins.
- **Ribosomes.** Ribosomes are structures the cell uses to make needed proteins.
- **Endoplasmic reticulum (ER).** The endoplasmic reticulum is important in the synthesis of proteins and lipids and in the storage of the mineral calcium. The ER looks like a maze of interconnected channels.
- **Mitochondria.** Often called the cell's powerhouse, mitochondria produce the energy molecule ATP (adenosine triphosphate) from basic food components. ATP can be thought of as a stored form of energy, drawn upon as we need it. Cells that have high energy needs contain more mitochondria than cells with lower energy needs.

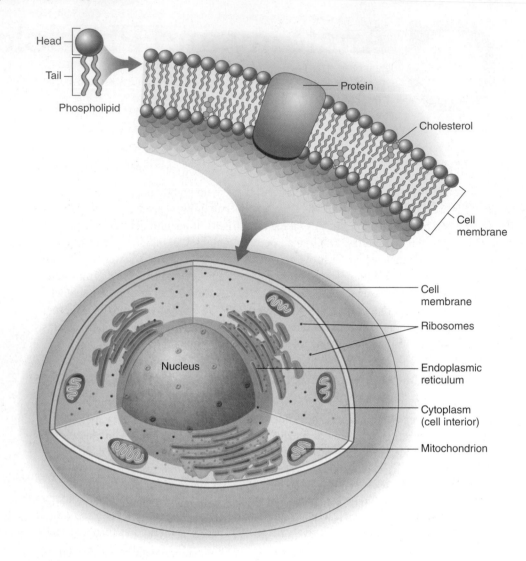

FIGURE C.1 Representative cell of the small intestine, showing the cell membrane and a variety of organelles.

Molecules Cross the Cell Membrane in Several Ways

Recall that the cell membrane is the gatekeeper that, along with its proteins, determines what goes into and out of the cell. This means that cell membranes are *selectively permeable*, allowing only some compounds to enter and leave the cell.

Passive Transport: Principles of Diffusion and Osmosis

Passive transport is "passive" because it transports a molecule without requiring the cell to expend any energy. Passive transport relies on the mechanism of diffusion.

Molecules in a gas or a liquid move about randomly, colliding with other molecules and changing direction. The movement of molecules from one region to another as the result of this random motion is known as diffusion.

If there are more molecules in one region than in another, then strictly by chance more molecules will tend to diffuse away from the area of high concentration and toward the region of low concentration. In other words, the *net* diffusion of molecules requires that there be a difference in concentration, called a *concentration gradient*, between two points. Once the concentration of molecules is the same throughout the solution, a state of equilibrium exists in which molecules are diffusing randomly but equally in all directions.

Not all substances diffuse readily into and out of living cells. The cell membrane is selectively permeable, meaning that it allows some substances to cross by diffusion but not others. It is highly permeable to water, but not to all ions or molecules. The net diffusion of water across a selectively permeable membrane is called *osmosis*. Osmosis and osmotic pressure are discussed in more detail in Chapter 9.

Most substances cross cell membranes by passive transport. Passive transport always proceeds "downhill" with respect to the concentration gradient, meaning that it relies on diffusion in some way. Three forms of passive transport across the cell membrane are (1) diffusion through the lipid bilayer, (2) diffusion through channels, and (3) facilitated transport.

Diffusion through the Lipid Bilayer   The lipid bilayer structure of the cell membrane allows the free passage of some molecules while restricting others. For instance, small uncharged nonpolar molecules can diffuse right through the lipid bilayer as if it did not exist. Such molecules simply dissolve in the lipid bilayer, passing through it as one might imagine a ghost walking through a wall. Polar or electrically charged molecules, on the other hand, cannot cross the lipid bilayer because they are not soluble in lipids.

Two important lipid-soluble molecules are oxygen (O_2), which diffuses into cells and is used up in the process of metabolism, and carbon dioxide (CO_2), a waste product of metabolism, which diffuses out of cells and is removed from the body by the lungs. Another substance that crosses the lipid bilayer by diffusion is urea, a neutral waste product removed from the body by the kidneys.

Diffusion through Channels   Water and many ions diffuse through channels in the cell membrane. The channels are constructed of proteins that span the entire lipid bilayer. The sizes and shapes of these protein channels, as well as the electrical charges on the various amino acid groups that line the channel, determine which molecules can pass through.

Some channels are open all the time (typical of water channels). The diffusion of any molecule through the membrane is largely determined by the number of channels through which the molecule can fit. Other channels are "gated," meaning that they can open and close under certain conditions. Gated channels are particularly important in regulating the transport of ions (sodium, potassium, and calcium) in cells that are electrically excitable, such as nerves.

Facilitated Transport   In facilitated transport, also called *facilitated diffusion*, the molecule does not pass through a channel at all. Instead, it attaches to a membrane protein, triggering a change in the protein's shape or orientation that transfers the molecule to the other side of the membrane and releases it there. Once the molecule is released, the protein returns to its original form. A protein that carries a molecule across the plasma membrane in this manner, rather than opening a channel through it, is called a transport protein (or carrier protein).

Facilitated transport is highly selective for particular substances. The direction of movement is always from a region of high concentration to one of lower concentration, and thus it does not require the cell to expend energy. The normal process of diffusion is simply being "facilitated" by the transport protein. Glucose and other simple sugars enter most cells by this method.

Active Transport Requires Energy

All methods of passive transport allow substances to move only down their concentration gradients, in the direction they would normally diffuse if there were no barrier. However, active transport can move substances through the plasma membrane *against* their concentration gradient. Active transport allows a cell to accumulate essential molecules even when their concentration outside the cell is relatively low and to get rid of molecules that it does not need. Active transport requires the expenditure of energy.

Like facilitated transport, active transport is accomplished by proteins that span the plasma membrane. The difference is that active transport proteins must have some source of energy in order to transport certain molecules. Some active transport proteins use the high-energy molecule ATP for this purpose. They break ATP down to ADP and a phosphate group (P_i) and use the released energy to transport one or more molecules across the plasma membrane against their concentration gradient. Figure 3.15 on page 92 provides an overview of active and passive transport.

From Cells to Organ Systems

Cells of a single type, such as muscle cells, join together to form functional groupings of cells called tissues. In general, several types of tissues join together to form organs, which are sophisticated structures that perform a unique body function. The stomach and small intestine are examples of organs.

Organs are further grouped into systems that perform integrated functions. The stomach, for example, is an organ that is part of the gastrointestinal system. It holds and partially digests a meal, but it cannot perform all system functions—digestion, absorption, and elimination—by itself. These functions require several organs working together in an integrated system. The following sections provide a review of some other body systems.

The Muscular System

Muscle cells are found in every organ and tissue in the body and participate in every activity that requires movement. The most obvious are the *skeletal muscles* that attach to the skeleton and give us strength and mobility. There are two other types of muscle in the body besides skeletal muscle. Rhythmic contractions of the *cardiac muscle* of the heart pump blood throughout the body. Powerful, intermittent contractions of *smooth muscle* in the walls of the uterus contribute to childbirth. Slower waves of smooth muscle contractions push food through the digestive tract and transport urine from the kidney to the bladder. Steady, sustained contractions of smooth muscle in the walls of blood vessels regulate blood flow to every living cell in the body.

A Muscle Is Composed of Many Muscle Cells

A single *muscle* (sometimes referred to as a "whole muscle") is a group of individual muscle cells, all with the same function. In cross section, a muscle appears to be arranged in bundles called *fascicles*, each enclosed in a sheath of a type of fibrous connective tissue called *fascia*. Each fascicle contains from a few dozen to thousands of individual muscle cells, or *muscle fibers*. The outer surface of the whole muscle is covered by several more layers of fascia. At the ends of the muscle all of the fasciae (plural) come together, forming the tendons that attach the muscle to bone (**Figure C.2**).

Individual muscle cells are tube shaped, larger, and usually longer than most other human cells. The entire interior of each muscle cell is packed with long cylindrical structures arranged in parallel, called *myofibrils*. The myofibrils are packed with contractile proteins called *actin* and *myosin*. When myofibrils contract (shorten), the muscle cell also shortens.

The Contractile Unit Is a Sarcomere

Sarcomeres are segments of myofibrils. A single myofibril within one muscle cell in the biceps muscle may contain more than 100,000 sarcomeres arranged end to end. The microscopic shortening of these 100,000 sarcomeres all at once is what produces contraction (shortening) of the muscle cell and of the whole muscle. Understanding muscle shortening, then, is simply a matter of understanding how a single sarcomere works.

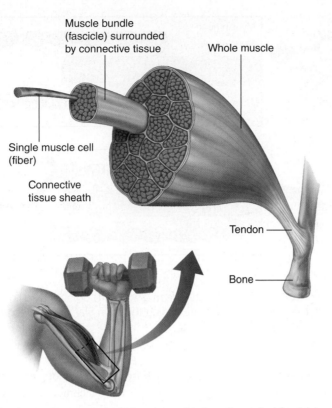

FIGURE C.2 Muscle structure. A muscle is arranged in bundles called fascicles, each composed of many muscle cells and each surrounded by a sheath of connective tissue called fascia. Surrounding the entire muscle are several more layers of fascia. The fascia join together to become the tendon, which attaches the muscle to bone.

A sarcomere consists of two kinds of protein filaments. Thick filaments composed of *myosin* are interspersed at regular intervals within filaments of *actin*. Muscle contractions depend on the interaction between these actin and myosin filaments.

Nerves Activate Skeletal Muscles

Skeletal muscle cells are stimulated to contract by certain nerve cells called motor neurons. The motor neurons secrete a chemical substance called *acetylcholine (ACh)*. Acetylcholine is a neurotransmitter, a chemical released by nerve cells that has either an excitatory or an inhibitory effect on another excitable cell (another nerve cell or a muscle cell). In the case of skeletal muscle, acetylcholine excites (activates) the cells.

When a muscle cell is activated, an electrical impulse races down the inside of the muscle cell. The arrival of that impulse triggers the release of calcium ions from the sarcoplasmic reticulum (a structure similar to other cells' smooth endoplasmic reticulum). The calcium diffuses into the cell cytoplasm and then comes into contact with the myofibrils, where it sets in motion a chain of events that leads to contraction. Muscles contract when sarcomeres shorten, and sarcomeres shorten when the thick and thin filaments slide past each other, a process known as the sliding filament mechanism of contraction (**Figure C.3**).

Muscles Require Energy to Contract and to Relax

Muscle contraction requires a great deal of energy. Like most cells, muscle cells use ATP as their energy source. In the presence of calcium, myosin acts as an enzyme, splitting ATP into ADP and inorganic phosphate and releasing energy to do work.

The energy is used to "energize" the myosin head so that it can form a cross-bridge and undergo bending. Once the bending has occurred, another molecule of ATP binds to the

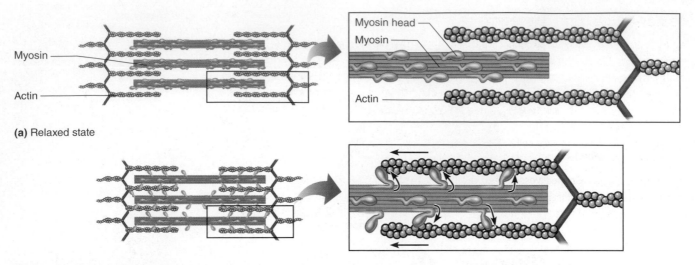

(a) Relaxed state

(b) Contracted state

FIGURE C.3 Sliding filament mechanism of contraction. **(a)** In the relaxed state, the myosin heads do not make contact with actin. **(b)** During contraction, the myosin heads form cross-bridges with actin and bend, pulling the actin filaments toward the center of the sarcomere.

myosin, which causes the myosin head to detach from actin. As long as calcium is present, the cycle of ATP breakdown, attachment, bending, and detachment is repeated over and over again in rapid succession. The result is a shortening of the sarcomere.

At the end of the contractile period (when nerve impulses end), energy from the breakdown of ATP is used to transport calcium back into the sarcoplasmic reticulum so that relaxation can occur. However, a second requirement for relaxation is that an intact molecule of ATP must bind to myosin before myosin can finally detach from actin.

Muscle Cells Obtain ATP from Several Sources   Muscle cells store only enough ATP for about 10 seconds' worth of maximal activity. Once this is used up, the cells must produce more ATP from other energy sources, including creatine phosphate, glycogen, glucose, and fatty acids.

An important pathway for producing ATP involves creatine phosphate (creatine-P), a high-energy molecule with an attached phosphate group. Creatine phosphate can transfer a phosphate group and energy to ADP and therefore create a new ATP quickly. This reaction is reversible: If ATP is not needed to power muscle contractions, the excess ATP can be used to build a fresh supply of creatine phosphate, which is stored until needed.

The combination of previously available ATP plus stored creatine phosphate produces only enough energy for up to 30 to 40 seconds of heavy activity. Beyond that, muscles must rely on stored glycogen. For the first 3 to 5 minutes of sustained activity, a muscle cell draws on its internal supply of stored glycogen. Glucose molecules are converted from the stored glycogen, and their energy is used to synthesize ATP. Part of the process of the breakdown of glucose can be done without oxygen (called anaerobic metabolism) fairly quickly, but it only yields two ATP molecules per glucose molecule.

The most efficient long-term source of energy is the aerobic metabolism of glucose, fatty acids, and other high-energy molecules such as lactic acid. Aerobic metabolism takes place in mitochondria and requires oxygen. The next time you engage in strenuous exercise, note that it may take you a few minutes to start breathing heavily. The increase in respiration indicates that aerobic metabolism is now taking place. Until aerobic metabolism kicks in, however, cells are relying on stored ATP, creatine phosphate, and anaerobic metabolism of glycogen. Weight lifters can rely on stored energy because their muscles perform for relatively short periods. Long-distance runners start out by depending on stored energy, but in less than a minute they are relying almost exclusively on aerobic metabolism. If they could not, they would collapse in exhaustion.

The Cardiovascular System

The heart and blood vessels are known collectively as the cardiovascular system (*cardio* comes from the Greek word for "heart," and vascular derives from the Latin word for "small vessel"). The heart provides the power to move the blood, and the vascular system represents the network of branching conduit vessels through which the blood flows. The cardiovascular system is essential to life because it supplies every region of the body with just the right amount of blood.

Blood Vessels Transport Blood

We classify the body's blood vessels into three major types: *arteries, capillaries*, and *veins*. Thick-walled arteries transport blood to body tissues under high pressure. Microscopic capillaries participate in exchanging solutes and water with the cells of the body. Thin-walled veins store blood and return it to the heart.

As blood leaves the heart it is pumped into large, muscular, thick-walled arteries. Arteries transport blood away from the heart. The larger arteries have a thick layer of muscle because they must be able to withstand the high pressures generated by the heart. Arteries branch again and again, so the farther blood moves from the heart, the smaller in diameter the arteries become. Eventually blood reaches the smallest arteries, called arterioles (literally, "little arteries").

Where an arteriole joins a capillary is a band of smooth muscle called the precapillary sphincter. The precapillary sphincters serve as gates that control blood flow into individual capillaries. Extensive networks of capillaries, called *capillary beds*, can be found in all areas of the body, which is why you are likely to bleed no matter where you cut yourself. Capillaries' branching design and thin, porous walls enable blood to exchange oxygen, carbon dioxide, nutrients, and waste products with tissue cells. In fact, capillaries are the *only* blood vessels that can exchange materials with the interstitial fluid.

Figure C.4 illustrates the general pattern of how water and substances move across a capillary. At the beginning of a capillary, fluid is filtered out of the vessel into the interstitial fluid, accompanied by oxygen, nutrients, and raw materials needed by the cell. The filtered fluid is essentially like plasma except that it contains very little protein because most protein molecules are too large to be filtered. Filtration of fluid is caused by the blood pressure generated by the heart. Waste materials such as carbon dioxide and urea diffuse out of the cells and back into the blood.

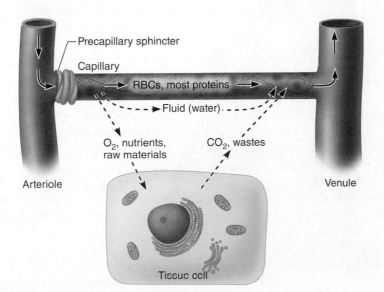

FIGURE C.4 The general pattern of movement between capillaries, the interstitial fluid, and cells. For simplicity, only a single tissue cell is shown, but a single capillary may supply many nearby cells.

From the capillaries, blood flows back to the heart through *venules* (small veins) and veins. Like the walls of arteries, the walls of veins consist of three layers of tissue. However, the outer two layers of the walls of veins are much thinner than those of arteries. Veins also have a larger lumen (that is, are larger in diameter) than arteries.

The Heart Pumps Blood Through the Vessels

The heart is a muscular, cone-shaped organ slightly larger than your fist, located in the thoracic cavity between the lungs and behind the sternum (breastbone). The heart consists mostly of cardiac muscle. Unlike skeletal muscle, cardiac muscle does not connect to bone. Instead, it pumps ceaselessly in a squeezing motion to propel blood through the blood vessels.

The heart consists of four separate chambers. The two chambers on the top are the atria (singular *atrium*), and the two more muscular bottom chambers are the ventricles. A muscular partition called the septum separates the right and left sides of the heart (**Figure C.5**).

The Pulmonary Circuit Provides for Gas Exchange

Review Figure 3.16 on page 93, which shows the general structure of the entire cardiovascular system. Note that the heart is pumping blood through the lungs (the pulmonary circuit) and through the rest of the body to all the cells (the systemic circuit) simultaneously. Each circuit has its own set of blood vessels. Let's follow the pulmonary circuit first:

1. When blood returns to the heart from the veins, it enters the right atrium. The blood that returns to the heart is deoxygenated—it has given up oxygen to tissue cells and taken up carbon dioxide.
2. From the right atrium, blood passes through the right atrioventricular valve into the right ventricle.
3. The right ventricle pumps blood through the pulmonary semilunar valve into the pulmonary trunk (the main pulmonary artery) leading to the lungs. The pulmonary trunk divides into the right and left pulmonary arteries, which supply the right and left lungs, respectively.

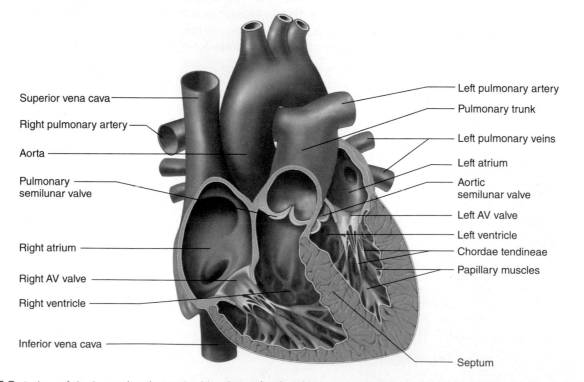

FIGURE C.5 A view of the heart showing major blood vessels, chambers, and valves. The pulmonary vessels are shown in purple to distinguish them from systemic arteries and veins.

4. At the pulmonary capillaries, blood gives up carbon dioxide and receives a fresh supply of oxygen from the air we inhale. It is now oxygenated.
5. The freshly oxygenated blood flows into the pulmonary veins leading back to the heart. It enters the left atrium and flows through the left atrioventricular valve into the left ventricle.

The Systemic Circuit Serves the Rest of the Body

When blood enters the left ventricle, it begins the *systemic circuit*, which takes it to the rest of the body.

1. The left ventricle pumps blood through the aortic semilunar valve into the aorta, the largest artery.
2. From the aorta, blood travels through the branching arteries and arterioles to the capillaries, where it delivers oxygen and nutrients to all of the body's tissues and organs and removes waste products. Even some tissues of the lungs receive their nutrient blood supply from the systemic circulation.
3. From the capillaries, blood flows to the venules, veins, and then back again to the right atrium.

The Lymphatic System

The lymphatic system is closely associated with the cardiovascular system. The lymphatic system performs three important functions:

1. It helps maintain the volume of blood in the cardiovascular system.
2. It transports lipids and fat-soluble vitamins absorbed from the digestive system.
3. It defends the body against infection and injury.

Lymphatic Vessels Transport Lymph

The lymphatic system begins as a network of small, blind-ended *lymphatic capillaries* in the vicinity of the cells and blood capillaries. The lymphatic system helps maintain blood volume and interstitial fluid volume by absorbing excess fluid that has been filtered out of the capillaries and returning it to the cardiovascular system. Lymphatic capillaries in the small intestine are called lacteals and pick up most lipids and fat-soluble vitamins absorbed in the small intestine and eventually send them to the bloodstream.

Lymph capillaries have wide spaces between overlapping cells. Their structure allows them to take up substances (including bacteria) that are too large to enter a blood capillary.

The fluid in the lymphatic capillaries is *lymph*, a milky body fluid that contains white blood cells, proteins, fats, and the occasional bacterium. Lymphatic capillaries merge to form the *lymphatic vessels*. Located at intervals along the lymphatic vessels are small organs called lymph nodes, described in the following section. Like veins, lymphatic vessels contain one-way valves to prevent backflow of lymph. The lymphatic vessels merge to form larger and larger vessels, eventually creating two major lymphatic ducts: the *right lymphatic duct* and the *thoracic duct*. The two lymph ducts join the subclavian veins near the shoulders, thereby returning the lymph to the cardiovascular system.

Lymph Nodes Cleanse the Lymph

Lymph nodes remove microorganisms, cellular debris, and abnormal cells from the lymph before returning it to the cardiovascular system. There are hundreds of lymph nodes, clustered in the areas of the digestive tract, neck, armpits, and groin. They vary in diameter from about 1 mm to 2.5 cm. Each node is enclosed in a dense capsule of connective tissue pierced by lymphatic vessels. Inside each node are connective tissue and two types of white blood cells, known as macrophages and lymphocytes.

The largest lymphatic organ, the spleen, is a soft, fist-sized mass located in the upper- left abdominal cavity. The spleen has two main functions: It controls the quality of circulating red blood cells by removing the old and damaged ones, and it helps fight infection. Note that the main distinction between spleen and lymph nodes is *which* fluid they cleanse—the spleen cleanses the blood, and the lymph nodes cleanse lymph. Together, they keep the circulating body fluids relatively free of damaged cells and microorganisms.

The thymus gland is located in the lower neck, behind the sternum and just above the heart. Encased in connective tissue, the gland contains lymphocytes and epithelial cells. The thymus gland secretes two hormones, thymosin and thymopoietin, that cause certain lymphocytes called *T lymphocytes* (T cells) to mature and take an active role in specific defenses.

The *tonsils* are masses of lymphatic tissue near the entrance to the throat. Lymphocytes in the tonsils gather and filter out many of the microorganisms that enter the throat in food or air.

The Respiratory System

For the sake of convenience, the respiratory system can be divided into the upper and lower respiratory tracts. The *upper respiratory tract* comprises the nose (including the nasal cavity) and pharynx—structures above the "Adam's apple" in men's necks. The *lower respiratory tract* starts with the larynx and includes the trachea, the two bronchi that branch from the trachea, and the lungs themselves (**Figure C.6**).

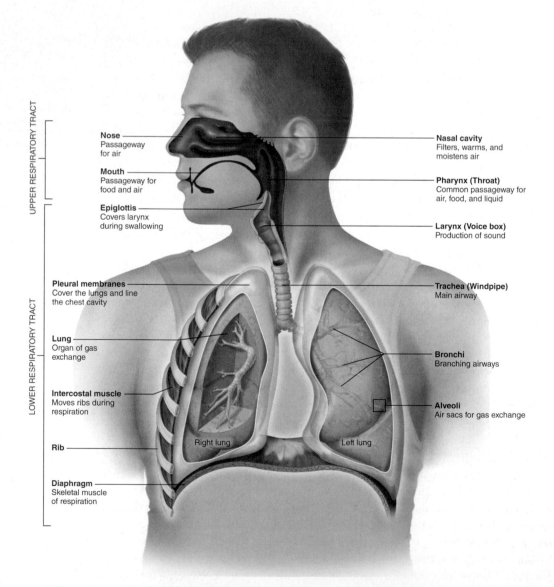

FIGURE C.6 The human respiratory system. The functions of each of the anatomical structures are included.

The Upper Respiratory Tract Filters, Warms, and Humidifies Air

During inhalation, air enters through the nose or mouth. The internal portion of the nose is called the nasal cavity. The mucus in the nasal cavity traps dust, pathogens, and other particles in the air before they get any farther into the respiratory tract.

Incoming air next enters the pharynx (throat), which connects the mouth and nasal cavity to the larynx (voice box). The upper pharynx extends from the nasal cavity to the roof of the mouth. The lower pharynx is a common passageway for both food and air. Food passes through on its way to the esophagus, and air flows through to the lower respiratory tract.

The Lower Respiratory Tract Exchanges Gases

The lower respiratory tract includes the larynx, the trachea, the bronchi, and the lungs with their bronchioles and alveoli. The larynx extends about 5 cm (2 in.) below the pharynx. The larynx contains two important structures: the epiglottis and the vocal cords. The epiglottis is a flexible flap of cartilage located at the opening to the larynx. When air is flowing into the larynx, the epiglottis remains open. But when we swallow food or liquids, the epiglottis tips to block the opening temporarily. This "switching mechanism" routes food and beverages into the esophagus and digestive system, rather than into the trachea. This is why it is impossible to talk while you are swallowing.

As air continues down the respiratory tract, it passes to the trachea, the "windpipe" that extends from the larynx to the left and right bronchi. If a foreign object lodges in the trachea, respiration is interrupted and choking occurs. If the airway is completely blocked, death can occur within minutes. Choking often happens when a person carries on an animated conversation while eating. The risk of choking provides a good reason beyond good manners not to eat and talk at the same time.

The trachea branches into two airways called the right and left bronchi (singular *bronchus*) as it enters the lung cavity. Like the branches of a tree, the two bronchi divide into a network of smaller and smaller bronchi. The smaller airways that lack cartilage are called bronchioles. The smallest bronchioles are 1 mm or smaller in diameter and consist primarily of a thin layer of smooth muscle surrounded by a small amount of elastic connective tissue.

The bronchi and bronchioles also clean the air, warm it to body temperature, and saturate it with water vapor before it reaches the delicate gas exchange surfaces of the lungs.

The Lungs Are Organs of Gas Exchange

The lungs are organs consisting of supportive tissue enclosing the bronchi, bronchioles, blood vessels, and the areas where gas exchange occurs. If you could touch a living lung, you would find that it is very soft and frothy. In fact, most of it is air. The lungs are basically a system of branching airways that end in 300 million tiny air-filled sacs called alveoli (singular *alveolus*). It is here that gas exchange takes place. Alveoli are arranged in clusters at the end of every terminal bronchiole, like grapes clustered on a stem. A single alveolus is a thin bubble of living squamous epithelial cells only one cell layer thick. Their combined surface area is nearly 800 ft^2, approximately forty times the area of a person's skin. The tremendous surface area and thinness facilitate gas exchange with nearby capillaries.

The Nervous System

The nervous system comprises the central nervous system (CNS) and the peripheral nervous system (PNS). The CNS consists of the brain and the spinal cord. It receives, processes, stores, and transfers information. The PNS represents the components of the nervous system that lie outside the CNS. The PNS has two functional subdivisions: The sensory division carries information to the brain and spinal cord, and the motor division carries information from the CNS (**Figure C.7**).

The motor division of the peripheral nervous system is further subdivided along functional lines. The *somatic division* of the PNS controls skeletal muscles, and the autonomic division of the PNS controls smooth muscles, cardiac muscles, and glands.

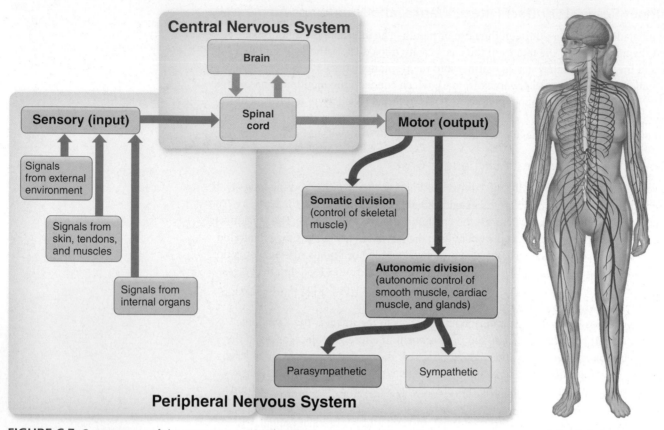

FIGURE C.7 Components of the nervous system. The CNS receives input from the sensory component of the PNS, integrates and organizes the information, and then sends output to the periphery via the motor components of the PNS.

In turn, the *autonomic division* has two subdivisions called the *sympathetic* and *parasympathetic* divisions. In general, the actions of the sympathetic and parasympathetic divisions oppose each other. They work antagonistically to accomplish the automatic, subconscious maintenance of homeostasis within the body.

Neurons

Neurons are cells specialized for communication. They generate and conduct electrical impulses, also called *action potentials*, from one part of the body to another. The longest neurons extend all the way from your toes to your spinal cord.

There are three types of neurons in the nervous system:

1. Sensory neurons of the PNS are specialized to respond to a certain type of stimulus, such as pressure or light. They transmit information about this stimulus to the CNS in the form of electrical impulses. In other words, sensory neurons provide input to the CNS.
2. Interneurons within the CNS transmit impulses between components of the CNS. Interneurons receive input from sensory neurons, integrate this information, and influence the functioning of other neurons.
3. Motor neurons of the PNS transmit impulses away from the CNS. They carry the nervous system's output, still in the form of electrical impulses, to all of the tissues and organs of the body.

All neurons consist of a cell body, one or more dendrites, and an axon. The main body of a neuron is called the cell body. Slender extensions of the cell body, called dendrites, receive information from receptors or incoming impulses from other neurons. Interneurons and motor neurons have numerous dendrites that are fairly short and extend in many directions from the cell body. Sensory neurons are an exception, for their dendrites connect directly to an axon.

An axon is a long, slender tube of cell membrane containing a small amount of cytoplasm. Axons are specialized to conduct electrical impulses. Axons of sensory neurons originate from a dendrite, whereas the axons of interneurons and motor neurons originate from a cone-shaped area of the cell body called the *axon hillock*. At its other end, the axon branches into slender extensions called *axon terminals*. Each axon terminal ends in a small rounded tip called an *axon bulb*.

Action Potentials

An action potential occurs as a sequence of three events: (1) depolarization, (2) repolarization, and (3) reestablishment of the resting potential.

1. *Depolarization: Sodium moves into the axon.* Voltage-sensitive Na^+ channels in the axon's membrane open briefly and Na^+ ions diffuse rapidly into the cytoplasm of the axon. This influx of positive ions causes *depolarization*, meaning that the membrane potential shifts from negative (-70 mV) to positive (about $+30$ mV).

2. *Repolarization: Potassium moves out of the axon.* After a short delay, the Na^+ channels close automatically. But the reversal of the membrane polarity triggers the opening of K^+ channels. This allows more K^+ ions than usual to diffuse rapidly out of the cell. The loss of positive ions from the cell leads to *repolarization*, meaning that the interior of the axon becomes negative again.

3. *Reestablishment of the resting potential.* Because the K^+ channels are slow to close, there is a brief overshoot of membrane voltage during which the interior of the axon is slightly hyperpolarized. Shortly after the K^+ channels close, the resting potential is reestablished. At this point the axon is prepared to receive another action potential. The entire sequence of three steps takes about 3 ms.

Once an action potential is initiated, it sweeps rapidly down the axon until it reaches the axon terminals.

Synaptic Transmission

Once an action potential reaches the axon terminals of a neuron, the information inherent in it must be converted to another form for transmittal to its target. In essence, the action potential causes the release of a chemical that crosses a specialized junction between the two cells called a synapse. This chemical substance is called a neurotransmitter because it transmits a signal from a neuron to its target.

Figure C.8 illustrates the structure of a typical synapse and the events that occur during synaptic transmission. At a synapse, the *presynaptic membrane* is the cell membrane of the neuron that is sending the information. The *postsynaptic membrane* refers to the membrane of the cell that is about to receive the information. The small, fluid-filled gap that separates the presynaptic and postsynaptic membranes is the *synaptic cleft*.

The Endocrine System and Hormones

The endocrine system is a collection of specialized cells, tissues, and glands that produces and secretes circulating chemical messenger molecules called hormones. Most hormones are secreted by endocrine glands—ductless organs that secrete their products into interstitial fluid, lymph, and blood (*endocrine* means "secreted internally"). In contrast, *exocrine* glands secrete products such as mucus, sweat, tears, and digestive fluids into ducts that empty into the appropriate sites. There are approximately fifty known hormones circulating in the human bloodstream, and new ones are still being discovered. Hormones are bloodborne units of information, just as nerve impulses are units of information carried in nerves.

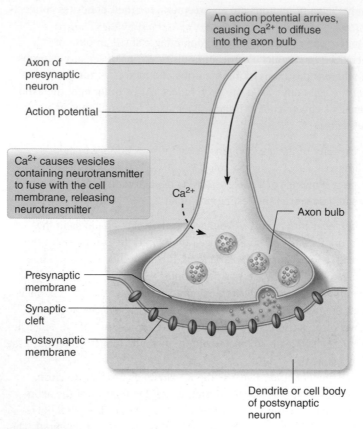

FIGURE C.8 Summary of synaptic transmission.

The endocrine system has certain characteristics that set it apart from the nervous system as a communications system:

1. Hormones of the endocrine system reach nearly every living cell.
2. Each hormone acts only on certain cells.
3. Endocrine control tends to be slower than nervous system control.
4. The endocrine and nervous systems can (and often do) interact with each other.

Hormones Are Classified as Steroid or Nonsteroid

Hormones generally are classified into two basic categories based on their structure and mechanism of action. Steroid hormones are structurally related to cholesterol; in fact, all of them are synthesized from cholesterol and all are lipid soluble. Nonsteroid hormones consist of, or at least are partly derived from, the amino acid building blocks of proteins. In general, they are lipid insoluble. The differences in lipid solubility explain most of the important differences in how the two categories of hormones work. Steroid hormones usually enter the cell, bind to an intracellular receptor, and activate genes that produce new proteins. Nonsteroid hormones generally bind to receptors on the cell's surface. Their binding either opens or closes cell membrane ion channels or activates enzymes within the cell.

The Hypothalamus and the Pituitary Gland

The hypothalamus is a small region in the forebrain that plays an important role in homeostatic regulation. It monitors internal environmental conditions such as water and solute balance, temperature, and carbohydrate metabolism.

The hypothalamus also produces hormones and monitors the pituitary gland, a small endocrine gland located beneath the hypothalamus and connected to it by a stalk of tissue (review Figure 3.1 on page 73). The pituitary gland is sometimes called the "master gland" because it secretes eight different hormones and regulates many of the other endocrine glands.

The Urinary System

Excretion refers to processes that remove wastes and excess materials from the body. **Figure C.9** provides a review of the systems involved in managing metabolic wastes and maintaining homeostasis of water and solutes.

Because the excretory capacity of the other organs is limited, the urinary system has primary responsibility for homeostasis of water and most of the solutes in blood and other body fluids. The urinary system consists of the organs (kidneys, ureters, bladder, and urethra) that produce, transport, store, and excrete urine.

Urine is essentially water and solutes. Among the solutes excreted in urine are excess elements and ions, drugs, vitamins, toxic chemicals, and waste products produced by the liver or by cellular metabolism. Some substances, such as water and sodium chloride (salt), are excreted to regulate body fluid balance and salt levels. About the only major solutes *not* excreted by the kidneys under normal circumstances are the three classes of macronutrients. The kidneys keep these nutrients in the body for other organs to regulate.

Water is the most abundant molecule in the body, accounting for at least half of body weight. The urinary system plays a large role in regulating water levels in the blood and body fluids.

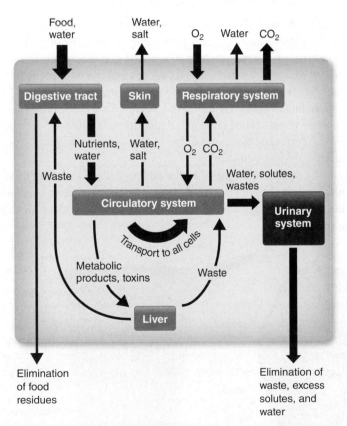

FIGURE C.9 Organ systems involved in removing wastes and maintaining homeostasis of water and solutes. With the large tan box representing the body, this diagram maps the inflow and outflow of key compounds we consume. The kidneys of the urinary system are the organs primarily responsible for the maintenance of homeostasis of water and solutes and for the excretion of most waste products.

Even though many solutes in the body are essential for life, we continually acquire more of them than we can use. The primary solutes excreted by the urinary system are nitrogenous wastes, excess ions, and trace amounts of other substances.

Nitrogenous wastes are formed during the metabolism of proteins. The major nitrogenous waste product in urine is urea. The metabolism of protein initially liberates ammonia (NH_3). Ammonia is quite toxic to cells; however, it is quickly detoxified by the liver. In the liver, two ammonia molecules are combined with a molecule of carbon dioxide to produce a molecule of urea ($H_2N\text{-}CO\text{-}NH_2$) plus a molecule of water. Although far less toxic than ammonia, urea is also dangerous in high concentrations. A small amount of urea appears in sweat, but most of it is excreted by the urinary system.

Dozens of different ions are ingested with food or liberated from nutrients during metabolism. The most abundant ions in the body are sodium (Na^+) and chloride (Cl^-), which are important in determining the volume of the extracellular fluids, including blood. The volume of blood, in turn, affects blood pressure. Other important ions include potassium (K^+), which maintains electrical charges across membranes; calcium (Ca^{2+}), important in nerve and muscle activity; and hydrogen (H^+), which maintains acid–base balance. The rate of urinary excretion of each of these ions is regulated by the kidneys in order to maintain homeostasis.

Trace amounts of many other substances are excreted in proportion to their daily rate of gain by the body. Among them are *creatinine*, a waste product that is produced during the metabolism of creatine phosphate in muscle, and various waste products that give the urine its characteristic yellow color.

Kidneys: The Principal Urinary Organs

The main organs of the urinary system are the two kidneys. The kidneys are located on either side of the vertebral column, near the posterior body wall (**Figure C.10a**). Each kidney is a dark-reddish-brown organ about the size of your fist and shaped like a kidney bean. A *renal artery* and a *renal vein* connect each kidney to the aorta and inferior vena cava, respectively (*renal* comes from the Latin *ren*, meaning "kidney").

Seen in a longitudinal section (Figure C.10b), each kidney consists of inner pyramid-shaped zones of dense tissue (called renal pyramids) that constitute the medulla and an outer zone called the cortex. At the center of the kidney is a hollow space, the *renal pelvis*, where urine collects after it is formed.

A closer look at a section of the renal cortex and medulla reveals that it contains long, thin, tubular structures called *nephrons* (Figure C.10c). Nephrons share a common final section called the *collecting duct*, through which urine produced by the nephrons is delivered to the renal pelvis.

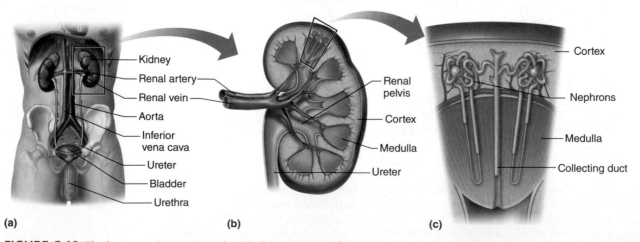

(a)   (b)   (c)

FIGURE C.10 The human urinary system (male). **(a)** Locations of the components of the urinary system within the body. **(b)** Internal structure of a kidney. **(c)** The cortex and medulla of the kidney are composed of numerous nephrons.

In addition to being the primary organs of the urinary system, the kidneys regulate the production of red blood cells in the bone marrow, through the secretion of the hormone erythropoietin, activate the inactive form of vitamin D from the liver, and help maintain blood pressure, volume, and pH.

The Integumentary System

The proper name for the skin and its accessory structures such as hair, nails, and glands is the integumentary system (from the Latin *integere*, meaning "to cover").

The skin has several different functions related to its role as the outer covering of the body: protection from dehydration (helps prevent our bodies from drying out), protection from injury (such as abrasion), defense against invasion by bacteria and viruses, regulation of body temperature, synthesis of an inactive form of vitamin D, and sensation (provides information about the external world via receptors for touch, vibration, pain, and temperature).

The outer layer of the skin's tissue is the epidermis and the inner layer of connective tissue is the dermis (**Figure C.11**).

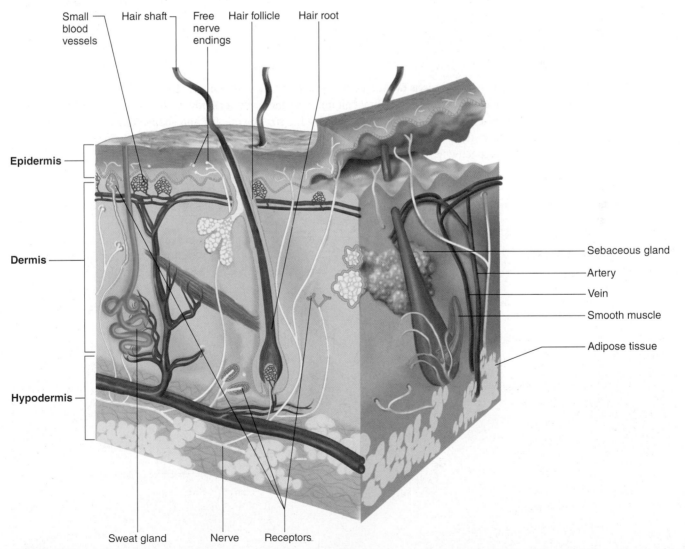

FIGURE C.11 The skin. The two layers of skin (epidermis and dermis) rest on a supportive layer (hypodermis). Although not part of the skin, the hypodermis provides the important functions of cushioning and insulation.

The skin rests on a supportive layer called the *hypodermis* (*hypo-* means "under"), consisting of loose connective tissue containing fat cells. The hypodermis is flexible enough to allow the skin to move and bend. The fat cells in the hypodermis insulate against excessive heat loss and cushion against injury.

As discussed in Chapter 11, skin synthesizes an inactive form of vitamin D. A cholesterol compound in the skin becomes an inactive form of vitamin D when it is exposed to the ultraviolet rays of sunlight. The inactive form must then be modified in the liver and kidneys before it becomes active (see Figure 11.8 on page 437).

Appendix

D Calculations and Conversions

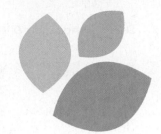

Calculation and Conversion Aids

Commonly Used Metric Units

millimeter (mm):	one-thousandth of a meter (0.001)
centimeter (cm):	one-hundredth of a meter (0.01)
kilometer (km):	one-thousand times a meter (1,000)
kilogram (kg):	one-thousand times a gram (1,000)
milligram (mg):	one-thousandth of a gram (0.001)
microgram (µg):	one-millionth of a gram (0.000001)
milliliter (ml):	one-thousandth of a liter (0.001)

International Units

Some vitamin supplements may report vitamin content as International Units (IU).

To convert IU to

- Micrograms of vitamin D (cholecalciferol), divide the IU value by 40 or multiply by 0.025.
- Milligrams of vitamin E (alpha-tocopherol), divide the IU value by 1.5 if vitamin E is from natural sources. Divide the IU value by 2.22 if vitamin E is from synthetic sources.
- Vitamin A: 1 IU = 0.3 µg retinol or 3.6 µg beta-carotene.

Retinol Activity Equivalents

Retinol Activity Equivalents (RAE) are a standardized unit of measure for vitamin A. RAE account for the various differences in bioavailability from sources of vitamin A. Many supplements will report vitamin A content in IU, as just shown, or Retinol Equivalents (RE).

1 RAE =	1 µg retinol
	12 µg beta-carotene
	24 µg other vitamin A carotenoids

To calculate RAE from the RE value of vitamin carotenoids in foods, divide RE by 2.

For vitamin A supplements and foods fortified with vitamin A, 1 RE = 1 RAE.

Folate

Folate is measured as Dietary Folate Equivalents (DFE). DFE account for the different factors affecting bioavailability of folate sources.

1 DFE =	1 µg food folate
	0.6 µg folate from fortified foods
	0.5 µg folate supplement taken on an empty stomach
	0.6 µg folate as a supplement consumed with a meal

To convert micrograms of synthetic folate, such as that found in supplements or fortified foods, to DFE:

$$\mu g \text{ synthetic} \times \text{folate } 1.7 = \mu g \text{ DFE}$$

For naturally occurring food folate, such as spinach, each microgram of folate equals 1 microgram DFE:

$$\mu g \text{ folate} = \mu g \text{ DFE}$$

Conversion Factors

Use the following table to convert U.S. measurements to metric equivalents:

Original Unit	Multiply By	To Get
ounces avdp	28.3495	grams
ounces	0.0625	pounds
pounds	0.4536	kilograms
pounds	16	ounces
grams	0.0353	ounces
grams	0.002205	pounds
kilograms	2.2046	pounds
liters	1.8162	pints (dry)
liters	2.1134	pints (liquid)
liters	0.9081	quarts (dry)
liters	1.0567	quarts (liquid)
liters	0.2642	gallons (U.S.)
pints (dry)	0.5506	liters
pints (liquid)	0.4732	liters
quarts (dry)	1.1012	liters
quarts (liquid)	0.9463	liters
gallons (U.S.)	3.7853	liters
millimeters	0.0394	inches
centimeters	0.3937	inches
centimeters	0.03281	feet
inches	25.4000	millimeters

Original Unit	Multiply By	To Get
inches	2.5400	centimeters
inches	0.0254	meters
feet	0.3048	meters
meters	3.2808	feet
meters	1.0936	yards
cubic feet	0.0283	cubic meters
cubic meters	35.3145	cubic feet
cubic meters	1.3079	cubic yards
cubic yards	0.7646	cubic meters

Length: U.S. and Metric Equivalents

¼ inch = 0.6 centimeter
1 inch = 2.5 centimeters
1 foot = 0.3048 meter
        30.48 centimeters
1 yard = 0.91144 meter
1 millimeter = 0.03937 inch
1 centimeter = 0.3937 inch
1 decimeter = 3.937 inches
1 meter = 39.37 inches
        1.094 yards
1 micrometer = 0.00003937 inch

Weights and Measures

Food Measurement Equivalencies from U.S. to Metric

Capacity

1/5 teaspoon = 1 milliliter
¼ teaspoon = 1.25 milliliters
½ teaspoon = 2.5 milliliters
1 teaspoon = 5 milliliters
1 tablespoon = 15 milliliters
1 fluid ounce = 28.4 milliliters
¼ cup = 60 milliliters
1/3 cup = 80 milliliters
½ cup = 120 milliliters
1 cup = 225 milliliters
1 pint (2 cups) = 473 milliliters
1 quart (4 cups) = 0.95 liter
1 liter (1.06 quarts) = 1,000 milliliters
1 gallon (4 quarts) = 3.84 liters

Weight

0.035 ounce = 1 gram
1 ounce = 28 grams
¼ pound (4 ounces) = 114 grams
1 pound (16 ounces) = 454 grams
2.2 pounds (35 ounces) = 1 kilogram

U.S. Food Measurement Equivalents

3 teaspoons = 1 tablespoon
½ tablespoon = 1½ teaspoons
2 tablespoons = 1/8 cup
4 tablespoons = ¼ cup
5 tablespoons + 1 teaspoon = 1/3 cup
8 tablespoons = ½ cup
10 tablespoons + 2 teaspoons = 2/3 cup
12 tablespoons = ¾ cup
16 tablespoons = 1 cup
2 cups = 1 pint
4 cups = 1 quart
2 pints = 1 quart
4 quarts = 1 gallon

Volumes and Capacities

1 cup = 8 fluid ounces
        ½ liquid pint
1 milliliter = 0.061 cubic inch
1 liter = 1.057 liquid quarts
        0.908 dry quart
        61.024 cubic inches
1 U.S. gallon = 231 cubic inches
        3.785 liters
        0.833 British gallon
        128 U.S. fluid ounces
1 British Imperial gallon = 277.42 cubic inches
        1.201 U.S. gallons
        4.546 liters
        160 British fluid ounces
1 U.S. ounce, liquid or fluid = 1.805 cubic inches
        29.574 milliliters
        1.041 British fluid ounces
1 pint, dry = 33.600 cubic inches
        0.551 liter
1 pint, liquid = 28.875 cubic inches
        0.473 liter
1 U.S. quart, dry = 67.201 cubic inches
        1.101 liters
1 U.S. quart, liquid = 57.75 cubic inches
        0.946 liter
1 British quart = 69.354 cubic inches
        1.032 U.S. quarts, dry
        1.201 U.S. quarts, liquid

Energy Units

1 kilocalorie (kcal) = 4.2 kilojoules
1 millijoule (MJ) = 240 kilocalories
1 kilojoule (kJ) = 0.24 kcal
1 gram carbohydrate = 4 kcal
1 gram fat = 9 kcal
1 gram protein = 4 kcal

Temperature Standards

	°Fahrenheit	°Celsius
Body temperature	98.6°	37°
Comfortable room temperature	65–75°	18–24°
Boiling point of water	212°	100°
Freezing point of water	32°	0°

Temperature Scales

To Convert Fahrenheit to Celsius:

$$[(°F - 32) \times 5]/9$$

1. Subtract 32 from °F.
2. Multiply (°F − 32) by 5; then divide by 9.

To Convert Celsius to Fahrenheit:

$$[(°C \times 9)/5] + 32$$

1. Multiply °C by 9; then divide by 5.
2. Add 32 to (°C × 9/5).

Appendix

E Foods Containing Caffeine

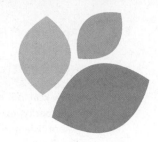

Source: USDA Nutrient Database for Standard Reference, Release 24, by the U.S. Department of Agriculture, Agricultural Research Service, from the Nutrient Data Laboratory Home Page, 2011.

Beverages

Food Name	Serving	Caffeine/Serving (mg)
Beverage mix, chocolate flavor, dry mix, prepared w/milk	1 cup (8 fl. oz)	7.98
Beverage mix, chocolate malt powder, fortified, prepared w/milk	1 cup (8 fl. oz)	5.3
Beverage mix, chocolate malted milk powder, no added nutrients, prepared w/milk	1 cup (8 fl. oz)	7.95
Beverage, chocolate syrup w/o added nutrients, prepared w/milk	1 cup (8 fl. oz)	5.64
Beverage, chocolate syrup, fortified, mixed w/milk	1 cup milk and 1 tbsp. syrup	2.63
Cocoa mix w/aspartame and calcium and phosphorus, no sodium or vitamin A, low kcal, dry, prepared	6 fl. oz water and 0.53 oz packet	5
Cocoa mix w/aspartame, dry, low kcal, prepared w/water	1 packet dry mix with 6 fl. oz water	1.92
Cocoa mix, dry mix	1 serving (3 heaping tsp. or 1 envelope)	5.04
Cocoa mix, dry, w/o added nutrients, prepared w/water	1 oz packet with 6 fl. oz water	4.12
Cocoa mix, fortified, dry, prepared w/water	6 fl. oz H_2O and 1 packet	6.27
Cocoa, dry powder, high-fat or breakfast, plain	1 piece	6.895
Cocoa, hot, homemade w/whole milk	1 cup	5
Coffee liqueur, 53 proof	1 fl. oz	9.048
Coffee liqueur, 63 proof	1 fl. oz	9.05
Coffee w/cream liqueur, 34 proof	1 fl. oz	2.488
Coffee mix w/sugar (cappuccino), dry, prepared w/water	6 fl. oz H_2O and 2 rounded tsp. mix	74.88
Coffee mix w/sugar (French), dry, prepared w/water	6 fl. oz H_2O and 2 rounded tsp. mix	51.03
Coffee mix w/sugar (mocha), dry, prepared w/water	6 fl. oz and 2 round tsp. mix	33.84
Coffee, brewed	1 cup (8 fl. oz)	94.8
Coffee, brewed, prepared with tap water, decaffeinated	1 cup (8 fl. oz)	2.37
Coffee, instant, prepared	1 cup (8 fl. oz)	61.98
Coffee, instant, regular, powder, half the caffeine	1 cup (8 fl. oz)	30.99
Coffee, instant, decaffeinated	1 cup (8 fl. oz)	1.79
Coffee and cocoa (mocha) powder, with whitener and low-calorie sweetener	1 cup	405.48
Coffee, brewed, espresso, restaurant-prepared	1 cup (8 fl. oz)	502.44
Coffee, brewed, espresso, restaurant-prepared, decaffeinated	1 cup (8 fl. oz)	2.37
Energy drink, with caffeine, niacin, pantothenic acid, vitamin B6	1 fl. oz	9.517
Milk beverage mix, dairy drink w/aspartame, low kcal, dry, prep	6 fl. oz	4.08
Milk, lowfat, 1% fat, chocolate	1 cup	5
Milk, whole, chocolate	1 cup	5
Soft drink, cola w/caffeine	1 fl. oz	2
Soft drink, cola, w/higher caffeine	1 fl. oz	8.33
Soft drink, cola or pepper type, low kcal w/saccharin and caffeine	1 fl. oz	3.256
Soft drink, cola, low kcal w/saccharin and aspartame, w/caffeine	1 fl. oz	4.144
Soft drink, lemon-lime soda, w/caffeine	1 fl. oz	4.605

Food Name	Serving	Caffeine/Serving (mg)
Soft drink, low kcal, not cola or pepper, with aspartame and caffeine	1 fl. oz	4.44
Soft drink, pepper type, w/caffeine	1 fl. oz	3.07
Tea mix, instant w/lemon flavor, w/saccharin, dry, prepared	1 cup (8 fl. oz)	16.59
Tea mix, instant w/lemon, unsweetened, dry, prepared	1 cup (8 fl. oz)	26.18
Tea mix, instant w/sugar and lemon, dry, no added vitamin C, prepared	1 cup (8 fl. oz)	28.49
Tea mix, instant, unsweetened, dry, prepared	1 cup (8 fl. oz)	30.81
Tea, brewed	1 cup (8 fl. oz)	47.36
Tea, brewed, prepared with tap water, decaffeinated	1 cup (8 fl. oz)	2.37
Tea, instant, unsweetened, powder, decaffeinated	1 tsp.	1.183
Tea, instant, w/o sugar, lemon-flavored, w/added vitamin C, dry prepared	1 cup (8 fl. oz)	26.05
Tea, instant, with sugar, lemon-flavored, decaffeinated, no added vitamin	1 cup	9.1

Cake, Cookies, and Desserts

Food Name	Serving	Caffeine/Serving (mg)
Brownie, square, large (2-3/4" 3 7/8")	1 piece	1.12
Cake, chocolate pudding, dry mix	1 oz	1.701
Cake, chocolate, dry mix, regular	1 oz	3.118
Cake, German chocolate pudding, dry mix	1 oz	1.985
Cake, marble pudding, dry mix	1 oz	1.985
Candies, chocolate-covered, caramel with nuts	1 cup	35.34
Candies, chocolate-covered, dietetic or low-calorie	1 cup	16.74
Candy, milk chocolate w/almonds	1 bar (1.45 oz)	9.02
Candy, milk chocolate w/rice cereal	1 bar (1.4 oz)	9.2
Candy, raisins, milk-chocolate-coated	1 cup	45
Chocolate chips, semisweet, mini	1 cup chips (6 oz package)	107.12
Chocolate, baking, unsweetened, square	1 piece	22.72
Chocolate, baking, Mexican, square	1 piece	2.8
Chocolate, sweet	1 oz	18.711
Cookie Cake, Snackwell Fat Free Devil's Food, Nabisco	1 serving	1.28
Cookie, Snackwell Caramel Delights, Nabisco	1 serving	1.44
Cookie, chocolate chip, enriched, commercially prepared	1 oz	3.118
Cookie, chocolate chip, homemade w/margarine	1 oz	4.536
Cookie, chocolate chip, lower-fat, commercially prepared	3 pieces	2.1
Cookie, chocolate chip, refrigerated dough	1 portion, dough spooned from roll	2.61
Cookie, chocolate chip, soft, commercially prepared	1 oz	1.985
Cookie, chocolate wafers	1 cup, crumbs	7.84
Cookie, graham crackers, chocolate-coated	1 oz	13.041
Cookie, sandwich, chocolate, cream-filled	3 pieces	3.9
Cookie, sandwich, chocolate, cream-filled, special dietary	1 oz	0.85
Cupcake, chocolate w/frosting, low-fat	1 oz	0.86
Doughnut, cake, chocolate w/sugar or glaze	1 oz	0.284
Doughnut, cake, plain w/chocolate icing, large (3-1/2")	1 each	1.14
Fast food, ice cream sundae, hot fudge	1 sundae	1.58
Fast food, milk beverage, chocolate shake	1 cup (8 fl. oz)	1.66
Frosting, chocolate, creamy, ready-to-eat	2 tbsp. creamy	0.82
Frozen yogurt, chocolate	1 cup	5.58
Fudge, chocolate w/nuts, homemade	1 oz	1.984
Granola bar, soft, milk-chocolate-coated, peanut butter	1 oz	0.85
Granola bar, w/coconut, chocolate-coated	1 cup	5.58

Food Name	Serving	Caffeine/Serving (mg)
Ice cream, chocolate	1 individual (3.5 fl. oz)	1.74
Ice cream, chocolate, light	1 oz	0.85
Ice cream, chocolate, rich	1 cup	5.92
M&M's Peanut Chocolate	1 cup	18.7
M&M's Plain Chocolate	1 cup	22.88
Milk chocolate	1 cup chips	33.6
Milk-chocolate-coated coffee beans	1 NLEA serving	48
Milk dessert, frozen, fat-free milk, chocolate	1 oz	0.85
Milk shake, thick, chocolate	1 fl. oz	0.568
Pastry, éclair/cream puff, homemade, custard-filled w/chocolate	1 oz	0.567
Pie crust, chocolate-wafer-cookie-type, chilled	1 crust, single 9"	11.15
Pie, chocolate mousse, no bake mix	1 oz	0.284
Pudding, chocolate, instant dry mix prepared w/reduced-fat (2%) milk	1 oz	0.283
Pudding, chocolate, regular dry mix prepared w/reduced-fat (2%) milk	1 oz	0.567
Pudding, chocolate, ready-to-eat, fat-free	4 oz can	2.27
Syrups, chocolate, genuine chocolate flavor, light, Hershey	2 tbsp.	1.05
Topping, chocolate-flavored hazelnut spread	1 oz	1.984
Yogurt, chocolate, nonfat milk	1 oz	0.567
Yogurt, frozen, chocolate, soft serve	0.5 cup (4 fl. oz)	2.16

F Stature-for-Age Charts

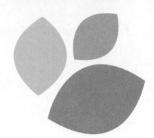

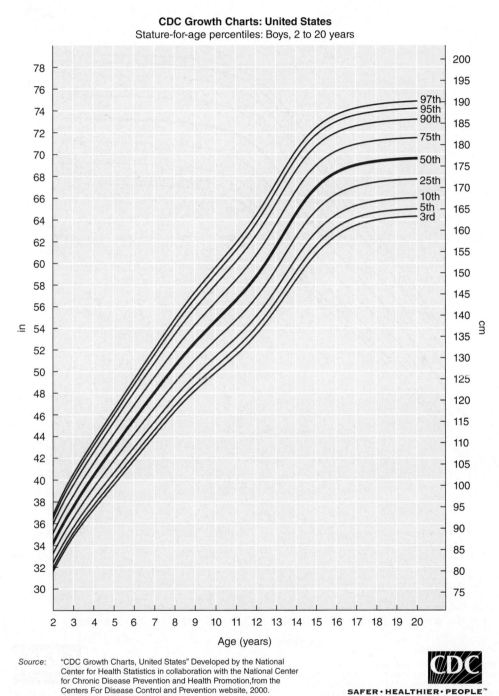

CDC Growth Charts: United States
Stature-for-age percentiles: Boys, 2 to 20 years

Source: "CDC Growth Charts, United States" Developed by the National Center for Health Statistics in collaboration with the National Center for Chronic Disease Prevention and Health Promotion, from the Centers For Disease Control and Prevention website, 2000.

CDC
SAFER · HEALTHIER · PEOPLE™

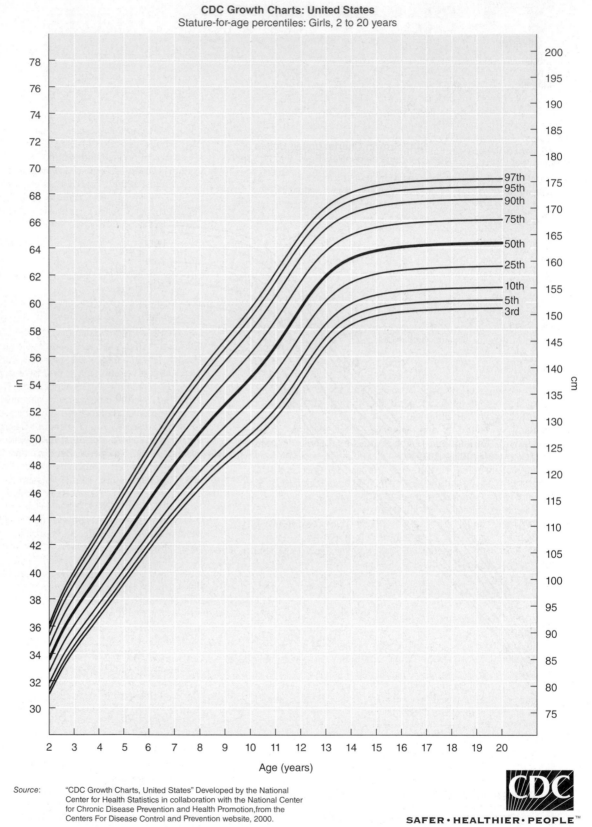

CDC Growth Charts: United States
Stature-for-age percentiles: Girls, 2 to 20 years

Age (years)

Source: "CDC Growth Charts, United States" Developed by the National
Center for Health Statistics in collaboration with the National Center
for Chronic Disease Prevention and Health Promotion,from the
Centers For Disease Control and Prevention website, 2000.

SAFER · HEALTHIER · PEOPLE™

References

Chapter 1

1. Lim, S. S., T. Vos, A. D. Flaxman, G. Danaei, K. Shibuya, H. Adair-Rohani, … , and Z. A. Memish. 2012. A comparative risk assessment of burden of disease and injury attributable to 67 risk factors and risk factor clusters in 21 regions, 1990-2010: a systematic analysis for the Global Burden of Disease Study 2010. Lancet. 380(9859):2224–2260.
2. U.S. Department of Health and Human Services. Updated January 13, 2015. HealthyPeople.gov. http://www.healthypeople.gov/2020/About-Healthy-People. Accessed March 14, 2015.
3. Institute of Medicine, Food and Nutrition Board. 2003. Dietary Reference Intakes: Applications in Dietary Planning. Washington, DC: National Academies Press.
4. Institute of Medicine, Food and Nutrition Board. 2002. Dietary Reference Intakes for Energy, Carbohydrates, Fiber, Fat, Protein and Amino Acids (Macronutrients). Washington, DC: National Academies Press.
5. Cochrane Bias Methods Group. Addressing reporting bias. https://bmg.cochrane.org/addressing-reporting-biases. Accessed March 14, 2015.
6. Winterfeldt, E. A., M. L. Bogle, and L. L. Ebro. 2013. Dietetics. Practice and Future Trends. 4th edn. Sudbury, MA: Jones and Bartlett.

Chapter 2

1. Ogden, C. L., M. D. Carroll, B. K. Kit, and K. M. Flegal. 2014. Prevalence of childhood and adult obesity in the United States, 2011–2012. *JAMA* 311(8):806–814.
2. Academy of Nutrition and Dietetics. 2013. Position of the Academy of Nutrition and Dietetics: functional Foods. *J. Acad. Nutr. Diet*. 113(8):1096–1103.
3. U.S. Department of Health and Human Services and U.S. Department of Agriculture. *2015–2020 Dietary Guidelines for Americans*. 8th Edition. December 2015. Available at http://health.gov/dietaryguidelines/2015/guidelines.
4. Nielsen, S. J., and B. M. Popkin. 2003. Patterns and trends in food portion sizes, 1977–1998. *JAMA* 289(4):450–453.
5. Young, L. R., and M. Nestle. 2002. The contribution of expanding portion sizes to the U.S. obesity epidemic. *Am. J. Pub. Health*. 92(2):246–249.
6. U.S. Department of Agriculture, Economic Research Service. 2014. *Data Products. Food Expenditures*.http://www.ers.usda.gov/data-products/food-expenditures.aspx#26636.
7. Mandala Research, LLC. 2011. LivingSocial dining out survey. Key findings. http://mandalaresearch.com/index.php/purchase-reports/download_form/24-livingsocial-dining-out-survey-key-findings
8. Swartz, J. J., D. Braxton, and A. J. Viera. 2011. Calorie menu labeling on quick-service restaurant menus: an updated systematic review of the literature. *Int. J. Behav. Nutr. Phys. Act.* 8:135.
9. Sinclair, S. E., M. Cooper, and E. D. Mansfield. 2014. The influence of menu labeling on calories selected or consumed: a systematic review and meta-analysis. *J. Acad. Nutr. Diet*. 114:1375–1388, e15.
10. Bleich, S. N., C. L. Barry, T. L. Gary-Webb, and B. J. Herring. 2014. Reducing sugar-sweetened beverage consumption by providing caloric information: how black adolescents alter their purchases and whether the effects persist. *Am. J. Public Health*. 104(12):2417–2424.

Chapter 3

1. Pesta, D. H. and Samuel, V. T. 2014. A high-protein diet for reducing body fat: mechanisms and possible caveats. *Nutr. Metab. (Lond)*. 11(1):53. doi: 10.1186/1743-7075-11-53.

2. Agency for Healthcare Research and Quality. October 2014. Safety of Probiotics Used to Reduce Risk and Prevent or Treat Disease. AHRQ, Rockville, MD. http://www.ahrq.gov/research/findings/evidence-based-reports/er200-abstract.html
3. National Institute of Diabetes and Digestive and Kidney Diseases (NIDDK). 2013, September. Gastroesophageal Reflux (GER),and Gastroesophageal Reflux Disease (GERD) in Adults. NIH Publication No. 13–0882. http://digestive.niddk.nih.gov/ddiseases/pubs/gerd/index.htm.
4. National Digestive Diseases Information Clearinghouse (NDDIC). 2014, August. *Peptic Ulcer Disease and* H. pylori. NIH Publication No. 14–4225. http://www.niddk.nih.gov/health-information/health-topics/digestive-diseases/peptic-ulcer/Documents/hpylori_508.pdf
5. Trasande, L., J. Blustein, M. Liu, E. Corwin, L. M. Cox, and M. J. Blaser 2013. Infant antibiotic exposures and early-life body mass. *Intl. J. Obesity*. 37(1):16–23.
6. Bezmin Abadi, A. T. 2014. *Helicobacter pylori*: a Beneficial Gastric Pathogen? *Front Med (Lausanne)*. 1: 26. Published online Aug 25, 2014. doi: 10.3389/fmed.2014.00026
7. U.S. Food and Drug Administration (FDA). 2014, October 23. Food Allergies: What You Need to Know. www.fda.gov/food/resourcesforyou/consumers/ucm079311.htm.
8. National Digestive Diseases Information Clearinghouse (NDDIC). 2012. Celiac Disease. NIH Publication No. 12-4269. http://digestive.niddk.nih.gov/ddiseases/pubs/celiac/.
9. Tian, N., G. Wei , D. Schuppan, and E. J. Helmerhorst 2014. Effect of Rothia mucilaginosa enzymes on gliadin (gluten) structure, deamidation, and immunogenic epitopes relevant to celiac disease. Am J Physiol: Gastrointest Liver Physiol. 15;307(8):G769–76. doi: 10.1152/ajpgi.00144.2014.
10. Fasano, A., A. Sapone, V. Zevallos, and D. Schuppan, D. 2015. Non-celiac gluten sensitivity. *Gastroenterology*. pii: S0016-5085(15)00029-3. doi: 10.1053/j.gastro.2014.12.049
11. Ludvigsson, J. F., D. A. Leffler, J. C. Bai, F. Baiqi, A. Fasano, P. H. Green…C. Ciacci. (2013). The Oslo definitions for coeliac disease and related terms. *Gut*;62:43–52. doi:10.1136/gutjnl-2011-301346.
12. Mansueto, P., A. Seidita, A. D'Alcamo, and A. Carrocio. 2014. Non-celiac gluten sensitivity: a literature review. *J. Am. Coll. Nutr.* 33(1):39–54. doi: 10.1080/07315724.2014.869996.
13. National Digestive Diseases Information Clearinghouse (NDDIC). 2014, February. Cyclic Vomiting Syndrome. NIH Publication No. 14-4548. http://www.niddk.nih.gov/health-information/health-topics/digestive-diseases/cyclic-vomiting-syndrome/Documents/CyclicVomitingSyndrome_508.pdf.
14. National Digestive Diseases Information Clearinghouse (NDDIC). 2014, September. Crohn's Disease. NIH Publication No. 14-3410. http://www.niddk.nih.gov/health-information/health-topics/digestive-diseases/crohns-disease/Documents/Crohns_508.pdf.
15. National Digestive Diseases Information Clearinghouse (NDDIC). 2014, September. Ulcerative Colitis. NIH Publication No. 14-1597. http://www.niddk.nih.gov/health-information/health-topics/digestive-diseases/ulcerative-colitis/Documents/Ulcerative Colitis_508.pdf.
16. National Digestive Diseases Information Clearinghouse (NDDIC). Update November 25, 2013. Diarrhea. NIH Publication No. 11-5176. http://www.niddk.nih.gov/health-information/health-topics/digestive-diseases/diarrhea/Pages/ez.aspx.
17. National Digestive Diseases Information Clearinghouse (NDDIC). 2013, September. Irritable Bowel Syndrome. NIH Publication No. 13-693. http://www.niddk.nih.gov/health-information/health-topics/digestive-diseases/ibs/Documents/ibs_508.pdf.
18. American Cancer Society. 2014. *Cancer Facts & Figures 2014*. Atlanta: American Cancer Society. http://www.cancer.org/acs/groups/content/@research/documents/webcontent/acspc-042151.pdf

Chapter 4

1. TODAY Study Group. 2012. A clinical trial to maintain glycemic control in youth with type 2 diabetes. *N. Engl. J. Med.* 366:2247–2256.
2. Imperatore G., J. P. Boyle, T. J. Thompson, D. Case, D. Dabelea, R. F. Hamman,..., and SEARCH for Diabetes in Youth Study Group. 2012. Projections of type 1 and type 2 diabetes burden in the U.S. population aged < 20 years through 2050: dynamic modeling of incidence, mortality, and population growth. *Diab Care.* 35(12):2515–2520.
3. Sears, B. 1995. *The Zone. A Dietary Road Map.* New York: HarperCollins.
4. Steward, H. L., M. C. Bethea, S. S. Andrews, and L. A. Balart. 1995. *Sugar Busters! Cut Sugar to Trim Fat.* New York: Ballantine Books.
5. Atkins, R. C. 1992. *Dr. Atkins' New Diet Revolution.* New York: M. Evans & Company.
6. Institute of Medicine, Food and Nutrition Board. 2002. *Dietary Reference Intakes for Energy, Carbohydrates, Fiber, Fat, Protein and Amino Acids (Macronutrients).* Washington, DC: National Academy of Sciences.
7. Humphreys, K. J., M. A. Conlon, G. P. Young, D. L. Topping, Y. Hu, J. M. Winter, A.R. Bird, L. Cobiac, N. A. Kennedy, M. Z. Michael, and R. K. Le Leu. 2014. Dietary manipulation of oncogenic microRNA expression in human rectal mucosa: a randomized trial. *Cancer Prev. Res.* 7(8):786–795.
8. US Department of Agriculture and US Department of Health and Human Services. 2010. *Dietary Guidelines for Americans,* 2010. 7th Edn. Washington, DC: US Government Printing Office. www.cnpp.usda.gov/dietaryguidelines.htm.
9. Goff, L. M., D. E. Cowland, L. Hooper, and G. S. Frost. 2013. Low glycaemic index diets and blood lipids: a systematic review and meta-analysis of randomized controlled trials. *Nut. Metab. Cardiovasc. Dis.* 23(1):1–10.
10. De Koning, L., V. S. Malik, M. D. Kellogg, E. B. Rimm, W. C. Willett, and F. B. Hu. 2012. Sweetened beverage consumption, incident coronary heart disease, and biomarkers of risk in men. *Circulation* 125:1735–1741.
11. Yang Q., Z. Zhang, E. W. Gregg, W. D. Flanders, R. Merritt, and F. B. Hu. 2014. Added sugar intake and cardiovascular diseases mortality among US adults. *JAMA Intern. Med.* 174(4):516–524.
12. Basu, S., P. Yoffee, N. Hills, and R. H. Lustig. 2013. The relationship of sugar to population-level diabetes prevalence: an econometric analysis of repeated cross-sectional data. *PLoS ONE* 8(2):e57873. doi:10.1371/journal.pone.0057873.
13. Te Moranga, L., S. Mallard, and J. Mann. 2013. Dietary sugars and body weight: systematic review and meta-analyses of randomized controlled trials and cohort studies. *BMJ* 346:e7492.
14. Astrup A., A. Raben, and N. Geiker. 2015. The role of higher protein diets in weight control and obesity-related comorbidities. *Int. J. Obes,* epub ahead of print, 20 January 2015. doi: 10.1038/ijo.2014.216.
15. International Food Information Council Foundation. 2014. Facts about Low-Calorie Sweeteners. http://www.foodinsight.org/articles/facts-about-low-calorie-sweeteners.
16. International Food Information Council Foundation. 2014. Everything You Need to Know about Aspartame. http://www.foodinsight.org/Everything_You_Need_to_Know_About_Aspartame
17. Miller, P. E., and V. Perez. 2014. Low-calorie sweeteners and body weight and composition: a meta-analysis of randomized controlled trials and prospective cohort studies. *Am. J. Clin. Nutr.* 100(3):765–777.
18. Peters, J., H. R. Wyatt, G. D. Foster, Z. Pan, A. C. Wojtanowski, S. S. Vander Veur, S.J. Herring, C. Brill, and J. O. Hill. 2014. The effects of water and non-nutritive sweetened beverages on weight loss during a 12-week weight loss treatment program. *Obesity* 22(6):1415–1421.
19. CDC National Center for Chronic Disease Prevention and Health Promotion, Division of Diabetes Translation. 2014. National Diabetes Statistics Report, 2014. http://www.cdc.gov/diabetes/pubs/statsreport14/national-diabetes-report-web.pdf.
20. American Diabetes Association. 2014. Genetics of Diabetes. http://www.diabetes.org/diabetes-basics/genetics-of-diabetes.html.
21. American College Health Association (ACHA). National College Health Assessment (NCHA). 2014. ACHA NCHA II. Reference Group Executive Summary Spring 2014. http://www.acha-ncha.org/docs/ACHA-NCHA-II_ReferenceGroup_ExecutiveSummary_Spring2014.pdf
22. American College of Sports Medicine and the American Diabetes Association. 2010. Exercise and type 2 diabetes: American College of Sports Medicine and American Diabetes Association joint position statement. *Med. Sci. Sports Exerc.* 42(12):2282–2303.
23. Academy of Nutrition and Dietetics. 2014. Diabetes and Diet. http://www.eatright.org/resource/health/diseases-and-conditions/diabetes/diabetes-and-diet
24. National Digestive Diseases Information Clearinghouse. 2014. Lactose Intolerance. NIH Publication No. 14-7994. http://www.niddk.nih.gov/health-information/health-topics/digestive-diseases/lactose-intolerance/Pages/facts.aspx

Chapter 4.5

1. Centers for Disease Control and Prevention. 2015. Alcohol Poisoning Deaths. Available at http://www.cdc.gov/media/dpk/2015/dpk-vs-alcohol-poisoning.html (Accessed February 2015).
2. Hogenkamp, P. S., C. Benedict, P. Sjögren, L. Kilander, L. Lind, and H. B. Schiöth. 2012. Late-life alcohol consumption and cognitive function in elderly men. *Age* 36:243–249.
3. Poli, A., F. Marangoni, A. Avogaro, G. Barba, S. Bellentani, M. Bucci,...and F. Visioli. 2013. Moderate alcohol use and health: a consensus document. *Nutr., Metab Cardiovasc Dis* 23:487–504.
4. Limin Xiang, L., L. Xiao, Y. Wang, H.Li, Z.Huang, and X.He. 2014. Health benefits of wine: don't expect resveratrol too much. *Food Chem* 156:258–263.
5. Park, S-Y., L. N. Kolonel, U. Lim, K. K. White, B. E. Henderson, and L. R. Wilkens. 2014. Alcohol consumption and breast cancer risk among women of five ethnic groups with light to moderate intakes: the Multiethnic Cohort Study. *Interntl. J. Cancer* 134:1504–1510.
6. Jimenez, M., S. E. Chiuve, R. J. Glynn, M. J. Stampfer, C. A. Camargo, W. C. Willett, J. E. Manson, and K. M. Rexrode. 2012. Alcohol consumption and risk of stroke in women. *Stroke* 43:939–945.
7. Chakraborty, S. 2014. Analysis of NHANES 1999-2002 data reveals noteworthy association of alcohol consumption with obesity. *Ann. Gastroenterol.* 27:250–257.
8. NIAAA. 2014. Alcohol Facts and Statistics. www.niaaa.nih.gov/alcohol-health/overview-alcohol-consumption/alcohol-facts-and-statistics. (Accessed February 2015)
9. Centers for Disease Control and Prevention. 2014. Fact Sheets—Binge Drinking. www.cdc.gov/alcohol/fact-sheets/binge-drinking.htm. (Accessed February 2015).
10. White, A., and R. Hingson. 2014. The burden of alcohol use: excessive alcohol consumption and related consequences among college students. *Alcohol Res.* 35:201–218. Available at http://pubs.niaaa.nih.gov/publications/arcr352/201-218.htm (Accessed February 2015).
11. NIAAA. 2014. Harmful Interactions: mixing Alcohol with Medicines. NIH Publication No. 13-5329. Revised 2014. http://pubs.niaaa.nih.gov/publications/Medicine/medicine.htm

12. Feldstein Ewing, S.W., A. Sakhardande, and S-J. Blakemore. 2014. The effect of alcohol consumption on the adolescent brain: a systematic review of MRI and fMRI studies of alcohol-using youth. *NeuroImage: Clinical* 5:420–437.

13. Parada, M., M. Corral, N. Mota, A. Crego, S. Rodríguez Holguín, and F. Cadaveira. 2012. Executive functioning and alcohol binge drinking in university students. Addict. Behav 37:167–172.

14. Molina, P. E., J. D. Gardner, F. M. Souza-Smith, and A. M. Whitaker. 2014. Alcohol abuse: critical pathophysiological processes and contributions to disease burden. *Physiology* 29:203–215.

15. Bagnardi, V., M. Rota, E. Botteri, I. Tramacere, F. Islami F, V. Fedirko, … and C. La Vecchia. 2014. Alcohol consumption and site-specific cancer risk: a comprehensive dose-response. *Brit. J. Cancer* doi:10.1038/bjc.2014.579. 12:580-593

16. Stahre, M., J. Roeber, D. Kanny, R. D. Brewer, and X. Zhang. 2014. Contribution of excessive alcohol consumption to deaths and years of potential life lost in the U.S. *Prev. Chronic. Dis.* doi:10.5888/pcd11.130293.

17. National Institute on Alcohol Abuse and Alcoholism. A Snapshot of Annual High-Risk College Drinking Consequences. 2013, www.collegedrinkingprevention.gov/statssummaries/snapshot.aspx (Accessed February 2015).

18. National Institute on Alcohol Abuse and Alcoholism. Rethinking Drinking: How to Reduce Your Risks. http://.rethinkingdrinking.niaaa.gov/Strategies/TipsToTry.asp. (Accessed February 2015)

Chapter 5

1. Marieb, E. N., and K. Hoehn. 2013. *Human Anatomy and Physiology*. 9th Edn. San Francisco: Benjamin Cummings, p. 46.

2. Brouwer, I. A., A. J. Wanders and M. B. Katan (2013). "Trans fatty acids and cardiovascular health: research completed?" *European journal of clinical nutrition* 67(5): 541–547.

3. Harvey RA., and D.R. Ferrier, 2013. *Lippincott's Illustrated Reviews: Biochemistry*. 5th ed. Philadelphia: Lippincott Williams & Wilkins.

4. Gropper, S. S. and J. L. Smith. 2013. Advanced Nutrition and Human Metabolsim. 6th ed. Belmont, CA: Thompson Wadsworth. Grudy, S. M. 2006. Nutrition in the management of disorders of serum lipids andlipoproetins. IN: Shils. M.E., M. Shike, A. C. Ross, B. Babllero, and R. J. Cousins, eds. *Modern Nutrition in Health and Disease*. 10th Edn. Philadelphia: Lippincott Williams & Wilkins.

5. Pan, A., M. Chen, R. Chowdhury, J. H. Wu, Q. Sun, H. Campos, D. Mozaffarian and F. B. Hu (2012). "a-Linolenic acid and risk of cardiovascular disease: a systematic review and meta-analysis." *Am J Clin Nutr* 96(6): 1262–1273.

6. Lane, K., E. Derbyshire, W. Li and C. Brennan (2014). "Bioavailability and potential uses of vegetarian sources of omega-3 fatty acids: a review of the literature." *Critical reviews in food science and nutrition* 54(5): 572–579.

7. Kaleta, C., L. F. de Figueiredo, S. Werner, R. Guthke, M. Ristow, and S. Schuster. 2011. In silico evidence for gluconeogenesis-from fatty acids in humans. *PLoS Computational Biology* 7(7):e1002116.

8. Gerstein, D. E., G. Woodward-Lopez, A. E. Evans, K. Kelsey, and A. Drewnowski. 2004. Clarifying concepts about macronutrients' effects on satiation and satiety. *J. Am. Diet.* Assoc. 104:1151–1153

9. Howe, S. M., T. M. Hand and M. M. Manore (2014). "Exercise-Trained Men and Women: Role of Exercise and Diet on Appetite and Energy Intake." *Nutrients* 6(11): 4935–4960.

10. Rolls, B. J. (2012). "Dietary strategies for weight management." *Nestlé Nutrition Institute workshop series* 73: 37–48.

11. Rolls, B. J. 2009. The relationship between dietary energy density and energy intake. *Physiol. Behav.* 97(5):609–615.

12. *Institute of Medicine (IOM), Food and Nutrition Board*. 2005. Dietary Reference Intakes for Energy, Carbohydrate, Fiber, Fat, Fatty Acids, Cholesterol, Protein, and Amino Acids (Macronutrients). Washington, DC: National Academies Press.

13. Rodriguez, N. R., N. M. DiMarco, and S. Langley. 2009. Position of the American Dietetic Association, Dietitians of Canada, and the American College of Sports Medicine: nutrition and athletic performance. *J. Am. Diet. Assoc.* 109(3):509–527.

14. Lichtenstein, A. H., and L. Van Horn. 1998. Very low fat diets. *Circulation* 98:935–939.

15. National Institutes of Health, Expert Panel on Detection, Evaluation, and Treatment of High Blood Cholesterol in Adults, 2002. Third report of the National Cholesterol Education Program (NCEP) Expert Panel on Detection, Evaluation, and Treatment of High Blood Cholesterol in Adults (Adult Treatment Panel III) final report. *Circulation* 106:3143–3421. www.nhlbi.nih.gov/guidelines/cholesterol/atp3xsum.pdf

16. United States Department of Agriculture (USDA), Agriculture Research Service (ARS). 2008. Weighing in on Fats. www.ars.usda.gov/is/AR/archive/mar08/fats308.htm (Accessed, January 2015)

17. Ratnayake, W., M. R. L'Abbe, S. Farnworth, et al. 2009. Trans fatty acids: current contents in Canadian foods and estimated intake levels for the Canadian opulation. *Journal of AOAC International* 92(5):1258–1276.

18. Teegala, S. M., W. C. Willett, and D. Mozaffarian. 2009. Consumption and health effects of trans fatty acids: a review. *Journal of AOAC International* 92(5):1250–1257.

19. Clapp, J., C. J. Curtis, A. E. Middleton and G. P. Goldstein (2014). "Prevalence of Partially Hydrogenated Oils in US Packaged Foods, 2012." *Preventing Chronic Disease* 11: E145.

20. Mozaffarian, D., M. B. Katan, A. Ascherio, M. J. Stampfer and W. C. Willett (2006). "Trans fatty acids and cardiovascular disease." *The New England journal of medicine* 354(15): 1601–1613.

21. Willett, W. C. (2012). "Dietary fats and coronary heart disease." *Journal of internal medicine* 272(1): 13–24.

22. Othman, R. A., M. H. Moghadasian and P. J. Jones (2011). "Cholesterol-lowering effects of oat b-glucan." *Nutr Rev* 69(6): 299–309.

23. Baum, S. J., P. M. Kris-Etherton, W. C. Willett, A. H. Lichtenstein, L. L. Rudel, K. C. Maki, J. Whelan, C. E. Ramsden and R. C. Block (2012). "Fatty acids in cardiovascular health and disease: a comprehensive update." *Journal of clinical lipidology* 6(3): 216–234.

24. Flock, M. R., M. H. Green and P. M. Kris-Etherton (2011). "Effects of adiposity on plasma lipid response to reductions in dietary saturated fatty acids and cholesterol." *Advances in Nutrition.* 2(3): 261–274.

25. Grudy, S. M. 2006. Nutrition in the management of disorders of serum lipids andlipoproetins. IN: Shils. M.E., M. Shike, A. C. Ross, B. Babllero, and R. J. Cousins, eds. *Modern Nutrition in Health and Disease*. 10th Edn. Philadelphia: Lippincott Williams & Wilkins.

26. Fernandez, M. L. and M. Calle (2010). "Revisiting dietary cholesterol recommendations: does the evidence support a limit of 300 mg/d?" *Current atherosclerosis reports* 12(6): 377–383.

27. Sabastian R., C. Enns, J. Goldman, and A. Moshfegh. 2008. Effect of fast food consumption on dietary intake and likelihood of meeting MyPyramid recommendations in adults: results from What We Eat in America, NHANES 2003–2004. *FASEB Journal* 22:868.7.

28. Tucker, R. M. and R. D. Mattes (2012). "Are free fatty acids effective taste stimuli in humans? *Journal of food science* 77(3): S148–151.

29. Center for Disease Control and Prevention (CDC) (2010). *How tobacco smoke causes disease: The biology and behavioral basis for smoking-attributable disease: A report of the surgeon general*, Centers for Disease Control and Prevention (US).

30. K.D. Kochanek, S.L. Murphy, J. Xu, and E. Arias. "Mortality in the United States, 2013,"*NCHS Data Brief* No. 178 (December, 2014), data table for Figure 3, http://www.cdc.gov/nchs/data/databriefs/db178.pdf

31. Heidenreich, P. A., J. G. Trogdon, O. A. Khavjou, J. Butler, K. Dracup, M. D. Ezekowitz, E. A. Finkelstein, Y. Hong, S. C. Johnson, A. Khera, D. M. Lloyd-Jones, S. A. Nelson, G. Nichol, D. Orenstein, P. W. F. Wilson, and J. Y. Woo. 2011. Forecasting the future of cardiovascular disease in the United States: a policy statement from the American Heart Association. *Circulation* 123. DOI: 10.1161/CIR.0b013e31820a55f5.

32. Mizuno, Y., F. R. Jacob, and R. P. Mason. 2011. Inflammation and the development of atherosclerosis. *Journal of Atherosclerosis and Thrombosis* 28(5):351–358.

33. Rippe, J. M., T. J. Angelopoulos, and L. Zukley. 2007. The rationale for intervention to reduce the risk of coronary heart disease. *Am. J. Lifestyle Med.* 1(1):10–19.

34. Marwick, T. H., M. D. Hordern, T. Miller, D. A. Chyun, A. G. Bertoni, R. S. Blumenthal, G. Philippides, and A. Rocchini. 2009. Exercise training for type 2 diabetes mellitus: impact on cardiovascular risk: a scientific statement from the American Heart Association. *Circulation* 119:3244–3262.

35. United States Department of Agriculture (USDA) and Department of Health and Human Services (DHHS). 2010. *Dietary Guidelines for Americans 2010.* 7th ed. Washington, DC: US Government Printing Office.

36. Libby, P. (2012). "Inflammation in atherosclerosis." *Arteriosclerosis, thrombosis, and vascular biology* 32(9): 2045–2051.

37. Department of Health and Human Services (DHHS). 2008. *Physical Activity Guidelines Advisory Committee Report.* Washington, DC:US Government Printing Office.

38. Department of Health and Human Services (DHHS). 2010. How Tobacco Smoke Causes Disease: The Biology and Behavioral Basis for Smoking-Attributable Disease: A Report of the Surgeon General. Atlanta, GA: US Department of Health and Human Services, Centers for Disease Control and Prevention, *National Center for Chronic Disease Prevention and Health Promotion*, Office on Smoking and Health.

39. National Cancer Institute. 2011. Harms of Smoking and Health Benefits of Quitting. www.cancer.gov/ (Accessed, December 2014).

40. Hohensinner, P. J., A. Niessner, K. Huber, C. M. Weyand, and J. Wojta. 2011. Inflammation and cardiac outcome. *Current Opinion in Infectious Diseases* 24(3):259–264.

41. Navab, M., S. T. Reddy, B. J. Van Lenten and A. M. Fogelman (2011). "HDL and cardiovascular disease: atherogenic and atheroprotective mechanisms." *Nature reviews Cardiology* 8(4): 222–232.

42. Flock, M. R., W. S. Harris and P. M. Kris-Etherton (2013). "Long-chain omega-3 fatty acids: time to establish a dietary reference intake." *Nutr Rev* 71(10): 692–707.

43. Kromhout, D., & de Goede, J. (2014). Update on cardiometabolic health effects of -3 fatty acids. *Current Opinion In Lipidology*, 25(1), 85–90. doi: http://dx.doi.org/10.1097/MOL.0000000000000041

44. Harris, W. S., D. Mozffarian, E. Rimm, P. Kris-Etherton, L. L. Rudel, L. J. Appel, M. M. Engler, M. B. Engler, and F. Sacks. 2009. Omega-6 fatty acids and risk for cardiovascular disease. *Circulation* 119. DOI: 10.1161/CIRCULATIONAHA.108.19167.

45. National Center for Chronic Disease Prevention and Health Promotion. 2011. Division for Heart Disease and Stroke Prevention addressing the nation's leading killers. At a glance 2011. http://www.cdc.gov/chronicdisease/resources/publications/aag/pdf/2011/heart-disease-and-stroke-aag-2011.pdf (Accessed, December 2014).

46. Lichtenstein, A. H., L. J. Appel, M. Brands, M. Carnethon, S. Daniels, H. A. Franch, B. Franklin, P. Kris-Etherton, W. S. Harris, B. Howard, N. Karanja, M. Lefevre, L. Rudel, F. Sacks, L. Van Horn, M. Winston, and J. Wylie-Rosett. 2006. Diet and lifestyle recommendations revision 2006: scientific statement from the American Heart Association Nutrition Committee. *Circulation* 114:82–96.

47. Gidding, S. S., A. H. Lichtenstein, M. S. Faith, A. Karpyn, J. A. Mennella, B. Popkin, J. Rowe, L. Van Horn, and L. Whitsel. 2009. Implementing American Heart Association Pediatric and Adult Nutrition Guidelines. *Circulation* 119:1161–1175.

48. Flock, M. R. and P. M. Kris-Etherton (2011). "Dietary Guidelines for Americans 2010: implications for cardiovascular disease." *Current atherosclerosis reports* 13(6): 499–507.

49. Eckel, R. H., J. M. Jakicic, J. D. Ard, J. M. de Jesus, N. Houston Miller, V. S. Hubbard, I. M. Lee, A. H. Lichtenstein, C. M. Loria, B. E. Millen, C. A. Nonas, F. M. Sacks, S. C. Smith, Jr., L. P. Svetkey, T. A. Wadden and S. Z. Yanovski (2014). "2013 AHA/ACC guideline on lifestyle management to reduce cardiovascular risk: a report of the American College of Cardiology/American Heart Association Task Force on Practice Guidelines." *Journal of the American College of Cardiology* 63(25): 2960–2984.

50. Rideout, T. C., and P. J. H. Jones. 2010. Plant sterols: an essential component of preventive cardiovascular medicine. *SCAN Pulse* 29(1):1–6.

51. Despres, J. P., and I. Lemieux. 2006. Abdominal obesity and metabolic syndrome. *Nature* 444(14):881–887.

52. Lumeng, C. N. and A. R. Saltiel (2011). "Inflammatory links between obesity and metabolic disease." *The Journal of clinical investigation* 121(6): 2111–2117.

53. Appel, L. J., M. W. Brands, S. R. Daniels, N. Karaja, P. J. Elmer, and F. M. Sacks. 2006. Dietary approaches to prevent and treat hypertenesion: a scientific statement from the American Heart Association. *Hypertension* 47:296–308.

54. American Cancer Society (ACS). 2013. *Body Weight and Cancer Risk.* http://www.cancer.org/acs/groups/content/documents/image/acspc-043765.pdf (Accessed December, 2014)

55. Alexander, D. D., L. M. Morimoto, P. J. Mink, and K. A. Lowe. 2010. Summary and meta-analysis of prospective studies of animal fat intake and breast cancer. *Nutrition Research Reviews* 23(1):169–179.

56. Chlebowski, R. T. (2013). "Nutrition and physical activity influence on breast cancer incidence and outcome." *Edinburgh, Scotland* 22 Suppl 2: S30–37.

57. Meyerhardt, J. A., D. Niedzwiecki, D. Hollis, L. B. Saltz, F. B. Hu, R. J. Mayer, H. Nelson, R. Whittom, A. Hantel, J. Thomas, and C. S. Fuchs. 2007. Association of dietary patterns with cancer recurrence and survival in patients with stage III colon cancer. *JAMA* 298(7):754–764.

58. Chan, A. T. and E. L. Giovannucci (2010). "Primary prevention of colorectal cancer." *Gastroenterology* 138(6): 2029–2043.

59. American Cancer Society (ACS). October 2014. What Are the Risk Factors for Prostate Cancer? http://www.cancer.org/cancer/prostatecancer/overviewguide/prostate-cancer-overview-what-causes (Accessed, December 2014).

60. Ma, R. W., and K. Chapman. 2009. A systemic review of the effect of diet in prostate cancer prevention and treatment. *Journal of Human Nutrition and Dietetics* 22(3):187–199.

61. American Institute for Cancer Research (AICR) World Cancer Research Fund. 2007. *Food, Nutrition, Physical Activity, and the Prevention of Cancer: A Global Perspective.* Washington, DC: AICR.

Chapter 6

1. Vegetarian Resource Group. May 30, 2014. How many teens and other youth are vegetarian and vegan? The Vegetarian Resource Group Asks in a 2014 National Poll. *Vegetarian Resource Group Blog,*http://www.vrg.org/blog/2014/05/30/how-many-teens-and-other-youth-are-vegetarian-and-vegan-the-vegetarian-resource-group-asks-in-a-2014-national-poll/

2. Rafii, M., M. Chapman, J. Owens, R. Elango, W. W. Campbell, R. O. Ball, P. B. Pencharz, and G. Courtney-Martin. 2015. Dietary protein requirement of female adults > 65 years determined by the indicator amino acid oxidation technique is higher than current recommendations. *J. Nutr.* 145(1):18–24.

3. Wright, J. D., and C-Y. Wang. 2010. Trends in intake of energy and macronutrients in adults from 1999–2000 through 2007–2008. *NCHS Data Brief*, no. 49. Hyattsville, MD: National Center for Health Statistics.

4. Phillips, S. M., and L. J. van Loon. 2011. Dietary protein for athletes: from requirements to optimum adaptation. *J. Sports Sci.* 29 Suppl 1:S29–S38.

5. Chowdhury, R., S. Warnakula, S. Kunutsor, F. Crowe, H. A. Ward, L. Johnson, …, and E. Di Angelantonio. 2014. Association of dietary, circulating, and supplement fatty acids with coronary risk: a systematic review and meta-analysis. *Ann. Intern. Med.* 160(6):398–406.

6. van Bussel, B. C. T., R. M. A. Henry, I. Ferreira, M. M. J. van Greevenbroek, C. J. H. van der Kallen, J. W. R. Twisk, …, and C. D. A. Stehouwer. 2015. A healthy diet is associated with less endothelial dysfunction and less low-grade inflammation over a 7-year period in adults at risk of cardiovascular disease. *J. Nutr.* E-pub ahead of print: jn.114.201236.

7. Calvez, J., N. Poupin, C. Chesneau, C. Lassale, and D. Tomé. 2012. Protein intake, calcium balance and health consequences. *Eur. J. Clin. Nutr.* 66:281–295.

8. Evert, A. B., J. L. Boucher, M. Cypress, S. A. Dunbar, M. J. Franz, E. J. Mayer-Davis, …, and W. S. Yancy, Jr. 2013. Nutrition therapy recommendations for the management of adults with diabetes. *Diabetes Care* 36:3821–3842.

9. Martin, W. F., L. E. Armstrong, and N. R. Rodriguez. 2005. Dietary protein intake and renal function. *Nutr. Metabol.* 2:25. www.nutritionandmetabolism.com/content/2/1/25.

10. Bao, Y., J. Han, F. B. Hu, E. L. Giovannucci, M. J. Stampfer, W. C. Willett, and C. S. Fuchs. 2013. Association of nut consumption with total and cause-specific mortality. *N. Engl. J. Med.* 369:2001–2011.

11. Lu, H. N., W. J. Blot, Y.-B. Xiang, H. Cai, M. K. Hargreaves, H. Li, …, and X-O. Shu. 2015. Prospective evaluation of the association of nut/peanut consumption with total and cause-specific mortality. *JAMA Intern. Med.* Epub ahead of print, doi:10.1001/jamainternmed.2014.8347.

12. Pan, A., Q. Sun, J. E. Manson, W. C. Willett, and F. B. Hu. 2013. Walnut consumption is associated with lower risk of type 2 diabetes in women. *J. Nutr.* 143:512–518.

13. World Cancer Research Fund and the American Institute for Cancer Research. 2012. Continuous Update Project. Colorectal Cancer. *Latest Evidence.* www.dietandcancerreport.org/cup/-current_progress/colorectal_cancer.php.

14. Bardone-Cone, A. M., E. E. Fitzsimmons-Craft, M. B. Harney, C. R. Maldonado, M. A. Lawson, R. Smith, and D. P. Robinson. 2012. The inter-relationships between vegetarianism and eating disorders among females. *J. Acad. Nutr. Diet.* 112(8):1247–1252.

15. Institute of Medicine, Food and Nutrition Board. 2005. *Dietary Reference Intakes for Energy, Carbohydrate, Fiber, Fat, Fatty Acids, Cholesterol, Protein, and Amino Acids (Macronutrients).* Washington, DC: National Academies Press.

16. Smith, M. I., T. Yatsunenko, M. J. Manary, I. Trehan, R. Mkakosya, J. Cheng, …, and J. I. Gordon. 2013. Gut microbiomes of Malawian twin pairs discordant for kwashiorkor. *Science* 339:548–554.

Chapter 7

1. Nei, M., J. I. Sirvenand, and M. R. Sperling. 2014. Ketogenic diet in adolescents and adults with epilepsy. *Seizure* 23:439–442.

2. O'Connor, S. E., C. Richardson, W. H. Trescher, D. L. Byler, J. D. Sather, E. H. Michael,…, and B. Zupec-Kania. 2014. The ketogenic diet for the treatment of pediatric status epilepticus. *Ped. Neurology.* 50:101–103.

3. Durazzo, M., R. Belci, A. Collo, V. Prandi, E. Pistone, M. Martorana, R. Bambino, and S. Bo. 2014. Gender specific medicine in liver diseases: a point of view. *World J Gastroenterology* 20:2127–2135.

Chapter 7.5

1. Institute of Medicine, Food and Nutrition Board. 2001. *Dietary Reference Intakes for Vitamin A, Vitamin K, Arsenic, Boron, Chromium, Copper, Iodine, Iron, Manganese, Molybdenum, Nickel, Silicon, Vanadium, and Zinc.* Washington, DC: National Academies Press.

2. Mursu, J., K. Robien, L. J. Harnack, K. Park, and D. R. Jacobs Jr. 2011. Less is more: dietary supplements and mortality rate in older women: the Iowa Women's Health Study. *Arch. Intern. Med.* 171:1625–1633.

3. Burckhardt, P. 2015. Vitamin A and bone health. In: M. F. Holick and J. W. Nieves, eds. *Nutrition and Bone Health.* New York, NY:Springer.

4. Pollan, M. 2007. The age of nutritionism. *New York Times Magazine,* January 28.

5. Pollan, M. 2008. *In Defense of Foods.* New York: Penguin Press.

6. Nazki, F. H., A. S. Sameer, and A. G. Bashir. 2014. Folate: metabolism, genes, polymorphisms and the associated diseases. *Gene* 533:11–20.

Chapter 8

1. Bernstein, L. 2000, February. Dementia without a cause: lack of vitamin B12 can cause dementia. *Discover.* http://discovermagazine.com/2000/feb/featdementia (Accessed March 2004).

2. Bettendorff, L. 2012. Thiamin. In: Erdman J W., I. A. Macdonald, and S. H. Zeisel, eds. *Present Knowledge in Nutrition*, 10th Edn, pp. 261–279. Washington, DC: ILSI Press.

3. Manore, M. N., N. A. Meyer, and J. T. Thompson. 2009. *Sport Nutrition for Health and Performance,* 2nd Edn. Champaign, IL: Human Kinetics, pp. 109–131.

4. Institute of Medicine (IOM), Food and Nutrition Board. 1998. *Dietary Reference Intakes for Thiamin, Riboflavin, Niacin, Vitamin B_6, Folate, Vitamin B_{12}, Pantothenic Acid, Biotin, and Choline.* Washington, DC: National Academy Press.

5. Woolf, K., D. L. LoBuono, and M. M. Manore. 2012. B-vitamins and physical activity: is need increased? In: Beals, K. A., ed. *Nutrition and the Female Athlete: From Research to Practice.* Baton Rouge, FL: CRC Press.

6. Wilken, K. G., and V. Juneja. 2008. Medical nutrition therapy for renal disorders. In: Mahan, K. L., and S. Escott-Stump, eds. *Krause's Food and Nutrition Therapy.* Philadelphia: W. B. Saunders, pp. 921–958.

7. McCormick, D. B. 2006. Niacin, riboflavin, and thiamin. In: M. H. Stipanuk, ed. *Biochemical and Physiological Aspects of Human Nutrition*, 2nd edn. Philadelphia: W. B. Saunders, pp. 665–691.

8. Gropper. S. S. and Smith, J. L. 2013. *Advanced Nutrition and Human Health.* 6th Edn. Belmont, CA: Wadsworth.

9. Hochholzer, W., D. D. Berg, and R. P. Giugliano. 2011. The facts behind niacin. *Ther. Adv. Cardiovasc. Dis.* 5(5):227–240.

10. DaSilva V, Mackey, A. D., S. R. Davis, and J. F. Gregory III. 2014. Vitamin B6. In: Ross, A. C., B. Caballero, R. Cousins, Tucker K.L, and Ziegler T. R. eds. *Modern Nutrition in Health and Disease*, 11th Edn. Philadelphia: *Lippincott Williams & Wilkins*, pp. 341–350

11. Huang, S. C., J. C. Wei, D. J. Wu, and Y. C. Huang. 2010. Vitamin B6 supplementation improves pro-inflammatory responses in patients with rheumatoid arthritis. *Eur. J. Clin. Nutri.* 64(9):1007–1013.

12. Stover, P. J. 2014. Folic Acid. In: Ross, A. C., B. Caballero, R. Cousins, K. L. Tucker, and T. R. Ziegler, eds. *Modern Nutrition in Health and Disease*, 11th Edn. Philadelphia: Lippincott Williams & Wilkins, pp. 358–368.

13. Shane, B. 2006. Folic acid, vitamin B12, and vitamin B6. In: M. H. Stipanuk, ed. *Biochemical, Physiological, and Molecular Aspects of Human Nutrition.* Philadelphia: W. B. Saunders, pp. 693–732.

14. Carmel, R. 2014. Cobalamin (Vitamin B_{12}). In: Ross, A. C., B. Caballero, R. Cousins, K. L. Tucker, and T. R. Ziegler, eds. *Modern Nutrition in Health and Disease*, 11th edn. Philadelphia: Lippincott Williams & Wilkins, pp. 369–389.

15. United States Department of Agriculture, Agriculture Research Service, National Nutrient Database for Standard Reference Release 27. Available at: http://ndb.nal.usda.gov/ndb/nutrients/index. Accessed Feb, 2015.

16. Laurberg, P. 2014. Iodine. In: Ross, A. C., B. Caballero, R. Cousins, K. L. Tucker, and T. R. Ziegler, eds. *Modern Nutrition in Health and Disease*, 11th edn. Philadelphia: Lippincott Williams & Wilkins, pp. 217–224.

17. Institute of Medicine, Food and Nutrition Board. 2001. *Dietary Reference Intakes for Vitamin A, Vitamin K, Arsenic, Boron, Chromium, Copper, Iodine, Iron, Manganese, Molybdenum, Nickel, Silicon, Vanadium, and Zinc*. Washington, DC: National Academy Press.

18. World Health Organization. 2014. WHO I Guideline: Fortification of food-grade salt with iodine for the prevention and control of iodine deficiency disorders. Geneva: WHO. Available at: http://apps.who.int/iris/bitstream/10665/136908/1/9789241507929_eng.pdf?ua = 1 (accessed February, 2015).

19. World Health Organization. 2007. Assessment of iodine deficiency disorders and monitoring their elimination. Geneva: WHO. Available at: http://whqlibdoc.who.int/publications/2007/9789241595827_eng.pdf?ua = 1&ua = 1 (accessed February, 2015).

20. Zimmermann M. B. 2012. Iodine and iodine deficiency disorders. In: J. W. Erdman, I. A. Macdonald, and S. H. Zeisel, eds. *Present Knowledge in Nutrition*, 10th Edn, pp. 554–567. Washington, DC: ILSI Press.

21. World Health Organization. 2014. WHO I Guideline: Fortification of food-grade salt with iodine for the prevention and control of iodine deficiency disorders. Geneva: WHO. Available at: http://apps.who.int/iris/bitstream/10665/136908/1/9789241507929_eng.pdf?ua = 1 (accessed February, 2015).

22. Andersson, M., V. Karumbunathan, and M. B. Zimmerman. 2012. Global iodine status in 2011 and trends over the past decade. *J. Nutr.* DOI:10.3945/jn.111.149393.

23. Aburto N. J., M. Abudou, T. Candeias, Wu. 2014. Effect and safety of salt iodization in prevent iodine deficiency disorders: a systematic review with meta-analyses. Geneva: WHO. Available at: http://apps.who.int/iris/bitstream/10665/148175/1/9789241508285_eng.pdf?ua = 1 (accessed Feb, 2015).

24. National Institutes of Health (NIH) Office of Dietary Supplements. 2013. Chromium Dietary Supplement Fact Sheet. http://ods.od.nih.gov/factsheets/Chromium-HealthProfessional/ (Accessed Feb 2015).

25. van der Beek, E. J., W. van Dokkum, J. Schrijver, M. Wedel, A. W. K. Gaillard, A. Wesstra, H. van de Weerd, and R. J. J. Hermus. 1988. Thiamin, riboflavin, and vitamins B_6 and C: impact of combined restricted intake on functional performance in man. *Am. J. Clin. Nutr.* 48:1451–1462.

26. van der Beek, E. J., W. van Dokkum, M. Wedel, J. Schrijver, and H. van den Berg. 1994. Thiamin, riboflavin and vitamin B6: impact of restricted intake on physical performance in man. *J. Am. Coll. Nutr.* 13:629–640

27. Vaz, M., Pauline, M., Unni, U. S., Parikh, P., Thomas, T., Bharathi, A. Avadhany S, Muthayya S, Mehra R, Kurpad, A. V. (2011). Micronutrient supplementation improves physical performance measures in Asian Indian school-age children. *J. Nutr.*, 141(11), 2017-2023. doi: http://dx.doi.org/10.3945/jn.110.135012

Chapter 9

1. Center for Food Safety and Applied Nutrition Adverse Event Reporting System. 2012. Voluntary and Mandatory Reports on 5-Hour Energy, Monster Energy, and Rockstar Energy Drink. Available at www.fda.gov/downloads/AboutFDA/CentersOffices/Officeof Foods/CFSAN/CFSANFOIAElectronicReadingRoom/UCM328270.pdf. (Accessed April, 2015)

2. Zhang, Y., A. Coca, D. J. Casa, J. Antonio, J. M. Green, and P. A. Bishop. 2014. Caffeine and dieresis during rest and exercise: a meta-analysis. *J. Sci. Med. Sport.*http://dx.doi.org/10.1016/j.jsams.2014.07.017.

3. Institute of Medicine. 2004. *Dietary Reference Intakes for Water, Potassium, Sodium, Chloride, and Sulfate*. Washington, D.C.: National Academies Press.

4. Beis, L. Y., M. Wright-Whyte, B. Fudge, T. Noakes, and Y. Pitsiladis. 2012. Drinking behaviors of elite male runners during marathon competition. *Clin. J. Sport Med.* 22:254–261.

5. Duffield, R., A. McCall, A. J. Coutts, and J. J. Peiffer. 2012. Hydration, sweat and thermoregulatory responses to professional football training in the heat. *J. Sport Sci.* 30:957–965.

6. Mesirow, M. S. C., and J. A. Welsh. 2015. Changing beverage consumption patterns have resulted in fewer liquid calories in the diets of US children: National Health and Nutrition Examination Survey 2001–2010. *J. Acad. Nutr. Diet.* 115:559–566.

7. International Bottled Water Association. 2014. Bottled Water Sales and Consumption Projected to Increase in 2014, Expected to be the Number One Packaged Drink by 2016. www.bottledwater.org/bottled-water-sales-and-consumption-projected-increase-2014-expected-be-number-one-packaged-drink. (Accessed April 2015)

8. Ding, M., S. N Bhupathiraju, M. Chen, R. M. van Dam, and F. B. Hu. 2014. Caffeinated and decaffeinated coffee consumption and risk of type 2 diabetes: a systematic review and a dose-response meta-analysis. *Diabetes Care* 37:569–586.

9. Larsson, S. C. 2014. Coffee, tea and cocoa and risk of stroke. *Stroke* 45:309–314.

10. Panza, F., V. Solfrizzi, M. R. Barulli, C. Bonfiglio, V. Guerra, A. Osella,..., and G. Logroscino. 2015. Coffee, tea, and caffeine consumption and prevention of late-life cognitive decline and dementia: a systematic review. *J. Nutr. Health Aging* 19:313–328.

11. Yarmolinsky, J., G. Gom, and P. Edwards. 2015. Effect of tea on blood pressure for secondary prevention of cardiovascular disease: a systematic review and meta-analysis of randomized controlled trials. *Nutr. Rev.* 73:236–246.

12. Petrone, A. B., J. M. Gaziano, and L. Djoussé. 2014. Chocolate consumption and risk of heart failure in the Physicians Health Study. *Eur. J. Heart Failure* 16:1372–1376.

13. Rath, M. 2012. Energy drinks: what is all the hype? The dangers of energy drink consumption. *Am. Acad. Nurse Practitioners* 24:70–76.

14. The DAWN Report. Update on emergency department visits involving energy drinks: a continuing public health concern. 2013. Available at http://archive.samhsa.gov/data/2k13/DAWN126/sr126-energy-drinks-use.pdf

15. Ng, S. W., M. M. Slining, and B. M. Popkin. 2014. Turning point for US diets? Recessionary effects or behavioral shifts in foods purchased and consumed. *Am. J. Clin. Nutr.* 99:609–616.

16. U.S. Department of Health and Human Services and U.S. Department of Agriculture. *2015–2020 Dietary Guidelines for Americans*. 8th Edition. December 2015. Available at http://health.gov/dietaryguidelines/2015/guidelines.

17. Graudal, N., G. Jürgens, B. Baslund, and M. H. Alderman. 2014. Compared with usual sodium intake, low- and excessive-sodium diets are associated with increased mortality: a meta-analysis. *Am. J. Hypertension* 27:1129–1137.

18. Nicoll, R., and J. M. Howard. 2014. The acid-ash hypothesis revisited: a reassessment of the impact of dietary acidity on bone. *J. Bone Mineral Metab.* 32:469–475.

19. Institute of Medicine. Food and Nutrition Board. 1999. *Dietary Reference Intakes for Calcium, Phosphorus, Magnesium, Vitamin D, and Fluoride*. Washington, D.C.: National Academies Press.

20. Meyer, N. L., M. M. Manore, and J. Berning. 2012. Fueling for fitness: food and fluid recommendations for before, during, and after exercise. *ACSM's Health & Fitness J.* 16:7–12.

21. Kucera, K. L, D. Klossner, B. Colgate, and R. C. Cantu. 2014. *Annual Survey of Football Injury Prevention*. Available at http://nccsir.unc.edu/files/2014/06/Annual-Football-2013-Fatalities-Final.pdf (Accessed May 2015)

22. Centers for Disease Control and Prevention. 2015. *High Blood Pressure: High Blood Pressure Facts.* Available at http://www.cdc.gov/bloodpressure/facts.htm (Accessed April 2015).

23. Madhur, M. S., K. Riaz, A. W. Dreisbach, and D. G. Harrison. 2014. *Hypertension: Practice essentials.* Available at http://emedicine.medscape.com/article/241381-overview#showall (Accessed May 2015)

24. Mayo Clinic Staff. 2014. *Ten Ways to Control Blood Pressure without Medication.* Available at http://www.mayoclinic.org/diseases-conditions/high-blood-pressure/in-depth/high-blood-pressure/art-20046974?pg = 1. (Accessed April 2015.)

25. Siervo, M., J. Lara, S. Chowdhury, A. Ashor, C. Oggioni, and J. C. Mathers. 2015. Effects of the Dietary Approach to Stop Hypertension (DASH) diet on cardiovascular risk factors: a systematic review and meta-analysis. *Brit. J. Nutr.* 113:1–15.

26. Saneei, P., A. Salehi-Abargouei, A. Esmaillzadeh, and L. Azadbakht. 2014. Influence of Dietary Approaches to Stop Hypertension (DASH) diet on blood pressure: a systematic review and meta-analysis on randomized controlled trials. *Metab. Nutr. Cardiovasc. Dis.* 24:1253–1261.

27. Boggs, D. A., Y. Ban, J. R. Palmer, and L. Rosenberg. 2015. Higher diet quality is inversely associated with mortality in African-American women. *J. Nutr.* 145(3):547–554

Chapter 10

1. The HOPE and HOPE-TOO Trial Investigators. 2005. Effects of long-term vitamin E supplementation on cardiovascular events and cancer. A randomized controlled trial. *JAMA* 293:1338–1347.

2. Bjelakovic, G., D. Nikolova, L. L. Gluud, R. G. Simonetti, and C. Gluud. 2012. Antioxidant supplements for prevention of mortality in healthy participants and patients with various diseases. *Cochrane Database Syst. Rev.* Issue 3. Art. No.: CD007176. DOI: 10.1002/14651858.CD007176.pub2.

3. Klein, E. A., I. M. Thompson Jr., C. M. Tangen, J. J. Crowley, M. S. Lucia, P. J. Goodman,..., and L. H. Baker. 2011. Vitamin E and the risk of prostate cancer: the Selenium and Vitamin E Cancer Prevention Trial (SELECT). *JAMA* 306:1549–1556.

4. Institute of Medicine, Food and Nutrition Board. 2000. *Dietary Reference Intakes for Vitamin C, Vitamin E, Selenium, and Carotenoids.* Washington, DC: National Academy of Sciences, National Academies Press.

5. Fulgoni III, V. L., D. R. Keast, R. L. Bailey, and J. Dwyer. 2011. Foods, fortificants, and supplements: where do Americans get their nutrients? *J. Nutr.* 141(10):1847–1854.

6. U.S. National Library of Medicine. *National Institutes of Health.* 2014. MedlinePlus. Beta-carotene. http://www.nlm.nih.gov/medlineplus/druginfo/natural/999.html.

7. U.S. Department of Agriculture (USDA), Agricultural Research Service. 2014. USDA *National Nutrient Database for Standard Reference*, Release 27. http://www.ars.usda.gov/

8. Albanes, D., O. P. Heinonen, J. K. Huttunen, P. R. Taylor, J. Virtamo, B. K. Edwards,..., and P. Greenwald. 1995. Effects of a-tocopherol and a-carotene supplements on cancer incidence in the Alpha-Tocopherol Beta-Carotene Cancer Prevention Study. *Am. J. Clin. Nutr.* 62(suppl.):1427S–1430S.

9. Omenn, G. S., G. E. Goodman, M. D. Thornquist, J. Balmes, M. R. Cullen, A. Glass, J. P. Keogh, F. L. Meyskens Jr., B. Valanis, J. H. Williams Jr., S. Barnhart, and S. Hammar. 1996. Effects of a combination of beta carotene and vitamin A on lung cancer and cardiovascular disease. *N. Engl. J. Med.* 334:1150–1155.

10. Druesne-Pecollo, N., P. Latino-Martel, T. Norat, E. Barrandon, S. Bertrais, P. Galan, and S. Hercberg. 2010. Beta-carotene supplementation and cancer risk: a systematic risk and meta-analysis of randomized controlled trials. *Int. J. Cancer* 127(1):172–184.

11. El-akawi, Z., N. Abdel-Latif, and K. Abdul-Razzak. 2006. Does the plasma level of vitamins A and E affect acne condition? *Clin. Experimen. Dermatol.* 31:430–434.

12. Institute of Medicine. Food and Nutrition Board. 2001. *Dietary Reference Intakes for Vitamin A, Vitamin K, Arsenic, Boron, Chromium, Copper, Iodine, Iron, Manganese, Molybdenum, Nickel, Silicon, Vanadium, and Zinc.* Washington, DC: National Academy Press.

13. World Health Organization (WHO). 2015. Micronutrient Deficiencies. Vitamin A Deficiency. www.who.int/nutrition/topics/vad/en/.

14. American Cancer Society. 2015. *Cancer Facts and Figures, 2015.* Atlanta: American Cancer Society. http://www.cancer.org/acs/groups/content/@editorial/documents/document/acspc-044552.pdf.

15. Tomasetti, C., and B. Vogelstein. 2015. Variation in cancer risk among tissues can be explained by the number of stem cell divisions. *Science* 347(6217):78–81.

16. International Agency for Research on Cancer. World Health Organization. 2015. Most types of cancer not due to "bad luck." IARC responds to scientific article claiming that environmental and lifestyle factors account for less than one third of cancers. Press Release No 231, 13 January 2015. http://www.iarc.fr/en/media-centre/pr/2015/pdfs/pr231_E.pdf.

17. American Cancer Society. 2015. *Stay Healthy.* http://www.cancer.org/healthy/index.

18. Lazovich, D., R. I. Vogel, M. Berwick, M. A. Weinstock, K. E. Anderson, and E. M. Warshaw. 2010. Indoor tanning and risk of melanoma: a case-control study in a highly exposed population. *Cancer Epidemiol. Biomarkers Prev.* 19:1557–1568.

19. Shukla, S., and S. Gupta. 2010. Apigenin: a promising molecule for cancer prevention. *Pharm. Res.* 27(6):962–978.

20. Arango, D., K. Morohashi, A. Yilmaz, K. Kuramochi, A. Parihar, B. Brahimaj, E. Grotewold, and A. I. Doseff. 2013. Molecular basis for the action of a dietary flavonoid revealed by the comprehensive identification of apigenin human targets. *Proc. Natl. Acad. Sci.* 110(24):E2153–E2162.

21. Abdull Razis, A. F. and N. M. Noor. 2013. Cruciferous vegetables: dietary phytochemicals for cancer prevention. *Asian Pac. J. Cancer Prev.* 14(3):1565–1570.

22. Bjelakovic, G., D. Nikolova, L. L. Gluud, R. G. Simonetti, and C. Gluud. 2012. Antioxidant supplements for prevention of mortality in healthy participants and patients with various diseases. *Cochrane Database Syst. Rev.*, Issue 3. Art. No.: CD007176. DOI: 10.1002/14651858.CD007176.pub2.

23. Centers for Disease Control and Prevention. 2015. *Heart Disease Facts.* http://www.cdc.gov/heartdisease/facts.htm.

24. Centers for Disease Control and Prevention. *Division for Heart Disease and Stroke Prevention.* 2015. Heart Disease Fact Sheet. http://www.cdc.gov/dhdsp/data_statistics/fact_sheets/fs_heart_disease.htm.

25. Egger, G. 2012. In search of a germ theory equivalent for chronic disease. *Prev. Chronic Dis.* 9:110301. Doi: http://dx.doi.org/10.5888/pcd9.110301.

26. Calder, P. C., N. Ahluwalia, F. Brouns, T. Buetler, K. Clement, K. Cunningham,..., and B. M. Winklhofer-Roob. 2011. Dietary factors and low-grade inflammation in relation to overweight and obesity. *Br. J. Nutr.* 106(S3):S1–S78.

27. Puchau, B., M. A. Zulet, A. G. de Echávarri, H. H. M. Hermsdorff, and J. A. Martínez. 2010. Dietary total antioxidant capacity is negatively associated with some metabolic syndrome features in healthy young adults. *Nutrition* 26(5):534–541.

Chapter 10.5

1. American Institute for Cancer Research. (2013, April 10). *Phytochemicals: The Cancer Fighters in the Foods We Eat.* http://www.aicr.org/reduce-your-cancer-risk/diet/elements_phytochemicals.html.

2. Rodriguez-Casado, A. 2014. The health potential of fruits and vegetables phytochemicals: notable examples. *Crit. Rev. Food.*

Sci. Nutr. [Epub ahead of print] DOI:10.1080/10408398.2012.7
55149

3. Bellik, Y., S. M. Hammoudi, F. Abdellah, M. Iguer-Ouada, and
L. Boukraa. 2012. Phytochemicals to prevent inflammation and
allergy. *Recent Pat. Inflamm. Allergy Drug Discov.* 6(2):147–58.

4. Bonaccio, M., C. Cerletti, L. Iacoviello, and G. D. Gaetano. 2014.
Mediterranean Diet and sub-clinical chronic inflammation:
the MOLI-SANI Study. *Endocr. Metab. Immune. Disord. Drug.
Targets.* [Epub ahead of print] DOI: EMIDDT-EPUB-62924

5. Mena, P., R. Domínguez-Perles, A. Gironés-Vilaplana, N. Baenas, C.
García-Viguera, and D. Villaño. 2014. Flavan-3-ols, anthocyanins,
and inflammation. *IUBMB Life.* 66(11):745–758. DOI: 10.1002/
iub.1332. Epub 2014 Dec 11.

6. Nabavi, S. M., S. Habtemariam, M. Daglia, and S. F. Nabavi.
2015. Apigenin and breast cancers: from chemistry to medicine.
Anticancer Agents Med. Chem. 2015 Mar 4. [Epub ahead of print]

7. T. Rossi, C. Gallo, B. Bassani, S. Canali, A. Albini, and A. Bruno.
2014. Drink your prevention: beverages with cancer preventive
phytochemicals. *Pol. Arch. Med. Wewn.* 2014; 124(12):713-722.
Available at http://pamw.pl/sites/default/files/PAMW%20
2014_12_Albini_0.pdf

8. Luo W. P., Y. J. Fang, M. S. Lu, X. Zhong, Y. M. Chen, and C.
X. Zhang. 2015. High consumption of vegetable and fruit colur
groups is inversely associated with the risk of colorectal cancer:
a case-control study. *Br. J. Nutr.* 16:1-10. [Epub ahead of print]

9. Gostner, J. M., K. Becker, F. Ueberall, and D. Fuchs. 2015.
The good and bad of antioxidant foods: an immunological
perspective. *Food Chem Toxicol..* pii: S0278-6915(15)00058-7.
DOI: 10.1016/j.fct.2015.02.012. [Epub ahead of print]

10. Ryu S., H. J. You, Y. W. Kim, A. Lee, G. P. Ko, S. J. Lee, and M. J.
Song. 2015. Inactivation of norovirus and surrogates by natural
phytochemicals and bioactive substances. *Mol. Nutr. Food. Res.*
59(1):65–74. DOI: 10.1002/mnfr.201400549. Epub 2014 Dec 16.

11. Vasanthi, H. R., N. Shrishrimal, and D. K. Das. 2012.
Phytochemicals from plants to combat cardiovascular disease.
Curr. Med. Chem. 19(14):2242–2251.

12. Mattson, M. P. 2014. Challenging oneself intermittently to improve
health. *Dose Response.* 12(4):600–618. Available at http://www.
ncbi.nlm.nih.gov/pmc/articles/PMC4267452/

13. American Heart Association. 2014, March 18. *Phytochemicals
and Cardiovascular Disease.* http://www.heart.org/HEARTORG/
GettingHealthy/NutritionCenter/Phytochemicals-and-
Cardiovascular-Disease_UCM_306020_Article.jsp

14. Ban J. O., D. H. Lee, E. J. Kim, J. W. Kang, M. S. Kim, M. C.
Cho,..., and do Y. Yoon. 2012. Antiobesity effects of a sulfur
compound thiacremenone mediated via down-regulation of
serum triglyceride and glucose levels and lipid accumulation
in the liver of db/db mice. *Phytother. Res.* DOI 10.1002/ptr.3729
[e-pub ahead of print].

15. Huang, B., H. D. Yuan, Y. Kim do, H. Y. Quan, and S. H. Chung.
2011. Cinnamaldehyde prevents adipocyte differentiation and
adipogenesis via regulation of peroxisome proliferators–activated
receptor-Y (PPARy) and AMP-activated protein kinase (AMPK)
pathways. *J. Agric. Food Chem.* 59(8):3666–3673.

16. Wenwen, X., J. J. Huang, and P. C. K. Cheung. 2012. Extract
of Pleurotus pulmonarius suppresses liver cancer development
and progression through inhibition of VEGF-induced P13K/AKT
signaling pathway. *PLoS One* 7(3):e34406.

17. Ohene-Agyei, T., R. Mowla, T. Rahman, and H. Venter. 2014.
Phytochemicals increase the antibacterial activity of antibiotics
by acting on a drug efflux pump. *MicrobiologyOpen.* 3(6):885–
896. DOI: 10.1002/mbo3.212. Epub 2014 Sep 16.

18. Panel on Dietary Antioxidants and Related Compounds.
Food and Nutrition Board. Institute of Medicine. 2011, May
10. Antioxidants Panel: Activity. www.iom.edu/Activities/
Nutrition/-AntioxidantsPanel.aspx.

19. Chen, F. P., M. H. Chien, and I. Y. Chern. 2015. Impact of lower
concentrations of phytoestrogens on the effects of estradiol in
breast cancer cells. *Climacteric.* 5:1–8. [Epub ahead of print] DO
I:10.3109/13697137.2014.1001357

20. National Center for Complementary and Integrative Health.
2013. *Antioxidants and Health: An Introduction.* November,
2013. NCCIH Pub No. D483. https://nccih.nih.gov/health/
antioxidants/introduction.htm

21. National Cancer Institute. 2014, January 16. *Antioxidants
and Cancer Prevention.* http://www.cancer.gov/cancertopics/
causes-prevention/risk/diet/antioxidants-fact-sheet

22. The Alpha-Tocopherol, Beta-Carotene Cancer Prevention Study
Group. 1994. The effect of vitamin E and beta carotene on the
incidence of lung cancer and other cancers in male smokers. *N.
Engl. J. Med.* 330(15):1029–1035.

23. Omenn G. S., G. E. Goodman, M. D. Thornquist, J. Balmes, M. R.
Cullen, A. Glass,..., and S. Hammar. 1996. Risk factors for lung
cancer and for intervention effects in CARET, the Beta-Carotene
and Retinol Efficacy Trial. *J. Natl. Cancer Inst.* 88(21):1550–1559.

24. Moyer, V. A., for the U.S. Preventive Services Task Force. 2014.
Vitamin, mineral, and multivitamin supplements for the primary
prevention of cardiovascular disease and cancer: U.S. Preventive
Services Task Force recommendation statement. *Ann. Intern.
Med.* 160(8):558–564. DOI:10.7326/M14-0198

Chapter 11

1. *NIH Osteoporosis and Related Bone Diseases National Resource
Center.* 2012. Osteoporosis: peak bone mass in women. http://
www.niams.nih.gov/Health_Info/Bone/Osteoporosis/bone_
mass.asp. Accessed April 14, 2015.

2. Institute of Medicine, Food and Nutrition Board. 1997. *Dietary
Reference Intakes for Calcium, Phosphorus, Magnesium, Vitamin
D, and Fluoride.* Washington, DC: National Academy Press.

3. Mangano, K. M., S. J. Walsh, K. L. Insogna, A. M. Kenny, and
J. E. Kerstetter. 2011. Calcium intake in the United States from
dietary and supplemental sources across adult age groups: new
estimates from the National Health and Nutrition Examination
Survey 2003–2006. *J. Acad. Nutr. Diet.* 111(5):687–695.

4. U.S. Department of Health and Human Services, National Kidney
and Urologic Diseases Information Clearinghouse. 2013. *Diet for
kidney stone formation.* NIH Publication No. 13-6425.

5. Institute of Medicine, Food and Nutrition Board. 2010. *Dietary
Reference Intakes for Calcium and Vitamin D.* Washington, DC:
National Academy Press.

6. Vimaleswaran, V. S., D. J. Berry, C. Lu, E. Tikkanen, S. Pilz, L. T.
Hiraki,..., and E. Hyppönen. 2013. Causal relationship between
obesity and vitamin D status: bi-directional Mendelian randomization
analysis of multiple cohorts. **PLOS Med.** 10(2):e1001383.

7. Thacher, T. D., P. R. Fischer, P. J. Tebben, R. J. Singh, S. S.
Cha, J. A. Maxson, and B. P. Yawn. 2013. Increasing incidence of
nutritional rickets: a population-based study in Olmsted County,
Minnesota. *Mayo Clin. Proc.* 88(2):176–183.

8. Institute of Medicine, Food and Nutrition Board. 2002. *Dietary
Reference Intakes for Vitamin A, Vitamin K, Arsenic, Boron,
Chromium, Copper, Iodine, Iron, Manganese, Molybdenum,
Nickel, Silicon, Vanadium, and Zinc.* Washington, DC: National
Academy Press.

9. Fang, Y., C. Hu, X. Tao, Y. Wan, and F. Tao. 2012. Effect
of vitamin K on bone mineral density: a meta-analysis of
randomized controlled trials. *J. Bone Miner. Metab.* 30(1):60–68.

10. Fodor, D., A. Albu, L. Poantă, and M. Porojan. 2010. Vitamin K
and vascular calcifications. *Acta Physiol. Hung.* 97(3):256–266.

11. Chang, A. R., M. Lazo, L. J. Appel, O. M. Gutiérrez, and M. E. Grams.
2014. High dietary phosphorus intake is associated with all-cause
mortality: results from NHANES III. *Am. J. Clin. Nutr.* 99:320–327.

12. McNaughton, S. A., N. Wattanapenpaiboon, J. D. Wark, and
C. A. Nowson. 2011. An energy-dense, nutrient-poor dietary
pattern is inversely associated with bone health in women. *J.
Nutr.* 141(8):1516–1523.

13. Mooren, F. C., K. Krüger, K. Völker, S. W. Golf, M. Wadepuhi, and A. Kraus. 2011. Oral magnesium supplementation reduces insulin resistance in non-diabetic subjects—a double-blind, placebo-controlled, randomized trial. *Diabes. Obes. Metab.* 13(3):281–284.

14. Chen, G. C., Z. Pang, and Q. F. Liu. 2012. Magnesium intake and risk of colorectal cancer: a meta-analysis of prospective studies. *Eur. J. Clin. Nutr.* 66(11):1182–1186.

15. Klaus, J., M. Reinshagen, K. Herdt, G. Adler, G. B. T. von Boyen, and C. von Tirpitz. 2011. Intravenous ibandronate or sodium-fluoride—a 3.5 years study on bone density and fractures in Chrohn's disease patients with osteoporosis. *J. Gastrointestin. Liver Dis.* 20(2):141–148.

16. National Cancer Institute, National Institutes of Health. 2012. *National Cancer Institute FactSheet.* Fluoridated Water. www.cancer.gov/cancertopics/factsheet/Risk/fluoridated-water.

17. Centers for Disease Control and Prevention. 2013. Community Water Fluoridation: Questions and Answers. http://www.cdc.gov/fluoridation/faqs/index.htm.

18. National Osteoporosis Foundation. 2015. *Debunking the Myths.* http://nof.org/articles/4.

19. International Osteoporosis Foundation. 2015. *Osteoporosis & Musculoskeletal Disorders.* Osteoporosis in Men. http://www.iofbonehealth.org/osteoporosis-men.

20. *National Osteoporosis Foundation.* 2015. Just for Men. http://nof.org/articles/236

21. Urano, T. and S. Inoue. 2015. Recent genetic discoveries in osteoporosis, sarcopenia and obesity. *Endocr. J.* epub ahead of print, April 11 2015, doi:10/1507/endocrj.EJ15-0154.

22. Maurel, D. B., N. Boisseau, C. L. Benhamou, and C. Jaffre. 2012. Alcohol and bone: review of dose effects and mechanisms. *Osteoporos. Int.* 23(1):1–16.

23. Body, J. J., P. Bergmann, S. Boonen, Y. Boutsen, O. Bruyere, J.-P. Devogelaer,..., and J.-Y. Reginster. 2011. Non-pharmacological management of osteoporosis: a consensus of the Belgian Bone Club. *Osteoporos. Int.* 22:2769–2788.

24. Xie, H. L., B. H. Wu, W. Q. Xue, M. G. He, F. Fan, W. F. Ouyang,..., and Y.M. Chen. 2013. Greater intake of fruit and vegetables is associated with a lower risk of osteoporotic hip fractures in elderly Chinese: a 1:1 matched case-control study. *Osteoporos. Int.* 24(11):2827–2836.

25. Boeing, H., A. Bechthold, A. Bub, S. Ellinger, D. Haller, A. Kroke,..., and B. Watzl. 2012. Critical review: vegetables and fruit in the prevention of chronic diseases. *Eur. J. Nutr.* 51(6):637–663.

26. Dawson-Hughes, B., and S. S. Harris. 2002. Calcium intake influences the association of protein intake with rates of bone loss in elderly men and women. *Am. J. Clin. Nutr.* 75:773–779.

27. Rizzoli, R., M. L. Bianchi, M. Garabédian, H. A. McKay, and L. A. Moreno. 2010. Maximizing bone mineral mass gain during growth for the prevention of fractures in the adolescents and the elderly. *Bone* 46(2):294–015.

28. Doyle, M. E., and K. A. Glass. 2010. Sodium reduction and its effect on food safety, food quality, and human health. *Comp. Rev. Food Sci. Food Safety* 9(1):44–56.

29. Howe, T. E., B. Shea, L. J. Dawson, F. Downie, A. Murray, C. Ross,..., and Creed. 2011. Exercise for preventing and treating osteoporosis in postmenopausal women. *Cochrane Database Syst. Rev.* 2011, Issue 7. Art. No.:CD000333. DOI:10.1002/14651858. CD000333.pub.2.

30. National Institute of Arthritis and Musculoskeletal and Skin Diseases. NIH Osteoporosis and Related Bone Diseases National Resource Center. 2012. *Exercise for Your Bone Health.* http://www.niams.nih.gov/Health_Info/Bone/Bone_Health/Exercise/default.asp.

31. Real J., G. Galindo, L. Galván, M. A. Lafarga, M. D. Rodrigo, and M. Ortega. 2015. Use of oral bisphosphonates in primary prevention of fractures in postmenopausal women: a population-based cohort study. *PLoS ONE* 10(4):e0118178.

32. Black, D. M., M. P. Kelly, H. K. Genant, L. Palermo, R. -Eastell, C. Bucci-Recthweg,..., and D. C. Bauer for the Fracture Intervention Trial and HORIZON Pivotal Fracture Trial Steering Committees. 2010. Bisphosphonates and fractures of the subtrochanteric or diaphyseal femur. *N. Engl. J. Med.* 362:1761–1777.

33. Schilcher, J., K. Michaëlsson, and P. Aspenberg. 2011. Bisphosphonate use and atypical fractures of the femoral shaft. *N. Engl. J. Med.* 364:1728–1737.

34. Lee, S., R. V. Yin, H. Hirpara, N. C. Lee, A. Lee, S. Llanos, and O. J. Phung. 2015. Increased risk for atypical fractures associated with bisphosphonate use. *Fam. Pract.* Epub ahead of print, April 5, 2015. pii:cmu088.

35. Writing Group for the Women's Health Initiative Investigators. 2002. Risks and benefits of estrogen plus progestin in healthy postmenopausal women. Principal results from the Women's Health Initiative randomized control trial. *JAMA* 288:321–332.

36. U.S. Preventive Services Task Force. 2013. Understanding task force recommendations. Menopausal hormone therapy for the primary prevention of chronic conditions: U.S. Preventive Services Task Force recommendation statement. *Ann. Intern. Med.* 158(1):47–54.

Chapter 12

1. World Health Organization (WHO) Nutrition. 2015. *Micronutrient Deficiencies: Iron Deficiency Anemia*http://www.who.int/nutrition/topics/ida/en/#. Accessed February, 2015.

2. *World Health Organization (WHO) Nutrition.* 2014. Global Nutrition Targets 2025: Anemia Policy Brief (WHO/NMH/NHD/14.4). http://www.who.int/nutrition/topics/ida/en/http://www.who.int/nutrition/publications/globaltargets2025_policybrief_anaemia/en/. Accessed March, 2015.

3. Crichton R.R. 2006. Iron. In: Stipanuk MH, Ed. Biochemical, Physiological, and Molecular Aspects of Human Nutrition. Philadelphia: WB Sanders, pp. 1001–1042.

4. Collings, R., L. J. Harvey, L. Hooper, R. Hurst, T. J. Brown, J. Ansett, M. King, S. J. Fairweather-Tait. 2013. The absorption of iron from whole diets: a systematic review. *Am J Clin Nutr* 98(1):65–81.

5. Institute of Medicine (IOM), Food and Nutrition Board. 2002. *Dietary Reference Intakes for Vitamin A, Vitamin K, Arsenic, Boron, Chromium, Copper, Iodine, Iron, Manganese, Molybdenum, Nickel, Silicon, Vanadium, and Zinc.* Washington, DC: National Academy Press.

6. Gropper. S. S. and J. L. Smith. 2013. *Advanced Nutrition and Human Health.* 6th Edn. Belmont, CA: Wadsworth.

7. *National Institutes of Health (NIH),* Office of Dietary Supplements. 2015. Iron fact sheet. http://ods.od.nih.gov/pdf/factsheets/Iron-HealthProfessional.pdf. Accessed February, 2015.

8. Sharp, P. A. 2010. Intestinal iron absorption: regulation by dietary and systemic factors. *Int. J. Vitam. Nutr. Res.* 80(4–5): 231–242.

9. Hunt, J. R. 2010. Algorithms for iron and zinc bioavailability: are they accurate? *Int. J. Vitam. Nutr. Res.* 80(4-5):257–262.

10. Coates, T. D. 2014. Physiology and pathophysiology of iron in hemoglobin-associated diseases. *Free Radical Biol.* Med. 72:23–40.

11. Spanierman, C. S. 2014. Iron Toxicity. Medscape Reference. *Drugs, Diseases and Procedures.* http://emedicine.medscape.com/article/815213-overview. Accessed February, 2015.

12. Duchini, A. 2014. Hemochromatosis. Medscape Reference. *Drugs, Disease and Procedures.* http://emedicine.medscape.com/article/177216-overview Accessed February, 2015.

13. Ganz, T., and E. Nameth. 2011. Hepcidin and disorders of iron metabolism. *Ann. Rev. Med.* 62:347–360.

14. Tussing-Humphreys, L., C. Pustacioglu, E. Nemeth, and C. Braunschweig. 2012. Rethinking iron regulation and assessment in iron deficiency, anemia of chronic disease, and obesity: introducing hepcidin. *J. Acad. Nutri. Diet.* 112:381–400.

15. Hinton, P. S., C. Giordano, T. Brownlie, and J. D. Hass. 2000. Iron supplementation improves endurance after training in iron-depleted, nonanemic women. *J. Appl. Physiol.* 88:1103–1111.

16. McClung, J. P., and L. E. Murray-Kolb. 2013. Iron nutrition and premenopausal women: effects of poor iron status on physical and neuropsychological performance. *Annu Rev Nutr.* 33: 271–288.

17. DellaValle, D. M. 2013. Iron supplementation for female athletes: effects on iron status and performance outcomes. *Curr. Sports Med. Rep.* 12(4):234–239.

18. Prasad, A. S. 2014. Impact of the discovery of human zinc deficiency on health. *GMS* 28(4):357–363. DOI: http://dx.doi.org/10.1016/j.jtemb.2014.09.002

19. Holt, R. R., J. Y. Uriu-Adams, and C. L. Keen 2012. Zinc. In: Erdman J. W., I. A. Macdonald, S. H. Zeisel, eds. *Present Knowledge in Nutrition*, 10th Edn, pp. 521–539. Washington, DC: ILSI Press.

20. Gropper S.S. and J.L. Smith. (2013). *Advanced Nutrition and Human Metabolism*. Belmont, CA: Wadsworth Cengage Learning, pp. 481–546

21. Mayo-Wilson, E., J. A. Junior, A. Imdad, S. Dean, X. H. Chan, E. S. Chan,…, and Z. A. Bhutta. 2014. Zinc supplementation for preventing mortality, morbidity, and growth failure in children aged 6 months to 12 years of age. *Cochrane Database Syst. Rev.*. 5. DOI: http://dx.doi.org/10.1002/14651858.CD009384.pub2.

22. Beulens, J. W., S. L. Booth, E. G. van den Heuvel, E. Stoecklin, A. Baka, and C. Vermeer, C. 2013. The role of menaquinones (vitamin K2) in human health. *Br. J. Nutr.* 110(8):1357–1368.

23. Hamidi, M. S., O. Gajic-Veljanoski, and A. M. Cheung. 2013. Vitamin K and bone health. *J. Clin. Densitomet.* 16(4):409–413.

24. Ferland G. 2012. Vitamin K. In: Erdman, J.W., I. A. Macdonald, S. H. Zeisel, eds. *Present Knowledge in Nutrition*, 10th Edn, pp. 230–247. Washington, DC: ILSI Press.

25. Institute of Medicine (IOM), Food and Nutrition Board. 1998. *Dietary Reference Intakes for Thiamin, Riboflavin, Niacin, Vitamin B6, Folate, Vitamin B12, Pantothenic Acid, Biotin, and Choline.* Washington, DC: National Academy Press.

26. Mahan L. K, S. Escot-Stump, J. L. Raymond. 2012. *Krause's Food and the Nutrition Care Process.* 13th Edn, pp.725–741. St. Louis, MO: Elsevier Sanders.

27. National Institutes of Health (NIH) Office of Dietary Supplements. 2013. Vitamin B12. *Dietary Supplement Fact Sheet.* http://ods.od.nih.gov/pdf/factsheets/VitaminB12-HealthProfessional.pdf. Accessed February, 2015.

28. Herrmann, W., and R. Obeid, R. 2012. Cobalamin deficiency. IN: Stanger, O., Ed. *Water Soluble Vitamins. Series: Subcellular Biochemistry* 56, pp. 301–322. Springer Science+Business Media:New York, NY.

29. Ahmed, T., and N. Haboubi, N. 2010. Assessment and management of nutrition in older people and its importance to health. *Clin. Interventions Aging* 5:207–216.

30. Beck, M. A., J. Handy, and O. A. Levander. 2004. Host nutri-tional-status: the neglected virulence factor. *Trends Microbiol.* 12:417–423.

31. Calder P. P., and Yaqoob P. 2012. Nutrient Regulation of the Immune Response. In: Erdman, J.W., I. A. Macdonald, S. H. Zeisel, eds. *Present Knowledge in Nutrition*, 10th Edn, pp. 688–708. Washington, DC: ILSI Press.

32. Scrimshaw, N. S. 2003. Historical concepts of interactions, synergism and antagonism between nutrition and infection. *J. Nutr.* 133:316S–321S.

33. Jones, K. D., J. Thitiri, M. Ngari, and J. A. Berkley. 2014. Childhood malnutrition: toward an understanding of infections, inflammation, and antimicrobials. *Food Nutr Bull* 35(2):S64–70.

34. Calder, P. P. 2014. Nutrition and Inflammatory Processes. In: Ross, A. C., B. Caballero, R. Cousins, K. L. Tucker, and T. R. Ziegler, eds. *Modern Nutrition in Health and Disease*, 11th Edn. Philadelphia:Lippincott Williams & Wilkins, pp. 837–848.

35. Lucas, S. 2010. Predictive clinicopathological features derived from systematic autopsy examination of patients who died with A/H1N1 influenza infection in the UK 2009-10 pandemic. *Health Technol Assess* 14(55):83–114.

36. Catalán, V., J. Gómez-Ambrosi, A. Rodríguez, and G. Frühbeck, G. 2013. Adipose tissue immunity and cancer. *Frontiers Physiol.* 4:275.

37. Sunde R. A. 2014. Selenium. In: Ross, A. C., B. Caballero, R. Cousins, K. L. Tucker, and T. R. Ziegler, eds. *Modern Nutrition in Health and Disease*, 11th Edn. Philadelphia: Lippincott Williams & Wilkins, pp. 225–237.

38. Stephensen C. B., and S. J. Zunino. 2014. Nutrition and the Immune System. In: Ross, A. C., B. Caballero, R. Cousins, K. L. Tucker, and T. R. Ziegler, Eds. *Modern Nutrition in Health and Disease* 11th Edn. Philadelphia: Lippincott Williams & Wilkins, pp. 601–610.

Chapter 13

1. 60 Minutes Overtime Staff. (2012, February 12). Adele Talks About Her Body Image and Weight. *CBS News.* www.cbsnews.com/8301-504803_162-57376080-10391709/adele-talks-about-her-body-image-and-weight/. (Accessed February 2012.)

2. Flegal, K. M., B. K. Kit, H. Orpana, and B. I. Graubard. 2013. Association of all-cause mortality with overweight and obesity using standard body mass index categories. A systematic review and meta-analysis. *JAMA* 309(1):71–82.

3. Willett, W. C., Hu, F. B., and Thun, M. 2013. Letters. Overweight, obesity and all-cause mortality. *JAMA* 309(16):1681–1682.

4. Hughes, V. 2013. The big fat truth. *Nature* 497:428–430. http://www.nature.com/news/the-big-fat-truth-1.13039#/b9

5. Hu, F. B. 2011. Globalization of Diabetes. The role of diet, lifestyle, and genes. *Diab. Care* 34(6):1249–1257.

6. Shai, I., R. Jiang, J. E. Manson, M. J. Stampfer, W. C. Willett, G. A. Colditz, and F. B. Hu. 2006. Ethnicity, obesity, and risk of type 2 diabetes in women. *Diab. Care.* 29:1585–1590.

7. Galgani, J., and E. Ravussin. 2008. Energy metabolism, fuel selection and body weight regulation. *Int. J. Obes.* 32:S109–S119.

8. O'Rahilly S, Farooqi IS. 2013. The Genetics of Obesity in Humans. In: De Groot L. J., P. Beck-Peccoz , Chrousos, et al., eds. Endotext [Internet]. *South Dartmouth (MA): MDText.com, Inc.*; 2000-. Available from: http://www.ncbi.nlm.nih.gov/books/NBK279064/

9. Bouchard, C. 2010. Defining the genetic architecture of the predisposition to obesity: a challenging but not insurmountable task. *Am. J. Clin. Nutr.* 91:5–6.

10. Bloss, C. S., N. J. Stork, and E. J. Topol. 2011. Effect of direct-to-consumer genomewide profiling to assess disease risk. *N. Engl. J. Med.* 364(6):524–534.

11. Razquin, C., A. Marti, and J. A. Martinez. 2011. Evidences on three relevant obesogenes: MC4R, FTO, and PPARR. *Mol. Nutr. Food Res.* 55(1):136–149.

12. Kilpeläinen, T. O., L. Qi, S. Brage, S. J. Sharp, E. Sonestedt, E. Demerath,…, and R. J. Loos. 2011. Physical activity attenuates the influence of FTO variants on obesity risk: a meta-analysis of 218,166 adults and 19,268 children. *PLoS Med.* 8(11)e1001116, Epub 2011 Nov 1.

13. Centers for Disease Control and Prevention. 2015. *Adolescent and School Health.* Childhood Obesity Facts. http://www.cdc.gov/healthyyouth/obesity/facts.htm. (Accessed May 2015).

14. Bouchard, C., A. Tremblay, J. P. Després, A. Nadeau, P. J. -Lupien, G. Thériault, J. Dussault, S. Moorjani, S. Pinault, and G. Fournier. 1990. The response to long-term overfeeding in identical twins. *N. Engl. J. Med.* 322:1477–1482.

15. National Institute of Diabetes and Digestive and Kidney Diseases. Weight-control Information Network. 2012. *Understanding Adult Overweight and Obesity.* NIH Publication No. 06-3680.

http://www.niddk.nih.gov/health-information/health-topics/weight-control/understanding/Pages/understanding-adult-overweight-and-obesity.aspx. (Accessed May 2015.)

16. Sumithran, P., L. A. Prendergast, E. Delbridge, K. Purcell, A. Shulkes, A. Kriketos, and J. Proietto. 2011. Long-term persistence of hormonal adaptations to weight loss. *N. Engl. J. Med.* 365:1597–1604.

17. Castañeda, T. R., J. Tong, R. Datta, M. Culler, and M. H. Tschöp. 2010. Ghrelin in the regulation of body weight and metabolism. *Frontiers Neuroendocrinol.* 31(1):44–60.

18. Suzuki, K., C. N. Jayasena, and S. R. Bloom. 2011. The gut hormones in appetite regulation. *J. Obes.* www.hindawi.com/journals/jobes/2011/528401/.

19. Sacks, H., and M. E. Symonds. 2013. Anatomical locations of human brown adipose tissue. Functional relevance and implications in obesity and type 2 diabetes. *Diabetes* 62(6):1783–1790.

20. Im, E.-O., B. Lee, H. Hwang, K. H. Yoo, W. Chee, A. Stuifbergen, L. Walker, A. Brown, C. McPeek, M. Miro, and E. Chee. 2010. "A Waste of Time": Hispanic women's attitudes toward physical activity. *Women & Health* 50(6):563–579.

21. Wilcox, S., P. A. Sharpe, D. Parra-Medina, M. Granner, and B. Hutto. 2011. A randomized trial of a diet and exercise intervention for overweight and obese women from economically disadvantaged neighborhoods: Sisters Taking Action for Real Success (STARS). *Contemp. Clin. Trials* 32(6):931–945.

22. Levine, J. A. 2011. Poverty and obesity in the U.S. *Diabetes* 60(11):2667–2668.

23. Jerrett, M., R. McConnell, J. Wolch, R. Chang, C. Lam, G. Dunton, F. Gilliland, F. Lurmann, T. Islam, and K. Berhane. 2014. Traffic-related air pollution and obesity formation in children: a longitudinal, multilevel analysis. *Env Health* 13:49, http://www.ehjournal.net/content/13/1/49

24. Zeki Al Hazzouri, A., M. N. Haan, W. R. Robinson, P. Gordon-Larsen, L. Garcia, E. Clayton, and A. E. Aiello. 2015. Associations of intergenerational education with metabolic health in U.S. Latinos. *Obesity* 23(5):1097–1104.

25. Robinson, W. R., K. N. Kershaw, B. Mezuk, J. Rafferty, H. Lee, V. Johnson-Lawrence, M. J. Seamans, and J. S. Jackson. Coming unmoored: disproportionate increases in obesity prevalence among young, disadvantaged white women. *Obesity* 23(1):213–219.

26. Ding, D., T. Sugiyama, and N. Owen. 2012. Habitual active transport, TV viewing and weight gain: a four-year follow-up study. *Prev. Med.* 54:201–204.

27. Lumeng, J. C., P. Forrest, D. P. Appugliese, N. Kaciroti, R. F. Corwyn, and R. H. Bradley. 2010. Weight status as a predictor of being bullied in third through sixth grades. *Pediatrics* 125(6):1301–1307.

28. Ogden, C. L., M. D. Carroll, B. K. Kit, and K. M. Flegal. 2014. Prevalence of childhood and adult obesity in the United States, 2011–2012. *JAMA* 311(8):806–814.

29. Kassi, E., P. Pervanidou, G. Kaltsas, and G. Chrousos. 2011. Metabolic syndrome: definitions and controversies. *BMC Med.* 9:48, http://www.biomedcentral.com/1741-7015/9/48

30. MyHealthyWaist.org. 2015. The Concept of CMR. www.myhealthywaist.org/the-concept-of-cmr/index.html. (Accessed May 2015.)

31. Agency for Healthcare Research and Quality, National Guideline Clearinghouse. 2011. *Cardiometabolic risk management in primary care.* http://www.guideline.gov/content.aspx?id=34113&search=cardiometabolic+risk+management+in+primary+care. (AccessedMay 2015).

32. Beltrán-Sánchez H., M. O. Harhay, M. M. Harhay, and S. McElligott. 2013. Prevalence and trends of metabolic syndrome in the adult U.S. population, 1999–2010. *J. Am. Coll. Cardiol.* 62(8):697–703.

33. Foresight. Government Office for Science. 2007. *Tackling Obesities: Future Choices—Project Report.* 2nd Edition.

https://www.gov.uk/government/uploads/system/uploads/attachment_data/file/287937/07-1184x-tackling-obesities-future-choices-report.pdf

34. Phelan, S., R. R. Wing, C. M. Loria, Y. Kim, and C. E. Lewis. 2010. Prevalence and predictors of weight-loss maintenance in a bi-racial cohort. Results from the CARDIA study. *Am. J. Prev. Med.* 39(6):546–554.

35. Institute of Medicine, Food and Nutrition Board. 2002. *Dietary Reference Intakes for Energy, Carbohydrate, Fiber, Fat, Fatty Acids, Cholesterol, Protein, and Amino Acids (Macronutrients).* Washington, DC: National Academies Press.

36. Mayo Clinic. 2015. Healthy Lifestyle. Weight loss. *Prescription weight loss drugs.* http://www.mayoclinic.org/healthy-lifestyle/weight-loss/in-depth/weight-loss-drugs/art-20044832. Accessed May 2015.

37. National Institutes of Health. Office of Dietary Supplements. 2015. Dietary Supplements for Weight Loss. *Fact Sheet for Health Professionals.* http://ods.od.nih.gov/factsheets/WeightLoss-HealthProfessional/#en8. (Accessed May, 2015).

38. Chang, S.-H., C. R. T. Stoll, J. Song, J. E. Varela, C. J. Eagon, and G. A. Colditz. 2014. The effectiveness and risks of bariatric surgery. An updated systematic review and meta-analysis, 2003-2012. *JAMA Surg.* 149(3):275–287.

39. Academy of Nutrition and Dietetics. 2014. *Staying Away from Fad Diets.* February 4, 2014. http://www.eatright.org/resource/health/weight-loss/fad-diets/staying-away-from-fad-diets. (Accessed May 2015.)

40. Prentice, R. L., B. Caan, R. T. Chlebowski, R. Patterson, L. H. Kuller, J. Ockene,..., and M. M. Henderson. 2006. Low-fat dietary pattern and risk of invasive breast cancer: the Women's Health Initiative Randomized Controlled Dietary Modification Trial. *JAMA* 295:629–642.

41. Beresford, S. A., K. C. Johnson, C. Ritenbaugh, N. L. Lasser, L. G. Snetselaar, H. R. Black,..., and E. Whitlock. 2006. Low-fat dietary pattern and risk of colorectal cancer: the Women's Health Initiative Randomized Controlled Dietary Modification Trial. *JAMA* 295:643–654.

42. Howard, B. V., L. Van Horn, J. Hsia, J. E Manson, M. L. Stefanick, S. Wassertheil-Smoller,..., and J. M. Kotchen. 2006. Low-fat dietary pattern and risk of cardiovascular disease: the Women's Health Initiative Randomized Controlled Dietary Modification Trial. *JAMA* 295:655–666.

43. Howard, B. V., J. E. Manson, M. L. Stefanick, S. A. Beresford, G. Frank, B. Jones,..., and R. Prentice. 2006. Low-fat dietary pattern and weight change over 7 years: the Women's Health Initiative Dietary Modification Trial. *JAMA* 295:39–49.

44. Hu, T, K. T. Mills, L. Yao, K. Demanelis, M. Eloustaz, W. S. Yancy Jr., T. N. Kelly, J. He, and L. A. Bazzano. 2012. Effects of low-carbohydrate diets versus low-fat diets on metabolic factors: a meta-analysis of randomized controlled clinical trials. *Am. J. Epidemiol.* 176(Suppl 7):S44–S54.

45. Piernas, C., and B. M. Popkin. 2011. Food portion patterns and trends among U.S. children and the relationship to total eating occasion size, 1977–2006. *J. Nutr.* 141(6):1159–1164.

46. Freedman, M. R. and C. Brochado. 2012. Reducing portion size reduces food intake and plate waste. *Obesity* 18(9):1864–1866.

47. Centers for Disease Control and Prevention. Nutrition Resources for Health Professionals. 2011. *Weight Management Research to Practice Series.* Low-Energy-Dense Foods and Weight Management: Cutting Calories While Controlling Hunger – Research to Practice Series No. 5. http://www.cdc.gov/nutrition/professionals/researchtopractice/index.html?s_cid=.

48. The National Weight Control Registry. *NWCR Facts.* http://www.nwcr.ws/Research/default.htm

49. Timmerman, G. M., and A. Brown. 2012. The effect of a Mindful Restaurant Eating intervention on weight management in women. *J. Nutr. Educ. Behav.* 44:22–28.

50. Dalen, J., B. W. Smith, B. M. Shelley, A. L. Sloan, L. Leahigh, and D. Begay. 2010. Pilot study: mindful Eating and Living (MEAL): weight, eating behaviour, and psychological outcomes associated with a mindfulness-based intervention for people with obesity. *Complement. Ther. Med.* 18:260–264.

51. Miller, C. K., J. L. Kristeller, A. Headings, H. Nagaraja, and W. F. Miser. 2012. Comparative effectiveness of a mindful eating intervention to a diabetes self-management intervention among adults with type 2 diabetes: a pilot study. *J. Acad. Nutr. Diet.* 112:1835–1842.

Chapter 13.5

1. Grave, R. D. 2011. Eating disorders: progress and challenges. *Europ. J. Internal. Med.* 22:153–160.

2. Treasure, J., A. M. Claudino, and N. Zucker. 2010. Eating disorders. *Lancet* 375:583–593.

3. Treasure, J., A. R. Sepulved, P. MacDonald, W. Whitaker, C. Lopez, M. Zabala, O. Kyracou, and G. Todd. 2008. The assessment of the family of people with eating disorders. *Europ. Eating Disorder Rev.* 16:247–255.

4. Strasburger, V. C., A. B. Jordan, and E. Donnerstein. 2010. Health effects of media on children and adolescents. *Pediatrics.* 125(4):756–767.

5. Strasburger, V. C., E. Donnerstein, and B. J. Bushman. 2014. Why is it so hard to believe that media influence children and adolescents? *Pediatrics,* 133(4):571–573.

6. Costa-Font, J., and M. Jofre-Bonet. 2011, November. Anorexia, Body Image, and Peer Effects: Evidence from a Sample of European Women. *Centre for Economic Performance*: CEP discussion paper No. 1098. http://cep.lse.ac.uk/pubs/download/dp1098.pdf. (Accessed March 2015.)

7. Fitzsimmons-Craft, E. E. 2011. Social psychological theories of disordered eating in college women: review and integration. *Clin. Psychol. Rev.* 31(7):1224–1237.

8. Young, S., P. Rhodes, S. Touyz, and P. Hay, P. 2013. The relationship between obsessive-compulsive personality disorder traits, obsessive-compulsive disorder and excessive exercise in patients with anorexia nervosa: a systematic review. *J. Eat. Disord.,* 1:16.

9. Koven, N. S., and A. W. Abry. 2015. The clinical basis of orthorexia nervosa: emerging perspectives. *Neuropsychiatr. Dis. Treat.* 11:385–394.

10. Keel, P. K., T. A. Brown, L. A. Holland, and L. D. Bodell. 2012. Emperical classification of eating disorders. *Ann. Rev. Clin. Psychol.* 8:381–404.

11. U.S. Department of Human Services, Office of Women's Health. 2009. *Anorexia Nervosa.* http://womenshealth.gov/publications/our-publications/fact-sheet/anorexia-nervosa.pdf. (Accessed March 2015).

12. National Association of Anorexia Nervosa and Associated Disorders. 2015. *Eating Disorder Statistics.* www.anad.org/get-information/about-eating-disorders/eating-disorders-statistics/. (Accessed March 2015.)

13. Jones, W.R., and J. F. Morgan. 2010. Eating disorders in men: a review of the literature. *J. Public Ment. Health.* 9(2):23–31

14. American Psychiatric Association (APA). 2013. *Diagnostic and Statistical Manual of Mental Disorders (DSM-5)*, 5th Edn. Washington, DC.

15. Beals, K. A. 2004. *Disordered Eating in Athletes: A Comprehensive Guide for Health Professionals.* Champaign, IL: Human Kinetics.

16. American Psychiatric Association (APA). 2005. *Let's Talk Facts About Eating Disorders.* http://www.psychiatry.org/mental-health/lets-talk-facts-brochures. (Accessed March 2015).

17. American Psychiatric Association (APA). 2015. *Eating Disorders.* http://www.psychiatry.org/eating-disorders. (Accessed March 2015).

18. National Institute of Mental Health (NIMH). 2014. *Eating Disorders: About More than Food.* NIH Publication No. (TR 14-4901). http://www.nimh.nih.gov/health/publications/eating-disorders-new-trifold/index.shtml. (Accessed March 2015.)

19. Grilo, C. M. 2002. Binge eating disorder. In: Fairburn, D. G., and K. D. Brownell, eds. *Eating Disorders and Obesity: A Comprehensive Handbook*, 2nd Edn. New York:Guilford Press, pp.178–182.

20. Vander Wal, J. S. 2012. Night eating syndrome: a critical review of the literature. *Clin. Psychol. Rev..* 32:49–59.

21. Gallant, A. R., Lundgren, J., and Drapeau, V. 2012. The night-eating syndrome and obesity. *Obes. Rev.,* 13(6), 528–536.

22. Nattiv A., A. B. Loucks, M. M. Manore, C. F. Sanborn, J. Sundgot-Borgen, and M. P. Warren. 2007. The female athlete triad. *Med. Sci. Sport Exer.* 39(10):1867–1882.

23. Reiter, S. C., and L. Graves. 2010. Nutrition therapy for eating disorders. *Nutr. Clin. Prac..* 25:122–136.

24. National Eating Disorders Association. 2013. What Should I Say? Tips for Talking to a Friend Who May Be Struggling with an Eating Disorder. http://www.nationaleatingdisorders.org/what-should-i-say. (Accessed March 2015.)

Chapter 14

1. U.S. Department of Health and Human Services. 1996. *Physical Activity and Health: A Report of the Surgeon General.* Atlanta: US Department of Health and Human Services, Centers for Disease Control and Prevention, National Centers for Chronic Disease Prevention and Health Promotion.

2. Caspersen, C. J., K. E. Powell, and G. M. Christensen. 1985. Physical activity, exercise, and physical fitness: definitions and distinctions for health-related research. *Public Health Rep.* 100:126–131.

3. Heyward, V. H. and A. Gibson. 2014. *Advanced Fitness Assessment and Exercise Prescription.* 7th Edn. Champaign, IL: Human Kinetics.

4. *Centers for Disease Control and Prevention.* 2014. Facts about Physical Activity. http://www.cdc.gov/physicalactivity/data/facts.html.

5. Centers for Disease Control and Prevention. Office of Surveillance, Epidemiology, and Laboratory Services. Behavioral Risk Factor Surveillance System. 2012. *Prevalence and Trends Data.* Exercise - 2012. http://apps.nccd.cdc.gov/brfss/list.asp?cat = EX&yr = 2012&qkey = 8041&state = All.

6. Centers for Disease Control and Prevention. 2014. Youth risk behavior surveillance—United States, 2013. *Morbid. Mortal. Weekly Rev.* 63:SS-4. http://www.cdc.gov/healthyyouth/physicalactivity/facts.htm.

7. Institute of Medicine, Food and Nutrition Board. 2002. *Dietary Reference Intakes for Energy, Carbohydrates, Fiber, Fat, Protein and Amino Acids (Macronutrients).* Washington, DC: National Academy of Sciences.

8. U.S. Department of Health and Human Services. 2009. *2008 Physical Activity Guidelines for Americans.* http://health.gov/paguidelines/guidelines/default.aspx#toc.

9. Arem, H., S. C. Moore, A. Patel, P. Hartge, A. Berrington de Gonzalez, K. Visvanathan,…, and C. E. Matthews. 2015. Leisure time physical activity and mortality: a detailed pooled analysis of the dose-response relationship. *JAMA Intern. Med.* 175(6):959–967.

10. Gebel, K., D. Ding, T. Chey, E. Stamatakis, W. J. Brown, and A. E. Bauman. 2015. Effect of moderate to vigorous physical activity on all-cause mortality in middle-aged and older Australians. *JAMA Intern. Med.* 175(6):970–977.

11. Silva, M. N., D. Markland, E. V. Carraça, P. N. Vieira, S. R. Coutinho, C. S. Minderico, M. G. Matos, L. B. Sardinha, and P. J. Teixeira. 2011. Exercise autonomous motivation predicts 3-yr weight loss in women. *Med. Sci. Sports Exerc.* 43(4):728–737.

12. Teixeira, P. J., M. N. Silva, J. Mata, A. L. Palmeira, and D. Markland. 2012. Motivation, self-determination, and long-term weight control. *Int. J. Behav. Nutr. Phys. Activ.* 9:22, http://www.ijbnpa.org/content/9/1/22.

13. Centers for Disease Control and Prevention. 2011. Physical Activity for Everyone. Measuring Physical Activity Intensity. *Target Heart Rate and Estimated Maximum Heart Rate*. www.cdc.gov/physicalactivity/everyone/measuring/heartrate.html.

14. Gibala, M. J., J. P. Little, M. J. MacDonald, and J. A. Hawley. 2012. Physiological adaptations to low-volume, high-intensity interval training in health and disease. *J. Physiol.* 590:1077–1084.

15. Burke, L. 2010. Nutrition for recovery after competition and training. In: Burke, L., and V. Deakin, eds. *Clin. Sports Nutr.* 4th Edn. New York: McGraw-Hill, pp. 358–392.

16. Pritchett, K. and R. Pritchett. 2013. Chocolate milk: a post-exercise recovery beverage for endurance sports. *Med. Sport Sci.* 59:127–134.

17. Phillips, S. M., and L. J. C van Loon. 2011. Dietary protein for athletes: from requirements to optimum adaptation. *J. Sports Sci.* 29(S1):S29–S38.

18. Sears, B. 1995. *The Zone: A Dietary Road Map*. New York: HarperCollins.

Chapter 15

1. U.S. Centers for Disease Control and Prevention (CDC). 2014, January 8. *Estimates of Foodborne Illness in the United States*. www.cdc.gov/foodborneburden/index.html.

2. U.S. Government Accountability Office. 2015. *Improving Federal Oversight of Food Safety*. http://www.gao.gov/highrisk/revamping_food_safety/why_did_study#t = 0.

3. U.S. Centers for Disease Control and Prevention (CDC). 2013, January 29. Contribution of Different Food Commodities (Categories) to Estimated Domestically Acquired Illnesses and Deaths, 1998–2008. http://www.cdc.gov/foodborneburden/attribution-image.html#foodborne-illnesses.

4. U.S. Centers for Disease Control and Prevention (CDC). 2014. *Food Safety Progress Report for 2013*. http://www.cdc.gov/media/releases/2014/images/p0417-2013-foodborne-infections.pdf.

5. U.S. Centers for Disease Control and Prevention (CDC). 2014, December 30. *Norovirus*. http://www.cdc.gov/norovirus/index.html.

6. U.S. Centers for Disease Control and Prevention (CDC). 2014, September 18. *Viral Hepatitis*. http://www.cdc.gov/hepatitis/.

7. U.S. Centers for Disease Control and Prevention (CDC). 2014, October 3. Top pathogens contributing to domestically acquired foodborne illnesses and deaths, 2000–2008. http://www.cdc.gov/Features/dsFoodborneEstimates/.

8. U.S. Centers for Disease Control and Prevention (CDC). 2015, March 26. *Parasites—Toxoplasmosis: Epidemiology and Risk Factors*. http://www.cdc.gov/parasites/toxoplasmosis/epi.html.

9. U.S. Centers for Disease Control and Prevention (CDC). 2012, July 13. *Parasites—Giardia: Epidemiology and Risk Factors*. http://www.cdc.gov/parasites/giardia/epi.html.

10. U.S. Centers for Disease Control and Prevention (CDC). 2014, October 7. *vCJD (Variant Creutzfeldt-Jakob Disease)*. http://www.cdc.gov/ncidod/dvrd/vcjd/qa.htm.

11. U.S. Centers for Disease Control and Prevention (CDC). 2014, April 25. *Botulism*. http://www.cdc.gov/nczved/divisions/dfbmd/diseases/botulism/.

12. U.S. Centers for Disease Control and Prevention (CDC). 2010, July 20. *Marine Toxins*. www.cdc.gov/nczved/divisions/dfbmd/diseases/marine_toxins.

13. Horowitz, B. Z. 2013, April 3. *Mushroom Toxicity*. Medscape Reference. http://emedicine.medscape.com/article/167398-overview 10.

14. National Institutes of Health. 2013, October 21. *Potato Plant Poisoning: Green Tubers and Sprouts*. MedlinePlus. www.nlm.nih.gov/medlineplus/ency/article/002875.htm.

15. U.S. Department of Health & Human Services. (n.d.) Clean: Wash Hands and Surfaces Often. Accessed March 31, 2015. http://www.foodsafety.gov/keep/basics/clean/index.html.

16. U.S. Department of Health & Human Services. (n.d.) Separate: Don't Cross-Contaminate. Accessed March 31, 2015. http://www.foodsafety.gov/keep/basics/separate/index.html.

17. U.S. Department of Health & Human Services. (n.d.) Chill: Refrigerate Promptly. Accessed March 31, 2015. http://www.foodsafety.gov/keep/basics/chill/index.html.

18. U.S. Department of Agriculture Food Safety and Inspection Service. 2015, March 24. Food Product Dating. http://www.fsis.usda.gov/wps/portal/fsis/topics/food-safety-education/get-answers/food-safety-fact-sheets/food-labeling/food-product-dating/food-product-dating.

19. U.S. Department of Health & Human Services. (n.d.) Frozen Food and Power Outages: When to Save and When to Throw Out. Accessed March 31, 2015. http://www.foodsafety.gov/keep/charts/frozen_food.html.

20. U.S. Department of Agriculture Food Safety and Inspection Service. 2013, August 22. Molds on Food: Are They Dangerous? http://www.fsis.usda.gov/wps/portal/fsis/topics/food-safety-education/get-answers/food-safety-fact-sheets/safe-food-handling/molds-on-food-are-they-dangerous_/.

21. U.S. Department of Agriculture Food Safety and Inspection Service. 2013, May. Is It Done Yet? http://www.fsis.usda.gov/wps/wcm/connect/c825bac8-c024-4793-be76-159dfb56a88f/IsItDoneYet_Brochure.pdf?MOD = AJPERES.

22. Center for Science in the Public Interest (CSPI). 2014. Chemical Cuisine. Learn About Food Additives. www.cspinet.org/reports/chemcuisine.htm.

23. U.S. Department of Agriculture Economic Research Service. 2014, July 14. Adoption of Genetically Engineered Crops in the US: Recent Trends in GE Adoption. http://www.ers.usda.gov/data-products/adoption-of-genetically-engineered-crops-in-the-us/recent-trends-in-ge-adoption.aspx.

24. U.S. Environmental Protection Agency (EPA). 2014, June 12. *Persistent Organic Pollutants: A Global Issue, a Global Response*. http://www2.epa.gov/international-cooperation/persistent-organic-pollutants-global-issue-global-response.

25. National Institute of Environmental Health Sciences. 2014, September 22. Mercury. http://www.niehs.nih.gov/health/topics/agents/mercury/index.cfm.

26. National Institute of Environmental Health Sciences. 2014, August 14. Lead. http://www.niehs.nih.gov/health/topics/agents/lead/index.cfm.

27. Bae, S., J. H. Kim, Y. H. Lim, H. Y. Park, and Y. C. Hong. 2012. Associations of bisphenol A exposure with heart rate variability and blood pressure. *Hypertension*. 60(3):786–793. doi: 10.1161/HYPERTENSIONAHA.112.197715. Epub 2012 Jul 30.

28. National Institute of Environmental Health Sciences. 2015, January 25. *Endocrine Disruptors*. http://www.niehs.nih.gov/health/topics/agents/endocrine/index.cfm.

29. U.S. Environmental Protection Agency (EPA). 2012, March 14. *Phthalates Action Plan*. http://www.epa.gov/oppt/existingchemicals/pubs/actionplans/phthalates_actionplan_revised_2012-03-14.pdf.

30. National Institute of Environmental Health Sciences. 2015, January 21. *Bisphenol A (BPA)*. http://www.niehs.nih.gov/health/topics/agents/sya-bpa/index.cfm.

31. National Institute of Environmental Health Sciences. 2014, May 22. *Dioxins*. http://www.niehs.nih.gov/health/topics/agents/dioxins/index.cfm.

32. International Agency for Research on Cancer. 2015, March 20. IARC Monographs Volume 112: Evaluation of five organ ophosphate insecticides and herbicides. http://www.iarc.fr/en/media-centre/iarcnews/pdf/MonographVolume112.pdf.

33. National Institutes of Health. 2014. *Agricultural Health Study (AHS): 2014 Study Update*. http://aghealth.nih.gov/news/2014.html.

34. American Academy of Pediatrics. 2012, November 26. AAP Makes Recommendations to Reduce Children's Exposures to Pesticides.

https://www.aap.org/en-us/about-the-aap/aap-press-room/pages/AAP-Makes-Recommendations-to-Reduce-Children's-Exposure-to-Pesticides.aspx.

35. U.S. Environmental Protection Agency (EPA). 2015, March 19. *Pesticides and Food: Healthy, Sensible Food Practices*. www.epa.gov/pesticides/food/tips.htm.

36. American Cancer Society. 2014, September 10. Recombinant Bovine Growth Hormone. www.cancer.org/cancer/cancercauses/othercarcinogens/athome/recombinant-bovine-growth-hormone.

37. Environmental Working Group. 2013. Superbugs invade American supermarkets. www.ewg.org/meateatersguide/superbugs/.

38. U.S. Centers for Disease Control and Prevention (CDC). 2015, January 8. Methicillin-Resistant *Staphylococcus aureus* (MRSA) Infections. www.cdc.gov/mrsa/.

39. U.S. Department of Agriculture Agricultural Marketing Service. National Organic Program. Organic Standards. 2013, April 4. http://www.ams.usda.gov/AMSv1.0/NOPOrganicStandards.

40. Organic Trade Association. 2015. Media: Quick Stats. https://ota.com/media/quick-stats.

41. Brandt, K., C. Leifert, R. Sanderson, and C. J. Seal, Agroecosystem management and nutritional quality of plant foods: the case of organic fruits and vegetables. *Crit. Rev. Plant Sci.*. 30(1–2):177–197.

42. Smith-Spangler, C., M. L. Brandeau, G. E. Hunter, J. C. Bavinger, M. Pearson, P. J. Eschbach,…, and D. M. Bravata. Are organic foods safer or healthier than conventional alternatives? A systematic review. *Ann. Intern. Med.* 157(5):348–366. doi:10.7326/0003-4819-157-5-201209040-00007.

43. Benbook, C. M., G. Butler, M. A. Latif, C. Leifert, and D. R. Davis. 2013. Organic production enhances milk nutritional quality by shifting fatty acid composition: a United States-wide, 18-month study. *PLoS One*. 8(12):e82429. doi: 10.1371/journal.pone.0082429. eCollection 2013.

44. Baranski, M., D. Srednicka-Tober, N. Volakakis, C. Seal, R. Sanderson, G. B. Stewart,…, and C. Leifert. 2014. Higher antioxidant and lower cadmium concentrations and lower incidence of pesticide residues in organically grown crops: a systemic literature review and meta-analyses. *Br. J. Nutr.* 26:1–18.

45. Forman, J., and J. Silverstein. 2012. Organic foods: health and environmental advantages and disadvantages. *Pediatrics*. 130(5):e1406–e1415. doi: 10.1542/peds.2012-2579

Chapter 16

1. James, S. W., and Friel, S. 2015. An integrated approach to identifying and characterising resilient urban food systems to promote population health in a changing climate. *Public Health Nutr.* 10:1–11. [Epub ahead of print]

2. Food and Agricultural Organization of the United Nations (FAO). 2014. FAO Hunger Map 2014. Available at http://www.fao.org/fileadmin/templates/ess/foodsecurity/poster_web_001_WFS.jpg.

3. Central Intelligence Agency. 2015. *The World Factbook*. Available at https://www.cia.gov/library/publications/the-world-factbook/

4. U.S. Centers for Disease Control and Prevention (CDC). 2014, September 3. Childhood Obesity Facts. Available at http://www.cdc.gov/obesity/data/childhood.html.

5. Wang H, A. E. Schumacher, C. E. Levitz, A. H. Mokdad, and C. J. Murray. 2013. Left behind: widening disparities for males and females in U.S. county life expectancy, 1985–2010. *Population Health Metrics*. 11:8.

6. Food and Agricultural Organization of the United Nations (FAO). 2015. *The State of Food Insecurity in the World*. Available at http://www.fao.org/3/a-i4646e.pdf.

7. Economic Research Service. 2015, January 12. *Food Security Status of U.S. Households in 2013*. United States Department of Agriculture. Available at http://www.ers.usda.gov/topics/food-nutrition-assistance/food-security-in-the-us.aspx.

8. World Hunger Education Service. 2015. *2015 World Hunger and Poverty Facts and Statistics*. Available at http://www.worldhunger.org/articles/Learn/world%20hunger%20facts%202002.htm.

9. United States Census Bureau. 2013, December 4. World Population. www.census.gov/population/international/data/.

10. Kinsella, B. 2011, November 17. Secondary education for females: a primary way to prevent overpopulation. *Harvard College Global Health Review*. Available at http://www.hcs.harvard.edu/hghr/online/secondary-education-women/.

11. World Health Organization. 2014, July 21. *Global Summary of the AIDS Epidemic: 2013*. Available at http://www.who.int/hiv/data/epi_core_dec2014.png?ua = 1.

12. U.S. Environmental Protection Agency. 2014, March 18. Climate Change: Basic Information. Available at http://www.epa.gov/climatechange/basics/.

13. U.S. Environmental Protection Agency. 2013, September 9. Glossary of Climate Change Terms. http://www.epa.gov/climatechange/glossary.html.

14. Fischer, E. M., and R. Knutti, R. 2015. Anthropogenic contribution to global occurrence of heavy-precipitation and high-temperature extremes. *Nature*. 27 April 2015. doi: 10.1038/NCLIMATE2617

15. Porter, J. R., L. Xie, A. J. Challinor, K. Cochrane, S. M. Howden, M. M. Iqbal, D. B. Lobell, and M. I. Travasso. 2014. Food security and food production systems. In: Field, C. B., V. R. Barros, D. J. Dokken, K. J. Mach, M. D. Mastrandrea, T. E. Bilir,…, and L. L. White. eds. *Climate Change 2014: Impacts, Adaptation, and Vulnerability. Part A: Global and Sectoral Aspects. Contribution of Working Group II to the Fifth Assessment Report of the Intergovernmental Panel on Climate Change* Cambridge, United Kingdom and New York, NY, USA: Cambridge University Press, *pp.* 485–533.

16. Suweis, S., Carr, J.A., Maritan, A., Rinaldo, A., and D'Odorico, P. 2015. Resilience and reactivity of global food security. *Proceedings of the National Academy of Sciences*, 2015; 201507366 DOI: 10.1073/pnas.1507366112

17. Briend, A. 2014, August 13. Measuring the Burden of Severe Acute Malnutrition: Current Challenges. *Global Nutrition Report*. Available at http://globalnutritionreport.org/2014/08/13/measuring-the-burden-of-severe-acute-malnutrition/

18. World Health Organization. 2012. Child Malnutrition: A Hidden Crisis Which Threatens the Global Economy. www.who.int/pmnch/media/news/2012/20120215_stc_pr_children_malnutrition/en/.

19. World Health Organization. 2015. Micronutrient deficiencies. Available at http://www.who.int/nutrition/topics/

20. Iodine Global Network. 2015. About the Iodine Global Network. Available at http://www.ign.org/p142000253.html

21. World Health Organization. 2015, January. Obesity and Overweight. Fact Sheet No311. Available at http://www.who.int/mediacentre/factsheets/fs311/en/

22. Sarmiento, O. L., D. C. Parra, S. A. Gonzalez, I. González-Casanova, A. Y. Forero, and J. Garcia. 2014. The dual burden of malnutrition in Colombia. *Am J. Clin. Nutr.* 100(6):1628S–35S. doi: 10.3945/ajcn.114.083816. Epub 2014, October 29.

23. Freire, W. B., K. M. Silva-Jaramillo, M. J. Ramirez-Luzuriaga, P. Belmont, and W. F. Waters. 2014. The double burden of undernutrition and excess body weight in Ecuador. *Am. J. Clin. Nutr.* 100(6):1636S-43S. doi: 10.3945/ajcn.114.083766. Epub 2014, October 29.

24. Demment, M. M., J. D. Haas, and C. M. Olson. 2014. Changes in family income status and the development of overweight and obesity from 2 to 15 years: a longitudinal study. *BMC Public Health*. 14:417. doi: 10.1186/1471-2458-14-417.

25. Oddo, V. M., and J. C. Jones-Smith. 2015. Gains in income during early childhood are associated with decreases in BMI z scores among children in the United States. *Am. J. Clin. Nutr.* 2015 Jun;101(6):1225-31. pii: ajcn096693. [Epub ahead of print]

26. U.S. Department of Agriculture Agricultural Marketing Service. n.d. Food Deserts. Available at http://apps.ams.usda.gov/fooddeserts/fooddeserts.aspx.

27. Fair Food Network. 2015. The Food System: Equity. Available at http://www.fairfoodnetwork.org/food-system/equity.

28. Hruschka, D. J. 2012. Do economic constraints on food choice make people fat? A critical review of two hypotheses for the poverty-obesity paradox. *Am. J. Hum. Bio.* 24:277–285.

29. Hemmingsson, E. 2014. A new model of the role of psychological and emotional distress in promoting obesity: conceptual review with implications for treatment and prevention. *Obesity Reviews.* 2014 Sep; 15(9):769-79. doi: 10.1111/obr.12197.

30. Haushofer, J., and E. Fehr. 2014. On the psychology of poverty. *Science* 344(6186):862–867. doi: 10.1126/science.1232491.

31. Tryon, M. S., K. L. Stanhope, E. S. Epel, A. E. Mason, R. Brown, V. Medici, P. J. Havel, K. D. Laugero. 2015. Excessive sugar consumption may be a difficult habit to break: a view from the brain and body. *J. Clin. Endocrinol. Metab.*. 100(6):2239:2247. Available at http://press.endocrine.org/doi/abs/10.1210/jc.2014-4353.

32. Rockefeller Foundation. 2012, August. *Social and Economic Equity in U.S. Food and Agriculture Systems.* Available at http://www.fsg.org/Portals/0/Uploads/Documents/PDF/Equity_in_US_Food_Agriculture_Systems.pdf?cpgn = WP%20DL%20-%20Social%20and%20Economic%20Equity%20in%20U.S.%20Food%20and%20Agriculture%20Systems.

33. McCluskey, M., T. McGarity, S. Shapiro, and M. Shudtz. 2013, January. *At the Company's Mercy: Protecting Contingent Workers from Unsafe Working Conditions.* Center for Progressive Reform. White Paper #1301. Available at http://www.progressivereform.org/articles/contingent_workers_1301.pdf.

34. U.S. Centers for Disease Control and Prevention. 2014, December 15. *Agricultural Safety.* http://www.cdc.gov/niosh/topics/aginjury/.

35. United States Department of Labor. 2015, January 1. *State Child Labor Laws Applicable to Agriculture.* Available at http://www.dol.gov/whd/state/agriemp2.htm.

36. Bureau of Labor Statistics. 2014, January 8. *Food and Beverage Serving and Related Workers.* Available at http://www.bls.gov/ooh/food-preparation-and-serving/food-and-beverage-serving-and-related-workers.htm.

37. U.S. Department of Agriculture. n.d. *Census of Agriculture: Historical Archive.* Available at http://agcensus.mannlib.cornell.edu/AgCensus/homepage.do.

38. U.S. Department of Agriculture. May 2, 2014. Census of Agriculture: 2012. Available at http://www.agcensus.usda.gov/Publications/2012/.

39. Foley, J. 2013, March 5. It's Time to Rethink America's Corn System. *Scientific American.* Available at http://www.scientificamerican.com/article/time-to-rethink-corn/.

40. Khoury, C. K., A. D. Bjorkman, H. Dempewolf, J. Ramirez-Villegas, L. Guarino, A. Jarvis, L. H. Rieseberg, and P. C. Struik. 2014. Increasing homogeneity in global food supplies and the implications for food security. *Proc. Natl. Acad. Sci. U.S.A.* 111(11):4001–4006. doi:10.1073/pnas.1313490111.

41. Center for Responsive Politics. 2015, March. PACs: Agribusiness Sector. Available at http://www.opensecrets.org/pacs/sector.php?txt = A01&cycle = 2014.

42. U.S. Department of Agriculture (USDA). 2015, April 16. Dairy Research and Promotion Program. Available at http://www.ams.usda.gov/AMSv1.0/ams.fetchTemplateData.do?template = TemplateN&leftNav = IndustryMarketingandPromotion&page = DairyProducerCheckoffPrograms&description = Dairy + Producer + Checkoff + Programs.

43. Yale Rudd Center for Food Policy & Obesity. 2013, November. *Fast Food F.a.c.t.s. 2013: Measuring Progress in Nutrition and Marketing to Children and Teens.* Available at http://fastfoodmarketing.org/media/FastFoodFACTS_Report_Summary.pdf.

44. Nestle, M. 2013. *Food Politics: How the Food Industry Influences Nutrition and Health: Revised and Expanded* 10th *Anniversary Edition.* Berkeley: University of California Press, p. 13.

45. United Nations. 2014. The Millennium Development Goals Report 2014. 14-27027. Available at http://www.un.org/millenniumgoals/2014%20MDG%20report/MDG%202014%20English%20web.pdf.

46. LocalHarvest. 2014. Community Supported Agriculture. www.localharvest.org/csa/.

47. U.S. Department of Agriculture (USDA). 2015, March 23. Farmers Markets and Direct-to-Consumer Marketing. Available at www.ams.usda.gov/AMSv1.0/farmersmarkets.

48. Slow Food USA. 2015. About Us. Accessed April 29, 2015 at http://www.slowfoodusa.org/about-us.

49. Fair Trade USA. (2015). What Is Fair Trade? Accessed April 29, 2015 at www.fairtradeusa.org/what-is-fair-trade.

50. Moore Lappé, F. 2011, September 14. The Food Movement: Its Power and Possibilities. *The Nation.* www.thenation.com/article/163403/food-movement-its-power-and-possibilities.

Chapter 17

1. Martin, J. A., B. E. Hamilton, M. J. K. Osterman, S. C. Curtin, and T. J. Mathews. 2015. Births: final data for 2013. *Natl Vital Stat Rep* 64:1–68.

2. MacDorman, M. F., and T. J. Mathews. 2014. International comparisons of infant mortality and related factors: United States and Europe, 2010. *Natl Vital Stat Rep* 63:1–6.

3. U.S. Department of Health and Human Services. Healthy People 2020 Objectives and Topics. www.healthypeople.gov/2020/-topicsobjectives2020/default.aspx. Accessed May 1, 2015.

4. March of Dimes. 2014. Low Birthweight. Available at http://www.marchofdimes.org/baby/low-birthweight.aspx#. Accessed April 2015.

5. Rasmussen, K. M., and A. L. Yaktine, eds. 2009. *Weight Gain During Pregnancy: Reexamining the Guidelines.* Washington, DC: National Academy Press.

6. Gaillard, R., E. A. P. Steegers, L. Duijts, J. F. Felix, A. Hofman, O. H. Franco, and V. W. V. Jaddoe. 2014. Childhood cardiometabolic outcomes of maternal obesity during pregnancy—the generation R study. *Hyperten* 63:683–691.

7. Barbour, L. A. 2012. Weight gain in pregnancy: is less truly more for mother and infant? *Obstetric Medicine* 5:58–64.

8. Institute of Medicine, Food and Nutrition Board. 2002. *Dietary Reference Intakes for Energy, Carbohydrate, Fiber, Fat, Fatty Acids, Cholesterol, Protein, and Amino Acids.* Washington, DC: National Academy Press.

9. Food and Drug Administration. 2014. Food Safety for moms-to-be: while you're pregnant – methylmercury. Available at http://www.fda.gov/Food/ResourcesForYou/HealthEducators/ucm083324.htm. Accessed April 2015.

10. Food and Drug Administration 2015. New Advice: Pregnant Women and Young Children Should Eat More Fish. Available at: http://www.fda.gov/forconsumers/consumerupdates/ucm397443.htm

11. Spina Bifida Association. Folic Acid. Available at: http://www.spinabifidaassociation.org/site/c.evKRI7OXIoJ8H/b.8090137/k.8D22/Folic_Acid_Facts.htm. Accessed April 2015.

12. Institute of Medicine, Food and Nutrition Board. 1998. *Dietary Reference Intakes for Thiamin, Riboflavin, Niacin, Vitamin B$_6$, Folate, Vitamin B$_{12}$, Pantothenic Acid, Biotin, and Choline.* Washington, DC: National Academy Press.

13. Institute of Medicine, Food and Nutrition Board. 2001. *Dietary Reference Intakes for Vitamin A, Vitamin K, Arsenic, Boron, Chromium, Copper, Iodine, Iron, Manganese, Molybdenum, Nickel, Silicon, Vanadium, and Zinc.* Washington, DC: National Academy Press.

14. Institute of Medicine, Food and Nutrition Board. 2011. *Dietary Reference Intakes for Calcium and Vitamin D.* Washington, DC: National Academy Press.

15. Rosen, C. J., J. S. Adams, D. D. Bikle, D. M. Black, M. B. Demay, J. E. Manson, M. H. Murad, and C. S. Kovacs. 2012. The nonskeletal effects of vitamin D: an endocrine society scientific statement. *Endocrine Rev.* 33:456–492.

16. Mayo-Wilson, E., A. Imdad, J. Junior, S. Dean and Z. A. Bhutta. 2014. Preventive zinc supplementation for children, and the effect of additional iron: a systematic review and meta-analysis. *BMJ Open 4:e004647.* doi:10.1136/bmjopen-2013-004647.

17. Institute of Medicine, Food and Nutrition Board. 2004. *Dietary Reference Intakes for Water, Potassium, Sodium, Chloride, and Sulfate.* Washington, DC: National Academy Press.

18. Matthews, A., D. M. Haas, D. P. O'Mathuna, T. Dowswell, and M. Doyle. 2014. Interventions for nausea and vomiting in early pregnancy. The Cochrane Library. doi: 10.1002/14651858. CD007575.pub3.

19. DeSiston, D. C. L., S. Y. Kim, and A. J. Sharma. 2014. Prevalence estimates of gestational diabetes mellitus in the United States, Pregnancy Risk Assessment Monitoring System (PRAMS), 2007-2009. *Prev Chronic Dis* 11:130415. Available at http://www.cdc.gov/pcd/issues/2014/13_0415.htm. Accessed April 2015.

20. Mitanchez, D., A. Burguet, and U. Simeoni. 2014. Infants born to mothers with gestational diabetes mellitus: mild neonatal effects, a long-term threat to global health. *J Ped* 164:445–450.

21. Schoenaker, D. A. J. M., S. S. Soedamah-Muthu, and G. D. Mishra. 2014. The association between dietary factors and gestational hypertension and pre-eclampsia: a systematic review and meta-analysis of observational studies. *BMC Med* 12:157–174.

22. Barton, J. R., S. D. Joy, D. J. Rhea, A. J. Sibai, and B. M. Sibai. 2014. The influence of gestational weight gain on the development of gestational hypertension in obese women. *Amer J Perinatol.* 32(7):615–620. doi:10.1055/s-0034-1386634.

23. Centers for Disease Control and Prevention. 2015. Listeria (Listeriosis). Available at http://www.cdc.gov/listeria/. Accessed May 2015.

24. U.S. Food and Drug Administration. 2014. *Food Safety for Moms-to-Be: At-a-Glance.* Available at www.fda.gov/Food/ResourcesForYou/HealthEducators/ucm081819.htm. Accessed April 2015.

25. U.S. Food and Drug Administration. 2014. Food Safety for Moms-to-Be: Safe Eats – Eating Out & Bringing In. Available at www.fda.gov/Food/FoodBorneIllnessContaminants/PeopleAtRisk/ucm082539.htm. Accessed April 2015.

26. Office of Adolescent Health. 2015. Trends in teen pregnancy and childbearing. U.S. Department of Health & Human Services. Available at http://www.hhs.gov/ash/oah/adolescent-health-topics/reproductive-health/teen-pregnancy/trends.html. Accessed April 2015.

27. Mayo Clinic. 2014. Pregnancy after 35: healthy moms, healthy babies. Available at http://www.mayoclinic.org/healthy-lifestyle/getting-pregnant/in-depth/pregnancy/art-20045756. Accessed April 2015.

28. Centers for Disease Control and Prevention. 2014. First births to older women continue to rise. *NCHS Data Brief.* No. 152. Available at http://www.cdc.gov/nchs/data/databriefs/db152.pdf Accessed May 2015.

29. Balasch, J., and E. Gratacós. 2011. Delayed childrearing: effects on fertility and the outcome of pregnancy. *Fetal Diagn Ther* 29:263–273.

30. American College of Obstetricians and Gynecologists. 2014. Later Childbearing. Available at http://www.acog.org/-/media/For-Patients/faq060.pdf?dmc = 1&ts = 20150505T0917505782. Accessed May 2015.

31. Piccoli, G. B., R. Clari, F. N. Vigotti, F. Leone, R. Attini, G. Cabiddu, G. Mauro,..., and P. Avagnina. 2015. Vegan-vegetarian diets in pregnancy: danger or panacea? A systematic narrative review. *BJOG* 122:623–633.

32. Price, B. B., S. B. Amini, and K. Kappeler. 2012. Exercise in pregnancy: effect on fitness and obstetric outcomes—a randomized trial. *Med Sci Sports Exerc* 44:2263–2269.

33. Downs, D. S., L. Chasan-Taber, K. R. Evenson, J. Leiferman, and S. Yeo. 2012. Physical activity and pregnancy: past and present evidence and future recommendations. *Res Quarterly Exerc Sport* 83:485–502.

34. American College of Sports Medicine. Exercise during Pregnancy. (undated). Available at https://www.acsm.org/docs/current-comments/exerciseduringpregnancy.pdf. Accessed April 2015

35. Academy of Nutrition and Dietetics. 2014. Position of the Academy of Nutrition and Dietetics: Nutrition and lifestyle for a healthy pregnancy outcome. 114:1099–1103.

36. Greenwood, D. C., N. J. Thatcher, J. Ye, L. Garrard, G. Keogh, L. G. King, and J. E. Cade. 2014. Caffeine intake during pregnancy and adverse birth outcomes: a systematic review and dose-response meta-analysis. *Eur J Epidemiol* 29:725–734.

37. Pope, E., G. Koren, and P. Bozzo. 2014. Sugar substitutes during pregnancy. *Canadian Family Physician* 60:1003–1005.

38. May, P. A., A. Baete, J. Russo, A. J. Elliot, J. Blankenship, W. O. Kalberg,..., H. E. Hoyme. 2014. Prevalence and characteristics of fetal alcohol spectrum disorders. *Pediatrics* 134:855–866.

39. Jully-Martens, K., K. Denys, S. Treit, S. Tamana, and C. -Rasmussen. 2012. A review of social skills deficits in individuals with fetal alcohol spectrum disorders and prenatal alcohol exposure: Profiles, mechanisms, and interventions. *Alcoholism: Clin. Exper. Res.* 36:568–576.

40. Pineles, B. L., E. Park, and J. M. Samet. 2014. Systematic review and meta-analysis of miscarriage and maternal exposure to tobacco smoke during pregnancy. *Am J Epidemiol* 179:807–823.

41. Bottorff, J. L., N. Poole, M. T. Kelly, L. Greaves, L. Marcellus, and M. Jung. 2014. Tobacco and alcohol use in the context of adolescent pregnancy and postpartum: a scoping review of the literature. *Health and Social Care in the Community* 22:561–574.

42. Centers for Disease Control and Prevention. 2014. Tobacco Use and Pregnancy. www.cdc.gov/reproductivehealth/-tobaccouse pregnancy/. Accessed April 2015.

43. Varner, M. W., R. M. Silver, C. J. Rowland Hogue, M. Willinger, C. B. Parker, V. R. Thorsten,..., Eunice Kennedy Shriver National Institute of Child Health and Human Development Stillbirth Collaborative Research Network. 2014. Association between stillbirth and illicit drug use and smoking during pregnancy. *Obstet Gynecol* 123:113–125.

44. Worley, J. 2014. Identification and management of prescription drug abuse in pregnancy. *J Perinatal & Neonatal Nursing* 28:196–203.

45. Servey, J. and J. Chang. 2014. Over-the-counter medications in pregnancy. *Am Fam Physician* 90:548–555.

46. Smeriglio, A., A. Tomaino, and D. Trombetta. 2014. Herbal products in pregnancy: experimental studies and clinical reports. *Phytotherapy Res* 28:1107–1116.

47. Centers for Disease Control and Prevention. 2014. Breastfeeding Report Card: United States/2014. Available at www.cdc.gov/breastfeeding/pdf/2014breastfeedingreportcard.pdf Accessed April 2015.

48. Colen, C. G. and D. M. Ramey. 2014. Is breast truly best? Estimating the effects of breastfeeding on long-term child health and wellbeing in the United States using sibling comparisons. *Soc Sci & Med* 109:55–65.

49. McGuire, S. 2014. Centers for Disease Control and Prevention. 2013. Strategies to prevent obesity and other chronic diseases: the CDC guide to strategies to support breastfeeding mothers and babies. Atlanta, GA: U.S. Department of Health and Human Services, 2013. *Adv Nutr* 5:291–292.

50. Raju, T. N. K. 2014. Reasonable break time for nursing mothers: a provision enacted through the Affordable Care Act. *Pediatrics* 134:423–424.

51. Goodman, K., and E. DiFrisco. 2012. Achieving baby-friendly designation; step-by-step. *MCN Am. J. Matern. Child Nurs.* 37:146–152.

52. Urwin, H. J. E., A. Miles, P. S. Noakes, L. S. Kremmyda, M. Vlachava, N. D. Diaper,..., and P. Yaqoob. 2012. Salmon

consumption during pregnancy alters fatty acid composition and secretory IgA concentration in breast milk. *J Nutr.* 142(8):1603–1610. doi:10.3945/jn.112.160804.

53. American Academy of Pediatrics, Section on Breastfeeding. 2012. Breastfeeding and the use of human milk policy statement. *Pediatrics* 129:e827–841.

54. U.S. Food and Drug Administration. 2015, January 6. Bisphenol A (BPA): Use in Food Contact Application: Update. Available at http://www.fda.gov/food/ingredientspackaginglabeling/foodadditivesingredients/ucm064437.htm#regulations.

55. Kotsopoulos, J., J. Lubinshi, L. Salmena, H. T. Lynch, C. -Kim-Sing, W. D. Foulkes,…, and S. A. Narod for the Hereditary Breast Cancer Clinical Study Group. 2012. Breastfeeding and the risk of breast cancer in BRAC1 and BRAC2 mutation carriers. *Breast Cancer Research* 14:R42.

56. Kindra, G., A. Coutsoudis, F. Exposito, and T. Esterhuizen. 2012. Breastfeeding in HIV exposed infants significantly improves child health: a prospective study. *Matern. Child Health J.* 16:632–640.

57. Turcksin, R., S. Bel, S. Galjaard, and R. Devlieger. 2014. Maternal obesity and breastfeeding intention, initiation, intensity and duration: a systematic review. *Maternal and Child Nutrition* 10:166–183.

58. Merewood, A., S. D. Mehta, X. Grossman, T. C. Chen, J. -Mathieu, M. F. Holick, and H. Bauchner. 2012. Vitamin D status among 4-month-old infants in New England: a prospective cohort study. *J. Human Lactation.* 28:159–166.

59. McWilliams, L., T. Mousallem, and W. Burks. 2012. Future therapies for food allergy. *Human Vaccines & Immunotherapeutics* 8:etext prior to publication. www.landesbioscience.com/journals/vaccines/article/20868/?show_full_text = true&.

Chapter 18

1. Institute of Medicine, Food and Nutrition Board. 2002. *Dietary Reference Intakes for Energy, Carbohydrates, Fiber, Fat, Protein and Amino Acids (Macronutrients)*. Washington, DC: The National Academy of Sciences.

2. American Academy of Pediatrics. 2011. Healthy Children, Fit Children: Answers to Common Questions from Parents About Nutrition and Fitness. Elk Grove Village, IL. *American Academy of Pediatrics*.

3. Kranz, S., M. Brauchla, J. L. Slavin, and K. B. Miller. 2012. What do we know about dietary fiber intake in children and health? The effects of fiber intake on constipation, obesity, and diabetes in children. *Adv. Nutr.* 3:47–53.

4. Dror, D. K., and L. H. Allen. 2014. Dairy product intake in children and adolescents in developed countries: trends, nutritional contribution, and a review of association with health outcomes. *Nutr. Rev.* 72:68–81.

5. Ross, A. C., C. L. Taylor, A. L. Yaktine, and H. B. Del Valle, eds. 2011. *Dietary Reference Intakes for Calcium and Vitamin D.* Washington, DC: National Academy Press.

6. Institute of Medicine, Food and Nutrition Board. 2001. *Dietary Reference Intakes for Vitamin A, Vitamin K, Arsenic, Boron, Chromium, Copper, Iodine, Iron, Manganese, Molybdenum, Nickel, Silicon, Vanadium, and Zinc.* Washington, DC: National Academy Press.

7. Institute of Medicine, Food and Nutrition Board. 2004. *Dietary Reference Intakes for Water, Potassium, Sodium, Chloride, and Sulfate.* Washington, DC: National Academy Press.

8. Wallace, T. C., M. McBurney, and V. L. Fulgoni III. 2014. Multivitamin/mineral supplement contribution to micronutrient intakes in the United States, 2007–2010. *J. Am. Coll. Nutr.* 33:94–102.

9. Palfreyman, Z., E. Haycraft, and C. Meyer. 2014. Development of the parental modeling behaviours scale (PARM): links with food intake among children and their mothers. *Matern. Child Nutr.* 10:617–629.

10. Leitzmann, C. 2014. Vegetarian nutrition: past, present, future. *Am. J. Clin. Nutr.* 100:496S–502S.

11. Gibson, R. S., A. L. M. Heath, and E. A. Szymlek-Gay. 2014. Is iron and zinc nutrition a concern for vegetarian infants and young children in industrialized countries? *Am. J. Clin. Nutr.* 100:459S–468S.

12. Academy of Nutrition and Dietetics. 2015. Position of the Academy of Nutrition and Dietetics: vegetarian Diets. *J. Am. Acad. Nutr. Diet* 115:801–810.

13. Keast, D. R., K. M. Hill Gallant, A. M. Albertson, C. K. Gugger, and N. M. Holschuh. 2015. Associations between yogurt, dairy, calcium, and vitamin D intake and obesity among U.S. children aged 8-18 years: NHANES 2005-2008. *Nutrients* 7:1577–1593.

14. Branum, A. M., L. M. Rossen, and K. C. Schoendorf. 2014. Trends in caffeine intake among U.S. children and adolescents. *Pediatrics* 133(3):386–393. doi: 10.1542/peds.2013-2877. Epub 2014 Feb 10.

15. Schwartz, D. L., K. Gilstad-Hayden, A. Carroll-Scott, S. A. Grilo, C. McCaslin, M. Schwartz, and J. R. Ickovics. 2015. Energy drinks and youth self-reported hyperactivity/inattention symptoms. *Acad. Pediatr.* 15(3):297–304. doi: 10.1016/j.acap.2014.11.006. Epub 2015 Feb 9.

16. Flattum, C., M. Draxten, M. Horning, J. A. Fulkerson, D. Neumark-Sztainer, A. Garwick, M. Y. Kubik, and M. Story. 2015. HOME Plus: program design and implementation of a family-focused, community-based intervention to promote the frequency and healthfulness of family meals, reduce children's sedentary behavior, and prevent obesity. *Int. J. Behav. Nutr. Phys. Activ.* 12(1):53. doi: 10.1186/s12966-015-0211-7

17. Harrison, M. E., M. L. Norris, N. Obeid, M. Fu, H. Weinstangel, and M. Sampson. 2015. Systematic review of the effects of family meal frequency on psychosocial outcomes in youth. *Can. Fam. Physician.* 61(2):e96–106.

18. Powers, J. M., and G. R. Buchanan. 2014. Iron deficiency anemia in toddlers to teens: how to manage when prevention fails. *Contemporary Pediatrics.* Available at http://contemporarypediatrics.modernmedicine.com/contemporary-pediatrics/content/tags/american-academy-pediatrics/iron-deficiency-anemia-toddlers-tee. (Accessed May 2015).

19. Feeding America. 2015. *Map the Meal Gap 2015: Highlights of Findings for Overall and Child Food Insecurity.* Available at http://www.feedingamerica.org/hunger-in-america/our-research/map-the-meal-gap/2013/map-the-meal-gap-2013-exec-summ.pdf. (Accessed May 2015).

20. Rausch, R. 2013. Nutrition and academic performance in school-age children: the relation to obesity and food insufficiency. *J. Nutr. Food Sci.* 3:190–192.

21. Kohn, M. J., J. F. Bell, H. M. G. Grow, and G. Chan. 2013. Food insecurity, food assistance and weight status in US youth: new evidence from NHANES 2007–08. *Ped. Obesity* 9:155–166.

22. Hunsberger, M., P. McGinnis, J. Smith, B. A. Beamer, and J. O'Malley. 2014. Elementary school children's recess schedule and dietary intake at lunch: a community-based participatory research partnership pilot study. *BMC Public Health* 14:156–162.

23. Imberman, S. A., and A. D. Kugler. 2012. *The Effect of Providing Breakfast on Student Performance: Evidence from an In-Class Breakfast Program.* NBER Working Paper No.17720. Cambridge, MA: National Bureau of Economic Research.

24. Cohen, J. F.W., S. Richardson, E. Parker, P. J. Catalano, and E. B. Rimm. 2014. Impact of the new U.S. Department of Agriculture school meal standards on food selection, consumption, and waste. *Am. J. Prev. Med.* 46:388–394.

25. Loth, K. A., R. F. MacLehose, J. A. Fulkerson, S. Crow, and D. Neumark-Sztainer. 2013. Are food restriction and pressure-to-eat parenting practices associated with adolescent disordered eating behaviors? *Int. J. Eat. Disord.* 47:310–314.

26. Balantekin, K. N., J. S. Savage, M. E. Marini, and L. L. Birch. 2014. Parental encouragement of dieting promotes daughters' early dieting. *Appetite* 80:190–196.

27. Caperton, C., S. Block, M. Viera, J. Keri, and B. Berman. 2014. Double-blind, placebo-controlled study assessing the effect

of chocolate consumption in subjects with a history of acne vulgaris. *J. Clin. Aesthet. Dermatol.* 7:19–23.

28. Burris, J., W. Rietkerk, and K. Woolf. 2013. Acne: the role of medical nutrition therapy. *J. Acad. Nutr. Dietet.* 113:416–430.

29. Bhate, K., and H. C. Williams. 2014. What's new in acne? An analysis of systemic reviews published in 2011–2012. *Clin. Exp. Dermatol.* 39:273–278.

30. Melnik, B. C. 2012. Diet in acne: further evidence for the role of nutrient signaling in acne pathogenesis. *Acta Derm. Venereol.* 92:228–231.

31. Lange, K., S. Thamothoran, M. Racine, C. Hirko, and S. Fields. 2014. The relationship between weight and smoking in a national sample of adolescents: role of gender. *J. Health Psychol* doi:10.1177/1359105313517275 Available at http://hpq.sagepub.com/content/early/2014/01/09/1359105313517275.long (Accessed July 2015)..

32. Arnold, E. M., E. Greco, K. Desmond, and M. J. Rotheram-Borus. 2014. When life is a drag: depressive symptoms associated with early adolescent smoking. *Vulnerable Child Youth Stud.* 9:1–9.

33. Centers for Disease Control and Prevention. 2012. Teen Drinking and Driving. Available at http://www.cdc.gov/vitalsigns/teendrinkinganddriving/index.html. (Accessed May 2015).

34. Skinner, A. C., and J. A. Skelton. 2014. Prevalence and trends in obesity and severe obesity among children in the United States, 1999–2012. *JAMA Pediatr.* 168:561–566.

35. Expert Panel on Integrated Guidelines for Cardiovascular Health and Risk Reduction in Children and Adolescents: National Heart, Lung, and Blood Institute. 2011. Expert panel on integrated guidelines for cardiovascular health and risk reduction in children and adolescents: summary report. *Pediatr.* 128(suppl):S213–S256.

36. Kit, B. K., E. Kuklina, M. D. Carroll, Y. Ostchega, D. S. Freedman, and C. L. Ogden. 2015. Prevalence of and trends in dyslipidemia and blood pressure among US children and adolescents, 1999-2012. *JAMA Pediatr.* 169:272–279.

37. Gary-Webb, T. L., A. L. Maisonet Giachello, K. Maier, and H. Skrabak. 2014. Socioecological determinants of prediabetes and type 2 diabetes: agenda for action. *Clin. Diabetes* 32:140–143.

38. Rank, M., M. Siegrist, D. C. Wilks, H. Langhof, B. Wolfarth, B. Haller, W. Koenig, and M. Halle. 2013. The cardio-metabolic risk of moderate and severe obesity in children and adolescents. *J. Pediatr.* 163:137–142.

39. Zenlea, I. S., E. T. Burton, N. Askins, E. I. Pluhar, and E. T. Rhodes. 2015. The burden of psychosocial stressors and urgent mental health problems in a pediatric weight management program. *Clin. Pediatr..* pii: 0009922815574077. Available at http://cpj.sagepub.com/content/early/2015/03/12/0009922815574077.long (Accessed July 2015).

40. Dietz, W. H. 2015. The response of the US Centers for Disease Control and Prevention to the obesity epidemic. *Ann Rev Public Health* 36:575–596.

41. Arsenault, L. N., K. Xu, E. M. Taveras, and K. A. Hacker. 2014. Parents' obesity-related behavior and confidence to support behavioral change in their obese children: data from the STAR study. *Acad. Pediatr.* 14:456–462.

42. Wells, N. M., B. M. Myers, and C. R. Henderson Jr. 2014. School gardens and physical activity: a randomized controlled trial of low-income elementary schools. *Prev. Med.* 69:S27–S33.

43. Affenito, S. G., D. Thompson, A. Dorazio, A. M. Albertson, A. Loew, and N. M. Holschuh. 2013. Ready-to-eat cereal consumption and the School Breakfast Program: relationship to nutrient intake and weight. *J. School Health* 83:28–35.

44. Centers for Disease Control and Prevention. 2015. Physical activity: How much physical activity do children need? Available from http://www.cdc.gov/physicalactivity/everyone/guidelines/children.html. (Accessed May 2015).

45. American Academy of Pediatrics Council on Communications and Media. 2011. Policy statement: media use by children younger than 2 years. *Pediatr.* 128:1040–1045.

46. Herrick, K. A., T. H. I. Fakhouri, S. A. Carlson, and J. E. Fulton. TV watching and computer use in U.S. youth aged 12-15, 2012. *NCHS Data Brief* 157 Hyattsville, MD. National Center for Health Statistics. 2014.

47. Hale, L., and S. Guan. 2015. Screen time and sleep among school-aged children and adolescents: a systematic literature review. *Sleep Med. Rev.* 21:50–58.

48. Thompson, D., D. Cantu, R. Bhatt, T. Baranowski, W. Rodgers, R. Jago,…, and R. Buday. 2014. Texting to increase physical activity among teenagers (TXT ME!); rationale, design, and methods proposal. *JMIR Res. Protoc.* 3:e14.

49. Goodell, S., and C. H. Williams. 201 The built environment and physical activity: What is the relationship? Available at: http://www.rwjf.org/en/library/research/2007/04/the-built-environment-and-physical-activity.html. (Accessed May 2015).

50. Mayne, S. L., A. H. Auchincloss, and Y. L. Michael. 2015. Impact of policy and built environment changes on obesity-related outcomes: a systematic review of naturally occurring experiments. *Obes. Rev.* 16:362–375.

51. Robbins, L. B., K. A. Pfeiffer, S. M. Wesolek, and Y-J. Lo. 2014. Process evaluation for a school-based physical activity intervention for 6th- and 7th-grade boys: reach, dose, and fidelity. *Eval. Program Plan.* 42:21–31.

52. Barlow, S. E. 2007. Expert committee recommendations regarding the prevention, assessment, and treatment of child and adolescent overweight and obesity: summary report. *Ped.* 120:S164-S192.

53. Hoelscher, D. M., K. Kirk, L. Ritchie, L. Cunningham-Sabo, and Academy Positions Committee. 2013. Position of the Academy of Nutrition and Dietetics: interventions for the prevention and treatment of pediatric overweight and obesity. 113:1375–1394.

54. Kelly, A. S., S. E. Barlow, G. Rao, T. H. Inge, L. L. Hayman, J. Steinberger,…, and Council on Clinical Cardiology. 2013. Severe obesity in children and adolescents: identification, associated health risks, and treatment approaches. A scientific statement from the American Heart Association. *Circulation* 128:1689–1712.

55. Nobili, V., P. Vajro, A. Dezsofi, B. Fischler, N. Hadzic, J. Jahnel,…, and U. Baumann. 2015. Indications and limitations of bariatric intervention in severely obese children and adolescents with and without nonalcoholic steatohepatitis: ESPGHAN Hepatology Committee position statement. *JGM* 60:550–561.

56. Dietz, W. H., L. A. Baur, K. Hall, R. M. Puhl, E. M. Taveras, R. Uauy, and P. Kopelman. 2015. Management of obesity: improvement of health-care training and systems for prevention and care. *Lancet. Lancet* 9986:2521-2533.

57. Wickham, E. P. III, and M. D. DeBoer. 2015. Evaluation and treatment of severe obesity in childhood. *Clin. Pediatr.* doi:10.1177/0009922814565886. Available at http://cpj.sagepub.com/content/early/2015/01/06/0009922814565886.long (Accessed July 2015).

58. Adeyemo, M. A., J. R. McDuffie, M. Kozlosky, J. Krakoff, K. A. Calis, S. M. Brady, and J. A. Yanovski. 2015. Effects of metformin on energy intake and satiety in obese children. *Diabetes Obes. Metab.* 17:363–370.

59. McDonagh, M., S. Selph, A. Ozpinar, and C. Foley. 2014. Systematic review of the benefits and risks of metformin in treating obesity in children aged 18 years and younger. *JAMA Pediatr.* 168:178–184.

60. Zitsman, J. L., T. H. Inge, K. W. Reichard, A. F. Browne, C. M. Harmon, and M. P. Michalsky. 2014. Pediatric and adolescent obesity: management, options for surgery, and outcomes. *J. Pediatr. Surg.* 49:491–494.

61. Wulkan, M. L., and S. M. Walsh. 2014. The multi-disciplinary approach to adolescent bariatric surgery. *Seminars Pediatr. Surg.* 23:2–4.

Chapter 19

1. U.S. Census Bureau. *2014 National Population Projections.* Available at www.census.gov/population/projections/data/national/2014.html. Accessed June 2015.

2. Ortman, J. M., V. A. Velkoff, and H. Hogan. An Aging Nation: The Older Population in the United States: Population estimates and projections. U.S. Department of Commerce, U.S. Census Bureau. 2014. Available at www.census.gov/prod/2014pubs/p25-1140.pdf. Accessed June 2015.

3. Forman, J. B. 2014. What do we know about the oldest old? *In The Public Interest* 9:9–13.

4. Xu, J. Q., K. D. Kochanek, S. L. Murphy, E. Arias. 2014. Mortality in the United States, 2012. NCHS data brief, no 168. Hyattsville, MD: National Center for Health Statistics.

5. National Center for Health Statistics. Health, United States, 2013: With Special Feature on Prescription Drugs. Hyattsville, MD. 2014.

6. Gerontology Research Group. 2014. Current Validated Living Supercentenarians. Available at www.grg.org/Adams/E.HTM. Accessed June 2015.

7. Scott, D., K. M. Sanders, D. Aitken, A. Hayes, P. R. Ebeling, and G. Jones. 2014. Sarcopenic obesity and dynapenic obesity: 5-year associations with falls risk in middle-aged and older adults. *Obesity* 22:1568–1574.

8. Pahor, M., J. M. Guralnik, W. T. Ambrosius, S. Blair, D. E. Bonds, T. S. Church,…, and LIFE Study Investigators. 2013. Effect of structured physical activity on prevention of major mobility disability in older adults: the LIFE study randomized clinical trial. *JAMA* 311:2387–2396.

9. Öhman, H., N. Savikko, T. E. Strandberg and K. H. Pitkälä. 2014. Effect of physical exercise on cognitive performance in older adults with mild cognitive impairment or dementia: a systematic review. *Dement. Geriatr. Cogn. Disord.* 38:347–365.

10. Attems, J., L. Walker, and K. A. Jellinger. 2015. Olfaction and aging: a mini-review. *Gerontol..* doi: 10.1159/000381619. Available at www.Karger.com/Article/Pdf/381619. Accessed June 2015.

11. Croy, I., S. Nordin, and T. Hummel. 2014. Olfactory disorders and quality of life—an updated review. *Chem. Senses* 39:185–194.

12. Feng, P., L. Huang, and H. Wang. 2014. Taste bud homeostasis in health, disease, and aging. *Chem. Senses* 39:3–16.

13. Abrams, A. P., and L. A. Thompson. 2014. Physiology of aging of older adults: systemic and oral health considerations. *Dent. Clin. North Am.* 58:729–738.

14. Lakshminarayanan, B., C. Stanton, P. W. O'Toole, and R. P. Ross. 2015. Compositional dynamics of the human intestinal microbiota with aging: implications for health. *J. Nutr., Health Aging* 18:773–786.

15. Batsis, J. A., T. A. Mackenzie, L. K. Barre, F. Lopez-Jimenez, and S. J. Bartels. 2014. Sarcopenia, sarcopenic obesity and mortality in older adults: results from the National Health and Nutrition Examination Survey III. *Eur. J. Clin. Nutr.* 68:1001–1007.

16. Anunciacão, P. C., R. C. L. Ribeiro, M. Q. Pereira, and M. Comunian. 2014. Different measurements of waist circumference and sagittal abdominal diameter and their relationship with cardiometabolic risk factors in elderly men. *J. Human Nutr. Dietet.* 27:162–167.

17. Deutz, N. E. P., J. M. Bauer, R. Barazzoni, G. Biolo, Y. Boirie, A. Bosy-Westphal,…, and P. C. Calder. 2014. Protein intake and exercise for optimal muscle function with aging: recommendations from the ESPEN Expert Group. *Clin. Nutr.* 33:929–936.

18. Institute of Medicine, Food and Nutrition Board. 2002. *Dietary Reference Intakes for Energy, Carbohydrates, Fiber, Fat, Protein and Amino Acids (Macronutrients)*. Washington, DC: National Academy of Sciences.

19. Paddon-Jones, D., W. W. Campbell, P. F. Jacques, S. B. Kritchevsky, L. L. Moore, N. R. Rodriguex, and L. J. C. van Loon. 2015. Protein and healthy aging. *Am. J. Clin. Nutr.* 101(Suppl):1339S–1345S.

20. Marinia, J. C. 2015. Protein requirements: are we ready for new recommendations? *J. Nutr.* 145:5–6.

21. Rafii, M., K. Chapman, J. Owens, R. Elango, W. W. Campbell, R. O. Ball, P. B. Pencharz, and G. Courtney-Martin. 2015. Dietary protein requirement of female adults >65 years determined by the indicator amino acid oxidation technique is higher than current recommendations. *J. Nutr.* 145:18–24.

22. Layman, D. K., T. G. Anthony, B. B. Rasmussen, S. H. Adams, C. J. Lynch, G. D. Brinkworth, and T. A. Davis. 2015. Defining meal requirements for protein to optimize metabolic roles of amino acids. *Am. J. Clin. Nutr.* 101(Suppl):1330S–1338S.

23. Deer, R. R., and E. Volpi. 2015. Protein intake and muscle function in older adults. *Curr. Opin. Clin. Nutr. Metab. Care.* 18:248–253.

24. Hoffmann, M. R., P. A. Senior, and D. R. Mager. 2015. Vitamin D supplementation and health-related quality of life: a systematic review of the literature. *J. Acad. Nutr. Diet* 115:406–418.

25. Bruyére, O., J. Slomian, C. Beaudart, F. Buckinx, E. Cavalier, S. Gillain, J. Petermans, and J. V. Reginster. 2014. Prevalence of vitamin D inadequacy in European women aged over 80 years. *Arch. Gerontol. Geriatr.* 59:78–82.

26. Institute of Medicine. 2011. *Dietary Reference Intakes for Calcium and Vitamin D*. Washington, DC: National Academy Press.

27. Institute of Medicine, Food and Nutrition Board. 2001. *Dietary Reference Intakes for Vitamin A, Vitamin K, Arsenic, Boron, Chromium, Copper, Iodine, Iron, Manganese, Molybdenum, Nickel, Silicon, Vanadium, and Zinc*. Washington, DC: National Academy Press.

28. Institute of Medicine, Food and Nutrition Board. 2000. *Dietary Reference Intakes for Vitamin C, Vitamin E, Selenium, and Carotenoids*. Washington, DC: National Academy Press.

29. Michaëlsson, K., A. l. Wolk, L. Byberg, J. Ärnlöv, and H. Melhus. 2014. Intake and serum concentrations of ⊠-tocopherol in relation to fractures in elderly women and men: 2 cohort studies. *Am. J. Clin. Nutr.* 99:107–114.

30. Christen, W. G., R. J. Glynn, J. M. Gaziano, A. K. Darke, J. E. Crowley, P. J. Goodman,…, and E. A. Klein. 2015. Age-related cataract in men in the selenium and vitamin E cancer prevention trial eye endpoints study. *JAMA Opthalmol.* 133:17–24.

31. Institute of Medicine, Food, and Nutrition Board. 1998. *Dietary Reference Intakes for Thiamin, Riboflavin, Niacin, Vitamin B6, Folate, Vitamin B12, Pantothenic Acid, Biotin, and Choline*. Washington, DC: National Academy Press.

32. Lachner, C., C. Martin, D. John, S. Nekkalapu, A. Sasan, N. Steinle, and W. T. Regenold. 2014. Older adult psychiatric in patients with non-cognitive disorders should be screened for vitamin B12 deficiency. *J. Nutr. Health Aging* 18:209–212.

33. The Age-Related Eye Disease Study 2 (AREDS2) Research Group. 2014. Secondary analysis of the effects of lutein/zeaxanthin on age-related macular degeneration progression—AREDS2 Report No. 3. *JAMA Ophthalmol.* 132:142–149.

34. Fairweather-Tait, S. J., A. A. Wawer, R. Gillings, A. Jennings, and P. K. Myint. 2014. Iron status in the elderly. *Mech. Ageing Dev.* 136–137:22–28.

35. Institute of Medicine, Food and Nutrition Board. 2004. *Dietary Reference Intakes for Water, Potassium, Sodium, Chloride, and Sulfate*. Washington, DC: National Academy Press.

36. Waters, D. L., A. L. Ward, and D. T. Villareal. 2013. Weight loss in obese adults 65 years and older: a review of the controversy. *Exp. Gerontol.* 48:1054–1061.

37. Gebhart, A., M. T. Young, and N. T. Nguyen. 2015. Bariatric surgery in the elderly: 2009-2013. *Surg. Obes. Relat. Dis.* 11:393–398.

38. Loy, J. J., H. A. Youn, B. Schwack, M. S. Kuriamn, G. A. Fielding, and C. J. Ren-Fielding. 2014. Safety and efficacy of laparoscopic adjustable gastric banding in patients aged seventy and older. *Surg. Obes. Relat. Dis.* 10:284–289.

39. Batsis, J. A., and K. M. Dolkart. 2015. Evaluation of older adults with obesity for bariatric surgery: geriatricians' perspective. *J. Clin. Gerontol. Geriatr.* 6:45–53.

40. National Osteoporosis Foundation. 2014. *54 Million Americans Affected by Osteoporosis and Low Bone Mass.* Available at http://nof.org/news/2948. Accessed June 2015.

41. American Academy of Orthopaedic Surgeons/American Association of Orthopaedic Surgeons. 2014. AAOS Position Statement: Osteoporosis/Bone Health in Adults as a National Public Health Policy. Available at www.aaos.org/about/papers/position/1113.asp. Accessed June 2014.

42. Cosman, F., S. J. de Beur, M. S. LeBoff, E. M. Lewiecki, B. Tanner, S. Randall, and R. Lindsay. 2014. Clinician's guide to prevention and treatment of osteoporosis. *Osteoporos. Int.* 25:2359–2381.

43. Centers for Disease Control and Prevention. 2014. Arthritis-Related Statistics. Available at: http://www.cdc.gov/arthritis_related_stats.htm/. Accessed June 2015.

44. Academy of Nutrition and Dietetics. 2013. Oral health and nutrition. *J. Acad. Nutr. Diet.* 113:693–701.

45. National Eye Institute. 2015. Facts about age-related macular degeneration. Available at https://nei.nih.gov/health/maculardegen/armd_facts. Accessed June 2015.

46. Hobbs, R. P, and P. S. Bernstein. 2014. Nutrient supplementation for age-related macular degeneration, cataract, and dry eye. *J. Ophthalmic. Vis. Res.* 9:487–493.

47. Wei, L., C. Cai, and J. Lv. 2015. Association of vitamin C with the risk of age-related cataract: a meta-analysis. *Acta. Ophthalmol.* doi: 10.1111/aos.12688. Available at http://onlinelibrary.wiley.com/enhanced/doi/10.1111/aos.12688/ (Accessed July 2015)

48. Zhang, Y., W. Xie, W. Wu, and D. Zhang. 2015. Vitamin E and risk of age-related cataract: a meta-analysis. *Publ. Health Nutr.* doi: 10.1017/S1368980014003115.

49. Glaser, T.S., L.E. Doss, G. Shih, D. Nigam, R.D. Sperduto, F.L. Ferris 3rd,..., and Age-Related Eye Disease Study Research Group. 2015. The association of dietary lutein plus zeaxanthin and B vitamins with cataracts in the Age-Related Eye Disease Study. *Ophthalmol.* 122:1471-1479.

50. Alzheimer's Association. 2014. 2014 Alzheimer's disease facts and figures. *Alzheim. Dement.* 10:1–75.

51. Barnard, N. D., A. I. Bush, A. Ceccarelli, J. Cooper, C. A. de Jager, K. I. Ericksonj,..., R. Squitti. 2014. Dietary and lifestyle guidelines for the prevention of Alzheimer's disease. *Neurobiol. Aging* 35:S74–S78.

52. Erickson, K. I., R. L. Leckie, and A. M. Weinstein. 2014. Physical activity, fitness, and gray matter volume. *Neurobiol. Aging* 35:S20–S28.

53. Beckett, M. W., C. I. Ardern, and M. A. Rotondi. 2015. A meta-analysis of prospective studies on the role of physical activity and the prevention of Alzheimer's disease in older adults. *BMC Geriatr.* 15:9–15.

54. Vélez-Díaz-Pallarés, M., I. Lozano-Montoya, I. Abraha, A. Cherubini, R. L. Soiza, D. O'Mahony,..., and A. J. Cruz-Jentoft. 2015. Nonpharmacologic interventions to heal pressure ulcers in older patients: an overview of systematic reviews (The SENATOR-ONTOP Series). *JAMDA* 16:448–469.

55. Posthauer, M. E., M. Banks, B. Dorner, and J. M. G. A. Schols. 2015. The role of nutrition for pressure ulcer management: National Pressure Ulcer Advisory Panel, European Pressure Ulcer Advisory Panel, and Pan Pacific Pressure Injury Alliance White Paper. *Adv. Skin Wound Care* 28:175–188.

56. National Institute on Drug Abuse. 2014. Prescription drug abuse: older adults. Available at www.drugabuse.gov/publications/research-repots/prescription-drugs/trends-in-prescription-drug-abuse/older-adults. Accessed June 2015.

57. Health Research Funding. 2014. 12 Incredible polypharmacy statistics. Available at www.healthresearchfunding.org/polypharmacy-statistics/. Accessed June 2015.

58. Boullata, J. I., and L. M. Hudson. 2012. Drug-nutrient interactions: a broad view with implications for practice. *J. Acad. Nutr. Diet.* 112: 506–517.

59. FamilyDoctor. 2014. Drug-nutrient interactions and drug-supplement interactions: what you need to know. Available at www.familydoctor.org/familydoctor/en/drugs-procedures-devices/over-the-counter/drug-nutrient-drug-supplement-interactions.html. Accessed June 2015.

60. Manrique, Y. J., D. J. Lee, F. Islam, L. M. Nissen, J. A. Y. Cichero, J. R. Stokes, and K. J. Steadman. 2014. Crushed tablets: does the administration of food vehicles and thickened fluids to aid medication swallowing alter drug release? *J. Pharm. Pharm. Sci.* 17:207–219.

61. National Council on Aging. (undated) FAQs on elder abuse. Available at www.ncoa.org/public-policy-action/elder-justice/faqs-on-elder-abuse.html. Accessed June 2015.

62. U.S. Department of Agriculture Economic Research Service. (January, 2015). Food security in the United States: 2013. http://www.ers.usda.gov/topics/food-nutrition-assistance/food-security-in-the-us/key-statistics-graphics.aspx. Accessed June 2015.

63. Goldberg, S.L. and B.E. Mawn. 2014. Predictors of food insecurity among older adults in the United States. *Publ. Health Nurs.* doi:10.1111/phn.12173. Available at http://onlinelibrary.wiley.com/enhanced/doi/10.1111/phn.12173/ (Accessed July 2015)

64. Berkowitz, S. A., H. K. Seligman, and N. K. Choudhry. 2014. Treat or eat: food insecurity, cost-related medication underuse, and unmet needs. *Am. J. Med.* 127:303–310.

65. Hanson, K. L., and L. M. Connor. 2014. Food insecurity and dietary quality in U.S. adults and children: a systematic review. *Am. J. Clin. Nutr.* 100:684–692.

66. U.S. Department of Agriculture, Food and Nutrition Service, Office of Policy Support. *Characteristics of Supplemental Nutrition Assistance Program Households: Fiscal Year 2013.* Alexandria, VA, 2014.

67. U.S. Department of Agriculture. Senior Farmers' Market Nutrition Program. Available from www.fns.usda.gov/sfmnp/overview. Accessed June 2015.

68. Feeding America. Hunger and poverty fact sheet. 2015. Available at www.feedingamerica.org. Accessed June 2015.

69. Centers for Disease Control and Prevention. 2014. QuickStats: life expectancy at birth by race/ethnicity—United States, 2011. *MMWR* 63:776.

70. Academy of Nutrition and Dietetics. 2015. Ethical decisions for withholding/withdrawing medically assisted nutrition and hydration. *J. Acad. Nutr. Diet.* 115:440–443.

Answers to Review Questions

Chapter 1

1. **c.** identifying and preventing nutrient-deficiency diseases. Contemporary nutrition research focuses on associations between diet and chronic disease. Although nutrition science contributes to improving the nutritional quality of food crops, agricultural science and technology works to improve yields. Botany is the science most concerned with identifying and classifying plants.

2. **a.** Scurvy is caused by a nutrient deficiency. More specifically, scurvy is the name given to the set of signs and symptoms that develop in a person whose diet is deficient in vitamin C. Although nutrition may influence the risk for osteoporosis, heart disease, and some forms of diabetes, it does not directly cause these complex disorders.

3. **d.** micronutrients. Of the nutrients listed, only vitamin C and thiamin are water-soluble vitamins, and only vitamin A is a fat-soluble vitamin. Calcium and magnesium are minerals. The nutrients listed are not energy nutrients as they do not provide kilocalories.

4. **b.** the RDA for vitamin C. The EAR is the average daily nutrient intake level estimated to meet the requirement of half of the healthy individuals in a group; thus, the recommended intake (the RDA) is always higher. The UL is the highest daily intake level likely to pose no risk of adverse health effects; however, there is no benefit to meeting the UL for any nutrient, and considerable risk in exceeding it. The AMDR identifies a range of intake for the energy nutrients only; therefore, there is no AMDR for vitamin C.

5. **a.** Measurement of height. Height is an anthropometric measurement which provides objective data; that is, the data can be verified by repeating the measurement. Assessment of a client's history of illness, injuries, and surgeries, of current symptoms such as fatigue, and of dietary intake, all elicit subjective information; that is, information that cannot be verified.

6. **d.** overt signs and symptoms. Jane is experiencing weight loss and exhaustion, which are overt signs and symptoms of malnutrition. Overnutrition is characterized by excessive weight gain, not loss. A primary deficiency results from a failure to consume adequate amounts of a nutrient, but Jane's condition has resulted from a severe digestive disorder, not a poor diet. A subclinical deficiency demonstrates no obvious signs and symptoms, but Jane is experiencing both weight loss and exhaustion.

7. **b.** "A high-protein diet increases the risk for porous bones" is an example of a valid hypothesis. It is a possible explanation for an observation, and can be tested by conducting a research study. In contrast, the statement "One hundred inactive residents of the Sunshine Care Home have high blood pressure, and 32 inactive residents have normal blood pressure" is an example of an observation. Although data from a single experiment and even multiple experiments may support a hypothesis, that hypothesis is not confirmed as fact; however, it may be proposed as a theory.

8. **c.** randomized clinical trial. This is an example of a randomized clinical trial, in which volunteers were randomly assigned by surname to an intervention group (who got the treatment) or a control group (who got a placebo). The study is not, however, a double-blind study because the researchers—who knew the participants' names—knew which group each participant belonged to. Thus, when speaking to them over the phone, they could have subtly influenced the participants' responses. It is not an observational study, because observational studies look at phenomena already present within large populations to determine the factors that may be associated with these phenomena. A case-control study is a type of observational study that compares a large group of individuals with a certain condition to a similar group without this condition.

9, **b.** a conflict of interest. The study described in question 8 exhibits a conflict of interest because the researchers were being paid by the company whose product they were evaluating. This could bias them toward findings supporting the product's effectiveness. A peer review is a critique of a research article by other specialists working in the same scientific field. Transparency is a principle by which researchers fully disclose their funding sources and other potential sources of bias. Quackery is the promotion of an unproven remedy.

10. **c.** the website of the National Institutes of Health. The websites of other agencies of the U.S. Department of Health and Human Services are also sources of accurate nutrition information. Because the term *nutritionist* has no definition or laws governing it, the nutritionist on the staff of your local supermarket may be a registered dietitian and thus trustworthy, or a person with no training whatsoever in nutrition and health. Without verifying his or her credentials, you would be unwise to assume that this person was a source of reliable and accurate nutrition information. Although the personal trainer at your campus fitness center may be passionate about health and nutrition, there's no guarantee that the information he or she provides is reliable or accurate. Although it might seem that everything printed in a reputable national newspaper like the *New York Times* must be true, this is a dangerous assumption. A paid advertisement in the *New York Times* is no more trustworthy than one in a tabloid publication.

11. **False.** Fat provides 9 kcal per gram, and is required for the fat-soluble vitamins to be transported in the body, but neither fat-soluble nor water-soluble vitamins provide energy.

12. **False.** The Tolerable Upper Intake Level (UL) meets this definition. In contrast, the RDA is the average daily intake level estimated to meet the needs of almost all healthy people in a given population group.

13. **True.** Unlike a blood test result or a measurement of body weight, a food-frequency questionnaire elicits subjective data; that is, data that cannot be independently verified.

14. **False.** An epidemiological study is a study that examines patterns, causes and effects of health and disease conditions in defined populations.

15. **True.** This journal is published by the *Academy of Nutrition and Dietetics*, the largest organization of food and nutrition professionals in the world.

16. The Estimated Average Requirement, or EAR, represents the average daily nutrient intake level estimated to meet the requirement of half of the healthy individuals in a particular life stage or gender group. The Recommended Dietary Allowance, or RDA, represents the average daily nutrient intake level that meets the nutrient requirements of 97% to 98% of healthy individuals in a particular life stage or gender group. The EAR is used to estimate the RDA.

17. In a well-designed experiment, a control group allows a researcher to compare between treated and untreated individuals, and thereby to determine whether or not a particular treatment has exerted a significant effect.

18. I would explain to Marilyn that the term *nutritionist* does not guarantee that the person who suggested the supplements is qualified to give nutritional guidance. I would recommend that she would be better off talking with a qualified healthcare professional about her fatigue. To find reliable nutrition information, I would suggest she talk with a registered dietitian. She can find registered dietitians in her local area by contacting the American Dietetic Association. She can also access free, reliable information from the websites of organizations such as the American Dietetic Association, the National Institutes of Health, and the Centers for Disease Control and Prevention.

19. Seven ounces.

20. 24.5% of Kayla's diet comes from fat; this percentage is within the AMDR for fat.

Chapter 2

1. **b.** provides enough of the energy, nutrients, and fiber needed to maintain a person's health. Meeting energy needs is important, of course, but sufficient energy alone doesn't make a diet adequate. A variety of foods and balance in combinations of nutrients are also important characteristics of a healthful diet, but these responses don't define an adequate diet.

2. **d.** the % Daily Values of selected nutrients in a serving of the packaged food. It does not identify all of the nutrients and Calories in the package of food, nor does it identify the RDA for every nutrient found in the food. The footnote, if present, is always the same statement of general information. It does not identify the UL for nutrients found in the food.

3. **a.** is an example of an FDA-approved nutrient claim. Label claims for packaged foods such as crackers are regulated by the FDA, not the USDA, and *reduced fat* is a nutrient claim, not a health claim. *Reduced fat* and *low fat* do not have the same meaning: *reduced fat* means at least 25% less fat than the standard version of the food, whereas *low fat* means 3 g of fat per serving or less. A food with less than 0.5 g of fat per serving would qualify as fat free.

4. **b.** Foods with a lot of nutrients per Calorie, such as fish, are more nutritious choices than foods with fewer nutrients per Calorie, such as candy, which should be limited. The actual density of a food is not a reliable indicator of its nutritional profile, nor is its color. Fat in foods doesn't necessarily make foods less nutrient-dense; for example, some fatty fish, such as salmon, are excellent, nutrient-dense choices because they provide abundant nutrients for their number of Calories.

5. **c.** increasing your intake of fruits and vegetables. They encourage limiting your sodium intake, but not choosing and preparing entirely sodium-free foods. They do not recommend any precise level of alcohol consumption; instead, those who drink are encouraged to do so in moderation, which is defined as no more than one drink per day for women and two for men. The DGAs do not recommend following the Mediterranean diet or any other specific diet plan.

6. **a.** make half your grains whole; that is, make at least half of your grain choices whole grain foods. You should also go lean with protein, and vary your veggies. Although you should focus on fruit, you should go easy on the fruit juices.

7. **d.** does not make specific recommendations for protein food choices. The Mediterranean diet recommends red meat only monthly, fish weekly, and legumes and nuts as daily sources of protein.

8. **c.** Calories from solid fats and added sugars that provide few or no nutrients. The USDA recommends you limit your empty Calorie intake to a small number per day, but this small allowance is not in itself the definition of empty Calories. Water is Calorie-free. Empty Calories are not defined as Calories in a portion of food larger than the serving size indicated on the packaging.

9. **c.** MyPlate Supertracker. The NuVal System is an in-store nutritional guidance product-rating system. The exchange system is a diet planning tool that organizes exchanges, or portions, according to the amount of carbohydrate,

fat, protein, and Calories in the food. MyDietAnalysis is available to students using this text, but not to the general public.

10. **d.** One way to reduce the Calorie content of a restaurant meal is to order an appetizer instead of an entrée. Although eating healthfully while eating out can be challenging, it's not impossible. Calorie-labelling on restaurant menus has not been shown to increase the likelihood that patrons will make more healthful, lower-Calorie menu choices. When ordering meat, grilled or broiled meats are more healthful choices than breaded or fried meats.

11. **True.**

12. **False.** Nutrient and health claims require FDA approval, but not structure-function claims.

13. **True.**

14. **False.** No standardized definition for a serving size exists.

15. **False.** Plain tomato sauce is rich in vitamins, minerals, and fiber, and is likely to be very low in fat. It's a healthful choice. Cheese sauces are typically very high in fat and Calories.

16. As humans, we are all different in terms of body size, physical activity level, religious and ethnic beliefs, and disease risk factors. No single diet can meet the needs of every human being, as our needs are very different. It is necessary to vary a diet based on individual needs.

17. Answers will vary. Be sure labels contain all five of the primary components of information identified in Figure 2.1.

18. At least 5 grams per serving.

19. It is not accurate. The Mediterranean diet is actually relatively high in fat, not low in fat. However, this diet recommends consuming foods that contain more healthful mono- and polyunsaturated fats. Bread and pasta are a daily part of the Mediterranean diet, but this diet does not recommend unlimited consumption of these foods. If Sylvia eats more energy than she expends, even while consuming the Mediterranean diet, she will not be able to lose weight.

20. The USDA Food Patterns suggest a range in the number of daily servings of each food group because our energy needs are dependent upon our physical activity level and body size, and therefore are different for everyone. The lower end of the range applies to inactive women and small individuals, while the higher end of the range applies to more active people and larger men. In fact, highly active people may need to eat even more servings than those recommended at the higher end of the range. People should not eat fewer than the lowest recommended number of servings, because this could lead to nutritional deficiencies.

21. Total Calories = 646; Total fat content = 33 g; Percentage of Calories from fat = 46%; item contributing the highest amount of fat to the lunch = ranch salad dressing. Hannah can skip the salad dressing or ask for a low-fat dressing, if available, to make a healthier change to this lunch.

Chapter 3

1. **c.** hypothalamus. It is a region above the pituitary gland in the forebrain. The satiety center is a cluster of cells in the hypothalamus that, when stimulated, cause us to feel satiated (full). *Hypo*-means below, and the hypothalamus is below the thalamus.

2. **b.** the duodenum, then the jejunum, and then the ileum. These are the three regions of the small intestine in order from the pyloric sphincter to the ileocecal valve. The esophagus does not encounter chyme. Food is churned into chyme by the stomach. The liver, gallbladder, and pancreas are not part of the GI tract. The jejunum empties into the ileum, not the transverse colon. From the ileum, chyme leaving the small intestine at the ileocecal valve first enters the ascending colon, then moves through the transverse colon, the sigmoid colon, and the rectum before leaving the body at the anus.

3. **a.** begins to denature proteins. Protein digestion is not possible without the contribution of digestive enzymes from the stomach, pancreas, and small intestine. Carbohydrate digestion begins in the mouth, with the action of salivary amylase. Hydrochloric acid is more acidic than vinegar or lemon juice, but it is not more acidic than battery acid.

4. **d.** Upon release into the GI tract, digestive enzymes typically facilitate hydrolysis reactions. Hormones, not enzymes, are chemical messenger molecules. Hormones are typically produced by endocrine glands, and released into the bloodstream in which they travel to their target cells. Most hormones act only on their target cells, and most enzymes are specific to the substance they act upon.

5. **d.** emulsifies lipids. Bile is produced by the liver and stored in the gallbladder. Intrinsic factor, not bile, is necessary for the absorption of vitamin B_{12}.

6. **c.** has fingerlike projections called villi that contain capillaries and a lacteal that pick up absorbed nutrients. Rugae are a feature of the stomach, not the small intestine. Lymphatic vessels are studded with lymph nodes, which filter lymph during its transport to the cardiovascular system. Enterocytes end in hairlike projections called microvilli; that is, enterocytes do not line microvilli.

7. **b.** facilitated diffusion. Passive diffusion requires neither a carrier protein nor energy. Active transport requires both a transport protein and energy derived from ATP. Endocytosis is a form of active transport.

8. **b.** peristalsis. Segmentation is active in the small intestine, and haustration and mass movements occur in the large intestine.

9. **a.** by pooling of gastric juice in the lower esophagus. Gastroesophageal reflux is not mediated by the immune system. Ulcerative colitis causes ulceration of the lining of the colon. Irritable bowel syndrome, not GERD, is linked to stress.

10. **d.** can be detected with a screening test before it produces signs or symptoms. Colorectal cancer is diagnosed in more than 136,000 Americans annually, which is more than one-third of all gastrointestinal system cancers annually. Colorectal cancer is not the most common cancer in both men and women. The most common cancer in men is prostate cancer. The most common cancer in women is breast cancer. The second most common cancer in both men and women is lung cancer. Although precancerous polyps can be successfully removed during a colonoscopy, true colorectal cancer requires surgery.

11. **True.**
12. **False.** Vitamins and minerals require no digestion.
13. **True.**
14. **False.** The central nervous system includes the brain and spinal cord. The enteric nerves of the GI tract are part of the peripheral nervous system.
15. **True.**
16. Our bodies are composed of cells, which are the smallest units of matter that exhibit the properties of living things. That is, cells can grow, reproduce themselves, and perform certain basic functions, such as taking in nutrients, transmitting impulses, producing chemicals, and excreting wastes. The human body is composed of billions of cells that are constantly replacing themselves, destroying worn or damaged cells, and manufacturing new ones. To support this constant demand for new cells, we need a ready supply of nutrient molecules, such as simple sugars, amino acids, and fatty acids, to serve as building blocks. These building blocks are the molecules that come from the breakdown of foods. All cells, whether of the skin, bones, or brain, are made of the same basic molecules of amino acids, sugars, and fatty acids, which are also the main components of the foods we eat. Thus, we are what we eat in that the building blocks of our cells are comprised of the molecules contained in the foods we eat.

17. The stomach does not digest itself because it secretes mucus that protects the lining from being digested by the hydrochloric acid it secretes.

18. No. The main function of the small intestine is to absorb nutrients and transport them into the bloodstream or the lymphatic system. In order to do this effectively, the surface area of the small intestine needs to be as large as possible. The inside of the lining of the small intestine, referred to as the mucosal membrane, is heavily folded. This feature increases the surface area of the small intestine and allows it to absorb more nutrients than if it were smooth. The villi are in constant movement, which helps them encounter and trap nutrient molecules. Covering the villi are specialized cells covered with hairlike structures called microvilli (also called the brush border). These intricate folds increase the surface area of the small intestine by more than 500 times, which tremendously increases the absorptive capacity of the small intestine.

19.

Digestive Disorder	Area of Inflammation	Symptoms	Treatment Options
Celiac disease	Small intestine	▪ Fatty stools ▪ Diarrhea or constipation ▪ Cramping ▪ Anemia ▪ Pallor ▪ Weight loss ▪ Fatigue ▪ Irritability	Modified diet that excludes foods that contain gluten or gliadin (for example, wheat, rye, and barley)
Crohn's disease	Usually ileum of small intestine but can affect any area of gastrointestinal tract	▪ Diarrhea ▪ Abdominal pain ▪ Rectal bleeding ▪ Weight loss ▪ Fever ▪ Anemia ▪ Delayed physical and mental development in children	Combination of prescription drugs, nutritional supplements, and surgery
Ulcerative	Mucosa of large intestine (or colon)	▪ Diarrhea (which may be bloody) ▪ Abdominal pain ▪ Weight loss ▪ Anemia ▪ Fever ▪ Severe urgency to have bowel movement	▪ Anti-inflammatory medications ▪ Surgery if medications are not effective

20. Your roommate could be suffering from heartburn or gastroesophageal reflux disease (GERD). Eating food causes the stomach to secrete hydrochloric acid to start the digestive process. In many people, the amount of HCl secreted is occasionally excessive or the gastroesophageal sphincter opens too soon. In either case, the result is that HCl seeps back up into the esophagus. Although the stomach is protected from HCl by a thick coat of mucus, the esophagus does not have this mucus coating. Thus, the HCl burns it. When this happens, a person experiences a painful sensation in the region of his or her chest above the sternum (breastbone). This condition is commonly called heartburn.

If your roommate experiences this painful type of heartburn more than twice per week, he may be suffering from GERD. Similar to heartburn, GERD occurs when HCl flows back into the esophagus. Although people who experience occasional heartburn usually have no structural abnormalities, many people with GERD have an overly relaxed or damaged esophageal sphincter or a damaged esophagus itself. Symptoms of GERD include persistent heartburn and acid regurgitation. Some people have GERD without heartburn and instead experience chest pain, trouble swallowing, burning in the mouth, the feeling that food is stuck in the throat, or hoarseness in the morning.

21. The difference between pH 9 and pH 2 is 7. The alkalinity of baking soda as compared to gastric juice can be expressed as: 7 = log10 (10,000,000). Baking soda is 10 million times more alkaline than gastric juice.

Chapter 4

1. **a.** monosaccharides. Disaccharides such as sucrose are formed by the bonding of two monosaccharides. Oligosaccharides are made up of 3 to 10 monosaccharides and polysaccharides contain more than 10.

2. **d.** all of the above. Because of its beta bond, lactose requires sufficient levels of the lactase enzyme for digestion. Their beta bonds make resistant starches and cellulose indigestible.

3. **c.** are generally found in whole grains, as well as many vegetables and some fruits. Unlike soluble fibers, they are not viscous and cannot be fermented by colonic bacteria. Types of insoluble fiber include lignins, cellulose, and hemicelluloses, whereas pectins, fructans, gums, and mucilages are soluble.

4. **b.** the potential of foods to raise blood glucose and insulin levels. Although pancreatic amylase promotes the digestion of carbohydrates, the glycemic index does not rate the potential of foods to prompt the secretion of pancreatic amylase. Although insulin, cortisol, and certain other hormones do assist the body with maintaining blood glucose, the glycemic index does not rate their ratios in the blood following a carbohydrate-rich meal. Although diet is thought to play a role in risk for type 2 diabetes, the glycemic index does not rate the potential of a given diet for increasing diabetes risk.

5. **d.** can be metabolized for energy very quickly either with or without oxygen. Fat, not glucose, is the predominant energy source used by our bodies at rest. Between meals, our bodies draw on liver glycogen reserves—not muscle glycogen—to maintain blood glucose levels. When carbohydrate intake is low, the body begins to break down stored fat, not ketones. In fact, ketones are the alternative fuel produced by this process.

6. **b.** The AMDR for carbohydrates is 45% to 65% of total energy intake. The current RDA for carbohydrate—not the AI for fiber—for adults 19 years of age and older is 130 g per day. The RDA for carbohydrates does not cover the amount of carbohydrate needed to support daily activities; it covers only the amount of carbohydrate needed to supply adequate glucose to the brain. Make half your grains whole is a message from the USDA Food Patterns. It is not a DRI.

7. **b.** a high-sugar diet and obesity. Although many people believe that sugar causes children to become hyperactive, research studies have not yielded evidence supporting such a hypothesis. Actually, consumption of high-fructose corn syrup negatively affects our metabolism and storage of body fat; this can cause body cells to become more resistant—not more sensitive—to the normal actions of insulin. Although a diet high in added sugars is associated with unhealthful changes in blood lipids and an increased risk for heart disease, the Institute of Medicine has not set an upper tolerable intake limit for sugar.

8. **a.** legumes and other vegetables, fruits, whole grains, and nuts and seeds. Like most vegetables, potatoes are a good source of fiber if you eat the skin; however, fruit juices, unless they are unstrained, and grains, unless they are whole grains, are not high in fiber. Although dairy foods (including fermented dairy foods), meat, fish, poultry, tofu, and eggs provide protein and other nutrients, they are not good sources of fiber. Brown rice, whole grain pasta, and chunky peanut butter are good sources of fiber, but not white rice and pasta or smooth peanut butter.

9. **a.** phenylketonuria. People who have phenylketonuria cannot metabolize phenylalanine, one of the components of aspartame. Aspartame is considered safe to consume in moderation for other population groups, including people with diabetes, lactose intolerance, milk allergy, and other health concerns.

10. **c.** is characterized by autoimmune destruction of the beta cells of the pancreas. Type 1 diabetes typically arises in adolescence. Type 2 diabetes typically arises in middle and older adulthood, and is a progressive disorder in which body cells become less responsive to insulin. The risk for type 2 diabetes—not type 1—can be reduced by maintaining a healthful body weight, but obesity does not directly cause type 2 diabetes.

11. **True.**

12. **False.** Insulin is a pancreatic hormone that assists cells to take up glucose; however, inulin is a soluble fiber in the fructans group.

13. **False.** Although it is true that manufacturers are required to replace some of the vitamins and minerals lost from breads made with white flour, this process is enrichment, not fortification.

14. **False.** Sugar alcohols, such as mannitol, sorbitol, isomalt, and xylitol, are nutritive sweeteners.

15. **True.**

16.

Carbo-hydrate	Molecular Composition	Food Sources
Glucose	Six carbon atoms, twelve hydrogen atoms, six oxygen atoms	Fruits, vegetables, grains, dairy products; does not generally occur alone in foods but attaches to other sugars to form disaccharides and complex carbohydrates
Fructose	Six carbon atoms, twelve hydrogen atoms, six oxygen atoms	Fruits and some vegetables
Lactose	One glucose molecule and one galactose molecule	Milk and other dairy products
Sucrose	One glucose molecule and one fructose molecule	Honey, maple syrup, fruits, vegetables, table sugar, brown sugar, powdered sugar

17. Grain-based foods contain carbohydrates, and sometimes these foods are processed, meaning that many of the important nutrients we need for health are taken out of them. Fiber-rich carbohydrates contain not only more fiber, which is important for the health of our digestive tract, but also many vitamins and minerals that we need to be healthy. The foods you listed here are examples of foods in the "grains" group that are processed. Examples of healthier fiber-rich alternative choices include whole-wheat saltine crackers, whole-wheat or pumpernickel bagels, brown rice, and whole-wheat spaghetti.

18. Insulin is a hormone secreted by the beta cells of the pancreas in response to increased blood levels of glucose. When we eat a meal, our blood glucose level rises. But glucose in our blood cannot help the nerves, muscles, and other tissues function unless it can cross into them. Glucose molecules are too large to cross the cell membranes of our tissues independently. To get in, glucose needs assistance from insulin. Insulin is transported in the blood to the cells of tissues throughout the body, where it stimulates special molecules located in the cell membrane to transport glucose into the cell. Insulin can be thought of as a key that opens the gates of the cell membrane and carries the glucose into the cell interior, where it can be used for energy. Insulin also stimulates the liver and muscles to take up glucose.

19. a. Fiber adds bulk to the stools, which aids in efficient excretion of feces.
b. Fiber keeps stools moist and soft, helping prevent hemorrhoids and constipation.

c. Fiber gives the gut muscles something to push on, making it easier to eliminate stools. Diverticulosis can result in part from trying to eliminate small, hard stools.
d. Fiber may bind with cancer-causing agents and speed their elimination from the colon, which could in turn reduce the risk for colon cancer.

20. Diabetes more commonly runs in families, but just because no one in the family has diabetes does not mean that someone cannot get it. Being obese or overweight increases a person's risk for developing type 2 diabetes. Overweight and obesity trigger insulin insensitivity, or insulin resistance, which in turn causes the pancreas to produce greater amounts of insulin, so that glucose can enter the cells and be used for energy. Eventually, type 2 diabetes develops because (1) there is an increasing degree of insulin insensitivity; (2) the pancreas can no longer secrete enough insulin; or (3) the pancreas has entirely stopped producing insulin.

21. a) 3,500 kcal per day × 0.45 = 1,575 kcal per day to 3,500 kcal per day × 0.65 = 2,275 kcal per day. Thus Simon should consume between 1,575 and 2,275 kcal per day of carbohydrate, preferably from fiber-rich sources; and b) 1,575 kcal per day ÷ 4 kcal per gram of carbohydrate = 393.75 grams to 2,275 kcal per day ÷ 4 kcal per gram of carbohydrate = 568.75 grams. Thus Simon should consume between 394 and 569 grams of carbohydrate per day.

Chapter 5

1. a. triglycerides. *Trans* fatty acids are only found naturally in small amounts in meats and full-fat dairy products. The majority of *trans* fatty acids in our diet are found in some processed foods, but their use has declined dramatically in the past decade because of associated health concerns. Phospholipids and sterols are two types of lipids found in foods, but they are present in much smaller amounts than triglycerides.

2. b. monounsaturated. Saturated fatty acids have no double carbon bonds, and polyunsaturated fatty acids have more than one double bond. Steroids are not fatty acids but sterols with an OH group attached.

3. d. increase the blood's level of the lipids associated with cardiovascular disease. *Trans* fatty acids have double carbon bonds, but the hydrogen atoms are attached on diagonally opposite sides of the double carbon bond, not on the same side, as in *cis* fatty acids. Cholesterol—not *trans* fatty acids—is synthesized in the liver and intestine.

4. d. found in leafy green vegetables, flaxseed oil, and fatty fish. Alpha-linolenic acid (ALA) is not a precursor to linoleic acid; instead, it is a distinct essential fatty acid that must be consumed in the diet. ALA is not a metabolic

derivative of EPA and DHA; rather, EPA and DHA are metabolic derivatives of ALA. ALA is not known as arachidonic acid. Linoleic acid is metabolized in the body to arachidonic acid.

5. **a.** lipoprotein lipase. Gastric lipase digests some triglycerides in the stomach. Bile and pancreatic lipase act in the small intestine to emulsify and break down dietary triglycerides into free fatty acids and monoglycerides.

6. **b.** are a major source of fuel for the body both during physical activity and at rest. Fats provide more than twice the energy, gram for gram, than carbohydrates. Fats enable the absorption of fat-soluble vitamins: neither water-soluble nor fat-soluble vitamins require digestion. Fats don't keep foods from turning rancid; rather, it is the oxidation of the fats in rancid foods that causes their unpleasant odor and taste.

7. **c.** 20% to 35% of total energy. Fat intakes lower than 20% of total energy do not confer additional health benefits and are not recommended for the general population.

8. **c.** vegetables, fish, and seeds. Although skim milk, fruits, oats, broth-based soups, red wine, and egg whites are healthful foods, they contain only small amounts of fat of any kind, or none at all. Lamb and whole milk contain saturated fat and a small amount of *trans* fat, and some brands of stick margarine also contain *trans* fats.

9. **d.** high-density lipoproteins. HDL-cholesterol is sometimes referred to as "good cholesterol." High blood levels of triglycerides, very-low-density lipoproteins, or low-density lipoproteins would increase the risk for cardiovascular disease.

10. **d.** engage in regular physical activity. Smokers have a two- to six-fold greater chance of developing cardiovascular disease than nonsmokers. There appears to be no direct link between dietary cholesterol and cardiovascular disease. Consumption of a moderate amount of alcohol is associated with a reduced risk for cardiovascular disease; however, moderate drinking is defined as no more than two alcoholic drinks per day for men and one drink per day for women, and the alcoholic beverage consumed does not have to be red wine.

11. **False.** Although lecithin is found in egg yolks, it is a phospholipid and is the primary emulsifier in bile.

12. **False.** *Trans* fatty acids are present in very small amounts in meats and full-fat dairy products.

13. **True.** During aerobic exercise, such as running or cycling, lipids can be mobilized from muscle tissue, adipose tissue, and blood lipoproteins.

14. **False.** Although reduced-fat versions of foods often do have fewer Calories than full-fat versions—as is the case, for example, with cow's milk—many reduced-fat foods have nearly the same number of Calories as full-fat versions.

15 **True.** Spacing smaller meals and snacks throughout the day decreases the load of fat entering the body at any one time.

16. Dietary fat enables the transport of the fat-soluble vitamins, specifically vitamins D and K. Vitamin D is important for regulating blood calcium and phosphorus concentrations and keeping them within the normal range, which indirectly helps maintain bone health. If vitamin D is low, blood calcium levels will drop below normal, and the body will draw calcium from the bones to maintain blood levels. Vitamin K is also important for proteins involved in maintaining bone health.

17. This is not particularly good advice for someone doing a 20-mile walk-a-thon. The energy sources used will depend partly on how fast you walk. If you are walking at a slow (2–3 miles/hour) to moderate (4 miles/hour) pace, fat will be the predominate energy source. Fat is a primary source of energy during rest and during less intense exercise. In addition, we use predominantly more fat as we perform longer-duration exercise. This is because we use more carbohydrate earlier during the exercise bout, and once our limited carbohydrate sources are depleted during prolonged exercise, we rely more on fat as an energy source. Although carbohydrates are an important source of energy during exercise, loading up on carbohydrates is typically only helpful for individuals who are doing longer-duration exercise at intensities higher than those experienced during walking at a slow to moderate pace. As the primary goal of this walk-a-thon is to raise money and not to finish in record time, you can walk at a pace that matches your current fitness level. Thus, it would be prudent to consume adequate carbohydrate prior to and during the walk-a-thon, but loading up on carbohydrates is not necessary. If you walked the event at a very fast pace (race-walking), carbohydrate loading could be beneficial.

18. Caleb's father probably had a blood test to determine his blood lipid levels, including total cholesterol, low-density lipoprotein cholesterol (LDL-C), high-density lipoprotein cholesterol (HDL-C), and triglycerides. Unfortunately, switching to cottage cheese and margarine may not improve his blood lipid values. Margarines can be high in *trans* fatty acids, which negatively impact blood lipids and increase our risk for heart disease. In addition, full-fat cottage cheese is a high-fat food, and it contains saturated fatty acids, which also negatively alter blood lipid levels. Both *trans* and saturated fatty acids will increase Caleb's father's risk for heart disease. Dietary changes that improve blood lipids include decreasing intake of saturated and *trans* fats, and switching to monounsaturated or polyunsaturated fatty acid products. A nondietary lifestyle choice that might improve his health is regular physical activity. Regular physical activity can help people maintain a more healthful body weight, can increase HDL-C, and can cause other changes that reduce our risk for heart disease.

19.

Type of Fat	Maximum Recommended Intake (% of total energy intake)	Maximum Recommended Calorie Intake
Saturated fat	7%	140 Calories/d
Linoleic acid	10%	200 Calories/d
Alpha-linolenic acid	1.2%	24 Calories/d
Trans fatty acids	0%	0 Calories/d
Unsaturated fat	None; amount equal to remainder of total fat Calories after you account for intake of saturated fat and linoleic and alpha-linolenic acids	336 Calories/d

Calculations used:
- Total energy needs = 2,000 Calories per day
- Maximum AMDR for fat = 35% of total energy intake = 0.35 × 2,000 = 700 Calories
- Saturated fat = 7% of total energy intake = 0.07 × 2,000 = 140 Calories
- Linoleic acid = 10% of total energy intake × 0.10 × 2,000 = 200 Calories
- Alpha-linolenic acid = 1.2% of total energy intake = 0.012 × 2,000 = 24 Calories
- *Trans* fatty acids = 0 Calories

20. **1.** The first rule for weight loss is that energy (kcal) matters. Thus, Hannah needs to consider total energy intake in addition to total fat intake. Weight loss programs often focus on reducing fat intake because fat has the highest number of kcal/g, but all calories count. Thus, Hannah needs to consider the number of calories in her nonfat yogurt and topping.
2. The total amount of energy (kcal) in her after-class treat adds up to 168 kcal.
3. There are a number of snacks Hannah can select that would be healthier and make her feel satisfied. Some examples, which are all low in saturated fat, include:
- Yogurt (6oz low fat) with 1/2 c berries (155 kcals, 9 g protein, 23 g carbohydrate, 2.5g fat)
- Apple (medium) and 1 T peanut butter (194 kcals, 4 g protein, 29 g carbohydrate, 8 g fat)
- Banana (medium) and milk (6oz skim) (163 kcals, 7 g protein, 35 g carbohydrate, < 1g fat)
- 1/2 Peanut butter (1T) sandwich on whole wheat bread (1 slice) (200 kcal, 8.5 g protein, 24 g carbohydrate, 9.5 g fat)

Chapter 6

1. **b.** amine group. The side chain varies for each amino acid. The acid group contains carbon, hydrogen, and oxygen. No portion of an amino acid is known as a nitrate cluster.

2. **c.** amino acids that the body is able to synthesize in sufficient quantities to meet its needs. The body needs these amino acids as much as it needs essential amino acids, which are those it is unable to synthesize and that must be consumed in the diet. Except in people with metabolic diseases such as PKU, the body is able to metabolize all 20 amino acids, including phenylalanine.

3. **d.** mutual supplementation. Vegetarians typically practice mutual supplementation, but vegetarianism is a consistent practice of restricting the diet mostly or entirely to food substances of plant origin. Deamination is the process by which an amine group is removed from an amino acid. Transamination is the process of transferring the amine group from one amino acid to another.

4. **c.** proteases. Hydrochloric acid and pepsin play roles in protein digestion in the stomach. Phosphofructokinase is an enzyme that influences the rate at which we break down glucose and use it for energy during exercise.

5. **b.** are taken from the blood and body tissues when needed for energy. Carbohydrates and fats are the body's two primary sources of energy. Nitrogen released from deamination bonds with hydrogen, creating ammonia, which the liver combines with carbon dioxide to make urea, which is then transported to the kidneys for excretion. Proteins contribute very little to an average adult's energy needs.

6. **a.** 1.3 to 1.5 grams per kilogram of body weight. Non-vegetarian endurance athletes need to consume slightly less protein, about 1.2 to 1.4 grams per kilogram of body weight. People who are more moderately active, especially if they are vegetarian, need slightly more than 0.8 grams of protein per kilogram of body weight, which is the amount recommended for sedentary adults.

7. **c.** Research suggests that higher intakes of animal and soy protein protect bone in older women. There is no consensus on the role of high-protein diets in increasing the risk for heart attacks, strokes, or bone fractures.

8. **d.** walnuts. Red meat and skim milk are good sources of protein, but are low in fiber and unsaturated fats. Skim milk by definition is fat-free. Green, leafy vegetables are nutrient-rich food choices; however, they are not a good source of protein.

9. **a.** rice, pinto beans, acorn squash, soy butter, and almond milk. Vegans avoid all animal products, including eggs and dairy; therefore, neither a yogurt milkshake nor egg salad would be appropriate items in a vegan meal. A meal consisting solely of brown rice and green tea would be vegan, but it would be neither balanced nor adequate.

10. **d.** all of the above are true. A change in a single amino acid in the hemoglobin protein changes the shape of the red blood cells from disc-like to sickle-shaped. Sickle-shaped cells are sticky and clump together, disrupting blood flow through smaller vessels.

11. **False.** Both shape and function are lost when a protein is denatured.
12. **True.**
13. **False.** Some hormones are made from lipids.
14. **True.**
15. **False.** Depending on the type of sport, athletes may require the same amount of or up to two times as much protein as nonactive people.
16. Use Figure 6.4 as a guide. Amino acids should be joined at the acid group of one amino acid and the amino group of the next amino acid. Multiple amino acids joined in this way make a protein.
17. mRNA, or messenger RNA, transcribes or copies genetic information from DNA in the nucleus and carries this information to the ribosomes in the cytoplasm. Once this genetic information reaches the ribosomes, it is translated into the language of amino acid sequences, or proteins. tRNA, or transfer RNA, binds with select amino acids dissolved in the cytoplasm and transfers these amino acids to the ribosome, so that they can be assembled into proteins. The specific amino acids that are transferred to the ribosome from tRNA are dictated by the amino acid sequence presented by mRNA.
18. In general, only people who are susceptible to kidney disease or who have kidney disease suffer serious consequences when eating a high-protein diet. Consuming a high-protein diet increases protein metabolism and urea production. Individuals with kidney disease or those who are at risk for kidney disease cannot adequately flush urea and other by-products of protein metabolism from the body through the kidneys. This inability can lead to serious health consequences and even death.
19. There are various classifications of vegetarianism. Many people feel that, if a person eats any meat or products from animals (such as dairy or eggs), he or she cannot be a vegetarian. People who eat only plant-based foods are classified as vegans. If you believe this, then you would argue that your Dad is not a true vegetarian. However, there are others who believe a vegetarian is someone who can eat dairy foods, eggs, or both in addition to plant-based foods. There are also people who classify themselves as pesco-vegetarians, meaning they eat fish along with plant-based foods. Semi-vegetarians may eat lean meats, such as poultry, on occasion in addition to plant-based foods, eggs, and dairy products. If you believe in these broader definitions of vegetarianism, you would agree with your Dad's opinion that he is now a vegetarian.
20. Adequate protein is needed to maintain the proper balance of fluids inside and outside the cells. When a child suffers from kwashiorkor, the protein content of the blood is inadequate to maintain this balance. Fluid seeps from inside the cells out to the tissue spaces and causes bloating and swelling of the abdomen.

21. **a.** The AMDR for protein is 10% to 35% of total daily energy intake. Barry's protein intake in g must be converted to kcal to answer this question. Remember that the energy content of protein is 4 kcal/g. Thus: 190 g of protein × 4 kcal/g = 760 kcal protein
To calculate the percentage of protein Barry is eating in his diet = (760 kcal ÷ 3000 kcal) × 100 = 25.3% of Barry's total energy intake comes from protein. This amount meets the AMDR for protein.
b. The RDA for protein is 0.8 g per kg body weight per day. Barry's weight is 182 lbs. You must first convert Barry's weight to kg = 182 lbs ÷ 2.2 lbs/kg = 82.7 kg. Barry's protein intake is 190 g. To calculate whether he meets the RDA for protein, divide his protein intake in g by his body weight = 190 g ÷ 82.7 kg = 2.3 g per kg body weight per day. This amount exceeds the RDA for protein, and is more than sufficient to support Barry even if he is an endurance or strength athlete.

Chapter 7

1. **d.** is composed of one molecule of adenosine bonded to one phosphate group. Adenosine monophosphate is produced when two phosphate groups are released from ATP. High-energy phosphate bonds occur between phosphate groups. Since AMP has only one phosphate group, it has no high-energy phosphate bonds. It is, in fact, a low-energy compound.
2. **a.** hydrolysis. Dehydration synthesis is anabolic, not catabolic, and releases a molecule of water. Oxidation is a chemical reaction during which electrons are lost. Phosphorylation reactions involve the addition of one or more phosphate groups to a chemical compound.
3. **a.** lactate. In an aerobic environment where oxygen is plentiful, pyruvate is converted to acetyl CoA. Oxaloacetate is a metabolic intermediate within the TCA cycle. Pyruvate is not converted to NADH; rather, NADH donates hydrogen to lactate, leaving NAD^+.
4. **c.** acetyl CoA is blocked from entering the TCA cycle. This is more likely to occur when people follow a very-low-carbohydrate diet, not a high-carbohydrate diet, because oxaloacetate, a carbohydrate derivative, reacts with acetyl CoA to produce citrate, the event that initiates the TCA cycle. Thus, oxaloacetate depletion, not build-up, prompts ketone production.
5. **b.** they contain nitrogen, which must be removed before the remaining compound can be used for energy. Glucogenic amino acids are converted to glucose in the process of gluconeogenesis. Amino acids contain nitrogen, not ammonia. Removal of an amino acid's amine group leaves a carbon skeleton and ammonia, which the liver, not the kidneys, converts to urea. When consumed to excess, amino acids prompt increased synthesis of fatty acids.

6. **d.** None of the above statements is true. Gastric ADH can reduce the absorption of alcohol by as much as 20%, not 30% to 35%. Most of the alcohol consumed by an individual is rapidly absorbed into the bloodstream and transported to the liver. It is not taken up by muscles. Finally, because Anya rarely drinks alcohol, it is highly unlikely that the MEOS system would be activated by her consumption of a glass of wine.

7. **b.** about 85% is from triglycerides, and most of the remaining 15% is from protein. Glycogen accounts for only a small percentage of energy reserves. Water provides no energy.

8. **c.** occurs in liver cells. Most lipogenesis occurs in liver cells, when individuals consume an excess of carbohydrate, alcohol, or ketogenic—not glucogenic—amino acids. In lipogenesis, acetyl CoA is converted into fatty acid chains, not into glycerol. The fatty acid chains are then attached to glycerol. Lipogenesis does not occur in adipose cells; however, triglycerides are stored in adipose cells.

9. **d.** catabolic hormones. Insulin is an anabolic hormone. Coenzymes are organic cofactors, which are not hormones at all, but substances that facilitate the action of enzymes.

10. **b.** liver glycogen for glucose for red blood cells, brain cells, and other body cells. Muscle glycogen is used as a fuel source for muscle cells. Only when fasting is prolonged does the body convert fatty acids—not glycerol—to ketone bodies, or break down body proteins for gluconeogenesis.

11. **True.**

12. **False.** Glycolysis requires two ATP and produces four ATP, thus yielding a net of two ATP that can be used as energy for the cell.

13. **True.**

14. **False.** The body stores only enough liver glycogen to provide glucose for red blood cells and other body needs for less than one day. Although muscle glycogen stores are larger, they fuel only muscle cells and would be depleted within 1 to 2 days.

15. **True.**

16. The final stage of glucose oxidation is called oxidative phosphorylation and occurs in the electron transport chain of the mitochondria. In this step, a series of enzyme-driven reactions occur in which electrons are passed down a "chain." As the electrons are passed from one carrier to the next, energy is released. In this process, NADH and FADH2 are oxidized and their electrons are donated to O2, which is reduced to H2O (water). The energy released when water is formed generates ATP.

17. Fatty acids released from the adipose tissue or fatty acids that come from the foods we eat are transported on albumin in the blood. They are then transported to the cells that need energy, such as the muscle cells. The fatty acids move across the cell membrane into the cytosol, where they are activated by the addition of CoA and then transported to the mitochondria, where fatty acid oxidation occurs. Once in the mitochondria, the fatty acid is systematically broken down into two-carbon units that lead to the formation of acetyl-CoA, which can enter the TCA cycle for energy production.

18. Without insulin, the body cannot utilize the glucose derived from food. Since glucose cannot enter the cells, the body begins the process of breaking down body fats to fatty acids, which can be used to produced ketones and alternative fuel for the brain when glucose is not available. These ketones are acidic and can build up in the blood, leading to ketoacidosis. Under these conditions more ketones are produced than can be utilized or eliminated from the body, so they build up in the blood.

19. When children with PKU go off their diets, they increase the levels of the amino acid phenylalanine in the body. They cannot metabolize phenylalanine correctly due to a genetic enzyme disorder that can result in the toxic buildup of phenylalanine in the body, which causes organ tissue damage.

20. We can assume that Aunt Winifred has been eating so little food that her need for carbohydrate (to maintain blood glucose) has not been met. Since the brain, red blood cells, and other types of cells, are all dependent on glucose for fuel, her body has no doubt been breaking down muscle protein in order to use some of the amino acids—known as glucogenic amino acids—to synthesize new glucose (gluconeogenesis). So not only has Aunt Winifred been losing body fat, but she has also been losing muscle mass, our main pool of body protein.

21. **(a)** To calculate Chris' weight in kg: 170 lb ÷ 2.2 lb/kg = 77.3 kg To estimate Chris' need for protein: 77.3 kg = 0.8 g protein/ kg = 61.8 g protein per day (round to 62 g).
    (b) To calculate how much protein is in 3 servings of the supplement: 1800 mg amino acids/serving × 3 servings/d = 5400 mg amino acids = 5.4 g protein from the supplement. To calculate what percent of Chris' daily need for protein is met by the supplement: [5.4 g protein from the supplement ÷ 62 g total protein need] × 100 (to convert to percentage) = 8.7% of Chris' total protein need is met by 3 servings of the supplement.

    If eggs cost $1.80/dozen, each egg costs 15 cents. You could buy ten eggs for $1.50, providing a total of 60 g protein (each egg provides about 6 g protein).

Chapter 8

1. **b.** act as coenzymes to promote energy metabolism. The B-vitamins do not themselves act as enzymes, but combine with enzymes to facilitate their action. They do not yield energy but help to convert macronutrients to energy. The mineral iodine is essential to the synthesis of thyroid hormones, which regulate metabolic rate.

2. **d.** thiamin, riboflavin, and niacin.

3. **c.** pellagra. Flushing is actually associated with niacin toxicity. Marasmus is a severe protein-deficiency disease. Thiamin-deficiency disease is called beriberi.

4. **a.** vitamin B_6. Both folate and vitamin B_{12} play many essential roles in the body, but these are not among them.

5. **c.** an increased risk for cardiovascular disease. High homocysteine is likely to occur with low blood levels of the amino acid methionine and with vitamin B_6, folate, and B_{12} deficiency. Folate deficiency increases the risk for neural tube defects.

6. **b.** folate is critical for cell division, which is rapid in the developing embryo. Folate toxicity, not deficiency, can mask a simultaneous vitamin B_{12} deficiency. Maternal iodine deficiency, not folate deficiency, increases the risk for cretinism. Vitamin B_{12}, not folate, helps maintain the myelin sheath coating nerve fibers.

7. **d.** Choline is a vitamin-like compound necessary for homocysteine metabolism and the synthesis of bile. It is found in a wide variety of foods, including plant foods such as certain legumes and other vegetables. It is not a neurotransmitter, although it accelerates the synthesis and release of acetylcholine, which is a neurotransmitter.

8. **b.** chromium. Iodine is a trace mineral necessary for the synthesis of thyroid hormones. Manganese plays roles in metabolism of carbohydrates, fats, and proteins, helps synthesize bone protein and cartilage, and is part of an antioxidant enzyme system. Sulfur is a major mineral.

9. **a.** iodine deficiency. Although chromium deficiency can damage the brain and nervous system, chromium is widely distributed in foods and deficiency is rare. Neither manganese nor sulfur deficiency is associated with neurological impairment.

10. **c.** have a reduced ability to perform most types of physical activity, including both intense and endurance activities. An increased risk of musculoskeletal injury with physical activity is more closely associated with a low-energy diet in general.

11. **True.**

12. **False.** Riboflavin occurs naturally in milk, and macrocytic anemia is associated with deficiency of folate or vitamin B_{12}, not riboflavin. Riboflavin-deficiency disease is ariboflavinosis.

13. **True.**

14. **False.** Iodine is necessary for the synthesis of thyroid hormones.

15. **True.**

16. Dialysis can remove water-soluble vitamins from the blood, which need to be replaced with either foods high in these nutrients or supplements.

17. Vitamin B6 is important in the transamination of essential amino acids to nonessential amino acids.

18. Mr. Katz's doctor probably did not give him the vitamin in pill form because Mr. Katz is 80 years of age, and it is more likely that he suffers from low stomach acid secretion. This is a condition known as atrophic gastritis, and it is estimated that about 10% to 30% of adults older than 50 years have this condition. Stomach acid separates food-bound vitamin B12 from dietary proteins. If the acid content of the stomach is inadequate, we cannot free up enough vitamin B12 from food sources alone. Because atrophic gastritis can affect almost one-third of the older adult population, it is recommended that people older than 50 years of age consume foods fortified with vitamin B12, take a vitamin B12–containing supplement, or have periodic B12 injections. Because Mr. Katz's condition was so severe, it was critical to treat him with a form of vitamin B12 that would be guaranteed to enter his system as quickly and effectively as possible; thus, his physician opted to use a vitamin B12 injection.

19. People from inland regions are more prone to goiter because they consumer fewer seafoods, which are high in iodine.

20. Researchers have designed studies in which they identify individuals with poor B vitamin status and then determine the impact of the low status on the individuals' ability to perform exercise. They have also performed controlled metabolic studies to determine whether athletes need higher levels of B-vitamins as compared to sedentary adults to maintain their vitamin status. They have also conducted cross-sectional studies that compare the nutritional status of trained athletes to sedentary individuals to determine the frequency of poor B-vitamin status in each group.

21. DFEs = 70 µg/day + 1.7 (224 µg/day) = 451 µg/day. This individual is getting 85% of his or her DFE from fortified foods.

Chapter 9

1. **a.** extracellular fluid. Intracellular fluid is held within the cell membrane. Tissue fluid is extracellular fluid in the body's tissue spaces, whereas plasma is intravascular fluid. Metabolic water is water produced as a byproduct of normal metabolism.

2. **a.** is freely permeable to water, but not to electrolytes. Osmotic pressure draws water across the cell membrane to equalize the concentration of solutes on either side.

3. **b.** secrete renin. In a mildly dehydrated state, the receptors in the kidneys sense the reduced blood volume and blood pressure, and secrete renin, which triggers a cascade of reactions that result in vasoconstriction. The pituitary gland, not the kidneys, secretes ADH. The adrenal glands, not the kidneys, secrete aldosterone. In response to dehydration, the kidneys will attempt to increase—not decrease—water reabsorption.

4. **d.** all of the above.

5. **c.** an individual is likely to hyperventilate, forcing carbon dioxide out of the respiratory system. In a state of alkalosis—not acidosis—the blood pH is elevated above 7.45 and blood proteins release hydrogen ions.

6. **c.** chocolate milk. Red wine and fresh-squeezed orange juice contain natural sugars, not added sugars. Sparkling waters, whether plain or flavored, typically do not contain any sweeteners, although a few brands may be made with artificial sweeteners.

7. **b.** It can be found in fresh fruits and vegetables. Phosphorus—not potassium—is a critical component of bone. Potassium is an intracellular cation. The major cation in the extracellular fluid is sodium, and the major anion in the extracellular fluid is chloride.

8. **d.** is a significant risk in an individual experiencing severe and persistent vomiting. Hyponatremia is characterized by low—not excessive—blood sodium. People who take prescription diuretics are at risk for hypokalemia, not hyponatremia. People with congestive heart failure are at increased risk for hypernatremia, not hyponatremia.

9. **c.** is a greater risk for older adults than for younger adults, because older adults have a lower total amount of body water and their thirst mechanism is less effective. Dehydration is characterized by dark—not colorless— urine, and may decrease—not increase—appetite. Heat stroke—not dehydration—is due to failure of the body's heat-regulating mechanisms.

10. **b.** For people who are overweight and hypertensive, losing 10 pounds can reduce blood pressure. More than 40%— not 70%—of African American adults have hypertension. A blood pressure reading of 120 over 80 is not normal. Prehypertension is defined as a systolic blood pressure of 120 or higher, or a diastolic blood pressure of 80 or higher.

11. **True.**

12. **False.** An increased concentration of blood electrolytes stimulates the thirst mechanism.

13. **True.**

14. **True.**

15. **False.** Drinking lots of plain water throughout a marathon may actually prompt hyponatremia, low blood sodium.

16. Water is a solvent; in blood and lymph, water acts as a transport mechanism; water contributes to the volume of blood and thereby to blood pressure; its high capacity for heat, together with the process of evaporative cooling, helps maintain a normal body temperature; water protects tissues such as the brain and spinal cord; and water lubricates tissues, such as the joints and lungs.

17. Most over-the-counter weight-loss pills are diuretics, which means that they cause fluid loss from the body. Your cousin should avoid diuretics, as she needs to maintain her fluid levels at a higher-than-normal level due to breastfeeding. If she becomes dehydrated, she cannot produce adequate milk for her infant. In addition, the substances in the weight-loss pills could be passed along to her infant in her breast milk, which could cause serious health consequences for the infant.

18. Although there are many things to consider when consuming foods prior to exercise, one important factor is consuming an optimal balance of fluid and electrolytes. In this case, lunch (b) would be the better choice. Lunch (a) is very high in sodium. While our bodies need adequate sodium to function properly, lunch (a) is filled with very high-sodium foods, such as chicken soup, ham, and tomato juice. It is likely that consuming lunch (a) will lead to excessive thirst due to a rise in blood sodium levels. This excessive thirst could cause distraction or even lead to consuming so much fluid that you feel nauseous during practice. Lunch (b) has a more desirable balance of sodium and fluid, should not cause excessive thirst, and should provide ample energy for hockey practice.

19. Chronic diarrhea in a young child can lead to severe dehydration very quickly due to his or her small body size. Diarrhea causes excessive fluid loss from the intestinal tract and extracellular fluid compartment. This fluid loss causes a rise in extracellular electrolyte concentration, and intracellular fluid leaves the cells in an attempt to balance the extracellular fluid loss. These alterations in fluid and electrolyte balance change the flow of electrical impulses through the heart and can lead to abnormal heart rhythms and eventual death if left untreated.

20. Her muscle cramps may be prompted by an electrolyte imbalance brought on by dehydration.

21. To estimate total fluid loss: 3 lb weight loss × 2 cups fluid lost/lb weight loss = 6 cups fluid lost during practice. To estimate total fluid needed for rehydration: 6 cups fluid lost × 1.5 = 9 cups fluid needed for full rehydration.

Chapter 10

1. **b.** an atom loses an electron. A mutation in DNA occurs in the initiation stage of cancer, and can occur randomly, be inherited, or occur as a result of exposure to a carcinogen. Two atoms exchange electrons in exchange reactions in which one is oxidized and the other is reduced. Hydrolysis is a process in which a complex compound is broken apart with the addition of water.

2. **d.** It protects the lipid molecules in cell membranes from oxidation. Vitamin C enhances the absorption of iron. Vitamin A can be manufactured from beta-carotene. Selenium is a critical component of the glutathione peroxidase system.

3. **a.** It is required for the formation of collagen. Vitamin C does not regenerate glutathione to its antioxidant form, but is regenerated by glutathione. It does not reduce the incidence of the common cold in the general population, nor has it been shown to reduce its severity. It has been shown to modestly reduce the duration of a cold if taken

before the onset of symptoms. Cleavage of beta-carotene results in the formation of two molecules of vitamin A; vitamin C is not involved in this process.

4. **b.** iron. Iodine is not a trace mineral with antioxidant properties. Copper and manganese are part of the structure of superoxide dismutase, not catalase.

5. **d.** all of the above. Beta-carotene is a weak antioxidant phytochemical in the carotenoid group. The body converts it to retinol; therefore, it acts as a provitamin for vitamin A.

6. **c.** is a key component of the pigment in rod cells that enables us to perceive black-and-white images. Iodopsin is a pigment in cone cells; it is not converted to rhodopsin, the pigment in rod cells. Vitamin A is not conclusively known to have antioxidant functions. Although vitamin A plays a role in enabling humans to see in dim light, humans cannot see in the dark.

7. **c.** xerophthalmia and hyperkeratosis—as well as night blindness, impaired immunity, and many other health problems. Scurvy and anemia occur with vitamin C deficiency, and erythrocyte hemolysis and impaired movement are associated with deficiency of vitamin E. Carotenosis and carotenodermia are synonyms for the yellowing of skin seen in people who consume excess amounts of beta-carotene.

8. **d.** none of the above is true. Initiation is the first stage in cancer. It is followed by progression, which typically lasts many years as malignant cells multiply into a mass large enough to be clinically detected. The third and final stage of cancer is progression, and is characterized by invasion, establishment of a blood supply, and metastasis.

9. **c.** tobacco use. Smoking directly causes cancer and is the single greatest cause of cancer deaths. Neither random mutation nor heredity is a modifiable factor. Poor nutrition is modifiable, but its role in cancer risk is difficult to separate from the role of overweight/obesity and physical inactivity; moreover, it is associated with cancer, but there is no evidence that it directly causes cancer.

10 **b.** protecting endothelial cell membranes and reducing inflammation and coagulation. Non-malignant body cells with mutated DNA have internal mechanisms by which they typically self-repair or, if unable to self-repair, self-destruct. This behavior is helpful in avoiding cancer, not CVD. A high concentration of either homocysteine or CRP in the blood is associated with an increased risk—not a decreased risk—for CVD, and a diet rich in antioxidants does not promote either factor.

11. **True.**

12. **False.** Vitamin C helps regenerate vitamin E.

13. **True.**

14. **False.** Liver is high in vitamin A, which is toxic to a developing fetus. Pregnant women should not consume it daily or weekly.

15. **True.** According to the National Cancer Institute, human papillomaviruses cause virtually all cervical cancers.

16. Free radicals steal electrons from the stable lipid molecules in our cell membranes. This stealing can destroy the integrity of the membrane and lead to membrane dysfunction and potential cell death.

17. Vitamin E may help reduce our risk for cardiovascular disease in a number of ways. Vitamin E protects LDLs from oxidation, thus helping reduce the buildup of plaque in our blood-vessel walls. Vitamin E may also help reduce low-grade inflammation. Vitamin E is known to reduce blood coagulation and the formation of blood clots, which will reduce the risk of a blood clot clogging a blood vessel and causing a stroke or heart attack.

18. Trace minerals such as selenium, copper, iron, zinc, and manganese are part of the antioxidant enzyme systems that convert free radicals to less damaging substances that are excreted by our bodies. Selenium is part of the glutathione peroxidase enzyme system. Copper, zinc, and manganese are part of the superoxide dismutase enzyme complex, and iron is a part of the structure of catalase.

19. Nico should advise his father not to purchase the supplement. Antioxidant supplementation does not reduce cancer risk; in fact, it may increase risks for various cancers and other chronic diseases. Nico should specifically advise his father against beta-carotene supplementation, since 30 mg of beta-carotene is associated with an increased risk of lung cancer and lung cancer death in multiple studies. Finally, Nico should advise his father to consult his physician for help to quit smoking; to lose weight; and to begin a regular program of physical activity.

20. Cancer development has three primary steps: initiation, promotion, and progression. During the initiation step, the DNA of normal cells is mutated, causing permanent changes in the cell. During the promotion step, the genetically altered cells repeatedly divide, locking the mutated DNA into each new cell's genetic instructions. During the progression step, the cancerous cells grow out of control and invade surrounding tissues. These cells then metastasize, or spread, to other sites of the body.

21. a) Each tablet contains 400 IU of the synthetic form of vitamin E. In supplements containing the synthetic form of vitamin E, 1 IU is equal to 0.45 mg α-TE. To convert IU to mg α-TE = 400 IU × 0.45 = 180 mg α-TE, which is equal to 180 mg of active vitamin E.

b) The RDA for vitamin A is 15 mg alpha-tocopherol per day. To calculate the percentage of the RDA for vitamin E coming from the supplements = (180 mg α-TE ÷ 15 mg α-TE) × 100 = 1200%.

The tolerable upper intake level is 1,000 mg alpha-tocopherol per day, and thus the amount coming from the supplement is relatively small at 180 mg. Although in the past up to 18 times the RDA has been shown to be safe (18 × 15 mg = 270 mg of alpha-tocopherol per day), recent evidence suggests that even 400 IU per day could increase the risk for premature mortality. Thus it would be safest for Joey's mother to obtain adequate vitamin E from her diet. If she is taking aspirin each day as prescribed, it is imperative that she stop taking vitamin E supplements, as aspirin is an anticoagulant and taking vitamin E supplements could enhance its action and result in uncontrollable bleeding and hemorrhaging.

Chapter 11

1. **d.** It provides the scaffolding for cortical bone. Trabecular bone accounts for about 20%—not 80%—of the skeleton, and forms the core of many, but not all, bones. It is also called spongy bone.

2. **b.** bone modeling. The size of bone increases during bone growth. Bone resorption, together with bone formation, are the two components of bone remodeling, which is a bone recycling process that occurs throughout life.

3. **c.** normal bone density. Low bone density begins at a score of −1, and a score more negative than −2.5 indicates osteoporosis. A score of +1.0 is not abnormally high.

4. **d.** the body's regulation of acid-base balance. For this reason, the body maintains blood calcium levels at all costs. Calcium contributes to the mineralization—not demineralization—of bone. Vitamin D is necessary for the regulation of calcium levels, and calcium helps initiate, not oppose, blood clotting.

5. **a.** a cup of cooked kale. We absorb about 106 mg of calcium from this food. In contrast, cauliflower has less calcium per serving, and spinach, although very high in calcium, has binding factors that greatly reduce its absorption: we absorb only about 14 mg of calcium per serving of these foods. Although red leaf lettuce is high in other nutrients, it is not a good source of calcium, providing only about 9 mg per serving.

6. **c.** a dark-skinned retiree living in Illinois. There are four reasons: darker skin pigmentation reduces the absorption of sunlight required for skin synthesis of vitamin D; older adults typically have reduced capacity for skin synthesis of vitamin D; a retiree may be less likely to spend sufficient time outdoors for vitamin D synthesis; and Illinois is a northern state where skin synthesis of vitamin D during winter months is not possible. People who have fair skin, are younger, are outdoors more frequently, and live in more southern states are less likely than this individual to require vitamin D supplements.

7. **c.** both a and b. Both phosphorus and magnesium are major components of bone. About 85% of the body's phosphorus and 50% to 60% of the body's magnesium is stored in bone.

8. **a.** stimulates new bone growth. Although research is ongoing, fluoride is not currently used as a treatment for osteoporosis. Excessive fluoride causes fluorosis, which is characterized by pitting and staining of teeth; however, it is not known to impair the function of teeth.

9. **a.** smoking. High-impact exercise may reduce the risk. Chronic alcohol abuse is indeed detrimental to bone health, but bone density may be higher in people who are light or *moderate* drinkers.

10. **b.** Hormone replacement therapy is effective in preventing and treating osteoporosis. The most effective exercise programs for the treatment of osteoporosis involve weight-bearing exercise such as walking and running. Bisphosphonates and selective estrogen receptor modulators work by slowing, not increasing, bone resorption. Aspirin and other anti-inflammatory drugs are primary drug therapies for osteoarthritis, not osteoporosis.

11. **True.**

12. **True.**

13. **False.** Sunlight is not a direct source of vitamin D; rather, the body can use the energy from sunlight to convert 7-dehydrocholesterol to a precursor of vitamin D.

14. **False.** The beneficial bacteria in the large intestine produce vitamin K.

15. **False.** Fractures caused by osteoporosis often result in premature death.

16. The two processes behind this phenomenon are bone resorption and bone formation. The combination of these processes is referred to as bone remodeling. To preserve bone density, our bodies attempt to achieve a balance between the breakdown of older bone tissue and the formation of new bone tissue.

      One of the primary reasons that bone is broken down is to release calcium into the bloodstream. We also want to break down bone when we fracture a bone and need to repair it. During resorption, osteoclasts erode the bone surface by secreting enzymes and acids that dig grooves into the bone matrix. Their ruffled surface also acts much as a scrubbing brush to assist in the erosion process. Once bone is broken down, the products are transported into the bloodstream and utilized for various body functions.

      Osteoblasts work to form new bone. These cells help synthesize new bone matrix by laying down the collagen containing organic component of bone. Within this substance, the hydroxapatites crystallize and pack together to create new bone where it is needed.

      In young, healthy adults, the processes of bone resorption and formation are equal, so that just as much bone is broken down as is being built. The result is that bone mass is maintained. At around 40 years of age, bone resorption begins to occur more rapidly than bone formation, and this imbalance results in an overall loss in bone density. This loss of bone density affects all bones, including the vertebrae of the spine, and thus results in a loss of height as we age.

17. This meal does not ensure that your calcium needs for the day are met because our bodies can absorb only about 500 mg of calcium at one time. Although this meal contains more than 100% of the DRI for calcium, you cannot absorb all of the calcium present. To meet your daily calcium needs, it is recommended that you eat multiple servings of calcium-rich foods throughout the day and try to consume no more than 500 mg of calcium at one time.

18. The sunlight is not sufficient in Buffalo, New York, during the winter to provide adequate vitamin D for anyone. Thus, all people living in this climate in winter need to consume vitamin D in foods and/or supplements to meet their needs.

19. Because vitamin D is a fat-soluble vitamin, it is absorbed with the fat we consume in our diets. If a person has a disease that does not allow for proper absorption of dietary fat, there will also be a malabsorption of the fat-soluble vitamins, which includes vitamin D.

20. The pediatrician would be unlikely to prescribe fluoride supplements because Hans is already consuming fluoride in his drinking water and is also getting some fluoride from his toothpaste, even though he doesn't swallow it. Adding fluoride supplements would increase the risk that Hans might develop fluorosis, a staining and pitting of his developing teeth.

21. The amount of calcium absorbed from 1 cup of skim milk is 96 mg. The amount of calcium absorbed from 1 cup of broccoli is 37 mg. Thus skim milk has 96 mg ÷ 37 mg = 2.6 times the amount of absorbable calcium as compared to broccoli. You would have to eat 1 cup × 2.6 = 2.6 cups of broccoli to absorb the same amount of calcium as in 1 cup of skim milk.

Chapter 12

1. **b.** lack a nucleus and mitochondria, and are filled with hemoglobin, which is essential for oxygen transport. Glucose, albumin, and other solutes travel in the blood plasma. Leukocytes are involved in immunity. All three cellular elements of blood are produced in the bone marrow.

2. **b.** Iron is a component of hemoglobin, the oxygen-transport protein within red blood cells. Every molecule of hemoglobin contains four atoms of iron; however, the myoglobin molecule contains one iron atom. Iron in myoglobin accounts for about 10% of total body iron.

3. **c.** an iron-fortified breakfast bar with a glass of orange juice. The vitamin C in the juice will boost her absorption of the non-heme iron in the breakfast bar. In contrast, the calcium in cow's milk and cheese, the soy protein (and, if fortified, the calcium) in soy milk, coffee, and tea all inhibit iron absorption. A cheese croissant and a diet coke provide very little iron to begin with.

4. **a.** reduced levels of circulating ferritin. Stage II iron deficiency is characterized by an increase in total iron binding capacity. Iron-deficiency anemia, stage 3, is characterized by smaller than normal red blood cells that are pale in color, as well as exhaustion, impaired cognitive functions, and increased risk for infection.

5. **a.** heme synthesis. Zinc helps maintain the structural integrity of proteins, not iron, which is an element. Rather than preventing copper deficiency, zinc is sometimes prescribed as a supplement to treat copper toxicity. Pernicious anemia is associated with vitamin B_{12} deficiency, not zinc deficiency.

6. **d.** organ meats, seafood, nuts, and seeds. Grain products are not fortified with copper. Dairy products are not good sources of copper. Red, orange, and yellow fruits and vegetables are likely to be rich in beta-carotene, not copper.

7. **b.** blood clotting. Iron and vitamin B_6 contribute to heme synthesis. Folate is essential to formation of the neural tube. Vitamin B_{12} helps maintain the myelin sheath.

8. **c.** erythropoiesis: the production of erythrocytes. Only vitamin B_6, is associated with formation of the porphyrin rings in heme. Platelets are cell fragments—mostly cytoplasm surrounded by a cell membrane—that function in clotting. They do not require vitamin B_6, folate, and vitamin B_{12} for their functioning. Hemochromatosis is a genetic disorder characterized by excessive absorption of iron.

9. **a.** plasma cells. In contrast, NK cells, macrophages, and neutrophils are all cells active in nonspecific immunity.

10. **d.** decreased immunocompetence. Although nausea and vomiting reduce nutrient intake and absorption, they can resolve quickly and are not sensitive indicators of reduced nutritional status. Fatigue, weakness, and inflammation (which is an immune response) are common signs and symptoms associated with many disorders. They are not sensitive indicators of reduced nutritional status.

11. **True.**

12. **False.** Iron deficiency, if prolonged and severe, causes iron-deficiency anemia, a type of microcytic anemia. Pernicious anemia is a type of macrocytic anemia associated with vitamin B_{12} deficiency.

13. **False.** Wilson's disease is a genetic disorder characterized by copper toxicity, and zinc supplementation is used in its treatment.

14. **True.**

15. **True.**

16. Jessica is at a higher risk for iron-deficiency anemia due to her menstrual status and the fact that she consumes only plant-based foods. Plant-based foods contain only the non-heme form of iron, which is more difficult to absorb. Consuming vitamin C enhances the absorption of iron from our foods; thus, it is imperative that Jessica's parents encourage her to eat good plant-based food sources of iron with a vitamin C source to optimize her iron absorption and reduce her risk for iron-deficiency anemia.

17. Vitamin K is available from only a few foods, such as leafy green vegetables. Fortunately, it is also synthesized by

healthful bacteria residing in the large intestine; however, these bacteria are not present in the GI tract in sufficient numbers immediately after birth. Thus, healthcare providers give newborns an injection of vitamin K to meet their needs until their bacterial flora are established.

18. **a.** Janine is of childbearing age. It is recommended that all women of childbearing age consume adequate folate even if they do not plan to become pregnant. This recommendation is made to reduce the risk for neural tube defects in the developing fetus in case a woman does become pregnant.

    b. Janine is avoiding foods that are excellent sources of folate, including many vegetables and enriched grain products. Thus, it is likely that her intake of folate is inadequate. If she continues to avoid these folate-rich foods, a folate supplement may be warranted.

19. Both underweight and obese people have an increased risk for infection and, if they are infected, an increased risk that the infection will be severe. Undernutrition reduces defense against infection because micronutrient deficiencies impair immune function. In obese individuals, most studies show a lower ability of B and T cells to multiply in response to infection. Obese individuals also appear to maintain a low-grade inflammatory state, currently thought to increase the likelihood that they will develop asthma, type 2 diabetes, and other disorders that would increase the severity of infection.

20. This statement is false. Although 20 mg/day × 100 days = 2000 mg, or 2 g, zinc absorption rates range from just 10–35% of dietary intake.

Chapter 13

1. **d.** none of the above. First, remember that a healthful weight has six characteristics, not one or two. Moreover, although a healthful weight is based on your genetic background and family history, it isn't necessarily going to be close to the current body weight of other members of your immediate family if they are all underweight or obese. Also, a healthful body weight is one you can achieve and sustain without severely curtailing your food intake or constantly dieting, whereas keeping your kcal intake no higher than your BMR is very challenging and, unless prescribed by a healthcare provider, unhealthful. Finally, one characteristic of a healthful weight is that it is acceptable to you, not your peers.

2. **a.** body mass index. The fat distribution pattern is the apple- or pear-shaped pattern of distribution of body fat and is not a ratio of weight to height. The apple-shaped pattern is associated with an increased risk for chronic disease. Basal metabolic rate is the energy the body expends to maintain its physiologic functions and is not a ratio of weight to height. An individual's fat-to-lean tissue ratio is a measure of body composition, not weight to height.

3. **b.** take in more energy than they expend. The energy balance equation is not solely dictated by the nutrient composition of the diet, but is greatly influenced by the number of kcals the diet provides in relation to the number of kcals expended; for example, eating > 35% of the diet as fat is not going to cause all people to gain weight, since some people may be expending huge amounts of energy in athletic training or competition, vigorous physical labor, and so on. Failing to exercise is certainly likely to promote weight gain if the individual also consumed more energy than expended in basal metabolism and other daily activities; however, many people have jobs that demand a high level of physical activity, and even people with a very sedentary lifestyle will not gain weight if they consume only the energy they do expend. Consuming more energy, on average, than a person did the previous year might seem as if it would lead to weight gain, but not if the individual also increased his or her physical activity to a level that compensated for the extra energy intake.

4. **a.** energy expended via basal metabolism, the thermic effect of food, and physical activity equals energy intake. Temperature regulation is part of basal metabolism, not an independent factor; moreover, when energy expenditures from basal metabolism and exercise are greater than energy intake, weight loss—not energy balance—occurs. The body mass index is a ratio of weight to height, not a component of energy expenditure.

5. **b.** ghrelin. Its level increases before a meal and decreases after a meal, indicating that it may contribute to both hunger and satiety. Leptin and PYY tend to discourage food intake, and uncoupling proteins promote energy expenditure and reduce energy storage.

6. **c.** a low-income single mother who provides child care to other families in her urban apartment block. This is the individual most likely to have reduced access to healthcare, nourishing food, and opportunities for safe and regular physical activity. The other three individuals are likely to have more resources than the single mother, including income, healthcare, educational attainment, and opportunities to purchase healthful foods and engage in physical activity. Moreover, although many people who are obese smoke, smoking itself curbs appetite and may reduce energy intake.

7. **d.** all of the above. Obesity increases the risk for certain types of cancer, dementia, cardiovascular disease, type 2 diabetes, depression, and many other diseases. It also increases the risk for premature death.

8. **c.** is justified if the immediate threat of serious obesity-related disease and death is more dangerous than the associated risks. Only about one-third to one-half of people who undergo bariatric surgery lose significant amounts of weight and maintain the loss. Bariatric surgery

is not necessarily considered too risky for people with morbid obesity; in fact, people with morbid obesity are the primary candidates for this surgery.

9. **a.** a realistic, achievable goal. Behavioral counseling or enrollment in a support group can be a helpful step toward achieving your goal, but is not a first step and is not necessary for everyone. Neither a low-fat diet nor a low-carb diet is necessary for weight loss. Macronutrient composition of the diet is not as important as reduction in energy intake.

10. **c.** a peanut-butter sandwich on whole-grain bread with an apple. A slice of pepperoni pizza with extra cheese would be energy dense, but most of its Calories would be from saturated fat. Four chocolate chip cookies would also be high in empty Calories from saturated fats and added sugars. Flavored milks such as strawberry milk are very high in added sugars, and it is not necessary to use protein powders or any other form of supplement to gain weight healthfully.

11. **False.** Apple-shaped fat patterning, or upper-body obesity, increases the individual's risk for many chronic diseases.

12. **True.**

13. **True.**

14. **False.** Prescription weight-loss medications are associated with side effects and a certain level of risk, and are therefore advised only for people who are obese (BMI greater than or equal to 30 kg/m^2). They are also advised for people who have a BMI greater than or equal to 27 kg/m^2 who also have other significant health risk factors.

15. **False.** Weight-gain programs should include both aerobic exercise for a healthy cardiovascular system and resistance training to build muscle mass.

16. A weight that is appropriate for your age and physical development; a weight that you can achieve and sustain without restraining your food intake or constantly dieting; a weight that is acceptable to you; a weight that is based on your genetic background and family history of body shape and weight; a weight that promotes good eating habits and allows you to participate in regular physical activity.

17. You can increase your basal metabolic rate by increasing your lean body mass or by using drugs such as stimulants, caffeine, and tobacco. Stress and certain illnesses can also increase BMR. The most healthful way to increase BMR is to increase your lean body mass by participating in regular strength-training exercises. Attempting to increase your BMR by using drugs or by increasing your stress is not wise and can be dangerous to your health.

18. Abdominal obesity is one of the five risk factors collectively referred to as metabolic syndrome, which greatly increases an individual's risk for heart disease and type 2 diabetes. Metabolic syndrome in turn is a key component of cardiometabolic risk, a cluster of risk factors that also includes elevated LDL cholesterol, smoking, inflammation, and insulin resistance.

19. **a.** Greater access to inexpensive, high-fat, high-Calorie foods (for example, fast foods, vending machine foods, and snack/convenience foods).
b. Significant increases in portion sizes of foods.
c. Increased reliance on cars instead of bicycles, public transportation, or walking.
d. Use of elevators and escalators instead of stairs.
e. Increased use of computers, dishwashers, televisions, and other time-saving devices.
f. Lack of safe, accessible, and affordable places to exercise.

20. *Dietary recommendations for a sound weight-loss program include the following:*
a. Set reasonable weight-loss goals. Reasonable weight loss is defined as 0.5 to 2 pounds per week. To achieve this rate of weight loss, energy intake should be reduced approximately 250 to no more than 1,000 kcal/d of present intake. A weight-loss plan should never provide less than a total of 1,200 kcal/d.
b. Eat a diet that is relatively low in fat and high in complex carbohydrates. Total fat intake should be 15% to 25% of total energy intake. Saturated fat intake should be 5% to 10% of total energy intake. Monounsaturated fat intake should be 10% to 15% of total energy intake. Polyunsaturated fat intake should be no more than 10% of total energy intake. Carbohydrate intake should be around 55% of total energy intake, with less than 10% of energy intake coming from simple sugars, and fiber intake should be 25 to 35 g/day.
Physical activity recommendation: Set a long-term goal for physical activity that is at least 30 minutes of moderate physical activity most, or preferably all, days of the week. Doing 45 minutes or more of an activity such as walking at least 5 days per week is ideal.
Behavior modification recommendations include:
a. Eliminating inappropriate behaviors by shopping when you are not hungry, only eating at set times in one location, refusing to buy problem foods, and avoiding vending machines, convenience stores, and fast-food restaurants.
b. Suppressing inappropriate behaviors by taking small food portions, eating foods on smaller serving dishes so they appear larger, and avoiding feelings of deprivation by eating regular meals throughout the day.
c. Strengthening appropriate behaviors by sharing food with others, learning appropriate serving sizes, planning healthful snacks, scheduling walks and other physical activities with friends, and keeping clothes and equipment for physical activity in convenient places.
d. Repeating desired behaviors by slowing down eating, always using utensils, leaving food on your plate, moving more throughout the day, and joining groups who are physically active.

e. Rewarding yourself for positive behaviors with nonfood rewards.

f. Using the "buddy" system by exercising with a friend or relative and/or calling this support person when you need an extra boost to stay motivated.

g. Refusing to punish yourself if you deviate from your plan.

21. To calculate Misty's BMI, first convert her weight in lb to kg: 148 lb/2.2 lb per kg = 67.3 kg.

Then convert her height in inches to meters = 5'8" = 68 in × 0.0254 m/in = 1.73 m.

Then square her height in meters = 1.73 m × 1.73 m = 2.99 m2.

Then calculate her BMI by dividing her weight in kg by height in square meters = 67.3 kg/2.99 m2 = 22.5 kg/m2.

Based on this BMI value, it is clear that Misty is not overweight.

One primary question for Misty is, What is her idea of her ideal weight? It sounds as if Misty might have significant body image concerns. If this is the case, it is important that she meet with a healthcare provider or nutrition professional who can assist her with improving her body image perceptions.

Another question is, What weight can she achieve and sustain without trying so hard (in other words, without restricting her food intake or constantly dieting)? The fact that she must try so hard and is still not losing weight is a good indication that she may already be at the weight that is healthful.

A third question is, How does her current weight and body shape compare to her genetic background and family history? If her body weight and shape are consistent with her genetic makeup and family history, she may have unrealistic expectations of reducing her body weight or significantly altering her shape.

A final question Misty should consider is whether she is able to maintain her current weight by being regularly active and by eating a healthful, balanced diet. If not, then this is another indication that her body weight goals are unrealistic.

To calculate how many kcal she needs to maintain her current body weight, you first need to calculate Misty's BMR. This can be done in two steps:

1. To estimate how many kcal per hour Misty expends at her present body weight, multiply her body weight in kg by 0.9 kcal/kg body weight/hour = 0.9 kcal/kg body weight/hr × 67.3 kg = 60.57 kcal/hour.

2. To calculate her BMR for the total day (or 24 hours) = 60.57 kcal/hour × 24 hours = 1454 kcal/day.

Misty's activity level is classified as moderately active. According to the values presented in the chapter, the energy cost of Misty's activities ranges from 50% to 70% of her BMR. Thus the range of energy that Misty expends at her current activity level is equal to:

- 1454 kcal/day × 0.50 (or 50%) = 727 kcal/day
- 1454 kcal/day × 0.70 (or 70%) = 1018 kcal/day

To calculate Misty's total energy expenditure in kcal each day, add together BMR and the energy needed to perform her daily activities:

- 1454 kcal/day + 727 kcal/day = 2181 kcal/day
- 1454 kcal/day + 1018 kcal/day = 2472 kcal/day

Assuming Misty is maintaining weight at her current activity level, she needs between 2181 and 2472 kcal/day to stay in energy balance.

Chapter 14

1. a. increases our ability to carry out daily tasks with vigor and alertness, without undue fatigue. Regular physical activity may reduce our risk for colon cancer, but this association is not conclusive, and a benefit of regular physical activity in reducing the risk of other forms of cancer also is unknown. Although regular physical activity can be helpful in treating mild to moderate depression, it is not an effective treatment for severe depression.

2. c. cardiorespiratory fitness, musculoskeletal fitness, flexibility, and body composition. Aerobic capacity, aerobic fitness, cardiovascular fitness, and respiratory fitness are all part of cardiorespiratory fitness. Similarly, resistance, strength, and tone are aspects of musculoskeletal fitness and lean body mass is one component of body composition. An increased ability to resist chronic disease is a benefit of regular physical activity, not a component of fitness.

3. c. for at least 150 minutes a week. His sessions can be as short as 10 minutes each, as long as he achieves a minimum of 150 minutes. He should also engage in resistance training at least 2 days a week. The 1996 physical activity recommendation of the U.S. Surgeon General is 30 minutes most days of the week, and the Institute of Medicine recommendation is 60 minutes a day. No guidelines recommend 150 minutes a day.

4. d. includes a cool-down period to help prevent injury and muscle soreness. Typically, a preliminary assessment by a cardiopulmonary specialist would be recommended only for someone with a history of cardiopulmonary disease. For most children and adults, a program of moderate exercise is healthful and safe. The initiation phase of a sound fitness program is a period of time in which you start to incorporate relatively brief bouts of physical activity into your daily life and reduce the time you spend in sedentary activities. Your goal during this phase is to build up to 30 minutes a day. A sound fitness program appropriately overloads the body and promotes muscle hypertrophy, not atrophy.

5. **b.** 50% to 70% of your estimated maximal heart rate. A target heart rate of 30% to 60% of your estimated maximal heart rate would be less effective in achieving moderate-intensity physical activity. A target heart rate of 70% to 85% of your estimated maximal heart rate would be appropriate to achieve vigorous-intensity physical activity. Competitive athletes typically train at 80% to 95% of their estimated maximal heart rate.

6. **a.** about 1 to 3 seconds. ATP and creatine phosphate together can fuel activity for up to 15 seconds. After that time, the body must rely on other fuels, such as carbohydrate and fat.

7. **c.** 1.8 g/kg body weight. The RDA for protein for sedentary adults is 0.8 g/kg. Moderately active people need about 1.0 g/kg. Based on recent evidence, an intake of 2.8 g/kg body weight is likely too high for nearly all people and is not necessary to support training and recovery.

8. **c.** It involves altering both exercise duration and carbohydrate intake to maximize the amount of muscle glycogen. The practice does not support performance in baseball or other non-endurance activities. The schedule concludes with rest—not vigorous training—the day before the competition, and the intake of carbohydrate does not exceed 10 g per kg body weight. Even in endurance events, carbohydrate loading does not always improve performance, and there are many adverse effects, such as diarrhea and sluggishness, that can reduce performance.

9. **b.** a beverage containing carbohydrates and sodium and other electrolytes. Plain water, cooler than the environmental temperature, and flavored to promote consumption, is appropriate for activity lasting 1 hour or less. Beverages high in fructose, such as 100% fruit juice, may cause gastrointestinal distress, and beverages containing caffeine may increase fluid excretion; thus, both should be avoided.

10. **d.** all of the above.

11. **True.** Although the overload must be appropriate to gradually progress toward your fitness goals while avoiding injury, a sound fitness program does overload the body.

12. **True.**

13. **False.** A fat intake of 20% to 35% of total energy intake is generally recommended for most athletes, with less than 10% of total energy intake as saturated fat. This is the same as the AMDR for non-athletes.

14. **False.** Sports anemia is not true anemia but a transient decrease in iron stores that occurs at the start of an exercise program as plasma volume increases ahead of increases in hemoglobin.

15. **True.**

16. Factors that assist Marisa in maintaining a normal, healthful weight include the following:
    - Walking to/from school each day.

    - Covering the lunch shift at her college's day care center, which requires that she be on her feet, walk, and perform light lifting 2 hours each day.
    - Walking on the weekends.
    Factors that contribute to Conrad's weight gain include the following:
    - Driving to school each day.
    - Working an office job 2 hours each day.
    - Going to the movies on the weekends instead of doing some form of physical activity.

17. There are an infinite number of correct answers to this question. The plan outlined here is for a 40-year-old woman who is interested in maintaining a healthful body weight, optimizing her blood lipid profile, reducing her stress, and maintaining aerobic fitness, flexibility, and upper body strength. She works full-time as a research scientist, and most of her occupational activities are sedentary.
    - **Monday and Wednesday:** 60 minutes of fitness walking (including 5-minute warm-up and 5-minute cooldown).
    - **Tuesday and Thursday:** 75 minutes of power/ashtanga yoga (including warm-up and cool-down); 45 minutes of morning swimming (substitute with bicycling in the summer months).
    - **Friday:** 60 minutes of fitness walking (including warmup and cool-down); 30 minutes of gardening.
    - **Saturday:** 75 minutes of hatha yoga (including warmup and cool-down); 120 minutes of gardening.
    - **Sunday:** 30 minutes of hatha yoga (including warm-up and cool-down); 180 minutes of hiking with a light daypack.

18. Gustavo is 69 years of age, has high blood pressure, and has a family history of colon cancer. He manages a vineyard. You would need to know a little bit more about his occupation to determine his level of activity at work. However, based on his health status, Gustavo could most likely benefit from participating in a planned exercise program of low to moderate intensity. This type of program will help keep his blood pressure under better control; will reduce his risk for cardiovascular disease, stroke, and type 2 diabetes; will help Gustavo maintain a healthful body weight; and will assist in maintaining bone density. This type of program may also reduce his risk for colon cancer. Before Gustavo begins an exercise program, he should get a thorough physical exam by his physician because of his older age and his high-blood-pressure status. His physician can then determine the safest forms of physical activity for Gustavo.

19. The most helpful strategy you might consider is the use of sports beverages. Sports beverages were designed for people who exercise for more than 60 minutes at a time and are specially formulated to replenish the fluid and micronutrients that are lost during intense, long-duration

exercise. By consuming sports beverages during training for a marathon, you can ensure that you are maintaining adequate hydration levels and can avoid hyponatremia by replenishing sodium.

20. Dehydration significantly increases an athlete's risk for heat illnesses. This is because the body's production of heat surges during heavy exercise, and the primary mechanism through which this heat is dissipated is evaporative cooling—commonly called sweating—which requires and results in the loss of a significant amount of fluid. When body fluid levels are limited, such as when a person is dehydrated, blood volume and flow may be inadequate to effectively cool the body. As such, this puts the athlete at greater risk for heat stroke than if he or she had been adequately hydrated prior to starting the training session.

21. **a)** Liz's suggested intake for protein is identified as 1.5 grams per kg body weight. Her body weight is equal to 105 lbs ÷ 2.2 = 47.7 kg. Her protein intake (in grams) is equal to 1.5 grams protein/kg body weight × 47.7 kg = 71.6 grams
b) Liz's preferred fat intake is 20% of her total daily energy intake, thus 1,800 kcal × 0.20 = 360 kcal. As the energy value of fat is 9 kcal per gram, her total intake of fat in grams = 360 kcal ÷ 9 kcal/gram = 40 grams of fat.
c) To calculate Liz's carbohydrate intake, you must first determine the amount of kcal of her total energy intake that remains once her protein and fat intake are accounted for.

- Liz's protein intake is 71.6 grams; as the energy value of protein is 4 kcal per gram, her kcal intake from protein = 71.6 grams × 4 kcal/gram = 286.4 kcal
- Liz's fat intake has already been calculated as 360 kcal
- As Liz's total energy intake is 1,800 kcal per day, the amount of kcal she'll consume from carbohydrate = 1,800 kcal – 286.4 kcal – 360 kcal = 1153.6 kcal of carbohydrate.
- The energy value of carbohydrates is 4 kcal per gram, and thus Liz's intake of carbohydrate in grams is equal to 1153.6 kcal ÷ 4 kcal/gram = 288.4 grams

To determine if Liz's carbohydrate intake falls within the AMDR = (1153.6 kcal of carbohydrate ÷ 1,800 kcal) × 100 = 64%. Thus her carbohydrate intake does fall within the AMDR.

Chapter 15

1. **c.** federal oversight of food safety is fragmented among 15 different agencies. An estimated 48 million Americans—not 4.8 million—experience foodborne illness each year, and about 3,000—not 300—die. Food additives are tested before introduction into the U.S. food supply, and are not a significant cause of foodborne illness. Rather, microbial contamination of produce typically accounts for the greatest percentage of foodborne illness, and contaminated

meats and poultry account for the most deaths. The CDC's most recent food safety progress report indicates no progress in reducing foodborne illness from six specific pathogens, not from any and all sources; moreover, the report is produced by the CDC, not the Food Safety Working Group, which has not met since 2011.

2. **d.** *Toxoplasma gondii* is the only species of protozoa. Five—not six—of culprits are bacteria, and one is a virus, norovirus, which is responsible for the greatest number of illnesses. *Salmonella,* not Shiga toxin-producing *E. coli,* is responsible for the most deaths.

3. **a.** between 40°F and 140°F. This range of temperature is known as the danger zone. Most foodborne microorganisms thrive in slightly acidic to neutral pH environments, and most require an aerobic environment. One exception is *C. botulinum,* which prefers an alkaline, anaerobic (oxygen-free) environment.

4. **c.** within a maximum of 1 hour after serving. Even on a hot day, it is not necessary to refrigerate leftovers immediately after serving or within 30 minutes; however, it is not harmful to do so. Leaving food out for longer than 1 hour in a hot environment is unsafe.

5. **b.** modified atmosphere packaging. Aseptic packaging is similar to canning in that foods and beverages are heated, then cooled, then placed in sterile containers. High-pressure processing subjects food to an extremely high pressure. Irradiation exposes food to gamma rays that kill or disable any microorganisms present.

6. **b.** sulfites and nitrites. Sodium chloride is salt and beta-carotene is an antioxidant phytochemical; the former is used for flavoring and the latter for coloring. Alpha-tocopherol is vitamin E and ascorbic acid is vitamin C; they are used as preservatives.

7. **a.** confer tolerance to herbicides. HT GMOs can tolerate increased application of stronger chemicals than could otherwise be used. Although crops are also genetically modified to protect them from disease, enable them to grow in challenging environmental conditions, and boost their concentration of nutrients, these are not the top uses of genetic modification in the United States.

8. **d.** Industrial contaminants become more concentrated in animal tissues as they move up the food chain. Although fertilizers, pesticides, industrial pollutants, and animal wastes can contaminate soil, air, and water, these events are not definitive of biomagnification.

9. **c.** they can act as neurotoxins, carcinogens, or endocrine disruptors. Indiscriminate use of antibiotics causes antibiotic to develop in livestock. Although certain chemicals can prompt allergies, asthma, or migraine headaches in certain susceptible individuals, these health problems are not the specific threats to public health posed by residues from POPs and some pesticides. Incidents of foodborne illness, not POP and pesticide residues, are associated with nausea, vomiting, and diarrhea.

10. **a.** contain only organically produced ingredients, excluding water and salt. They may display the USDA's—not the EPA's—organic seal. Some organic foods are produced with pesticides, as certain biopesticides and other non-toxic, nonpersistent pesticides are approved for organic farming. Organic foods include meats, poultry, fish, and eggs and dairy, not just plants.

11. **True.**

12. **False.** Washing these foods does not kill the microorganisms that might be present, and could in fact spread them to your sink and other surfaces. The only way to keep these foods safe to eat is to cook them to the proper temperature.

13. **False.** The gamma rays kill or disable any microorganisms that may be present in the food, but do not make the food radioactive.

14. **False.** The FDA has imposed a voluntary ban on the use of antibiotics, not recombinant bovine growth hormone (rBGH).

15. **True.**

16. **a.** Failure to wash your hands before you removed chicken from the freezer. You touched the chicken when you placed it in the bowl to thaw in the refrigerator.
    b. Failure to wash your hands with hot water and soap prior to putting the chicken breasts on the cutting board.
    c. Failure to wash the chicken breasts thoroughly prior to putting them on the clean cutting board.
    d. Failure to wash your hands with hot water and soap after handling the chicken breasts just prior to touching and rinsing the lettuce, red pepper, and scallions.
    e. Failure to check the temperature of the chicken breasts. Even though they were no longer pink in color, they may not have been cooked to a high enough temperature to kill bacteria.

17. There are a few different processes of pickling, but this process requires the use of vinegar and salt. The vinegar used works to destroy microbes that cause food-borne illness (particularly the *Clostridium botulinum* bacterium). The salt used not only adds flavor but also inhibits spoilage and the growth of harmful bacteria.

18. The safest choice is to select the pasteurized juice. Unpasteurized beverages (such as juices and milk) may contain a significant number of microbes that can cause food-borne illnesses. Pasteurization does not eliminate all microbes but significantly decreases the numbers of heat-sensitive microorganisms, which tend to be the most harmful. The amount of pesticides found in juice is most likely very low or zero, as the pesticides would have been applied to the trees and oranges with the peel on the fruit. It is highly likely that this juice contains none of the pesticides that may have been used, because the peel is not used to make the juice.

19. Based on this brief description, it sounds as if the cause of this disease was mercury poisoning. Mercury, a naturally occurring element, is found in soil, rocks, lakes, streams, and oceans. It is also released into the environment by pulp and paper processing and the burning of garbage and fossil fuels. As mercury is released into the environment, it falls from the air, eventually finding its way into streams, lakes, and oceans. Fish absorb mercury as they feed on aquatic organisms. This mercury is passed on to people when they consume the fish. As mercury accumulates in the body, it has a toxic effect on the nervous system. Mercury is especially toxic to the developing nervous systems of fetuses and growing children. Thus, pregnant and breastfeeding women and young children are advised to avoid eating fish that may be contaminated with mercury.

Based on an Internet search, it appears that Minamata disease was caused by mercury poisoning. A variety of heavy metals were used in a highly successful industrial plant on Minamata Bay. After careful study and elimination of other toxic chemicals used in this industrial plant, it was discovered that the disease experienced by these people was a result of mercury poisoning.

20. No, this food is not 100% organic. This is because it contains whey, which is a protein from cow's milk. This item is not designated as organic. Remember that to be considered 100% organic a food must contain only organically produced ingredients, excluding water and salt. This food also contains food additives; in this case, the additive is salt.

21. $145°F - 32 = 113; 113 \times 5/9 = 63°C$
    $160°F - 32 = 128; 128 \times 5/9 = 71°C$
    $165°F - 32 = 133; 133 \times 5/9 = 74°C$

Chapter 16

1. **a.** Asia. South Africa does not have an unusually high prevalence of hunger, and is not large enough or densely populated enough to account for the majority of the world's hungry people. As a region, sub-Saharan Africa has the greatest prevalence of hunger, but accounts for about 28% of the world's hungry people. Less than 2% of the world's hungry people live in the developed nations of the world.

2. **c.** unequal distribution of food, largely because of poverty. Famine and war often prompt acute food shortages, but are not leading causes of longstanding hunger in a region. Overpopulation increases pressure on a region's food supply, but even developing nations currently produce sufficient food for their populations overall.

3. **c.** Worldwide, the probability of extreme heat events has been five times higher over the past 60 years than prior to the Industrial Age. Recall that climate change is defined as a significant change in the measures of climate—such as temperature, precipitation, or wind patterns—that occurs

over several decades or longer. Natural disasters such as earthquakes and climate events such as heat waves are individual events. Greenhouse gas emissions by definition trap heat and contribute to global warming, but do not in themselves qualify as an example of climate change.

4. **d.** all of the above.

5. **d.** a geographic area where people lack access to fresh, healthy, and affordable food. Food deserts are typically found in remote areas or in inner-city neighborhoods rather than in suburbs. Although many inner-city food deserts are indeed served by fast-food restaurants and convenience stores, rural food deserts may not have any food vendors for many miles. Although more than half of the 23.5 million people who live in food deserts are low-income, about 10 million are not.

6. **b.** The majority of farm and food service workers live below the poverty line. In many states in the United States, food service workers who receive more than $30 in tips—not all food service workers and not farm workers—may lawfully be paid just $2.13 an hour. On average, many more than 100 workers (372 in 2012) die each year from farm-labor injuries. This includes more than 100 youths (under age 20).

7. **b.** It has dramatically increased food security throughout South America, Asia, and Africa. It has not increased global production of organic foods, as organic farmers do not use methods such as genetic modification and synthetic fertilizers that are hallmarks of industrial agriculture. The Green Revolution has actually increased the erosion of topsoil and the depletion and pollution of ground water.

8. **c.** The U.S. food industry produces about twice as many Calories per capita per year than Americans require. American farmers receive subsidies to grow several crops, including not only corn but also soybeans, wheat, and rice. The fast-food industry alone spends $4.6 billion a year on advertising.

9. **a.** the Supplemental Nutrition Assistance Program. In contrast, the Special Supplemental Nutrition Program for Women, Infants, and Children serves pregnant women, infants, and children to age 5, and the Commodity Supplemental Food Program serves Americans age 60 years and older.

10. **d.** a pint of strawberries you pick yourself at an organic farm. These would be not only organic and local but also healthful, and picking them yourself might help raise your consciousness of the physical labor involved in harvesting America's food. Because it isn't a food, a fair-trade certified t-shirt, while an equitable purchase, is not likely to support food equity, sustainability, and quality. A cup of hot apple cider you buy at a farmer's market is likely to have been made from local apples, but it is not necessarily organic, and there is no guarantee that the farm workers who picked the apples had safe working conditions or

were equitably compensated. A certified organic beef burger on a whole-grain bun from an organic foods restaurant is still beef, which depletes more natural resources and releases more greenhouse gases than plant foods. Also, there is no guarantee that the beef hasn't been flown in from a distant state, incurring the environmental costs of transportation, and the food server may be paid as little as $2.13 an hour before tips.

11. **False.** Those at higher risk for food insecurity are households with incomes below 185% of the official U.S. poverty threshold (which was $23,634 for a family of four in 2013), families consisting of single mothers or single fathers and their children, African American households, and Hispanic households. Adults over age 65 years, in part because of Social Security and Medicare benefits, are not at unusually high risk for food insecurity.

12. **False.** The high prevalence of obesity in low-income populations is called the poverty–obesity paradox. In contrast, the nutrition paradox is the coexistence of aspects of both stunting and overweight/obesity within the same region, household, family, or person.

13. **True.** Under federal law, children as young as 12 are allowed to work on farms with parental permission after school hours, on weekends, and during school vacations.

14. **True.**

15. **True.**

16. Women with access to education are more likely to have increased earning potential, access to information about contraception, and information to use better health practices. These circumstances lead to smaller, healthier, more economically stable families.

17. When undernutrition is endemic throughout an area, growth stunting becomes the norm. In such a population, a person who is of average height by U.S. standards would be considered unusually tall.

18. Mexico is a country experiencing economic growth and the nutrition transition. Obesity is becoming a serious problem for both adults and children. Because of obesity, type 2 diabetes is being diagnosed at younger and younger ages in the Hispanic population. The best solution to diabetes is prevention, and a concerned pediatrician is likely to be able to make a tremendous beneficial difference in the lives of the children he sees.

19. The food industry employs lobbyists who attempt to persuade lawmakers and food agency executives (at the FDA, USDA, etc.) to adopt policies favorable to the industry. Food companies and associations also attempt to purchase influence by contributing to political campaigns. They also fund campaigns to persuade voters to vote against measures to which they're opposed, such as taxes on sugary drinks, and judicial challenges to laws unfavorable to their products. Finally, they spend many billions of dollars each year on food advertising.

20. Breast milk contains antibodies that protect against infections. In addition, there is a danger in developing countries of feeding infants with formula, because the use of unsanitary water for mixing batches of formula results in diarrheal diseases. Another problem is that overdilution of formula by families who cannot afford adequate amounts results in inadequate intake for the infant, whereas breast milk is likely to contain adequate amounts of the nutrients needed.

21. Steve earns \$15,080 annually (\$7.25/hour × 40 hours a week × 52 weeks a year). He and his family are currently living far below the federal poverty line. If Diane were to return to work for 40 hours a week, their annual income would double to \$30,160 (\$15,080 × 2 = \$30,160). As you learned in this chapter, families earning at or below 185% of the federal poverty level are at increased risk for food insecurity. The federal poverty threshold in 2015 was \$20,090 for a family of three: 185% of \$20,090 = \$37,167 (\$20,090 × 1.85 = \$37,167). Even if Steve and Diane both worked full time (80 hours a week combined), they would still be at high risk for food insecurity (\$30,160 is less than \$37,167).

Chapter 17

1. **b.** neural tube defects, in which the embryonic neural tube (the primitive structure that becomes the brain and spinal cord) fails to close. FASD (fetal alcohol spectrum disorders) is related to maternal alcohol use, not folate deficiency. Maternal overweight and obesity, not folate deficiency, are associated with an increased risk for gestational diabetes and birth of a large for gestational age (LGA) newborn.

2. **d.** the third trimester. Throughout the first trimester, both in the embryonic and early fetal periods, the mother's energy needs do not substantively increase above her pre-pregnancy needs. Although energy needs do increase in the second trimester, fetal growth, and the requirement for increased Calorie intake to support that growth, is greatest during the third trimester.

3. **b.** women who begin their pregnancy underweight. Women who begin their pregnancy at a normal weight should strive to gain between 25 and 35 lb. Women who begin their pregnancy overweight should gain 15 to 25 lb, and women who are obese should gain no more than 11 to 20 lb.

4. **a.** protein. The RDA for protein for pregnant women increases from 0.8 g/kg of body weight for nonpregnant women, to 1.1 g/kg during pregnancy. Vitamin D and calcium are important to maintain maternal bone and build fetal bone, but the RDA for these micronutrients does not change for pregnant women because the amount of vitamin D transferred from the mother to the fetus is relatively small, and calcium is absorbed more efficiently during pregnancy.

5. **c.** more common in overweight and obese women compared to women of normal weight. Gestational hypertension, not preeclampsia, is likely to be diagnosed in a pregnant woman with high blood pressure but no other signs or symptoms. Eclampsia, not preeclampsia, is a medical emergency characterized by seizures and kidney failure. Preeclampsia is typically managed by bed rest and strict monitoring, not by exercise and a reduced Calorie diet.

6. **a.** exercise. Drinking more than about a cup of brewed coffee a day is not recommended because a caffeine intake as low as 100 mg/day has been shown in some studies to increase the risk for miscarriage, stillbirth, preterm birth, and low birth weight. Saccharin accumulates in fetal tissues and is not appropriate to consume in pregnancy.

7. **c.** oxytocin. Progesterone and estrogen are reproductive hormones that, among many other roles, foster the preparation of breast tissue for lactation and, during pregnancy, suppress the effects of prolactin, a pituitary hormone responsible for milk synthesis.

8. **c.** Breastfeeding can help the mother more easily lose the weight she gained during pregnancy. Breastfeeding actually suppresses ovulation and thus fertility. Breast milk does not provide all of the nourishment an infant needs for the first year of life. Beginning at about 6 months of age, infants begin to have a physiologic need for solid food in addition to breast milk.

9. **d.** iron. Breast milk is an excellent source of the fatty acids arachidonic acid (AA) and docosahexaenoic acid (DHA), and these fatty acids are now added to many infant formulas; thus, it is not necessary to supplement these nutrients for either breast-fed or formula-fed infants. All infants are given an injection of vitamin K shortly after birth, then, as their beneficial GI tract bacteria become established, they produce vitamin K; thus, supplemental vitamin K is not needed. Breast milk is low in vitamin D; however, supplementation is typically prescribed throughout infancy, not just for older infants.

10. **d.** puréed peas. Many infants experience allergic reactions to wheat and dairy; moreover, cow's milk is too concentrated in minerals and protein and contains too little carbohydrate for infants. Small fruits such as grapes and raisins are choking hazards and should not be offered to infants or toddlers.

11. **False.** Exposure to teratogens and nutrient deficiencies is most likely to cause developmental errors and birth defects when it occurs during the first trimester of pregnancy.

12. **False.** Because they receive too much glucose during fetal development, newborns of mothers with gestational diabetes are likely to be large for gestational age.

13. **True.**

14. **True.**

15. **True.**

16. It is possible that your cousin is partly right and partly wrong. If she is very careful and consumes a wide variety of nutrient-dense foods, she is likely consuming adequate amounts of the macronutrients and many of the micronutrients she needs to support her pregnancy. However, there are some nutrients that are extremely difficult to consume in adequate amounts in the diet during pregnancy, as a woman's needs are very high for these nutrients. One of these nutrients is iron. During pregnancy, the demand for red blood cells increases to accommodate the needs of the growing uterus, the placenta, and the fetus itself. Thus, more iron is needed. Fetal demand for iron increases even further during the last trimester, when the fetus stores iron in the liver for use during the first few months of life. This iron storage is protective, because breast milk is low in iron. Because of these risks, the RDA for iron for pregnant women is 27 mg per day, compared to 18 mg per day for non-pregnant women. Even though your cousin feels her eating habits are sufficient, it is highly likely that she had low iron stores prior to pregnancy, as this is a common problem in many women. Women have a difficult time consuming 18 mg of iron per day in their diets; consuming twice this amount is extremely difficult, if not impossible, for most women. Thus, women of childbearing age typically have poor iron stores, and the demands of pregnancy are likely to produce deficiency. To ensure adequate iron stores during pregnancy, an iron supplement (as part of, or distinct from, a total prenatal supplement) is routinely prescribed during the last two trimesters. In addition, consuming vitamin C will enhance iron absorption, as do dietary sources of heme iron.

17. After reviewing the girl's typical dietary intake, I would discuss the importance of appropriate prenatal weight gain (not too much, not too little); the importance of taking folic acid, iron, and possibly calcium supplements; and the need to avoid alcohol, street drugs, and (unless prescribed by her healthcare provider) medications.

18. *Advantages:* offers optimal nutritional quality; protects infants from infections and allergies; reduces risk for sudden infant death syndrome; quickens the return of the uterus in the mother to pre-pregnancy size and reduces post-pregnancy bleeding; suppresses ovulation, which lengthens the time between pregnancies and gives the mother's body time to recover before conceiving again; provides for mother–infant bonding and attachment; is more convenient than bottle-feeding; is less expensive than bottle-feeding.
Disadvantages: allows passage of drugs (caffeine, prescription drugs), alcohol, and irritating components of foods such as onion or garlic; causes allergic reactions to foods mother eats, such as wheat, peanuts, and cow's milk; transmits HIV from mother to infant in mothers who are HIV-positive; creates the need for the mother to balance the challenges of regular breastfeeding with job duties; causes sleep deprivation for the mother due to feeding every 2 to 3 hours; is associated with social concerns, such as exposing breasts in public and discomfort of others who may observe breastfeeding in public.

19. The primary information to share with this woman is that breastfeeding is recommended for all children up to at least 2 years (24 months) of age. Thus, an 11-month-old child is not too old to be breastfed. In addition, it is also possible that this woman is offended by seeing your sister breastfeed in public. If this is the case, it is important to point out that all women have the right to breastfeed in a public place. If this woman is offended, she can leave the area or choose not to observe your sister as she breastfeeds her child.

20. Based on this description, it is possible that Katie has a condition referred to as colic. Overstimulation of the nervous system, feeding too rapidly, swallowing of air, and intestinal gas pain are considered possible culprits, but the precise cause is unknown. As with allergies, if a colicky infant is breastfed, breastfeeding should be continued, but the parents should try to determine whether eating certain foods seems to prompt crying and, if so, eliminate the offending food(s) from her diet. Formula fed infants may benefit from a change in type of formula. In the worst cases of colic, a physician may prescribe medication. Fortunately, most cases disappear spontaneously, possibly because of maturity of the gastrointestinal tract, around 3 months of age. It is important that Katie's parents discuss her condition with her pediatrician before making any decisions about changing her diet.

21. **a)** To calculate the % of kcal in breast milk that come from fat:
First convert grams of fat to fat kcal: 35 g fat/liter × 9 kcal/g = 315 fat kcal/liter.
Then calculate the % of total breast milk kcal from fat: [315 fat kcal divided by 700 total kcal] × 100 (to convert to percentage) = 45% of kcal in breast milk are from fat.
b) To calculate the % of kcal in breast milk that come from protein:
First convert grams of protein to protein kcal: 9 g protein × 4 kcal/g = 36 protein kcal. Then calculate the % of total breast milk kcal from protein: [36 kcal divided by 700 total kcal] × 100 (to convert to percentage) = 5% of kcal from protein.

    45% of kcal from fat is much higher than the range that is recommended for healthy young adults (20–35% of total kcal from fat), but a high fat diet is needed to meet the energy needs of rapidly growing infants. 5% of kcal from protein is much lower that what is recommended for most young adults (10–35% of total kcal from protein), but the kidneys of young infants are immature and not able to excrete large amounts of nitrogen. The small gastric capacity of infants and their relatively immature kidneys explain why the proportions of Calories from fat and protein in breast milk are ideally suited for young infants.

Chapter 18

1. **c.** about 7 mg of iron per day. Toddlers need about 1.1 g/kg of body weight of protein, and about 130 g/day of carbohydrate. Toddlers need about 4 cups of beverages—not 7—per day.

2. **b.** 2 tablespoons of plain full-fat yogurt, 2 tablespoons of applesauce, 2 tablespoons of iron-fortified cooked cereal, and ½ cup of calcium-fortified orange juice. Toddlers need age-appropriate portions of foods that provide a healthful balance of nutrients and do not put them at risk for choking. A cup of oatmeal is too large a portion for a 22-month-old child, as are two eggs and two slices of toast. Both low-fat and skim milk are inappropriate for a 22-month-old child. Cubed pineapple is a choking hazard, as are cherry tomatoes and link sausages cut in 1-inch pieces.

3. **c.** 45% to 65%. A carbohydrate range beginning at either 25% or 35% is too low. Fat should make up 25% to 35% of a child's diet. No single macronutrient should make up 55% to 75% of the diet.

4. **b.** food insecurity; as many as one in five U.S. children is food insecure. Children need less fat per unit of body weight as they mature, and inappropriately low fat intake is not a common problem. As children's GI tracts become populated with beneficial bacteria, their risk for botulism—a problem in infants who eat contaminated honey or corn syrup—declines. Vegetarian diets, including vegan diets, are considered safe and healthful for both toddlers and school-age children, as long as the diets are carefully planned.

5. **a.** Under these programs, students must be offered both fruits and vegetables every day. Sources of competitive foods are allowed if the food they sell meets certain nutritional standards. Although children from families with incomes at or below 185% of the federal poverty threshold do qualify for free or reduced-price meals, not all food-insecure households meet this guideline. In fact, in some U.S. counties, one-third or more of food-insecure families have incomes over 185% of the poverty threshold and therefore do not qualify for either SNAP benefits or free or low-cost school meals.

6. **d.** greater than that for young children, adults, and pregnant adults. This is because adolescence is a critical time for increasing bone density and reducing the risk for osteoporosis.

7. **a.** Cigarette smoking can interfere with the metabolism of nutrients. Consumption of alcohol and the use of certain illegal drugs typically promote food cravings, whereas smoking commonly depresses appetite. The iPLEDGE program is an FDA-mandated program used to ensure that no woman who is pregnant begins using the prescription medication 13-cis retinoic acid (isotretinoin; trade name Accutane) and no woman using the drug becomes pregnant.

8. **b.** Pediatric obesity increases a child's risk for liver disease and type 2 diabetes. About 32% of U.S. children are classified as overweight, not obese. Children whose parents are both overweight/obese are actually four times as likely to be overweight as those with no overweight/obese parent. Toddlers are indeed classified as obese; in fact, currently, 8% of U.S. toddlers are classified as obese.

9. **d.** Take a one-hour hike together on a nearby trail popular with families. Restaurant meals are fine for occasional treats, but they tend to be very high in total energy, saturated fat, and often added sugars, so a more healthful choice would be to prepare a nutritious meal together. Although playing outdoors or taking Lyra and Lyla to scheduled activities would certainly be healthful for the girls, it wouldn't promote their parents' health, nor give them the opportunity to role model the enjoyment to be derived from physical activity. Hiking together would thus be the best choice.

10. **a.** regular sessions with an exercise specialist. Neither orlistat nor metformin has FDA-approval for use in a 7-year-old child, and bariatric surgery is most commonly reserved for adults and older teens, and only rarely has been used in patients as young as age 11, not 7.

11. **True.**

12. **False.** Toddlers mimic older children and adults: if they see their parents enjoying a variety of healthful foods, they will be likely to do so as well. Adults have a significant impact on the nutritional quality of toddler's food choices.

13. **False.** Program meals must meet nutritional standards, but students may or may not eat the foods provided.

14. **True.**

15. **False.** The Institute of Medicine recommends that children participate in aerobic physical activity for at least an hour each day.

16. Toddlers are relatively picky eaters, and they are small individuals and can only consume small amounts of food at any given time. In consuming a vegan diet, the primary sources of quality proteins are restricted to legumes, meat substitutes, and various combinations of vegetables and whole grains. It is highly likely that a vegan diet will be too low in protein for toddlers, as their protein needs are relatively high. Few toddlers can consume enough legumes and whole grains to provide sufficient protein, and many may not prefer the taste of vegetables and meat substitutes. In addition, certain staples of the vegan diet that are high in protein, such as wheat, soy, and nuts, commonly provoke allergic reactions in children. When this happens, finding a plant-based substitute that contains adequate protein and other nutrients can be challenging.

17. There are numerous correct answers to this question. The key to designing a menu for this age group is to keep in mind that these children need adequate fluid, and they

do not eat large amounts of food. The foods should also look fun and attractive to encourage regular snacking and should be easy to eat when the children are active. Here are some foods you may want to offer to these children:

- Ample water in small, colored plastic cups.
- Whole-grain crackers that are small and easy to eat.
- Small chunks of different colors and flavors of cheese to eat with the crackers (or you could make peanut butter/whole-grain cracker "sandwiches").
- Baby carrot sticks.
- Orange slices.

18. Here are three of many lunch choices that you could offer to these students:

- Menu 1: bean burrito with salsa; rice; low/no-fat milk; fresh fruit.
- Menu 2: grilled turkey and muenster cheese sandwich on whole-wheat bread; assorted raw vegetables; pineapple/ orange yogurt fruit smoothie.
- Menu 3: chicken and vegetable teriyaki rice bowl; fruit skewers; low/no-fat milk.

19. A registered dietitian would be concerned about (1) Lydia's monotonous and unbalanced diet, (2) her lack of physical activity, and (3) Lydia's potential homesickness and isolation. Her poor dietary habits are probably contributing to a lack of protein as well as most vitamins and minerals. Her poor diet and the fact that she lives in a northern region almost certainly mean that she is vitamin D deficient, and her consumption of soda rather than milk or a calcium-fortified beverage further increases her risk for low bone density. These deficiencies may also account for some of her lethargy and lack of physical activity. By guiding Lydia toward more healthful meals and menus, she would feel more energetic and be more likely to ride a bicycle, take an activity class, or join a gym. A regular routine of physical activity would probably stimulate Lydia's appetite, encouraging her to consume greater amounts of food, hopefully healthy food! Lydia's move from Vermont to New York could account for her isolation; she may need additional guidance in finding and developing new friendships. If Lydia had always lived at home, where someone else prepared the meals, she would benefit from specific sessions on planning menus, shopping for healthful foods, and preparing daily meals.

20. *Advantages:* improved access to a wider variety of affordable fresh, healthful foods from around the United States and the world; improved access to nutrition and health information from a variety of sources, including television and Internet sources; improved access to interactive nutrition and healthful lifestyle programs that encourage family participation.

Disadvantages: reduced energy expenditure due to increased television viewing and computer use leading to obesity; lower fitness levels and higher risk for chronic diseases due to the lack of physical activity; increased exposure to advertisements promoting junk foods and less healthful foods; failure to acquire important physical skills because not much time is spent engaged in physical activities; inhibition of imagination and creativity in young children because they do not have to develop skills necessary for creative play.

21. 1/3 of 1,300 mg is 433 mg. She would get 230 mg Ca from spinach, 100 mg from the tofu, and 225 mg from the orange juice for a total of 555 mg. Yes, she would meet 1/3rd of her calcium RDA.

Chapter 19

1. **d.** 122 years. This is the oldest age known to have been achieved by a human being. Life expectancy at birth is currently 78.8 years. This is the average age to which a child born in 2012 can be expected to live, and is thus a very different measure from life span, which is the oldest age a human has ever achieved.

2. **c.** glycosylation. This is one of the "errors" identified in the error theories of aging. Xerostomia is dry mouth due to decreased saliva production. Macular degeneration is an age-related vision disorder. Achlorhydria is inadequate hydrochloric acid secretion by the stomach. These are age-related health problems, but not errors that help to explain the process of aging.

3. **a.** smoking. Alcohol consumption, at moderate levels, is not associated with accelerated aging. Excessive consumption of alcohol, excessive energy intake, and a sedentary lifestyle all promote aging, but not as dramatically as smoking.

4. **a.** dysgeusia. The prefix *dys-* means difficult or abnormal. Dysphagia is difficulty swallowing. Dyspnea is difficulty breathing. Dysmorphia is an abnormality in the shape or size of a body structure.

5. **d.** protein. Energy needs are lower in older adults. There is no RDA for adults. The RDA for carbohydrate is the same for adults of all ages.

6. **b.** vitamin D. The requirement for vitamin D is higher because of an age-related reduction in dietary absorption and in the production of vitamin D in the skin. Older adults do not have a higher RDA for vitamin B_{12}; however, it is recommended they consume B_{12} in supplements or fortified foods; alternatively, their healthcare provider may prescribe periodic B_{12} injections. Older adults have the same RDA for vitamin A as younger adults; however, older adults are at increased risk for vitamin A toxicity. Whereas older males have the same RDA for iron as younger males, older females have a greatly decreased RDA for iron.

7. **b.** macular degeneration. Supplements most commonly prescribed for osteoporosis provide calcium and vitamin D. Alzheimer's disease is invariably progressive. Although a nutritious diet might play a limited role in prevention, there is no research suggesting that antioxidant supplements delay the progression.

8. **a.** Consumption of iron supplements can reduce the absorption of certain antibiotics. Actually, consumption of yogurt and other probiotics is commonly recommended when taking antibiotics to help maintain the protective GI flora. Vitamin E supplementation should be avoided by people who are taking "blood thinning" medications such as warfarin, as vitamin E also has an anticlotting activity and therefore taking both simultaneously can increase the risk for bleeding.

9. **c.** food insecurity. The facts that they take advantage of the senior center's free baked goods every week and that their clothing is worn suggest that they may not be able to afford enough nourishing food. They walk together to the senior center, and thus are not immobile. Their independence, demonstrations of affection and caring for each other, and care for their personal appearance suggest that they are not experiencing elder abuse or neglect or social isolation.

10. **c.** palliative care; that is, the care is meant to comfort rather than cure the patient. Long-term care is care provided in a setting meant for rehabilitation or health maintenance, not in a hospital—which is an acute-care setting. Geriatric care is simply care of older adults, and can range from medical and surgical treatment to palliative care. Providing foods and beverages for comfort rather than nutrition is appropriate for terminally ill patients unless contraindicated for another reason.

11. **True.** Nutrition may, however, indirectly reduce some factors in aging, such as by helping to preserve immune function.

12. **True.**

13. **False.** The Institute of Medicine recommends that older adults obtain the DRI for vitamin B_{12} by consuming foods fortified with B_{12} or a B_{12}-containing supplement.

14. **True.**

15. **True.**

16. Lack of adequate stomach acid can lower the absorption of vitamin B12, calcium, iron, and zinc, increasing the risk for deficiencies of these nutrients.

17. Older adults may purposefully limit fluid intake to avoid embarrassing "accidents" due to poor bladder control; they may be taking medications that act as diuretics, increasing urinary output; many elderly fail to perceive thirst and may not drink adequate amounts of fluid during the day; and some elderly may not be able to drink enough fluids due to physical limitations related to a stroke, Parkinson's disease, or other neuromuscular disorders.

18. Osteoarthritis is a condition in which stress on joints over time wears away the protective tissues at the ends of the articulating bones. Obesity increases the load on joints and therefore the risk for osteoarthritis. A weight-loss diet and regular exercise would help Margaret lose weight, which in turn would reduce the stress to her joints. Because water buoys body structures, exercise in water would not increase the stress to Margaret's joints. Swimming is, however, an excellent aerobic activity and would help increase Margaret's cardiorespiratory fitness while expending significant calories.

19. It been shown that this approach can increase or decrease the rate of drug absorption, the rate at which the crushed pill dissolves, and the blood concentration (thus therapeutic effect) of a given medication. Moreover, the high fat content of the milkshake will slow gastric emptying, potentially also increasing or decreasing these factors.

20. **a.** If not fluent in English, an elderly immigrant woman may not be confident enough to go out to shop for food on a regular basis, or she may not qualify for a driver's license, which would affect her ability to obtain food. In both cases, she might have to purchase food from the nearest convenience store (not the best source), and/or simply run low on food, possibly leading to malnutrition. **b.** If isolated, with no Southeast Asian friends or relatives nearby, the woman could easily become depressed, which often results in poor food intake and rapid onset of nutrient deficiencies.

21. To calculate the total vitamin A intake of Kristina's grandmother, add up the amount of Vitamin A in one dose of each of the three supplements: 3333 + 1500 + 2200 = 7033 µg of vitamin A/d.

    To calculate the % of the RDA consumed by Kristina's grandmother, take her daily total intake, divide by the RDA, and multiply by 100 to convert to a percent: [7033 µg ÷ 700 µg] × 100 = 1005% of the RDA, or, 10 times more than the recommended amount.

    To calculate the % of the vitamin A UL consumed by Kristina's grandmother each day, take her daily total intake, divide by the UL, and multiply by 100 to convert to a percent: [7033 µg ÷ 3000 µg] × 100 = 234% of the UL or more than twice the recommended upper limit. This amount of vitamin A, taken on a regular basis, could certainly lead to vitamin A toxicity over time. The UL for adults, including the elderly, is 3,000 µg/day.

    NOTE: These calculations reflect % of the RDA, not % above the RDA.

Glossary

A

Absorption   The process by which molecules of food are taken from the gastrointestinal tract into the circulation.

Acceptable Daily Intake (ADI)   An estimate made by the Food and Drug Administration of the amount of a non-nutritive sweetener that someone can consume each day over a lifetime without adverse effects.

Acceptable Macronutrient Distribution Range (AMDR)   A range of intakes for a particular energy source that is associated with reduced risk of chronic disease while providing adequate intakes of essential nutrients.

Accessory organs of digestion   The salivary glands, liver, pancreas, and gallbladder, which contribute to GI function but are not anatomically part of the GI tract.

acetyl CoA   Coenzyme A (CoA) is derived from the B-vitamin pantothenic acid; it readily reacts with two-carbon acetate to form the metabolic intermediate acetyl CoA; sometimes referred to as *acetyl coenzyme A*.

acetylcholine   A neurotransmitter that is involved in many functions, including muscle movement and memory storage.

achlorhydria   Severely reduced hydrochloric acid secretion by the parietal cells of the stomach.

Acidosis   A disorder in which the blood becomes acidic; that is, the level of hydrogen in the blood is excessive. It can be caused by respiratory or metabolic problems.

Active transport   A transport process that requires the use of energy to shuttle ions and molecules across the cell membrane in combination with a carrier protein.

Added sugars   Sugars and syrups that are added to food during processing or preparation.

adenosine diphosphate (ADP)   A metabolic intermediate that results from the removal of one phosphate group from ATP.

adenosine monophosphate (AMP)   A low-energy compound that results from the removal of two phosphate groups from ATP.

adenosine triphosphate (ATP)   A high-energy compound made up of the purine adenine, the simple sugar ribose, and three phosphate units; it is used by cells as a source of metabolic energy.

Adequate diet   A diet that provides enough of the energy, nutrients, and fiber to maintain a person's health.

Adequate Intake (AI)   A recommended average daily nutrient intake level based on observed or experimentally determined estimates of nutrient intake by a group of healthy people.

aerobic exercise   Exercise that involves the repetitive movement of large muscle groups, increasing the body's use of oxygen and promoting cardiovascular health.

albumin   A serum protein, made in the liver, that transports free fatty acids from one body tissue to another.

Alcohol abuse   A pattern of alcohol consumption, whether chronic or occasional, that results in harm to one's health, functioning, or interpersonal relationships.

Alcohol   Chemically, a compound characterized by the presence of a hydroxyl group; in common usage, a beverage made from fermented fruits, vegetables, or grains and containing ethanol.

alcohol dehydrogenase (ADH)   An enzyme that converts ethanol to acetaldehyde in the first step of alcohol oxidation.

Alcohol dependence   A disease state characterized by alcohol craving, loss of control, physical dependence, and tolerance.

Alcohol hangover   A consequence of drinking too much alcohol; symptoms include headache, fatigue, dizziness, muscle aches, nausea and vomiting, sensitivity to light and sound, extreme thirst, and mood disturbances.

Alcohol poisoning   A potentially fatal condition in which an overdose of alcohol results in cardiac and/or respiratory failure.

Alcoholic hepatitis   A serious condition of inflammation of the liver caused by alcohol.

aldehyde dehydrogenase (ALDH)   An enzyme that oxidizes acetaldehyde to acetate.

aldosterone   A hormone released from the adrenal glands that signals the kidneys to retain sodium and chloride, which in turn results in the retention of water.

Alkalosis   A disorder in which the blood becomes basic; that is, the level of hydrogen in the blood is deficient. It can be caused by respiratory or metabolic problems.

Alpha bond   A type of chemical bond that can be digested by enzymes found in the human intestine.

alpha-linolenic acid (ALA)   An essential fatty acid found in leafy green vegetables, flaxseed oil, soy oil, fish oil, and fish products; an omega-3 fatty acid.

amenorrhea   The absence of menstruation. In females who had previously been menstruating, it is defined as the absence of menstrual periods for 3 or more continuous months.

Amino acids   Nitrogen-containing molecules that combine to form proteins.

amniotic fluid   The watery fluid within the innermost membrane of the sac containing the fetus. It cushions and protects the growing fetus.

anabolic   The characteristic of a substance that builds muscle and increases strength.

anabolism   The process of synthesizing larger molecules from smaller ones.

anencephaly   A fatal neural tube defect in which there is partial absence of brain tissue, most likely caused by failure of the neural tube to close.

angiotensin II   A potent vasoconstrictor that constricts the diameter of blood vessels and increases blood pressure; it also signals the release of the hormone aldosterone from the adrenal glands.

anorexia nervosa   A serious, potentially life-threatening eating disorder that is characterized by self-starvation, which eventually leads to a deficiency in the energy and essential nutrients required by the body to function normally.

Antibodies   Defensive proteins of the immune system. Their production is prompted by the presence of bacteria, viruses, toxins, and allergens.

antidiuretic hormone (ADH)   A hormone released from the pituitary gland in response to an increase in blood solute concentration. ADH stimulates the kidneys to reabsorb water and to reduce the production of urine.

antigens   Parts of a molecule, usually large proteins, from microbes, toxins, or other substances that are recognized by immune cells and activate an immune response.

antioxidant   A compound that has the ability to prevent or repair the damage caused by oxidation.

antiserum   Human or animal serum that contains antibodies to a particular antigen because of previous exposure to the disease or to a vaccine containing antigens from that infectious agent.

Appetite   A psychological desire to consume specific foods.

ariboflavinosis   A condition caused by riboflavin deficiency.

atherosclerosis   A disease in which arterial walls accumulate deposits of lipids and scar tissue, which build up to a point at which they impair blood flow.

atrophic gastritis   A condition, frequently seen in people over the age of 50, in which stomach-acid secretions are low.

atrophy   A decrease in the size and strength of muscles that occurs when they are not worked adequately.

B

B cells White blood cells that can become either antibody-producing plasma cells or memory cells.

bacteria Microorganisms that lack a true nucleus and reproduce by division or by spore formation.

Balanced diet A diet that contains the combinations of foods that provide the proper nutrient proportions.

bariatric surgery Procedure in which the stomach and often the small intestine are surgically altered to induce weight loss.

bariatric surgery Surgical alteration of the gastrointestinal tract performed to promote weight loss.

basal metabolic rate (BMR) The energy the body expends to maintain its fundamental physiologic functions.

Behavioral Risk Factor Surveillance System (BRFSS) The world's largest telephone survey that tracks lifestyle behaviors that increase our risk for chronic disease.

beriberi A disease caused by thiamin deficiency, characterized by muscle wasting and nerve damage.

Beta bond A type of chemical bond that cannot be easily digested by enzymes found in the human intestine.

Bile Fluid produced by the liver and stored in the gallbladder; it emulsifies lipids in the small intestine.

Binge drinking The consumption of five or more alcoholic drinks on one occasion for a man, or four or more drinks for a woman.

binge eating Consumption of a large amount of food in a short period of time, usually accompanied by a feeling of loss of self-control.

binge-eating disorder A disorder characterized by binge eating an average of twice a week or more, typically without compensatory purging.

bioavailability The degree to which the body can absorb and use any given nutrient.

biologic age Physiologic age as determined by health and functional status; often estimated by scored questionnaires.

biomagnification The process by which persistent organic pollutants become more concentrated in animal tissues as they move from one creature to another through the food chain.

biopesticides Primarily insecticides, these chemicals use natural methods to reduce damage to crops. Peeling a fruit reduces its level of pesticide residue; however, you should still scrub fruits before peeling.

bleaching process A reaction in which the rod cells in the retina lose their color when rhodopsin is split into retinal and opsin.

blood volume The amount of fluid in blood.

body composition The ratio of a person's body fat to lean body mass.

body fat mass The amount of body fat, or adipose tissue, a person has.

body image A person's perception of his or her body's appearance and functioning.

body mass index (BMI) A measurement representing the ratio of a person's body weight to his or her height (kg/m^2).

Bolus A mass of food that has been chewed and moistened in the mouth.

bone density The degree of compactness of bone tissue, reflecting the strength of the bones. Peak bone density is the point at which a bone is strongest.

b-oxidation (fatty acid oxidation) A series of metabolic reactions that oxidize free fatty acids, leading to the end products of water, carbon dioxide, and ATP.

brown adipose tissue A type of adipose tissue that has more mitochondria than white adipose tissue and can increase energy expenditure by uncoupling oxidation from ATP production. It is found in significant amounts in animals and newborn humans.

Brush border The microvilli of the small intestine's lining. These microvilli tremendously increase the small intestine's absorptive capacity.

Buffers Proteins that help maintain proper acid–base balance by attaching to, or releasing, hydrogen ions as conditions change in the body.

bulimia nervosa A serious eating disorder characterized by recurrent episodes of binge eating and recurrent inappropriate compensatory behaviors in order to prevent weight gain, such as self-induced vomiting, fasting, excessive exercise, or misuse of laxatives, diuretics, enemas, or other medications.

C

calcitriol The primary active form of vitamin D in the body.

calcium rigor A failure of muscles to relax, which leads to a hardening or stiffening of the muscles; caused by high levels of blood calcium.

calcium tetany A condition in which muscles experience twitching and spasms due to inadequate blood calcium levels.

calorimeter A special instrument in which food can be burned and the amount of heat that is released can be measured; this process demonstrates the energy (caloric) content of the food.

cancer A group of diseases characterized by cells that reproduce spontaneously and independently and may invade other tissues and organs.

carbohydrate loading A process that involves altering training and carbohydrate intake so that muscle glycogen storage is maximized; also known as *glycogen loading*.

Carbohydrates One of the three macronutrients, a compound made up of carbon, hydrogen, and oxygen that is derived from plants and provides energy.

carbon skeleton The unique "side group" that remains after deamination of an amino acid; also referred to as a *keto acid*.

cardiovascular disease A general term that refers to abnormal conditions involving dysfunction of the heart or blood vessels, including coronary heart disease, stroke, and hypertension.

carnitine A small, organic compound that transports free fatty acids from the cytosol into the mitochondria for oxidation.

carotenoid A fat-soluble plant pigment that the body stores in the liver and adipose tissues. The body is able to convert certain carotenoids to vitamin A.

Case-control studies Complex observational studies with additional design features that allow us to gain a better understanding of factors that may influence disease.

cash crops Crops grown to be sold rather than eaten, such as cotton or tobacco.

catabolism The breakdown, or degradation, of larger molecules to smaller molecules.

cataract A damaged portion of the eye's lens, which causes cloudiness that impairs vision.

Celiac disease A disorder characterized by an immune reaction that damages the lining of the small intestine when the individual is exposed to a component of a protein called gluten.

cell differentiation The process by which immature, undifferentiated stem cells develop into highly specialized functional cells of discrete organs and tissues.

Centers for Disease Control and Prevention (CDC) The leading federal agency in the United States that protects the health and safety of people. Its mission is to promote health and quality of life by preventing and controlling disease, injury, and disability.

cephalic phase The earliest phase of digestion, in which the brain thinks about and prepares the digestive organs for the consumption of food.

ceruloplasmin A copper-containing protein that transports copper in the body. It also plays a role in oxidizing ferrous to ferric iron (Fe^{2+} to Fe^{3+}).

Chemical score A method used to estimate a food's protein quality; it is a comparison of the amount of the limiting amino acid in a food to the amount of the same amino acid in a reference food.

cholecalciferol   Vitamin D3, a form of vitamin D found in animal foods and the form we synthesize from the sun.

Chronic disease   A disease characterized by a gradual onset and long duration, with signs and symptoms that are difficult to interpret and that respond poorly to medical treatment.

chylomicron   A lipoprotein produced in the mucosal cell of the intestine; transports dietary fat out of the intestinal tract.

Chyme   A semifluid mass consisting of partially digested food, water, and gastric juices.

Cirrhosis of the liver   End-stage liver disease characterized by significant abnormalities in liver structure and function; may lead to complete liver failure.

climate change   Any significant change in the measures of climate— such as temperature, precipitation, or wind patterns— that occurs over several decades or longer.

Clinical trials   Tightly controlled experiments in which an intervention is given to determine its effect on a certain disease or health condition.

coenzyme   Organic (carboncontaining) cofactor; many coenzymes are derived from B-vitamins.

cofactor   A small, nonprotein substance that enhances or is essential for enzyme action; trace minerals such as iron, zinc, and copper function as cofactors.

colic   A condition of unconsolable infant crying of unknown origin that can last for hours at a time.

collagen   A protein found in all connective tissues in the body.

colostrum   The first fluid made and secreted by the breasts from late in pregnancy to about a week after birth. It is rich in immune factors and protein.

Complementary proteins   Proteins contained in two or more foods that together contain all nine essential amino acids necessary for a complete protein. It is not necessary to eat complementary proteins at the same meal.

Complete proteins   Foods that contain sufficient amounts of all nine essential amino acids.

Complex carbohydrates   A nutrient compound consisting of long chains of glucose molecules, such as starch, glycogen, and fiber.

conception   The uniting of an ovum (egg) and sperm to create a fertilized egg, or zygote; also called fertilization.

Conditionally essential amino acid   Amino acids that are normally considered nonessential but become essential under certain circumstances when the body's need for them exceeds the ability to produce them.

cone cells   Light-sensitive cells found in the retina that contain the pigment iodopsin and react to bright light and interpret color images.

Conflict of interest   A situation in which a person is in a position to derive personal benefit and unfair advantage from actions or decisions made in their official capacity.

Constipation   A condition characterized by the absence of bowel movements for a period of time that is significantly longer than normal for the individual.

cool-down   Activities done after an exercise session is completed; should be gradual and allow your body to slowly recover from exercise.

cortical bone (compact bone)   A dense bone tissue that makes up the outer surface of all bones, as well as the entirety of most small bones of the body.

Covert   A sign or symptom that is hidden from a client and requires laboratory tests or other invasive procedures to detect.

creatine phosphate (CP)   A highenergy compound that can be broken down for energy and used to regenerate ATP.

cretinism   A unique form of mental retardation that occurs in infants when the mother experiences iodine deficiency during pregnancy.

Crohn's disease   A chronic disease that causes inflammation in the small intestine, leading to diarrhea, abdominal pain, rectal bleeding, weight loss, and fever.

crop rotation   The practice of alternating crops in a particular field to prevent nutrient depletion and erosion of the soil and to help with control of crop-specific pests.

cross-contamination   Contamination of one food by another via the unintended transfer of microorganisms through physical contact.

Cystic fibrosis   A genetic disorder that causes an alteration in chloride transport, leading to the production of thick, sticky mucus that causes life threatening respiratory and digestive problems.

cytotoxic T cells   Activated T cells that kill infected body cells.

D

danger zone   The range of temperature (about 40°F to 140°F, or 4°C to 60°C) at which many microorganisms capable of causing human disease thrive.

DASH diet   The Dietary Approaches to Stop Hypertension diet plan emphasizing fruits and vegetables, whole grains, low/no-fat milk and dairy, and lean meats.

***de novo* synthesis**   The process of synthesizing a compound "from scratch."

Deamination   The process by which an amine group is removed from an amino acid. The nitrogen is then transported to the kidneys for excretion in the urine, and the carbon and other components are metabolized for energy or used to make other compounds.

dehydration synthesis   An anabolic process by which smaller, chemically simple compounds are joined and a molecule of water is released; also called *condensation*.

dehydration   The depletion of body fluid, which results when fluid excretion exceeds fluid intake.

dementia   A decline in brain function.

Denaturation   The process by which proteins uncoil and lose their shape and function when they are exposed to heat, acids, bases, heavy metals, alcohol, and other damaging substances.

Diabetes   A chronic disease in which the body can no longer regulate glucose.

Diarrhea   A condition characterized by the frequent passage of loose, watery stools.

Dietary fiber   The nondigestible carbohydrate parts of plants that form the support structures of leaves, stems, and seeds.

Dietary Guidelines for Americans   A set of principles developed by the U.S. Department of Agriculture and the U.S. Department of Health and Human Services to assist Americans in designing a healthful diet and lifestyle.

Dietary Reference Intakes (DRIs)   A set of nutritional reference values for the United States and Canada that applies to healthy people.

Digestion   The process by which foods are broken down into their component molecules, either mechanically or chemically.

direct calorimetry   A method used to determine energy expenditure by measuring the amount of heat released by the body.

Disaccharide   A carbohydrate compound consisting of two monosaccharide molecules joined together.

disordered eating   A general term used to describe a variety of abnormal or atypical eating behaviors that are used to keep or maintain a lower body weight.

diuretic   A substance that increases fluid loss via the urine. Common diuretics include alcohol and prescription medications for high blood pressure and other disorders.

docosahexaenoic acid (DHA)   A metabolic derivative of alpha-linolenic acid; together with EPA, it appears to reduce the risk of heart disease.

doubly labeled water   A form of indirect calorimetry that measures total daily energy expenditure through the rate of carbon dioxide production. It requires the consumption of water that is labeled with nonradioactive isotopes of hydrogen (deuterium, or 2H) and oxygen (18O).

Drink   The amount of an alcoholic beverage that provides approximately 0.5 fl. oz of pure ethanol.

dual-energy x-ray absorptiometry (DXA, DEXA)   Currently the most accurate tool for measuring bone density.

dysgeusia   Abnormal taste perception.

dysphagia   Abnormal swallowing.

E

eating disorder   A clinically diagnosed psychiatric disorder characterized by severe disturbances in body image and eating behaviors.

Edema   A potentially serious disorder in which fluids build up in the tissue spaces of the body, causing fluid imbalances and a swollen appearance.

eicosapentaenoic acid (EPA)   A metabolic derivative of alpha-linolenic acid.

electrolyte   A compound that disassociates in solution into positively and negatively charged ions and is thus capable of conducting an electrical current; the ions in such a solution.

electron transport chain   A series of metabolic reactions that transports electrons from NAHD or FADH2 through a series of carriers, resulting in ATP production.

Elimination   The process by which the undigested portions of food and waste products are removed from the body.

embryo   The human growth and developmental stage lasting from the third week to the end of the eighth week after fertilization.

Empty Calories   Calories from solid fats and/or added sugars that provide few or no nutrients.

Endocytosis   A transport process in which ions and molecules are engulfed by the cell membrane, which folds inwardly and is released in the cell interior (also called pinocytosis).

energy cost of physical activity   The energy that is expended on body movement and muscular work above basal levels.

energy expenditure   The energy the body expends to maintain its basic functions and to perform all levels of movement and activity.

energy intake   The amount of energy a person consumes; in other words, the number of kcal consumed from food and beverages.

Enriched foods   Foods in which nutrients that were lost during processing have been added back, so that the food meets a specified standard.

Enteric nervous system (ENS)   The autonomic nerves in the walls of the GI tract.

Enterocytes   Specialized absorptive cells in the villi of the small intestine.

Enzymes   Small chemicals, usually proteins, that act on other chemicals to speed up bodily processes but are not changed during those processes.

Epidemiological studies   Studies that examine patterns, causes, and effects of health and disease conditions in defined populations.

epiphyseal plates   Plates of cartilage located toward the end of long bones that provide for growth in the length of long bones.

ergocalciferol   Vitamin D2, a form of vitamin D found exclusively in plant foods.

ergogenic aids   Substances used to improve exercise and athletic performance.

error theories of aging   Aging is a cumulative process determined largely by exposure to environmental insults; the fewer the environmental insults, the slower the aging process.

erythrocyte hemolysis   The rupturing or breakdown of red blood cells, or erythrocytes.

erythrocytes   Red blood cells; they transport oxygen in the blood.

Esophagus   A muscular tube of the GI tract connecting the back of the mouth to the stomach.

Essential amino acid   Amino acids not produced by the body, or not produced in sufficient amounts, so they must be obtained from food.

essential fatty acids (EFAs)   Fatty acids that must be consumed in the diet because they cannot be made by the body. The two essential fatty acids are linoleic acid and alpha linolenic acid (ALA).

Estimated Average Requirement (EAR)   The average daily nutrient intake level estimated to meet the requirement of half of the healthy individuals in a particular life stage or gender group.

Estimated Energy Requirement (EER)   The average dietary energy intake that is predicted to maintain energy balance in a healthy individual.

Ethanol   A specific alcohol compound (C_2H_5OH) formed from the fermentation of dietary carbohydrates and used in a variety of alcoholic beverages.

evaporative cooling   Sweating, which is the primary way in which the body dissipates heat.

exercise   A subcategory of leisuretime physical activity; any activity that is purposeful, planned, and structured.

extracellular fluid   The fluid outside of the body's cells, either in the body's tissues (interstitial fluid) or as the liquid portion of the blood or lymph (intravascular fluid).

F

Facilitated diffusion   A transport process in which ions and molecules are shuttled across the cell membrane with the help of a carrier protein.

failure to thrive (FTT)   A condition in which an infant's weight gain and growth are far below typical levels for age and previous patterns of growth, for reasons that are unclear or unexplained.

fair trade   A trading partnership promoting equity in international trading relationships and contributing to sustainable development by securing the rights of marginalized producers and workers.

famine   A severe food shortage affecting a large percentage of the population in a limited geographic area at a particular time.

fat-soluble vitamins   Vitamins that are not soluble in water but are soluble in fat; these include vitamins A, D, E, and K.

Fat-soluble vitamins   Vitamins that are not soluble in water but soluble in fat. These include vitamins A, D, E, and K.

fatty acid   An acid composed of a long chain of carbon atoms bound to each other as well as to hydrogen atoms, with a carboxyl group at the alpha end of the chain

Fatty liver   An early and reversible stage of liver disease often found in people who abuse alcohol, characterized by the abnormal accumulation of fat within liver, and cells; also called alcoholic steatosis.

female athlete triad   A syndrome that consists of three clinical conditions in some physically active females: low energy availability (with or without eating disorders), menstrual dysfunction, and low bone density.

Fermentation   The anaerobic process in which an agent causes an organic substance to break down into simpler substances and results in the production of ATP.

ferritin   A storage form of iron found primarily in the intestinal mucosa, spleen, bone marrow, and liver.

ferroportin   An iron transporter that helps regulate intestinal iron absorption and the release of iron from the enterocyte into the general circulation.

Fetal alcohol spectrum disorders (FASD)   An umbrella designation for a wide range of clinical outcomes that can result from prenatal exposure to alcohol. Fetal alcohol syndrome (FAS), alcohol-related neurodevelopmental disorder (ARND), and alcohol-related birth defects (ARBD) are components of FASD.

Fetal alcohol syndrome (FAS)   A set of serious, irreversible alcohol-related birth defects characterized by certain physical and mental abnormalities, including malformations of the face, limbs, heart, and nervous system; impaired growth; and a spectrum of mild to severe cognitive, emotional, and physical problems.

fetus The human growth and developmental stage lasting from the beginning of the ninth week after conception to birth.

Fiber-rich carbohydrates A group of foods containing either simple or complex carbohydrates that are rich in dietary fiber. These foods, which include most fruits, vegetables, and whole grains, are typically fresh or moderately processed.

FITT principle The principle used to achieve an appropriate overload for physical training; FITT stands for *f*requency, *i*ntensity, *t*ime, and *t*ype of activity.

flavin adenine dinucleotide (FAD) A coenzyme derived from the B-vitamin riboflavin; FAD readily accepts electrons (hydrogen) from various donors.

fluid A substance composed of molecules that move past one another freely. Fluids are characterized by their ability to conform to the shape of whatever container holds them.

fluorohydroxyapatite A mineral compound in human teeth that contains fluoride, calcium, and phosphorus and is more resistant to destruction by acids and bacteria than hydroxyapatite.

fluorosis A condition characterized by staining and pitting of the teeth; caused by an abnormally high intake of fluoride.

food additive A substance or mixture of substances intentionally put into food to enhance its appearance, safety, palatability, and quality.

Food allergy An allergic reaction to food, caused by a reaction of the immune system.

food desert A geographic area where people lack access to fresh, healthy, and affordable food.

food diversity The variety of different species of food crops available.

food insecurity Unreliable access to a sufficient supply of nourishing food.

Food intolerance Gastrointestinal discomfort caused by certain foods that is not a result of an immune system reaction

Food The plants and animals we consume.

foodborne illness An illness transmitted by food or water contaminated by a pathogenic microorganism, its toxic secretions, or a toxic chemical.

Fortified foods Foods in which nutrients are added that did not originally exist in the food or existed in insignificant amounts.

free radical A highly unstable atom with an unpaired electron in its outermost shell, or the molecule in which such an atom occurs.

frequency Refers to the number of activity sessions per week you perform.

Fructose The sweetest natural sugar; a monosaccharide that occurs in fruits and vegetables; also called *levulose*, or *fruit sugar*.

Functional fiber The nondigestible forms of carbohydrate that are extracted from plants or manufactured in the laboratory and have known health benefits.

Functional foods Foods that may have biologically active ingredients with the potential to provide health benefits beyond providing energy and nutrients necessary to sustain life.

fungi Plantlike, spore-forming organisms that can grow as either single cells or multicellular colonies.

G

Galactose A monosaccharide that joins with glucose to create lactose, one of the three most common disaccharides.

Gallbladder A pear-shaped organ beneath the liver that stores bile and secretes it into the small intestine.

Gastric juice Acidic liquid secreted within the stomach; it contains hydrochloric acid, pepsin, and other compounds.

Gastroesophageal reflux disease (GERD) A painful type of heartburn that occurs more than twice per week.

Gastrointestinal (GI) system The body system responsible for digestion, absorption, and elimination. It includes the organs of the GI tract and the accessory organs.

Gastrointestinal (GI) tract A long, muscular tube consisting of several organs: the mouth, pharynx, esophagus, stomach, small intestine, and large intestine.

Gene expression The process of using a gene to make a protein.

Generally Recognized as Safe (GRAS) A list established by Congress to identify substances used in foods that are generally recognized as safe based on a history of long-term use or on the consensus of qualified research experts.

genetic modification The process of changing an organism by manipulating its genetic material.

gestation The period of intrauterine development from conception to birth.

gestational diabetes Insufficient insulin production or insulin resistance that results in consistently high blood glucose levels, specifically during pregnancy; the condition typically resolves after birth occurs.

ghrelin A protein synthesized in the stomach that acts as a hormone and plays an important role in appetite regulation by stimulating appetite.

global warming The increase of about 1.4°F (0.8°C) in temperature that has occurred near the Earth's surface over the past century.

Glucagon A hormone secreted by the alpha cells of the pancreas in response to decreased blood levels of glucose; it stimulates the liver to convert stored glycogen into glucose, which is released into the bloodstream and transported to cells for energy.

glucogenic amino acid An amino acid that can be converted to glucose via gluconeogenesis.

glucokinase An enzyme that adds a phosphate group to a molecule of glucose.

gluconeogenesis The synthesis of glucose from noncarbohydrate precursors, such as glucogenic amino acids and glycerol.

Glucose The most abundant sugar molecule, a monosaccharide generally found in combination with other sugars; the preferred source of energy for the brain and an important source of energy for all cells.

glutathione (GSH) A tripeptide composed of glycine, cysteine, and glutamic acid that assists in regenerating vitamin C into its antioxidant form.

Glycemic index A rating of the potential of foods to raise blood glucose and insulin levels.

Glycemic load The amount of carbohydrate in a food multiplied by the glycemic index of the carbohydrate.

glycerol An alcohol composed of three carbon atoms; it is the backbone of a triglyceride molecule.

Glycogen The storage form of glucose (as a polysaccharide) in animals.

glycolysis A sequence of chemical reactions that converts glucose to pyruvate.

glycosylation The addition of glucose to blood and tissue proteins; typically impairs protein structure and function.

goiter Enlargement of the thyroid gland; can be caused by iodine toxicity or deficiency.

grazing Consistently eating small meals throughout the day; done by many athletes to meet their high energy demands.

Green Revolution The tremendous increase in global productivity between 1944 and 2000 due to selective cross-breeding or hybridization to produce highyield grains and industrial farming techniques.

H

Haustration Involuntary, sluggish contraction of the haustra of the proximal colon, which moves wastes toward the sigmoid colon.

Healthful diet A diet that provides the proper combination of energy and nutrients and is adequate, moderate, balanced, and varied.

Heartburn The painful sensation that occurs over the sternum when gastric juice backs up into the lower esophagus.

heat cramps Muscle spasms that occur several hours after strenuous exercise; most often occur when sweat losses and fluid intakes are high, urine volume is low, and sodium intake is inadequate.

heat exhaustion A heat illness characterized by excessive sweating, weakness, nausea, dizziness, headache, and difficulty concentrating. Unchecked, heat exhaustion can lead to heat stroke.

heat stroke A potentially fatal heat illness characterized by hot, dry skin; rapid heart rate; vomiting; diarrhea; elevated body temperature; hallucinations; and coma.

heat syncope Dizziness that results from blood pooling in the lower extremities; often results from standing too long in hot weather, standing rapidly from a lying position, or stopping suddenly after physical exertion.

helminth A multicellular microscopic worm.

helper T cells Activated T cells that secrete chemicals needed to recruit, promote, or activate other immune cells. Natural killer (NK) cells are part of our nonspecific defenses. Here, an NK cell attacks two cancer cells.

heme The iron-containing molecule found in hemoglobin and myoglobin.

heme iron Iron that is a part of hemoglobin and myoglobin; it is found only in animal-based foods, such as meat, fish, and poultry.

hemoglobin The oxygen-carrying protein found in red blood cells; almost two-thirds of all of the iron in the body is found in hemoglobin.

hemosiderin A storage form of iron found primarily in the intestinal mucosa, spleen, bone marrow, and liver.

hephaestin A copper-containing protein that oxidizes Fe^{2+} to Fe^{3+} once iron is transported across the basolateral membrane by ferroportin.

high-density lipoprotein (HDL) A lipoprotein made in the liver and released into the blood. HDLs function to transport cholesterol from the tissues back to the liver; often called "good cholesterol."

high-fructose corn syrup A type of corn syrup in which part of the sucrose is converted to fructose, making it sweeter than sucrose or regular corn syrup; most high-fructose corn syrup contains 42% to 55% fructose.

high-yield varieties Semi-dwarf varieties of plants that are unlikely to fall over in wind and heavy rains and thus can carry larger amounts of seeds, greatly increasing the yield per acre.

homocysteine An amino acid that requires adequate levels of folate, vitamin B6 and vitamin B12 for its metabolism. High levels of homocysteine in the blood are associated with an increased risk for cardiovascular disease.

Hormones A chemical messenger that is secreted into the bloodstream by one of the many endocrine glands of the body. Hormones act as regulators of physiologic processes at sites remote from the glands that secreted them.

hospice Supportive care provided to individuals at end-of-life; a program providing such care.

Hunger A physiologic sensation that prompts us to eat.

hydrogenation The process of adding hydrogen to unsaturated fatty acids, making them more saturated and thereby more solid at room temperature.

hydrolysis A catabolic process by which a large, chemically complex compound is broken apart with the addition of water.

hypercalcemia A condition characterized by an abnormally high concentration of calcium in the blood.

Hyperglycemia A condition in which blood glucose levels are higher than normal.

hyperkalemia A condition in which blood potassium levels are dangerously high.

hyperkeratosis A condition resulting in the excess accumulation of the protein keratin in the follicles of the skin; this condition can also impair the ability of epithelial tissues to produce mucus.

hypermagnesemia A condition marked by an abnormally high concentration of magnesium in the blood.

hypernatremia A condition in which blood sodium levels are dangerously high.

hypertension A chronic condition characterized by above-average blood pressure readings—specifically, systolic blood pressure over 140 mm Hg or diastolic blood pressure over 90 mm Hg.

hyperthyroidism A condition characterized by high blood levels of thyroid hormone.

hypertrophy The increase in strength and size that results from repeated work to a specific muscle or muscle group.

hypocalcemia A condition characterized by an abnormally low concentration of calcium in the blood.

Hypoglycemia A condition marked by blood glucose levels that are below normal fasting levels.

hypokalemia A condition in which blood potassium levels are dangerously low.

hypomagnesemia A condition characterized by an abnormally low concentration of magnesium in the blood.

hyponatremia A condition in which blood sodium levels are dangerously low.

Hypothalamus A region of the brain below (*hypo-*) the thalamus and cerebral hemispheres and above the pituitary gland and brain stem where visceral sensations such as hunger and thirst are regulated.

Hypothesis An educated guess as to why a phenomenon occurs.

hypothyroidism A condition characterized by low blood levels of thyroid hormone.

I

immunocompetence The body's ability to adequately produce an effective immune response to an antigen.

Impaired fasting glucose Fasting blood glucose levels that are higher than normal but not high enough to lead to a diagnosis of type 2 diabetes.

Incidence The rate of new (or newly diagnosed) cases of a disease within a period of time.

Incomplete proteins Foods that do not contain all of the essential amino acids in sufficient amounts to support growth and health.

indirect calorimetry A method used to estimate energy expenditure by measuring oxygen consumption and carbon dioxide production.

infant mortality A population's rate of death of infants between birth and 1 year of age.

Inorganic A substance or nutrient that does not contain carbon and hydrogen.

insensible fluid loss The unperceived loss of body fluid, such as through evaporation from the skin and exhalation from the lungs during breathing.

Insoluble fibers Fibers that do not dissolve in water.

Insulin A hormone secreted by the beta cells of the pancreas in response to increased blood levels of glucose that facilitates uptake of glucose by body cells.

intensity The amount of effort expended during an activity, or how difficult the activity is to perform.

interstitial fluid The fluid that flows between the cells that make up a particular tissue or organ, such as muscle fibers or the liver.

intracellular fluid The fluid held at any given time within the walls of the body's cells.

intravascular fluid The fluid in the bloodstream and lymph.

intrinsic factor A protein secreted by cells of the stomach that binds to vitamin B12 and aids its absorption in the small intestine.

invisible fats Fats that are hidden in foods, such as the fats found in baked goods, regular-fat dairy products, marbling in meat, and fried foods.

iodopsin A color-sensitive pigment found in the cone cells of the retina.

ion   Any electrically charged particle, either positively or negatively charged.

iron depletion (stage I)   The first phase of iron deficiency, characterized by a decrease in stored iron, which results in a decrease in blood ferritin levels.

iron-deficiency anemia (stage III)   A form of anemia that results from severe iron deficiency.

iron-deficiency erythropoiesis (stage II)   The second stage of iron deficiency, characterized by a decrease in the transport of iron in the blood and an increase in total iron binding capacity.

irradiation   A sterilization process in which food is exposed to gamma rays or high-energy electron beams to kill microorganisms. Irradiation does not impart any radiation to the food being treated.

Irritable bowel syndrome (IBS)   A stress-related disorder that interferes with normal functions of the colon. Symptoms are abdominal cramps, bloating, and constipation or diarrhea.

K

Keshan disease   A heart disorder caused by selenium deficiency. It was first identified in children in the Keshan province of China.

keto acid   The chemical structure that remains after deamination of an amino acid.

Ketoacidosis   A condition in which excessive ketones are present in the blood, causing the blood to become very acidic, which alters basic body functions and damages tissues. Untreated ketoacidosis can be fatal. This condition is often found in individuals with untreated diabetes mellitus.

ketogenic amino acid   An amino acid that can be converted to acetyl CoA for the synthesis of free fatty acids.

ketone bodies   Three- and fourcarbon compounds (acetoacetate, acetone, and ⊠- or 3-hydroxybutyrate) derived when acetyl CoA levels become elevated.

Ketones   Substances produced during the breakdown of fat when carbohydrate intake is insufficient to meet energy needs. They provide an alternative energy source for the brain when glucose levels are low.

Ketosis   The process by which the breakdown of fat during fasting states results in the production of ketones.

Kwashiorkor   A form of protein– energy malnutrition that is typically seen in developing countries in infants and toddlers who are weaned early. Denied breast milk, they are fed a cereal diet that provides adequate energy but inadequate protein.

L

Lactase   A digestive enzyme that breaks lactose into glucose and galactose.

lactate (lactic acid)   A three-carbon compound produced from pyruvate in oxygen-deprived conditions.

lactation   The production of breast milk.

Lacteal   A small lymphatic vessel located inside the villi of the small intestine.

Lactose   Also called *milk sugar,* a disaccharide consisting of one glucose molecule and one galactose molecule; found in milk, including human breast milk.

Lactose intolerance   A disorder in which the body does not produce sufficient lactase enzyme and therefore cannot digest foods that contain lactose, such as cow's milk.

large for gestational age (LGA)   A birth weight that falls above the 90th percentile for gestational age.

Large intestine   The final organ of the GI tract, consisting of the cecum, colon, rectum, and anal canal and in which most water is absorbed and feces are formed.

lean body mass   The amount of fat-free tissue, or bone, muscle, and internal organs, a person has.

leisure-time physical activity   Any activity not related to a person's occupation; includes competitive sports, recreational activities, and planned exercise training.

leptin   A hormone, produced by body fat, that acts to reduce food intake and to decrease body weight and body fat.

leukocytes   White blood cells; they are important to immune functions.

Levulose   Another term for fructose,or fruit sugar.

life expectancy   The expected number of years remaining in one's life; typically stated from the time of birth. Children born in the United States in 2012 can expect to live, on average, 78.8 years.

life span   The highest age reached by any member of a species; currently, the human life span is 122 years.

Limiting amino acid   The essential amino acid that is missing or in the smallest supply in the amino acid pool and is thus responsible for slowing or halting protein synthesis.

linoleic acid   An essential fatty acid found in vegetable and nut oils; an omega-6 fatty acid.

lipids   A diverse group of organic substances that are insoluble in water; lipids include triglycerides, phospholipids, and sterols.

lipogenesis   The synthesis of free fatty acids from nonlipid precursors, such as ketogenic amino acids or ethanol.

lipolysis   The enzyme-driven catabolism of triglycerides into free fatty acids and glycerol.

lipoprotein   A spherical compound in which fat clusters in the center and phospholipids and proteins form the outside of the sphere.

lipoprotein lipase   An enzyme that sits on the outside of cells and breaks apart triglycerides, so that their fatty acids can be removed and taken up by the cell.

Listeriosis   Potentially fatal foodborne illness caused by infection with the bacterium *Listeria monocytogenes.*

Liver   The largest accessory organ of the GI tract and one of the most important organs of the body. Its functions include the production of bile and processing of nutrient-rich blood from the small intestine.

long-chain fatty acids   Fatty acids that are 14 or more carbon atoms in length.

low birth weight   An infant weight of less than 5.5 lb at birth.

low-density lipoprotein (LDL)   A lipoprotein formed in the blood from VLDLs that transports cholesterol to the cells of the body; often called "bad cholesterol."

low-intensity activities   Activities that cause very mild increases in breathing, sweating, and heart rate.

M

macrocytic anemia   A form of anemia manifested as the production of larger than normal red blood cells containing insufficient hemoglobin; also called megaloblastic anemia. Macrocytic anemia can be caused by folate deficiency or vitamin B12 deficiency.

Macronutrients   Nutrients that the body requires in relatively large amounts to support normal function and health. Carbohydrates, lipids, proteins, and water are macronutrients.

macular degeneration   A vision disorder caused by deterioration of the central portion of the retina and marked by loss or distortion of the central field of vision.

Major minerals   Minerals we need to consume in amounts of at least 100 mg per day and of which the total amount in our body is at least 5 g (5,000 mg).

Malnutrition   A nutritional status that is out of balance; an individual is either getting too much or not enough of a particular nutrient or energy over a significant period of time.

Maltase   A digestive enzyme that breaks maltose into glucose.

Maltose   A disaccharide consisting of two molecules of glucose; does not generally occur independently in foods but results as a by-product of digestion; also called *malt sugar.*

Mannitol   A type of sugar alcohol.

Marasmus   A form of protein–energy malnutrition that results from grossly inadequate intakes of protein, energy, and other nutrients.

Mass movement   Involuntary, sustained, forceful contraction of the colon that occurs two or more times a day to push wastes toward the rectum.

maternal mortality   A population's rate of deaths of a woman during pregnancy, childbirth, or in the immediate postpartal period.

matrix Gla protein   A vitamin K–dependent protein located in the protein matrix of bone and in cartilage, blood-vessel walls, and other soft tissues.

maximal heart rate   The rate at which the heart beats during maximal-intensity exercise.

meat factor   A special factor found in meat, fish, and poultry that enhances the absorption of nonheme iron.

medium-chain fatty acids   Fatty acids that are 6 to 12 carbon atoms in length.

megadosing   Taking a dose of a nutrient that is ten or more times greater than the recommended amount.

memory cells   White blood cells that recognize a particular antigen and circulate in the body, ready to respond if the antigen is encountered again. The purpose of vaccination is to create memory cells.

menaquinone   The form of vitamin K produced by bacteria in the large intestine.

menarche   The onset of menstruation, or the menstrual period.

metabolic syndrome   A clustering of risk factors that increase one's risk for heart disease, type 2 diabetes, and stroke, including abdominal obesity, higher-than-normal triglyceride levels, lower-than-normal HDL-cholesterol levels, higher-than-normal blood pressure (greater than or equal to 130/85 mm Hg), and elevated fasting blood glucose levels.

metabolic water   The water formed as a by-product of the body's metabolic reactions.

metabolism   The sum of all the chemical and physical processes by which the body breaks down and builds up molecules.

metallothionein   A zinc-containing protein within the enterocyte; it assists in the regulation of zinc homeostasis.

micelle   A spherical compound made up of bile salts and biliary phospholipids that transports lipid digestion products to the intestinal mucosal cell.

microcytic anemia   A form of anemia manifested as the production of smaller than normal red blood cells containing insufficient hemoglobin, which reduces the red blood cell's ability to transport oxygen; it can result from iron deficiency or vitamin B6 deficiency.

Micronutrients   Nutrients needed in relatively small amounts to support normal health and body functions. Vitamins and minerals are micronutrients.

microsomal ethanol oxidizing system (MEOS)   A liver enzyme system that oxidizes ethanol to acetaldehyde; its activity predominates at higher levels of alcohol intake.

mindful eating   The nonjudgmental awareness of the emotional and physical sensations one experiences while eating or in a food-related environment.

Minerals   Naturally occurring elements essential for the formation of blood, bone, many enzymes, and other critical compounds; classified as major, trace, or ultra-trace.

Moderate drinking   Alcohol consumption of up to one drink per day for women and up to two drinks per day for men.

moderate-intensity activities   Activities that cause moderate increases in breathing, sweating, and heart rate.

Moderation   Eating any foods in moderate amounts—not too much and not too little.

Monosaccharide   The simplest of carbohydrates; consists of one sugar molecule, the most common form of which is glucose.

monounsaturated fatty acids (MUFAs)   Fatty acids that have two carbons in the chain bound to each other with one double bond; these types of fatty acids are generally liquid at room temperature.

morbid obesity   A condition in which a person's body weight exceeds 100% of normal, putting him or her at very high risk for serious health consequences; a BMI = 40 kg/m^2.

morning sickness   A condition characterized by varying degrees of nausea and vomiting associated with pregnancy, most commonly in the first trimester.

multifactorial disease   A disease that may be attributable to one or more of a variety of causes.

muscle cramps   Involuntary, spasmodic, and painful muscle contractions that last for many seconds or even minutes; electrolyte imbalances are often the cause of muscle cramps.

Mutual supplementation   The process of combining two or more incomplete protein sources to make a complete protein.

myoglobin   An iron-containing protein found in muscle cells.

MyPlate   The visual representation of the USDA Food Patterns.

N

National Health and Nutrition Examination Survey (NHANES)   A survey conducted by the National Center for Health Statistics and the CDC; this survey tracks the nutrient and food consumption of Americans.

National Institutes of Health (NIH)   The world's leading medical research center and the focal point for medical research in the United States.

neonatal   Referring to a newborn.

neural tube   Embryonic tissue that forms a tube, which eventually becomes the brain and spinal cord.

Neurotransmitters   Chemical messengers that transmit messages from one nerve cell to another.

nicotinamide adenine dinucleotide (NAD)   A coenzyme form of the B-vitamin niacin; NAD readily accepts electrons (hydrogen) from various donors.

night blindness   A vitamin A– deficiency disorder that results in loss of the ability to see in dim light.

night-eating syndrome   Disorder characterized by intake of the majority of the day's energy between 8:00 pm and 6:00 am. Individuals with this disorder also experience mood and sleep disorders.

Nonessential amino acids   Amino acids that can be manufactured by the body in sufficient quantities and therefore do not need to be consumed regularly in our diet.

nonheme iron   The form of iron that is not a part of hemoglobin or myoglobin; it is found in animal based and plant-based foods.

Non-nutritive sweeteners   Also called *alternative sweeteners;* manufactured sweeteners that provide little or no energy.

nonspecific immune function   Generalized body defenses including tissues, mechanisms, and cells that protect against the entry or reproduction of non-self agents, such as microbes, toxins, and body cells with mutated DNA; also called innate immunity.

normal weight   Having an adequate but not excessive level of body fat for health.

Nucleotide   A molecule composed of a phosphate group, a pentose sugar called deoxyribose, and one of four nitrogenous bases: adenine (A), guanine (G), cytosine (C), or thymine (T).

Nutrient density   The relative amount of nutrients per amount of energy (number of Calories).

Nutrientdense foods   Foods that provide the highest level of nutrients for the least amount of energy (Calories).

Nutrients   Chemicals found in foods that are critical to human growth and function.

Nutrition   The scientific study of food and how it nourishes the body and influences health.

Nutrition Facts panel   The label on a food package containing the nutrition information required by the FDA.

nutrition paradox   The coexistence of aspects of both stunting and overweight/obesity within the same region, household, family, or person.

Nutritive sweeteners   Sweeteners, such as sucrose, fructose, honey, and brown sugar, that contribute Calories (energy).

O

obesity   Having an excess of body fat that adversely affects health, resulting in a person having a weight that is substantially greater than some accepted standard for a given height; a BMI of 30 to 39.9 kg/m².

Observational studies   Types of epidemiological studies that indicate relationships between nutrition habits, disease trends, and other health phenomena of large populations of humans.

Oligosaccharides   Complex carbohydrates that contain 3 to 10 monosaccharides.

opsin   A protein that combines with retinal in the retina to form rhodopsin.

Organic   A substance or nutrient that contains the elements carbon and hydrogen.

osmosis   The movement of water (or any solvent) through a semipermeable membrane from an area where solutes are less concentrated to areas where they are highly concentrated.

osmotic pressure   The pressure that is needed to keep the particles in a solution from drawing liquid toward them across a semipermeable membrane.

osteoblasts   Cells that prompt the formation of new bone matrix by laying down the collagen-containing component of bone, which is then mineralized.

osteocalcin   A vitamin K–dependent protein that is secreted by osteoblasts and is associated with bone turnover.

osteoclasts   Cells that erode the surface of bones by secreting enzymes and acids that dig grooves into the bone matrix.

osteomalacia   A vitamin D– deficiency disease in adults, in which bones become weak and prone to fractures.

osteoporosis   A disease characterized by low bone mass and deterioration of bone tissue, leading to increased bone fragility and fracture risk.

Ounce-equivalent (oz-equivalent)   A serving size that is 1 ounce, or equivalent to an ounce, for the grains and the protein foods sections of MyPlate.

overhydration   The dilution of body fluid. It results when water intake or retention is excessive.

overload principle   Placing an extra physical demand on your body in order to improve your fitness level.

Overnutrition   A situation in which too much energy or too much of a given nutrient is consumed over time, causing conditions such as obesity, heart disease, or nutrient-toxicity symptoms.

overpopulation   Condition in which a region's available resources are insufficient to support the number of people living there.

Overt   A sign or symptom that is obvious to a client, such as pain, fatigue, or a bruise.

overweight   Having a moderate amount of excess body fat, resulting in a person having a weight that is greater than some accepted standard for a given height but is not considered obese; a BMI of 25 to 29.9 kg/m².

oxidation   A chemical reaction in which molecules of a substance are broken down into their component atoms. During oxidation, the atoms involved lose electrons.

oxidation–reduction reactions   Reactions in which electrons are lost by one compound (it is oxidized) and simultaneously gained by another compound (it is reduced).

P

palliative care   Patient care aimed at reducing an individual's pain and discomfort without attempting to treat or cure.

Pancreas   A gland located behind the stomach that secretes digestive enzymes.

Pancreatic amylase   An enzyme secreted by the pancreas into the small intestine that digests any remaining starch into maltose.

parasite   A microorganism that simultaneously derives benefit from and harms its host.

parathyroid hormone (PTH)   A hormone secreted by the parathyroid gland when blood calcium levels fall. It is also known as parathormone, and it increases blood calcium levels by stimulating the activation of vitamin D, increasing reabsorption of calcium from the kidneys, and stimulating osteoclasts to break down bone, which releases more calcium into the bloodstream.

Passive diffusion   A transport process in which ions and molecules, following their concentration gradient, cross the cell membrane without the use of a carrier protein or the requirement of energy.

pasteurization   A form of sterilization using high temperatures for short periods of time.

pellagra   A disease that results from severe niacin deficiency.

Pepsin   An enzyme in the stomach that begins the breakdown of proteins into shorter polypeptide chains and single amino acids.

Peptic ulcer   An area of the GI tract that has been eroded away by the acidic gastric juice of the stomach. The two main causes of peptic ulcers are *Helicobacter pylori* infection and the use of non-steroidal anti-inflammatory drugs.

Peptide bond   Unique types of chemical bond in which the amine group of one amino acid binds to the acid group of another in order to manufacture dipeptides and all larger peptide molecules.

peptide YY (PYY)   A protein produced in the gastrointestinal tract that is released after a meal in amounts proportional to the energy content of the meal; it decreases appetite and inhibits food intake.

Percent daily values (%DVs)   Information on a Nutrition Facts panel that identifies how much a serving of food contributes to your overall intake of nutrients listed on the label; based on an energy intake of 2,000 Calories per day.

Peristalsis   Waves of squeezing and pushing contractions that move food, chyme, and feces in one direction through the length of the GI tract.

pernicious anemia   A form of macrocytic anemia that is the primary cause of a vitamin B12 deficiency; occurs at the end stage of an autoimmune disorder that causes the loss of various cells in the stomach.

persistent organic pollutants (POPs)   Chemicals released as a result of human activity into the environment, where they persist for years or decades.

pesticides   Chemicals used either in the field or in storage to decrease destruction and crop losses by weeds, predators, or disease.

phospholipids   A type of lipid in which a fatty acid is combined with another compound that contains phosphate; unlike other lipids, phospholipids are soluble in water.

phosphorylation   The addition of one or more phosphate groups to a chemical compound.

Photosynthesis   A process by which plants use sunlight to fuel a chemical reaction that combines carbon and water into glucose, which is then stored in their cells.

phylloquinone   The form of vitamin K found in plants.

physical activity   Any movement produced by muscles that increases energy expenditure; includes occupational, household, leisure-time, and transportation activities.

physical fitness   The ability to carry out daily tasks with vigor and alertness, without undue fatigue, and with ample energy to enjoy leisuretime pursuits and meet unforeseen emergencies.

phytic acid   The form of phosphorus stored in plants.

phytochemicals   Compounds found in plants and believed to have health-promoting effects in humans.

pica   An abnormal craving to eat various nonfood substances, such as clay, chalk, or soap.

placenta   A pregnancy-specific organ formed from both maternal and embryonic tissues. It is responsible for oxygen, nutrient, and waste exchange between mother and fetus.

plasma   The fluid (noncellular) portion of the blood.

plasma cells   White blood cells that have differentiated from activated B cells and produce millions of antibodies to an antigen during an infection.

platelets   Cell fragments that aggregate to form blood clots that help slow or stop bleeding.

polypharmacy   The concurrent use of five or more medications.

Polysaccharides   A complex carbohydrate consisting of long chains of glucose.

polyunsaturated fatty acids (PUFAs)   Fatty acids that have more than one double bond in the chain; these types of fatty acids are generally liquid at room temperature.

Portal venous system   A system of blood vessels that drains blood and various products of digestion from the digestive organs and spleen and delivers them to the liver.

poverty–obesity paradox   The high prevalence of obesity in low-income populations.

prediabetes   A term used synonymously with *impaired fasting glucose;* it is a condition considered to be a major risk factor for both type 2 diabetes and heart disease.

preeclampsia   High blood pressure that is pregnancy-specific and accompanied by protein in the urine, edema, and unexpected weight gain.

preterm   The birth of a baby prior to 38 weeks of gestation.

Prevalence   The percentage of the population that is affected with a particular disease at a given time.

Primary deficiency   A deficiency that occurs when not enough of a nutrient is consumed in the diet.

prion   A pathogenic form of a normal and protective protein that misfolds and becomes infectious and destructive; prions are not living cellular organisms or viruses.

Probiotics   Microorganisms, typically bacteria, theorized to benefit human health.

Processed foods   Includes foods that are fortified, enriched, or enhanced, such as orange juice with added calcium and vitamin D, or bread enriched with folate.

programmed theories of aging   Aging is biologically determined, following a predictable pattern of physiologic changes, although the timing may vary from one person to another.

Proof   A measure of the alcohol content of a liquid; 100-proof liquor is 50% alcohol by volume, 80-proof liquor is 40% alcohol by volume, and so on.

prooxidant   A nutrient that promotes oxidation and oxidative damage of cells and tissues.

Proteases   Enzymes that continue the breakdown of polypeptides in the small intestine.

Protein digestibility corrected amino acid score (PDCAAS)   A measurement of protein quality that considers the balance of amino acids as well as the digestibility of the protein in the food.

Protein–energy malnutrition   A disorder caused by inadequate consumption of protein. It is characterized by severe wasting.

Proteins   Large, complex molecules made up of amino acids and found as essential components of all living cells.

proteolysis   The breakdown of dietary proteins into single amino acids or small peptides that are absorbed by the body.

protozoa   Single-celled, mobile parasites.

provitamin   An inactive form of a vitamin that the body can convert to an active form. An example is beta-carotene.

puberty   The period in life in which secondary sexual characteristics develop and the body becomes biologically capable of reproduction.

purging   An attempt to rid the body of unwanted food by vomiting or other compensatory means, such as excessive exercise, fasting, or laxative abuse.

Q

Quackery   The promotion of an unproven remedy, such as a supplement or other product or service, usually by someone unlicensed and untrained.

R

Raffinose   An oligosaccharide composed of galactose, glucose, and fructose. Also called melitose, it is found in beans, cabbage, broccoli, and other vegetables.

recombinant bovine growth hormone (rBGH)   A genetically engineered hormone injected into dairy cows to enhance their milk output.

recombinant DNA technology   A type of genetic modification in which scientists combine DNA from different sources to produce a transgenic organism that expresses a desired trait.

Recommended Dietary Allowance (RDA)   The average daily nutrient intake level that meets the nutrient requirements of 97% to 98% of healthy individuals in a particular life stage and gender group.

Registered dietitian (RD)   A professional designation that requires a minimum of a bachelor's degree in nutrition, completion of a supervised clinical experience, a passing grade on a national examination, and maintenance of registration with the Academy of Nutrition and Dietetics (in Canada, the Dietitians of Canada). RDs are qualified to work in a variety of settings.

remodeling   The two-step process by which bone tissue is recycled; includes the breakdown of existing bone and the formation of new bone.

renin   An enzyme secreted by the kidneys in response to a decrease in blood pressure. Renin converts the blood protein angiotensinogen to angiotensin I, which eventually results in an increase in sodium reabsorption.

residues   Chemicals that remain in foods despite cleaning and processing.

resistance training   Exercise in which our muscles act against resistance.

resorption   The process by which the surface of bone is broken down by cells called osteoclasts.

Resveratrol   A chemical known to play a role in limiting cell damage from the by-products of metabolic reactions. It is found in red wine and certain other plant-based foods.

retina   The delicate, light-sensitive membrane lining the inner eyeball and connected to the optic nerve. It contains retinal.

retinal   An active, aldehyde form of vitamin A that plays an important role in healthy vision and immune function.

retinoic acid   An active, acid form of vitamin A that plays an important role in cell growth and immune function.

retinol   An active, alcohol form of vitamin A that plays an important role in healthy vision and immune function.

rhodopsin   A light-sensitive pigment found in the rod cells that is formed by retinal and opsin.

Ribose   A five-carbon monosaccharide that is located in the genetic material of cells.

rickets   A vitamin D–deficiency disease in children. Symptoms include deformities of the skeleton, such as bowed legs and knocked knees.

rod cells   Light-sensitive cells found in the retina that contain rhodopsin and react to dim light and interpret black-and-white images.

S

Saliva   A mixture of water, mucus, enzymes, and other chemicals that moistens the mouth and food, binds food particles together, and begins the digestion of carbohydrates.

Salivary amylase An enzyme in saliva that breaks starch into smaller particles and eventually into the disaccharide maltose.

Salivary glands A group of glands found under and behind the tongue and beneath the jaw that releases saliva continually as well as in response to the thought, sight, smell, or presence of food.

salt resistant A condition in which certain people do not experience changes in blood pressure with changes in salt intake.

salt sensitivity A condition in which certain people respond to a high salt intake by experiencing an increase in blood pressure; these people also experience a decrease in blood pressure when salt intake is low.

sarcopenia Age-related, progressive loss of muscle mass, muscle strength, and muscle function.

sarcopenic obesity A condition in which increased body weight and body fat mass coexist with inappropriately low muscle mass and strength.

saturated fatty acid (SFA) Fatty acids that have no carbons joined together with a double bond; these types of fatty acids are generally solid at room temperature.

Secondary deficiency A deficiency that occurs when a person cannot absorb enough of a nutrient, excretes too much of a nutrient from the body, or cannot utilize a nutrient efficiently.

Segmentation Rhythmic contraction of the circular muscles of the small intestine, which squeezes chyme, mixes it, and enhances the digestion and absorption of nutrients from the chyme.

seizures A sudden episode of abnormal electrical activity in the brain that can result from electrolyte imbalances or a chronic disease, such as epilepsy.

selenocysteine An amino acid derivative that is the active form of selenium in the body.

selenomethionine An amino acid derivative that is the storage form for selenium in the body.

senescence The progressive deterioration of bodily functions over time, resulting in increased risk for disability, disease, and death. As people age, their ability to smell foods often declines.

sensible fluid loss Body fluid loss that is noticeable, such as through urine output and sweating.

set-point theory A theory suggesting that the body raises or lowers energy expenditure in response to increased and decreased food intake and physical activity. This action maintains an individual's body weight within a narrow range.

severe acute malnutrition (SAM) A state of severe energy deficit defined as a weight for height more than 3 standard deviations below the mean, or the presence of nutrition-related edema.

short-chain fatty acids Fatty acids fewer than six carbon atoms in length.

Sickle cell anemia A genetic disorder that causes red blood cells to be shaped like a sickle or crescent. These cells cannot travel smoothly through blood vessels, causing cell breakage and anemia.

Simple carbohydrates A monosaccharide or disaccharide, such as glucose; commonly called *sugar*.

small for gestational age (SGA) A birth weight that falls below the 10th percentile for gestational age.

Small intestine The longest portion of the GI tract, where most digestion and absorption takes place.

Soluble fibers Fibers that dissolve in water.

solvent A substance that is capable of mixing with and breaking apart a variety of compounds. Water is an excellent solvent.

Sorbitol A type of sugar alcohol.

specific immune function The strongest defense against pathogens. It requires adaptation of white blood cells that recognize antigens and that multiply to protect against the pathogens carrying those antigens; also called adaptive immunity or acquired immunity.

Sphincter A tight ring of muscle separating some of the organs of the GI tract and opening in response to nerve signals indicating that food is ready to pass into the next section.

spina bifida An embryonic neural tube defect that occurs when the spinal vertebrae fail to completely enclose the spinal cord, allowing it to protrude.

spontaneous abortion The natural termination of a pregnancy and expulsion of pregnancy tissues because of a genetic, developmental, or physiologic abnormality that is so severe that the pregnancy cannot be maintained; also called *miscarriage*.

Stachyose An oligosaccharide composed of two galactose molecules, a glucose molecule, and a fructose molecule; found in the Chinese artichoke and various beans and other legumes.

Starch The storage form of glucose (as a polysaccharide) in plants.

sterols A type of lipid found in foods and the body that has a ring structure; cholesterol is the most common sterol that occurs in our diets.

Stomach A J-shaped organ where food is partially digested, churned, and stored until released into the small intestine.

stretching Exercise in which muscles are gently lengthened using slow, controlled movements.

stunted growth A condition of shorter stature than expected for chronological age, often defined as 2 or more standard deviations below the mean reference value.

Subclinical deficiency A deficiency in its early stages, when few or no symptoms are observed.

Sucrase A digestive enzyme that breaks sucrose into glucose and fructose.

Sucrose A disaccharide composed of one glucose molecule and one fructose molecule; sweeter than lactose or maltose.

sustainability The ability to meet or satisfy basic economic, social, and security needs now and in the future without undermining the natural resource base and environmental quality on which life depends.

sustainable agriculture Term referring to techniques of food production that preserve the environment indefinitely.

T

T cells White blood cells that are of several varieties, including cytotoxic T cells and helper T cells.

TCA cycle The tricarboxylic acid (TCA) cycle is a repetitive series of eight metabolic reactions, located in cell mitochondria, that metabolizes acetyl CoA for the production of carbon dioxide, high-energy GTP, and reduced coenzymes NADH and FADH2.

Teratogen A substance or compound known to cause fetal harm or birth defects.

Theory A scientific consensus, based on data drawn from repeated experiments, as to why a phenomenon occurs.

thermic effect of food (TEF) The energy expended as a result of processing food consumed.

thirst mechanism A cluster of nerve cells in the hypothalamus that stimulates our conscious desire to drink fluids in response to an increase in the concentration of salt in our blood or a decrease in blood pressure and blood volume.

thrifty gene theory A theory suggesting that some people possess a gene (or genes) that causes them to be energetically thrifty, resulting in their expending less energy at rest and during physical activity.

time of activity How long each exercise session lasts.

tocopherols A family of vitamin E that is the active form in our bodies.

tocotrienols A family of vitamin E that does not play an important biological role in our bodies.

Tolerable Upper Intake Level (UL) The highest average daily nutrient intake level likely to pose no risk of adverse health effects to almost all individuals in a particular life stage and gender group.

Total fiber The sum of dietary fiber and functional fiber.

toxin Any harmful substance; in microbiology, a chemical produced by a microorganism that harms tissues or causes harmful immune responses.

trabecular bone (spongy bone)   A porous bone tissue that makes up only 20% of the skeleton and is found within the ends of the long bones, inside the spinal vertebrae, inside the flat bones (sternum, ribs, and most bones of the skull), and inside the bones of the pelvis.

Trace minerals   Minerals we need to consume in amounts less than 100 mg per day and of which the total amount in our body is less than 5 g (5,000 mg).

Transamination   The process of transferring the amine group from one amino acid to another in order to manufacture a new amino acid.

Transcription   The process through which messenger RNA copies genetic information from DNA in the nucleus.

transferrin   The primary iron transport protein in the blood; transports iron to body cells.

Translation   The process that occurs when the genetic information carried by messenger RNA is translated into a chain of amino acids at the ribosome.

Transport proteins   Protein molecules that help transport substances throughout the body and across cell membranes.

triglyceride   A molecule consisting of three fatty acids attached to a three-carbon glycerol backbone.

trimester   Any one of three stages of pregnancy, each lasting approximately 13 to 14 weeks.

T-score   A numerical score comparing an individual's bone density to the average peak bone density of a 30-year-old healthy adult, to determine the risk for osteoporosis.

tumor   Any newly formed mass of immature, undifferentiated cells with no physiologic function.

Type 1 diabetes   A disorder in which the pancreas cannot produce enough insulin.

Type 2 diabetes   A progressive disorder in which body cells become less responsive to insulin.

type of activity   The range of physical activities a person can engage in to promote health and physical fitness.

U

Ulcerative colitis (UC)   A chronic disease of the colon, indicated by inflammation and ulceration of the mucosa, or innermost lining, of the colon.

ultra-trace minerals   Minerals we need to consume in amounts less than 1 mg per day.

umbilical cord   The cord containing arteries and veins that connects the baby (from the navel) to the mother via the placenta.

Undernutrition   A situation in which too little energy or too few nutrients are consumed over time, causing significant weight loss or a nutrient deficiency disease.

underweight   Having too little body fat to maintain health, causing a person to have a weight that is below an acceptable defined standard for a given height; a BMI less than 18.5 kg/m².

urinary tract infection   A bacterial infection affecting any portion of the urinary tract, but most commonly affecting the bladder or the urethra, the tube leading from the bladder to the body exterior.

V

vaccination   The method of administering a small amount of antigen to elicit an immune response for the purpose of developing memory cells that will protect against the disease at a later time.

Variety   Eating a lot of different foods each day.

Vegetarianism   The practice of restricting the diet mostly or entirely to foods of plant origin, including vegetables, fruits, grains, and nuts.

very-low-density lipoprotein (VLDL)   A lipoprotein made in the liver and intestine that functions to transport endogenous lipids, especially triglycerides, to the tissues of the body.

vigorous-intensity activities   Activities that produce significant increases in breathing, sweating, and heart rate; talking is difficult when exercising at a vigorous intensity.

viruses   A group of infectious agents that are much smaller than bacteria, lack independent metabolism, and are incapable of growth or reproduction outside of living cells.

Viscous   Having a gel-like consistency; viscous fibers form a gel when dissolved in water.

visible fats   Fats we can see in our foods or see added to foods, such as butter, margarine, cream, shortening, salad dressings, chicken skin, and untrimmed fat on meat.

Vitamins   Micronutrient compounds that contain carbon and assist us in regulating our body's processes; classified as water soluble or fat soluble.

Vomiting   The involuntary expulsion of the contents of the stomach and duodenum from the mouth.

W

warm-up   Also called preliminary exercise; includes activities that prepare you for an exercise bout, including stretching, calisthenics, and movements specific to the exercise bout.

wasting   A physical condition of very low body-weight-for-height or extreme thinness.

Water-soluble vitamins   Vitamins that are soluble in water. These include vitamin C and the B-vitamins.

water-soluble vitamins   Vitamins that are soluble in water; these include vitamin C and the B-vitamins.

Wellness   A multidimensional, lifelong process that includes physical, emotional, and spiritual health.

Whole foods   Foods in their natural state such as nuts, oats, and blueberries, that can also be classified as functional foods.

X

xerophthalmia   An irreversible blindness due to hardening of the cornea and drying of the mucous membranes of the eye.

xerostomia   Dry mouth due to decreased saliva production.

Z

zygote   A fertilized egg (ovum) consisting of a single cell.

Index

Credits

p. iv: Courtesy of Janice Thompson; p. vi: Courtesy of Melinda Manroe; p. vi: Courtesy of Linda Vaughn; p. vii: Rubberball/Getty Images; p. vii: George Doyle/Ciaran Griffin/Getty Images; p. vii: Fuse/Getty Images; p. xxi: Gekaskr/Fotolia; p. xxii: Africa Studio/Fotolia; p. xxii: Sage Brousseau/Snapwire/Corbis; p. xxiii: Mike Berceanu/Getty Images; p. xxiv: Ziggy Spray/Snapwire/Corbis; p. xxv: Volff/Fotolia; p. xxv: Jag_cz/Fotolia; p. xxvi: Koss13/Fotolia; p. xxviii: Columbus Leth/All Over Press/Corbis; p. xxviii: Tim E. Klein /EyeEm/Getty Images; p. xxix: Bergamont/Fotolia; p. xxx: Raphye Alexius/Image Source/Corbis; p. xxxi: Ben North/Snapwire/Corbis; p. xxxi: Karaidel/Fotolia; p. xxxii: Maryellen Baker/Getty Images; p. xxxii: Westend61/Getty Images; p. xxxiii: Yuri Arcurs/Getty Images; p. xxxiv: Martin Barraud/Getty Images; p. xxxv: Radius Images/Corbis; p. xxxv: Ingrid Rasmussen/Design Pics/Getty Images; p. xxxvi: Zoranm/Getty Images; p. xxxvii: WavebreakMediaMicro/Fotolia; p. xxxviii: Ronnie Kaufman/Larry Hirshowitz/Getty Images

Chapter 1

p. 2: Gekaskr/Fotolia; p. 4: Peangdao/Fotolia; p. 5: Dr. M.A. Ansary/Science Source; p. 5: Kraut, A. Dr. Joseph Goldberger and the War on Pellagra. National Institutes of Health, Office of NIH History. http://history.nih.gov/exhibits/Goldberger/index.html; p. 6: Yeko Photo Studio/Shutterstock; p. 7: Kochanek, K.D., S.L. Murphy, J. Xu, and E. Arias. "Mortality in the United States, 2013,"NCHS Data Brief No. 178 (December, 2014). Print; p. 8: U.S. Department of Health and Human Services. Updated January 13, 2015. HealthyPeople.gov. http://www.healthypeople.gov/2020/About-Healthy-People; p. 8: Data from "Healthy People 2020" (U.S. Department of Health and Human Services); p. 8: Graphics from Centers for Disease Control and Prevention, Obesity Prevalence Maps 1985 to 2010.); p. 14: Lidante/Shutterstock; p. 19: Blair Seitz/Science Source; p. 21: Marcin Balcerzak/Shutterstock; p. 24: Monkey Business Images/Shutterstock; p. 24: Simone van den Berg/Fotolia; p. 24: Monkey Business Images/Shutterstock; p. 24: Alexander Raths/Shutterstock; p. 34: Reprinted with permission of Randy L. Jirtle.

Chapter 2

pp. 2-2: Pearson Education, Inc; p. 40: Africa Studio/Fotolia; p. 42: Alamy; p. 43: Photosani/Shutterstock; p. 43: Forest Badger/Shutterstock; p. 44: B.A.E. Inc/Alamy; p. 45: Pearson Education, Inc.; p. 47: Sky Bonillo/PhotoEdit, Inc.; p. 47: Pearson Education, Inc.; p. 48: U.S. Food and Drug Administration ; p. 49: U/S/ Food and Drug Administration ; p. 51: Pearson Education, Inc.; p. 52: Alexander Walter/Getty Images; p. 53: Carla9/Fotolia; p. 55: ALEAIMAGE/E + /Getty Images; p. 55: Kelly Cline/E + /Getty Images; p. 55: AbbieImages/E + /Getty Images; p. 55: Hurst Photo/Shutterstock; p. 55: Pearson Education, Inc.; p. 56: United States Department of Agriculture; p. 58: Pearson Education, Inc.; p. 58: Pearson Education, Inc.; p. 58: Pearson Education, Inc.; p. 58: Pearson Education, Inc.; p. 58: Pearson Education, Inc.; p. 58: Pearson Education, Inc.; p. 58: Pearson Education, Inc.; p. 58: Pearson Education, Inc.; p. 58: Pearson Education, Inc.; p. 58: Pearson Education, Inc.; p. 58: Pearson Education, Inc.; p. 58: Pearson Education, Inc.; p. 58: Pearson Education, Inc.; p. 58: Pearson Education, Inc.; p. 58: Pearson Education, Inc.; p. 58: Pearson Education, Inc.; p. 58: Pearson Education, Inc; p. 58: Pearson Education, Inc; p. 59: Alamy; p. 59: Qstock/Fotolia; p. 59: Getty Images; p. 59: Ragnar Schmuck/Getty Images; p. 60: United States Department of Agriculture; p. 62: Ed Ou/Associated Press; p. 63: Evgeny Litvinov/Shutterstock; p. 65: Physicians Committee for Responsible Medicine.

Chapter 3

p. 70: Sage Brousseau/Snapwire/Corbis; p. 72: Howord Kingsnorth/Getty Images; p. 75: Jon Riley/The Image Bank/Getty Images; p. 75: Photomadnz/Alamy; p. 79: Michael Flippo/Fotolia; p. 86: SPL/Science Source; p. 91: Maridav/Shutterstock; p. 91: David Musher/Science Source; p. 91: Steve Gschmeissner/Science Source; p. 91: Don W. Fawcett/Science Source; p. 98: Dr. E. Walker/Science Source; p. 100: David Murray/Jules Selmes /Dorling Kindersley Ltd.; p. 100: Bill Grove/Getty Images; p. 103: Data from National Digestive Diseases Information Clearinghouse (NDDIC). Update 2013, November 25. Diarrhea. NIH Publication No. 11–5176. http://www.niddk.nih.gov/health-information/health-topics/digestive-diseases/diarrhea/Pages/ez.aspx; p. 104: Nataliya Peregudova/Fotolia; p. 105: CDC Small Business Finance; p. 106: Pearson Education, Inc.

Chapter 4

p. 110: Mike Berceanu/Getty Images; p. 113: Brocreative/Shutterstock; p. 116: U.S. Department of Agriculture, Agricultural Research Service. 2014. USDA National Nutrient Database for Standard Reference, Release 27; p. 116: Foodcollection/Getty; p. 116: Danny Smythe/Shutterstock; p. 117: Pearson Education, Inc; p. 118: Monkey Business Images/Shutterstock; p. 122: George Doyle/Stockbyte/Getty; p. 123: Shutterstock; p. 123: Flashon Studio/Shutterstock; p. 124: Steve Shott/Dorling Kindersley; p. 124: Ryan McVay/Photodisc/Getty; p. 125: Figure data adapted from the "Regulation of endogenous fat and carbohydrate metabolism in relation to exercise intensity and duration" by Romijn et al., from American Journal of Physiology, September 1, 1993. Copyright © 1993 by The American Physiological Society. Reprinted with permission.; p. 125: Mr.markin/Fotolia; p. 125: Bernd Leitner/Fotolia; p. 125: Doug Menuez/Photodisc/Getty; p. 126: Maridav/Fotolia; p. 126: Dorling Kindersley; p. 128: Justin Sullivan/Getty; p. 129: Institute of Medicine, Food and Nutrition Board. 2005. Dietary Reference Intakes for Energy, Carbohydrates, Fiber, Fat, Fatty Acids, Cholesterol, Protein, and Amino Acids (Macronutrients). Washington, DC: The National Academy of Sciences. Reprinted by permission.†US Department of Health and Human Services and US Department of Agriculture. 2010. Dietary Guidelines for Americans; p. 130: Joe Raedle/Getty; p. 131: Dorling Kindersley; p. 133: Data from U.S. Department of Agriculture, Agricultural Research Service. 2014. USDA National Nutrient Data base for Standard Reference, Release 27. Nutrient Data Laboratory home page. www.ars.usda.gov/ba/bhnrc/ndl.); p. 133: Alex459/Shutterstock; p. 134: Andy Crawford/Dorling Kindersley; p. 135: Pearson Education, In.; p. 135: Pearson Education, Inc; p. 135: Pearson Education, Inc.; p. 135: Pearson Education, Inc; p. 135: Pearson Education, Inc; p. 136: Pearson Education, Inc; p. 136: Giuseppe_R./Shutterstock; p. 136: Vidady/Fotolia; p. 137: Pearson Education, Inc.; p. 138: Data from "Aspartame" from The Calorie Control website, 2015. http://www.caloriecontrol.org/sweeteners-and-lite/sugar-substitutes/aspartame; p. 140: CDC National Center for Chronic Disease Prevention and Health Promotion, Division of Diabetes Translation. 2014. National Diabetes Statistics Report, 2014. http://www.cdc.gov/diabetes/pubs/statsreport14/national-diabetes-report-web.pdf; p. 142: Data from U.S. Dept. of Health and Human Services, National Diabetes Information Clearinghouse (NDIC). Available online at http://diabetes.niddk.nih.gov/dm/pubs/type1and2/index.aspx#signs and from Centers for Disease Control and Prevention, Basics about Diabetes, available at http://www.cdc.gov/diabetes/basics/diabetes.html; p. 143: Data from American Diabetes Association. 2014. Diagnosing Diabetes and Learning About Prediabetes. http://www.diabetes.org/diabetes-basics/diagnosis/; p. 143: Dmitry Lobanov/Shutterstock; p. 144: Sandy Young/Alamy; p. 145: Dorling Kindersley; p. 146: Brian Buckley/Alamy; p. 146: isifa Image Service s.r.o./Alamy; p. 147: Andre Jenny/Alamy.

Chapter 4.5

p. 152: Ziggy Spray/Snapwire/Corbis; p. 153: Pearson Education, Inc; p. 153: U.S. Department of Agriculture and U.S. Department of Health and Human Services. Dietary Guidelines for Americans, 2010. 7th Edition, Washington, DC: U.S. Government Printing Office, December 2010; p. 154: Bikeriderlondon/Shutterstock; p. 157: National Institutes of Health; p. 157: National Institute on Alcohol Abuse and Alcoholism; p. 159: Science Source; p. 159: Martin M. Rotker/Science Source; p. 160: Enigma/Alamy; p. 161: Streissguth, AP, Landesman-Dwyer S, Martin, JC, & Smith, DW (1980). Teratogenic effects of alcohol in humans and laboratory animals. Science, 209, 353-361. Courtesy of University of Washington Fetal Alcohol & Drug Unit.

Chapter 5

p. 163: Steve Gorton/Dorling Kindersley Limited; p. 164: Volff/Fotolia; p. 168: Nikolych/Fotolia; p. 168: Oriori/Shutterstock; p. 171: Stephen VanHorn/Shutterstock; p. 173: Hurley, J., and B. Liebman. 2009. Covering the Spreads. Tracking down the butters and margarines. Nutrition Action Health Letter, September 13–15. Food Processor-SQL, Version 10.3, ESHA Research, Salem, OR; Websites of various margarine manufacturers; p. 178: Elenathewise/Fotolia; p. 181: Quest/Science Source; p. 182: Andersen Ross/Getty Images; p. 183: Data from Coyle, E. F. 1995. Substrate utilization during exercise in active people. Am. J. Clin. Nutr. 61[Suppl.]:968S–979S; p. 183: Doug Pensinger/Getty Images; p. 184: Amy Myers/Shutterstock; p. 185: Danny E Hooks/Shutterstock; p. 186: Jeff Greenberg/AGE Fotostock America Inc; p. 187: ESHA Research; p. 190: Wilmy van Ulft/Shutterstock; p. 191: Pearson Education, Inc; p. 191: Pearson Education, Inc; p. 191: Pearson Education, Inc; p. 191: Pearson Education, Inc; p. 191: Pearson Education, Inc; p. 191: B.O'Kane/Alamy; p. 192: Data from Food Processor-SQL, Version 9.9, ESHA Research, Salem, OR; p. 193: AlexAvich/Shutterstock; p. 193: AlexAvich/Shutterstock; p. 194: Richard Megna/Fundamental Photographs; p. 195: 14ktgold/Fotolia; p. 197: Rich Kareckas/AP Images; p. 200: National Institutes of Health. 2002. Third Report of the National Cholesterol Education Program: Detection, Evaluation and Treatment of High Blood Cholesterol in Adults (ATP III). Bethesda, MD: National Cholesterol Education Program, National Heart, Lung, and Blood Institute, NIH. Available at www.nhlbi.nih.gov/guidelines/cholesterol/atp3xsum. pdf.; p. 201: Bonchan/Shutterstock; p. 202: Altafulla/Shutterstock; p. 202: Pearson Education, Inc.

Chapter 6

p. 210: Jag_cz/Fotolia; p. 219: Andrew Syred/Science Source; p. 220: Pearson Education, Inc; p. 220: Pearson Education, Inc; p. 220: Pearson Education, Inc; p. 220: Pearson Education, Inc; p. 220: Sea Wave/Fotolia; p. 223: Ian O Leary/Dorling Kindersley; p. 225: Fotolia; p. 225: Mediscan/Alamy; p. 229: Jupiterimages/Getty Images; p. 229: Mike Goldwater/Alamy; p. 230: Data from Food and Nutrition Board, Institute of Medicine. 2005. Dietary Reference Intakes for Energy, Carbohydrate, Fiber, Fat, Fatty Acids, Cholesterol, Protein, and Amino Acids (Macronutrients). Washington, DC: National Academies Press. Available at http://www.nap.edu/openbook. php?isbn = 0309085373. 2 Data American College of Sports Medicine, American Dietetic Association, and Dietitians of Canada.2009. Joint position statement. Nutrition and athletic performance. Med. Sci. Sports Exerc. 41(3): 709–731; p. 232: Rubberball/Alan K. Bailey/Getty Images; p. 232: Pearson Education, Inc; p. 232: Pearson Education, Inc; p. 232: Pearson Education, Inc; p. 232: Pearson Education, Inc; p. 232: Pearson Education, Inc; p. 232: Pearson Education, Inc; p. 233: Ranald MacKechnie/Dorling Kindersley; p. 234: Values obtained from U.S. Department of Agriculture, Agricultural Research Service. 2013. USDA National Nutrient Database for Standard Reference, Release 26. Available online at http://ndb.nal.usda.gov/; p. 236: Ekaterina Nikitina/Shutterstock; p. 236: Elena Elisseeva/Shutterstock; p. 237:

Pearson Education, Inc.; p. 237: Dorlinkg Kindersley; p. 239: Alamy; p. 242: Paul Almasy/Corbis; p. 242: Christine Osborne Pictures/Alamy; p. 243: CDC/ Sickle Cell Foundation of Georgia: Jackie George, Beverly Sinclair.

Chapter 7

p. 250: Koss13/Fotolia; p. 252: David Sacks/The Image Bank/Getty Images; p. 255: YouTube Video: Mitochondria ATP Synthesis by biologyR120. Found at: www.youtube.com/watch?v = TgJt4KgKQJI&feature = related; p. 259: Foodfolio/Alamy; p. 260: YouTube Video:Glycolysis by garlandscience. Found at: https://www.youtube.com/watch?v = O5eMW4b29rg; p. 269: Fred Vogelstein. "Epilepsy's Big Fat Miracle," New York Times Magazine. 17 November 2010; p. 270: Ian O'Leary/Dorling Kindersley; p. 273: NatUlrich/Fotolia; p. 274: Barry Gregg/Corbis; p. 274: Female figure based on "BAC Chart Female" from Pennsylvania Liquor Control Board Website, Pennsylvania Liquor Control Board. Male figure based on "BAC Chart Male" from Pennsylvania Liquor Control Board Website, Pennsylvania Liquor Control Board; p. 275: Nyul/Fotolia; p. 277: Jaroslaw Grudzinski/Fotolia; p. 281: Rudchenko Liliia/Shutterstock; p. 283: april_89/Fotolia; p. 283: Sniegirova Mariia/Shutterstock; p. 285: Opolja/Shutterstock; p. 285: Maks Narodenko/Shutterstock; p. 291: BioMed Central Ltd. Part of Springer Science + Business Media.

Chapter 7.5

p. 29: Simon Smith/Dorling Kindersley; p. 292: Columbus Leth/All Over Press/Corbis; p. 294: Paul Prescott/Shutterstock; p. 299: Perry Correll/Shutterstock; p. 299: Sozaijiten; p. 300: Kristin Piljay/Pearson Education, Inc.; p. 300: Kristin Piljay/Pearson Education, Inc.; p. 300: Kristin Piljay/Pearson Education, Inc.; p. 300: Kristin Piljay/Pearson Education, Inc.; p. 300: Kristin Piljay/Pearson Education, Inc.; p. 301: Nancy R.Cohen/Getty Images; p. 302: Suzannah Skelton/Getty Images; p. 303: NIH Video "MAKING DECISIONS" found at http://ods.od.nih.gov/HealthInformation/makingdecisions.sec.aspx; p. 303: FDA Website: Dietary Supplements; www.fda.gov/food/dietarysupplements/default.htm; p. 303: USDA: Dietary Supplements [http://fnic.nal. usda.gov/dietary-supplements]; p. 303: NIH: Dietary Supplement Fact Sheets; www.ods.od.nih.gov; p. 303: Linus Pauling Institute, Oregon State University.

Chapter 8

p. 304: Tim E. Klein /EyeEm/Getty Images; p. 310: Data from U.S. Department of Agriculture, Agricultural Research Service. 2009. USDA Nutrient Database for Standard Reference, Release 22. Nutrient Data Laboratory Home Page. www.ars.usda.gov; p. 310: Fuat Kose/Pearson Education, Inc; p. 310: Olga Nayashkova/Shutterstock; p. 312: Data from U.S. Department of Agriculture, Agricultural Research Service. 2009. Nutrient Data Laboratory Home Page. www.ars.usda.gov; p. 312: MaraZe/Shutterstock; p. 313: Data from U.S. Department of Agriculture, Agricultural Research Service. 2009. USDA Nutrient Database for Standard Reference, Release 22. Nutrient Data Laboratory Home Page. www.ars.usda.gov; p. 313: Alex Staroseltsev/Shutterstock; p. 316: youlian/Shutterstock; p. 317: Data from U.S. Department of Agriculture,- Agricultural Research Service. 2009. USDA Nutrient Database for Standard Reference, Release 22. Nutrient Data Laboratory Home Page. www.ars.usda.gov; p. 317: Madlen/Shutterstock; p. 319: Data from U.S. Dept of Agriculture, Agriculture Research Services. 2009. USDA Nutrient Database for Standard Reference, Release 22. Nutrient Data Laboratory Home Page. www.ars.usda.gov; p. 319: Motorolka/Shutterstock; p. 321: From GROPPER/SMITH/GROFF. Advanced Nutrition and Human Metabolism (with InfoTrac®), 4E. © 2005 Brooks/Cole, a part of Cengage Learning, Inc. Reproduced by permission. www.cengage.com/permissions; p. 322: Data from U.S. Department of Agriculture, Agriculture Research Services. 2009.

USDA Nutrient Data Base for Standard Reference, Release 22. Nutrient Data Laboratory Home Page. www.ars.usda.gov; p. 322: Oocoskun/Fotolia; p. 322: Alamy; p. 323: David Murray/Dorling Kindersley; p. 325: Data from U.S. Department of Agriculture, Agriculture Research Services. 2009. USDA Nutrient Data Base for Standard Reference, Release 22. Nutrient Data Laboratory Home Page. www.ars.usda.gov; p. 325: Dave King/Dorling Kindersley; p. 326: Duncan Smith/Corbis; p. 328: Bruce Coleman Inc./Alamy; p. 328: Pearson Education, Inc.; p. 330: Data from U.S. Department of Agriculture, Agriculture Research Service. 2009. USDA Nutrient Data Base for Standard Reference, Release 22. Nutrient Data Laboratory Home Page. www.ars.usda.gov; p. 330: Viktar Malyshchyts/Shutterstock; p. 330: Dorling Kindersley; p. 331: Kati Molin/Shutterstock; p. 332: Alamy; p. 333: Crepesoles/Shutterstock; p. 334: Jupiterimages/Getty Images; p. 335: Kashanian, M., R. Mazinani, and S. Jalalmanesh. 2007. Pyridoxine (vitamin B6) therapy for premenstrual syndrome. Int. J. Gynaecol. Obstet. 96:43–44; p. 335: Pearson Education, Inc.

Chapter 9

p. 340: Bergamont/Fotolia; p. 342: Vinicius Tupinamba/Shutterstock; p. 344: www.nlm.nih.gov, Informative video on blood pressure, National Institutes of Health (NIH); p. 346: Jupiterimages/Getty Images; p. 346: www.npr.org, Proteins in body tissues, National Public Radio.; p. 347: Shkind/Shutterstock; p. 348: WavebreakmediaMicro/Fotolia; p. 351: Photo25th/Shutterstock; p. 351: Stockbyte/Getty Images; p. 354: Photodisc/Getty Images; p. 354: Ted Levine/Corbis; p. 355: Fotogiunta/Shutterstock; p. 356: Network Productions/The Image Works; p. 357: Viktor/Fotolia; p. 357: Silberkorn/Shutterstock; p. 360: Andrea Skjold Mink/Shutterstock; p. 362: Wiktory/Shutterstock; p. 362: Valentyn Volkov/Shutterstock; p. 364: Foodcollection/Shutterstock; p. 365: Peter Zijlstra/Shutterstock; p. 366: Susanna Price/DK Images; p. 367: Arthur Tilley/Getty Images; p. 368: George Doyle/Getty Images; p. 368: www.nhlbi.nih.gov, Comprehensive guide to the DASH diet, National Institutes of Health; p. 369: Clive Streeter/DK Images; p. 369: "Healthier Eating with DASH," National Institutes of Health from National Heart, Lung and Blood Institute website; p. 372: Rido/Shutterstock; p. 377: www.water.epa.gov, Drinking water quality, standards, and safety, United States Environmental Protection Agency; p. 377: www.bottledwater.org, For more information about bottled water here, International Bottled Water Association; p. 377: www.nim.nih.gov/medlineplus, Dehydration and heat stroke, National Institute of Health; p. 377: www.nhlbi.nih.gov, Heart disease and how to prevent high blood pressure, National Heart, Lung, and Blood Institute; p. 377: www.americanheart.org, Tips on how to lower your blood pressure, American Heart Association; p. 377: www.nih.gov, DASH Diet, National Institutes of Health (NIH).

Chapter 10

p. 378: Raphye Alexius/Image Source/Corbis; p. 381: Trekandphoto/Fotolia; p. 385: Oriori/Shutterstock; p. 385: Hemilä, H., and E. Chalker. 2013. Vitamin C for preventing and treating the common cold. Cochrane Database of Systematic Reviews. Issue 1. Art. No. CD000980. DOI: 10.1002/14651858.CD000980.pub4; p. 385: Data from U.S. Department of Agriculture, Agricultural Research Service, 2014. USDA National Nutrient Database for Standard Reference, Release 27. www.ars.usda.gov/ba/bhnrc/ndl; p. 386: Valentyn Volkov/Shutterstock; p. 388: Pia Tryde/Dorling Kindersley, Ltd; p. 389: David Murray/Dorling Kindersley, Ltd; p. 390: Bluestocking/Getty Images; p. 390: Data from U.S. Department of Agriculture, Agricultural Research Service, 2014. USDA National Nutrient Database for Standard Reference, Release 27. http://www.ars.usda.gov/ba/bhnrc/ndl; p. 392: Dorling Kindersley, Ltd; p. 393: Bernardo De Niz/MCT/Newscom; p. 393: Dream79/Fotolia; p. 393: Data from U.S. Department of Agriculture, Agricultural Research Service, 2014. USDA National Nutrient Database for Standard Reference, Release 27. www.ars.usda.gov/ba/bhnrc/ndl; p. 394: Bozeman Science; p. 395: Philip

Wilkins/Dorling Kindersley, Ltd; p. 396: USDA (U.S. Department of Agriculture); p. 396: Dionisvera/Shutterstock; p. 396: Data from U.S. Department of Agriculture, Agricultural Research Service, 2014. USDA National Nutrient Database for Standard Reference, Release 27. www.ars.usda.gov/ba/bhnrc/ndl; p. 399: Siri Stafford/Digital Vision/Getty Images; p. 400: Pearson Education, Inc; p. 400: Pearson Education, Inc; p. 400: Pearson Education, Inc; p. 400: Pearson Education, Inc; p. 402: Dorling Kindersley, Ltd; p. 403: Tim UR/Fotolia; p. 403: Data from U.S. Department of Agriculture, Agricultural Research Service, 2014. USDA National Nutrient Database for Standard Reference, Release 27. www.ars.usda.gov/ba/bhnrc/ndl; p. 404: MD Anderson; p. 406: Dave King/Dorling Kindersley, Ltd.; p. 407: St Bartholomew's Hospital/Science Source; p. 407: NIH Custom Medical Stock Photo/Newscom; p. 408: Dr. P. Marazzi/Science Source; p. 408: Suzannah Skelton/Getty Images; p. 409: WavebreakmediaMicro/Fotolia; p. 409: Monkey Business/Fotolia; p. 409: Hear the real stories of people living with smoking-related diseases and disability by going to the Centers for Disease Control and Prevention "Tips from Former Smokers at http://www.cdc.gov/tobacco/campaign/tips/; p. 410: Cordelia Molloy/Science Source; p. 413: Data from NIH National Center for Complementary and Integrative Health. 2015. Herbs At a Glance. https://nccih.nih.gov/health/herbsataglance.htmand WebMD. 2015. Vitamins & Supplements. http://www.webmd.com/vitamins-supplements/.

Chapter 10.5

p. 418: Ben North/Snapwire/Corbis; p. 419: Ian O'Leary/Dorling Kindersley, Ltd; p. 420: Southern Illinois University/Science Source; p. 420: DJM-photo/Shutterstock; p. 420: Joy Brown/Shutterstock; p. 421: HG Photography/Fotolia; p. 422: Valentyn Volkov/Shutterstock; p. 422: National Center for Complementary and Integrative Health.

Chapter 11

p. 424: Karaidel/Fotolia; p. 426: Â© Ed Geller/ZUMA Press/Alamy; p. 429: Amgen, www.bonebiology.amgen.com; p. 429: WebMD, LLC, www.webmd.com; p. 430: Phanie Agency/Science Source; p. 430: Phanie Agency/Science Source; p. 431: Shutterstock; p. 433: Dave King/Dorling Kindersley; p. 434: Peter Anderson/Dorling Kindersley; p. 434: Data from U.S. Department of Agriculture, Agricultural Research Service, 2014, USDA Nutrient Database for Standard Reference, Release 27. Nutrient Data Laboratory Home Page, www.ars.usda.gov/ba/bhnrc/ndl; p. 434: Healthy Eating, www.healthyeating.com; p. 434: Constantinos/Fotolia; p. 435: Pearson Education, Inc; p. 435: Brand Z Food/Alamy; p. 435: Pearson Education, Inc; p. 435: Comstock/Getty Images; p. 435: Ramon Espelt/Shutterstock; p. 435: Dorling Kindersley; p. 435: BW Folsom/Shutterstock; p. 436: Pearson Education, Inc; p. 438: Cyrille Gibot/Alamy; p. 440: Dorling Kindersley; p. 441: Jiri Hera/Shutterstock; p. 441: Science Source; p. 441: Data from U.S. Department of Agriculture, Agricultural Research Service, 2014, USDA Nutrient Database for Standard Reference, Release 27. Nutrient Data Laboratory Home Page, www.ars.usda.gov/ba/bhnrc/ndl; p. 443: Data from U.S. Department of Agriculture, Agricultural Research Service, 2014, USDA Nutrient Database for Standard Reference, Release 27. Nutrient Data Laboratory Home Page, www.ars.usda.gov/ba/bhnrc/ndl; p. 443: Mates/Fotolia; p. 444: Dorling Kindersley; p. 444: Dorling Kindersley; p. 444: Catherine Ledner/Getty Images; p. 445: Spencer Jones/Getty Images; p. 446: CanuckStock/Shutterstock; p. 446: Data from U.S. Department of Agriculture, Agricultural Research Service, 2014, USDA Nutrient Database for Standard Reference, Release 27. Nutrient Data Laboratory Home Page, www.ars.usda.gov/ba/bhnrc/ndl; p. 447: Subbotina Anna/Fotolia; p. 448: National Institute of Dental Research; p. 449: Michael Klein/Getty Images; p. 449: Robert Destefano/Alamy; p. 449: Neil Borden/Science Source; p. 449: Newscom; p. 450: Larry Mulvehill/Science Source; p. 450: Information adapted from the National Osteoporosis Society. 2014. Factors that increase your risk of osteoporosis and fractures.

https://www.nos.org.uk/healthy-bones-and-risks/are-you-at-risk; accessed April 14, 2015; p. 451: Sergey Lukianov/Fotolia; p. 451: Methodist Health System, www.methodisthealthsystem.org ; p. 452: Christopher Edwin Nuzzaco/Shutterstock; p. 452: Marc Romanelli/Getty Images; p. 453: International Osteoporosis Foundation, www.osteofound.org; p. 454: Bsip Sa/Alamy; p. 455: Pearson Education, Inc; p. 456: Paul Reid/Shutterstock; p. 457: UV Safety: The Global Solar Ultraviolet Index from the Environmental Protection Agency, May 2004.

Chapter 12

p. 462: Maryellen Baker/Getty Images; p. 465: National Library of Medicine video at www.nlm.nih.gov/medlineplus/ency/anatomyvideos/000104.htm; p. 468: From Gropper/Smith. Advanced Nutrition and Human Metabolism, 6E. © 2013 Brooks/Cole, a part of Cengage Learning, Inc. Reproduced by permission. www.cengage.com/permissions; p. 469: Jupiterimages/Getty Images; p. 470: Shawn Pecor/Shutterstock; p. 471: Data from Institute of Medicine, Food and Nutrition Board. 2002. Dietary Reference Intakes for Vitamin A, Vitamin K, Arsenic, Boron, Chromium, Copper, Iodine, Iron, Manganese, Molybdenum, Nickel, Silicon, Vanadium, and Zinc. Washington, DC: National Academies Press. © 2002 by the National Academy of Sciences; p. 472: zcw/Shutterstock; p. 472: Data from U.S. Department of Agriculture, Agricultural Research Service, 2009, USDA Nutrient Database for Standard Reference, Release 22. Nutrient Data Laboratory Home Page, www.ars.usda.gov/ba/bhnrc/ndl; p. 476: National Heart, Lung, and Blood Institute video at www.nhlbi.nih.gov/health/health-topics/topics/ida/; p. 479: OlegD/Shutterstock; p. 479: Isabelle Rozenbaum & Frederic Cirou/Getty Images; p. 479: Data from U.S. Department of Agriculture, Agricultural -Research Service, 2009, USDA Nutrient Database for Standard Reference, Release 22. Nutrient Data Laboratory Home Page, www.ars.usda.gov/ba/bhnrc/ndl.); p. 479: From Gropper/Smith. Advanced Nutrition and Human Metabolism, 6E. © 2013 Brooks/Cole, a part of Cengage Learning, Inc. Reproduced by permission. www.cengage.com/permissions; p. 481: Dorling Kindersley, Ltd; p. 481: Data from U.S. Department of Agriculture, Agricultural Research -Service. 2005. USDA Nutrient Database for Standard Reference, Release 21. www.ars.usda.gov/Services/docs.htm?docid = 8964; p. 481: Melinda Fawver/Shutterstock; p. 482: Sebastian Kaulitzki/Shutterstock; p. 482: Shutterstock; p. 482: National Library of Medicine video at http://www.nlm.nih.gov/medlineplus/ency/anatomyvideos/000011.htm; p. 483: Ian O'Leary/Dorling Kindersley, Ltd; p. 484: Steve Moss/Alamy; p. 486: Centers for Disease Control and Prevention, Spina bifida, data and statistics, 2011.; p. 486: Gary Carlson/Science Source; p. 487: Eye of Science/Science Source; p. 487: Dr. Andrejs Liepins/Science Source; p. 488: Aaron Haupt/Science Source; p. 488: Horizon International Images Limited/Alamy; p. 489: United States Department of Agriculture; p. 490: Pearson Education, Inc; p. 491: Color Day Production/Getty Images; p. 495: Nutrient Data Laboratory, www.ars.usda.gov/ba/bhnrc/ndl; p. 495: Web MD, www.webmd.com; p. 495: Medline Plus, U.S. National Library of Medicine, National Institutes of Health, www.nlm.nih.gov/medlineplus; p. 495: Kidshealth, www.kidshealth.org/parent; p. 495: U.S. Food and Drug Administration FDA, www.fda.gov; p. 495: Office of Dietary Supplements (ODS), www.dietary-supplements.info.nih.gov.

Chapter 13

p. 496: Westend61/Getty Images; p. 498: CBS News, http://www.cbsnews.com/; p. 498: PAUL BUCK/EPA/Newscom; p. 500: Robert Harding World Imagery; p. 501: U.S. Centers for Disease Control, www.CDC.gov; p. 502: Peter Menzel/Science Source; p. 502: May/Science Source; p. 502: May/Science Source; p. 502: Science Source; p. 502: Photo provided courtesy of COSMED USA, Inc., Concord, CA; p. 503503: Pearson Education, Inc; p. 504: U.S. Centers for Disease Control, www.CDC.gov; p. 504: Peter Anderson/Dorling Kindersley Limited; p. 505: Pearson Education, Inc.; p. 505: Helder Almeida/Shutterstock; p. 505: Maga/Shutterstock; p. 505: Lightpoet/Shutterstock; p. 505: Kenneth Man/Shutterstock; p. 505: Kenneth Man/Shutterstock; p. 505: Zurijeta/Shutterstock; p. 505: Brian A Jackson/Shutterstock; p. 506: Science Source; p. 507: Getty Images; p. 509: U.S. Centers for Disease Control, www.CDC.gov; p. 511: U.S. Centers for Disease Control, www.CDC.gov; p. 512: Alvis Upitis/Getty Images; p. 513: JackJelly/Getty Images; p. 515: Philip Dowell/Dorling Kindersley Limited; p. 516: Bruce Dale/Getty Images; p. 517: Mark Douet/Getty Images; p. 518: Chad Baker/Jason Reed/Ryan McVay/Getty Images; p. 520: Amble Design/Shutterstock; p. 520: Auremar/Shutterstock; p. 520: Africa Studio/Fotolia; p. 520: Epictura/Alamy; p. 521: U.S. Centers for Disease Control, www.CDC.gov; p. 521: U.S. Centers for Disease Control, www.cdc.gov; p. 524: Newscom; p. 526: Daniel Padavona/Shutterstock; p. 528: National Institutes of Health (NIH), www.nhlbi.nih.gov/; p. 530: Pearson Education, Inc; p. 530: Pearson Education, Inc; p. 530: Pearson Education, Inc; p. 530: Pearson Education, Inc; p. 530: Pearson Education, Inc; p. 530: Pearson Education, Inc; p. 532: JJAVA/Fotolia; p. 533: Food Alan King/Alamy; p. 534: Chuck Place/Alamy; p. 539: Federal Trade Commission, www.ftc.gov; p. 539: USDA, www.nutrition.gov/weight-management; p. 539: USDA, www.nutrition.gov/weight-management; p. 539: Academy of Nutrition and Dietetics, www.eatright.org; p. 539: National Institute of Diabetes and Digestive and Kidney Diseases (NIDDK), http://www.niddk.nih.gov/health-information/Pages/default.aspx; p. 539: National Institute of Diabetes and Digestive and Kidney Diseases (NIDDK), http://www.niddk.nih.gov/health-information/Pages/default.aspx; p. 539: Overeaters Anonymous, www.oa.org.

Chapter 13.5

p. 540: Yuri Arcurs/Getty Images; p. 541: Eugenio Savio/AP Images; p. 543: National Institute of Mental Health, www.nimh.nih.gov; p. 543: Pearson Education, Inc; p. 544: Data from Smiley, L., L. King, and H. Avery. University of Arizona Campus Health Service. Original Continuum, C. Shlaalak. Preventive Medicine and Public Health. Copyright © 1997 Arizona Board of Regents.); p. 544: Angela Hampton/Bubbles Photolibrary/Alamy; p. 545: Blake Little/Getty Images; p. 547: Blickwinkel/Dautel/Alamy; p. 548: D. Hurst/Alamy; p. 549: Photodisc/Getty Images; p. 549: National Eating Disorders Association, www.nationaleatingdisorders.org p. 550: Harris Center for Education and Advocacy in Eating Disorders, www.massgeneral.org p. 550: Disordered Eating, National Institute of Mental Health (NIMH) Office of Communications and Public Liaison, www.nimh.nih.gov; p. 550: National Association of Anorexia Nervosa and Associated Disorders, www.anad.org.

Chapter 14

p. 552: Martin Barraud/Getty Images; p. 554: My Good Images/Shutterstock; p. 555: Mayo Clinic, www.mayoclinic.com; p. 556: Blue Jean Images/Alamy; p. 556: Centers for Disease Control and Prevention. 2014. Facts about Physical Activity, http://www.cdc.gov/physicalactivity/data/facts.html and Centers for Disease Control and Prevention. Office of Surveillance, Epidemiology, and Laboratory Services. Behavioral Risk Factor Surveillance System. 2012. Prevalence and Trends Data. Exercise - 2012. http://apps.nccd.cdc.gov/brfss/list.asp?cat = EX&yr = 2012&qkey = 8041&state = All; p. 557: Stockbyte/Getty Images; p. 559: Mark Lennihan/AP Images; p. 560: Endostock/Fotolia; p. 560: Tatyana Vyc/Shutterstock; p. 560: Martin Novak/Shutterstock; p. 561: Will/Deni McIntyre/Science Source; p. 561: Mayo Clinic, www.mayoclinic.com; p. 561: Centers for Disease Control and Prevention. 2011. Physical Activity for Everyone. Measuring Physical Activity Intensity. Target Heart Rate and Estimated Maximum Heart Rate. www.cdc.gov/physicalactivity/everyone/measuring/heartrate.html; p. 563: Moodboard/Alamy; p. 563: University of Pittsburgh Physical Activity Resource Center for Public Health, www.parcph.org; p. 564: Livestrong; p. 567: Ariwasabi/Shutterstock; p. 567: Peter

Bernik/Shutterstock; p. 567: Koji Aoki/Getty Images; p. 567: Nigel Roddis/EPA/Newscom; p. 567: Maho/Fotolia; p. 567: Colin Underhill/Alamy; p. 567: Maridav/Shutterstock; p. 568: Alamy; p. 569: Source: Data from Brooks, G. A., and J. Mercier. 1994. Balance of carbohydrate and lipid utilization during exercise: the "crossover" concept. J. Appl. Physiol. 76[6]:2253–2261.); p. 572: Dorling Kindersley, Ltd; p. 572: Jens Schlueter/AFP/Getty Images; p. 573: Pearson Education, Inc; p. 573: Pearson Education, Inc; p. 573: Pearson Education, Inc; p. 573: Pearson Education, Inc; p. 573: Pearson Education, Inc; p. 573: Pearson Education, Inc; p. 574: Data from Costill, D. L., and J. M. Miller. 1980. Nutrition for endurance sport: CHO and fluid balance. Int. J. Sports Med. 1:2–14. Copyright 1980 Georg Thieme Verlag; p. 575: Getty Images; p. 575: Data from Manore, M. M., N. L. Meyer, and J. L. Thompson. 2009. Sport Nutrition for Health and Performance. 2nd edn. Champaign, IL: Human Kinetics; p. 578: Val Thoermer/Shutterstock; p. 578: Dorling Kindersley, Ltd.; p. 579: Zhukov Oleg/Shutterstock; p. 579: Dburke/Alamy; p. 579: Denkou Images/Getty Images; p. 580: Data adapted from Murray, R. 1997. Drink more! Advice from a world class expert. ACSM's Health and Fitness Journal 1:19–23; American College of Sports Medicine Position Stand. 2007. Exercise and fluid replacement. Med. Sci. Sports Exerc. 39(2):377–390; and Casa, D. J., L. E. Armstrong, S. K. Hillman, S. J. Montain, R. V. Reiff, B. S. E. Rich, W. O. Roberts, and J. A. Stone. 2000. National Athletic Trainers' Association position statement: fluid replacement for athletes. J. Athlet. Train. 35:212–224; p. 582: Istvan Csak/Shutterstock; p. 583: Derek Hall/Dorling Kindersley, Ltd; p. 584: U.S. Food and Drug Administration, www.fda.gov; p. 589: American Heart Association www.heart.org; p. 589: American College of Sports Medicine www.acsm.org; p. 589: U.S. Department of Health and Human Services www.hhs.gov; p. 589: Weight-Control Information Network www.win.niddk.nih.gov; p. 589: NIH Office of Dietary Supplements www.ods.od.nih.gov; p. 589: Food and Nutrition Information Center www.fnic.nal.usda.gov; p. 589: The President's Challenge Adult Fitness test www.adultfitnesstest.org.

Chapter 15

p. 590: Radius Images/Corbis; p. 592: Monkey Business Images/Shutterstock; p. 593: Joe Sohm/VisionsofAmerica/SuperStock; p. 593: Avatar444/Fotolia; p. 593: David Wei/Alamy; p. 593: Frank Rumpenhorst/Deutsch Presse Agentur/Newscom; p. 593: Huntstock/Alamy; p. 595: Laguna Design/Science Source; p. 596: Tony Brain/Science Source; p. 596: Centers for Disease Control and Prevention, http://www2c.cdc.gov; p. 597: Andrew Syred/Science Source; p. 597: Data from Iowa State University Extension, Food Safety. 2015. What Are the Most Common Foodborne Pathogens? http://www.extension.iastate.edu/foodsafety/L1.7; U.S. Food and Drug Administration, Foodborne Illnesses: What You Need to Know, Updated January 29, 2015, from http://www.fda.gov/Food/FoodborneIllnessContaminants/FoodborneIllnessesNeedToKnow/default.htm; and L. H. Gould, et al., 2013. Surveillance for Foodborne Disease Outbreaks—United States, 1998–2008, MMWR, 62(SS02):1–34; p. 598: Miguel A. Muñoz/Alamy; p. 598: Dorling Kindersley, Ltd.; p. 600: U.S. Department of Health and Human Services; p. 601: Planet5D LLC/Shutterstock; p. 601: U.S. Department of Health and Human Services, http://www.foodsafety.gov/; p. 602: Data from U.S. Department of Agriculture, Food Safety and Inspection Service. May, 2010. Food Safety Information. Refrigeration and Food Safety. http://www.fsis.usda.gov/shared/PDF/Refrigeration_and_Food_Safety.pdf; p. 603: U.S. Department of Health and Human Services, http://www.foodsafety.gov/; p. 604: BlueOrange Studio/Shutterstock; p. 604: Data from U.S. Food and Drug Administration. 2014, July 2. Barbecue Basics: Tips to Prevent Foodborne Illness. http://www.fda.gov/forconsumers/ucm094562.htm; p. 606: New York Times Co/Getty Images; p. 608: Nikreates/Alamy; p. 608: U.S. Food and Drug Administration; p. 609: Getty Images; p. 61: Ron Sutherland/Science Source; p. 610: Corbis; p. 612: Incinereight/Fotolia; p. 612: Ionescu Bogdan/Fotolia; p. 612: Natural Resources Defense Council, www.nrdc.org; p. 613: Frank Boston/Fotolia; p. 613: National Institute of Environmental Health Sciences. 2015, January 21. Bisphenol A (BPA). http://www.niehs.nih.gov/health/topics/agents/sya-bpa/index.cfm; p. 614: Vanessa Davies/Dorling Kindersley, Ltd; p. 615: Paul Gunning/Science Source; p. 616: United States Food and Drug Administration - Organic Food Seal; p. 617: Newscom; p. 617: Environmental Working Group. 2015. EWG's Shopper's Guide to Pesticides in Produce. http://www.ewg.org/foodnews/; p. 619: Toby Talbot/AP Images; p. 619: James Laurie/Shutterstock; p. 625: U.S. Department of Health and Human Services, www.foodsafety.gov; p. 625: Centers for Disease Control and Prevention, www.cdc.gov/foodsafety/index.html; p. 625: U.S. Food and Drug Administration, www.fsis.usda.gov/food_safety_education/index.asp; p. 625: U.S. Environmental Protection Agency: Pesticides www.epa.gov/pesticides; p. 625: U.S. Food and Drug Administration, www.ams.usda.gov.

Chapter 16

p. 626: Ingrid Rasmussen/Design Pics/Getty Images; p. 628: Antony Njuguna/Reuters; p. 628: Food and Agricultural Organization, www.fao.org/.; p. 629: Source: Based on Food and Agricultural Organization of the United Nations (FAO). 2014. FAO Hunger Map 2014. Available at http://www.fao.org/fileadmin/templates/ess/foodsecurity/poster_web_001_WFS.jpg; p. 629: Economic Research Service. 2015, January 12. Food Security Status of U.S. Households in 2013. United States Department of Agriculture. Available at http://www.ers.usda.gov/topics/food-nutrition-assistance/food-security-in-the-us/key-statistics-graphics.aspx#verylow; p. 630: Richard Wayman/Alamy; p. 631: Florian Kopp/imageBROKER/Newscom; p. 632: Joerg Boethling/Alamy; p. 632: Heine/imageBROKER/Alamy; p. 633: AP Images; p. 634: Neil Cooper/Alamy; p. 635: Based on World Health Organization. 2015, January. Obesity and Overweight. Fact Sheet No311. Available at http://www.who.int/mediacentre/factsheets/fs311/en/; p. 636: Norma Joseph/Alamy; p. 637: David White/Alamy; p. 637: U.S. Department of Agriculture, http://ams.usda.gov/ p. 638: Mikeledray/Shutterstock; p. 642: World Food Programme, www.wfp.org; p. 643: Mike Harrington/Iconica/Getty Images; p. 643: Yann Layma/Getty Images; p. 644: U.S. Department of Agriculture, http://ams.usda.gov; p. 645: The Fair Trade Certified Logo, reprinted with permission from Fair Trade USA; p. 646: Corbis; p. 647: Clive Streeter/Dorling Kindersley, Ltd.; p. 647: Susanna Price/Dorling Kindersley, Ltd.; p. 647: Data from: Eshel, G., Shepon, A., Makov, T., and Milo, R. 2014. Land, irrigation water, greenhouse gas, and reactive nitrogen burdens of meat, eggs, and dairy production in the United States. PNAS August 19, 2014; vol. 111 no. 33:11996-12001. doi: 10.1073/pnas.1402183111; p. 647: CARE, www.care.org; p. 653: Freedom from Hunger, www.freefromhunger.org; p. 653: Heifer International, www.heifer.org; p. 653: National Student Campaign Against Hunger and Homelessness, www.studentsagainsthunger.org; p. 653: United Nations Children's Fund www.unicef.org/nutrition; p. 653: World Health Organization Nutrition www.who.int/nutrition/en; p. 653: Food Democracy Now, www.fooddemocracynow.org; p. 653: Slow Food USA, www.slowfoodusa.org/; p. 653: Fair Trade USA, www.fairtradeusa.org; p. 653: Meatless Monday, www.meatlessmonday.com/; p. 653: Environmental Protection Agency's Sustainability Tips, www2.epa.gov/learn-issues/green-living.

Chapter 17

p. 654: Zoranm/Getty Images; p. 656: Science Source; p. 657: U.S. National Library of Medicine, https://www.nlm.nih.gov/; p. 660: BIOPHOTO ASSOCIATES/PRI/Getty Images; p. 660: Claude Edelmann/Science Source; p. 660: Neil Bromhall/Science Source; p. 660: Kletr/Shutterstock; p. 662: Ian O'Leary/Getty Images; p. 662: Rasmussen, K.M., and A.L. Yaktine, eds. 2009. Weight Gain During Pregnancy: Reexamining the Guidelines. Institute of Medicine; National Research Council. Washington, DC: National Acaedmy

Chapter 18

Chapter 19

Appendix A

Appendix F

Appendix H

Tolerable Upper Intake Levels (ULs[*])

Life Stage Group	Vitamin A (µg/d)[a]	Vitamin C (mg/d)	Vitamin D (µg/d)	Vitamin E (mg/d)[b,c]	Niacin (mg/d)[c]	Vitamin B6 (mg/d)	Folate (µg/d)[c]	Choline (g/d)
Infants								
0–6 mo	600	ND[d]	25	ND	ND	ND	ND	ND
6–12 mo	600	ND	38	ND	ND	ND	ND	ND
Children								
1–3 y	600	400	63	200	10	30	300	1.0
4–8 y	900	650	75	300	15	40	400	1.0
Males								
9–13 y	1,700	1,200	100	600	20	60	600	2.0
14–18 y	2,800	1,800	100	800	30	80	800	3.0
19–30 y	3,000	2,000	100	1,000	35	100	1,000	3.5
31–50 y	3,000	2,000	100	1,000	35	100	1,000	3.5
51–70 y	3,000	2,000	100	1,000	35	100	1,000	3.5
>70 y	3,000	2,000	100	1,000	35	100	1,000	3.5
Females								
9–13 y	1,700	1,200	100	600	20	60	600	2.0
14–18 y	2,800	1,800	100	800	30	80	800	3.0
19–30 y	3,000	2,000	100	1,000	35	100	1,000	3.5
31–50 y	3,000	2,000	100	1,000	35	100	1,000	3.5
51–70 y	3,000	2,000	100	1,000	35	100	1,000	3.5
>70 y	3,000	2,000	100	1,000	35	100	1,000	3.5
Pregnancy								
≤18 y	2,800	1,800	100	800	30	80	800	3.0
19–50 y	3,000	2,000	100	1,000	35	100	1,000	3.5
Lactation								
≤18 y	2,800	1,800	100	800	30	80	800	3.0
19–50 y	3,000	2,000	100	1,000	35	100	1,000	3.5

Data from: Reprinted with permission from the Dietary Reference Intakes series. Copyright 1997, 1998, 2000, 2001, 2005, 2011 by the National Academies of Sciences, courtesy of the National Academies Press, Washington, D.C. These reports may be accessed via www.nap.edu.

[a] As preformed vitamin A only.

[b] As α-tocopherol; applies to any form of supplemental α-tocopherol.

[c] The ULs for vitamin E, niacin, and folate apply to synthetic forms obtained from supplements, fortified foods, or a combination of the two.

[d] ND=Not determinable due to lack of data of adverse effects in this age group and concern with regard to lack of ability to handle excess amounts. Source of intake should be from food only to prevent high levels of intake.

[*]Note: A Tolerable Upper Intake Level (UL) is the highest level of daily nutrient intake that is likely to pose no risk of adverse health effects to almost all individuals in the general population. Unless otherwise specified, the UL represents total intake from food, water, and supplements. Due to a lack of suitable data, ULs could not be established for vitamin K, thiamin, riboflavin, vitamin B12, pantothenic acid, biotin, and carotenoids. In the absence of a UL, extra caution may be warranted in consuming levels above recommended intakes. Members of the general population should be advised not to routinely exceed the UL. The UL is not meant to apply to individuals who are treated with the nutrient under medical supervision or to individuals with predisposing conditions that modify their sensitivity to the nutrient.

Tolerable Upper Intake Levels (ULs*)

Elements

Life Stage Group	Boron (mg/d)	Calcium (mg/d)	Copper (μg/d)	Fluoride (mg/d)	Iodine (μg/d)	Iron (mg/d)	Magnesium (mg/d)e	Manganese (mg/d)	Molybdenum (μg/d)	Nickel (mg/d)	Phosphorus (g/d)	Selenium (μg/d)	Vanadium (mg/d)f	Zinc (mg/d)	Sodium (g/d)	Chloride (g/d)
Infants																
0–6 mo	NDd	1,000	ND	0.7	ND	40	ND	ND	ND	ND	ND	45	ND	4	ND	ND
6–12 mo	ND	1,500	ND	0.9	ND	40	ND	ND	ND	ND	ND	60	ND	5	ND	ND
Children																
1–3 y	3	2,500	1,000	1.3	200	40	65	2	300	0.2	3	90	ND	7	1.5	2.3
4–8 y	6	2,500	3,000	2.2	300	40	110	3	600	0.3	3	150	ND	12	1.9	2.9
Males																
9–13 y	11	3,000	5,000	10	600	40	350	6	1,100	0.6	4	280	ND	23	2.2	3.4
14–18 y	17	3,000	8,000	10	900	45	350	9	1,700	1.0	4	400	ND	34	2.3	3.6
19–30 y	20	2,500	10,000	10	1,100	45	350	11	2,000	1.0	4	400	1.8	40	2.3	3.6
31–50 y	20	2,500	10,000	10	1,100	45	350	11	2,000	1.0	4	400	1.8	40	2.3	3.6
51–70 y	20	2,000	10,000	10	1,100	45	350	11	2,000	1.0	4	400	1.8	40	2.3	3.6
>70 y	20	2,000	10,000	10	1,100	45	350	11	2,000	1.0	3	400	1.8	40	2.3	3.6
Females																
9–13 y	11	3,000	5,000	10	600	40	350	6	1,100	0.6	4	280	ND	23	2.2	3.4
14–18 y	17	3,000	8,000	10	900	45	350	9	1,700	1.0	4	400	ND	34	2.3	3.6
19–30 y	20	2,500	10,000	10	1,100	45	350	11	2,000	1.0	4	400	1.8	40	2.3	3.6
31–50 y	20	2,500	10,000	10	1,100	45	350	11	2,000	1.0	4	400	1.8	40	2.3	3.6
51–70 y	20	2,000	10,000	10	1,100	45	350	11	2,000	1.0	4	400	1.8	40	2.3	3.6
>70 y	20	2,000	10,000	10	1,100	45	350	11	2,000	1.0	3	400	1.8	40	2.3	3.6
Pregnancy																
≤18 y	17	3,000	8,000	10	900	45	350	9	1,700	1.0	3.5	400	ND	34	2.3	3.6
19–50 y	20	2,500	10,000	10	1,100	45	350	11	2,000	1.0	3.5	400	ND	40	2.3	3.6
Lactation																
≤18 y	17	3,000	8,000	10	900	45	350	9	1,700	1.0	4	400	ND	34	2.3	3.6
19–50 y	20	2,500	10,000	10	1,100	45	350	11	2,000	1.0	4	400	ND	40	2.3	3.6

Data from: Reprinted with permission from the Dietary Reference Intakes series. Copyright 1997, 1998, 2000, 2001, 2005, 2011 by the National Academies of Sciences, courtesy of the National Academies Press, Washington, D.C. These reports may be accessed via www.nap.edu.

d ND=Not determinable due to lack of data of adverse effects in this age group and concern with regard to lack of ability to handle excess amounts. Source of intake should be from food only to prevent high levels of intake.

e The ULs for magnesium represent intake from a pharmacological agent only and do not include intake from food and water.

f Although vanadium in food has not been shown to cause adverse effects in humans, there is no justification for adding vanadium to food, and vanadium supplements should be used with caution. The UL is based on adverse effects in laboratory animals, and this data could be used to set a UL for adults but not children and adolescents.

*Note: A Tolerable Upper Intake Level (UL) is the highest level of daily nutrient intake that is likely to pose no risk of adverse health effects to almost all individuals in the general population. Unless otherwise specified, the UL represents total intake from food, water, and supplements. Due to a lack of suitable data, ULs could not be established for vitamin K, thiamin, riboflavin, vitamin B_{12}, pantothenic acid, biotin, and carotenoids. In the absence of a UL, extra caution may be warranted in consuming levels above recommended intakes. Members of the general population should be advised not to routinely exceed the UL. The UL is not meant to apply to individuals who are treated with the nutrient under medical supervision or to individuals with predisposing conditions that modify their sensitivity to the nutrient.